Modern Coronary Care

Modern Coronary Care

Edited by

GARY S. FRANCIS, M.D.

Professor of Medicine, University of Minnesota
Medical School; Director, Acute Cardiac Care,
University of Minnesota Hospital, Minneapolis

JOSEPH S. ALPERT, M.D.

Edward Budnitz Professor of Cardiovascular
Medicine, University of Massachusetts Medical
School; Director, Division of Cardiovascular
Medicine, University of Massachusetts Medical
Center, Worcester

Foreword by
Howard B. Burchell, M.D., Ph.D.
Emeritus Professor of Medicine, Cardiovascular
Division, University of Minnesota Medical School;
Emeritus Consultant in Medicine, Cardiovascular
Division, The Mayo Clinic, Rochester

Little, Brown and Company
Boston/Toronto/London

To our parents and teachers, without whom it would never have been started; and to our wives, Margaret and Helle, without whom it would never have been finished.

Contents

VII. Therapeutic Interventions During and After Acute Myocardial Infarction

VIII. Postmyocardial Infarction Considerations

Foreword

Twentieth century medicine may be remembered for its thorough understanding of coronary artery disease. Linked to the increase in understanding is the hope that this scourge would be brought under control. There are four cardinal coronary events, often separated for study but basically interconnected: namely, angina pectoris, sudden death with arrhythmia, acute necrosis of a portion of the myocardium, and chronic left ventricular dysfunction (heart failure). These conditions have occupied the attention of clinicians and basic research investigators over the past century.

Winnowed from the spectrum of clinical manifestations of coronary disease is acute myocardial infarction. About 75 years ago it was realized, largely from the reports of Dock and Herrick, that acute myocardial infarction and its corollary, acute coronary occlusion, were compatible with the patient's recovery. Since then, there have been cyclic bursts of interest in experimental coronary occlusion with interventional therapy to modify infarct size and arrhythmias. In addition to the studies of acute myocardial infarction, there have been periodic investigations into the precipitating cause of coronary artery obstruction. The mechanism of obstruction has become better understood.

The focus of interest in acute MI is mirrored by the frequency of symposia on the topic and by the plethora of listings in the *Index Medicus*. It is appropriate timing for *Modern Coronary Care*, edited by Gary Francis and Joseph Alpert, to appear. It presents the current thinking of American cardiologists on acute myocardial infarction and its aftermath. Each chapter identifies a milestone in the progress of our knowledge and accomplishment in the care of the patient. While the first few chapters present data and opinion on noncontroversial topics within the specialty, the latter chapters address subject matter where more turmoil and controversy exist.

The century of progress and advancement of knowledge has been characterized by an ascendancy of data over the opinions derived from clinical experience. With the melding of both clinical and statistical approaches, there is in this volume a formulation of conclusions that will be enduring.

Howard B. Burchell, M.D., Ph.D.

Preface

Today the rate at which people are dying from cardiovascular disease is declining, while knowledge in the cardiovascular sciences advances at an ever-increasing rate. The extent to which these two observations are related is unclear. Nevertheless, there is a perceived need to assess therapy, particularly with regard to how it might influence cardiovascular mortality. Perhaps nowhere is this need more challenging than in the patients with acute unstable coronary disease. Myocardial reperfusion therapy, angioplasty, and pharmacologic support of patients with acute coronary artery disease are improving constantly. Many uncertainties remain, however. What is clear is that therapy has changed from an entirely passive strategy to one of rapid intervention. With changing therapy comes new complications, additional costs, and conflicting data. Eventually, despite the rapid pace at which coronary care is evolving, there is a need to pause and review the progress made to date, realizing that the very latest information cannot always be included. We have perceived a need by physicians for a single, authoritative source encompassing diagnosis and management of patients with acute coronary syndromes. We hope this text will fulfill that need.

The purpose of this book is to update physicians and other health care personnel concerning acute coronary care. Contributing authors were requested to provide an up-to-date and balanced review of their topics, realizing that there still is substantial controversy and uncertainty in many areas such as thrombolytic therapy and emergent angioplasty. Diagnostic and therapeutic options are discussed in detail, with some overlap provided to emphasize varying points of view. For example, acute mitral regurgitation and ventricular septal rupture are presented from the perspective of the pathologist and the cardiologist. Approaches to the care of the patient with the acute coronary syndrome will continue to be refined, but our intent is that this text will serve as a reasonably current starting point for the new "modern" era of coronary care. Many chapters contain editorial comments to update readers or to present divergent points of view.

This text is not intended to be an exhaustive or entirely comprehensive review of the subject matter. For example, the electrocardiographic changes present in acute myocardial infarction are not presented in any detail. Myocardial imaging with positron emission tomography (PET) or magnetic resonance imaging (MRI) are not discussed. In the case of electrocardiography, there are many excellent textbooks available that discuss the subject thoroughly. The new imaging techniques of PET and MRI are still evolving, particularly in the context of acute myocardial infarction, and are not being routinely used to manage patients with unstable coronary disease. This may change in the upcoming decade.

Finally, we wish to express our gratitude to the many contributing authors who agreed to participate in this venture and provided critical reviews of subject matter related to their areas of expertise. This is truly their book. Nearly all contributors are actively involved in the day-to-day care of patients with acute myocardial infarction, and hopefully have provided useful and practical guidelines for readers. We give many thanks to our editors at

Little, Brown and Company, including Jim Krosschell, who initially solicited our interest, and more recently Laurie Anello and Katherine Arnoldi, who managed to keep the project flowing despite the ups and downs that invariably occur while taking on a task of this magnitude. Lastly, we thank our colleagues at our respective hospitals and universities for providing support and inspiration while freeing us up to carry on the project. For us, this has been a labor of love that began during our sharing of attending rounds in a coronary care unit in San Diego, California in 1974. We often made rounds together, seeing patients, fielding questions from students, house officers, and cardiology fellows. Their queries were often challenging and insightful, and our junior colleagues continue to challenge us as we enter the "modern" coronary care era of the 1990s. We have seen remarkable progress in coronary care through the years, and we now offer this book as a step toward the improved care of our patients.

G. S. F.
J. S. A.

Contributing Authors

Joseph S. Alpert, M.D.

Edward Budnitz Professor of Cardiovascular Medicine, University of Massachusetts Medical School; Director, Division of Cardiovascular Medicine, University of Massachusetts Medical Center, Worcester

William F. Armstrong, M.D.

Associate Professor of Medicine, Indiana University School of Medicine; Research Associate, Krannert Institute of Cardiology, Indianapolis

J. A. Bianco, M.D.

Associate Professor of Radiology, University of Wisconsin Medical School; Radiologist and Nuclear Cardiologist, University of Wisconsin Clinical Sciences Center, Madison

J. Thomas Bigger, Jr., M.D.

Professor of Medicine and Pharmacology, Columbia University College of Physicians and Surgeons; Attending Physician, Presbyterian Hospital in the City of New York, New York

Wanda M. Bride, R.N.

Head Nurse, Cardiac Care Unit, Duke University Medical Center, Durham

Robert P. Byington, Ph.D.

Assistant Professor of Epidemiology, Department of Public Health Sciences, Bowman Gray School of Medicine of Wake Forest University, Winston-Salem

Robert M. Califf, M.D.

Assistant Professor of Medicine, Duke University School of Medicine; Director, Cardiac Care Unit, Duke University Medical Center, Durham

Donald B. Canaday, M.D.

Department of Cardiology, Deaconess and Sacred Heart Medical Centers, Spokane

Kanu Chatterjee, M.B., F.R.C.P.

Lucie Stern Professor of Cardiology and Professor of Medicine, University of California, San Francisco, School of Medicine; Associate Chief, Division of Cardiology, Moffitt-Long Hospital, San Francisco

James H. Chesebro, M.D.

Professor of Medicine, Division of Cardiovascular Diseases, Mayo Medical School; Attending Cardiologist, Mayo Clinic, Rochester

Marc Cohen, M.D.

Assistant Professor of Medicine, Mount Sinai School of Medicine; Attending Cardiologist, Mount Sinai Medical Center, New York

Jay N. Cohn, M.D.

Professor of Medicine, University of Minnesota Medical School; Head, Cardiovascular Division, University of Minnesota Health Sciences Center, Minneapolis

James R. Corbett, M.D.

Associate Professor of Radiology, University of Texas Health Science Center at Dallas, Southwestern Medical School; Director of Nuclear Cardiology, University of Texas Health Science Center at Dallas

James E. Dalen, M.D.

Vice Provost for Medical Affairs, University of Arizona College of Medicine, Tucson

Charles A. Dennis, M.D.

Director of Cardiac Rehabilitation, Division of Cardiovascular Disease, Scripps Clinic and Research Foundation, La Jolla

Marcus A. DeWood, M.D.

Director, Cardiac Research, Deaconess and Sacred Heart Medical Centers, Spokane

Leonard A. Doerfler, Ph.D.

Assistant Professor of Medicine, Division of Preventive and Behavioral Medicine, University of Massachusetts Medical School, Worcester

Brooks S. Edwards, M.D.

Assistant Professor, Mayo Graduate School of Medicine; Senior Associate Consultant, Department of Medicine (Cardiology), Mayo Clinic, Rochester, Minnesota

Jesse E. Edwards, M.D.

Professor of Pathology, University of Minnesota Medical School; Senior Consultant, Registry of Cardiovascular Disease, United Hospital, St. Paul

Gordon A. Ewy, M.D.

Professor and Associate Head, Department of Medicine, University of Arizona College of Medicine; Chief, Cardiology Section, University Medical Center, Tucson

Joseph L. Fleiss, Ph.D.

Professor and Head, Division of Biostatics, Columbia University School of Public Health, New York

Gary S. Francis, M.D.

Professor of Medicine, University of Minnesota Medical School; Director, Acute Cardiac Care, University of Minnesota Hospital, Minneapolis

Curt D. Furberg, M.D., Ph.D.

Professor of Medicine and Director, Center for Prevention Research and Biometry, Bowman Gray School of Medicine of Wake Forest University, Winston-Salem

Valentin Fuster, M.D.

Arthur M. and Hilda A. Master Professor of Medicine, Mount Sinai School of Medicine; Chief, Division of Cardiology, Mount Sinai Medical Center, New York

William Ganz, M.D., C.Sc.

Professor of Medicine, University of California, Los Angeles, School of Medicine; Senior Scientist, Department of Cardiology, Cedars-Sinai Medical Center, Los Angeles

Joel M. Gore, M.D.

Associate Professor of Medicine, University of Massachusetts Medical School; Director, Coronary Care Unit, University of Massachusetts Medical Center, Worcester

Hartmut Henning, M.D.

Associate Professor of Medicine, University of British Columbia Faculty of Medicine; Director, Cardiac Care Unit, Vancouver General Hospital, Vancouver

Douglas H. Israel, M.D.

Clinical and Research Fellow in Cardiology, Mount Sinai School of Medicine and Mount Sinai Medical Center, New York

Stuart W. Jamieson, M.B., F.R.C.S.

Professor of Surgery, University of California, San Diego, School of Medicine; Head, Cardio-Thoracic Surgery, UCSD Medical Center, San Diego

Terrance P. Judge, M.D.

Department of Cardiology, Deaconess and Sacred Heart Medical Centers, Spokane

Joel S. Karliner, M.D.

Professor of Medicine, University of California, San Francisco, School of Medicine; Chief, Cardiology Section, Veterans Administration Medical Center, San Francisco

Karl B. Kern, M.D.

Assistant Professor of Medicine, University of Arizona College of Medicine; Director, Cardiac Catheterization Laboratory, Veterans Administration Medical Center, Tucson

Simon Lee, M.D.

Professor of Medicine, Ulsan Medical School, Ulsan, Korea; Director, Heart Center, Asan Medical Center, Seoul, Korea

Allan S. Lew, M.D., M.B., F.R.A.C.P.

Associate Cardiologist, Cedars-Sinai Medical Center, Los Angeles

Jay W. Mason, M.D.

Professor of Internal Medicine, University of Utah Medical School; Chief, Division of Cardiology, University of Utah Medical Center, Salt Lake City

Joel Morganroth, M.D.

Professor of Medicine and Pharmacology, Hahnemann University School of Medicine; Director of Cardiac Research and Development, Graduate Hospital, Philadelphia

James E. Muller, M.D.

Associate Professor of Medicine, Harvard Medical School; Associate Physician, Brigham and Women's Hospital, Boston

Margaret B. Munster, R.N., M.S.N.

Cardiology Clinical Nurse Specialist, Duke University Medical Center, Durham

Pasquale F. Nestico, M.D.

Assistant Professor of Medicine (Cardiology), Hahnemann University School of Medicine; Associate Director, Sudden Death Prevention Program, Likoff Cardiovascular Institute, Hahnemann Hospital, Philadelphia

Ira S. Ockene, M.D.

Professor of Medicine, University of Massachusetts Medical School; Associate Director, Division of Cardiovascular Medicine, University of Massachusetts Medical Center, Worcester

Judith K. Ockene, Ph.D.

Professor of Medicine, University of Massachusetts Medical School; Director, Division of Preventive and Behavioral Medicine, University of Massachusetts Medical Center, Worcester

Robert A. O'Rourke, M.D.

Charles Conrad Brown Distinguished Professorship in Cardiovascular Disease and Director, Division of Cardiology, University of Texas Health Science Center at San Antonio; Director, Division of Cardiology, Brady Green Hospital, Medical Center Hospital, and Audie L. Murphy Memorial Veterans Hospital, San Antonio

Milton Packer, M.D.	Professor of Medicine, Mount Sinai School of Medicine; Director, Cardiovascular Training, Mount Sinai Medical Center, New York
John J. Paris, S.J., Ph.D.	Professor, Department of Religious Studies, Holy Cross College, Boston; Clinical Professor of Community Health, Tufts Medical School, Boston; Adjunct Professor of Medicine, University of Massachusetts Medical School, Worcester
Eugene R. Passamani, M.D.	Director, Division of Heart and Vascular Diseases, National Heart, Lung, and Blood Institute, Bethesda
Robert W. Peters, M.D.	Associate Professor of Medicine, University of Maryland School of Medicine; Director, Coronary Care Unit, Veterans Administration Medical Center, Baltimore
Gordon L. Pierpont, M.D., Ph.D.	Associate Professor of Medicine, University of Minnesota Medical School; Medical Director, Coronary Care Unit, Veterans Administration Medical Center, Minneapolis
Bertram Pitt, M.D.	Professor of Internal Medicine and Director, Division of Cardiology, University of Michigan Medical School; Chief, Division of Cardiology, University of Michigan Medical Center, Ann Arbor
Eric N. Prystowsky, M.D.	Consulting Professor of Medicine, Duke University Medical Center, Durham; Director, Clinical Electrophysiology Laboratory, St. Vincent Hospital, Indianapolis
Peter R. Puleo, M.D.	Assistant Professor of Medicine, Bugher Foundation Center for Molecular Biology in the Cardiovascular System, Baylor College of Medicine; Director of Coronary Care, Ben Taub General Hospital, Houston
David A. Rawling, M.D.	Assistant Professor of Internal Medicine, University of Utah School of Medicine; Director, Electrophysiology Service, Veterans Administration Hospital, Salt Lake City
Frank E. Reardon, J.D., M.S.	Partner, Hassan and Reardon Law Offices, Brookline; Chairman, Board of Directors, St. Monica's Nursing Home, Roxbury; Formerly, House Counsel, Brigham and Women's Hospital, Boston

K. Nagendra Nath Reddy, Ph.D.

Assistant Professor of Biochemistry, University of Southern California School of Medicine, Los Angeles

A. Henry Reisig, M.D.

Department of Cardiology, Deaconess and Sacred Heart Medical Centers, Spokane

Robert Roberts, M.D.

Professor of Medicine, Baylor College of Medicine; Chief of Cardiology, The Methodist Hospital, Houston

Dan M. Roden, M.D.

Associate Professor of Medicine and Pharmacology, Vanderbilt University School of Medicine; Director, Vanderbilt Arrhythmia Service, Nashville

Linda M. Rolnitzky, M.D.

Biostatistician, Department of Medicine, Columbia University College of Physicians and Surgeons, New York

Prediman K. Shah, M.D., F.A.C.C.

Associate Professor of Medicine, University of California, Los Angeles, School of Medicine; Director, In-patient Cardiology and Cardiac Care Unit, and Co-Director, Cardiovascular Fellowship Training Program, Cedars-Sinai Medical Center, Los Angeles

J. Paul Shields, M.D.

Department of Cardiology, Deaconess and Sacred Heart Medical Centers, Spokane

David H. Spodick, M.D., D.Sc.

Professor of Medicine, University of Massachusetts Medical School; Lecturer in Medicine, Tufts University School of Medicine and Boston University School of Medicine; Director, Clinical Cardiology and Cardiology Fellowship Program, St. Vincent Hospital, Worcester

Bernardo Stein, M.D.

Research Fellow, Division of Cardiology, Mount Sinai School of Medicine and Mount Sinai Medical Center, New York

William F. Stifter, M.D.

Department of Cardiology, Deaconess and Sacred Heart Medical Centers, Spokane

Borys Surawicz, M.D.

Professor of Medicine, Indiana University School of Medicine; Senior Research Associate, Krannert Institute of Cardiology, Indianapolis

Heinrich Taegtmeyer, M.D., D.Phil.

Associate Professor of Medicine, University of Texas Medical School at Houston; Staff Physician, Hermann Hospital, Houston

Pierre Théroux, M.D.

Associate Professor of Medicine, University of Montreal Faculty of Medicine; Chief, Coronary Care Unit, Montreal Heart Institute, Montreal

Geoffrey H. Tofler, M.B.

Instructor in Medicine, Harvard Medical School and Brigham and Women's Hospital, Boston

Galen S. Wagner, M.D.

Associate Professor of Medicine, Duke University School of Medicine, Durham

Ann D. Walling, M.D.

Fellow, Cardiology Division, University of Texas Health Science Center at San Antonio

Richard A. Walsh, M.D.

Professor of Medicine and Director, Cardiac Catheterization Laboratory, University of Texas Health Science Center at San Antonio

James T. Willerson, M.D.

Professor of Internal Medicine, University of Texas Health Science Center at Dallas, Southwestern Medical School; Director, Cardiology Division, University of Texas Health Science Center at Dallas

Bruce C. Wilson, M.D.

Assistant Professor of Medicine, University of Pittsburgh School of Medicine; Director, Section of General Cardiology, Presbyterian-University Hospital and Director, Pittsburgh Heart Institute, Pittsburgh

Andrew A. Wolff, M.D.

Assistant Clinical Professor of Medicine, University of California, San Francisco, School of Medicine; Attending Physician, Cardiology Division, Veterans Administration Medical Center, San Francisco

Raymond L. Woosley, M.D., Ph.D.

Professor of Pharmacology and Medicine and Chairman, Department of Pharmacology, Georgetown University School of Medicine, Washington, D.C.

Peter L. Zwerner, M.D.

Assistant Professor of Medicine, University of Massachusetts Medical School; Director, Cardiac Catheterization Laboratory, Berkshire Medical Center, Pittsfield

I
Pathophysiology and Pathology of Acute Myocardial Infarction

1
Pathophysiology of Acute Myocardial Infarction

JOSEPH S. ALPERT

Nearly 80 years ago two Russian physicians, Obraztsov and Strazhesko, realized that coronary arterial thrombosis led to acute myocardial infarction [1]. Shortly thereafter, Herrick made similar observations in the United States [1]. Since these initial descriptions, enormous efforts have been expended to understand the pathophysiology of acute myocardial infarction (AMI) and its attendant complications. Controversy still surrounds a number of aspects of this pathophysiologic sequence, and our knowledge remains remarkably incomplete. Despite these shortcomings, much has been learned concerning the pathophysiology of AMI particularly during the 1980s.

Understanding the pathobiology of AMI is of considerable clinical importance. New therapeutic approaches to this common disease are based on an understanding of its pathophysiology. For example, thrombolytic therapy during the early hours after the onset of infarction is based on the recognition that coronary arterial thrombosis is a central feature during the initial phases of AMI. This chapter reviews the biochemical, ultrastructural, and functional precedents and consequences of AMI.

Atherosclerosis

In most patients with acute myocardial infarction, coronary atherosclerosis is the underlying etiology that eventually leads to infarction. Fatty streaks, the earliest lesions of atherosclerosis, can be found commonly in the coronary arteries of children [2]. With increasing age, fatty streaks evolve into fibromuscular, atherosclerotic plaques. The initial injury to the arterial endothelium that sets in motion the process leading to fatty streaks is apparently mediated by monocytes that adhere to the surface of the coronary arterial endothelium [3]. Platelet adherence, platelet aggregation, and release of smooth muscle growth factor causes the embryonic atherosclerotic plaque to increase in size. Adherent monocytes also migrate into the lesion and are transformed into macrophages, which also release smooth muscle and fibrous tissue growth factors [2, 3]. The disturbed endothelium is capable of releasing various growth factors as well (Fig. 1-1). The resultant fibrous/smooth muscle plaque demonstrates abnormal transport of lipid from the arterial lumen. Some of this lipid becomes deposited in the plaque, leading to further macrophage infiltration, growth factor release, and smooth muscle fibrous cellular proliferation. Late in this pathophysiologic sequence, necrosis and calcification may develop within the atherosclerotic plaque. A number of possible pathophysiologic events are being considered by various investigators as the first steps in the development of an atherosclerotic plaque. Each of these theories favors a different aspect of the above-mentioned sequence as the primary initiating factor (i.e., platelets, monocytes, lipids). It is possible, however, that all of these sequences are operative at different times and in different individuals, leading to atherosclerotic plaques that are therefore multifactorial in origin.

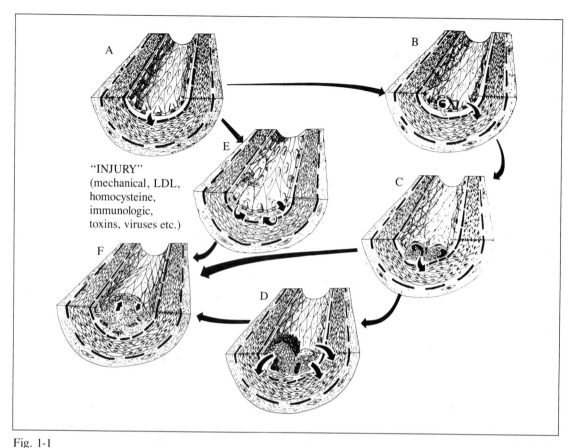

Fig. 1-1
Response of arterial wall to injury: a graphic hypothesis. Atherosclerotic lesions can begin by means of at least two pathways. The pathway demonstrated by the clockwise, long arrows is as follows: Injury to arterial endothelium (A) may induce growth factor secretion into the arterial media (*short arrows within drawings*). Monocytes attach to the injured endothelium (B), which continues to secrete growth factors into the arterial media. Monocytes migrate into the subendothelium and transform into macrophages (C), thereby leading to fatty streak formation and further release of growth factors. These fatty streaks may develop directly into fibrous plaques (*long arrow from C to F*) secondary to release of growth factors from macrophages or endothelial cells. Macrophages can also stimulate or injure overlying endothelium. At times, macrophages injure overlying endothelium to such a degree that the endothelium is lost, thereby exposing the underlying fatty streaks to blood flow. Platelet deposition results (D), providing yet another source for growth factor stimulation of the subendothelial region. In addition, smooth muscle cells in the proliferating lesion itself (F) may secrete growth factors and thereby increase the size of the fibrous plaques. An alternate pathway for the development of advanced atherosclerotic lesions is shown by the short, clockwise arrows: A–E–F. Here the endothelium is injured but remains intact. Endothelium secretes growth factor, which stimulates migration of smooth muscle cells from the media into the intima. Further growth factor is produced and released within this zone of injury and cellular migration (E). These interactions lead to fibrous plaque formation and further progression of the lesion (F). (Reprinted by permission from R. Ross, The pathogenesis of atherosclerosis—an update. *N. Engl. J. Med.* 314:488, 1986.)

Myocardial Ischemia

BIOCHEMISTRY AND ELECTROPHYSIOLOGY

When myocardial oxygen demand exceeds coronary arterial blood flow, myocardial ischemia develops. Cardiac muscle requires large amounts of oxygen and nutrients to function. Indeed, mitochondria, the organelle of oxidative metabolism where ATP is generated, make up 25 to 40 percent of the volume of left ventricular myocardial cells [4, 5]. With the onset of myocardial ischemia, aerobic mitochondrial function becomes markedly disturbed and ATP production falls off rapidly. Of course some anaerobic production of ATP is possible, but only small quantities are produced; and the end-products of glycolysis inhibit critical enzymes in the glycolytic pathway, thereby further reducing the production of ATP. Thus myocardial cells must have a constant supply of oxygen and nutrients to function.

When myocardial ischemia develops, normal systolic and diastolic function of the myocardium declines within a few seconds. High energy phosphate compounds (ATP and its "backup" system creatine phosphate) are the source of myocardial cellular energy. Although myocardial tissue ATP levels are maintained for several minutes following cessation of myocardial blood flow, tissue levels of creatine phosphate fall rapidly and are reduced to 20 percent of normal within 2 to 3 minutes of the onset of ischemia [6–8]. Systolic contraction declines rapidly with the onset of ischemia and loss of energy-rich phosphates, ceasing entirely approximately 90 seconds after the interruption of myocardial blood flow [9]. In addition to the loss of high energy phosphates, other intracellular events contribute to cessation of myocardial cellular function during ischemia. These events include acidosis, reduced sensitivity of contractile proteins to calcium, and accumulation of phosphate and lipid [10–12]. The end result of these intracellular disturbances is rapidly declining systolic and diastolic myocardial cellular function.

Another consequence of myocardial ischemia is alteration in the electrical properties of cardiac muscle. The monophasic action potential of the myocardial cell is altered approximately 16 beats after the onset of ischemia [13]. Ischemia causes myocardial cells to leak potassium into the surrounding extracellular space, resulting in changes in conduction velocity, rate of depolarization, resting membrane potential, and duration of the action potential. Some or all of these alterations in cellular electrophysiology may be involved in the genesis of arrhythmias that arise in the setting of myocardial ischemia.

Studies have documented biochemical alterations in human cardiac metabolism in the setting of myocardial ischemia [14, 15]. Under normal aerobic conditions, human myocardium metabolizes fatty acids and pyruvate in order to produce adenosine triphosphate (ATP). In the absence of oxygen, however, the myocardium is incapable of utilizing the latter substrates. In place of fatty acids and pyruvate, the myocardium takes up glucose for anaerobic (glycolytic) generation of ATP [14, 15]. The continued utilization of glucose by cardiac muscle that no longer contracts has been suggested as a marker for "stunned," or *reversibly* injured, myocardium (see below).

MYOCARDIAL METABOLIC DEMAND AND CORONARY BLOOD FLOW

Myocardial blood flow is coupled to myocardial metabolic demand under normal conditions. With the advent of coronary arterial stenosis or obstruction, myocardial blood flow can no longer increase in the face of myocardial metabolic demand. The result is myocardial ischemia.

Myocardial metabolic demands are dependent on heart rate, systolic blood pressure, left ventricular volume and wall thickness, and myocardial contractility. Increases in heart rate, systolic blood pressure, and myocardial contractility obviously increase myocardial metabolic demand. The product of heart rate and blood pressure are directly proportional to measured myocardial oxygen demand [16, 17]. Left ventricular wall stress is also a major determinant of myocardial oxygen demand [16, 17]. Wall stress increases (Laplace relation) with increasing ventricular volume and decreases with increasing wall thickness. However, hearts with left ventricular hypertrophy (increased wall thickness) have a larger quantity of functioning myocardium that requires oxygen and nutrients. Thus global left ventricular oxygen demand is augmented with increasing ventricular demand. If coronary arterial capacity for blood flow remains unchanged in the face of increasing myocardial mass, ischemia can result even in the absence of major atherosclerotic coronary arterial obstruction (e.g., hypertrophic cardiomyopathy).

There are two major determinants of coronary arterial blood flow: perfusion pressure and coronary vascular resistance. Perfusion pressure is the difference between aortic blood pressure and intramyocardial pressure, which compresses coronary blood vessels. Coronary blood flow is impeded during systole when collapsible vessels are compressed. Thus left ventricular myocardial blood flow occurs primarily during diastole because of high systolic intramyocardial wall tension. Because right ventricular systolic pressure and wall tension are much less than those in the left ventricle, systolic compressive forces are less in the right ventricular wall, and myocardial blood flow in the latter is of equal magnitude during systole and diastole. Because left ventricular blood flow occurs primarily during diastole, an increasing heart rate lessens left ventricular coronary blood flow by decreasing diastolic time.

Coronary vascular resistance is determined by blood viscosity and the diameter and length of the coronary arteries (Poiseuille's theorem). Blood viscosity and vessel length vary little from individual to individual. Hence it is the cross-sectional area of the coronary arteries and arterioles that determines coronary vascular resistance. Under normal circumstances, coronary arterial resistance is determined primarily by intramyocardial arterioles. However, when marked atherosclerotic obstruction develops in large epicardial coronary arteries, coronary vascular resistance is deter-

mined primarily by these lesions, which encroach on the arterial lumen [18].

Modest coronary arterial stenoses with moderate luminal encroachment do not alter resting coronary arterial blood flow. Stenosis severity must reach 80 to 90 percent luminal diameter reduction before resting blood flow is curtailed (Fig. 1-2). When the arterial pressure head beyond a coronary arterial stenosis falls below 55 mm Hg, subendocardial ischemia develops [19]. The more severe is the stenotic lesion, the more transmural in distribution is the resulting ischemia. Ischemia develops first in the subendocardium because myocardial compressive forces resisting myocardial blood flow are greatest here and because the subendocardium is the last site to receive blood flow from the coronary arterial tree, which originates on the epicardial surface of the heart. Therefore when a severe coronary arterial stenosis is present, blood flow

Fig. 1-2
Reduction in resting myocardial blood flow plotted against stenosis of the coronary arterial lumen. Myocardial blood flow is maintained at essentially control levels until the arterial lumen is reduced by approximately 80 percent or more. At this point, myocardial blood flow falls rapidly with increasing stenosis. (From J. S. Alpert. *Physiopathology of the Cardiovascular System.* Boston: Little, Brown, 1984. With permission.)

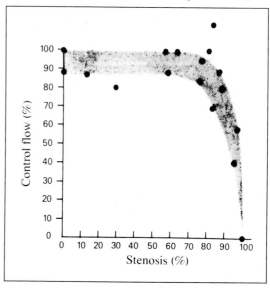

goes preferentially to the subepicardium [20, 21]. Imbalance between myocardial metabolic demand and coronary arterial blood flow results in myocardial ischemia. Most episodes of exertional angina are the result of myocardial metabolic demand outstripping blood flow. Episodes of rest or nocturnal angina (unstable angina) are thought to be the result of coronary arterial vasomotion or spasm with consequent marked reduction in coronary arterial blood flow (see below) [22–28].

SYSTOLIC AND DIASTOLIC MYOCARDIAL FUNCTION

Following abrupt cessation of myocardial blood flow, diastolic and systolic myocardial mechanical dysfunction develop rapidly [29, 30]. Within seconds, diastolic function decreases first as demonstrated by declining negative dP/dt, rising ventricular end-diastolic pressure, and less compliant pressure volume curves. Shortly thereafter, ventricular systolic function deteriorates, as judged from progressively abnormal positive dP/dt and cessation of regional myocardial contraction. All myocardial contraction ceases in the ischemic zone within 10 to 15 seconds of the onset of ischemia. Increases in heart rate and systemic arterial blood pressure usually follow, presumably as the result of activation of the sympathetic nervous system. Pulmonary arterial pressures increase pari passu with rising left ventricular diastolic pressure. If coronary blood flow is rapidly restored, diastolic and systolic hemodynamic abnormalities resolve. However, if ischemia is prolonged or occurs repetitively, diastolic or systolic function (or both) may remain abnormal for a more protracted period (see below).

TRANSITION FROM ISCHEMIA TO NECROSIS: STUNNED MYOCARDIUM

Following cessation of coronary arterial blood flow, myocardial ischemia appears first in the subendocardium. Thereafter, ischemia advances transmurally toward the subepicardium [31–35]. Initially, ischemic myocytes are reversibly injured. However, within 15 to 20 minutes of the onset of ischemia and continuing for 3 to 6 hours, a wave of irreversible myocardial cellular injury spreads from the subendocardium to the subepicardium. Along the leading edge of this wavefront of myocardial cellular necrosis lie cells that are seriously, but reversibly, injured. Cellular ATP and creatine phosphate levels are low in these injured cells, and cellular volume regulation is abnormal [35]. Overt membrane damage, however, judged by electron microscopy, is not observed in these reversibly injured cells. Cellular ischemic injury is reversible so long as ATP levels are not depleted below 70 percent of control levels.

Following reestablishment of myocardial blood flow, myocytes gradually replete adenine nucleotides. In general, recovery of myocardial systolic and diastolic function is inversely proportional to the duration of myocardial ischemia [36–42]. After prolonged periods of myocardial ischemia in experimental animals, complete recovery of diastolic and systolic function may take as long as 3 to 7 days. Indeed, myocardial ATP levels are still depressed 4 days after an episode of severe ischemia [43]. Ultrastructural cellular injury can also be observed 3 days after severe myocardial ischemia. Ultrastructural changes noted include the presence of abnormal vacuoles, intermyofibrillar and intermyofilamentous edema, and glycogen depletion [42]. Severely, but reversibly, injured myocardium that demonstrates a prolonged functional recovery phase has been referred to as *stunned myocardium* [42].

In light of the observations concerning stunned myocardium, the work of Geft and coworkers is of considerable interest. These investigators noted that brief, intermittent periods of myocardial ischemia (5, 10, or 15 minutes of ischemia followed by 15 minutes of reperfusion) produced small, but distinct areas of subendocardial necrosis in dogs. Thus stunned myocardium can be irreversibly injured by further episodes of ischemia [44].

Myocardial Infarction

ULTRASTRUCTURAL AND BIOCHEMICAL EVENTS

As noted earlier, marked biochemical and structural abnormalities develop in myocardial cells following cessation of coronary blood flow or reduction in flow below 15 percent of control values [31]. After approximately 20 to 40 minutes of myocardial ischemia, cellular derangement becomes irreversible and cell death or necrosis ensues. Cell death begins in the subendocardium 1 to 2 mm from the endocardial surface and extends to within 1 to 2 mm of the lateral edge of the ischemic vascular bed [33]. A wave front of cell death moves slowly *from* the subendocardial region *toward* the subepicardial zone where collateral blood is greatest. Approximately 3 to 6 hours are required for the wave front of cellular necrosis to reach the subepicardial zone, depending on the extent of collateral blood flow and myocardial oxygen demand (Fig. 1-3) [35].

As noted earlier, high energy phosphates are rapidly depleted in ischemic myocardial cells. Anaerobic glycolysis is initially employed to produce a modest amount of ATP, but these synthetic pathways are soon inhibited and ATP production ceases. [45, 46].

With the onset of irreversible myocardial cellular injury: (1) ATP is almost completely depleted (Fig. 1-4); (2) mitochondria are swollen and contain amorphous matrix densities composed of lipid and protein; and (3) the sarcolemmal membranes develop defects presumably leading to leakage of essential enzymes out of the cell and entrance of calcium ions and water into the cell. Reperfusion of irreversibly injured myocytes is associated with massive cellular edema and influx of Ca^{2+} [35]. Other ultrastructural changes associated with irreversible myocyte injury include clumping of nuclear chromatin plus further swelling and disruption of mitochondria and cell membranes. Intramitochondrial calcium crystals accumulate. The myofibrillar apparatus becomes disrupted with the formation of contraction bands. It has been hypothesized

Fig. 1-3
Wavefront progression of cell death over time following occlusion of the circumflex coronary artery in open-chested dogs. Necrosis occurs first in the subendocardium and then moves in a wavefront toward the subepicardium. Thus there is initially a large volume of ischemic but salvageable myocardium soon after coronary occlusion. As time passes, however, less and less viable myocardium remains. AP = anterior; PP = posterior. (From K. A. Reimer and R. B. Jennings, The "wavefront phenomenon" of myocardial ischemic cell death. II. Transmural progression of necrosis within the framework of ischemic bed size (myocardium at risk) and collateral flow. *Lab. Invest.* 40:633, 1979. With permission.)

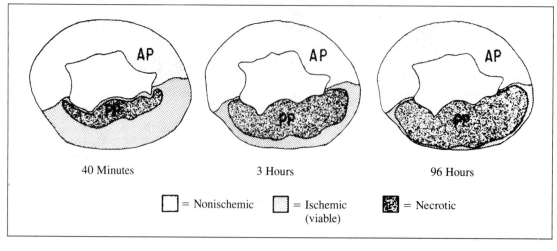

40 Minutes   3 Hours   96 Hours

☐ = Nonischemic   ☐ = Ischemic   ▨ = Necrotic
                          (viable)

that sarcolemmal injury is the critical event in determining irreversibility of cellular damage. Membrane damage may develop because of activation of endogenous phospholipases, detergent action of acyl carnitine and acyl coenzyme A, oxidation by oxygen free radicals, or failure to resynthesize portions of membranes lost through pinocytosis or other processes [35, 47].

Fig. 1-4
Adenine nucleotide contents of normal and severely ischemic myocardium of dogs following proximal occlusion of the circumflex coronary artery. After 40 minutes of ischemia, when most of the cells in the ischemic zone are irreversibly injured, only 6 percent of the original ATP content remains. Moreover, there was a 69 percent decrease in total adenine nucleotides. AMP = adenine monophosphate nucleotide; ADP = adenine diphosphate nucleotide; ATP = adenine triphosphate nucleotide. (From K. A. Reimer, et al. Pathobiology of acute myocardial ischemia: Metabolic, functional, and ultrastructural studies. *Am. J. Cardiol.* 52:72A, 1983. With permission.)

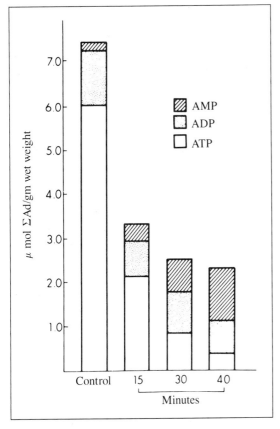

RELATION TO CORONARY ARTERIAL OBSTRUCTION

Although contested in the past, it is now generally agreed that coronary arterial thrombosis is the event that initiates myocardial infarction. Coronary thrombi are approximately 1 cm in length and are composed of platelets, fibrin, erythrocytes, and leukocytes [48]. The thrombus may vary in composition at different levels with white thrombus (composed of platelets and fibrin) mixed with red thrombus (composed of erythrocytes, fibrin, platelets, and leukocytes).

Early thrombi are usually nonocclusive and are composed primarily of platelets. Such early thrombi usually overlie a newly generated ulcer or fissure in a long-standing atherosclerotic plaque [49]. This fissuring or ulceration of the plaque apparently exposes underlying thrombogenic material to the circulating blood with resultant thrombogenesis (Fig. 1-5). Presumably, once thrombus formation is initiated, a series of dynamic reactions are set into motion, with endogenous thrombolysis opposing thrombogenesis. If thrombogenesis prevails, an occlusive thrombus totally occludes the coronary arterial lumen.

The process that causes a previously stable atherosclerotic plaque to rupture, fissure, or ulcerate is unknown at this time. A number of

Fig. 1-5
Initiation of myocardial infarction: current hypothesis for the sequence of events leading from a "benign," stable atherosclerotic plaque to a "complicated" plaque to complete coronary arterial obstruction by thrombus.

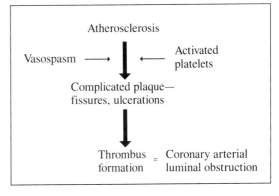

hypotheses have been suggested to explain the etiology of plaque disruption: (1) coronary arterial vasospasm; (2) stress fracture of the plaque secondary to repetitive bending during ventricular systole; (3) injury to coronary arterial vasa vasorum with resultant intramural hemorrhage or plaque necrosis; or (4) platelet aggregation with release of thromboxanes and other vasoactive substances [28, 48–53]. All or none of these processes may be operative simultaneously or sequentially in a particular individual.

A number of investigators have accumulated circumstantial evidence favoring a role for coronary arterial vasospasm in the genesis of coronary arterial thrombosis. Factor and Cho noted the presence of smooth muscle contraction bands consistent with coronary spasm in the medial layer of coronary arteries of patients with fatal myocardial infarction [54]. Angiographic studies in patients with unstable angina who developed coronary thrombosis and myocardial infarction during catheterization have documented the role of coronary vasospasm in the development of occlusive coronary thrombi [55–57].

Platelet aggregates in arteriosclerotic arteries are also thought to be important factors in the pathogenesis of acute myocardial infarction [58]. Severe coronary arterial stenosis causes turbulent blood flow and zones of stasis. In addition, the endothelial surface of atherosclerotic coronary arteries is capable of activating the platelet release reaction. Animal studies have documented the presence of platelet aggregates beyond critical coronary arterial stenoses [59, 60]. These platelet aggregates lead to periodic, cyclic reductions in coronary arterial blood flow. Evidence that similar events are occurring within atherosclerotic coronary arteries in man has come from a number of studies [61–63]. Elevated levels of thromboxane B_2, a stable metabolite of thromboxane A_2, have been observed in coronary venous blood of patients with unstable angina and acute myocardial infarction. Moreover, platelets in such individuals are more easily activated [64, 65], which may, in part, explain activation of platelets in patients with unstable angina despite normal plasma levels of cate-

cholamines. Further support for the concept that abnormal hemostatic function is a causative factor in the development of coronary arterial thrombosis is derived from studies documenting increased levels of fibrinogen and higher maximum rates of fibrin growth, as well as increased prothrombin time, thrombin time, and activated partial thromboplastin time in patients with acute myocardial infarction [66]. Leukocytes may also play a role in the genesis of coronary thrombosis via release of oxidative species or leukotrienes [67, 68]. Vasoactive substances such as the ones just mentioned in combination with thromboxanes may contribute to or initiate coronary arterial vasospasm. Thus a vicious spiral may be created with coronary vasospasm and vasoactive humoral factors reenforcing an ever-increasing reduction in coronary arterial luminal diameter. Activation of the clotting cascade leading to thrombogenesis further compromises luminal diameter. Eventually, the coronary artery is blocked by a combination of vasospasm and thrombus. Exactly which one of these factors is the primary event in this vicious spiral is unknown. It is even possible that a different factor initiates this process leading to thrombogenesis in different individuals.

In summary, angiographic, angioscopic, and pathological studies have repeatedly documented that patients with acute ischemic syndromes (unstable angina, acute myocardial infarction) have eccentric, irregular lesions in the involved coronary artery. These lesions represent plaque fissures with overlying partially occlusive thrombus. A sequence of events involving coronary arterial vasospasm, platelet activation, and thrombogenesis leads to ever-increasing coronary arterial obstruction. If the intrinsic thrombolytic system fails to counterbalance the forces favoring thrombogenesis, total arterial obstruction results [55–70], and myocardial ischemia and eventually necrosis develop.

A number of environmental factors are apparently involved in the genesis of the coronary arterial events just described. A recent respiratory viral infection is a common precursor of acute myocardial infarction [71, 72].

Moreover, there is a circadian rhythm present in the occurrence of myocardial infarction: The onset of infarction is most frequent during the early morning hours and least frequent in the evening [73]. Platelet aggregatory activity is also increased in the early morning hours, again supporting the role of platelets in the onset of acute myocardial infarction [74]. Finally, a number of weather parameters, such as season, barometric pressure, and humidity, correlate with the occurrence of acute myocardial infarction [75].

COLLATERAL BLOOD FLOW

It has been known since the 1930s that total occlusion of a coronary artery is not always followed by myocardial necrosis [76]. Indeed, the volume of collateral blood flow can be sufficient to maintain myocardial cellular viability despite coronary thrombosis. Normal hearts contain an extensive network of small, interarterial anastomotic blood vessels, 40 to 60 μm in diameter. This collateral circulation exists at birth, growing in size along with the rest of the coronary vascular bed. When obstructive coronary artery disease develops, these collateral channels gradually increase in size and blood flow capacity. Considerable variability exists from individual to individual with respect to potential collateral vascular development. Moreover, extensive collateral circulation requires time (perhaps years) to develop. Thus collateral blood flow is highest in older individuals with long-standing coronary artery disease. It is not surprising that well-developed collateral vessels are unusual in patients with acute myocardial infarction, as these patients represent a selected population [77]. The presence of infarction demonstrates that collateral blood flow was not sufficient to maintain myocardial cellular viability. However, significantly better ventricular function is present in regions of the left ventricle supplied by obstructed coronary arteries if extensive collateralization of the diseased coronary artery is present [78]. Congestive heart failure and cardiomegaly occur with greater frequency in infarct patients who lack

collateral blood vessels [79]. Moreover, it has frequently been observed in both animals and man that following coronary occlusion the zone of myocardial infarction is smaller than the area supplied by the occluded vessel if collateral blood vessels are present.

In summary, collateral blood vessels are present from birth and can enlarge in the presence of obstructive coronary artery disease. Collateral blood flow can limit infarct size when total occlusion of a coronary artery develops. Occasionally, the volume of collateral blood flow is sufficient to prevent infarction.

EFFECT OF INFARCTION ON REGIONAL AND GLOBAL VENTRICULAR FUNCTION

Abnormal systolic and diastolic myocardial cellular function develops within a few seconds of cessation of coronary arterial blood flow. Initially, ischemic myocardium expands passively during ventricular filling and emptying. Thus diastolic compliance is initially increased (decreased stiffness) [80–83]. Within a few minutes, however, ischemic myocardium becomes stiffer, and eventually its compliance is less than that of surrounding, viable myocardium [80–83]. This change in diastolic stiffness is probably the result of myocardial contracture, interstitial edema, and leukocyte infiltration during the early phases of AMI. Increased myocardial stiffness during the chronic phase of myocardial infarction is apparently caused by fibrous tissue proliferation and collagen deposition. The left ventricular diastolic pressure increases, and the pressure/volume relation is abnormally shifted by the increase in regional myocardial stiffness that develops post infarction.

Cessation of myocardial blood flow results in four sequential abnormal patterns of myocardial systolic contraction: (1) *dyssynchrony*, or dissociation over the time course of contraction of adjacent segments of myocardium; (2) *hypokinesis*, or reduction in the extent of myocardial shortening; (3) *akinesis*, or cessation of myocardial contraction in affected regions; and (4) *dyskinesis*, or paradoxical systolic expansion of affected myocardial segments [84]. All of these sequential contraction abnormalities occur within seconds to minutes of the cessation of myocardial blood flow.

When a substantial quantity of myocardium becomes ischemic or necrotic (>25 percent of left ventricular myocardium), global left ventricular function deteriorates sufficiently to reduce resting cardiac output, stroke volume, and peak dP/dt [85, 86]. Dyskinetic myocardial segments contribute to the reduction in ventricular stroke output. As edema, cellular infiltration, and ultimately fibrosis develop in ischemic and necrotic myocardial segments, the resultant increased stiffness of these myocardial zones improves left ventricular function by preventing systolic paradoxical wall motion (dyskinesis).

Rackely and coworkers observed a linear relation between left ventricular function and clinical symptoms [87]. The earliest observed abnormality in global left ventricular function is a reduction in diastolic compliance that occurs when 8 percent of the left ventricle is ischemic or necrotic. When the abnormal contracting segment exceeds 10 percent of the left ventricle, global ejection fraction is reduced; once 15 percent of the left ventricle is involved, ventricular end-diastolic pressure and volume increase. Clinical heart failure is evident when 25 percent of the left ventricle ceases to contract. Cardiogenic shock develops when 40 percent of the left ventricular myocardium becomes ischemic or necrotic [87].

Unless infarct extension or expansion develops (see below), some improvement or recovery of global left ventricular function is usually observed [88, 89]. Such improvement occurs over a period of days to weeks and may be the result of improved collateral blood flow, myocardial scar contraction, or myocardial hypertrophy. Such recovery of myocardial function is more common in patients with single-vessel disease than in individuals who have multivessel disease [88]. Patients in whom 20 to 25 percent of the left ventricle fails to contract manifest hemodynamic signs of left ventricular failure regardless of the age of their infarction [90].

Patients with AMI may demonstrate abnormally reduced wall motion in segments of the left ventricle remote from the acutely infarcted zone. Such remote wall motion abnormalities are the result of previous infarction or acute ischemia and are called *ischemia at a distance* [91, 92]. There are two reasons for ischemia at a distance: The noninfarcted myocardial zone is supplied by a critically stenotic coronary artery. Ischemia develops because of (1) increased compensatory myocardial work in the noninfarcted zone secondary to loss of working myocardial segments in the infarct zone, and (2) decreased collateral blood flow to the noninfarcted ischemic zone as a result of the acute coronary arterial thrombosis that produced the initial infarct.

INFARCTION EXPANSION AND VENTRICULAR DILATATION

After experimental infarction in dogs, the first 7 days of healing are associated with expansion of the infarct zone and dilatation of the left ventricular cavity [93]. Thereafter, the infarct zone contracts and thins as collagen is deposited. Similar changes have been observed in humans following AMI [94–97]. Marked infarct expansion and left ventricular cavity dilatation are associated with a poor prognosis, [94]. Noninfarcted zones develop volume-overload hypertrophy, thereby further contributing to remodeling of the left ventricle after acute infarction [95]. Large infarcts are more likely to expand than small infarcts [97]. Expansion of infarction is the result of slippage of intramural fibers within the infarct zone. In addition, infarct expansion contributes to left ventricular aneurysm formation.

ELECTRICAL INSTABILITY

Some form of arrhythmia is almost always present during the acute phase of myocardial infarction. Ventricular arrhythmias arise in ischemic peri-infarct zones as a result of: (1) increased myocardial cell electrical automaticity often resulting from delayed after-depolarizations; (2) slowing of conduction in specific areas of the heart with resultant reentry and reexcitation loops; and (3) variable shortening or lengthening of the refractory period combined with increased dispersion of refractoriness between ischemic and nonischemic zones [98]. Unidirectional abnormalities of conduction have been observed between ischemic and nonischemic zones of myocardium. Moreover, localized areas of ventricular fibrillation have been noted in experimental animals with AMI. It is thought that these localized zones of fibrillation can spread from the ischemic to the nonischemic segments. Atrial arrhythmias are the result of (1) ischemia or necrosis of atrial myocardium secondary to coronary thrombosis, and (2) atrial dilatation secondary to elevated ventricular filling pressures.

Metabolic products released from ischemic myocardium such as cyclic adenosine monophosphate (AMP), free fatty acids, long-chain fatty acid metabolites, lysophosphoglycerides, lactate, and pyruvate, to mention only a few, have electrophysiologic activity that can be arrhythmogenic [99]. A wide array of atrial and ventricular arrhythmias can occur.

MYOCARDIAL INFARCTION WITH NORMAL CORONARY ARTERIES

Approximately 4 percent of patients with AMI have normal coronary arteries documented by coronary angiography. This percentage is even higher, perhaps 10 to 15 percent, in patients under age 35. In some individuals the infarction is the result of a coronary artery disease other than atherosclerosis, for example, coronary arteritis, trauma, or embolism [100]. A number of theories have been developed to explain the etiology of infarction in individuals without an otherwise evident explanation. Coronary arterial vasospasm and small vessel coronary artery disease are two of the most popular theories. It seems likely that most of these patients do indeed have minimal atherosclerotic injury to the infarct-related coronary artery. This injury is so small that it is angiographically invisible [101]. Vasospasm with or without transient coronary arterial thrombosis with resultant infarction is thought to occur at the site of such minimal atherosclerotic change [101].

References

1. Muller, J. E. Coronary artery thrombosis: Historical aspects. *J. Am. Coll. Cardiol.* 3:893, 1983.
2. Ross, R. The pathogenesis of atherosclerosis—an update. *N. Engl. J. Med.* 314:488, 1986.
3. Joris, I., Zand, T., Nunnari, J. J., et al. Studies on the pathogenesis of atherosclerosis. I. Adhesion and emigration of mononuclear cells in the aorta of hypercholesterolemic rats. *Am. J. Pathol.* 113:341, 1983.
4. Sommer, J. R., and Johnson, E. A. Ultrastructure of cardiac muscle. In R. M. Berne and N. Sperelakis (eds.), *Handbook of Physiology, Sect. 2: The Cardiovascular System.* Bethesda: American Physiological Society, 1979, pp. 113–186.
5. Wollenberg, A. Responses of the heart mitochondria to chronic cardiac overload and physical exercise. In E. Bajusz and E. Rona (eds.), *Recent Advances in Studies on Cardiac Structure and Metabolism.* Baltimore: University Park Press, 1972. Pp. 213–222.
6. Braasch, W., Gudbjarnason, S., Puri, P. S., et al. Early changes in energy metabolism in the myocardium following acute coronary artery occlusion in anesthetized dogs. *Circ. Res.* 23:429, 1986.
7. Gudbjarnason, S., Mathes, P., and Ravens, K. G. Functional compartmentalization of ATP and creatine phosphate in heart muscle. *J. Mol. Cell. Cardiol.* 1:325, 1970.
8. Wollenberger, A., and Krause, E. G. Metabolic control characteristics of the acutely ischemic myocardium. *Am. J. Cardiol.* 22:349, 1968.
9. Tennant, R., and Wiggers, C. J. The effect of coronary occlusion on myocardial contraction. *Am. J. Physiol.* 112:351, 1935.
10. Tennant, R. Factors concerned in the arrest of contraction in an ischemic myocardial area. *Am. J. Physiol.* 113:677, 1935.
11. Serruys, P. W., Wijns, W., Van den Brond, M., et al. Left ventricular performance, regional blood flow, wall motion and lactate metabolism during transluminal angioplasty. *Circulation* 70:25, 1984.
12. Poole-Wilson, P. A. Haemodynamic and metabolic consequences of angina and myocardial infarction. In K. M. Fox (ed.), *Ischemic Heart*

Disease. Norwell, MA: MTP Press, 1987. Pp. 123–148.

13. Donaldson, R. M., Taggart, P., Bennett, J. G., et al. Study of electrophysiological ischemic events during coronary angioplasty. *Texas Heart Inst. J.* 11:23, 1984.

14. Schwaiger, M., Brunken, R., Grover-McKay, M., et al. Regional myocardial metabolism in patients with acute myocardial infarction assessed by positron emission tomography. *J. Am. Coll. Cardiol.* 8:800, 1986.

15. Camici, P., Araujo, L. I., Spinks, T., et al. Increased uptake of ^{18}F-fluorodeoxyglucose in postischemic myocardium of patients with exercise-induced angina. *Circulation* 74:81, 1986.

16. Sarnoff, S. J., Braunwald, E., Welch, G. H., et al. Haemodynamic determinants of oxygen consumption of the heart with special reference to the tension time index. *Am. J. Physiol.* 192:148, 1958.

17. Braunwald, E., Sarnoff, S. J., Case, R. B., et al. Hemodynamic determinants of coronary flow: Effect of changes in aortic pressure and cardiac output on the relationship between oxygen consumption and coronary flow. *Am. J. Physiol.* 192:157, 1958.

18. Sabbah, H. N., and Stein, P. D. Hemodynamics of multiple versus single 50 percent coronary arterial stenoses. *Am. J. Cardiol.* 50:278, 1982.

19. Wyatt, H. L., Forrester, J. S., Tyber, J. V., et al. Effect of graded reductions in the regional coronary perfusion on regional and total cardiac function. *Am. J. Cardiol.* 36:185, 1975.

20. Bache, R. J., and Schwartz, J. S. Effect of perfusion pressure distal to a coronary stenosis on transmural myocardial blood flow. *Circulation* 65:928, 1982.

21. Sabbah, H. N., and Stein, P. D. Effect of acute regional ischaemia in the subepicardium and subendocardium. *Am. J. Physiol.* 242:H240, 1982.

22. Buja, L. M., Hillis, L. D., Petty, C. S., et al. The role of coronary arterial spasm in ischemic heart disease. *Arch. Pathol. Lab. Med.* 105:221, 1981.

23. Gorlin, R. Role of coronary vasospasm in the pathogenesis of myocardial ischemia and angina pectoris. *Am. Heart. J.* 103:598, 1982.

24. Yasue, H., Omote, S., Takizawa, A., and Nagao, M. Coronary arterial spasm in ischemic heart disease and its pathogenesis: A review. *Circ. Res.* 52 (Suppl 1):147, 1983.

25. Maseri, A., L'Abbate, A., Baroldi, G., et al. Coronary vasospasm as a possible cause of myocardial infarction: A conclusion derived from the study of "preinfarction" angina. *N. Engl. J. Med.* 299:1271, 1978.

26. Oliva, P. B., and Breckenridge, N. C. Arter-

iographic evidence of coronary arterial spasm in acute myocardial infarction. *Circulation* 56:366, 1977.

27. MacAlpin, R. N. Relation of coronary arterial spasm to sites of organic stenosis. *Am. J. Cardiol.* 46:143, 1980.

28. Dalen, J. E., Ockene, I. S., and Alpert, J. S. Coronary spasm, coronary thrombosis, and myocardial infarction: A hypothesis concerning the pathophysiology of acute myocardial infarction. *Am. Heart. J.* 104:1119, 1982.

29. Maseri, A., Severi, S., Denes, M., et al. "Variant angina": One aspect of a continuous spectrum of vasospastic myocardial ischaemia. *Am. J. Cardiol.* 42:1019, 1978.

30. Chierchia, S., Burnelli, C., Simonett, I., et al. Sequence of events in angina at rest: Primary reduction in coronary flow. *Circulation* 61:759, 1980.

31. Jennings, R. B., Ganote, C. E., and Reimer, K. A. Ischemic tissue injury. *Am. J. Pathol.* 81:179, 1975.

32. Jennings, R. B., Somers, H. M., Smyth, G. A., et al. Myocardial necrosis induced by temporary occlusion of a coronary artery in the dog. *Arch. Pathol.* 70:68, 1960.

33. Reimer, K. A., and Jennings, R. B. The "wavefront phenomenon" of myocardial ischemic cell death. II. Transmural progression of necrosis within the framework of ischemic bed size (myocardium at risk) and collateral flow. *Lab. Invest.* 40:633, 1979.

34. Reimer, K. A., Lowe, J. E., and Rasmussen, M. M. The wavefront phenomenon of ischemic cell death. I. Myocardial infarct size v. duration of coronary occlusion in dogs. *Circulation* 56:786, 1977.

35. Reimer, K. A., Jennings, R., and Tatum, A. H. Pathobiology of acute myocardial ischemia: Metabolic, functional and ultrastructural studies. *Am. J. Cardiol.* 52:72A, 1983.

36. Heyndrickx, G. R., Baig, H., Nellers, P., et al. Depression of regional blood flow and wall thickening after brief coronary occlusion. *Am. J. Physiol.* 234:H653, 1978.

37. Jennings, R. B., Schaper, J., Hill, M. L., et al. Effect of reperfusion late in the phase of reversible ischemic injury. *Circ. Res.* 56:262, 1985.

38. Puri, P. S. Contractile and biochemical effects of coronary reperfusion after extended periods of coronary occlusion. *Am. J. Cardiol.* 36:244, 1975.

39. Weiner, J. M., Apstein, C. S., and Arthur, J. H. Persistence of myocardial injury following brief periods of coronary occlusion. *Cardiovasc. Res.* 10:678, 1976.

40. Wood, J. M., Hanley, H. G., Entman, M. L., et al. Biochemical and morphological correlates of acute experimental myocardial isch-

emia in the dog. IV. Energy mechanisms during very early ischemia. *Circ. Res.* 44:52, 1979.

41. Hess, M. L., Barnart, G. R., Crute, S., et al. Mechanical and biochemical effects of transient myocardial ischemia. *J. Surg. Res.* 26:175, 1979.

42. Braunwald, E., Kloner, R. A. The stunned myocardium: Prolonged postischemic ventricular dysfunction. *Circulation* 66:1146, 1982.

43. Reimer, K. A., Hill, M. L., and Jennings, R. B. Prolonged depletion of ATP and of the adenine nucleotide pool due to delayed resynthesis of adenine nucleotides following reversible myocardial ischemic injury in dogs. *J. Mol. Cell. Cardiol.* 13:229, 1981.

44. Geft, I. L., Fishbein, M. C., Ninomiya, K., et al. Intermittent brief periods of ischemia have a cumulative effect and may cause myocardial necrosis. *Circulation* 66:1150, 1982.

45. Gelet, T. R., Altschuld, R. A., and Weissler, A. M. Effects of acidosis on the performance and metabolism of the anoxic heart. IV. *Circulation* 39–40:60, 1969.

46. Wiliamson, J. R., Schaffer, S., Ford, C., et al. Contribution of tissue acidosis to ischemic injury in the perfused rat heart. *Circulation* 53(Suppl 1):I-13, 1976.

47. Hammond, B. and Hess, M. L. The oxygen free radical system: Potential mediation of myocardial injury. *J. Am. Coll. Cardiol.* 6:215, 1985.

48. Roberts, W. C. Coronary arteries in fatal acute myocardial infarction. *Circulation* 45:215, 1972.

49. Sherman, C. T., Litivack, F., Grundfest, W., et al. Coronary angioscopy in patients with unstable angina pectoris. *N. Engl. J. Med.* 315:913, 1986.

50. Mehta, J., Mehta, P., and Feldman, R. L. Thromboxane release in coronary artery disease: Spontaneous versus pacing-induced angina. *Am. Heart. J.* 107:286, 1984.

51. Bush, L. R., Campbell, W. B., Kern, K., et al. The effects of alpha adrenergic and serotonergic receptor antagonists on cyclic blood flow alternations in stenosed canine coronary arteries. *Circ. Res.* 55:642, 1984.

52. Lewis, H. D., Davis, J. W., Archibald, D. G., et al. Protective effects of aspirin against acute myocardial infarction and death in men with unstable angina. *N. Engl. J. Med.* 309:396, 1983.

53. Barger, A. C., Beeuwkes, R., Lainey, L. L., and Silverman, K. J. Hypothesis: Vasa vasorum and neovascularization of human coronary arteries, a possible role in the pathophysiology of atherosclerosis. *N. Engl. J. Med.* 310:175, 1984.

54. Factor, S. M., and Cho, S. Smooth muscle contraction bands in the media of coronary arteries: A postmortem marker of antemortem coronary spasm? *J. Am. Coll. Cardiol.* 6:1329, 1985.

55. Grollier, G., Scann, P., Commeau, P., et al. Role of coronary spasm in the genesis of myocardial infarction: Study of a case treated by isosorbide dinitrate in situ then by transluminal angioplasty. *Clin. Cardiol.* 8:644, 1985.

56. Naito, H., Yorozu, T., Matsuda, Y., et al. Coronary spasm producing coronary thrombosis in a patient with acute myocardial infarction. *Clin. Cardiol.* 10:275, 1987.

57. Feldman, R. L. Coronary thrombosis, coronary spasm and coronary atherosclerosis and speculation on the link between unstable angina and acute myocardial infarction. *Am. J. Cardiol.* 59:1187, 1987.

58. Conti, C. R., and Mehta, J. L. Acute myocardial ischemia: Role of atherosclerosis, thrombosis, platelet activation, coronary vasospasm, and altered arachidonic acid metabolism. *Circulation* 75(Suppl V):V-84, 1987.

59. Uchida, Y., Yoshoimoto, N., and Murao, S. Cyclic fluctuations in coronary blood pressure and flow induced by coronary artery constriction. *Jpn. Heart J.* 16:454, 1975.

60. Folts, J. D., Crowell, E. B., and Rowe, L. L. Platelet aggregation in partially obstructed vessels and its elimination with aspirin. *Circulation* 54:365, 1976.

61. Hirsh, P. H., Hillis, L. D., Campbell, W. B., et al. Release of prostaglandins and thromboxane into the coronary circulation in patients with ischemic heart disease. *N. Engl. J. Med.* 304:685, 1981.

62. Mehta, J., Mehta, P., and Horalek, C. Role of blood platelets and prostaglandins in coronary artery disease. *Am. J. Cardiol.* 48:366, 1981.

63. Mehta, J., Mehta, P., and Feldman, R. L. Severe intracoronary thromboxane release preceding acute coronary occlusion. *Prostaglandins Leukotrienes Med.* 8:599, 1982.

64. Mehta, J., Mehta, P., and Ostrowski, N. Increase in human platelet alpha-adrenergic receptor affinity for agonist in unstable angina. *J. Lab. Clin. Med.* 106:661, 1985.

65. Born, G. V. R., and Kratzer, M. A. A. Contribution of blood platelets to the pathogenesis of myocardial infarction. *Rev. Med. Brux.* 2:157, 1981.

66. Kostis, J. B., Gaughman, J., and Kuo, P. T. Association of recurrent myocardial infarction with hemostatic factors: A prospective study. *Chest* 81:571, 1982.

67. Werns, S. W., Shea, M. J., and Lucchesi, B. R. Free radical and myocardial injury: Pharmacologic implications. *Circulation* 74:1, 1986.

68. Lets, G. Leukotrienes: Role in cardiovascular physiology. *Cardiovasc. Clin.*, in press.
69. Ambrose, J. A., Winters, S. L., Stern, A., et al. Angiographic morphology and the pathogenesis of unstable angina pectoris. *J. Am. Coll. Cardiol.* 5:609, 1985.
70. Maseri, A., Chierchia, S., and Davies, G. Pathophysiology of coronary occlusion in acute infarction. *Circulation* 73:233, 1986.
71. Spodick, D. H., Flessas, A. P., and Johnson, M. M. Association of acute respiratory symptoms with onset of acute myocardial infarction: Prospective investigation of 150 consecutive patients and matched control patients. *Am. J. Cardiol.* 53:481, 1984.
72. Spodick, D. H. Acute viral (and other) infection in the onset, pathogenesis, and mimicry of acute myocardial infarction. *Am. J. Med.* 81:661, 1986.
73. Muller, J. E., Stone, P. H., Turi, Z. G., et al. Circadian variation in the frequency of onset of acute myocardial infarction. *N. Engl. J. Med.* 313:1315, 1985.
74. Toffler, G. H., Brezinski, D., Schafer, A. I., et al. Concurrent morning increase in platelet aggregability and the risk of myocardial infarction and sudden cardiac death. 316:1514, 1987.
75. Ruhenstroth-Bauer, G., Baumer, H., Burke, E. M., et al. Myocardial infarction and the weather: A significant positive correlation between the onset of heart infarct and 28 KHz atmospherics—a pilot study. *Clin. Cardiol.* 8:149, 1985.
76. Blumgart, H. L., Schlesinger, M. J., and David, D. Studies on the relation of the clinical manifestations of angina pectoris, coronary thrombosis, and myocardial infarction to the pathologic findings with particular reference to the significance of the collateral circulation. *Am. Heart J.* 19:1, 1940.
77. Schwartz, H., Leiboff, R. H., Bren, G. B., et al. Temporal evolution of the human coronary collateral circulation after myocardial infarction. *J. Am. Coll. Cardiol.* 4:1088, 1984.
78. Levin, D. C. Pathways and functional significance of the coronary collateral circulation. *Circulation* 50:831, 1974.
79. Hamby, R. I., Aintablian, A., and Schwartz, A. Reappraisal of the functional significance of the coronary collateral circulation. *Am. J. Cardiol.* 38:304, 1976.
80. Diamond, G., and Forrester, J. S. Effect of coronary artery disease and acute myocardial infarction on left ventricular compliance in man. *Circulation* 45:11, 1972.
81. Forrester, J. S., Diamond, G., Parmley, W., et al. Early increase in left ventricular compliance after myocardial infarction. *J. Clin. Invest.* 51:598, 1972.
82. Pirzada, F. A., Ekong, E. A., Vokonas, P. S., et al. Experimental myocardial infarction. XIII. Sequential changes in left ventricular pressure-length relationships in the acute phase. *Circulation* 53:970, 1976.
83. Smith, M., Ratshin, R. A., Harrel, F. E., et al. Early sequential changes in left ventricular dimensions and filling pressure in patients after myocardial infarction. *Am. J. Cardiol.* 33:363, 1974.
84. Herman, N. V., Heinle, R. A., Klein, M. D., et al. Localized disorders in myocardial contraction. *N. Engl. J. Med.* 227:222, 1967.
85. Pfeffer, M. A., Pfeffer, J. M., Fishbein, M. C., et al. Myocardial infarct size and ventricular function in rats. *Circ. Res.* 44:503, 1979.
86. Forrester, J. S., Wyatt, H. L. DaLuz, P. L., et al. Functional significance of regional ischemic contraction abnormalities. *Circulation* 54:64, 1976.
87. Rackely, C. E., Russell, R. O., Jr., Mantle, J. A., et al. Modern approach to the patient with acute myocardial infarction. *Curr. Probl. Cardiol.* 1:49, 1977.
88. Tamaki, N., Yasuda, T., Leinbach, R. C., et al. Spontaneous changes in regional wall motion abnormalities in acute myocardial infarction. *Am. J. Cardiol.* 58:406, 1986.
89. Sabbah, H. N., Gheorghiade, M., Smith, S. T., et al. Rate and extent of recovery of left ventricular function in patients following acute myocardial infarction. *Am. Heart J.* 114:516, 1987.
90. Klein, M. D., Herman, M. V., and Gorlin, R. G. A hemodynamic study of left ventricular aneurysm. *Circulation* 35:614, 1967.
91. Wynne, J., Sayres, M., Maddox, D. E., et al. Regional left ventricular function in acute myocardial infarction: Evaluation with quantitative radionuclide ventriculography. *Am. J. Cardiol.* 45:203, 1980.
92. Forrester, J. S., Diamond, G., Parmley, W., et al. Early increase in left ventricular compliance after myocardial infarction. *J. Clin. Invest.* 51:598, 1972.
93. Jugdutt, B. I., and Amy, R. W. Healing after myocardial infarction in the dog: Changes in infarct hydroxyproline and topography. *J. Am. Coll. Cardiol.* 7:91, 1986.
94. Eaton, L. W., Weiss, J. L., Bulkley, B. H., et al. Regional cardiac dilatation after acute myocardial infarction. *N. Engl. J. Med.* 300:57, 1979.
95. McKay, R. G., Pfeffer, M. A., Pasternak, R. C., et al. Left ventricular remodeling after myocardial infarction: A corollary to infarct expansion. *Circulation* 74:693, 1986.
96. Weisman, H. F., Bush, D. E., Mannisi, J. A., et al. Global cardiac remodeling after acute myocardial infarction: A study in the rat model. *J. Am. Coll. Cardiol.* 5:1355, 1985.

97. Pirolo, J. S., Hutchins, G. M., and Moore, G. W. Infarct expansion: Pathologic analysis of 204 patients with a single myocardial infarct. *J. Am. Coll. Cardiol.* 7:349, 1986.

98. Levites, R., Bank, V. S., and Helfant, R. H. Electrophysiological effects of coronary occlusion and reperfusion: Observations of dispersion of refractoriness and ventricular automaticity. *Circulation* 52:760, 1975.

99. Opie, L. H. Products of myocardial ischemia and electrical instability of the heart. *J. Am. Coll. Cardiol.* 5:162B, 1985.

100. Alpert, J. S., and Braunwald, E. Acute myocardial infarction: Pathological, pathophysiological, and clinical manifestations. In E. Braunwald (ed.), *Heart Disease* (2nd ed.). Philadelphia: Saunders, 1984. Pp. 1262–1300.

101. Lindsay, J., and Pichard, A. D. Acute myocardial infarction with normal coronary arteries. *Am. J. Cardiol.* 54:902, 1984.

2
Onset of Acute Myocardial Infarction: Possible Triggers

JAMES E. MULLER AND GEOFFREY H. TOFLER

Since 1985 information has been obtained indicating that in many cases there may be identifiable triggers of the onset of acute myocardial infarction. The primary data supporting this hypothesis are from epidemiologic studies showing a marked increase in frequency of the onset of myocardial infarction during the period from 6 A.M. to noon and, in some studies, a smaller, secondary increase during the period from 4 to 8 P.M. [1–16]. If the reasons for this timing of events can be identified, the potential for designing effective preventive therapy would be increased.

Morning Increase of Myocardial Infarction

The data supporting the contention that myocardial infarction is more likely to begin in the morning are contained in two studies that determined the onset of myocardial infarction objectively with creatine kinase (CK) timing [1, 2] and a larger number of older studies [3–16] that used onset of pain as a marker of time of myocardial infarction onset. The studies based on onset of pain received little attention because it was thought that the reported morning increase in incidence was simply the result of delayed reporting of the onset of a myocardial infarction that actually began during the night while the patient was sleeping but was not recognized because the pains were mild.

The first objective evidence of the morning increase of myocardial infarction was an unexpected by-product of the Multicenter Investigation of Limitation of Infarct Size (MILIS). The primary purpose of MILIS was to determine if propranolol or hyaluronidase limits the size of a myocardial infarction [17]. From 1978 until 1983, five centers screened almost 3000 patients and randomized 849 to therapy or placebo. MILIS demonstrated that neither agent limited infarct size when administered a mean of 8 hours after the onset of pain.

A secondary reason for conducting MILIS was to construct a database describing the natural history of myocardial infarction. The 100-megabyte database subsequently accumulated has produced information about numerous aspects of myocardial infarction. Documentation of the circadian variation of myocardial infarction resulted from use of the MILIS database to determine the time of year, day of the week, and hour of the day of the onset of the pain of myocardial infarction. Infarct onset was found to be randomly distributed among the months of the year and the days of the week, but there was a suggestion that the *onset of the pain* of myocardial infarction was more frequent during the 6 A.M. to noon period [1].

The obvious explanation that the observed morning increase resulted from delayed reporting of onset of pain could be tested by objective timing of the onset of myocardial infarction by CK-MB timing. In the MILIS study numerous CK-MB determinations were made to obtain an objective determination of the time of onset of myocardial infarction [18]. The onset of myocardial infarction was considered to have occurred 4 hours before the initial elevation of CK-MB.

The time of day of onset of myocardial in-

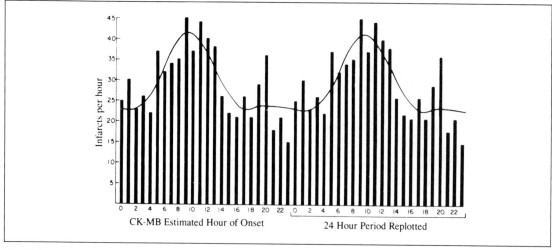

Fig. 2-1
Hourly frequency of onset of myocardial infarction as determined by the CK-MB
method in 703 patients. The number of infarctions beginning during each of the 24
hours of the day is plotted. A two-harmonic regression equation for the frequency
of onset of myocardial infarction has been fitted to the data (*curved line*). A
prominent circadian rhythm is present, with a primary peak incidence of
infarction at 9 A.M. and a secondary peak at 8 P.M. (Reprinted by permission from
J. E. Muller et al. Circadian variation in the frequency of onset of acute
myocardial infarction. *N. Engl. J. Med.* 313:1315, 1985.)

farction in the 703 patients in MILIS for whom
CK timing was available is shown in Figure 2-
1. The abscissa shows the hour of the day with
the same data replotted for a second day to
permit appreciation of the relation between
the end of one day and the beginning of the
next. The ordinate shows the number of infarcts per hour. The periodicity, as detected
by this more accurate, objective method, is
actually greater than that observed with reli-
ance on onset of pain for determination of onset, indicating that the subjective measure
tends to obscure, rather than simulate, a
pathologic rhythm.

By CK-MB timing a marked variation is apparent, with a maximum of 45 infarcts between 9 and 10 A.M. and a minimum of 15 between 11 P.M. and midnight. It is also of note
that this population was not standardized for
time of awakening. It is likely that these data
underestimate the morning increase, as at
least a few of the individuals who infarcted
during the afternoon worked unusual hours
and were actually arising at that time.

Thus objective timing of infarction indicated
that the infarcts *in the MILIS database* did occur more frequently in the morning. However,
because so many questions had been asked of
this database, it could have been a chance
occurrence not present in other databases.
Nevertheless, the finding is supported by 14
prior studies of the time of onset of the *pain*
of myocardial infarction [3–16], all but one of
which showed a peak onset of myocardial infarction during the 6 A.M. to noon period.

The objective evidence obtained in the
MILIS database has now been confirmed by
findings in an even larger database with CK
timing of onset [2]. Willich and colleagues examined the time of onset of myocardial infarction in the ISAM population—a database of
1741 patients randomly assigned to receive
placebo or streptokinase therapy [2]. This
database was studied with the prior hypothesis that a morning increase existed—in contrast to the MILIS experience in which the increase was found after numerous inquiries
into the data. In the ISAM population there

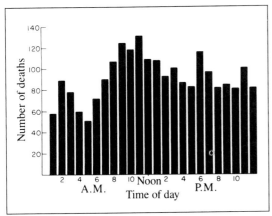

Fig. 2-2
Time of day of out-of-hospital sudden cardiac deaths for 2203 individuals dying in Massachusetts in 1983. A statistically significant ($p < .001$) circadian rhythm is present with a primary peak between 7 A.M. and 11 A.M. and a secondary peak between 5 P.M. and 6 P.M. (From J. E. Muller et al. Circadian variation in the frequency of sudden cardiac death. *Circulation* 75:131, 1987. By permission of the American Heart Association, Inc.)

was an even greater morning increase than that observed in the MILIS database. Infarcts were four times more likely to occur between 8 and 9 A.M. than between midnight and 1 A.M.

Thus the morning increase in onset of infarction is established by two large studies with CK timing of onset and supported by 14 additional studies that relied on symptoms to time the onset. It is also supported by data showing that the related conditions of sudden cardiac death (Fig. 2-2) [19, 20], transient myocardial ischemia [21], and stroke [22, 23] have similar morning increases.

Patients Receiving Prior Beta-Adrenergic Blockade Therapy

The time of onset was examined in various subgroups of patients in both the MILIS and ISAM databases. In MILIS, the morning peak of infarction was observed in both the older and younger halves of the population, men and women, smokers and nonsmokers, coffee drinkers and nondrinkers, and patients with and without a history of angina or myocardial

infarction. It is of note that a significant morning peak in incidence occurred in patients whose myocardial infarction began on a weekday (Monday to Friday) but *not* on Saturday or Sunday, days on which the population is less synchronized for time of awakening.

The subgroup of patients taking beta-adrenergic blocking agents during the 24 hours before the onset of myocardial infarction did not have a significant morning increase of onset of infarction. This finding was difficult to interpret because of the relatively small number of patients receiving beta-adrenergic blocking agents, the lack of a prior hypothesis, and the lack of information about other types of preinfarction medication.

The ISAM study has extended the knowledge obtained from the MILIS database. More extensive data about preinfarction medication were available in ISAM, and it was possible to test the prior hypothesis that the morning peak would be eliminated by beta blockade. When various subgroups were examined it was found that the group undergoing prior beta-adrenergic blockade was the only subgroup who did not demonstrate a morning increase. Patients taking calcium channel blocking agents prior to their infarction exhibited a typical morning increase—a finding consistent with the failure of relatively short-acting calcium blockers to provide secondary prevention against myocardial infarction [24].

Possible Causes of Morning Increase in Myocardial Infarction and Sudden Cardiac Death

The mechanisms through which physiologic changes occurring each morning could contribute to development of occlusive coronary thrombosis are summarized in Figure 2-3. First, the morning surge in systemic arterial pressure of 20 to 30 mm Hg could increase the likelihood of thrombogenic plaque rupture [25]. Second, coronary vascular tone is increased in the morning [26, 27]. Superimposed on a critical stenosis, such further narrowing could decrease coronary blood flow and pre-

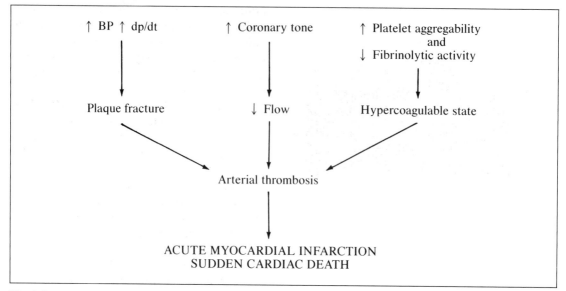

Fig. 2-3
Summary of physiologic changes occurring in the morning that could lead to the
onset of myocardial infarction.

dispose to thrombosis. Third, platelet aggregability is increased in the morning, and fibrinolytic activity is decreased [28, 29]; this combination may create a hypercoagulable state that may predispose a nonocclusive mural thrombus to extend and occlude the lumen. It is likely that a combination of events produces occlusive coronary thrombosis. Indeed, Constantinides demonstrated in dogs with experimental atherosclerosis that a combination of a sympathetic surge (produced by a catecholamine infusion) and endothelial dysfunction state (induced by injection of viper venom) was most effective in producing intraarterial thrombosis [30].

Beta-Adrenergic Blocking Agents and Prevention of Myocardial Infarction and Sudden Death

Consideration of the potential triggering mechanisms, together with the finding in the two databases that the morning increase in myocardial infarction is not observed in patients receiving beta-adrenergic blocking agents [1, 2], may provide a clue to the mechanism through which beta-blocking agents prevent myocardial infarction and sudden cardiac death. It has been known for some time that beta blockers reduce the incidence of recurrent myocardial infarction and sudden cardiac death following myocardial infarction [31, 32]. It has even been reported that these agents are capable of providing *primary* prevention against myocardial infarction [33].

Despite extensive study, the mechanism by which beta blockers exert their protective effect has not been identified. It has been particularly difficult to explain the ability of a beta blocker to prevent myocardial infarction, which is generally caused by coronary thrombosis, as most beta-adrenergic blocking agents have only minimal antiplatelet activity [34].

It is possible that the beta blockers exert their protective effect by blunting the morning increase in sympathetic activity. Such blunting would minimize increases in myocardial contractility and arterial pressure, which might increase the likelihood of plaque rupture.

A retrospective analysis of the time of day of out-of-hospital sudden cardiac death in the National Institute of Health (NIH)-sponsored Beta-Blocker Heart Attack Study (BHAT) adds further interest to the hypothesis that blockade of the morning surge in sympathetic activity may be beneficial [35]. An important finding of BHAT was that propanolol therapy reduced the incidence of sudden cardiac death; but as with myocardial infarction, the mechanism through which this beneficial effect was exerted has not been identified. Analysis of time of day of out-of-hospital sudden cardiac death in BHAT revealed that in the placebo group deaths were more frequent during the morning hours (from 2 A.M. to 2 P.M.) than during the remaining 12 hours of the day, indicating the presence of a morning increase similar to that observed in prior studies. However, in the group receiving propranolol, deaths during the morning period were 44 percent lower than in the placebo group.

An additional study suggesting a beneficial morning effect of beta-blockers has been reported [36]. Patients with silent myocardial ischemia were shown to have a distribution of transient ischemic periods that parallel sudden cardiac death and myocardial infarction (including a secondary evening peak). Treatment with beta blockers eliminated the morning peak, whereas calcium channel blockade was ineffective.

The accumulated indirect evidence suggesting a mechanism for the cardioprotective effect of beta blockers requires analysis of the time of myocardial infarction and death in other randomized studies of beta blockade.

Aspirin and Prevention of Myocardial Infarction and Sudden Cardiac Death

Two well-controlled, blinded, randomized studies of patients with unstable angina have demonstrated that, in patients with unstable angina, aspirin reduces the incidence of subsequent myocardial infarction, and sudden cardiac death by approximately 50 percent [37, 38]. In addition, combined analysis of six large studies of the administration of aspirin to patients post infarction indicates that aspirin reduces postinfarction mortality [39]. These studies of aspirin for secondary prevention have been supported by the results of the Physicians' Health Study in which the ability of aspirin to provide *primary* prevention against myocardial infarction was demonstrated [40].

At present there is no published information regarding the time of day of events in the placebo versus aspirin-treated groups, so the implication that an adverse morning process was blocked is less well supported for aspirin than for beta blockade. Because the primary effect of aspirin is to decrease platelet aggregability, it would be expected to eliminate the in vitro morning increase [28] in platelet responsiveness to epinephrine. It remains to be shown, however, that elimination of the in vitro response of platelets to a single agonist indicates that the in vivo response of platelets (in which multiple agonists participate) is diminished in the morning or that morning cardiac events are diminished.

"Circadian Variation" Versus "Morning Increase"

The original reports of the morning increase of myocardial infarction referred to a "circadian variation" in the incidence of the events. Subsequent study of processes likely to cause such events (increased platelet aggregability, increased sympathetic activity) indicated that the processes are not driven by an internal circadian pacemaker (as is cortisol secretion) but are a response to the daily activity cycle. Hence the accumulating evidence suggests that "morning increase" may be a more accurate descriptive term but it remains possible that there is an interaction between a true circadian rhythm and the daily activity cycle. Furthermore, the relation of onset to a morning activity (for which the population is synchronized) suggests that disease onset at other times of the day may be related to triggering activities that are randomly distributed throughout the day for a population and therefore produce no identifiable peak.

SIGNIFICANCE OF "MORNING INCREASE"

Awareness of this morning increase in onset of myocardial infarction leads to two practical questions: Is timing of medication important? Should exercise in the morning be avoided?

These questions can be answered for patients with symptoms of angina pectoris: The patient should be asked if angina occurs frequently in the morning, when the antianginal medications taken the night before may have lost their effect and the morning medications may not yet be active. Use of a long-acting nitrate, beta blocker, or calcium channel blocker the night before or of a rapidly acting agent in the morning may provide antianginal protection during a vulnerable period. Exercise that causes angina in the morning might be attempted at some other time of day.

For patients without morning angina and for the general population, these questions cannot yet be answered. It is possible that an agent effective against a potentially harmful morning physiologic process could prevent onset of myocardial infarction, sudden cardiac death, and stroke. Beta blockers could protect against the morning sympathetic surge, nitrates and calcium blockers against the morning increase in coronary tone, and aspirin against the morning increase in platelet aggregability; and a converting enzyme inhibitor could minimize the effects of assumption of the upright posture. There is at present no reason to administer any of these agents specifically for this purpose; but in patients taking the agents for other reasons, the night-time administration of long-acting preparations would be likely to provide protection during the morning. The available evidence suggests that beta blockers may be the most effective preventive agents, but additional studies are needed. Timing of aspirin administration is unlikely to be of significance, as the effect of aspirin on platelet aggregability lasts for days.

Exercise that does not cause angina appears to be beneficial, and at present there is no evidence that elimination of morning exercise is superior to no exercise at all.

The primary importance of the finding of morning increase of myocardial infarction is its use as a clue to investigate the cause of onset. The increased onset in the morning suggests that there are identifiable triggers that could also operate at other times of the day.

With such triggers in mind, a physician can elicit a history of a possible precipitating event in a surprisingly large number of patients with myocardial infarction. A precise quantitative study of the possible precipitants of myocardial infarction is needed so that increased information about triggering events can be obtained. Such information may lead to improved pharmacologic means to interrupt the linkage between a potentially triggering activity and its catastrophic consequences.

Acknowledgment

We are grateful for the assistance of Ms. Kathleen Carney in the preparation of the manuscript.

Editorial Comments

Examination of the MILIS database by Muller and colleagues has provided interesting and unique information regarding the onset of acute coronary events in the morning. The observations have obvious therapeutic implications with regard to the timing of antianginal drugs. More importantly, knowledge of these "triggers" of acute coronary syndromes may cast light on the underlying mechanisms. Vascular catastrophes, including stroke, myocardial infarction, and sudden death, appear to have a "morning increase." These observations provide further support for the unifying hypothesis that sympathetic nervous system activity and platelet aggregation are important processes in the pathophysiology of acute vascular "accidents." G. S. F.

References

1. Muller, J. E., Stone, P. H., Turi, Z. G., et al. Circadian variation in the frequency of onset of acute myocardial infarction. *N. Engl. J. Med.* 313:1315, 1985.
2. Willich, S. N., Linderer, T., Wegscheider, K., et al. Increased risk of myocardial infarction in the morning. *J. Am. Coll. Cardiol.* 11(Suppl A):28A, 1988.

3. Master, A. M. The role of effort and occupation (including physicians) in coronary occlusion. *J.A.M.A.* 174:942, 1960.

4. Pell, S., and D'Alonzo, C. A. Acute myocardial infarction in a large industrial population: Report of a 6-year study of 1,356 cases. *J.A.M.A.* 135:831, 1963.

5. Bock, K. D., and Kreuzenbeck, W. Spontaneous Blood Pressure Variations in Hypertension: The Effect of Antihypertensive Therapy and Correlations with the Incidence of Complications. In F. Gross (ed.), *Antihypertensive Therapy: Principles and Practice: An International Symposium.* New York: Springer-Verlag, 1966. Pp. 224–241.

6. Johansson, B. W. Myocardial infarction in Malmo 1960–1968. *Acta Med. Scand.* 191:505, 1972.

7. Myers, A., and Dewar, H. A. Circumstances attending 100 sudden deaths from coronary artery disease with coroner's necropsies. *Br. Heart J.* 37:1133, 1975.

8. Pedoe, H. T., Clayton, D., Morris, J. N., et al. Coronary heart attacks in East London. *Lancet* 2:833, 1975.

9. Churina, S. K., Ganelina, I. E., and Volpert, E. I. On the distribution of the incidence of acute myocardial infarction within a 24-hour period. *Kardiologiia* 15(7):115, 1975. [Russian].

10. Gyarfas, I., Csukas, A., and Horvath-Gaudi, I. Analysis of the diurnal periodicity of acute myocardial infarction attacks. *Sante Publique (Bucur.)* 19:77, 1976.

11. Myocardial Infarction Community Registers: Results of a WHO International Collaborative Study Coordinated by the Regional Office for Europe. In *Public Health in Europe* (No. 5, Vol. 1). Copenhagen: Regional Office for Europe (World Health Organization), 1976. P. 232.

12. Reinberg, A., and Smolensky, M. H. *Biological Rhythms and Medicine: Cellular, Metabolic, Physiopathologic, and Pharmacologic Aspects.* New York: Springer-Verlag, 1983.

13. Kaufmann, M. W., Gottlieb, G., Kahaner, K., et al. Circadian rhythm and myocardial infarct: A preliminary study. *IRCS J. Med. Sci. (Biochem.)* 9:557, 1981.

14. Ganelina, I. E., and Borisova, I. Y. Circadian rhythm of working capacity, sympathicoadrenal activity, and myocardial infarction. *Hum. Physiol.* 9(2):113, 1983.

15. Thompson, D. R., Blandford, R. L., Sutton, T. W., and Marchant, P. R. Time of onset of chest pain in acute myocardial infarction. *Int. J. Cardiol.* 7:139, 1985.

16. Dimitrov, I., and Khadzhikhristev, A. Dynamics of the incidence of myocardial infarction in Smoljan District for the period 1965–1979. *Vutr. Boles.* 22:40, 1983.

17. MILIS Study Group. National Heart, Lung, and Blood Institute Multicenter Investigation of the Limitation of Infarct Size (MILIS): Design and Methods of the Clinical Trial: An Investigation of Beta-Blockade and Hyaluronidase for Treatment of Acute Myocardial Infarction. In J. E. Muller (ed.), *American Heart Association Monograph No. 100.* Dallas: American Heart Association, 1984. Pp. 1–134.

18. Roberts, P., Gowda, K. S., Ludbrook, P. A., and Sobel, B. E. Specificity of elevated serum MB creatine phosphokinase with activity in the diagnosis of acute myocardial infarction. *Am. J. Cardiol.* 36:433, 1975.

19. Muller, J. E., Ludmer, P. L., Willich, S. N., et al. Circadian variation in the frequency of sudden cardiac death. *Circulation* 75:131, 1987.

20. Willich, S. N., Levy, D., Rocco, M. B., et al. Circadian variation in the incidence of sudden cardiac death in the Framingham Heart Study population. *Am. J. Cardiol.* 60:801, 1987.

21. Rocco, M. B., Barry, J., Campbell, S., et al. Circadian variation of transient myocardial ischemia in patients with coronary artery disease. *Circulation* 75:395, 1987.

22. Tsementzis, S. A., Gill, J. S., Hitchcock, E. R., et al. Diurnal variation of and activity during the onset of stroke. *Neurosurgery* 17:901, 1985.

23. Robertson, T., Marler, J., and Muller, J. E. Circadian variation in the frequency of onset of stroke. *J. Am. Coll. Cardiol.* 7(Suppl A):40A, 1986.

24. Moss, A. J. Long-term effect of diltiazem on mortality and reinfarction after myocardial infarction—the Multicenter Diltiazem Post-Infarction Research Group. *J. Am. Coll. Cardiol.* 11(Suppl A):27A, 1988.

25. Millar-Craig, M. W., Bishop, C. N., and Raftery, E. B. Circadian variation of blood pressure. *Lancet* 1:795, 1978.

26. Yasue, H., Omote, S., Takizawa, A., et al. Circadian variation of exercise capacity in patients with Prinzmetal's variant angina: Role of exercise-induced coronary arterial spasm. *Circulation* 59:938, 1979.

27. Fujita, M., and Franklin, D. Diurnal changes in coronary blood flow in conscious dogs. *Circulation* 76:488, 1987.

28. Tofler, G. H., Brezinski, D. A., Schafer, A. I., et al. Concurrent morning increase in platelet aggregability and the risk of myocardial infarction and sudden cardiac death. *N. Engl. J. Med.* 316:1514, 1987.

29. Rosing, D. R., Brakman, P., Redwood, D. R., et al. Blood fibrinolytic activity in man: Diurnal variation and the response to varying intensities of exercise. *Circ. Res.* 27:171, 1970.

30. Constantinides, P. Plaque fissure in human coronary thrombosis. *J. Atheroscler. Res.* 1:1, 1966.

31. Norwegian Multicenter Group. Timolol-induced

reduction in mortality and reinfarction in patients surviving acute myocardial infarction. *N. Engl. J. Med.* 304:801, 1981.

32. Beta-Blocker Heart Attack Trial Research Group. A randomized trial of propranolol in patients with acute myocardial infarction: Mortality results. *J.A.M.A.* 247:1707, 1982.

33. Wikstrand, J., Warnold, I., Olsson, G., et al. Primary prevention with metoprolol in patients with hypertension: Mortality results from the MAPHY study. *J.A.M.A.* 259:1976, 1988.

34. Frishman, W. H. Multifactorial actions of beta-adrenergic blocking drugs in ischemic heart disease: Current concepts. *Circulation* 67(Suppl I):I-11, 1983.

35. Peters, R. W., Muller, J. E., Goldstein, S., et al. Propranolol and the circadian variation in the frequency of sudden cardiac death: The BHAT experience. *Circulation* 76(Suppl IV):IV-364, 1988.

36. Mulcahy, D., Keegan, J., Park, A., et al. Effects of therapeutic interventions on the distribution of silent ischaemic episodes throughout the day. *J. Am. Coll. Cardiol.* 11(Suppl A):97A, 1988.

37. Lewis, H. D., Davis, J. W., Archibald, D. G., et al. Protective effects of aspirin against acute myocardial infarction and death in men with unstable angina: Results of a Veterans Administration cooperative study. *N. Engl. J. Med.* 309:396, 1983.

38. Canadian Cooperative Study Group. A randomized trial of aspirin and sulfinpyrazone in threatened stroke. *N. Engl. J. Med.* 299:53, 1978.

39. Peto, R., and Parish, S. Aspirin after myocardial infarction. *Lancet* 1:1172, 1980.

40. Physicians' Health Study Research Group. Aspirin for the primary prevention of myocardial infarction. *N. Engl. J. Med.* 318:262, 1988.

3
Biochemistry of Myocardial Infarction

HEINRICH TAEGTMEYER

For obvious reasons coronary arteries have long been the focus of research in ischemic heart disease. Only in recent years, in part due to the advent of techniques for myocardial reperfusion, has interest arisen in the rather complex biochemical derangements involving the ischemic and infarcting myocardium itself.

Cardiologists may find it difficult to digest the large amount of biochemical information without a brief recapitulation of the essence of energy metabolism in normal heart. This chapter therefore starts out with a description of the chemical supply side of a complex system, which is best defined by the heart's ability to convert chemical into mechanical energy. It then explores the consequences of the sudden interruption of this supply and their clinical implications. For the sake of clarity, concepts are emphasized, rather than details elaborated.

Heart Muscle as Site of Energy Conversion

The functions of metabolism in the heart are few in number and can be understood even without knowledge of chemical formulas. The main purpose of all biochemical reactions in the myocardial cell is to provide energy for contraction, ion transport, and synthesis as well as degradation of biomolecules. Like any other living tissue, heart muscle captures and utilizes this energy in the form of adenosine triphosphate (ATP). The tissue content of ATP is normally around 20 μmol/gm dry weight. At an oxygen consumption rate of about 4.5 μmol/min/gm dry weight [1] and a phosphorus/oxygen (P/O) ratio of 3, heart muscle utilizes and replenishes about 1500 μmol ATP/min/gm dry weight (25 μmol/sec/gm dry weight). This simple calculation illustrates that without replenishment intracellular stores of ATP would be exhausted within 1 second. Thus ATP must be resynthesized as quickly as it is broken down, a concept that finds its expression in the "ATP cycle," depicted in Figure 3-1. This concept and calculation are of course somewhat oversimplified, as they do not take into account the small stores of phosphocreatine that replenish ATP by the creatine kinase reaction (phosphocreatine + ADP → creatine + ATP) and the action of the adenylate kinase reaction, which restores 1 mol of ATP from 2 mol of adenosine diphosphate (ADP) (2 ADP → ATP + AMP) (vide infra). It can thus be gleaned that the rate of ATP turnover, rather than the steady-state concentrations of ATP, determines the energy state of the cell. Indeed, a number of studies have shown a lack of correlation between ATP tissue content and oxygen consumption as well as contractile function in reperfused myocardium [2–4].

The main sources of ATP in heart muscle are oxidative phosphorylation of ADP in the respiratory chain and, to a lesser extent, phosphorylation of ADP either by substrate-level phosphorylation in the glycolytic pathway and the Krebs cycle or by the action of creatine kinase. Because oxidative phosphorylation is quantitatively the major supplier of ATP and because the key enzymes of oxidative metabolism are located in mitochondria, myocardial cells are well endowed with these organelles,

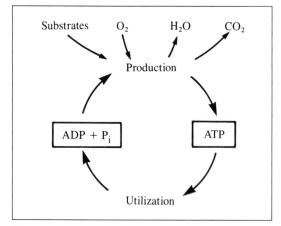

Fig. 3-1
Cycle of cardiac energy metabolism. The myocardial cell captures and utilizes energy in the phosphate bonds of ATP. Energy is captured in ATP by the conversion of substrates and oxygen to carbon dioxide and water. The energy is liberated through ATPase, causing hydrolysis of ATP to ADP and P_i; ATP is utilized for the various processes involved in contraction and maintenance of cellular homeostasis. An increase in energy utilization results in an instantaneous increase in energy production.

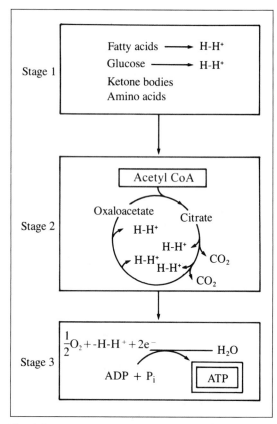

Fig. 3-2
Stages of normal cardiac energy metabolism. In the normal myocardium conversion of energy-providing substrates (fatty acids, glucose, ketone bodies, amino acids) to carbon dioxide and water occurs in a series of complex enzyme-catalyzed reactions, all of which ultimately lead to the production of reducing equivalents for reaction with molecular oxygen in the respiratory chain. All substrates are catabolized to acetyl CoA (stage 1). Acetyl CoA provides the substrate for the citrate synthesis reaction, which commits the compound to combustion in the citric acid cycle. This cycle is the main site for production of reducing equivalents (stage 2). Reducing equivalents react with oxygen in the respiratory chain, the site of oxidative phosphorylation of ADP to ATP (stage 3).

which make up more than 35 percent of the myocardial cell volume [5]. Not surprisingly, mitochondrial damage appears to be one of the main morphologic and functional consequences of myocardial ischemia [6–8].

In respiring tissues, oxidative phosphorylation of ADP depends on the production of reducing equivalents (protons) and the passage of electrons along the respiratory chain. Reducing equivalents are produced in the course of substrate catabolism to acetyl coenzyme A (CoA) and the subsequent oxidation of acetyl CoA in the Krebs cycle. As a matter of convenience, it seems reasonable to group the main energy (or proton) providing reactions into three stages (Fig. 3-2). The first stage comprises all reactions leading to acetyl CoA; the second stage comprises the oxidation of acetyl CoA in the Krebs cycle (producing carbon dioxide as by-product); and the third stage consists of the flow of electrons down the respiratory chain leading to the release of free energy (producing water as by-product),

which is conserved in the energy-rich phosphate bond of ATP (Figs. 3-1 and 3-2).

The heart's prodigious requirement for oxygen has been known for over 100 years. In 1885 Professor Yeo [9] at King's College in London provided the first direct demonstration of oxygen uptake by heart muscle when he perfused a frog heart in a chamber containing hemoglobin, which he analyzed by spectroscopy. Yeo observed not only the reduction of oxyhemoglobin by the heart but also a greater rate of hemoglobin reduction when the heart was electrically stimulated. "Indeed we may conclude," he summarized, "that the absorption of a considerable quantity of oxygen is one of the items essential to the life of the tissue. The greater amount of oxygen used by the contracting heart muscle is so constant that it would appear equally certain that during contraction the oxygen requirement of the tissue notably increases." Nearly 20 years later, Winterstein [10] demonstrated the oxygen requirement for the mammalian heart when he showed that isolated rabbit hearts resumed beating as oxygen was readmitted to the perfusion medium after a period of anoxia.

Although the heart plays only a minor role in the overall fuel balance of the body, it obeys the same general rules of metabolic regulation as do other tissues [11]. For instance, it has been known for a good number of years that in the fasting state the energy requirements of the heart are met largely by oxidation of fatty acids [12], and that after carbohydrate feeding the heart switches its preference to glucose [13]. The heart can therefore be regarded as an "omnivore"; that is, under aerobic conditions it is able to derive energy aerobically from a variety of fuel sources including fatty acids, ketone bodies, glucose, lactate, and even certain amino acids. Depending on the physiologic state of the individual, only plasma glucose levels are relatively constant, whereas levels of lactate, fatty acids, and ketone bodies may vary over a wide range. Thus it is expected, and has in fact been found, that the fuel for aerobic energy metabolism in heart muscle varies with the plasma concentration of individual substrates [13, 14] or hormones [15]. Given the large fluctuations in the plasma concentrations of exogenous fuels and the heart's ability to utilize a variety of fuels, Bing [11] has viewed the phenomenon as a safety mechanism for the survival of a vital organ.

Heart muscle itself is also capable of contributing to the fuels of respiration by releasing both fatty acids and glucose from their storage forms as triglycerides or glycogen. Rates of synthesis and degradation for either storage fuel have not been measured so far, but it is well known that starvation increases the tissue content of both triglycerides and glycogen [16] and that the heart utilizes endogenous triglycerides when perfused with nutrient-free medium [17] or under conditions of increased pressure development [18]. The most striking example of endogenous fuel utilization is of course seen with ischemia, when glycogen is rapidly broken down to lactate and alanine.

Metabolic Alterations of Myocardial Ischemia and Infarction

COUPLING OF CORONARY FLOW TO METABOLIC AND MECHANICAL ACTIVITY

It cannot be emphasized too strongly that the heart has a high rate of energy turnover. Another fact needs to be reiterated: Because almost all of the heart's energy is derived from aerobic metabolism, oxygen consumption of the heart is several times greater than oxygen consumption of other mammalian organs [1], and only a slight perturbance in the supply of oxygen may lead to disastrous consequences for the energy supply of the myocardial cell. Such events are best characterized as the reduced rates of ATP production (Fig. 3-3) and the buildup of intermediary metabolites, protons, carbon dioxide, and (under certain conditions) triglycerides.

Because even under resting conditions the heart extracts more than half of the oxygen delivered by arterial blood, there is a tight coupling between blood flow through the coronary arteries and myocardial oxygen consumption. Thus the heart's ability to produce energy aerobically depends on its ability to increase coronary flow in accordance with its energy needs. For example, under resting conditions coronary flow is about 1 ml/min/gm wet weight in humans, and it increases in parallel with myocardial oxygen consumption;

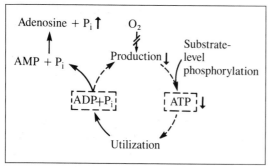

Fig. 3-3
Oxygen deprivation interrupts the cycle of cardiac energy metabolism at the level of energy production. Cellular stores of ATP are minimal, even when replenished by substrate-level phosphorylation. Because ADP is not phosphorylated, it is degraded further to AMP and adenosine.

that is, when oxygen consumption doubles, coronary flow doubles and so on.

Grading of Ischemia and Its Metabolic Response

The earliest forms of ischemia, defined as lack of oxygen supply due to inadequate blood flow, occur in patients unable to increase coronary flow in response to increased energy demands. Because resting coronary flow is normal in this setting, this form of ischemia is sometimes referred to as "normal flow" ischemia. By contrast, when coronary flow is reduced at rest, the term "low flow ischemia" has been used. The extreme form of ischemia is of course manifested as complete occlusion of a coronary artery with subsequent necrosis of the tissue supplied. Thus there is a continuum of ischemia, with mild, "normal flow" ischemia at one end and the extreme situation of a myocardial infarction at the other end of the spectrum. As discussed below, the concept of a continuum of ischemia is also borne out by the temporal progression and spatial architecture of an acute myocardial infarction [19], which indicates progression of the zone of irreversible tissue injury from the subendocardium to the subepicardium as the time of ischemia lengthens (see Fig. 1-3).

Ischemia affects myocardial energy metabolism by slowing down aerobic metabolism of substrates, reducing the tissue content of phosphocreatine and adenine nucleotides, and first increasing and then slowing down anaerobic metabolism of substrates (Table 3-1). Just as there is a continuum of the relative restriction of oxygen delivery, one might expect that there is a continuum of metabolic responses to ischemia. With "normal flow" ischemia, heart muscle is still capable of oxidizing fatty acids and glucose under resting conditions. Opie and coworkers [20] have shown that, as coronary blood flow decreases, the relative contribution of glucose to the residual oxidative metabolism increases and oxidation of glucose accounts for a greater percentage of aerobic ATP production (Table 3-2). Increased uptake of a glucose analog by ischemic myocardium has also been found when the energy demand for the heart was increased by pacing or exercise [14, 21]. There is increased lactate release from the stressed myocardium [21, 22] and increased glucose uptake, especially when fatty acid levels are low [23]. The possible reasons for increased glucose uptake with stress and ischemia are multiple: (1) Glucose makes better use of the restricted amounts of oxygen. If blood supply is mildly reduced, the heart switches from fatty acids to glucose as the preferred fuel for respiration. (2) Glycolysis yields a small amount of ATP through substrate-level phosphorylation in the cytosol independent of the availability of oxygen (2 mol of ATP/mol of glucose, whereas 36 mol of ATP are produced per mole of glucose oxidized). (3) Glucose transport is enhanced in oxygen-deprived tissue. Thus more glucose enters the cell, and glucose is preferred over fatty acids as substrate for energy production.

The regulation of intermediary metabolism

Table 3-1
Energy metabolism of myocardial ischemia

Aerobic metabolism	↓
Phosphocreatine	↓
Adenine nucleotides	↓
Anaerobic metabolism	↑ (first)
Anaerobic metabolism	↓ (later)

Table 3-2
Relative contributions of glucose, fatty acids, and lactate to ATP production of the aerobic and ischemic dog heart

Condition	ATP (μmol/min/gm)			
	From glucose	From fatty acids	From lactate	Total
Aerobic	1980	2224	468	4672
Mild ischemia	1008–1260	188–257	0	1265–1448
Severe ischemia	677	70	0	747
Total ischemia	0	0	0	0

Source: From L. H. Opie. Effects of regional ischemia on metabolism of glucose and fatty acids. *Circ. Res.* 38(Suppl I):I-52, 1976. With permission of the American Heart Association, Inc.

of glucose, fatty acids, and amino acids during ischemia is complex and requires further discussion with respect to accumulation of intermediary metabolites and reversibility of ischemic tissue damage.

When oxygen becomes limiting with respect to oxygen requirements for energy production, flux through the electron transport system of the respiratory chain slows down and the ratio of the reduced form of nicotinamide-adenine dinucleotide (NAD) to the oxidized form of NAD ([NADH]/[NAD$^+$]) increases. This reduced state indicates a lack of ATP production by oxidative phosphorylation, which is accompanied by a loss of contractile function.

The exact biochemical mechanisms responsible for the rapid loss of contractile function are not yet known with certainty. There are those who implicate loss of ATP [24] and others who implicate the accumulation of potentially toxic intermediary products such as hydrogen ions [25, 26] or lactate [4]. Kübler and Katz [27] suggested it is unlikely that decreased ATP supplies for energy-consuming reactions in the myocardial cell cause the observed decrease in myocardial contractility because of the low K_m for ATP at the substrate-binding sites of energy-consuming reactions in the heart. In other words, at prevailing concentrations of ATP in the ischemic, noncontracting tissue, enzymes such as myosin-ATPase should still operate at near-maximal velocity. However, Kübler and Katz speculated that small changes in ATP may already exert modulatory effects on ion fluxes,

and the large amount of inorganic phosphate may form insoluble calcium-phosphate precipitates that trap calcium in the sarcoplasmic reticulum and mitochondria [27]. Another possible explanation for the discrepancy between ATP content and ATP conversion into useful energy for the heart is the trapping, or "compartmentation," of ATP in a compartment not accessible to the enzymes of the contractile apparatus or ion pumps (e.g., mitochondria). Examining the acute effects of ischemia on phosphocreatine and ATP, Gudbjarnason et al. [28] found that breakdown of phosphocreatine was more rapid than the breakdown of ATP. The kinetic heterogeneity of ATP and phosphocreatine depletion seems to indicate an inhibition of transfer of ATP from mitochondria to the cytosol, and it has been speculated that the reduction in regeneration of cytosolic ATP causes the early cessation of contractile activity in ischemic myocardium. Given the uncertainty of the actual biochemical mechanism for contractile failure in the ischemic and infarcted myocardium, it appears reasonable to examine alterations in the metabolism of individual substrates next and to attempt a synthesis thereafter.

GLUCOSE METABOLISM DURING ISCHEMIA

Of all substrates used for energy production by the human myocardium, glucose is, with the possible exception of glutamate (vide infra), the only substrate yielding ATP by anaerobic substrate-level phosphorylation (Fig. 3-4). Intracellular glucose is derived from two sources: extracellular glucose in the plasma and interstitial space, and breakdown of intracellular glycogen (the storage form of glucose, which is also referred to as "emergency fuel").

Ischemia stimulates both glycogenolysis and glycolysis (Fig. 3-5). The sequence of events can be summarized as follows: Glycogen breakdown is increased as a result of phosphorylase activation (phosphorylation of phosphorylase b, giving rise to phosphorylase a). For example, with total ischemia in rat heart, glycogen stores fall by 50 percent within 5 minutes and by 70 percent within 20 minutes [2]. Similar observations have been made by many other investigators in many systems. With ischemia, transport of exogenous glucose is increased, and the hexokinase and phosphofructokinase activities are likewise increased. The rapid flux through the glycolytic pathway during early stages of ischemia leads to the intracellular accumulation of lactate, creating a bottleneck at the glyceraldehyde 3-phosphate dehydrogenase step, as evidenced by accumulation of metabolites arising from reactions leading to the glyceraldehyde 3-phosphate dehydrogenase reaction [29]. There is now good evidence that lactate and NADH inhibit the enzyme in both the intact heart [30] and the isolated enzyme preparation [31]. Thus in ischemic heart muscle, energy depletion is further complicated by the accumulation of a product that by itself inhibits the main pathway of anaerobic energy production. Another point needs to be kept in mind: Although ATP production via anaerobic glycolysis may be increased as much as tenfold during the early stages by ischemia, the amount of energy produced still falls short of 90 percent of the energy required for normal cardiac contraction [32].

During reperfusion of reversibly injured ischemic myocardium, lactate is rapidly oxidized, and cardiac function (including myocardial oxygen consumption) returns to normal before ATP or glycogen is restored to preischemic values in the tissue [2]. Thus upon return

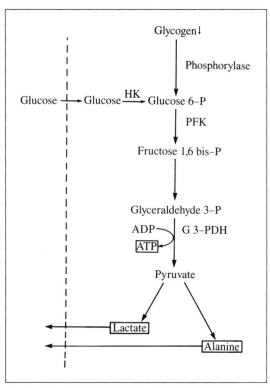

Fig. 3-4
Glucose metabolism in the ischemic heart. Glycogenolysis provides "emergency fuel." Ischemia increases glucose transport across the sarcolemma (*interrupted line*) and increases glycogen breakdown. Both glucose and glycogen are degraded in the glycolytic pathway to lactate and, to a lesser extent, alanine. Glycolysis yields 2 mol of ATP/mol of glucose (whereas the oxidative metabolism of glucose yields 36 mol of ATP). Regulatory enzymes: phosphorylase; HK = hexokinase; PFK = phosphofructokinase; G3-PDH = glyceraldehyde 3-phosphate dehydrogenase.

of oxidative metabolism in the reversibly ischemic myocardium, endogenous substrate (lactate) is utilized first. More importantly, at the high rates of oxygen consumption and substrate utilization found in the heart, the depressed steady-state content of ATP does not correlate with high rates of ATP turnover so long as there is no substantial loss of total adenine nucleotides. There have been numerous studies in the past that suggested a correlation between ATP content and ATP turnover, but they have not held up to more recent scrutiny [2, 4, 33].

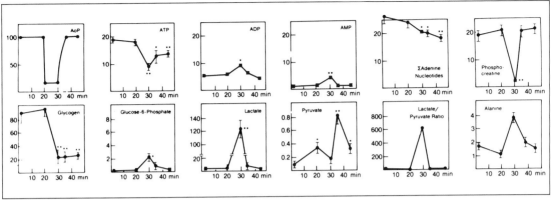

Fig. 3-5
Effects of short-term (10 minutes) ischemia on function and the metabolite content of isolated rat hearts. Hearts were perfused as "working hearts" and subjected to 10 minutes of normothermic total ischemia prior to reperfusion with an oxygenated medium. Recovery of function occurred within 93 seconds and was associated with a disappearance of lactate and restoration of phosphocreatine. Note that both ATP and glycogen levels remained depressed. (From H. Taegtmeyer et al. Energy metabolism in reperfused rat heart. *J. Am. Coll. Cardiol.* 6:864, 1985. With permission.)

FATTY ACID AND LIPID METABOLISM DURING ISCHEMIA

Oxygen deprivation affects fatty acid metabolism in an even more devastating way than glucose metabolism. In contrast to glucose, metabolism of fatty acids requires a net investment of ATP in the course of their activation that can only be reclaimed by oxidative metabolism (Fig. 3-6). Furthermore, unlike glycogen, fatty acids provide no "anaerobic fuel reserve" for any residual ATP production. As a result of decreased electron flux in the respiratory chain, reducing equivalents accumulate. This situation leads in turn to first a slowing and then the cessation of both β-oxidation and the citric acid cycle, as the rate of β-oxidation is controlled by the availability of (oxidated) NAD^+ [34]. As a consequence of decreased rates of β-oxidation, the tissue content of acetyl CoA declines and long-chain acyl CoA and long-chain acyl carnitine accumulate. The accumulation of long-chain acyl CoA in the cytosol provides substrate for esterification of fatty acids with α-glycerophosphate, resulting in increased synthesis of triglycerides and in a further decline in cytosolic ATP and accumulation of AMP plus PP_i (Fig.

3-6). Increased triglyceride synthesis in reversible damaged ischemic myocardium has been demonstrated in the border zone of myocardial infarctions [35] and with positron emission tomography using ^{11}C-palmitate residue curves [36].

The effects of fatty acids and their intermediates on membranes and enzyme activities are complex. Although not all of these effects are completely understood, a number of physiologically important observations have been made. High concentrations of fatty acyl CoA have been shown to specifically inhibit the adenine nucleotide translocator across the inner mitochondrial membrane [37, 38], although the amount of cytosolic long-chain acyl CoA required to significantly inhibit the transport of adenine nucleotides may be too high to be of physiologic importance. High levels of fatty acyl CoA inhibit the acyl CoA synthesis [39], which leads in turn to decreased uptake of fatty acids. It has further been suggested that the shuttle system for acetyl CoA between cytosol and mitochondria may also be impaired with ischemia [40].

The effects of elevated free fatty acid levels in the plasma on ischemic heart muscle are

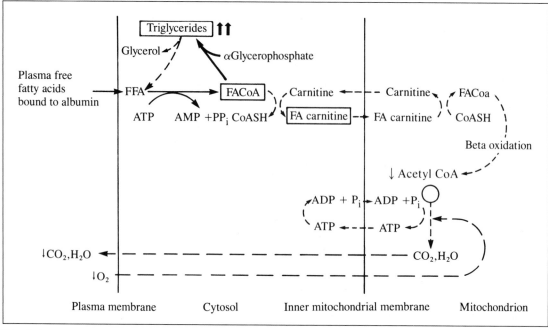

Fig. 3-6
Fatty acid metabolism in the ischemic heart. Lack of oxygen results in the inhibition of both β-oxidation and citric acid cycle activity. Free fatty acids (FFA), fatty acyl CoA (FACoA), fatty acyl carnitine (FA carnitine), and triglycerides accumulate in the ischemic myocardium.

deleterious in patients, where they may cause arrhythmias [41] as well as in the experimentally oxygen-deprived heart muscle, where they cause a decrease in myocardial contractility [40, 42–44].

There is increasing evidence that abnormalities in lipid metabolism participate in the pathogenesis of membrane damage in the ischemic myocardium [45–47]. Wood et al. [48] first reported inhibition of carnitine palmityl CoA transferase by ischemia and then proposed that accumulation of long-chain fatty acyl carnitines exert a detergent effect on ion pumps and possibly carrier systems as well [49]. Sobel et al. [50] reported that large amounts of lysophosphatides accumulated in the ischemic heart possibly causing arrhythmias. Chien et al. [51] demonstrated the accumulation of unesterified arachidonic acid in ischemic dog heart.

The increased concentrations of free fatty acids and fatty acids esters in the ischemic myocardium and their detergent action may

cause either reversible or irreversible membrane damage via inhibition of enzymes, uncoupling of oxidative phosphorylation, and permeability changes [45]. In addition to the detergent effects of lipid-derived substances from either endogenous or exogenous sources, the hydrolysis of membrane phospholipids in early myocardial ischemia has received considerable attention [45, 51]. Because arachidonic acid is a major component of phospholipids, its liberation during ischemia has been taken as a sign of membrane destruction. The significance of the early phospholipid degradation is still uncertain, however, because total myocardial phospholipid loss is small during the first 3 hours of ischemia [52, 53].

AMINO ACID METABOLISM IN MYOCARDIAL ISCHEMIA

Amino acid metabolism during myocardial ischemia has been studied by Mudge et al. [54]

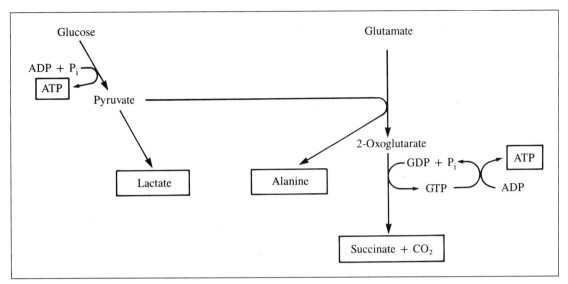

Fig. 3-7
Interaction of glucose and amino acid metabolism. Alanine, succinate, and carbon dioxide accumulate in ischemic myocardium together with lactate. Alanine arises from transamination of pyruvate with glutamate, which in turn is further degraded to succinate. Formation of succinate and carbon dioxide is linked to substrate-level phosphorylation of GDP, the only anaerobic source of energy other than lactate.

and Taegtmeyer et al. [55, 56]. Initially the possibility was considered that augmented release of alanine from heart muscle may serve as a marker of myocardial ischemia because of similarities in the release of amino acids from heart muscle [57] and the release of amino acids from skeletal muscle under conditions of relative oxygen deficiency [58]. As illustrated in Figure 3-7, the enzymes lactate dehydrogenase and alanine aminotransferase compete for the same substrate.

Following these observations, transmyocardial differences of amino acids in normal subjects and in patients with coronary artery disease demonstrated augmented myocardial alanine production and glutamate uptake in patients with coronary artery disease [54]. This finding has led to a more detailed study of myocardial amino acid metabolism during oxygen deprivation [55, 56, 59–62]. First, it was found that alanine did not arise from proteolysis but from enhanced rates of glucose breakdown [55, 56]. Second, it was learned that alanine production from glucose (Fig. 3-7) occurs not only in ischemic heart muscle but

also in the ischemic brain [63], ischemic rat liver [64], and the blood of diving vertebrates and man [65, 66]. Because oxygen deprivation is the most potent stimulus to glycolysis, it is plausible that the carbon skeleton of alanine arises from glucose breakdown during anaerobic glycolysis. A portion of alanine accumulating in ischemic heart muscle may also arise from aspartate via coupled transamination and decarboxylation of malate [67], but pyruvate production from other sources (e.g., from oxaloacetate via phosphoenol-pyruvate carboxykinase) seems unlikely under anaerobic conditions. Although quantitatively much less alanine is produced from pyruvate than lactate, the shunting of pyruvate to alanine might be of significance in order to reduce lactate levels in oxygen-deprived tissue and thus lessen the inhibition of glycolysis that occurs when lactate levels become too high [30]. The physiologic importance of this mechanism is not yet fully understood.

In the proposed scheme of alanine production from the transamination of glutamate and pyruvate, the glycolytic pathway is not in redox balance. If pyruvate is diverted to alanine instead of lactate, NAD^+ must be regenerated by a mechanism that is different from the lactate dehydrogenase reaction. Principally, two cytosolic reactions could be capable of restoring the altered redox balance: (1) the glycerol phosphate dehydrogenase reaction leading to the synthesis of glycerol phosphate and (2) the malate dehydrogenase reaction leading to the synthesis of malate from oxaloacetate. In the latter scheme oxaloacetate can be derived from aspartate, which in turn is transaminated to form glutamate, one of the substrates for alanine aminotransferase. This pathway would lead to formation of succinate from oxaloacetate via malate and fumarate and is thought to be one of the key factors in the tolerance of diving mammals to hypoxia [65, 66]. The quantitatively more important source of succinate accumulation during anoxia is glutamate (Fig. 3-7). As previously discussed, glutamate is transaminated with pyruvate to form alanine. The transamination product, 2-oxoglutarate, is oxidized, and subsequent formation of succinate is associated with substrate-level phosphorylation in the citric acid cycle and production of carbon dioxide. Formation of succinate from breakdown of the amino acids aspartate and glutamate has indeed been demonstrated in the isolated hypoxic papillary muscle of the rabbit [59, 60] and the ischemic isolated perfused rat heart [67]. Formation of carbon dioxide with ischemia and infarction has been demonstrated in dog hearts [68]. According to the scheme presented in Figure 3-7, the source of carbon dioxide is most likely glutamate.

Whereas heart mitochondria incubated under aerobic conditions rapidly and completely oxidize glutamate [69], oxygen-deprived heart muscle oxidizes glutamate only in the C1 position to succinyl CoA and succinate [60, 62]. The limited oxidation of glutamate is linked to substrate-level phosphorylation in the citric acid cycle and hence is a source of anaerobic energy.

There are two further observations supporting the view that succinate production by oxygen-deprived myocardium may be the result of anaerobic mitochondrial activity. First, oxidation of fumarate derived from aspartate has been observed to be coupled to the synthesis of ATP and succinate in cyanide-treated mitochondrial particles from rat heart [70]. Second, another energy-yielding reaction has been found to accompany oxidation of 2-oxoglutarate by mitochondria isolated from kidney and liver when these tissues are incubated under anaerobic conditions [71]. These two observations also support the hypothesis that anaerobic succinate formation is associated with energy production. Quantitative aspects of this nonglycolytic source of energy have not yet been fully evaluated. In hypoxic papillary muscles succinate and alanine production have been estimated to account for 16 percent of the ATP produced by glycolysis and lactate formation alone [59]. For the clinician the findings of enhanced glutamate uptake by ischemic myocardium are of interest [72], and most encouraging are the findings that addition of glutamate to the perfusate seems to lessen the damaging effects of ischemia during cardioplegia [73] and indeed may improve performance of the reperfused ischemic myocardium [74]. Other investigators, including those in our own laboratory [75], were unable to substantiate these findings.

PROTEIN SYNTHESIS AND DEGRADATION

Ever since Schoenheimer's classic observations on the "dynamic state of body constituents" [76] it has been recognized that proteins, the basic constituents of all organs in the mammalian body, are continuously synthesized and degraded. Heart muscle is no exception. Although each myocardial protein possesses a different life span, it has been estimated that the mean half-life of all myocardial proteins is only about 5 days and that the entire heart is completely exchanged once every 3 weeks [77].

Protein synthesis and degradation are energy-dependent processes that require ATP (Fig. 3-8). It is therefore not surprising that oxygen deprivation slows or inhibits both processes [55, 78, 79]. In ischemic rat heart protein synthesis and degradation, measured by

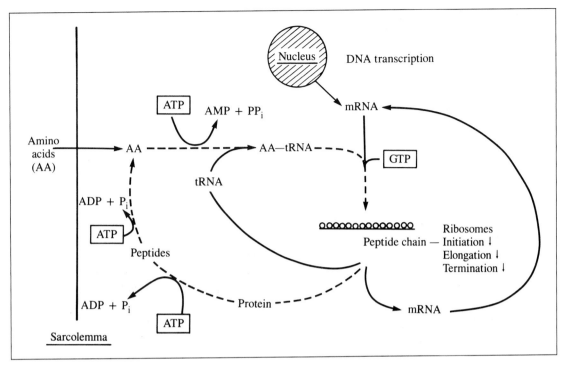

Fig. 3-8
Protein synthesis and degradation in ischemic myocardium. Protein sythesis and degradation are energy-dependent processes (see *squares*). Oxygen deprivation leads to a greater decrease in protein synthesis (transcription, peptide chain initiation, elongation, and termination) than protein degradation. With few exceptions, amino acids (AA) neither accumulate in nor disappear from ischemic myocardium. Broken lines show energy-dependent pathways.

incorporation and release of phenylalanine, were both reduced by 80 percent [80]. This observation might explain why release of amino acids from globally ischemic, autolyzing myocardium is delayed by 6 to 12 hours [55].

In oxygen-deprived muscle protein synthesis is inhibited more than protein degradation. According to Morgan et al. [81], such an imbalance between protein synthesis and degradation in energy-depleted heart muscle could lead to loss of those proteins with rapid rates of turnover and could be a major factor in irreversible damage to ischemic tissue. Indeed, one may take the case one step further and speculate that, in molecular terms, there is irreparable damage to the complex system of protein synthesis beginning with gene expression and ending with peptide chain termination, as well as in the ATP-dependent system of protein breakdown [82] (see Fig. 3-7). The

exact sites of these damages remains to be elucidated.

Although overall rates of protein degradation are decreased in oxygen-deprived myocardium, the release and activation of several lysosomal enzymes are known to increase [83]. Lysosomes are small cell organelles containing hydrolases and acid proteases, notably cathepsin D. The number of lysosomes in myocytes is relatively small, and specific activities of lysosomal enzymes are relatively low unless the organelle is disrupted by vigorous homogenization, detergent treatment, or, notably, ischemia [84]. The "lysosomal hypothesis of ischemic injury" states that ischemia leads to disruption of lysosomal membranes and release of the normally latent lysosomal hydrolases. This reaction results in abnormal degradation of certain cellular constituents because of abnormal contact between hydrolytic enzymes and substrates and lowering of the intracellular pH (i.e., nearer the pH optima of most lysosomal enzymes). If severe enough, this abnormal hydrolysis of cellular constituents could contribute to the development of further cell injury through degradation of structural and enzyme proteins and further activation of latent hydrolases [83]. In other words, a vicious cycle is set up. The "lysosomal hypothesis" has therefore been particularly attractive because drugs such as the tranquilizer chlorpromazine may limit lysosomal disruption in the liver [85], although the protective effect of chlorpromazine against ischemic damage in heart muscle seems to be small.

Although there is no doubt that lysosomes and lysosomal enzymes undergo major changes during myocardial ischemia, their role in the pathophysiology of early ischemic damage is still undefined. The "lysosomal hypothesis" may be a coincidental rather than a causal event [86], and more recent evidence suggests a particular role for lysosomal enzymes in the removal of abnormal, partially degraded proteins.

ADENINE NUCLEOTIDE METABOLISM

One of the most devastating effects of reduced oxygen delivery on the myocardium is the loss of adenine nucleotides from the total pool of ATP, ADP, and adenosine monophosphate (AMP). An increase in AMP levels leads to increased production of its degradation products adenosine, inosine, hypoxanthine, and xanthine (Fig. 3-9), as the activity of the rate-determining enzyme 5'-nucleotidase is far greater than that of adenylate deaminase, which competes for the same substrate [88]. The enzyme 5'-nucleotidase assumes a strategic position in the pathway of adenine nucleotide catabolism and deserves more detailed discussion. There are at least two isoforms of the enzyme. The soluble, sarcoplasmic form is physiologically more important than the membrane-bound, sarcolemmal form [89]. According to Swain and Holmes [33], ATP is a potent activator of cytosolic 5'-

nucleotidase. It follows that when ATP levels fall during ischemia the activity of 5'-nucleotidase would also fall. The whole process slows the rate of nucleotide hydrolysis and results in a halt to the drain of nucleotides from the cell. Thus it can easily be envisioned that inhibition of cytosolic 5'-nucleotidase and prevention of adenosine release into the interstitium (as described by Van Belle et al. [90]) may be a useful method to preserve myocardial adenine nucleotide pools.

Whereas rephosphorylation of the phosphorylated adenine nucleotides AMP and ADP to ADP and ATP occurs rapidly, the nonphosphorylated compound adenosine and its degradation products may enter a slower "salvage pathway" that eventually restores ATP [91]; more commonly, they leave the cell and appear in the bloodstream, which results in a net loss of adenine nucleotides. It seems that the supply-demand ratio for oxygen determines adenosine formation by the heart [92]. De novo synthesis of adenine nucleotides is a slow process [93], and it takes hours, if not days, for heart muscle to restore its adenine nucleotide pool [94].

As stated earlier, there is no correlation between adenine nucleotide content and turnover of ATP. Likewise, static measurements of nucleotide pools reflect only the balance between their rate of synthesis and degradation. With ischemia the rate of nucleotide breakdown exceeds their rate of synthesis, resulting first in a decline in the cellular content of nucleoside triphosphates (notably ATP) and shortly thereafter in a decline of all phosphorylated nucleosides and adenosine (Fig. 3-9). Because during ischemia the washout of catabolites is decreased, the metabolites further down in the pathway accumulate. During reperfusion following ischemia, the purine nucleotide content is depressed as a result of metabolite washout [2, 95, 96], although function may have returned to normal or evidence of myocardial necrosis is lacking [97]. It is, however, not to say that there is no close relation between a marked depletion in energy-rich phosphates (e.g., ATP less than 20 percent of control) and the development of irreversible ischemic injury and necrosis, as it has been

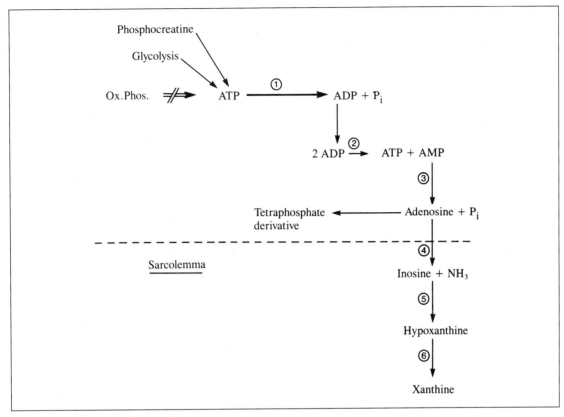

Fig. 3-9
Degradation of adenine nucleotides in ischemic myocardium. With interruption of
the main source of ATP (oxidative phosphorylation), ADP is not quantitatively
rephosphorylated. Instead, 1 mol of ATP is recovered from 2 mol of ADP, and
AMP is broken down to adenosine. A tetraphosphate derivative of adenosine has
been discovered in ischemic tissue [87], but most of the adenosine leaves the cell
and is further degraded. Key enzymatic steps: (1) ATPase; (2) adenylate kinase;
(3) 5'-nucleotidase; (4) adenosine deaminase; (5) nucleoside phosphorylase;
(6) xanthine oxidase.

described by Jennings et al. [98]. Thus *severe
adenine nucleotide depletion* is inevitably associated with cardiac cell death.

The initial, rapid hydrolysis of ATP to ADP
and P_i in response to ischemia is probably the
main source for protons accumulating in the
cytosol [99]. The link between ATP hydrolysis, intracellular acidosis, myocardial cell dysfunction, and cell death [25] awaits further exploration. Similarly, the attractive hypothesis
of Ca^{2+} chelation by phosphate, the hydrolysis product of ATP, advanced by Kübler and
Katz [27] and already mentioned, is still awaiting experimental proof.

OXYGEN-DERIVED FREE RADICALS

There has been increasing evidence suggesting
that oxygen-derived free radicals play an important role in several forms of tissue damage,
especially in injuries sustained with ischemia
and reperfusion but also in injuries associated
with intracellular drug metabolism (e.g., an-
thracycline antibiotics) and with inflammatory
responses [100]. A free radical is a molecule
or atom that possesses an unpaired electron.
Normally, free radicals are produced as intermediates in the mitochondrial electron transport system and during the metabolism of a

variety of lipids, including arachidonic acid. In heart muscle molecular oxygen (denoted as the superoxide anion O_2^-) is especially important as an acceptor of electrons in the mitochondrial electron transport system of the respiratory chain.

In an aqueous environment O_2^- is in equilibrium with its protonated form $HO_2\cdot$:

$$H^+ + O_2^- \rightleftharpoons HO_2\cdot$$

Whereas O_2^- is relatively unreactive, $HO_2\cdot$ and other of its derivative products are able to oxidize organic molecules such as membrane lipids and proteins. As shown in Table 3-3, H_2O_2 can be generated by spontaneous dismutation (i.e., rearrangement of electrons) of

Table 3-3
Formation of oxygen-derived free radicals

Step 1: Electron reduction of oxygen $O_2 + e^- \rightarrow O_2^-$
Step 2: Dismutation of O_2^- $2O_2^- + 2H^+ \rightarrow H_2O_2 + O_2$
Step 3: Haber-Weiss and/or Fenton reactions $H_2O_2 + O_2^- \rightarrow O_2 + OH^- + OH$

the reduced form of molecular oxygen (O_2^-) and the protonated form of the superoxide anion ($HO_2\cdot$). This reaction is in contrast to the xanthine oxidase reaction, in which H_2O_2 can be formed either by reduction of superoxide anions or the direct double reduction of O_2. Finally, H_2O_2 can also be generated by an enzyme-catalyzed dismutation of O_2^-. The enzyme superoxide dismutase is able to reduce two molecules of O_2^- to form H_2O_2 and O_2. Because these are different sources of oxygen-derived free radicals, there are also different mechanisms involved in maintaining low intracellular concentrations of oxygen-derived free radicals. Free radicals may be "quenched" by small molecules such as tocopherol, β-carotene, ascorbate, or glutathione. They may also react with lipids, proteins, or DNA. These reactions lead to impairment of cell function and to cell destruction, especially when there is a burst of oxygen-derived free radicals on reperfusion after ischemia. Lastly, a series of enzymes have evolved that "scavenge" superoxide and H_2O_2. They include superoxide dismutase, catalase, glutathione peroxidase, and glutathione reductase (Fig. 3-10). The latter system serves to lower

Fig. 3-10
Mechanisms of free radical scavenging. The superoxide anion O_2^-, an intermediate in mitochondrial electron transport systems, may undergo dismutation to O_2 and H_2O_2. H_2O_2 is converted to H_2O and O_2 by either catalase or glutathione peroxidase. GSSG = oxidized glutathione; GSH = reduced glutathione.

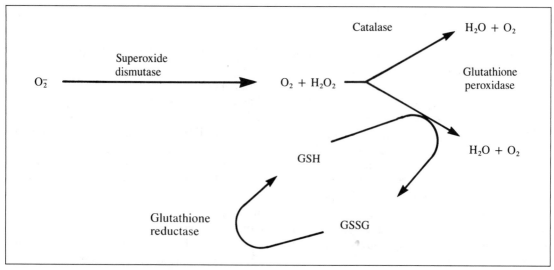

the steady-state concentrations of free radical species that might otherwise cause excessive damage to the membrane and enzyme systems of the cell.

Although the role of oxygen-derived free radicals in myocardial cell injury and cell death has not yet been completely characterized, a number of studies have shown that superoxide dismutase, catalase, and allopurinol (an inhibitor of the enzyme xanthine oxidase) offer a protective effect against the ravages of myocardial ischemia [101–103] and reperfusion injury after ischemia [104, 105]. Superoxide dismutase, catalase, and glutathione peroxidase can be considered free radical scavengers, because even though H_2O_2 is not a radical species it is a presursor of the highly toxic protonated form of the superoxide anion $OH\cdot$. The cytotoxic effect of H_2O_2 is therefore a function of intracellular catalase and glutathione peroxidase, which "scavenge" H_2O_2 on the one hand, and of the reactions that reduce H_2O_2 to $OH\cdot$ on the other hand. The direct mechanism of tissue damage induced by oxygen-derived free radicals most likely involves protein modifications by $OH\cdot$ (not O_2^-), rendering denatured substrates for accelerated intracellular proteolysis and lipid peroxidation [106, 107]. It can be expected that work in the near future will not only deepen the understanding of the physiologic role of oxygen-derived free radicals but also provide a basis on how protective mechanisms can be enhanced to defend cellular structures from damage caused by oxygen-derived free radicals, especially during reperfusion of ischemic myocardium.

CA^{2+} METABOLISM

The importance of Ca^{2+} for energy metabolism of the heart is easily understood: Ca^{2+} ions are the mediators of excitation-contraction coupling. In addition, most enzymes that hydrolyze ATP are stimulated by Ca^{2+}. Ca^{2+} is a cofactor for the actomyosin cross-bridge formation and for mitochondrial dehydrogenases. The cytosolic $[Ca^{2+}]$ changes in the course of the cardiac cycle by two orders of magnitude, from 10^{-7} M during diastole to 10^{-5} M during systole, respectively [108]. The plasma $[Ca^{2+}]$ is at 10^{-3} M, again two orders of magnitude greater than the highest physiologic cytosolic $[Ca^{2+}]$, indicating a $[Ca^{2+}]$ gradient between the extra- and intracellular spaces. Severe ischemia causes high permeability of the cell membrane to Ca^{2+} [109], decreased extrusion of Ca^{2+} through the sarcolemma, decreased Ca^{2+} uptake by the sarcoplasmic reticulum, decreased Ca^{2+} uptake by mitochondria (all of these, except Ca^{2+} entry into the cell, are energy-dependent processes), and intracellular Ca^{2+} overload leading to contractile failure and ultimately cell death [110–112] (Fig. 3-11).

As depicted in the algorithm in Figure 3-12, the effects of Ca^{2+} overload are overwhelmingly deleterious. Intracellular Ca^{2+} overload activates a number of enzymes (proteases, phospholipase, myofibrillar ATPase), disrupts lysosomal membranes, and "chokes" mitochondrial oxidative phosphorylation because damaged mitochondria accumulate Ca^{2+} in preference to oxidative phosphorylation [113–115]. Cell death occurs after a period of contractile failure. One of the earliest unequivocal signs of irreversible ischemic cell injury is the appearance of amorphous matrix densities and granular dense bodies of calcium phosphate. Accumulation of Ca^{2+} in mitochondria requires a partially functional respiratory chain and is lost after 90 minutes of ischemia [6]. However, if the injury condition disappears before the level of intramitochondrial calcium phosphate becomes too high, the excess Ca^{2+} is dissolved from the precipitates and is released at a rate compatible with the Ca^{2+}-exporting ability of the sarcolemmal systems. According to Carafoli and Bing [116], this process ensures survival of the injured heart cell.

As also discussed by Carafoli and Bing [116], disturbed Ca^{2+} transfer across the sarcolemma, sarcoplasmic reticulum, and mitochondrial membrane is just the "tip of the biochemical iceberg" of myocardial cell dysfunction. The primary target of ischemic tissue injury might well be the enzyme proteins involved in Ca^{2+} metabolism and, vice versa,

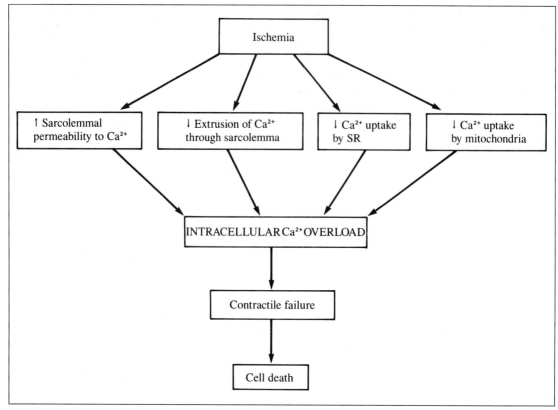

Fig. 3-11
Mechanisms of Ca²⁺ overload in ischemic myocardium. See text for explanation.
(Modified from G. N. Pierce et al. *Heart Dysfunction in Diabetes.* Boca Raton,
FL: CRC Press, 1988. With permission.)

the Ca^{2+} and cyclic AMP-mediated stimulation of protein kinases.

SYNTHESIS: PARADIGMS OF METABOLIC RESPONSES IN MYOCARDIAL ISCHEMIA AND INFARCTION; ENZYME RELEASE; REGIONAL MYOCARDIAL METABOLISM

The multiple metabolic responses to myocardial ischemia and infarction are listed in Table 3-4. It cannot be emphasized strongly enough that the relative contributions of individual factors (discussed earlier in the chapter) to myocardial cell injury in the presence of ischemia and infarction are not known. Each factor is not more than a paradigm. It is a matter of controversy how the paradigms relate to

each other. Even such nondestructive methods as magnetic resonance imaging have so far failed to determine whether, for example, depletion of energy-rich phosphates or intracellular acidosis is responsible for cell dysfunction [117, 118].

Irreversible cell damage and necrosis, on the other hand, are associated with virtual cessation of any form of energy metabolism and protein synthesis, the loss of nucleotides, accumulation of cystolic and mitochondrial Ca^{2+}, destruction of membranes, proteins, and nuclei, and release of enzyme proteins from myocardial cells into the bloodstream. Traditionally, only the latter phenomenon is available for direct analysis and has been used not only for the diagnosis but also for a quantitative assessment of myocardial cell necrosis [119–121]. Although time–activity curves of

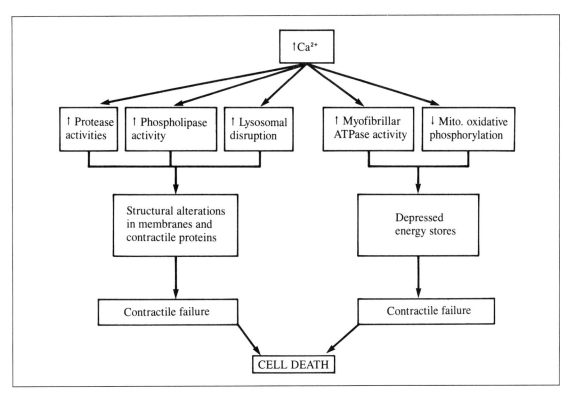

Fig. 3-12
Algorithm of the deleterious effects of Ca^{2+} overload in ischemic myocardium.
See text for explanation. (Modified from G. N. Pierce et al. *Heart Dysfunction in Diabetes.* Boca Raton, FL: CRC Press, 1988. With permission.)

Table 3-4
Loss and gain of metabolites and ions
during myocardial ischemia

Loss	Gain
Glycogen	Lactate, alanine
Phosphocreatine	P_i, PP_i
ATP	Adenosine, inosine, hypoxanthine, xanthine
Adenine nucleotides	Hydrogen ions, ammonia, fatty acyl CoA, triglycerides
Glutamate	Succinate, CO_2
K^+	Ca^{2+}
Phospholipids	Arachidonic acid and lysophosphatides, H_2O_2, free radicals
Structural proteins	Amino acids
Enzymes, myoglobin	
Mitochondrial cristae	Amorphous densities and granular dense bodies
Lysosomes	Cathepsin D and free lysosomal enzymes

enzyme release from the tissue are influenced by factors such as reperfusion, inactivation and degradation of enzymes in the lymphatic and systemic circulations, and membrane leakage not associated with irreversible cell damage, the liberation of cytosolic enzymes involved in myocardial energy metabolism such as creatine kinase (CK) MB, aspartate aminotransferase, alanine aminotransferase, and lactate dehydrogenase (specifically the LDH_1 isozyme) remains one of the three cornerstones for the clinical diagnosis of myocardial infarction, the other being the electrocardiogram (ECG). Given the complexity of myocardial energy metabolism, it is not surprising that damaged myocardial cells release a multitude of enzymes and low-molecular-weight proteins such as myoglobin (for review see Hearse [24]), but for practical purposes only the aforementioned enzymes have gained diagnostic importance. When the physical separation between the inside and the outside of the cell is removed, not only do enzymes leak out of the cell but substances normally excluded from the cell may gain access to the inside of the cell. Such substance is a labeled myosin antibody that binds to the principal protein of the myocardial cell and has been used to localize and quantitate necrotic tissue [122].

In vivo assessment of regional myocardial metabolism by positron emission tomography (PET) has gained increasing importance [123]. Unique features of this new imaging modality are the following: (1) tomographic, three-dimensional images of relatively high resolution; (2) availability of positron-emitting compounds to trace myocardial blood flow and specific metabolic pathways; and (3) the semi-quantitative nature of measuring radioactivity in defined regions of the myocardium [124]. When patients with acute myocardial infarction are studied within 72 hours of onset of chest pain or asymptomatic ECG changes, PET frequently reveals absent blood flow but persistent glucose-specific metabolic activity in infarcted regions [125]. When radioactivity of the glucose analog tracer ^{18}F-2-deoxyglucose (FDG) is measured, the tracer, which is phosphorylated but not further metabolized, accumulates to a greater extent in ischemic tissue than in the surrounding, normally perfused myocardium or in infarcted tissues [126]. Conversely, regional oxidation of ^{11}C-palmitate is decreased, presumably because of impaired oxidative metabolism and back-diffusion of tracer from ischemic tissue into the blood. Thus PET techniques are capable not only of tracing metabolic abnormalities but also of distinguishing the activity of different metabolic pathways in vivo. In a study by Tillisch and coworkers [127] enhanced FDG uptake by ischemic myocardium was a powerful predictor of tissue viability after revascularization. Future research will show if there are subsets of myocardial infarction with predominantly reversible tissue injury or predominantly irreversible tissue necrosis (as clinically suggested). Future research will also show if myocardial infarct size (and its reduc-

tion by therapeutic interventions) can be assessed by PET. Furthermore, as the ischemic myocardium cuts back on energy expenditure, PET metabolic tracer techniques may very well be able to distinguish between energy-deprived, surviving myocardium and energy-depleted, necrotic tissue.

Reversible Myocardial Ischemia, Reperfusion, and Reperfusion Injury

In contrast to the well-studied phenomenon of altered contractile function during ischemia and reperfusion dating back to the classic studies of Tennant and Wiggers during the 1930s [128] (which have shown that the rate of improvement of function in the ischemic segment is inversely related to the duration of the occlusion), the metabolic basis for reversible myocardial ischemia is still elusive. Progress in establishing early reperfusion in threatening myocardial infarction by clot-selective thrombolysis [129] has brought the concept of the "stunned myocardium" proposed by Braunwald and Kloner [130] into focus. Based on an extensive review of the literature, Braunwald and Kloner concluded that brief occurrences (usually less than 20 minutes) of myocardial ischemia are followed by metabolic and functional alterations that may last for days before function returns to normal. It is of interest that even during periods of ischemia longer than 20 minutes only the core of the tissue may undergo necrosis, whereas the surrounding tissue may be reversibly injured and committed to necrosis only if ischemia continues for a prolonged period [19]. Thus there is a metabolic "battlefield" surrounding the "bomb crater" of the infarction in the center, and the characterization of the "battlefield" is, since the discussion by Bing [131], the focus of much research activity.

According to Braunwald and Kloner [130], a myocardial infarction is characterized by a zone of reversibly injured cells surrounding the center of necrosis that shows delayed recovery of function. Because it is unlikely that any necrotic tissue may regain functional significance, it is reasonable to focus on the metabolic changes occurring in the reversibly injured, viable, yet functionally impaired myocardium. It is the current notion that metabolism in this reversibly injured myocardium can be restored to normal by reperfusion [132], although the return of function may be delayed by days or even weeks. Although associated with an increased uptake of the glucose analog FDG [127], few experimental data exist on the biochemical mechanism(s) underlying the slow recovery of tissue function in the zone of reversible ischemia.

More definitive data are available from reperfused heart muscle preparations after normothermic or hypothermic ischemia. For instance, numerous studies have shown rapid restoration of the phosphocreatine pool, whereas nucleotide pools remain depleted in functional, postischemic myocardium (for review see Swain and Holmes [33]). The rapid increase in phosphocreatine is thought to indicate that mitochondrial energy production is not limited, whereas resynthesis of adenine nucleotides is lagging behind. To date, no studies have unequivocally demonstrated a direct relation between repletion of adenine nucleotide pools and the return of cardiac function. The evidence for a relation between severe (>80 percent) depletion of adenine nucleotides and cell death is, however, convincing [98, 133], although the exact mechanism(s) remains to be defined.

The mechanisms of reperfusion injury are complex [134, 135] and still unexplainable. Some investigators have pointed out the similarities between reperfusion injury and the "calcium paradox" [136], a phenomenon observed in isolated rat hearts perfused with a Ca^{2+}-free medium. Once Ca^{2+} is readmitted to the perfusate, these hearts go into contracture and show evidence of intracellular Ca^{2+} overload. The exact mechanism(s) for the calcium paradox phenomenon is still unclear.

Other investigators have suggested the role of oxygen-derived free radicals as mediators for reperfusion damage [104, 137]. The possible mechanisms for the generation of oxygen-derived free radicals and their effects on cellular proteins were discussed earlier.

Still other investigators believe that lactate accumulation from glycogen breakdown impairs flux through the glycolytic pathway and return of function on reperfusion [4], whereas others have found that preservation of glycogen levels [138] or "glycogen loading" of the heart prior to ischemia [139] lessens the ischemic insult and preserves cardiac function on reperfusion. Decreased tissue content of pyrimidine nucleotide (NAD)—and not decreased activity of dehydrogenases—has been found to be not only a good correlate for the degree of ultrastructural injury but also the biochemical basis for negative tetrazolium staining of the irreversibly injured tissue [140].

Schaper and Schaper [141] concluded, probably correctly, that the effects of reperfusion depend on the severity of the ischemic insult at the time of reperfusion. In irreversibly injured myocardium, reperfusion leads to the accelerated demise of the tissue. In reversibly injured myocardium, reperfusion leads to an accelerated return of oxidative metabolism and contractile function. In other words, reperfusion seems beneficial to reversibly injured myocardium and deleterious to irreversibly injured myocardium. The most tantalizing question for both clinicians and biochemists remains how to distinguish the former from the latter while the patient is still alive.

Acknowledgment

The author is recipient of a NHLBI Research Career Development Award (No. 1K04-HL-01246).

Editorial Comments

As PET scanners become more widely available, the clinical cardiologist will be pushed to become more knowledgeable about myocardial metabolism and biochemistry. A major problem of contemporary cardiology is deciding whether hypokinetic myocardium is irreversibly necrotic or in a "hibernating" or stunned state and therefore capable of enhanced contractile function when coronary *perfusion is improved. PET scanning with tracers designed to measure myocardial blood flow ($^{13}NH_3$) and glucose metabolism (^{18}F-labeled 2-deoxyglucose, or ^{18}FDG) should prove useful in this regard. A mismatch between flow (reduced $^{13}NH_3$ uptake) and glucose utilization (increased ^{18}FDG uptake) should help localize areas of left ventricular dysfunction that are potentially able to recover with improved flow. G.S.F.*

References

1. Taegtmeyer, H., Hems, R., and Krebs, H. A. Utilization of energy-providing substrates in the isolated working rat heart. *Biochem. J.* 186:701, 1980.
2. Taegtmeyer, H., Roberts, A. F. C., and Rayne, A. E. G. Energy metabolism in reperfused rat heart: Return of function before normalisation of ATP content. *J. Am. Coll. Cardiol.* 6:864, 1985.
3. Hoffmeister, H. M., Mauser, M., and Schaper, W. Effect of adenosine and AICAR on ATP content and regional contractile function in reperfused canine myocardium. *Basic Res. Cardiol.* 80:445, 1985.
4. Neely, J. R., and Grotyohann, L. W. Role of glycolytic products in damage to myocardium: Dissociation of adenosine triphosphate levels and recovery of function of reperfused ischemic hearts. *Circ. Res.* 55:816, 1984.
5. Page, E., and McCallister, L. P. Quantitative electron microscopic description of heart muscle cells. *Am. J. Cardiol.* 31:172, 1973.
6. Jennings, R. B., and Ganote, C. E. Mitochondrial structure and function in myocardial ischemic injury. *Circ. Res.* 38(Suppl I):I-80, 1976.
7. Regitz, V., Raulson, D. J., Hodack, R. J., et al. Mitochondrial damage during myocardial ischemia. *Basic Res. Cardiol.* 79:207, 1984.
8. Schaper, J., Mulch, J., Winkler, B., and Schaper, W. Ultrastructural, functional and biochemical criteria for estimation of reversibility of ischemic injury: A study on the effect of global ischemia on the isolated dog heart. *J. Mol. Cell. Cardiol.* 11:521, 1979.
9. Yeo, G. F. An attempt to estimate the gaseous interchange of the frog's heart by means of the spectroscope. *J. Physiol. (Lond.)* 6:93, 1885.
10. Winterstein, H. Ueber die Sauerstoffatmung des isolieten Säugethierherzens. *Z. Allg. Physiol.* 4:333, 1904.
11. Bing, R. J. The metabolism of the heart. *Harvey Lect.* 50:27, 1955.
12. Goodale, W. T., and Hackel, D. B. Myocardial

carbohydrate metabolism in normal dogs, with effects of hyperglycemia and starvation. *Circ. Res.* 1:509, 1953.
13. Goodale, W. T., Olson, R. E., and Hackel, D. B. The effects of fasting and diabetes mellitus on myocardial metabolism in man. *Am. J. Med.* 27:212, 1959.
14. Schelbert, H. R. The Heart. In P. J. Ell and B. L. Holman (eds.), *Computed Emission Tomography.* Oxford: Oxford University Press, 1982. Pp. 91–133.
15. Merhige, M. E., Ekas, R., Mossberg, K., et al. Catecholamine stimulation, substrate competition, and myocardial glucose uptake in conscious dogs assessed with positron emission tomography. *Circ. Res.* 61(Suppl II):II-124, 1987.
16. Denton, R. M., and Randle, P. Concentration of glycerides and phospholipids in rat heart and gastrocnemius muscles. *Biochem. J.* 104:416, 1967.
17. Olson, R. E., and Hoeshen, R. J. Utilization of endogenous lipid by the isolated perfused rat heart. *Biochem. J.* 103:796, 1967.
18. Crass III, M. I., McCaskill, E. S., Shipp, J. C., and Murthy, V. K. Metabolism of endogenous lipids in cardiac muscle: Effect of pressure development. *Am. J. Physiol.* 220:428, 1971.
19. Reimer, K. A., Lowe, J. E., Rasmussen, M. M., and Jennings, R. B. The wave form phenomenon of ischemic cell death. I. Myocardial infarct size vs. duration of coronary occlusion in dogs. *Circulation* 56:786, 1977.
20. Opie, L. H., Owen, P., Thomas, M., and Samson, R. Coronary sinus lactate measurements in assessment of myocardial ischemia: Comparison with changes in lactate/pyruvate and beta-hydroxybutyrate/acetoacetate ratios and with release of hydrogen, phosphate and potassium from the heart. *Am. J. Cardiol.* 32:295, 1973.
21. Gertz, E. W., Wisneski, J. A., Neese, R., et al. Myocardial lactate metabolism: Evidence of lactate release during net chemical extraction in man. *Circulation* 63:1273, 1981.
22. Gertz, E. W., Wisneski, J. A., Neese, R., et al. Myocardial lactate extraction: Multidetermined metabolic function. *Circulation* 61:256, 1980.
23. Wisneski, J. A., Gertz, E. W., Neese, R. A., et al. Metabolic fate of extracted glucose in normal human myocardium. *J. Clin. Invest.* 76:1819, 1985.
24. Hearse, D. J. Myocardial enzyme leakage. *J. Mol. Med.* 2:185, 1977.
25. Katz, A. M., and Hecht, H. H. The early "pump" failure of the ischemic heart. *Am. J. Med.* 47:497, 1969.
26. Williamson, J. R., Schaffer, S. W., Ford, C., and Safer, B. Contribution of tissue acidosis to

ischemic injury in the perfused rat heart. *Circulation* 53:3, 1976.

27. Kübler, W., and Katz, A. M. Mechanism of early "pump" failure of the ischemic heart: Possible role of adenosine triphosphate depletion and inorganic phosphate accumulation. *Am. J. Cardiol.* 40:467, 1977.

28. Gudbjarnason, S., Mathes, P., and Ravens, K. G. Functional compartmentation of ATP and creatine phosphate in heart muscle. *J. Mol. Cell. Cardiol.* 1:325, 1970.

29. Williamson, J. R. Glycolytic control mechanisms. II. Kinetics of the intermediate changes during the aerobic-anaerobic transition in perfused rat heart. *J. Biol. Chem.* 241:5026, 1966.

30. Rovetto, M. J., Lamberton, W. F., and Neely, J. R. Mechanisms of glycolytic inhibition in ischemic rat hearts. *Circ. Res.* 37:742, 1975.

31. Mochizuki, S., and Neely, J. R. Control of glyceraldehyde 3-phosphate dehydrogenase in cardiac muscle. *J. Mol. Cell. Cardiol.* 11:221, 1979.

32. Morgan, H. E., Neely, J. R., and LaNoue, K. F. Biochemical Events in Ischemic Heart. In A. Hjalmarson and L. Wilhelmsen (eds.), *Acute and Long Term Management of Myocardial Ischemia.* Göteborg, Sweden: Astra, 1977. Pp. 10–22.

33. Swain, J. L., and Holmes, E. W. Nucleotide Metabolism in Cardiac Muscle. In H. A. Fozzard et al. (eds.), *The Heart and Cardiovascular System.* New York: Raven Press, 1986. Pp. 911–929.

34. Bremer, J., and Wojtczak, A. B. Factors controlling the role of fatty acid β-oxidation in rat liver mitochondria. *Biochim. Biophys. Acta* 280:515, 1972.

35. Biheimer, D. W., Buja, L. M., Parkey, R. W. et al. Fatty acid accumulation and abnormal lipid deposition in peripheral and border zones of experimental myocardial infarcts. *J. Nucl. Med.* 19:276, 1978.

36. Schwaiger, M., Fishbein, M. C., Block, M., et al. Metabolic and ultrastructural abnormalities during ischemia in canine myocardium: Noninvasive assessment by positron emission tomography. *J. Mol. Cell. Cardiol.* 19:259, 1987.

37. Shug, A. L., Shrago, E., Bittar, N., et al. Acyl-CoA inhibition of adenine nucleotide translocation in ischemic myocardium. *Am. J. Physiol.* 228:689, 1975.

38. Ho, C. H., and Pande, S. V. On the specificity of the inhibition of adenine nucleotide translocase by long-chain acyl-coenzyme A esters. *Biochim. Biophys. Acta* 369:86, 1974.

39. Oram, J. F., Bennetch, S. L., and Neely, J. R. Regulation of fatty acid utilization in isolated perfused rat hearts. *J. Biol. Chem.* 248:5299, 1973.

40. Liedtke, A. J. Alterations of carbohydrate and lipid metabolism in the acutely ischemic heart. *Prog. Cardiovasc. Dis.* 23:321, 1981.

41. Oliver, M. F., Kurien, V. A., and Greenwood, T. W. Relation between serum-free fatty acids and arrhythmias and death after acute myocardial infarction. *Lancet* 1:710, 1968.

42. Henderson, H. H., Most, H. S., and Parmley, W. W. Depression of myocardial contractility in rats by free fatty acids during hypoxia. *Circ. Res.* 26:439, 1970.

43. Kjekshus, J. K., and Mjos, O. D. Effect of free fatty acids on myocardial function and metabolism in the ischemic dog heart. *J. Clin. Invest.* 51:1767, 1972.

44. Liedtke, A. J., Nellis, S., and Neely, J. R. Effects of excess free fatty acids on mechanical and metabolic function in normal and ischemic myocardium in swine. *Circ. Res.* 43:652, 1978.

45. Katz, A. M. Membrane-derived lipids and the pathogenesis of ischemic myocardial damage. *J. Mol. Cell. Cardiol.* 14:627, 1982.

46. Katz, A. M., and Messineo, F. C. Lipid-membrane interactions and the pathogenesis of ischemic myocardial damage. *Circ. Res.* 48:1, 1981.

47. Katz, A. M., and Messineo, F. C. Fatty acid effects on membranes: Possible role in the pathogenesis of ischemic myocardial damage. *J. Mol. Cell. Cardiol.* 14(Suppl 3):119, 1982.

48. Wood, J. M., Sordahl, L. A., Lewis, R. M., and Schwartz, A. Effect of chronic myocardial ischemia on the activity of carnitine palmitylcoenzyme A transferase in isolated canine heart mitochondria. *Circ. Res.* 32:340, 1973.

49. Wood, J. M., Busch, B., Pitts, B. J. R., and Schwartz, A. Inhibition of bovine heart Na$^+$/K$^+$-ATPase by palmityl-carnitine and palmityl-CoA. *Biochem. Biophys. Res. Commun.* 74:677, 1977.

50. Sobel, B. E., Corr, R. B., Robison, A. K., et al. Accumulation of lysophosphoglycerides with arrhythmogenic properties in ischemic myocardium. *J. Clin. Invest.* 62:546, 1978.

51. Chien, K. R., Han, A., Sen, A. et al. Accumulation of unesterified arachidonic acid in ischemic canine myocardium. *Circ. Res.* 54:313, 1984.

52. Reimer, K. A., and Jennings, R. B. Failure of the xanthine oxidase inhibitor allopurinol to limit infarct site after ischemia and reperfusion in dogs. *Circulation* 71:1069, 1985.

53. Steenbergen, C., and Jennings, R. B. Relationship between lysophospholipid accumulation and plasma membrane injury during in vitro ischemia in dog heart. *J. Mol. Cell. Cardiol.* 16:605, 1984.

54. Mudge, G. H., Mills, R. M., Taegtmeyer, H., et al. Alterations of myocardial amino acid metabolism in chronic ischemic heart disease. *J. Clin. Invest.* 58:1185, 1976.

55. Taegtmeyer, H., Ferguson, A. G., and Lesch, M. Protein degradation and amino acid metabolism in autolyzing rabbit myocardium. *Exp. Mol. Pathol.* 26:52, 1977.

56. Taegtmeyer, H., Peterson, M. B., Ragavan, V. V., et al. De novo alanine synthesis in isolated oxygen deprived rabbit myocardium. *J. Biol. Chem.* 252:5010, 1977.

57. Carlsten, A., Hallgren, B., Jagenburg, R., and Werko, L. Myocardial metabolism of glucose, lactic acid, amino and fatty acids in healthy human individuals at rest and at different work loads. *Scand. J. Clin. Invest.* 13:418, 1961.

58. Felig, P., and Wahren, J. Amino acid metabolism in exercising man. *J. Clin. Invest.* 50:2703, 1971.

59. Taegtmeyer, H. Metabolic responses to cardiac hypoxia: Increased production of succinate by rabbit papillary muscles. *Circ. Res.* 43:808, 1978.

60. Sanborn, T., Gavin, W., Berkowitz, S., et al. Augmented conversion of aspartate and glutamate to succinate during anoxia in rabbit heart. *Am. J. Physiol.* 237:H535, 1979.

61. Rau, E. E., Shine, K. I., Gervais, A., et al. Enhanced mechanical recovery of anoxic and ischemic myocardium by amino acid perfusion. *Am. J. Physiol.* 236:H873, 1979.

62. Peschock, R., and Nunnally, R. L. Carbon-13 magnetic resonance of glutamate metabolism in intact perfused hearts (Abstract). *Circulation* 66(Suppl II):II-109, 1982.

63. Norberg, K., and Siesjo, B. K. Cerebral metabolism in hypoxic hypoxia. II. Citric acid cycle intermediates and associated amino acids. *Brain Res.* 86:45, 1975.

64. Brosnan, J. T., Krebs, H. A., and Williamson, D. H. Effects of ischemia on metabolic concentrations in rat liver. *Biochem. J.* 117:91, 1970.

65. Hochachka, P. W., Owen, T. G., Allen, J. F., and Whittow, G. C. Multiple end products of anaerobiosis in diving vertebrates. *Comp. Biochem. Physiol.* 508:17, 1975.

66. Hochachka, P. W., and Storey, K. B. Metabolic consequences of diving in animals and man. *Science* 187:613, 1975.

67. Peuhkurinen, K. J., Rakala, T. E. S., Nuutinen, E. M., and Hassinen, I. E. Tricarboxylic acid cycle metabolites during ischemia in isolated perfused rat heart. *Am. J. Physiol.* 244:H281, 1983.

68. Hillis, L. D., Khuri, S. F., Braunwald, E., et al. Assessment of the efficacy of interventions to limit ischemic injury by direct measurement of intramural carbon dioxide tension after coronary artery occlusion in the dog. *J. Clin. Invest.* 63:99, 1979.

69. Krebs, H. A., and Bellami, D. The interconversion of glutamic acid and aspartic acid in respiring tissues. *Biochem. J.* 75:523, 1960.

70. Wilson, M. A., and Cascarano, J. The energy-yielding oxidation of NADH by fumarate in submitochondrial particles of rat tissues. *Biochem. Biophys. Acta* 216:54, 1970.

71. Hunter, F. E. Anaerobic phosphorylation due to coupled oxidation-reduction between alpha-ketoglutaric acid and oxaloacetic acid. *J. Biol. Chem.* 177:361, 1949.

72. Zimmermann, R., Tillmanns, H., Knapp, W. H., et al. Regional myocardial nitrogen-13 glutamate uptake in patients with coronary artery disease: Inverse post-stress relation to thallium-201 uptake in ischemia. *J. Am. Coll. Cardiol.* 11:549, 1988.

73. Lazar, H. L., Buckberg, G. D., Manganaro, A. J., et al. Reversal of ischemic damage with amino acid substrate enhancement during reperfusion. *Surgery* 88:702, 1980.

74. Bittl, J. A., and Shine, K. I. Protection of ischemic rabbit myocardium by glutamic acid. *Am. J. Physiol.* 245:H406, 1983.

75. Taegtmeyer, H., and Russell III, R. R. Glutamate metabolism in rabbit heart: Augmentation by ischemia and inhibition with acetoacetate. *J. Appl. Cardiol.* 2:231, 1987.

76. Schoenheimer, R. *The Dynamic State of Body Constituents.* Cambridge, MA: Harvard University Press, 1942.

77. Morgan, H. E., and Neely, J. R. Metabolic Regulation and Myocardial Function. In J. W. Hurst (ed.), *The Heart* (6th ed.). New York: McGraw-Hill, 1986. Pp. 85–100.

78. Morgan, H. E., Rannels, D. E., and Kao, R. L. Factors controlling protein turnover in heart muscle. *Circ. Res.* 34 & 35(Suppl III):III-22, 1974.

79. Lesch, M., Taegtmeyer, H., Peterson, M. B., and Vernick, R. Studies on the mechanism of the inhibition of myocardial protein synthesis during oxygen deprivation. *Am. J. Physiol.* 230:120, 1976.

80. Chua, B., Kao, R. L., Rannels, D. E., and Morgan, H. E. Inhibition of protein degradation by anoxia and ischemia in perfused rat hearts. *J. Biol. Chem.* 254:6617, 1979.

81. Morgan, H. E., Rannels, D. E., and McKee, E. E. Protein Metabolism of the Heart. In R. E. Berne (ed.), *Handbook of Physiology. The Cardiovascular System I,* Washington, D.C.: American Physiological Society, 1979. Pp. 845–871.

82. Hershko, A., Ciechanover, A., Heller, H., et al. Proposed role of ATP in protein breakdown: Conjugation of proteins with multiple chains of the poly-peptide of ATP-dependent proteolysis. *Proc. Natl. Acad. Sci. U.S.A.* 77:1783, 1980.

83. Decker, R. S., and Wildenthal, K. Role of Lysosomes and Latent Hydrolytic Enzymes in Ischemic Damage and Repair of the Heart. In K. Wildenthal (ed.), *Degradative Processes in*

Heart and Skeletal Muscle. New York: Elsevier/North Holland, 1980. Pp. 389–418.

84. Wildenthal, K., and Crie, J. S. Lysosomes and Cardiac Protein Catabolism. In K. Wildenthal (ed.), *Degradative Processes in Heart and Skeletal Muscle*. New York: Elsevier/North Holland, 1980. Pp. 113–129.

85. Seglen, P. O., Grinde, B., and Solheim, A. Z. Inhibition of the lysosomal pathway of protein degradation in isolated rat hepatocytes by ammonia, methylamine, chloroquine and leupeptin. *Eur. J. Biochem.* 95:215, 1979.

86. Wildenthal, K. Lysosomal alterations in ischemic myocardium: Result or cause of myocardial damage? (Editorial). *J. Mol. Cell. Cardiol.* 10:595, 1978.

87. Mowbray, J., Hutchinson, W. L., Tibbs, G. R., and Morris, P. G. The discovery of a rapidly metabolized polymeric tetraphosphate derivative of adenosine in perfused rat heart. *Biochem. J.* 223:627, 1984.

88. Saleen, Y., Niveditha, T., and Sadasivudu, B. AMP-deaminase, 5'-nucleotidase and adenosine deaminase in rat myocardial tissue in myocardial infarction and hypothermia. *Experientia* 38:776, 1982.

89. Arch, J. R. S., and Newsholme, E. A. Activities and some properties of 5'-nucleotidase, adenosine kinase and adenosine deaminase in tissues from vertebrates and invertebrates in relation to the control of the concentration and the physiological role of adenosine. *Biochem. J.* 174:965, 1978.

90. Van Belle, H., Goossens, F., and Wynants, J. Formation and release of purine catabolites during hypoperfusion, anoxia, and ischemia. *Am. J. Physiol.* 252:H886, 1987.

91. Reibel, D. K., and Rovetto, M. Myocardial adenosine salvage rates and restoration of ATP content following ischemia. *Am. J. Physiol.* 237:H247, 1979.

92. Bardenheuer, H., and Schrader, J. Supply-to-demand ratio for oxygen determines formation of adenosine by the heart. *Am. J. Physiol.* 250:H173, 1986.

93. Zimmer, H. G., Trendelenburg, C., Kammermeier, H., and Gerlach, E. De novo synthesis of myocardial adenine nucleotides in the rat: Acceleration during recovery from oxygen deficiency. *Circ. Res.* 32:637, 1973.

94. Zimmer, H. G. Restitution of myocardial adenine nucleotides: Acceleration by administration of ribose. *J. Physiol. (Paris)* 76:769, 1980.

95. Swain, J. L., Sabina, R. L., McHale, P. A., et al. Prolonged myocardial nucleotide depletion after brief ischemia in the open-chest dog. *Am. J. Physiol.* 242:H818, 1982.

96. Reimer, K. A., Hill, M. L., and Jennings, R. B. Prolonged depletion of ATP and the adenine nucleotide pool due to delayed resynthesis of adenine nucleotides following reversible myocardial ischemia injury in dogs. *J. Mol. Cell. Cardiol.* 13:229, 1981.

97. DeBoer, L. W. V., Ingwall, J. S., Kloner, R. A., and Braunwald, E. Prolonged derangements of canine myocardial purine metabolism after a brief coronary artery occlusion not associated with curatomic evidence of necrosis. *Proc. Natl. Acad. Sci. U.S.A.* 77:5471, 1980.

98. Jennings, R. B., Hawkins, H. K., Lowe, J. E., et al. Relation between high energy phosphate and lethal injury in myocardial ischemia. *Am. J. Pathol.* 92:187, 1978.

99. Gevers, W. Generation of protons by metabolic processes in heart cells. *J. Mol. Cell. Cardiol.* 9:867, 1977.

100. Freeman, B. A., and Crapo, J. D. Biology of disease: Free radicals and tissue injury. *Lab. Invest.* 47:412, 1982.

101. Burton, K. P., McCord, J. M., and Ghai, G. Myocardial alterations due to free radical generation. *Am. J. Physiol.* 246:H776, 1984.

102. Chambers, D. E., Parks, P. A., Patterson, G., et al. Role of oxygen-derived free radicals in myocardial ischemia. *Fed. Proc.* 42:4696, 1983.

103. Shlafer, M., Kane, P. F., and Kirsh, M. M. Superoxide dismutase plus catalase enhance the efficacy of hypothermic cardioplegia to protect the globally ischemic reperfused heart. *J. Thorac. Cardiovasc. Surg.* 83:830, 1982.

104. Jolly, S. R., Kane, W. J., Bailie, M. B., et al. Canine myocardial reperfusion injury: Its reduction by the combined administration of superoxide dismutase and catalase. *Circ. Res.* 54:277, 1984.

105. McCord, J. M. Oxygen-derived free radicals in post ischemic tissue injury. *N. Engl. J. Med.* 312:159, 1985.

106. Davies, K. J. A. Protein damage and degradation by oxygen radicals. I. General aspects. *J. Biol. Chem.* 262:9895, 1987.

107. Davies, K. J. A., and Goldberg, A. L. Oxygen radicals stimulate intracellular proteolysis and lipid peroxidation by independent mechanisms in erythrocytes. *J. Biol. Chem.* 262:8220, 1987.

108. Fabiato, A., and Fabiato, F. Calcium release from the sarcoplasmic reticulum. *Circ. Res.* 40:110, 1977.

109. Shen, A. C., and Jennings, R. B. Kinetics of calcium accumulative in acute myocardial ischemic injury. *Am. J. Pathol.* 67:441, 1972.

110. Fleckenstein, A., Jahnke, J., Doring, H. J., and Leder, O. Myocardial biology. *Recent Adv. Stud. Cardiac Struct. Metab.* 4:563, 1974.

111. Katz, A. M., and Reuter, H. Cellular calcium and cell death. *Am. J. Cardiol.* 44:188, 1979.

112. Katz, A. M., and Tada, M. The "stone heart": A challenge to the biochemist. *Am. J. Cardiol.* 29:578, 1972.

113. Dhalla, N. S., Pierce, N. G., Panagia, V., et al. Calcium movements in relation to heart function. *Basic Res. Cardiol.* 77:117, 1982.

114. Lehninger, A. C. Mitochondria and calcium ion transport. *Biochem. J.* 119:129, 1970.

115. Slater, E. C., and Cleland, K. W. The effect of calcium on the respiratory and phosphorylative activities of heart muscle sarcosomes. *Biochem. J.* 55:566, 1953.

116. Carafoli, E., and Bing, R. J. Myocardial failure. *J. Appl. Cardiol.* 3:3, 1988.

117. Bailey, I. A., Radda, G. K., Seymour, A. M., and Williams, S. R. The effects of insulin on myocardial metabolism and acidosis in normoxia and ischemia: A ^{31}P-NMR study. *Biochim. Biophys. Acta* 720:1727, 1982.

118. Ross, B. D., and Freeman, D. Contributions to cardiac biochemistry from magnetic resonance. *J. Appl. Cardiol.* 1:75, 1986.

119. Roberts, R., Parker, C. W., and Sobel, B. E. Detection of acute myocardial infarction by radioimmunoassay for creatine kinase MB. *Lancet* 2:319, 1977.

120. Shell, W. E., Kjeushus, J. K., and Sobel, B. E. Quantitative assessment of the extent of myocardial infarction in the conscious dog by means of analysis of serial changes in serum creatine phosphokinase activity. *J. Clin. Invest.* 50:2614, 1971.

121. Sobel, B. E., Roberts, R., and Larson, K. B. Estimation of infarct size from serum MB creatine phosphokinase activity: Application and limitations. *Am. J. Cardiol.* 37:474, 1976.

122. Haber, E. In vivo diagnostic and therapeutic uses of monoclonal antibodies in cardiology. *Annu. Rev. Med.* 37:249, 1986.

123. Schelbert, H. R., Phelps, M. E., Hoffman, E., et al. Regional myocardium blood flow, metabolism and function assessed noninvasively with positron emission tomography. *Am. J. Cardiol.* 46:1269, 1980.

124. Schelbert, H. R., and Schwaiger, M. PET Studies of the Heart. In M. Phelps, J. Mazziotta, and H. Schelbert (eds.), *Positron Emission Tomography and Autoradiography: Principles and Applications for the Brain and Heart.* New York: Raven Press, 1986. P. 581.

125. Schwaiger, M., Brunken, R., Crover-McKay, M., et al. Detection of tissue viability in patients with acute myocardial infarction by positron emission tomography. *J. Am. Coll. Cardiol.* 8:800, 1986.

126. Marshall, R. C., Tillisch, J. H., Phelps, M. E., et al. Identification and differentiation of resting myocardial ischemia and infarction in man with positron computer tomography. ^{18}F-labeled-fluorodeoxyglucose and N-13 ammonia. *Circulation* 67:766, 1983.

127. Tillisch, J., Brunken, R., Marshall, R., et al. Prediction of reversibility of cardiac wall motion abnormality using positron tomography, ^{18}fluoro-deoxyglucose, and ^{13}NH$_3$. *N. Engl. J. Med.* 314:884, 1986.

128. Tennant, T., and Wiggers, C. J. Effect of coronary occlusion on myocardial contraction. *Am. J. Physiol.* 112:351, 1935.

129. Bergmann, S. R., Fox, K. A. A., Ter-Pogossian, M. M., et al. Clot-selective coronary thrombolysis with tissue-type plasminogen activator. *Science* 220:1181, 1983.

130. Braunwald, E., and Kloner, R. A. The stunned myocardium: Prolonged, postischemic ventricular dysfunction. *Circulation* 66:1146, 1982.

131. Bing, R. J. Reparative processes in heart muscle following myocardial infarction. *Cardiology* 50:314, 1971.

132. Bergmann, S. R., Lerch, R., Fox, K., et al. Temporal dependence of beneficial effects of coronary thrombolysis characterized by positron tomography. *Am. J. Med.* 73:573, 1982.

133. Vary, T. C., Angelakos, E. T., and Schaffer, S. W. Relationship between adenine nucleotide metabolism and irreversible ischemic tissue damage in isolated, perfused rat heart. *Circ. Res.* 45:218, 1979.

134. Becker, L. C., and Ambrosio, G. Myocardial consequences of reperfusion. *Prog. Cardiovasc. Dis.* 30:23, 1987.

135. Poole-Wilson, P. A. Reperfusion damage in heart muscle: Still unexplained but with new clinical relevance. *Clin. Physiol.* 7:439, 1987.

136. Zimmerman, A. N. E., and Hülsmann, W. C. Paradoxial influence of calcium ions on the permeability of the isolated rat heart. *Nature* 211:646, 1960.

137. Ambrosio, G., Weissfeldt, M. D., Jacobus, W. E., and Flaherty, J. T. Evidence of a reversible, radical-mediated component of reperfusion injury: Reduction by recombinant human superoxide dismutase administered at the time of reflow. *Circulation* 75:282, 1987.

138. Lagerstrom, C. F., Walker, W. E., and Taegtmeyer, H. Failure of glycogen depletion to improve left ventricular function of the rabbit heart after hypothermic ischemic arrest. *Circ. Res.*, 63:81, 1988.

139. McElroy, D. D., Taegtmeyer, H., and Walker, W. E. Effects of glycogen on function and energy metabolism of the isolated rabbit heart after hypothermic ischemic arrest. (Abstract). *Clin. Res.* 35:304A, 1987.

140. Klein, H. H., Puschmann, S., Schaper, J., and Schaper, W. The mechanism of the tetrazolium reaction in identifying experimental myocardial infarction. *Virchows Arch. [Pathol. Anat.]* 393:287, 1981.

141. Schaper, J., and Schaper, W. Reperfusion of ischemic myocardium: Ultrastructural and histochemical aspects. *J. Am. Coll. Cardiol.* 1:1037, 1983.

4
Pathology of Acute Myocardial Infarction

BROOKS S. EDWARDS AND JESSE E. EDWARDS

In considering the pathology of acute myocardial infarction (AMI) we have included the pathologic features that underlie the complications, both early and late, of the fundamental condition.

Pathologic Features of Myocardial Infarction

Acute myocardial infarction characteristically is observed in patients with chronic coronary arterial obstruction. In some of these, precipitation of the myocardial necrosis is associated with a superimposed acute coronary arterial occlusion from a thrombus. Infarcts so resulting are, in general, more extensive than are those in which acute coronary occlusion is not present.

Two degrees of involvement of the myocardium are recognized. The more extensive disease involves nearly the full thickness of the left ventricular myocardium in the distribution of the underlying coronary disease. Such infarcts tend to be conglomerate. The infarcts with less extensive involvement tend to lie in the subendocardial one-half or one-third of the myocardium, although patchy foci of involvement may lie in the subepicardial half of the myocardium. So-called subendocardial infarcts may be either multifocal or conglomerate. In most instances, regardless of the type of infarct, a layer of myocardium lying immediately underneath the mural endocardium is preserved.

The infarcts of the former type have generally been called transmural, and the latter have been termed subendocardial. Based on electrocardiography, infarcts have been categorized as Q wave infarcts and non-Q wave infarcts. Q wave infarcts tend to be transmural, and non-Q wave infarcts tend to be subendocardial [1]. Although it is beyond the scope of this chapter to enter into lengthy debate relative to the preferential use of the terms mentioned, it should be pointed out that the presence or absence of a Q wave in cases of AMI may be influenced not only by the extent of an infarct but also by its location, the presence or absence of earlier infarction, and delayed intraventricular conduction [2].

The earliest reliable manifestations of AMI, evident microscopically, usually appear at about 8 hours [3, 4]. Early changes include hypereosinophilia of the involved myocardial fibers (Fig. 4-1A); in addition, the ischemic myocytes may take on a "wavy" appearance. Thinning of fibers, nuclear loss, and cytoplasmic coagulation may occur within the first 24 hours. The next stage, namely interstitial infiltration with leukocytes, usually polymorphonuclear in nature, is seen at about 24 hours (Fig. 4-1B). The process of leukocytic infiltration occurs initially at the periphery of the myocardial infarct and proceeds toward the center of the infarct. In large infarcts leukocytic infiltration falls far short of involving the central part of the zone of infarction. After 2 days the leukocytes start showing signs of necrosis, leading to cytoplasmic disruption and nuclear fragmentation of these cells. After about 3 to 4 days, removal of infarcted myocardial fibers begins (Fig. 4-1C). At the early stages of removal the process cannot be identified grossly. Removal of necrotic myocardial fibers is the main process that occurs during

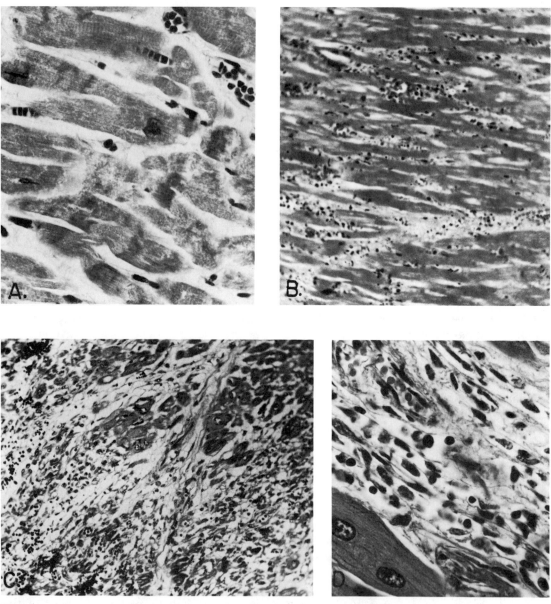

Fig. 4-1
Photomicrographs of myocardial infarcts of various ages. *A.* At 6 to 8 hours after
the onset of infarction some fibers have lost their nuclei. There are cytoplasmic
irregularities, including coagulation changes and contraction bands. H & E. ×
450. *B.* At 2 days, the myocardial fibers stain darkly because of
hypereosinophilia. Nuclei have been lost, and there is heavy infiltration
interstitially with polymorphonuclear neutrophils. H & E. × 200. *C.* Periphery of
the infarct at 5 days. Necrotic fibers are being removed, leaving a basketwork of
connective tissue and capillaries of the myocardium. H & E. × 100. *D.* Site of
removal of myocardial infarction at 2 weeks. At the center, myocardial fibers
have been removed, leaving the capillaries and connective tissue of myocardial
stroma. Some interstitial phagocytic cells are also present. H & E. × 450.

the latter half of the first week and all of the second week. The site of this process is identified histologically as a vascular basketwork representing myocardium from which the myocardial fibers have been removed, although the connective tissue and vascular stroma of the cardiac wall remain. Within this tissue may be found fragments of necrotic fibers, phagocytes containing "wear and tear" pigment (lipofuscin), and interstitial leukocytes, principally phagocytes (Fig. 4-1D).

During the third week the process of scar formation starts (Fig. 4-2A). It is characterized by fibroblastic proliferation and the laying down of delicate collagen. Additional removal of necrotic fibers may occur or is completed by this time. During the fourth week scar formation is evident, the scar having resulted from new production of connective tissue and condensation of stroma (Fig. 4-2B). Scattered phagocytes are present in the early scar.

In older scars, the collagen becomes compact; and at about 6 weeks after the onset of the infarct, elastic fibers may be noted in the scar tissue (Fig. 4-3A). In some scars dilated vessels are present and persist (Fig. 4-3B).

When the scar is established, the infarcted myocardium has usually been removed. Nevertheless, in some large infarcts necrotic muscle may remain for months or years enveloped by scar tissue (Fig. 4-3C). In such instances the remaining necrotic muscle may become calcified.

There are gross counterparts to the histologic stages reviewed. Within 6 hours or more the infarcted area may be identified as somewhat cyanotic in nature (Fig. 4-4A). By 1 day the necrotic area is tan, reflecting the color of infarcted myocardium and leukocytes (Fig. 4-4B). When removal of necrotic muscle is established, the zone of removal lying at the edge of the infarcted tissue is characteristically red to purple and depressed (Fig. 4-4C). During the third week the process of removal and early scar formation is represented by

Fig. 4-2
Photomicrographs of myocardial infarcts of various ages. *A*. At 3 weeks. Note the infarcted tissue at the right and the noninfarcted tissue at the left. Between the two zones is a zone from which necrotic myocardium has been removed. Early fibrous changes are occurring, and blood vessels are dilated. H & E. × 100. *B*. Endocardial half of the myocardium in healed myocardial infarction. The black streaks represent scarring. The mural endocardium is at the bottom. A strip of retained muscle is characteristically present immediately underneath the mural endocardium. Elastic tissue stain. × 5.

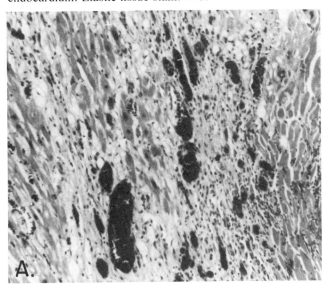
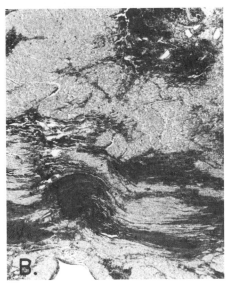

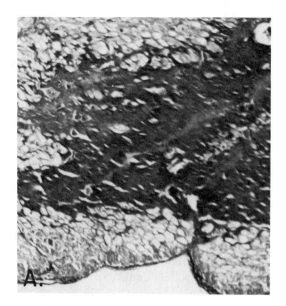

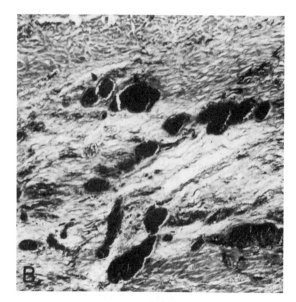

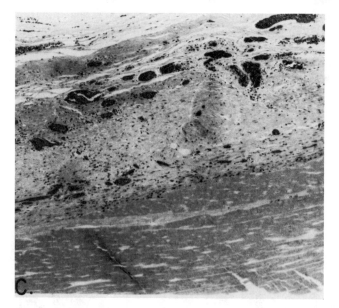

Fig. 4-3
Photomicrographs showing variations in healed myocardial infarction. *A.* Mural
endocardium is toward the bottom. Immediately underneath this layer is a zone of
retained myocardium. Some of the fibers are vacuolated. Underneath this area is
a black area representing dense scar following myocardial infarction. Elastic
tissue stain. × 100. *B.* Scar in old myocardial infarction in which numerous wide
blood vessels are present. *C.* The scar of the myocardial infarction (upper half) is
adjacent to an area of retained necrotic myocardial fibers (lowermost). H & E. ×
70.

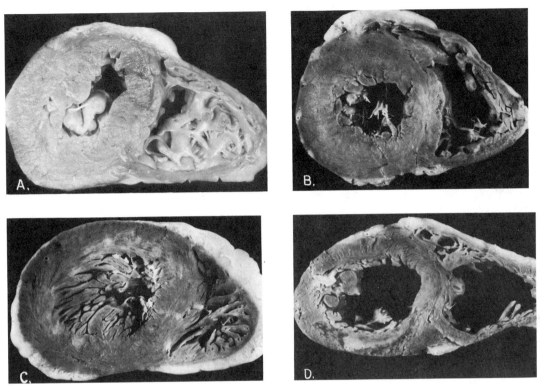

Fig. 4-4
Gross pathology of AMI. In each instance the ventricles have been cut in cross section and are viewed from the basal toward the apical aspect. The upper part of each illustration is anterior and the lower part inferior. The right ventricle lies to the right of the left ventricle in this perspective. *A.* Early anteroseptal infarction. The different texture of the anterior part of the septum and nearby anterior wall reflects a zone that in the fresh state yielded a cyanotic hue. *B.* Anterior infarction of about 4 days' duration. The pale area in the subendocardial half of the anterior wall and the nearby ventricular septum represents acute infarction. Removal is not yet apparent. *C.* Healing infarction in midportion of the ventricular septum. The dark, depressed area represents a zone of removed necrotic muscle. *D.* Transmural acute inferior infarction. The pale area in the inferior wall represents necrotic muscle yet to be removed. Peripheral to this zone is a dark, depressed area representing removal of tissue, characteristic of a 2- to 3-week-old infarct.

a depressed, translucent, ground-glass zone (Fig. 4-4D). The established scar is pale gray to white. Varying degrees of thinning of the wall occur in concert with the proportion of the myocardium that had been infarcted. In many cases scarring may be multifocal, indicating the frequent multifocal distribution of AMI. When the stage of scarring has been reached, thickening of the overlying mural endocardium by gray fibrous tissue (fibroelastosis) may be present. The larger the scar, the greater is the trend for fibroelastosis to develop (Fig. 4-5).

Complications

Hypotension and Congestive Heart Failure

The first week following AMI may be complicated by persistent or acute hypotension and

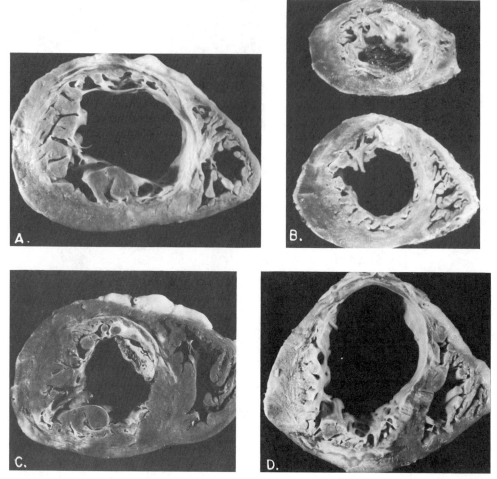

Fig. 4-5
Gross appearances of hearts with healed myocardial infarcts. *A.* Healed extensive
anteroseptal infarction. The involved part of the wall is thin. The mural
endocardium is thickened by virtue of fibroelastosis. *B.* Two levels of section
showing healed anterior infarction with mural thrombosis at the apex. There is
endocardial fibroelastosis as well. *C.* Healed conglomerate subendocardial
anterior infarction with endocardial fibroelastosis and a mural thrombosus
attached. In the inferolateral aspect there is scarring of healed infarction. The
papillary muscles are unaffected, however. *D.* Healed extensive anterior
infarction and healing inferior infarction. The thin wall and endocardial
fibroelastosis are characteristic of a healed extensive anterior infarct, which
suggests early aneurysm formation as well. In the inferior wall there is a
conglomerate infarct that is undergoing healing. The classic ground-glass
appearance of the zone of removal around the pale zone of retained necrotic
muscles suggests an age of about 3 weeks.

the syndrome of congestive heart failure. The etiology of this state ("pump failure") primarily relates to extensive myocardial ischemia and necrosis or unique sites of myocardial infarction with or without rupture.

Extensive Myocardial Ischemia or Necrosis

It has long been appreciated that extensive myocardial infarction results in severe hemodynamic disturbances and persistent congestive heart failure. The extent of infarction may result from a single AMI (Fig. 4-6); more commonly, though, this myocardial mass is lost during several distinct episodes of AMI (Fig. 4-5D). In the latter case, it has been demonstrated that the sequential loss of mass results in an additive effect. When a total of more than 40 percent of myocardial mass is lost, severe pump failure results, and the chances for recovery are remote [5, 6].

Attention has been focused on the so-called stunned myocardium. The stunned myocardium may be characterized by a reversible state of myocardial injury [7]. Under conditions in which perfusion is restored (either naturally or by intervention), that portion of myocardium may resume normal function. Although physiologic imaging devices may suggest the presence of stunned myocardium, there are no unique pathologic markers that identify this condition.

Right Ventricular Infarction

Infarction of the left ventricular inferior wall may extend into the right ventricle [8]. Usually the extent and consequences of this right ventricular infarction are minimal. The relative protection of the right ventricle from infarction may relate to the lower oxygen demands of the thin-walled chamber. Significant right ventricular infarction occurs more commonly in states where the oxygen demand of the right ventricle is increased, which may be seen where there is preexisting pulmonary hypertension and right ventricular hypertrophy. Usually the patients have a dominant right coronary artery with a high grade proximal stenosis or occlusion. Clinically, the patient may present as hypotensive and volume-depleted while undergoing spontaneous diuresis.

Rupture of Ventricular Septum

There are three general types of cardiac rupture that may complicate the acute stages of myocardial infarction [9]. Collectively, they constitute about 15 percent of all deaths resulting from AMI. Rupture may involve the left ventricular free wall (about 85 percent of all ruptures), a papillary muscle, or the ventricular septum, the latter two types constituting about 15 percent of ruptures. Rupture of the left ventricular free wall is considered in greater detail in the section dealing with hemopericardium. Rupture of a papillary muscle is covered in the section on mitral regurgitation.

Rupture of the ventricular septum leads to an acquired left-to-right shunt. Frequently, it is of overwhelming proportion, resulting in early shock followed by a rapidly deteriorating state. When the communication between the two ventricles is restricted in caliber, the

Fig. 4-6
Frontal section through the ventricular septum and ventricles. Extensive infarction of the apical area of the left ventricle extends into the lateral wall and ventricular septum. Note the overlying mural thrombosis.

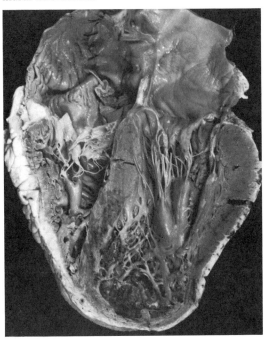

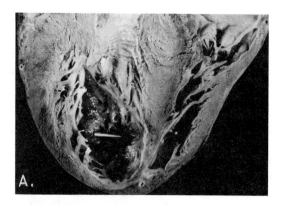

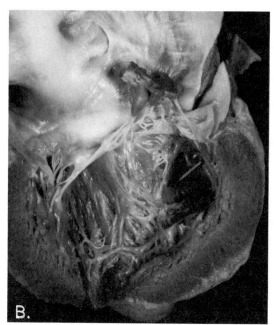

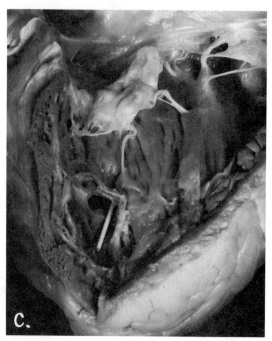

Fig. 4-7
Rupture of the ventricular septum: two types. *A*. Simple type. *B, C*. Complex
type. *A*. The ventricular septum has been sectioned in a frontal plane. The
ventricles are viewed from behind (left ventricle to the left). There is an acute
infarct involving the ventricular septum and the apical portion of the heart. A
simple through-and-through tract (probe) extends between the two ventricles. *B*.
Left ventricle and atrium. The rupture tract begins at the base of the ventricular
septum (probe). *C*. Right atrium and ventricle. The tract (probe) leads into the
right ventricle in a more apical location than the initial laceration in the left
ventricle.

shunt may be tolerated for varying periods of time.

There are two types of rupture of the ventricular septum, the simple and the complex [10]. As the name implies, the simple type represents a through-and-through, direct opening between the two ventricles (Fig. 4-7A). The complex type is represented by a tract or several tracts extending through the ventricular septum in a serpiginous manner (Fig. 4-7B, C). The opening(s) into the right ventricle may be some distance from the site of the primary tear. Although exceptions occur, it is usual that the simple type of septal rupture complicates infarcts in the apical half of the left ventricle (usually anterior), whereas the complex type tends to occur in basal infarcts (usually inferior).

Transmural myocardial infarction is virtually always present in individuals with rupture of the ventricular septum. Extensive right ventricular infarction in the presence of septal rupture negatively influences survival [11]. Although some have suggested that one-vessel coronary artery disease is common with this entity, one study reported significant three-vessel coronary artery disease in 48 of 53 autopsy cases studied [10].

Associated Conditions Leading to or Intensifying the Degree of Congestive Heart Failure

Especially among the relatively old with myocardial infarction, congestive heart failure, if present, may be caused by the loss of myocardial tissue through infarction (often recurrent) and by the effects of additional conditions. Among the common additional conditions are hypertension, aortic stenosis, chronic obstructive pulmonary disease, and, less commonly, extensive forms of senile (cardiac) amyloidosis [12].

MITRAL REGURGITATION

Mitral regurgitation may occur during the early phase following AMI and vary in severity from trivial to severe. Because the integrity of the mitral valve depends on the structure and function of not only the valve itself but also the mitral annulus, left atrial wall, left ventricular myocardium, and papillary muscles, mitral insufficiency may result from disruption or malfunction of one or more components [13].

Papillary Muscle Dysfunction or Infarction

Mild and often transient mitral regurgitation is associated with the entity "papillary muscle dysfunction," which may be the result of ischemia of either a papillary muscle or more commonly the left ventricular free wall from which the papillary muscles arise. Whether it represents transient ischemia or a stunned myocardium following infarction of adjacent tissue, the pathologic findings are often nonspecific.

More severe mitral regurgitation results from infarction of papillary muscle and underlying left ventricle (Fig. 4-8).

The posteromedial papillary muscle receives its blood supply from a branch of the posterior descending artery. Because it is an end-artery, collateral circulation is limited, and occlusion frequently results in infarction. The anterolateral papillary muscle commonly has dual blood supply from diagonal branches of the anterior descending artery and obtuse marginal branches of the left circumflex coronary artery. The dual supply provides some protective effect, making infarction of the anterolateral papillary muscle less frequent than that of the posteromedial papillary muscle.

Distortion in left ventricular geometry, which may occur following left ventricular infarction, may alter the relations between the two papillary muscles and result in mild to moderate mitral insufficiency. Chronic mitral insufficiency may lead to left atrial enlargement, annular dilatation, and progressively more severe mitral regurgitation [13].

Rupture of Papillary Muscle

Whereas infarction of a part of a papillary muscle system may lead to abnormal coaptation of the mitral leaflets and incompetence, rupture of part or all of a papillary muscle is associated with more severe mitral regurgitation [14, 15]. Each papillary muscle is composed of a number of heads. Rupture of an in-

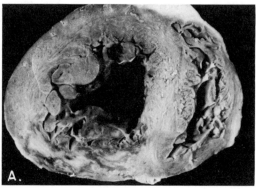
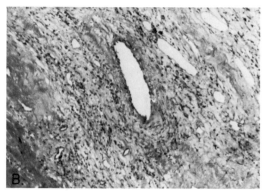

Fig. 4-8
Two examples of healing myocardial infarction without papillary muscle rupture
and with mitral regurgitation. *A.* Cross section of the ventricles. In the inferior
wall of the left ventricle is a healing transmural infarct. The related posteromedial
papillary muscle is also involved in infarction but is not ruptured. *B.*
Photomicrograph of a portion of the posteromedial papillary muscle from a
surgically excised mitral valve showing features of healing acute infarction.
Rupture of the papillary muscle had not been present. H & E. × 100.

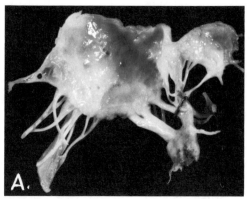
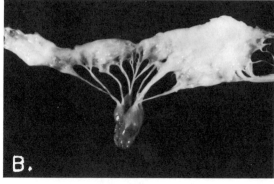

Fig. 4-9
Two examples of rupture of a papillary muscle from surgically excised specimens.
A. The posteromedial papillary muscle (ragged lower edge) has ruptured. *B.* The
anterolateral papillary muscle has ruptured.

dividual head may be well tolerated for some
time, whereas rupture of an entire papillary
muscle complex results in torrential mitral regurgitation and rapid hemodynamic collapse.
Rupture of a papillary muscle may occur following a "small," otherwise uncomplicated
myocardial infarction. Rupture typically occurs between days 3 and 7 following infarction. Rupture of the posteromedial muscle is

four times more common than rupture of the
anterolateral muscle (Fig. 4-9).

HEMOPERICARDIUM

One of the dramatic consequences of AMI is
hemopericardium causing acute cardiac tamponade. The most common cause of hemo-

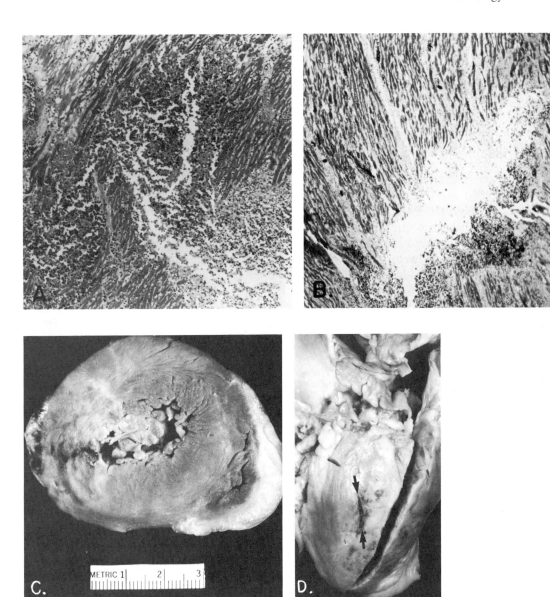

Fig. 4-10
A. Photomicrograph of AMI with unusually heavy leukocytic infiltration. H & E.
× 40. *B.* Photomicrograph of AMI with a microlaceration within the left
ventricular wall adjacent to a site of heavy leukocytic infiltration. H & E. × 40.
C. Cross section through the ventricles in an instance of acute lateral infarction
with rupture of the free wall. *D.* Acute lateral infarction with rupture of the left
ventricular free wall. External view of the heart. The laceration is linear (between
arrows).

pericardium following AMI is rupture of the free wall of the left ventricle [9]. Less commonly, fatal hemopericardium may result from the late effects of the pericarditis that may accompany transmural AMI [16].

Rupture of the Left Ventricular Free Wall

Rupture of the free wall is usually seen with transmural infarction and usually occurs within the first week after onset of acute infarction (so-called early rupture). The time peak occurs on about the third or fourth day.

Early rupture tends to occur at the periphery of the infarcted site and probably results from a shearing effect between the infarcted and the viable myocardium. It is common for cases with rupture to show histologic evidence of massive leukocytic infiltration. Such a process may cause liquefaction of infarcted myocardium and may represent the primary event leading to gross rupture (Fig. 4-10A,B). The rupture tract extends into and through the epicardium, leading to cardiac tamponade from hemopericardium (Fig. 4-10C). The epicardial lesion is usually a linear break in continuity (Fig. 4-10D).

Among a series of cases with rupture of the free wall, the underlying infarct was equally distributed among anterior, inferior, and lateral locations [9]. Because the lateral wall constitutes the least frequent site of primary infarction, it may be accepted that lateral infarction, once present, is more susceptible to the complication of rupture than are infarcts involving either the anterior or the inferior location. Women are more susceptible to the classic forms of left ventricular rupture than are men.

Uncommonly, rupture of the free wall may occur late, about 2 to 3 weeks after the onset of the underlying infarction. In such cases rupture is usually a complication of unusually early aneurysm formation (Fig. 4-11). The rupture site shows a "blow-out" type of defect at the center of the developing aneurysm.

Pericarditis

With AMI, pericarditis is first characterized by fibrinous exudation starting about the second day. The process tends to be localized

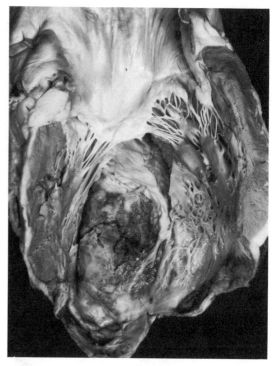

Fig. 4-11
Interior of the left ventricle with a developing aneurysm in early AMI. Rupture of the aneurysm occurred about 3 weeks after the onset of the infarction.

over the site of infarction and frequently remains in that position. In some cases the fibrinous exudation may be diffuse. In either case, the usual outcome of pericarditis is that it resolves or it becomes organized, the latter process leading to adhesions in the distribution of the fibrinous exudation.

Uncommonly, the process of organization may be a basis for hemopericardium (Fig. 4-12) [16]. The latter is derived from bleeding from capillaries of the organizing granulation tissue. The hemorrhagic effusion may be extensive, leading to cardiac tamponade.

This complication, if it appears, tends to occur 2 weeks or more after the onset of the myocardial infarction. It has been suggested that administration of anticoagulant drugs during the period of convalescence for the myocardial infarction makes pericardial hemorrhage more likely than were such drugs not used.

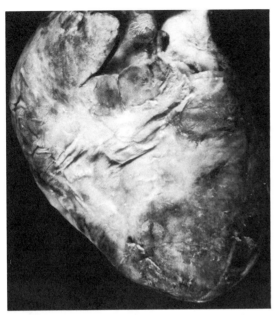

Fig. 4-12
Pericarditis associated with acute anterior
myocardial infarction from a case in which
infarction began 10 days earlier. The discoloration
over the apical region may represent early
hemorrhage into organizing pericarditis.

THROMBOEMBOLIC EVENTS

The thromboembolic events that complicate
AMI are so named because some are truly embolic, whereas others may be either thrombotic or the result of localized arterial disease.
In the latter case, ischemic disease of organs
supplied by the systemic circulation may result from localized obstructive disease complicated by hypotension related to myocardial
infarction.

During the early stage of AMI, ischemic disease of the various organs is likely a result of
inadequate perfusion by virtue of hypotension
and localized arterial disease. When myocardial infarction has existed for a week or
longer, it is likely that ischemic disease results
from embolism originating in mural thrombosis of the left ventricle or left atrium [17].
When left ventricular thrombosis complicates
myocardial infarction, the thrombosis tends to
occur at the apex of the left ventricle regardless of the location of the underlying infarct.

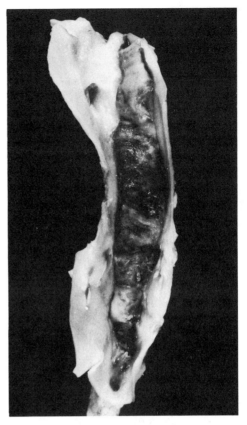

Fig. 4-13
Femoral vein containing thrombus as a
complication of congestive heart failure with a
potential for pulmonary embolism.

Among the exceptions is the occurrence of
thrombosis within an aneurysm occupying the
inferior aspect of the left ventricle.

Thromboembolic phenomena affecting the
lesser circulation are classically those of ileofemoral thrombophlebitis (Fig. 4-13) and
pulmonary embolism. With AMI such a phenomenon is now uncommon, probably the
consequence of early ambulation of patients
with AMI.

In contrast, with healed myocardial infarction the problem of ileofemoral thrombophlebitis and pulmonary embolism persists,
particularly in subjects with congestive heart
failure. In such patients thrombi may also occur in the right ventricle and, particularly, in
the right atrial appendage. Even in such in-

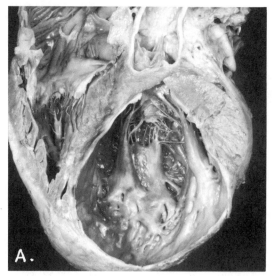
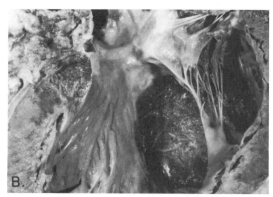

Fig. 4-14
Two examples of true left ventricular aneurysms. *A.* Aneurysm complicating an anterior infarction. The ventricular portion of the heart, cut in frontal section and viewed from in front, shows the left ventricle to the left of the right ventricle. The aneurysm is thin-walled and has a fibroelastic lining. *B.* Interior of the left ventricle with an aneurysm involving the inferior wall of the left ventricle. A large mural thrombus is contained within the aneurysm.

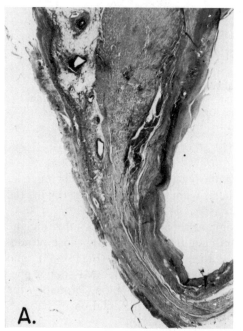
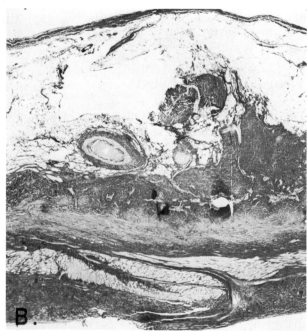

Fig. 4-15
Photomicrographs of true left ventricular aneurysms. *A.* Epicardium is to the left. This low-power view shows virtual molding of the aneurysm at the edge of an infarct. The aneurysm displays endocardial fibroelastosis and some mural thrombosis. Elastic tissue stain. × 5. *B.* Epicardium is above. Low-power view of the wall of the left ventricular aneurysm. Lowermost is a layer of thickened endocardium. Immediately above it, the light area represents a zone of preserved myocardium. More epicardially there is scar, and immediately under the fatty epicardium is a layer of preserved myocardial tissue. Elastic tissue stain. × 5.

stances the principal source of pulmonary embolism is venous thrombosis.

LEFT VENTRICULAR ANEURYSM

Aneurysms complicating myocardial infarction involve the left ventricle, and more commonly anteriorly than inferiorly. Men are more commonly affected than women. Aneurysms are of two types, true and false (pseudoaneurysm) [18].

True aneurysms are derived from extensive myocardial infarcts. As the healing process occurs, the left ventricular wall becomes thin and gradually dilates to become molded into a localized dilatation of the left ventricle (Fig. 4-14). Characteristically, the walls of true aneurysms are mostly fibrotic in nature as scar replaces infarcted wall. The mural endocardium at the aneurysm is thickened with collagen and elastic tissue, a process usually called *fibroelastosis* (Fig. 4-15). Underneath the thickened endocardium is a layer of preserved, noninfarcted myocardium. It is probable that the ventricular arrhythmias that occur in subjects with left ventricular aneurysm begin in this retained tissue.

False, or pseudo, aneurysms of the left ventricle result from contained rupture of the left ventricle complicating infarction without immediate hemopericardium (Fig. 4-16).

Left ventricular aneurysms, whether true or false, frequently harbor mural thrombi. Such thrombi tend to show limited or no organization and are subject to fragmentation and consequent systemic embolism.

Established old true aneurysms do not have

Fig. 4-16
A. Low-power photomicrograph of a false aneurysm of the left ventricle and adjacent tissues. There is an abrupt interruption in the continuity of the ventricular wall representing a site of previous rupture. The dark, thin wall of the false aneurysm represents organized hematoma. Elastic tissue stain. × 5. *B.* Interior of the left ventricle with a small false aneurysm at the apical area inferiorly. It had ruptured, leading to a fatal hemopericardium.

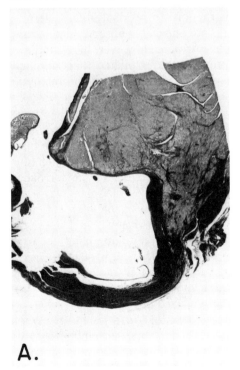

A.

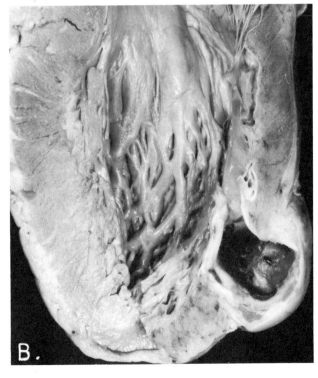

B.

a significant tendency to rupture. In contrast, false aneurysms are susceptible to rupture (Fig. 4-16B).

RECURRENT ANGINA OR INFARCTION

Postinfarction angina may result from residual ischemic tissue in the vicinity of the recent myocardial infarction, or it may indicate extensive coronary artery disease with myocardial ischemia remote from the site of recent infarction. An initial non-Q wave infarction may result in a relatively small area of tissue necrosis and typically is associated with a low incidence of coronary thrombosis [19]. However, this state should be regarded as unstable, possibly characterized by severe coronary artery disease with a large area of viable myocardium in jeopardy. Pathologically, one may observe a large transmural area of AMI with evidence of older subendocardial infarction. Extensive obstructive coronary artery disease is the rule in this situation. The occurrence of dilated vessels in some scars of healed myocardial infarction may represent a low resistance zone that may function as circulatory steal from intact myocardium. The syndrome of postinfarction angina may be an expression of such a steal.

POSTINFARCTION ARRHYTHMIAS AND SUDDEN DEATH

Following an AMI, arrhythmias of almost all types are known to occur. Some are merely coincidental to the infarct, whereas others are related to it.

Events of atrial fibrillation related to myocardial infarction may reflect left ventricular failure for one of many reasons. Any elevation of ventricular filling pressure with secondary atrial distention may provide the stimulus for atrial fibrillation.

Premature ventricular contractions are common. In instances of large infarcts or left ventricular aneurysm the site of origin of such

beats may be the preserved layer of myocardium immediately underneath the endocardium.

Sudden death is the most common type of coronary-related death [20]. In such subjects, the myocardium may be the site of acute ischemic disease with or without acute infarction. In most subjects dying of coronary-related ventricular fibrillation, scarring from a previous infarction is usually present. It should be pointed out that in many cases of sudden coronary death AMI is not present, a concept supported by a follow-up study of survivors of "sudden death," in whom acute infarction does not evolve. Such cases should be considered primary arrhythmogenic deaths and not classified as AMI.

PATHOLOGIC FEATURES FOLLOWING THROMBOLYTIC THERAPY

Selected autopsy studies have analyzed the pathologic findings following treatment with thrombolytic therapy [21–23]. As one would expect, even in vessels with successful lysis there often remains a significant degree of fixed obstruction. In residual atherosclerotic lesions it is not unusual to observe plaque rupture and hemorrhage; however, these findings may represent the stimulus that initiated thrombosis and not the effect of thrombolytic therapy.

A region of infarcted myocardium is typically present even in cases of successful thrombolysis. The infarcted myocardium may exhibit the classic findings of coagulation necrosis without significant hemorrhage; however, in other cases of spontaneous or drug-induced thrombolysis the infarcted myocardium may be hemorrhagic [21]. The observation of extensive contraction band necrosis following thrombolytic therapy suggests early reperfusion injury by free radical generation [23]. Caution should be employed when interpreting the presence of contraction bands, as they can be observed in a great variety of situations [24]. Hemorrhagic infarcts typically are observed in situations of delayed reperfusion where small vessel injury has occurred.

Editorial Comments

Pathologic examination of the heart following death from an acute coronary syndrome yields highly important information. Regrettably, there are fewer autopsies being performed at a time when we are perhaps most able to link clinical and morphologic findings. We hold a weekly conference at our hospital with Dr. Jesse Edwards or Dr. Jack Titus wherein the hearts of autopsied patients are described in great detail. The discussion and learning that occurs at these conferences is extraordinary. We cardiologists have much to learn from our colleagues in pathology and should strive to initiate and maintain this important collaborative effort. G. S. F.

References

1. Freifeld, A. G., Schuster, E. H., and Bulkley, B. H. Nontransmural versus transmural myocardial infarction: A morphologic study. *Am. J. Med.* 75:423, 1983.
2. Phibbs, B. "Transmural" versus "subendocardial" myocardial infarction: An electrocardiographic myth. *J. Am. Coll. Cardiol.* 1:561, 1983.
3. Mallory, G. K., White, P. D., and Salcedo-Salgar, J. The speed of healing of myocardial infarction: A study of the pathologic anatomy in seventy-two cases. *Am. Heart J.* 18:647, 1939.
4. Fishbein, M. C., Maclean, D., and Maroko, P. R. The histopathologic evolution of myocardial infarction. *Chest* 73:843, 1978.
5. Alonso, D. R., Scheidt, S., Post, M., and Killip, T. Pathophysiology of cardiogenic shock: Quantification of myocardial necrosis, clinical, pathologic and electrocardiographic correlations. *Circulation* 48:588, 1973.
6. Page, D. L., Caulfield, J. B., Kastor, J. A., et al. Myocardial changes associated with cardiogenic shock. *N. Engl. J. Med.* 285:133, 1971.
7. Buckberg, G. D. Studies of controlled reperfusion after ischemia. I. When is cardiac muscle damaged irreversibly? *J. Thorac. Cardiovasc. Surg.* 92:483, 1986.
8. Isner, J. M. Right ventricular myocardial infarction. *J.A.M.A.* 259:712, 1988.
9. Van Tassel, R. A., and Edwards, J. E. Rupture of heart complicating myocardial infarction: Analysis of 40 cases including nine examples of left ventricular false aneurysm. *Chest* 61:104, 1972.
10. Edwards, B. S., Edwards, W. D., and Edwards, J. E. Ventricular septal rupture complicating acute myocardial infarction: Identification of simple and complex types in 53 autopsied hearts. *Am. J. Cardiol.* 54:1201, 1984.
11. Moore, C. A., Nygaard, T. W., Kaiser, D. L., et al. Postinfarction ventricular septal rupture: The importance of location of infarction and right ventricular function in determining survival. *Circulation* 74:45, 1986.
12. Olson, L. J., Gertz, M. A., Edwards, W. D., et al. Senile cardiac amyloidosis with myocardial dysfunction: Diagnosis by endomyocardial biopsy and immunohistochemistry. *N. Engl. J. Med.* 317:738, 1987.
13. Edwards, J. E., and Burchell, H. B. Pathologic anatomy of mitral insufficiency. *Proc. Mayo Clin.* 33:497, 1958.
14. Nishimura, R. A., Schaff, H. V., Shub, C., et al. Papillary muscle rupture complicating acute myocardial infarction: Analysis of 17 patients. *Am. J. Cardiol.* 51:373, 1983.
15. Vlodaver, Z., and Edwards, J. E. Rupture of ventricular septum or papillary muscle complicating myocardial infarction. *Circulation* 55:815, 1977.
16. Anderson, M. W., Christensen, N. A., and Edwards, J. E. Hemopericardium complicating myocardial infarction in the absence of cardiac rupture: Report of three cases. *Arch. Intern. Med.* 90:634, 1952.
17. Visser, C. A., Kan, G., Lie, K. I., and Durrer, D. Incidence and one year follow up of left ventricular thrombus following acute myocardial infarction: An echocardiographic study of 96 patients (Abstract). *J. Am. Coll. Cardiol.* 1:648, 1983.
18. Nakajima, H., and Edwards, J. E. Factors favoring certain complications of acute myocardial infarction: Rupture, aneurysm and false aneurysm of left ventricle. *Minn. Med.* 68:291, 1985.
19. DeWood, M. A., Stifter, W. F., Simpson, C. S., et al. Coronary arteriographic findings soon after non-Q-wave myocardial infarction. *N. Engl. J. Med.* 315:417, 1986.
20. Vedin, A., Wilhelmsson, C., Elmfeldt, D., et al. Deaths and non-fatal reinfarctions during two years' follow-up after myocardial infarction: A follow-up study of 440 men and women discharged alive from hospital. *Acta Med. Scand.* 198:353, 1975.
21. Mathey, D. G., Schofer, J., Kuck, K-H., et al. Transmural, haemorrhagic myocardial infarction after intracoronary streptokinase: Clinical,

angiographic, and necropsy findings. *Br. Heart J.* 48:546, 1982.

22. Mattfeldt, T., Schwarz, F., Schuler, G., et al. Necropsy evaluation in seven patients with evolving acute myocardial infarction treated with thrombolytic therapy. *Am. J. Cardiol.* 54:530, 1984.

23. Matsuda, M., Fujiwara, H., Onodera, T., et al. Quantitative analysis of infarct size, contraction band necrosis, and coagulation necrosis in human autopsied hearts with acute myocardial infarction after treatment with selective intracoronary thrombolysis. *Circulation* 76:981, 1987.

24. Karch, S. B., and Billingham, M. E. Myocardial contraction bands revisited. *Hum. Pathol.* 17:9, 1986.

II
Clinical Diagnosis and
Routine Management of Acute
Myocardial Infarction

5
History and Physical Examination for Acute Myocardial Infarction

Ann D. Walling, Robert A. O'Rourke, and Richard A. Walsh

History

Among patients presenting with chest discomfort, a thorough history is often valuable for identifying those with evidence of myocardial ischemia. In fact, this evaluation, in conjunction with the physical examination, electrocardiogram (ECG), chest x-ray, and other noninvasive tests, often dictates important therapeutic decisions. The initial dilemma often faced by the physician is whether the pain is cardiac or noncardiac in origin (Fig. 5-1); and when the pain is cardiac, it must be defined as ischemic or nonischemic in etiology. Accordingly, the discussion here emphasizes the value and limitations of the history in the diagnosis of prolonged myocardial ischemia or infarction [1, 2].

CARDIAC CHEST PAIN

Ischemic Causes
Ischemic pain results from a transient or prolonged disparity between myocardial oxygen supply and oxygen demand due to the inability to increase myocardial blood flow sufficiently to meet an increment in myocardial oxygen demand, as occurs during exercise (e.g., severe coronary narrowing due to atherosclerosis), or to sudden decreases in coronary blood flow, as occur during coronary thrombosis or spasm. However, chest pain also may occur in the absence of coronary occlusive disease when coronary perfusion is low (e.g., hypotension) or when oxygen demands are greatly increased (e.g., aortic stenosis).

The precipitating events immediately prior to acute myocardial infarction (AMI) are poorly defined. A high percentage of patients have prodromal symptoms or have visited a physician during the weeks preceding the AMI; yet many die suddenly. Also, the relation of AMI to physical exertion, emotional stress, new symptoms, or altered anginal patterns preceding the event has not been well studied.

The clinical history may be straightforward and diagnostic or atypical and misleading. The typical patient is a middle-aged or older man or an older postmenopausal woman. The pain of myocardial ischemia is characterized by the abrupt or gradual onset of substernal discomfort, frequently described as deep, visceral, and squeezing in nature. Patients often use the following words: "pressure," "tightness," "heavy," "burning," "strangling," "aching," or "constricting." Importantly, many patients deny the presence of chest "pain" but readily admit the existence of severe chest "discomfort." Thus the clinician must realize the important influence of the patient's intelligence, education, and sociocultural background on the descriptive quality of precordial discomfort. Facial expressions and gestures [3] should be observed as they may provide additional diagnostic clues. The Levine sign (one or two clenched fists held by the patient over the sternal area) is much more suggestive of ischemic pain than is a pointed finger to localized discomfort in the left inframammary region [4]. Typically, the pain affects the retrosternal region, but it may involve the anterior chest wall, both shoulders or arms, the neck,

72

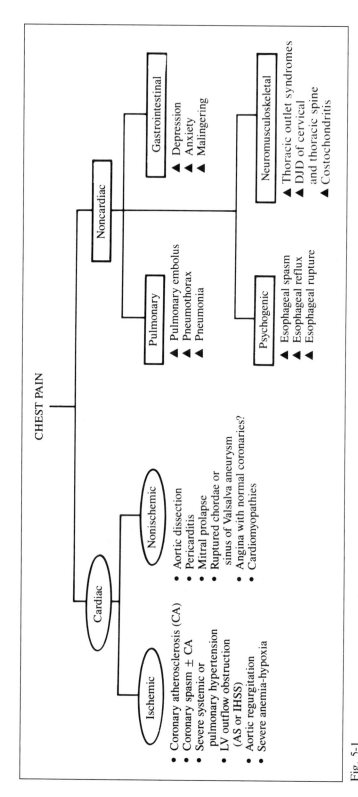

Fig. 5-1

Approach to the differential diagnosis of chest pain. AS = aortic stenosis; IHSS = idiopathic hypertrophic subaortic stenosis; DJD = degenerative joint disease. (From R. A. Walsh and R. A. O'Rourke. History and differential diagnosis of acute myocardial infarction. In J. Karliner and G. Gregoratos (eds.), *Coronary Care*. New York: Churchill Livingstone, 1981. P. 170. With permission.)

cheeks, teeth or chin, forearm or fingers, or the interscapular area. A well recognized presentation, particularly of inferior MI, is localized epigastric pain associated with a burning discomfort. Ischemic chest pain may remain localized to the chest or epigastrium, or it may radiate to one or both inner arms or the neck and jaw. Characteristically, the pain of angina pectoris is of short duration (<15 minutes), is related to exertion or emotion, and is promptly relieved by sublingual nitroglycerin. In contrast, pain associated with AMI is usually more severe, of longer duration (i.e., >30 minutes), unrelieved by nitroglycerin, and often associated with nausea, vomiting, and diaphoresis. However, it is often impossible to differentiate the pain of unstable angina from that of AMI. Patients who have suffered from angina pectoris frequently describe the pain of MI as similar in quality but of much greater intensity.

Associated findings of left ventricular (LV) dysfunction such as dyspnea and orthopnea are usually associated with large MIs. The patient who presents with a history of chest pain and syncope or presyncope presents a particularly perplexing problem for the physician. If this symptom complex is long-standing, the etiology is often functional. However, recurrent syncope associated with chest pain has been reported in the setting of symptomatic coronary disease with variant angina, and it may result from atrioventricular (AV) block due to myocardial ischemia affecting the conduction system [5, 6]. Transient, self-limited ventricular arrhythmias may also contribute to syncope in patients with AMI.

If the physician is present during an episode of rest pain, the response to various simple maneuvers may help discern the difference between ischemic and nonischemic causes of chest discomfort (Fig. 5-2). The Valsalva maneuver may relieve cardiac ischemic rest pain, presumably by a reduction of LV wall tension secondary to decreased systemic venous return during the strain phase [7]. Carotid sinus massage may also improve ischemic rest pain by decreasing myocardial oxygen demand during the reflex bradycardia. Sublingual nitroglycerin in the hypertensive or normotensive patient may provide complete or partial relief of ischemic pain. Failure to relieve chest pain by any of these three bedside maneuvers, ideally performed with ECG monitoring, suggests either a noncardiac etiology or pain secondary to AMI, rather than transient ischemia. These maneuvers should *not* be performed in patients with obvious AMI by history or ECG, in those with unstable hemodynamics, or in patients with bradycardia.

All interviews of patients with chest pain of potential ischemic etiology or with their relatives should include a careful search for the presence of known risk factors for coronary artery disease. Approximately 60 percent of patients presenting with AMI have a history of prior infarction or exertional angina [8]. A history of classic exertional angina accurately predicts arteriographic evidence of disease in 90 percent of patients. By contrast, a history of "rest" pain (pain while resting) alone that seems ischemic in origin has an accuracy of only 50 to 60 percent when correlated with angiography [9]. Established independent coronary risk factors include increasing age, male gender, cigarette smoking, diabetes, hypercholesterolemia, and hypertension. Potential risk factors include obesity, family history of premature coronary artery disease, sedentary life style, type A personality, hypertriglyceridemia, and hyperuricemia. The Framingham Study concluded that patients with the combination of increased serum cholesterol, hypertension, and a history of cigarette smoking have an incidence of coronary disease eight times that of the general population. However, some studies have suggested that as many as 40 percent of the patients presenting with AMI have no known risk factors. Thus negative information concerning risk factors may be of little value in the individual patient if the history otherwise suggests ischemic rest pain. Importantly, cardiac diseases other than fixed or vasospastic coronary artery disease may produce ischemic chest pain. For example, severe systemic or pulmonary hypertension, left ventricular outflow obstruction (e.g., aortic stenosis or hypertrophic cardiomyopathy), aortic regurgitation, hypoxia, or anemia may produce exertional chest pain, yet prolonged rest pain is uncommonly observed.

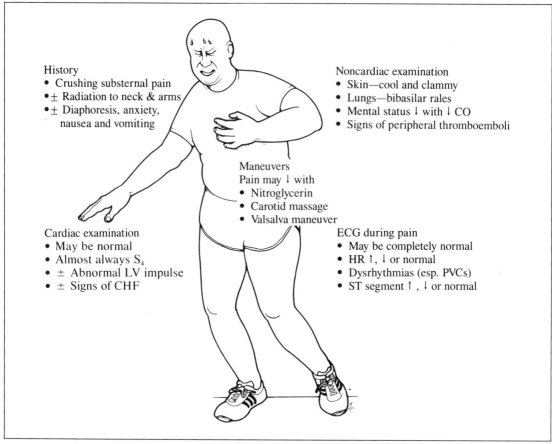

Fig. 5-2
Summary of baseline data that may be present in the typical patient with AMI.
S_4 = fourth heart sound; CHF = congestive heart failure; CO = cardiac output.
(From R. A. Walsh and R. A. O'Rourke. History and differential diagnosis of
acute myocardial infarction. In J. Karliner and G. Gregoratos (eds.), *Coronary
Care.* New York: Churchill Livingstone, 1981. P. 171 With permission.)

Atypical Presentations

Acute myocardial infarction may present as a variety of atypical syndromes that can obscure the correct diagnosis (Table 5-1). AMI must be considered in any patient presenting with pulmonary edema of unknown etiology, as severe respiratory distress may overshadow perception of chest pain. Extreme anxiety and nervousness are the predominant symptoms in certain patients, sometimes completely obscuring the chest discomfort of AMI. Syncope is occasionally the presenting symptom of and usually results from an acute episode of bradyarrhythmia or hypotension. Some patients present with profound fatigue, with or without syncope, due to severe ventricular arrhythmias or AV block. Others present with a stroke due to cerebral embolization from an LV mural thrombus. Nausea and vomiting with "indigestion" are relatively frequent symptoms due to acute inferior myocardial infarction (MI). Hypotension may accompany a "silent" infarct. Silent infarcts occur more commonly in elderly patients [10], in diabetics [11], and during surgical operations under general anesthesia. The only clue to the diagnosis in the latter setting may be the onset of pulmonary edema, ventricular arrhythmias, or hypotension unexplained by intravascular volume depletion. Infarction "without chest

Table 5-1
Atypical presentations of myocardial infarction

Nausea and vomiting alone
Atypical location of pain (e.g., arms, back, jaw,
  occiput only)
Profound fatigue of rapid onset ± syncope
Sudden onset of pulmonary edema
Cerebral or peripheral embolus
Pericarditis
Abnormal ECG in the mentally obtunded patient
  (e.g., perioperative infarct, diabetic
  ketoacidosis)
Severe ventricular dysrhythmias

Source: From R. A. Walsh and R. A. O'Rourke. History
and differential diagnosis of acute myocardial infarction. In J. Karliner and G. Gregoratos (eds.), *Coronary
Care.* New York: Churchill Livingstone, 1981. P. 174.
With permission.

pain" occurs in approximately 25 percent of
patients with myocardial infarction [11, 12].
Often the patient recalls no symptoms but has
ECG evidence of recent or remote transmural
infarction.

The mechanism of "silent" infarction in
most diabetics and nondiabetics is unknown.
In one study [8], only 4.8 percent of 250 consecutive patients with AMI had no chest pain
during the first 24 hours of observation.
However, 18 percent of the patients in the subgroup over age 60 had painless AMI. Among
elderly postinfarction patients, the prognosis
for those presenting without pain is similar to
that for those with characteristic prolonged
chest pain [12].

In elderly patients symptoms other than
pain or dyspnea frequently predominate, including confusion, syncope, stroke, vertigo,
weakness, general malaise, abdominal pain,
persistent vomiting, and even cough [10]. In
the elderly AMI patient, the sudden onset of
dyspnea often dominates the clinical picture;
chest pain is less common, and syncope is
more frequent. Infarction tends to occur at
rest and during sleep more commonly in the
elderly [13–16], and a history of prior myocardial infarction is also more common [10, 13,
14].

In patients 70 years of age or older, the
male-female ratio is nearly equal, whereas
among younger MI patients, men predominate
by 3:1 [10, 15, 16]. Among women, angina
pectoris is more likely to be the initial presentation of coronary heart disease [17]. Furthermore, women who sustain an AMI have a
more unfavorable prognosis while in hospital
[18, 19] and during 2-year follow-up [18]. In
addition, women are less responsive to cardiac
rehabilitation [19]. Because of these factors a
major goal with female patients is to detect
and aggressively treat angina pectoris in order
to prevent MI [17].

Nonischemic Causes

Nonischemic cardiac causes of chest pain at
rest (Fig. 5-1) are sometimes confused with
AMI. Most important in the differential diagnosis is acute aortic dissection. Typically, the
pain of aortic dissection occurs suddenly, with
the greatest severity at the onset of symptoms—in contrast with pain due to myocardial
ischemia, the intensity of which builds gradually with time. The pain is frequently described as excruciating, the most intense pain
ever experienced. It is also frequently described as "tearing" in quality. The pain may
radiate, depending on the location of the dissection and on the degree of luminal compression, to the neck, back, flanks, and legs. For
instance, syncope and neurologic symptoms
may occur when dissection involves the cerebral vessels. Most patients presenting with
aortic dissection have a history or clinical evidence of severe, long-standing hypertension.
Aortic dissection occurs commonly in Mar-
fan's syndrome, or idiopathic cystic medial
necrosis, and, although rare, it occurs more
frequently during pregnancy. Coronary luminal occlusion with resultant MI is a recognized complication of type I aortic dissection.

Either acute mitral regurgitation secondary
to ruptured chordae tendineae or acute aortic
regurgitation secondary to ruptured sinus of
Valsalva aneurysm may initially present with
features suggestive of AMI: a history of chest
pain and clinical findings of pulmonary or systemic venous congestion. However, the physical examination coupled with serial ECGs
and serum enzyme determinations should
readily distinguish these entities.

Acute massive pulmonary embolism with associated pulmonary hypertension and low cardiac output occasionally causes pain similar to that of AMI, as myocardial ischemia is present in both conditions. However, the associated signs of severe dyspnea, tachypnea, and intense diaphoresis associated with profound anxiety and agitation favor the diagnosis of pulmonary embolism. The clinical setting may be important because of the known association of pulmonary embolism with postpartum or postoperative states, long trips, congestive heart failure, hypercoagulable states, peripheral edema, or deep vein thrombophlebitis.

Acute pericarditis is another nonischemic cardiac cause of chest pain at rest. Although the pain is most often sharp and cutting in quality, it sometimes resembles ischemic pain. The diagnostic hallmark of pain due to pericardial disease is its aggravation by changes in body position, breathing, and occasionally swallowing. Radiation of the central precordial pain to the shoulders, upper back, and neck because of diaphragmatic pleural irritation may cause further diagnostic confusion. Because of the frequent association of acute pericarditis with MI and aortic dissection, proper diagnosis depends on careful synthesis of the history, physical, ECG, and often echocardiographic findings.

Finally, chest pain occurring as a feature of mitral valve prolapse syndrome is rarely confused with rest pain of ischemic origin because there is no exertional component to the pain, and the quality is usually atypical.

NONCARDIAC CHEST PAIN

Chest Pain of Gastrointestinal Origin
Diffuse esophageal spasm (DES) is the noncardiac condition most frequently confused with ischemic chest pain. The peak incidence is between the ages of 50 and 60 years. The pain is almost always substernal, may be squeezing or aching in quality, and frequently radiates to one or both arms. The pain may be precipitated by exercise, and many patients obtain relief with nitroglycerin or calcium channel blockers. A useful differential feature is the frequent association of DES with odynophagia (pain on swallowing), dysphagia, and regurgitation of gastric contents. The episodes of pain frequently are precipitated either by hot or cold drinks or an emotional upset. The definitive diagnosis of esophageal spasm depends on a demonstration of abnormal esophageal motility on esophagograms or by esophageal manometry.

Acute esophageal perforation may produce severe retrosternal pain secondary to chemical mediastinitis due to leakage of gastric contents. Esophageal rupture usually occurs in the setting of a prolonged bout of wretching or emesis and is a recognized complication of esophageal instrumentation. Finally, peptic ulcer disease and biliary colic are rarely confused with chest pain of cardiac origin, although the latter is relieved at times with nitroglycerin.

The patient with reflux esophagitis frequently describes indigestion or "heartburn" after meals or at bedtime while recumbent. Nocturnal or postprandial eructation and regurgitation of gastric juices are often noted by the patient. Many patients are obese and report relief of discomfort by food, antacids, or elevation of the head of the bed. The patient with significant lower esophageal sphincter incompetence may have had recurrent aspiration pneumonia, as also occurs in patients with achalasia or Zenker's diverticulum. Dysphagia may result from esophageal stricture secondary to long-standing esophageal reflux.

Chest Pain of Emotional Origin
By far the most common cause of chest discomfort is anxiety. Although anxiety can coexist with, and aggravate discomfort due to, myocardial ischemia, two features help to distinguish the two conditions. Chest pain of emotional nature is frequently sharp, left inframammary in location, and well circumscribed. Patients often use the following descriptive words: "needle-like," "knife-like," or "lightning-like." The duration of pain is helpful, as it is frequently either evanescent (seconds to 1 minute) or protracted (sometimes lasting for days). The pain is often noted

after, rather than during, activity, or it is experienced during the evening after work. The physician should actively search for indicators of underlying depression, such as a flat or saddened facial expression, retarded motor activity, and hand-wringing coupled with the history of insomnia, loss of appetite, and frequent crying spells. Associated symptoms such as air hunger, circumoral paresthesias, globus hystericus, and multiple somatic complaints suggest a psychogenic basis. Finally, many patients with mitral valve prolapse have atypical chest discomfort and often complain of chronic fatigue. A careful physical examination may disclose the presence of a midsystolic click or late systolic murmur, indicating that the atypical chest pain is part of the prolapsing mitral valve leaflet(s) syndrome.

Neuromusculoskeletal Chest Pain

Certain thoracic outlet syndromes may produce symptoms that are confused with cardiac chest pain. Compression of the neurovascular bundle by a cervical rib or the scalenus anterior muscle may cause discomfort radiating to the chest, neck, and ulnar surface of either arm. Helpful differential features from ischemic chest pain include the prominence of associated paresthesias, the lack of a clear association with exercise, and aggravation in certain body positions.

Tietze's syndrome, or idiopathic costochondritis, causes anterior chest wall pain that is aggravated by movement and deep breathing. This condition is frequently overdiagnosed because of localized tenderness to palpation of the costochondral junction; a more definitive diagnosis requires immediate relief of pain by local injection of lidocaine and salutory response to salicylates. Furthermore, demonstration of costochondral tenderness does not rule out the presence of coincident chest discomfort resulting from myocardial ischemia or infarction.

The degenerative arthritis of the cervical and thoracic vertebrae may cause band-like pain confined to the chest, neck, or back that often radiates to the arms. Radiologic evidence of degenerative disease of the cervical and thoracic vertebrae is often found in asymptomatic elderly patients. More valuable information to support the diagnosis of chest pain secondary to vertebral disease is the production or intensification of the pain by movement, sneezing, coughing, and various body positions coupled with a careful neuromusculoskeletal examination.

The prevesicular phase of herpes zoster may be characterized by band-like chest pain in a dermatomal distribution. The advanced age of the patient, the presence of hyperesthesia on physical examination, and eventual eruption of typical lesions 3 to 4 days after the onset of symptoms resolve any diagnostic dilemma.

LIMITATIONS OF THE HISTORY OF CHEST PAIN

Although a carefully acquired history is usually valuable for identifying the etiology of chest pain or for restricting the diagnostic possibilities, occasionally it is either not useful or frankly misleading. These limitations may result from the variable ability of physicians to elicit an accurate history or from the inability of the patient to clearly characterize symptoms because of intellectual, social, or cultural factors. In addition, patients often minimize symptoms for psychological (e.g., denial) or economic (e.g., job security) reasons. In contrast, other patients may magnify or manufacture symptoms to achieve disability compensation or other secondary gain. Finally, initial decisions concerning patient disposition should not be based on a normal resting ECG or on a history suggestive of angina at rest or AMI but, rather, on sound clinical judgment derived from synthesizing the information gained from the patient's history, physical examination, resting ECG, and chest x-ray (Fig. 5-2).

Physical Examination

The physical signs observed in patients during AMI are importantly determined by the temporal relation of the examination to the acute ischemic event and the presence or absence of electrical or mechanical complications. Therefore the physical findings associated with AMI are discussed in the following sequence: (1) early uncomplicated AMI; (2) early (<48 hours) complicated infarction; (3) late (>48 hours) complicated infarction; (4) often occurring noncardiac physical signs in patients with AMI [20].

EARLY UNCOMPLICATED MYOCARDIAL INFARCTION

The overall appearance of the patient presenting with AMI depends on whether pain persists and the patient's reaction to pain when it is present. Most patients do not appear markedly ill, although on close inspection they are usually quiet, fearful, and motionless. The clinical description of the pain is usually brief and is often associated with gestures toward the precordium with the hand or clenched fist. Occasionally, because of the intensity of pain or the reaction to it, the patient may appear restless and insists on walking about. Some appear to have acute indigestion, seeking relief by belching or vomiting. Finally, a few use the bedpan in an attempt to relieve the pain. Fowler [21] believed that the bedpan deaths in patients with AMI are coincidental rather than due to reflex vagal activity while straining. Autonomic dysfunction or transiently reduced LV performance may result in diaphoresis, nausea, vomiting, peripheral cyanosis, and dyspnea [21].

Vital Signs
The heart rate and blood pressure during AMI vary depending on when the patient is observed after the onset of symptoms and the extent of myocardial necrosis. Owing to use of mobile coronary care units (CCUs), patients are being seen much earlier in the course of their illness. In a study of 78 patients, Webb et al. [22] described autonomic dysfunction in 90 percent of those observed within 30 minutes from the onset of chest pain. Fifty-four percent of the patients with anterior infarcts (42

patients) had evidence of excess sympathetic tone as indicated by a heart rate of more than 100 beats per minute (bpm) and blood pressure more than 160/100 mm Hg, whereas most (77 percent) of the 44 patients with inferior or true posterior myocardial infarctions demonstrated excess parasympathetic tone (heart rate <60 bpm, systolic blood pressure <100 mm Hg, or AV block). AMI involving the inferior LV wall is often associated with transient hypotension and sinus bradycardia, which is seen in 30 percent of those examined within 30 minutes from onset of pain [23]. This response, the Bezold-Jarish reflex [24, 25], is due to chemical or mechanical stimulation [26] of inhibitory cardiac receptors, with vagal afferents and efferents located predominantly in the inferoposterior wall of the left ventricle. Hypotension is due to both parasympathetic activation and sympathetic withdrawal. In animal studies there is a reduction in arteriolar resistance as well as enhancement of venous capacitance so that both preload and afterload are reduced [27]. A third component of this reflex is nausea, vomiting, or both [28]. It is unclear whether the reflex is related to the cumulative effect of ischemia, giving rise to bulging of the affected myocardium during systole stimulating the mechanoreceptors [29], or reperfusion itself is the causative factor [30]. The Bezold-Jarish reflex may be manifest in a variety of other clinical situations, such as during thrombolytic therapy of AMI and resultant reperfusion [30], coronary angiography [31], and aortic stenosis syncope [32]. In addition, digitalis and nitroglycerin appear to facilitate the reflex directly or indirectly. Because hypotension and bradycardia should lessen myocardial oxygen demand the reflex may be beneficial for myocardial infarction. It has also been postulated to limit ischemia during episodes of variant angina [33]. In areas where mobile emergency CCUs are unavailable, the time between onset of symptoms and admission to the CCU is greater and the influence of autonomic imbalance on the initial physical signs is less. In such patients, the blood pressure and heart rate are more related to the size of the infarct, the presence of arrhythmias, and the existence of prior cardiovascular disease.

The patient is usually afebrile during the first 24 hours of acute infarction. Slight temperature elevation is common during the first week; it does not usually exceed 101°F, although with large infarctions it may reach 103°F. The fever due to myocardial necrosis must be differentiated from that due to other common causes of hyperthermia noted in the CCU setting, such as postcardiac arrest aspiration pneumonia, pyelonephritis from indwelling Foley catheters, thrombophlebitis, bacteremia from indwelling arterial or venous lines, pulmonary emboli, or pericarditis. The effect of elevated body temperature during infarct evolution is clinically important, as it increases the heart rate, cardiac workload, metabolic rate, and overall oxygen consumption. In a prospective, randomized, double-blind, controlled multicenter study to assess the effect of timolol treatment on infarct size, Risoe and collaborators [34] also studied the relation between increase in body temperatures and vectorcardiographic and enzymatic indices of ischemic injury. Maximal and mean temperatures obtained during the first 8 days were significantly lower in 33 patients randomized to beta-adrenergic blockade with timolol than those in the placebo group. In addition, mean and maximal body temperatures correlated significantly with a reduction in estimated infarct size. Thus early administration of beta blockers significantly reduced the response to pyrexia and appeared beneficial in reducing infarct extension. Further studies are required to confirm these results.

Precordial Palpation

In certain patients with AMI, the systolic apical impulse may be diffuse, sustained, or frankly dyskinetic. However, it may be difficult to distinguish a prominent apical impulse owing to abnormal wall motion in AMI from the sustained systolic impulse of LV pressure overload when coincident hypertension is present. In addition, a palpable LV presystolic filling wave (A wave) is often present that corresponds in timing to an audible fourth heart sound. Less frequently, an early LV diastolic rapid filling wave is palpated that is associated with an audible third heart sound. Lastly, patients with large transmural anterior infarcts often have transient early, mid, or late systolic impulses that are palpable medial and superior to the maximal impulse. Persistence of such dyskinetic areas for more than 8 weeks post MI may indicate the presence of an anteroapical aneurysm.

Jugular Venous Pulse

The jugular venous pulse (JVP) contour and pressure are usually normal in patients with early uncomplicated infarct (Fig. 5-3), except in the presence of cardiopulmonary disease or associated right ventricular infarction (see below). However, because the JVP reflects the atrial pressure, inspection of its contour may reveal the presence and nature of atrial or ventricular arrhythmias. For example, with some rhythm disorders, atrial systole (ECG p wave) may occur during ventricular systole (ECG Q–T interval) and produce cannon A waves because of right atrial contraction against a closed tricuspid valve. Cannon A waves may also be observed during ventricular tachycardia when there is AV dissociation or with premature ventricular beats [35].

The intensity of the first heart sound is diminished in approximately one-fourth of patients with AMI [21] (Fig. 5-3) and may be due to the presence of first-degree AV block or decreased LV dP/dt in patients with large infarcts. Paradoxical or reversed splitting of the second heart sound occurs during AMI or reversible ischemia [36]. The two possible mechanisms are transient LV conduction abnormalities and prolongation of electromechanical systole by ischemia or infarction. In our experience, reversed splitting of the second heart sound is rarely observed in ischemic heart disease in the absence of left bundle branch block. The true incidence of this auscultatory finding is unknown, and a frequent reason for misdiagnosis of reverse splitting is the disappearance of the pulmonic component of the second heart sound during inspiration in patients with chronic pulmonary disease and increased anteroposterior chest diameters.

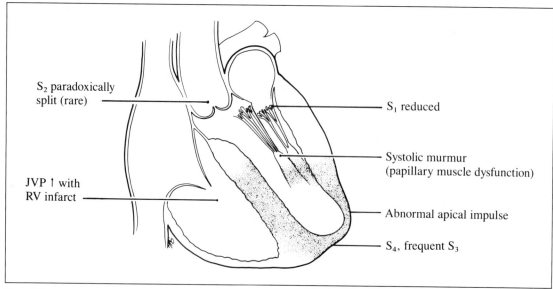

Fig. 5-3
Cardiac physical findings that may be present in uncomplicated AMI. S_1, S_2, S_3,
S_4 = first through fourth heart sounds, respectively; JVP = increase in jugular
venous pressure; RV = right ventricle. Right ventricular infarction is included to
indicate that it is a specific entity, even though it more commonly occurs in
patients with a complicated left ventricular infarction. (From R. A. Walsh and
R. A. O'Rourke. History and differential diagnosis of acute myocardial infarction.
In J. Karliner and G. Gregoratos (eds.), *Coronary Care*. New York: Churchill
Livingstone, 1981. P. 179. With permission.)

Left Ventricular Diastolic Gallop Sounds

Left ventricular diastolic gallop sounds are
frequently present during transient ischemia
or AMI (Fig. 5-3). These low-pitched sounds
are best heard with the bell of the stethoscope
lightly applied to the LV apex with the patient
turned to the left lateral decubitus position.
Right ventricular (RV) diastolic gallops may
be auscultated in the same manner; they are
loudest at the left sternal border or subxiphoid
area and frequently increase in intensity with
inspiration. In one study [37], the fourth heart
sound (S_4) was documented in 98 percent of
107 patients evaluated during the first 24 hours
after AMI by serial auscultation, phonocardiograms, and simultaneous apexcardiograms.
The S_4 is most likely due to reduced ventricular compliance resulting from ischemia or infarction. Thus the absence of the S_4 on careful
auscultation in a patient in sinus rhythm
makes the diagnosis of AMI less likely. Auscultation may be difficult, however, especially
in obese patients and in those with chronic air-

flow limitation; thus an S_4 may not be detected
despite acute infarction and sinus rhythm.

The third heart sound (S_3) frequently indicates heart failure and likely results from an
imbalance between the volume of LV inflow
during the rapid filling phase of diastole and
the ability of the ventricle to accommodate
this increment in volume flow. The S_3 is somewhat less common than the S_4 in AMI. Riley
and coworkers [38] noted the presence of an
S_3 in 40 percent of 156 patients at the time of
admission for AMI. The presence of S_3 was
predictive of an elevated pulmonary artery diastolic pressure or LV end-diastolic pressure
in 25 of 27 patients. However, a substantial
number of patients with elevated left-sided
filling pressures had no audible S_3. The prognostic importance was that patients with anterior AMI and S_3 had twice the mortality of
patients with anterior infarctions and no S_3 on
admission. The incidence of S_3 at the time of
initial examination in patients with AMI was
higher (65 percent) in another study [37],

in which serial phonocardiograms were performed in addition to auscultation. However, most (60 percent) of these S_3 sounds disappeared during the initial 3 days of hospitalization. Several techniques are available to accentuate an S_3 or S_4: (1) having the patient cough several times causes a transient rise in pulmonary venous pressure and a slight increase in heart rate; and (2) auscultation over the subclavian and carotid arteries may detect transmitted LV diastolic filling sounds in certain patients in whom precordial auscultation is limited by obesity, increased anteroposterior chest diameter, or respiratory sounds such as wheezing [39]. Up to 50 percent of left-sided fourth heart sounds (S_4) and 25 percent of third heart sounds (S_3) can be detected over the systemic arteries.

EARLY COMPLICATIONS OF MYOCARDIAL INFARCTION

The goals of CCU management during AMI include the prevention or prompt and effective treatment of cardiac arrhythmias and the early detection of surgically correctable (Fig. 5-4) mechanical complications. CCUs and continuous ECG monitoring have reduced considerably the mortality due to arrhythmic consequences of myocardial ischemia and infarction. Mechanical complications are now the most common cause of death in patients with AMI or recent MI. The availability of new inotropic agents, external and internal circulatory assist devices, and improved surgical techniques should encourage the early identification of these complications. Careful attention to the physical findings may provide the first clue to their presence.

Right and Left Ventricular Infarction

Right ventricular infarction associated with LV infarction has emerged as a distinct clinical entity (see Chapters 13, 16). The clinical hallmarks of predominant RV infarction must be promptly recognized in order to institute rapidly appropriate therapy. Studies using hemodynamic measurements and cardiac radionuclide imaging suggest that significant RV

Fig. 5-4
Summary of cardiac examination of a patient with complicated myocardial infarction. CHF = congestive heart failure; EM = electromechanical; VSD = ventriculoseptal defect. (From R. A. Walsh and R. A. O'Rourke. History and differential diagnosis of acute myocardial infarction. In J. Karliner and G. Gregoratos (eds.), *Coronary Care*. New York: Churchill Livingstone, 1981. P. 182. With permission.)

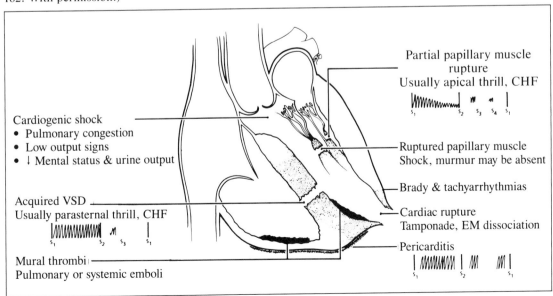

Partial papillary muscle rupture
Usually apical thrill, CHF

Ruptured papillary muscle
Shock, murmur may be absent

Brady & tachyarrhythmias

Cardiac rupture
Tamponade, EM dissociation

Pericarditis

Cardiogenic shock
• Pulmonary congestion
• Low output signs
• ↓ Mental status & urine output

Acquired VSD
Usually parasternal thrill, CHF

Mural thrombi
Pulmonary or systemic emboli

involvement may be present in as many as one-third of the patients presenting with inferior transmural AMI [40–43]. The physical examination may be of importance for ruling out significant RV involvement in patients with inferior AMI. Table 5-2 lists the physical examination findings that have been described in patients with RV infarction. Dell'Italia and colleagues [44] prospectively assessed whether the characteristic physical findings described in Table 5-2 could identify patients with and without RV infarction confirmed subsequently by hemodynamic measurements. The combination of physical findings listed in Table 5-2 was insensitive (25 percent) but was specific (96 percent) for RV infarction. In contrast, Kussmaul's sign (an increase in or failure to decrease the jugular venous pressure on inspiration) was observed clinically in all eight patients with hemodynamic evidence of RV infarction (group 1) and in none of the 45 patients (group II) with inferior MI and no hemodynamic evidence of RV involvement. Also, the combination of an elevated jugular venous pressure ($\geq$8 cm H_2O) and Kussmaul's sign was both sensitive (88 percent) and specific (100 percent) for identifying patients with hemodynamic evidence of RV infarction (Table 5-3).

A wide spectrum of hemodynamic findings have been described in patients with AMI involving the right ventricle [45]. This spectrum may range from patients in shock with markedly elevated and equalized ventricular filling pressures to patients with minimal RV dysfunction who may require volume loading to identify hemodynamics consistent with RV infarction. The hemodynamic parameters associated with significant RV infarction have been reported by Lopez-Sendon and coworkers [46].

In order to make the diagnosis of predominant RV infarction, the clinical and hemodynamic manifestations should be considered in conjunction with radionuclide assessment. An RV regional wall motion abnormality alone or in combination with an RV ejection fraction of less than 40 percent is a useful criterion for establishing the presence of hemodynamically significant RV infarction [47]. Echocardiogra-

Table 5-2
Clinical findings associated with RV infarction

Hypotension
Elevated jugular venous pressure
Kussmaul's sign
Abnormal jugular venous pressure pattern (y $\geq$ x descent)
Tricuspid regurgitation
Right-sided S_3 and S_4
Pulsus paradoxus
High-grade AV block

Source: From L. J. Dell'Italia and M. R. Starling. Right ventricular infarction: An important clinical entity. *Curr. Probl. Cardiol.* 9(9):16, 1984. With permission.

phy is useful for assessing RV cavity function and size, but most importantly it should be used to exclude cardiac tamponade as an alternative cause of equalized right and left heart filling pressure. One must also exclude pulmonary embolism and constrictive and restrictive cardiomyopathy by appropriate tests.

In summary, a careful history and physical examination can be important guides to initial therapy, as the presence of an elevated jugular venous pressure and Kussmaul's sign are strong evidence for the diagnosis of hemodynamically important RV infarction.

Left Ventricular Decompensation
The development of CCUs has resulted in a marked decline of deaths primarily attributable to cardiac arrhythmias, whereas LV failure has emerged as the prime factor responsible for most in-hospital deaths following AMI. Despite advances in coronary care, the incidence and mortality associated with cardiogenic shock are virtually unchanged. Cardiogenic shock is the most severe form of LV dysfunction secondary to acute infarction and occurs in 10 to 20 percent of patients with AMI (see Chapter 16). Cardiogenic shock is defined as a clinical syndrome in which the systolic blood pressure is 90 mm Hg or less and there is evidence of inadequate tissue perfusion manifested by cool, clammy skin, cyanosis, mental impairment, or oliguria. The physical findings are usually consistent with severe dysfunction, e.g., hypotension, diastolic gallops (S_3 and S_4), a laterally displaced

Table 5-3
Sensitivity and specificity of physical findings for hemodynamically important RV infarction in 53 patients

Parameter	Elevated JVP*	Kussmaul's sign	Elevated JVP and systemic blood pressure		
			Clear lungs	<100 mm Hg and clear lungs	Kussmaul's sign
Sensitivity (%)	88	100	50	25	88
Specificity (%)	69	100	82	96	100

*Jugular venous pressure: ⩾8 cm H₂O.
Source: From L. J. Dell'Italia et al. Physical examination of hemodynamically important right ventricular infarction. *Ann. Intern. Med.* 99:608, 1983. With permission.

and frequently dyskinetic apical impulse, and signs of pulmonary congestion. In patients with hypertensive disease, cardiogenic shock is defined as a drop in systolic blood pressure by at least 25 percent below prior levels accompanied by reflex-mediated signs of systemic arterial hypoperfusion. Clinical observations have failed to predict which patients will experience cardiogenic shock [48], but extension of the original infarction or necrosis of new areas of myocardium, regardless of whether clinically recognized, gradually reduces the amount of functioning muscle.

Two basic methods of classification have been used to describe the degree of LV failure in patients during AMI. Killip and Kimball used the initial clinical presentation to categorize MI patients into four subgroups: class 1—no pulmonary rales or S₃; class II—bibasilar rales that persist after coughing or S₃; class III—rales over one-half of the lung fields bilaterally with radiographic evidence for pulmonary edema; and class IV—cardiogenic shock. The 2-year mortality rates associated with this classification are 8, 30, 44, and 80 to 100 percent for classes I to IV, respectively [48].

Meanwhile, Forrester and coworkers [49] developed a classification that relates the clinical presentation to specific determinants of LV pump performance. Clinical subsets were defined by the manifestation of pulmonary congestion (reflecting increased pulmonary capillary pressure) and peripheral hypoperfusion (reflecting a decreased cardiac index). On the basis of these findings, four clinical subsets were defined (see Table 13-1). Further-

more, four comparable hemodynamic subsets were established using a pulmonary capillary wedge pressure (PCW) of more than 18 mm Hg as an index of increased pulmonary-capillary pressure and a cardiac index of less than 2.2 L/min/m² as an index of peripheral hypoperfusion. In this study, the clinical criteria were shown to predict the hemodynamic subset correctly in approximately 70 percent of the cases. Thus limitations exist in the clinical prediction of the hemodynamic profile. One-fourth of the patients designated clinically as not having hypoperfusion have a cardiac index of less than 2.2 L/min/m². Another important clinical limitation is the failure to recognize elevation of the pulmonary-capillary pressure (>18 mm Hg), which occurs in about 15 percent of patients. Thus in terms of LV dysfunction during AMI, the physical examination may be misleading [50]. For instance, a phase lag of as much as 48 hours may exist between invasively determined hemodynamic stabilization (PCW decreasing to normal) and the resolution of abnormal physical and radiologic signs [51]. Also, at times the differentiation of rales heard on auscultation during AMI may require hemodynamic evaluation for further assessment, especially in patients with chronic airflow limitation. However, certain clinical maneuvers may help differentiate cardiac from pulmonary rales. Cardiac rales occur as a result of transudation of fluid into pulmonary interstitial or interalveolar space secondary to the elevation of pulmonary venous pressure produced by ischemic LV dysfunction. The postural nature of these cardiac rales may be diagnosed by placing the patient on one side for 30 minutes and noting the increase in rales in the dependent lung fields. In contrast, rales of purely pulmonary origin frequently clear during coughing and are independent of posture.

A bedside clue to the presence of LV dysfunction, commonly severe, is the presence of *pulsus alternans*—an alternation in the amplitude of the arterial pulse on every other beat in the presence of regular sinus rhythm. In patients with LV failure, pulsus alternans is often present transiently after premature beats, although it may be sustained. It is best appreciated in the peripheral arterial pulses (e.g., radial or femoral) where the pulse pressure is usually greater than central pulses (e.g., carotids). The mechanism of pulsus alternans remains controversial. This phenomenon may be partially related to alternating end-diastolic volumes and result in alternation of the force of ventricular contraction (e.g., a Starling effect). Most evidence indicates an alternating failure or attenuation of electromechanical coupling due to diminished internal myocardial calcium stores, as the phenomenon may be produced in isolated cardiac muscle.

Pericarditis Following AMI

A pericardial friction rub associated with post-infarct pericarditis is detected clinically in 10 to 15 percent of patients (see Chapter 17). Yet at autopsy almost all patients with acute MI are found to have evidence of localized fibrinous pericarditis overlying the infarction. A characteristic history is obtained in approximately one-half of the patients with evidence of pericarditis. The pericardial rub usually develops during the first 4 days of hospitalization and most often occurs with large infarcts. The pericardial rub is best heard by applying firm pressure with the diaphragm of the stethoscope over the precordium while the patient is sitting up and leaning forward. The rub is influenced by respiratory variation and may be accentuated by having the patient either inhale or exhale maximally. The pericardial rub is characteristically leathery, scratching, or crunching in quality and may have three components. One component occurs during early

diastole at the time of rapid passive filling; another occurs during late diastole at the time of atrial contraction; and the third occurs during ventricular systole. A single systolic component heard near the apex may be confused with a murmur of mitral regurgitation due to papillary muscle dysfunction or rupture. Any or all of these components of a pericardial rub may be absent at various times. The hallmark of the pericardial rub associated with AMI is its evanescence. Thus serial auscultatory evaluation of patients in various positions in a quiet room is important for its detection. Postinfarction pericarditis must be differentiated from acute pulmonary embolism, peptic ulcer disease, and especially recurrent myocardial ischemia or infarction. Lastly, the appearance of a new friction rub more than 10 days after acute infarction probably represents Dressler's syndrome.

LATE COMPLICATIONS OF AMI

Cardiac Rupture

Rupture of the free wall of the heart is one of the most dreaded complications of AMI because the patient rarely survives. The incidence of cardiac rupture has been reported in approximately 10 percent of fatal cases of AMI [54–56], and it is listed third as a cause of death, after cardiogenic shock and cardiac arrhythmias (see Chapters 4, 16). The clinical profile associated with an increased risk for cardiac rupture is the elderly (80 years or older) hypertensive woman presenting with a first AMI that is usually complicated by recurrent chest pain without ECG changes suggestive of another infarct or extension [57]. Cardiac rupture usually occurs within the first postinfarct week and rarely after the second week.

The clinical symptoms and signs suggesting cardiac rupture may be categorized into three major patterns. The most common presentation is prolonged, recurring chest pain during the initial postinfarct week followed by an abrupt onset of dyspnea associated with hypotension and jugular neck vein distention that rapidly deteriorates to electromechanical dissociation (EMD) and death. EMD refers to a sudden loss of consciousness, not preceded by symptoms of respiratory failure or cardiac arrhythmias, associated with sinus rhythm on ECG without a palpable pulse or audible heart sounds. The prognosis of this underlying rhythm is poor [58], yet one must exclude other etiologies associated with EMD that may be reversible (i.e., severe hypovolemia and shock, cardiac tamponade, and pulmonary embolism). Failure to produce peripheral pulses during closed-chest resuscitation is also viewed as a terminal sign of cardiac rupture.

Less commonly, patients present with a more gradual onset of symptoms suggesting cardiac tamponade. These patients develop distended neck veins, tachycardia, systemic hypotension, and pulsus paradoxus. Pulsus paradoxus is an accentuation of the usual inspiratory decline in systolic arterial pressure, which is normally less than 10 mm Hg. It is best determined using the cuff sphygmomanometer during normal respiration and noting, first, the arterial pressure at which Korotkoff sounds are heard only with expiration and, second, the lower arterial pressure at which the sounds are heard during both inspiration and expiration. When the pulsus is more than 20 mm Hg, there is usually a palpable diminution in the peripheral arterial pulses during inspiration. Pulsus paradoxus may not be evident despite cardiac tamponade in the presence of profound systemic hypotension. It is important to recall that pulsus paradoxus may occur in patients with acute or chronic respiratory distress, hypovolemic shock, and massive pulmonary embolism as well as in intubated patients undergoing positive-pressure ventilation.

The final presentation of cardiac rupture occurs with formation of an LV pseudoaneurysm (see Chapter 4). The LV pseudoaneurysm represents a partially contained cardiac rupture that is usually connected to the left ventricle through a narrow neck. The to-and-fro movement of blood through the neck may produce systolic or diastolic murmurs. Rupture of false aneurysms (early or late) usually results in a rapidly accumulating hemopericardium and sudden, unexpected death. Cross-sectional (two-dimensional) echocardiography and radionuclide blood pool scans are valuable noninvasive techniques for confirming the diagnosis of ventricular pseudoaneurysm [59–62]. The presence of a pseudoaneurysm is an indication for early surgery because of the eminent risk of rupture and death.

Mitral Regurgitation

The development of a new systolic murmur during AMI is a common occurrence. Heikkila [63] described apical systolic murmurs consistent with mitral regurgitation (MR) in 55 percent of the patients admitted to hospital for AMI. In most of this group the MR was not hemodynamically significant, as judged by the absence of congestive heart failure and a stable clinical course. However, determination of the hemodynamic significance of a new systolic murmur in patients with congestive heart failure or shock becomes mandatory. Such a murmur may represent the acute development of a papillary muscle rupture or a ventricular septal rupture, two potentially serious but surgically correctable mechanical complications. In other cases, the murmur may indicate papillary muscle dysfunction due to papillary muscle ischemia or necrosis or spatial derangement of the papillary muscle or chordae tendineae system.

Papillary Muscle Dysfunction

The most commonly heard murmur following AMI is that of papillary muscle dysfunction. Burch and colleagues [64–66] were the first to recognize and describe the clinical manifestations of ischemic papillary muscle dysfunction. MR secondary to myocardial infarction reflects loss of the structural or functional integrity of the papillary muscle apparatus (see Chapters 4, 16). The function of the papillary muscle is to prevent retroversion of the mitral valve leaflets into the left atrium during systole. Inadequate papillary muscle contraction causes decreased chordae tension and allows retroversion of the mitral leaflets into the left atrium, often resulting in MR.

The posteromedial papillary muscle is more prone to ischemic injury than the anterolateral papillary muscle because of its single blood supply. Although the systolic murmur of papillary muscle dysfunction in AMI appears transient in most cases, its presence was associated with more mortality despite small infarct size in one study [67].

The murmur of papillary muscle dysfunction was originally described as "ejection" in type, with the first sound followed by a silent period that corresponds to isovolumic contraction. Subsequently, as the LV dimension diminished, the MR likely increased in severity as did the intensity of the murmur. Nevertheless, in many studies, the murmur of MR has been described as holosystolic and generally heard best at the apex. Radiation of the murmur toward the sternum or the aortic area often occurs in disorders affecting predominantly the posterior mitral leaflet. The murmur in this case may be confused with the murmur of ventricular septal defect or aortic stenosis. With predominant anterior leaflet involvement, the murmur often radiates to the back—to the thoracic and cervical spine. The murmur of MR shows little change in intensity despite the presence of large variations in LV stroke volume such as occurs with atrial fibrillation and with the systole after a premature ventricular beat [68]. By contrast, most mid-systolic murmurs, such as occur with aortic stenosis, increase in intensity during the cycle following a long diastole, because LV filling after a long R–R interval results in a greater contractile force and an increased gradient across the aortic valve. In the case of MR, the increased LV end-diastolic volume is partially dissipated during early systole by regurgitation into the left atrium. Also, the reduced aortic pressure resulting from the long diastolic period reduces the impedance of LV ejection; therefore the amount of MR may actually be decreased during the mid to later parts of systole. The murmur of MR varies little with respiration, being slightly louder during held expiration. However, with sudden standing and amyl nitrite inhalation the murmur decreases in intensity, whereas squatting or intravenous phenylephrine administration increases its loudness.

In an attempt to improve the identification of left-sided regurgitant murmurs, Lembo and coworkers [69] evaluated the effectiveness of transient arterial occlusion of both arms using blood pressure cuffs inflated to 20 to 40 mm Hg above systolic pressure for 20 seconds; they then compared their results to those obtained with isometric handgrip exercise, squatting, and amyl nitrite inhalation. They found transient arterial occlusion, which increases LV afterload; therefore increasing the intensity of left-sided murmurs was superior to squatting and did not differ from isometric handgrip exercise and amyl nitrite inhalation. This bedside maneuver can be done quickly and easily on all patients without any limitations or contraindications as described for the other standard techniques [70–74].

Papillary Muscle Rupture

Papillary muscle rupture occurs in 0.4 to 5.0 percent of patients dying with AMI [75–76]. Such rupture (see Chapters 4, 16) is 2.5 times as frequent in patients with inferior wall MI as in those with anterior wall infarction. Most patients developing cardiogenic shock secondary to papillary muscle rupture have less than 25 percent involvement of the LV myocardium at autopsy. Papillary muscle rupture usually occurs 2 to 4 days after the initial MI and is often associated with severe chest pain, shortness of breath, and a loud systolic murmur. However, the murmur of papillary muscle rupture may be unimpressive because of equalization of reduced LV pressure and elevated left atrial (LA) pressure early in systole, resulting from severe MR coupled with marked LV dysfunction. In fact, the velocity rather than the volume of mitral regurgitant flow determines the intensity of the murmur of MR [77]. Because diminished ventricular function is commonly found in the presence of myocardial ischemia, it is not surprising that many holosystolic murmurs are of low intensity even in the presence of considerable MR [78]. The clinical presentation is usually associated with intractable pulmonary edema and shock.

A second clinical manifestation may occur as a consequence of partial rupture of the papillary muscle or rupture of the head of a papillary muscle. The systolic murmur may have the characteristics that are observed with acute MR of any etiology. The murmur is usually holosystolic with decreasing intensity during late systole due to equilibration of LV and LA pressures at the time of the left atrial V wave. Other physical signs include the following: (1) A systolic parasternal lift may be detected at the lower left sternal border. If early and sustained, it may result from a right ventricular impulse due to severe pulmonary hypertension. If it is late and more dynamic, the parasternal lift may be secondary to distention of a noncompliant left atrium by the regurgitant jet. It corresponds in timing with a large left atrial V wave at cardiac catheterization. (2) Systolic thrills are rare, but if present they are usually felt at the apex. (3) A fourth heart sound is commonly heard with acute MR. It is usually ascribed to left atrial "overload" associated with diminished ventricular distensibility.

Ventricular Septal Rupture

Ventricular septal rupture [79–81], a rare complication, is found in 0.5 to 1.0 percent of cases of myocardial infarction. It generally occurs 2 to 3 days after the AMI (see Chapters 4, 16). In fact, the clinical presentation, time course, and auscultatory findings are similar to those in patients with papillary muscle rupture. If no acute surgical correction is undertaken, most patients die within a week. In contrast to congenital ventricular septal defects (VSD), acquired VSD always involves the muscular part of the ventricular septum and not the membranous septum. Associated ventricular aneurysm is present in one-half of the cases. Acquired VSD is more commonly associated with anterior MI, and the ECG frequently shows a right bundle branch block or conduction abnormalities. The systolic murmur is often accompanied by a thrill, which is maximal at the lower left sternal border. The thrill may be absent owing to severely impaired LV function or the large size of the regurgitant orifice or septal defect. Axillary transmission of the murmur is distinctly uncommon with VSD.

Mural Thrombi

Autopsy studies have shown that endocardial mural thrombosis is a frequent finding in patients dying of myocardial infarction [82–85]. Mural thrombi (see Chapters 4, 16) are fre-

quently recognized in patients with extensive anterior transmural infarction involving the left ventricle, especially in the presence of severe wall motion abnormalities involving the apex.

Clinically, the detection of mural thrombi is difficult without the help of ancillary tests, particularly two-dimensional echocardiography [86–90] (see Chapters 4, 16). Some patients are admitted initially to a neurology service because of a cerebrovascular accident. The presence of a recent, otherwise silent myocardial infarct may be evident only from the admission ECG. Other patients develop evidence for sudden arterial insufficiency in one or both lower extremities. The hallmark of arterial as opposed to venous insufficiency is the sudden onset of a cold extremity or digit associated with the "five Ps": pulselessness, pallor, paresthesias, pain, and paralysis [91]. While performing the physical examination one should search for evidence of an LV aneurysm. It can be recognized in some patients by the presence of an abnormal systolic impulse, medial and superior to the cardiac impulse. One may be able to determine if there is a prolonged systolic expansile pulsation at the site of this impulse. This persistent abnormal impulse must be distinguished from the occasional similar impulse found with acute infarction without aneurysm. The latter usually disappears within a few weeks. Patients with an LV aneurysm commonly have a ventricular gallop rhythm. Frequently there is a murmur of MR, which may be related in part to papillary muscle dysfunction.

IMPORTANT NONCARDIAC PHYSICAL FINDINGS IN THE POSTINFARCT PATIENT

Careful serial physical examinations are mandatory in the post-MI patient because of various noncardiac problems that may arise during the peri-infarct period (Fig. 5-5). At present, pulmonary embolism occurs much less frequently after AMI because of earlier mobilization of the patient, but it must be considered in the differential diagnosis of chest pain in the CCU. The most common auscultatory finding in patients with documented

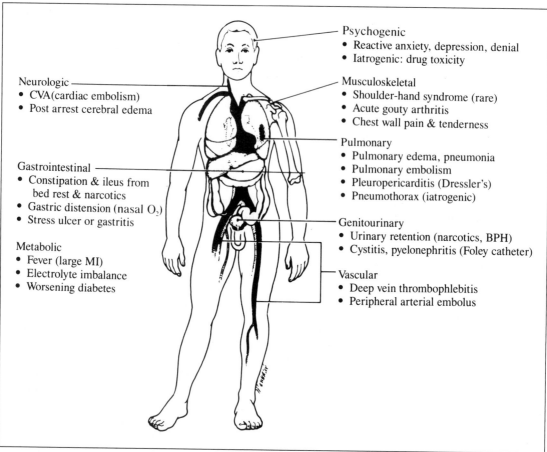

Fig. 5-5
Summary of important noncardiac physical findings that may develop during the peri-infarction period. CVA = cerebrovascular accident; MI = myocardial infarction; BPH = benign prostatic hypertrophy. (From R. A. Walsh and R. A. O'Rourke. History and differential diagnosis of acute myocardial infarction. In J. Karliner and G. Gregoratos (eds.), *Coronary Care*. New York: Churchill Livingstone, 1981. P. 186. With permission.)

pulmonary embolism is nonspecific atelectatic rales. Rarely, dullness to percussion at one or both lung bases due to pleural effusion is present in patients with pulmonary infarction. A pleural rub may be heard in this setting or with Dressler's syndrome (see Chapter 20). Nevertheless, the physical examination in the diagnosis of pulmonary embolism or infarction is much less helpful than are more specific laboratory tests, such as ventilation-perfusion lung scans, impedance plethysmography, and arterial blood gas determinations. The diagnosis of pulmonary embolism should be con-

sidered in any patient who has chest pain with associated tachypnea, tachycardia, or fever in the intensive care unit setting. It is of note that pulmonary infarction is a recognized complication of indwelling right heart balloon flotation catheters, particularly if the balloon has been inflated or the catheter has been in place for more than 72 hours [92]. Unilateral diminished or absent breath sounds may be the first clue to the presence of a pneumothorax produced by insertion of a subclavian venous line.

Gastrointestinal discomfort is common in

patients hospitalized in the CCU and may arise from multiple causes: (1) gastric distention from nasal oxygen administration; (2) improper endotracheal intubation (left upper quadrant tympany to percussion); (3) constipation and ileus due to bed rest and narcotic analgesics (decreased bowel sounds and fecal masses on abdominal palpation); (4) activation of peptic ulcer disease from stress or thrombolytic therapy; or (5) aggravation of esophageal reflux by recumbency (evidence of pyrosis, epigastric tenderness to palpation, and response to antacids).

Alterations in mental status are common in patients hospitalized in the CCU. Reactive anxiety, depression, denial, and hostility are frequent products of the psychogenic stress associated with AMI. These findings must be distinguished from iatrogenically induced mental status changes produced by drugs (e.g., lidocaine-induced hallucinations or seizures, digitalis toxicity, and paradoxical agitation from sedatives or hypnotics in the elderly). Focal neurologic symptoms may arise at any time during the peri-infarction period as a result of decreased cerebral perfusion from low cardiac output in patients with intrinsic cerebrovascular disease or from systemic embolization of a mural thrombus. At times, a reduction in mental alertness is the first sign of deteriorating LV function. Finally, patients who have been resuscitated successfully often have transient or global neurologic findings due to postarrest cerebral anoxia.

The clinical diagnosis of deep vein thrombosis (DVT) has a low specificity and sensitivity and is therefore inaccurate. Studies have shown that most patients who present with symptoms and signs of acute DVT (i.e., pain and tenderness, swelling, redness, palpable cord) do not have this condition confirmed when they are investigated by objective testing. The exception is the patient with clinical features typical of phlegmasia cerulea dolens, which is always caused by extensive iliofemoral thrombosis. Conversely, other patients may have extensive DVT and few clinical manifestations. Therefore management decisions in patients suspected of having DVT must always rely on objective testing. Objec-

tive tests for the diagnosis of DVT include (1) contrast venography; (2) impedance plethysmography, a noninvasive cost-effective technique highly sensitive and specific (95 percent) for detection of proximal DVT; (3) ^{125}I-fibrinogen leg scanning, a test that is highly sensitive (95 percent) for detection of calf DVT in patients who have had symptoms for fewer than 8 days; and (4) Doppler ultrasound, a useful tool to detect proximal DVT (cumulative sensitivity and specificity of approximately 90 percent).

With the advent of thrombolytic therapy (see Chapters 24, 25), bleeding has become the major and most serious noncardiac complication of MI. In general, gastrointestinal bleeding and bleeding at the arterial puncture sites are the most frequent complications. Intracranial, retroperitoneal, or other major bleeding episodes requiring transfusion occur in 0.4 to 2.0 percent of patients undergoing thrombolytic treatment for pulmonary embolism, deep venous thrombosis, or peripheral arterial occlusion. Less-major bleeding disorders include puncture site hematomas, ecchymoses, nosebleeds, purpura, and hematuria. The best approach to the hemorrhagic problem associated with thrombolytic therapy remains proper patient selection.

The most specific of the musculoskeletal complications of myocardial infarction, the shoulder-hand syndrome, is largely of historic interest and has rarely occurred since early mobilization of the infarction patient became commonplace therapy. However, a nonspecific "chest wall syndrome" has been noted in many patients with large infarcts. This poorly understood phenomenon is characterized by generalized tenderness over the left precordium and poorly characterized chest pain lasting seconds to days. The usual clinical manifestations associated with acute gouty arthritis and pseudogout may be precipitated by dehydration, medications, and stress experienced following myocardial infarction.

Genitourinary problems may be encountered because of drug administration or bladder instrumentation. Urinary retention in the elderly male patient with benign prostatic hypertrophy is frequently precipitated by narcotic analgesics. Careful suprapubic palpation and percussion may disclose a distended bladder in the patient with a "low" urine output. Cystitis and pyelonephritis are recognized complications of chronic indwelling Foley catheters. Suprapubic tenderness and costovertebral angle tenderness are helpful physical signs that should be elicited if an upper urinary tract infection is suspected.

Finally, metabolic complications are frequent and may be a spontaneous result of the physiologic stress of myocardial infarction or iatrogenically induced. For instance, polydipsia and polyuria may be the first clues to an aggravation of latent or previously controlled diabetes; leg cramps may be the first clue to the presence of diuretic-induced hypokalemia; and changes in mental status may indicate the presence of diuretic-induced hyponatremia.

Editorial Comments

In some patients with substantial mitral regurgitation, the systolic murmur is either soft or frankly inaudible. This situation may be the result of poor LV systolic function, obesity or a thick chest wall, or pulmonary disease. The clinician should not hesitate to perform a bedside echocardiographic Doppler study in the CCU in patients with unexplained or unexpected signs of LV failure in order to search for silent or near-silent mitral regurgitation. J.S.A.

References

1. Walsh, R. A., and O'Rourke, R. A. History and Differential Diagnosis of Acute Myocardial Infarction. In J. S. Karliner and G. Gregoratos (eds.), *Coronary Care*. New York: Churchill Livingstone, 1981. Pp. 169–176.
2. Walsh, R. A., and O'Rourke, R. A. Chest Pain. In J. H. Stein (ed.), *Internal Medicine* (2nd ed.). Boston: Little, Brown, 1987. Pp. 370–374.
3. Martin, W. B. Patient's use of gestures in the diagnosis of coronary insufficiency disease. *Minn. Med.* 40:691, 1957.
4. Levine, S. A. Coronary thrombosis—the variable clinical features. *Medicine (Baltimore)* 8:245, 1929.
5. Cheike, P., and Haist Steff, P. Angina pectoris with syncope due to transient atrioventricular block. *Br. Heart J.* 36:577, 1974.
6. Harper, R., Peter, R., and Hunt, P. Syncope in association with Prinzmetal's variant angina. *Br. Heart J.* 37:771, 1975.
7. Pepine, C. J., and Weiner, L. Effects of the Valsalva maneuver on myocardial ischemia in patients with coronary artery disease. *Circulation* 59:1304, 1979.
8. Chazov, E. I. Main Clinical Syndromes of Acute Myocardial Infarction. In E. I. Chazov (ed.), *Myocardial Infarction*. Moscow: MR Publishers, 1976. P. 140.
9. Proudfit, W. L., Shirey, E. K., and Sones Jr., F. M. Selective cine coronary angiography: Correlation with clinical findings in 1000 patients. *Circulation* 33:90, 1966.
10. Wei, J. Y., and Gersh, B. J. Heart disease in the elderly. *Curr. Probl. Cardiol.* 12(1):25, 1987.
11. Partamian, J., and Bradley, R. F. Acute myocardial infarction in 258 cases of diabetes: Immediate mortality and five year survival. *N. Engl. J. Med.* 273:455, 1965.
12. Kannel, W. B., and Abbot, R. D. Incidence and prognosis of unrecognized myocardial infarction: An update in the Framingham Study. *N. Engl. J. Med.* 311:1144, 1984.
13. Wei, J. Y. Heart disease in the elderly. *Cardiovasc. Med.* 9:971, 1984.
14. Gersh, B. J. Clinical manifestations of coronary heart disease in the elderly. In: *Working Conference on Recognition and Management of Coronary Heart Disease in the Elderly*, in press.
15. O'Rourke, R. A., Chatterjee, K., and Wei, J. Y. Coronary heart disease. *J. Am. Coll. Cardiol.* 10(2):52A, 1987.
16. Coodley, E. L., and Zebari, D. Characteristics of Myocardial Infarction in the Elderly. In E. L. Coodley (ed.), *Geriatric Heart Disease*. Littletown, MA: PSG Publishing, 1981. Pp. 334–345.
17. Murdaugh, C. L., and O'Rourke, R. A. Coronary heart disease in women—special considerations. *Curr. Probl. Cardiol.* in press.
18. Tofler, G. H., Stone, P. H., Muller, J. E., et al. Effects of gender and race in prognosis after myocardial infarction: Adverse prognosis for women, particularly black women. *J. Am. Coll. Cardiol.* 9:473, 1987.
19. Walling, A., Tremblay, G. J. L., Jobin, J., et al. Evaluating the rehabilitation potential of a large infarct population: Adverse prognosis for women. *J. Cardiac Rehabil.*, 8:99, 1988.
20. Walsh, R. A., and O'Rourke, R. A. The physical examination in acute uncomplicated and complicated myocardial infarction. In J. S. Karliner and G. Gregoratos (eds.), *Coronary Care*. New York: Churchill Livingstone, 1981. Pp. 177–188.
21. Fowler, N. O. Physical signs in acute myocar-

dial infarction and its complications. *Prog. Cardiovasc. Dis.* 10:287, 1968.
22. Webb, S. W., Adgey, A. A., and Pantridge, F. J. Autonomic disturbances at onset of acute myocardial infarction. *Br. Med. J.* 3:89, 1972.
23. Pantridge, J. F. Autonomic disturbance at the onset of acute myocardial infarction. In P. J. Schwartz, A. M. Brown, A. Malliani, and A. Zanchetti (eds.), *Neural Mechanisms in Cardiac Arrhythmias.* New York: Raven Press, 1978. Pp. 7–17.
24. Bezold, A., and Hirt, L. Uber die physiologischen Wirkungen des Essingsauren Veratrins. *Physiol. Lab. Wurzburg* 1:75, 1867.
25. Jarish, A., and Zotterman, Y. Depressor reflexes from the heart. *Acta Physiol. Scand.* 16:31, 1948.
26. Mark, A. L., Abboud, F. M., Heistad, D. D., et al. Evidence against the presence of ventricular chemoreceptors activated by hypoxia and hypercapnia. *Am. J. Physiol.* 227:178, 1974.
27. Rutlen, D. L., and Underwood, R. S. Reflex influence of selective coronary occlusion in the total capacitance vasculature in the dog. *J. Clin. Invest.* 73:241, 1984.
28. Sleight, P. Cardiac vomiting. *Br. Heart J.* 46:5, 1981.
29. Robertson, D., Hollister, A. S., Forman, M. B., and Robertson, R. M. Reflexes unique to myocardial ischemia and infarction. *J. Am. Coll. Cardiol.* 5:99B, 1985.
30. Wei, J. W., Markis, J. E., Malagold, M., and Braunwald, E. Cardiovascular reflexes stimulated by reperfusion of ischemic myocardium in acute myocardial infarction. *Circulation* 67:796, 1983.
31. Eckberg, D. L., White, C. W., Kioschos, J. M., and Abboud, F. M. Mechanisms mediating bradycardia during coronary arteriography. *J. Clin. Invest.* 54:1445, 1974.
32. Mark, A. L., Kioschos, J. M., Abboud, F. M., et al. Abnormal vascular responses to exercise in patients with aortic stenosis. *J. Clin. Invest.* 52:1138, 1973.
33. Robertson, R. M., and Robertson, D. The Bezold-Jarish reflex: Possible role in limiting myocardial ischemia. *Clin. Cardiol.* 4:75, 1981.
34. Risoe, C., Kerkey, O. J., Grottum, P., et al. Fever after acute myocardial infarction in patients treated with intravenous timolol or placebo. *Br. Heart J.* 57:28, 1987.
35. Harvey, W. P., and Ronan, J. A. Bedside diagnosis of arrhythmias. *Prog. Cardiovasc. Dis.* 8:419, 1966.
36. Yurchak, P. M., and Gorlin, R. Paradoxic splitting of the second heart sound in coronary artery disease. *N. Engl. J. Med.* 269:741, 1963.
37. Hill, J. C., O'Rourke, R. A., Lewis, R. P., and McGranahan, G. M. The diagnostic value of the atrial gallop in acute myocardial infarction. *Am.*

Heart J. 78:194, 1969.
38. Riley, C. P., Russel, R. O., and Rackly, C. E. Left ventricular gallop sound and acute myocardial infarction. *Am. Heart J.* 86:598, 1973.
39. DiDonna, G. J., Karliner, J. S., Peterson, K. L., and O'Rourke, R. A. Transmission of audible precordial gallop sounds to the right supraclavicular fossa. *Br. Heart J.* 37:1277, 1975.
40. Rigo, P., Murray, M., Taylor, D. R., et al. Right ventricular dysfunction detected by gated scintiphotography in patients with acute inferior myocardial infarction. *Circulation* 52:268, 1975.
41. Sharpe, D. N., Botvinick, E. H., Shames, O. M., et al. The non-invasive diagnosis of right ventricular infarction. *Circulation* 57:483, 1978.
42. Wackers, F. J., Lie, K. I., Sokole, E. B., et al. Prevalence of right ventricular involvement in inferior wall infarction assessed with myocardial imaging with thallium-201 and technetium-99m pyrophosphate. *Am. J. Cardiol.* 42:358, 1978.
43. Dell'Italia, L. J., Starling, M. R., Crawford, M. H., et al. Right ventricular infarction: Identification by hemodynamic measurements before and after loading and correlation with non-invasive techniques. *J. Am. Coll. Cardiol.* 4:931, 1984.
44. Dell'Italia, L. J., Starling, M. R., and O'Rourke, R. A. Physical examination for exclusion of hemodynamically important right ventricular infarction. *Ann. Intern. Med.* 99:608, 1983.
45. Dell'Italia, L. J., and Starling, M. R. Right ventricular infarction: An important clinical entity. *Curr. Probl. Cardiol.* 9(9):27, 1984.
46. Lopez-Sendon, J., Coma-Canella, I., and Gamallo, C. Sensitivity and specificity of hemodynamic criteria in the diagnosis of acute right ventricular infarction. *Circulation* 64:515, 1981.
47. Starling, M. R., Dell'Italia, L. J., Chaudhuri, T. K., et al. First transit and equilibrium radionuclide angiography in patients with inferior transmural myocardial infarction: Criteria for the diagnosis of associated hemodynamically significant right ventricular infarction. *J. Am. Coll. Cardiol.* 4:923, 1984.
48. Killip, T., and Kimball, J. T. Treatment of myocardial infarction in a coronary care unit: A two year experience with 250 patients. *Am. J. Cardiol.* 20:457, 1967.
49. Forrester, J. S., Diamond, G., Chatterjee, K., and Swan, H. J. C. Medical therapy of acute myocardial infarction by application of hemodynamic subsets. *N. Engl. J. Med.* 295:1356, 1976.
50. Abrams, D. S., Starling, M. R., Crawford, M. H., and O'Rourke, R. A. Value of noninvasive techniques for predicting early complications in patients with clinical class II acute myocardial infarction. *J. Am. Coll. Cardiol.* 2:818, 1983.

51. McHugh, T. J., Forrester, J. S., Alder, L., et al. Pulmonary vascular congestion in acute myocardial infarction; Hemodynamic and radiologic correlation. *Ann. Intern. Med.* 76:29, 1972.

52. Thadani, V., Chopra, M. P., and Aber Portal, R. W. Pericarditis after acute myocardial infarction. *Br. Med. J.* 2:135, 1971.

53. Lichstein, E. M., Lieu, H. M., and Gupta, P. Pericarditis complicating acute myocardial infarction: Incidence of complications and significance of electrocardiogram on admission. *Am. Heart J.* 87:246, 1974.

54. London, R. E., and London, S. B. Rupture of the heart: A critical analysis of 47 consecutive autopsy cases. *Circulation* 31:202, 1965.

55. Mundth, E. Rupture of the heart complicating myocardial infarction. *Circulation* 46:427, 1972.

56. Bates, R. J., Beutler, S., Resnekov, L., and Anagnostopoulous, C. E. Cardiac rupture—challenge in diagnosis and management. *Am. J. Cardiol.* 40:429, 1977.

57. Schuster, E. H., and Bulkey, B. H. Expansion of transmural myocardial infarction: A pathophysiologic factor in cardiac rupture. *Circulation* 60:1532, 1979.

58. Raizes, G., Wagner, G. S., and Hackel, D. B. Instantaneous non-arrythmic cardiac death in acute myocardial infarction: Role of electromechanical dissociation. *Am. J. Cardiol.* 39:1, 1977.

59. Gobel, F. L., Visudh-Arom, K., and Edwards, J. E. Pseudoaneurysm of the left ventricle leading to recurrent pericardial hemorrhage. *Chest* 59:23, 1971.

60. Vlodaver, Z., Coe, J. I., and Edwards, J. E. True and false left ventricular aneurysms: Propensity for the latter to rupture. *Circulation* 51:567, 1975.

61. Aher, B. R., Lewis, M. E., Vargas, A., et al. Non-invasive diagnosis of left ventricular pseudoaneurysm by radioangiography and echography. *Am. Heart J.* 101:236, 1981.

62. Levy, R., Rozanski, A., Charvzi, Y., et al. Complementary roles of two dimensional echocardiography and radionuclide ventriculography in ventricular pseudoaneurysm diagnosis. *Am. Heart J.* 102:1066, 1981.

63. Heikkila, J. Mitral incompetence complicating acute myocardial infarction. *Br. Heart J.* 29:162, 1967.

64. Phillips, J. H., Burch, G. E., and DePasquale, N. P. Syndrome of papillary muscle dysfunction. *Ann. Intern. Med.* 59:508, 1963.

65. Burch, G. E., De Pasquale, N. P., and Phillips, J. H. Clinical manifestations of papillary muscle dysfunction. *Arch. Intern. Med.* 112:112, 1963.

66. Burch, G. E., DePasquale, N. P., and Phillips, J. H. The syndrome of papillary muscle dys-

function. *Am. Heart J.* 75:399, 1968.

67. Maisel, A. S., Gilpin, E. A., Klein, L., et al. The murmurs of papillary muscle dysfunction in acute myocardial infarction: Clinical features and prognostic implications. *Am. Heart J.* 112:705, 1986.

68. Karliner, J. S., O'Rourke, R. A., Kearney, D. J., and Shabetai, R. Hemodynamic explanation of why the murmur of mitral regurgitation is independent of cycle length. *Br. Heart J.* 35:397, 1973.

69. Lembo, N., Dell'Italia, J. L., Crawford, M. H., and O'Rourke, R. A. Diagnosis of left-sided regurgitant murmurs by transient arterial occlusion: A new maneuver using blood pressure cuffs. *Ann. Intern. Med.* 105:368, 1986.

70. McGraw, D. B., Siegel, W., Stone Cipher, H. K., et al. Response of heart murmur intensity to isometric (handgrip) exercise. *Br. Heart J.* 34:605, 1972.

71. Fisher, M. L., Nutter, D. O., Jacobs, W., and Schlant, R. C. Hemodynamic responses to isometric exercise (handgrip) in patients with heart disease. *Br. Heart J.* 35:422, 1973.

72. Stefardourous, M. A., Grossman, W., El-Shahawy, M. E., and Witham, A. C. The effect of isometric exercise on the left ventricular volume in normal man. *Circulation* 49:1185, 1974.

73. Sharpey-Schafer, E. P. Effects of squatting on the normal and failing circulation. *Br. Med. J.* 1:1072, 1956.

74. Crawford, M. H., and O'Rourke, R. A. A systematic approach to the bedside differentiation of cardiac murmurs and abnormal sounds. *Curr. Probl. Cardiol.* 1:1, 1977.

75. Cederquist, L., and Soderstrom, J. Papillary muscle rupture in myocardial infarction: A study based upon an autopsy material. *Acta Med. Scand.* 176:287, 1964.

76. Wei, J. Y., Hutchins, G. M., and Bulkey, B. H. Papillary muscle rupture in fatal acute myocardial infarction, a potentially treatable form of cardiogenic shock. *Ann. Intern. Med.* 90:149, 1979.

77. Bruns, D. L. A general theory of the causes of murmurs in the cardiovascular system. *Am. J. Med.* 27:360, 1959.

78. DeBusk, R. F., and Harrison, D. C. The clinical spectrum of papillary muscle disease. *N. Engl. J. Med.* 281:1458, 1969.

79. Selzer, A., Gerln, K., and Kerth, W. J. Clinical, hemodynamic and surgical considerations of rupture of the ventricular septum after myocardial infarction. *Am. Heart J.* 78:59, 1969.

80. Vlodaver, Z., and Edwards, J. E. Rupture of ventricular septum or papillary muscle complicating myocardial infarction. *Circulation* 55:815, 1977.

81. Hutchins, G. M. Rupture of the interventricular septum complicating myocardial infarc-

tion: Pathological analysis of 10 patients with clinically diagnosed perforation. *Am. Heart J.* 97:165, 1979.

82. Hellerstein, H. K., and Martin, J. W. Incidence of thromboembolic lesions accompanying myocardial infarctions. *Am. Heart J.* 33:443, 1947.

83. Phares, W. S., Edwards, J. E., Burchell, H. B. Cardiac aneurysm: Clinicopathologic studies. *Mayo Clin. Proc.* 28:264, 1953.

84. Dubnow, M. H., Burchell, H. B., and Titus, J. L. Post-infarction ventricular aneurysm in a clinicopathologic and electrocardiographic study of cases. *Am. Heart J.* 70:753, 1969.

85. Davis, R. W., and Ebert, P. A. Ventricular aneurysm: A clinical pathologic correlation. *Am. J. Cardiol.* 29:1, 1972.

86. Van de Bos, A. A., Bletter, W. B., and Hagemeijer, F. Progressive development of left ventricular thrombus: Detection and evolution studied with echocardiographic techniques. *Chest* 74:307, 1978.

87. Stratton, J. R., Lighty, G. W., Jr., Pearlman, A. S., and Ritchie, J. L. Detection of left ventricular thrombosis in two-dimensional echocardiography: Sensitivity, specificity and causes of uncertainty. *Circulation* 66:156, 1982.

88. Reeder, G. S., Tajik, A. J., and Seward, J. B. Left ventricular mural thrombosis: Two-dimensional echocardiographic diagnosis. *Mayo Clin. Proc.* 56:82, 1981.

89. DeMaria, A. N., Neumann, A., Bomner, W., et al. Left ventricular thrombi identified by cross section echocardiography. *Ann. Intern. Med.* 90:14, 1979.

90. Asinger, R. W., Mikell, F. L., Elsperger, J., and Hudges, M. Incidence of left ventricular thrombosis after acute transmural infarction: Serial evaluation by two-dimensional echocardiography. *N. Engl. J. Med.* 305:297, 1981.

91. Thompson, J. E. Acute peripheral arterial occlusions. *N. Engl. J. Med.* 290:950, 1974.

92. Foote, G. A., Shabel, S. J., and Hodges, M. Pulmonary complications of the flow-directed balloon tipped catheter. *N. Engl. J. Med.* 290:927, 1974.

6
Plasma Enzymes in Acute Myocardial Infarction

PETER R. PULEO AND ROBERT ROBERTS

The utility of plasma enzymes as molecular markers of acute myocardial infarction (AMI) has undergone a steady evolution. During the 1960s an elevation of one or more of the "cardiac enzymes" was taken as supportive evidence for the diagnosis of AMI. The increased diagnostic specificity that resulted from the recognition and application of myocardium-specific isoenzymes during the 1970s greatly enhanced the clinical usefulness of these assays; today most clinicians would be reluctant to make the diagnosis of AMI if appropriately timed plasma samples failed to document a rise and fall in MB creatine kinase (CK). Serial analysis of plasma MB-CK has also been employed to accurately quantitate infarct size.

The advent of thrombolytic therapy during the 1980s has created the need for a sensitive and specific marker of AMI that is diagnostic during the initial hours of infarction. In addition, reliable noninvasive indicators of reperfusion might obviate the need for routine diagnostic catheterization following thrombolytic therapy. The subforms MM-CK and MB-CK show promise as early markers of AMI and of successful reperfusion.

Historical Perspective

Amylase was detected in the serum of normal individuals in 1908 [1]. However, it was not until 1936, when alkaline phosphatase was proposed as a marker of metastatic bone disease [2], that serum enzymes were used diagnostically. The first application of diagnostic enzymology to AMI was in 1954, when La

Due et al. [3, 4] reported a rise and fall in serum aspartate transaminase (AST; prior designation SGOT) activity following AMI. One year later, serum lactate dehydrogenase (LD) activity was also shown to be elevated following acute myocardial necrosis [5]. A drawback of using these enzymes as diagnostic markers of AMI is their lack of specificity for myocardial injury: Both are released into the blood with injury of muscle, liver, and other tissues. However, in 1957 several groups reported that LD activity in serum could be resolved into several peaks by electrophoresis [6–8], subsequently designated "isoenzymes" [9], with predominance of the fastest migrating peak being specific for AMI [7]. CK was shown to be elevated in the serum of patients with skeletal muscle disease (muscular dystrophy) in 1959 [10]. The following year, elevation of serum CK after AMI was detected [11]. The use of the MB isoenzyme of CK as a specific indicator of AMI was first reported in 1966 [12]. During the subsequent decade the sensitivity and specificity of plasma MB-CK elevation for acute myocardial necrosis was confirmed in many laboratories, and improved assays for the CK isoenzymes were developed. Today, assay of plasma MB-CK is universally accepted as the most reliable diagnostic test for AMI.

Biochemical Markers of AMI

Biochemical markers of AMI in current use have in common the property of being present in the intracellular compartment of cardiac myocytes, with release into the blood following the onset of infarction. In the absence of ischemia, the intact sarcolemma maintains the intracellular milieu; the membrane is impermeable to macromolecules, and movement of ions is tightly regulated by intramembrane gates and energy-dependent pumps. Shortly after the onset of ischemia, the ability of the membrane to maintain normal ionic gradients becomes impaired, and intracellular potassium is lost to the interstitium. Whether this reaction is a result of gate/channel dysfunction [13] or due to early loss of integrity of the lipid bilayer itself is unknown. It is also unclear if sufficient impairment of membrane integrity occurs during transient ischemia to allow some loss of macromolecular contents. Several studies have suggested that enzyme release in the animal model (at least in quantities sufficient to result in a discernible rise above baseline blood levels) occurs only with irreversible ischemia [14, 15]; however, the issue remains controversial and difficult to prove or disprove. We observed elevated levels of CK and glycogen phosphorylase in the lymph draining from the hearts of dogs following periods of occlusion as short as 10 to 15 minutes, followed by reperfusion. On histologic examination there was evidence of minute abnormalities, but not those typical of cardiac necrosis, suggesting release of enzymes in the absence of cell death. It is possible that reversible ischemia results in the release of intracellular macromolecules in quantities insufficient to raise plasma levels above the normal range [16]. However, if samples are analyzed from the nearby lymphatics, such release can be detected. Clinical studies have failed to demonstrate plasma enzyme elevations during transient ischemia (e.g., exercise stress with ischemia or unstable anginal episodes) [17, 18] despite coronary patency, which would favor the appearance of any released enzymes in the blood. In summary, it appears that if leakage of macromolecules from the cell occurs during transient ischemia it is in quantities insufficient to be detected by currently available assays.

Ischemia sustained for more than 30 to 40 minutes results in irreversible cellular injury and subsequent cell death. Membrane integrity is lost, and cellular contents, including macromolecules, are therefore in continuity with the interstitial space. A substantial proportion of cellular enzymes are denatured or degraded in situ; however, a predictable fraction gains entry to the cardiac lymphatics and is transported to the blood. Whether a significant quantity of these proteins enters the bloodstream directly via the cardiac capillaries is unknown; it would depend, among other factors, on the regional myocardial flow (which is usually minimal with a nonreperfused AMI), as well as the molecular size of the protein and the integrity of the capillaries in the infarct region.

It follows from the above discussion that the utility of a protein as a marker of AMI depends on certain factors.

1. Solubility: Molecules having low solubility, such as those that make up the contractile apparatus, move poorly out of the infarcted myocardium.
2. Baseline concentration of the marker molecule in myocardium and in blood: High concentration within myocardial cells and low concentration in normal lymph and blood result in a significant concentration gradient and rapid flux of the marker molecule into the blood following sarcolemma breakdown. Furthermore, a low ambient concentration in normal blood provides a background against which release of the marker molecule into the blood can be readily detected.
3. Molecular weight: Large molecules such as LD [molecular weight (MW) 135,000] diffuse slowly and appear in the blood relatively late, thus precluding early diagnosis; small molecules (e.g., myoglobin, MW 17,800) appear in the blood rapidly.
4. Detectability: The clinical utility of a diagnostic marker depends in part on the reliability, expense, and ease of detection of the marker in a clinical laboratory. The speed with which an assay can be performed is also a consideration for assays whose goal is the early diagnosis of AMI.
5. Specificity: Perhaps most importantly, the

usefulness of a marker is determined by the extent to which it is present in myocardium but not in other tissues, so that a rise in plasma levels is specific for myocardial injury.

6. Kinetics of clearance: Ideally, a biochemical marker is cleared from the blood quickly; however, if clearance is too rapid, the time frame during which the diagnosis of AMI can be made may be brief. This situation is the case for myoglobin, which is rapidly cleared into the urine; with small infarctions, serum levels may return to the normal range by 24 hours after AMI onset.

More than 20 muscle-associated proteins, including enzymes, myoglobin, and contractile proteins, have been evaluated as potential markers of AMI. Most have been of limited diagnostic value because their presence in noncardiac tissue results in elevated plasma levels in the absence of myocardial injury [19]. Three enzymes have been routinely used in the past for the diagnosis of AMI: AST, LD, and CK. Of these, CK and its isoenzymes have proved to be the most reliable and cost-effective biochemical markers of AMI.

CK

CHARACTERISTICS

CK catalyzes the reversible transfer of a high-energy phosphate group from adenosine triphosphate (ATP) to creatine (Cr):

$$\text{Cr} + \text{ATP} \xrightleftharpoons{\text{CK}} \text{Cr-P} + \text{ADP}$$

where Cr-P = creatine phosphate
ADP = adenosine diphosphate

The forward reaction is favored at pH 9.4, and the reverse reaction is favored at pH 7.4.

CK is a dimer [20] of MW 86,000. The cytosolic isoenzymes of CK are formed by the association of M and/or B CK polypeptide subunits in one of three possible combinations: (1) BB-CK, consisting of two B subunits, derives its name from brain tissue, where it is the most abundant form of cytosolic CK synthesized. (2) MM-CK, the predominant form of CK present in skeletal muscle, is composed of two M subunits. (3) MB-CK is a heterodimer composed of one of each of the cytosolic polypeptide chains. The mitochondrial isoenzyme is a homodimer whose two polypeptide chains differ from the M and B chains antigenically, biochemically, and by charge [21–23].

At pH 7.4, mitochondrial CK has a net positive charge, MM-CK is isoelectric, and BB-CK has a net negative charge; MB-CK has charge intermediate between MM-CK and BB-CK. These differences have been exploited to differentially assay the isoenzymes (see below), as well as for the purposes of isoenzyme purification.

Creatine kinase is enzymatically active only in the dimeric form. The three cytosolic isoenzymes can be induced to dissociate and randomly reassociate in solution by quick-freezing and thawing [20]; in this way, all three isoenzymes can be synthesized using any two isoenzymes as the initial substrate. However, mitochondrial CK monomers do not reassociate with the M-CK or B-CK polypeptide [24].

The M, B, and mitochondrial polypeptide chains are each encoded by a separate gene; available evidence suggests that each gene exists as a single copy per haploid human genome [25]. The cDNAs encoding both cytosolic human polypeptides have been cloned in our laboratory, and the full cDNA sequences determined [25, 26]. The genomic nucleotide sequence of the cytosolic forms is currently being elucidated.

Available data implicate CK in the coordination of ATP production in the mitochondria with cellular energy demand in the cytoplasm via the "creatine phosphate shuttle" [27–29]. In this facilitated diffusion model, creatine present in mitochondria is phosphorylated by the mitochondrial CK isoenzyme, utilizing ATP generated in the mitochondria by oxidative phosphorylation. The creatine phosphate thus formed diffuses across the mitochondrial membrane into the cytosol, where in the presence of ADP and cytosolic CK, ATP and creatine are regenerated in the reverse CK reaction. ATP is then used as an energy source in the cell; creatine diffuses back into the mitochondria. In addition to providing a link between cellular energy demand and ATP production, cytosolic creatine phosphate can act as an energy "buffer" against sudden bursts of energy utilization [29]. Although this model explains a great deal of accumulated experimental evidence [28], direct demonstration of ATP/ADP compartmentation is not yet available [29].

Immunohistochemical and cellular fractionation studies have demonstrated at least some degree of subcellular compartmentation of cytosolic CK. The tail portion of myosin has binding sites for MM-CK [30]; approximately 5 percent of cellular MM-CK activity is associated with the M-line of the sarcomere in both heart and skeletal muscle [31, 32]. In addition, antibodies directed against B-CK bind to the sarcomeric Z-line in heart muscle [33]. Small amounts of MM-CK have also been detected immunochemically and by differential centrifugation in association with the nuclear membrane [34], sarcolemma [35], and sarcoplasmic reticulum [36]. Subcellular compartmentation of "cytosolic" CK may provide optimum localization of ATP regeneration (e.g., at the contractile apparatus or adjacent to sarcolemmal Na^+/K^+-ATPase), in line with its function as the cytosolic limb of the "creatine phosphate shuttle." Mitochondrial CK is localized to the outer surface of the inner mitochondrial membrane [37].

The CK isoenzymes vary significantly in terms of their stability. The cytosolic isoenzymes have been shown to undergo two forms of inactivation [38]: (1) reversible inactivation due to oxidation of thiol groups, which may be prevented (or partially reversed) by storage with a thiol "activator" compound, which acts as a reducing agent; and (2) irreversible inactivation, probably as a consequence of thermal denaturation. MM-CK is the most stable of the isoenzymes; little loss of activity occurs even with storage at room temperature for several days. MB-CK loses activity quickly at room temperature but is stable at $-20°C$. However, because activity loss occurs with freezing and thawing, storage at 4°C is prefer-

able for preservation of activity for short to intermediate periods (less than 1 week). MB-CK is also subject to photoinactivation; consequently, samples should be shielded from direct light [38]. BB-CK and mitochondrial CK are labile molecules; substantial loss of activity occurs within hours of sample collection; therefore specimens stored without freezing are unlikely to demonstrate these isoenzymes unless assayed immediately after collection.

Samples for CK assay may be collected and stored as either plasma or serum. If an anticoagulant is employed for plasma collection, EGTA should be used rather than EDTA because the latter has a much higher affinity for Mg^{2+}, a required cation for CK activity. In our laboratory, samples are collected in tubes pretreated with β-mercaptoethanol and EGTA so that the final concentration after blood collection is approximately 10 mM for both compounds. β-Mercaptoethanol has been shown to be the most effective thiol "activator" agent and is most efficient when added to the sample at the time of collection rather than at the time of assay [38]. Glutathione should not be used as activator, as the serum enzyme glutathione reductase uses this molecule as a proton donor to reduce NADP, yielding false elevations in the CK assay (see below). In addition to serving as an anticoagulant, EGTA affords a protective effect on CK activity independent of mercaptoethanol. Finally, EGTA acts as an inhibitor of serum carboxypeptidase, an important consideration if MM-CK or MB-CK subforms are to be assayed; this subject is discussed at length in the final section.

Creatine kinase molecules of very high molecular weight have been detected in the blood. It is now clear that these "macro-CK" molecules consist of polymerized aggregates of CK. Macro-CK-1, which migrates between MM-CK and MB-CK on gel electrophoresis, is formed by antibody-induced polymerization of CK, most often involving the BB isoenzyme. The antibodies are usually of the immunoglobulin G (IgG) type [39]. Macro-CK-2 consists of polymerized molecules of mitochondrial CK [40]; the mechanism of polymerization is not known. CK-2 migrates close to MM-CK on gel electrophoresis. Both forms of macro-CK have been detected only in the blood of patients; they have not been recovered from cell extracts and therefore represent a post-translational modification rather than a distinct gene product. Other forms of CK include the modified subforms of MM-CK and MB-CK, which are discussed below.

ASSAY OF TOTAL AND ISOENZYME CK ACTIVITY

Total CK Activity

Assay of total CK enzymatic activity is achieved by a three-step, coupled enzyme system proposed by Oliver [41] and modified by Rosalki [42].

$$\text{Cr-P} + \text{ADP} \xrightleftharpoons{\text{CK}} \text{Cr} + \text{ATP}$$

$$\text{ATP} + \text{glucose} \xrightleftharpoons{\text{hexokinase}} \text{glucose-6-phosphate} + \text{ADP}$$

$$\text{Glucose-6-phosphate} + \text{NADP}$$

$$\xrightleftharpoons{\text{G-6-P-dH}} \text{6-phosphogluconate} + \text{NADPH}$$

where G-6-P-dH = glucose-6-phosphate dehydrogenase

Cr-P, ADP, glucose, hexokinase, NADP, and G-6-P-dH are the required substrates; in the presence of CK, ATP is generated, allowing the second and third steps to proceed (ADP formed during the second step is "recycled" to the first step). NADPH produced during the final step is detected by ultraviolet light absorption at 340 nm; the rate of change in absorption (after a several-minute "lag phase") is directly proportional to CK activity. Premixed lyophilized reagents are available from several commercial suppliers; reagent concentrations are preadjusted so that CK concentration is rate-limiting. In addition, an inhibitor of the enzyme adenylate kinase (AK), usually adenosine monophosphate (AMP) or 3′,5′-diadenylate phosphate, is included with the reagent mixture; adenylate kinase catalyzes the reaction.

$$\text{ADP} + \text{ADP} \xrightleftharpoons{\text{AK}} \text{AMP} + \text{ATP}$$

ATP thus generated can result in spuriously elevated values for CK activity. Because adenylate kinase is present in high concentration in erythrocytes, gross hemolysis can release sufficient adenylate kinase to overcome the inhibitor and produce falsely elevated CK activity.

Note that measurement of ATP generated in step 1 seems to provide a more direct index of CK activity; however, ATP is not readily detectable by any convenient method. Therefore the Rosalki system is employed by most clinical laboratories in the United States.

Results of the kinetic CK assay are expressed in international units of activity per liter (IU/L), with 1 IU defined by the International Convention on Biochemistry as the quantity of enzyme required to generate 1 micromole (μmol) of product from 1 μmol of substrate in 1 minute at 30°C. CK activity, like that of most enzymes, is temperature-dependent. Although the temperature at which CK activity is reported is not uniform among clinical laboratories, the relation of any given sample to the reference range is maintained regardless of temperature. CK activity at 37°C may be converted to standard temperature (30°C) by the formula

$$\text{Activity}_{37°} \times 0.577 = \text{activity}_{30°}$$

Isoenzyme Assays

The cytosolic CK isoenzymes may be assayed by a wide variety of techniques. The methods may be broadly categorized as those that separate the isoenzymes on the basis of charge differences and those that exploit the antigenic properties of the isoenzymes.

METHODS BASED ON ISOENZYME CHARGE DIFFERENCES

The most commonly employed CK isoenzyme assay is electrophoresis on agarose or cellulose acetate; this technique is used in more than 80 percent of the clinical laboratories in the United States [43]. Serum or plasma is diluted to a uniform total CK activity (usually 300 IU/L), and a small volume is applied to the well of a precast gel; constant voltage is then applied for 15 minutes. The gel acts as an inert support matrix, allowing free movement of water and CK molecules in the electrical field. Migration progresses according to molecular charge (Fig. 6-1); the negatively charged BB isoenzyme, if present in the sample, moves most rapidly toward the positive electrode. MB-CK, having a relative intermediate negative charge, also moves toward the anode, but less rapidly than BB-CK; MM-CK, with little net charge at physiologic pH, remains near the origin. An alternative nomenclature for the cytosolic isoenzymes is based on these charge

Fig. 6-1
Cytosolic CK isoenzymes detected by agarose gel electrophoresis. Right lane: Control containing heat-inactivated serum and all three purified isoenzymes. MM-CK remains near the origin; BB-CK, having a net negative change, shows the greatest migration toward the anode; and MB-CK is visible between MM-CK and BB-CK. Left lane: Serum from a patient with AMI. Although MM-CK predominates, a definite MB-CK band, constituting 12 percent of the total CK activity, is visible.

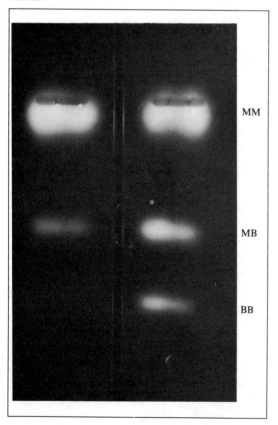

differences. By convention, isoenzymes are designated by speed of electrophoretic migration toward the positive electrode. Consequently, the most negative isoenzyme (BB-CK) is also designated CK-1, MB-CK as CK-2, and MM-CK as CK-3. After completion of electrophoresis, the gel is uniformly overlaid with the "Rosalki reagent," described above, and incubated for 5 minutes at 37°C. NADPH is generated in situ at the location of the CK isoenzymes on the gel. The intensity of fluorescence of the isoenzyme bands under ultraviolet light is compared by scanning densitometry and expressed as a relative percent. This technique has been improved significantly. Previously, difficulty with standardization of agarose side chains and electroendosmotic force, as well as lack of uniformity of pore size for cellulose acetate, resulted in significant lot-to-lot variability in gel performance. These problems have been resolved, and currently available "second generation" gels are uniform in thickness, agarose side chain characteristics, pore size, electroendosmotic force generation, and performance [44, 45]. In contrast to older systems, which were unable to detect MB-CK levels within the normal range (consequently, any detectable serum MB-CK was considered pathologic), present systems are sensitive for MB-CK at levels well within the normal range.

Nevertheless, electrophoresis still has several drawbacks compared with other available isoenzyme assays. One consistent problem has been an adequate definition of what constitutes a "normal" study. Because of the insensitivity of early electrophoretic systems, the appearance of any activity in the MB-CK range was associated with infarction in most cases. However, with the development of more sensitive systems, MB-CK bands were frequently detected in normal sera; as a result, the definition of a pathologic elevation of MB-CK has been selected as more than 3, 4, or 5 percent (depending on the author) of total CK activity [46]. These cutoff values are clearly adequate to distinguish patients suffering a moderate or large AMI from the normal population.

However, the significance of mild elevations of percent MB-CK (<10 percent of total CK activity) when total CK is only slightly elevated is not clear. In addition, because the electrophoretic assay is not kinetic, it is accurate only when conditions remain in the linear range for both MM-CK and MB-CK. If serum containing high total CK activity is assayed, MM-CK quickly exhausts the Rosalki substrate and the fluorescence "plateaus out," whereas MB-CK continues to generate NADPH. Consequently, serum having high total CK activity may yield artifactually elevated MB-CK values. Appropriate dilution of the sample to 300 to 500 IU/L prior to electrophoresis circumvents this problem. Another drawback of electrophoresis is artifact due to naturally fluorescing products in serum, such as albumin-bound bilirubin [47, 48]; a similar effect may be produced by certain drugs (see below). These artifacts do not interfere with kinetic assays, which determine CK activity by the change in ultraviolet absorbance over time; in contrast, electrophoresis provides only a "snapshot" of cumulative fluorescence. Non-CK artifact can usually be identified by inspection of the gel, as artifactual bands differ in color from the blue fluorescence of NADPH, and their migration on the gel usually does not correspond exactly with that of MM-CK or MB-CK. Such distinctions may be missed if gels are not examined by an experienced technician prior to densitometry.

The use of controls on each gel to define MB-CK position is helpful for defining artifact. If questions remain as to the source of a band, reagent containing all substrates required for the coupled Rosalki reactions except creatine phosphate, the specific CK substrate, is available; the persistence of a fluorescing band in a gel incubated with this modified reagent identifies its source as non-CK.

Finally, an important problem with electrophoretic detection of MB-CK is the need for individual sample processing by experienced personnel and the long time required to perform the assay (30–45 minutes). These factors are largely responsible for the limited frequency with which MB-CK assays are performed in most clinical laboratories; in most laboratories "stat" determinations are not available even though these results may be important for patient triage from the coronary care unit (CCU). "Third generation" high voltage systems with robotic sample application, rapid electrophoresis, and automated densitometry may overcome these problems.

Other MB-CK assays based on isoenzyme charge differences rely on the selective binding of the more negatively charged MB isoenzyme to an ion-exchange resin, consisting of a positively charged inert matrix equilibrated with buffer. In the minicolumn assay, sample is loaded onto a column packed with the positively charged resin; MB-CK and BB-CK electrostatically bind to the matrix, whereas the neutral MM-CK molecules pass directly through the column. Subsequent elutions with higher concentrations of sodium chloride displace MB-CK from the column by competition of the negatively charged B polypeptide with chloride ions for the resin-binding sites. BB-CK may be eluted in the same fashion. CK activity is then assayed in the collected eluate [49]. This assay has not achieved widespread clinical use, in large measure because of problems with carryover of MM-CK into the MB-CK fractions, especially when the applied sample contains high MM-CK activity [17].

The batch absorption assay of Henry et al. [50] employs glass beads coated with an ion-exchange resin. Plasma is mixed with the glass beads, and the resin binds MB-CK; MM-CK is removed by several rinses with low ionic strength buffer. MB-CK is then eluted from the beads by a high salt buffer, and CK activity is assayed by the Rosalki method. Carryover of MM-CK is not a problem because of the multiple low salt washes. This technique is sensitive (95 percent), efficient, precise, and reproducible (coefficient of variation ± 5 percent) [50, 51], and it can be completed in 5 minutes by personnel with minimal experience. In addition, results are quantitative rather than semiquantitative and are obtained in absolute MB-CK activity (IU/L), rather than as a percent of total CK. Because of these advantages over the more popular electrophoretic assays, we use this method as the standard CK isoenzyme assay at our institution. We now have experience with more than 200,000 assays using this system; sensitivity and specificity both exceed 95 percent. Samples are routinely analyzed eight times a day, with "stat" tests performed on request. This procedure has allowed more expeditious turnover of patients in the CCU, as patients having serial normal plasma MB-CK activities within 18 to 24 hours of the onset of symptoms may be transferred to less expensive non-CCU beds. It also reduces the incidence of "overflow" of coronary patients to other acute care units. A disadvantage of the glass bead assay is that BB-CK is measured along with MB-CK. However, BB-CK is rarely detectable in plasma by any available assay; when it has been detected by other methods, the level is almost always less than 5 IU/L. Thus even if it is erroneously measured as MB-CK, it is not a sufficient increment to lead to diagnostic confusion [52].

IMMUNOASSAYS

Immunoassays constitute the second major group of CK isoenzyme assays. The differences in charge, amino acid sequence, and conformation of the M and B polypeptide chains have permitted the development of antibodies that differentially recognize one chain or the other.

Immunoinhibition. Immunoinhibition assays measure MB-CK enzymatic activity by selectively inactivating M-CK subunits with an M-specific antibody. MM-CK and the M subunit of MB-CK are inhibited; consequently, residual activity is attributed to B subunit activity of the MB isoenzyme (as well as BB-CK, if present) [53].

Immunoprecipitation. Immunoprecipitation is similar to immunoinhibition except subunit-specific antibodies are used to precipitate rather than directly inhibit target CK. Anti-M-CK antibody is used to precipitate MM-CK and MB-CK; residual activity is attributed to serum BB-CK. In a separate aliquot, anti-B-CK antibody is employed to precipitate MB-CK and BB-CK; residual activity is due to MM-CK. These two results are then combined to determine MB-CK activity, as total CK activity minus MM-CK and BB-CK activity

must equal MB-CK activity [53]. This technique is obviously indirect, and substantial assay-to-assay variability [54] has led to its disuse.

Radioimmunoassay.   Radioimmunoassays (RIAs) constitute the most sensitive means available for detecting MB-CK. A radiolabeled ligand (e.g., ^{125}I-labeled BB-CK) is added to the serum sample. A B-subunit specific antibody is then added, and unlabeled serum MB-CK competes with the labeled BB-CK for antibody binding sites. Higher concentrations of MB-CK in the serum result in more competition with radiolabeled BB-CK for the antibody binding sites; thus less radioactivity is bound and precipitated by the anti-B-CK antibody. Patient samples are assayed in parallel with controls containing known quantities of unlabeled MB-CK. Unlike previously described assays, which quantitate CK in terms of its enzymatic function (expressed in IU/L), the RIA directly quantitates protein mass, expressed as micrograms of CK protein per milliliter (μg/ml). These assays are able to detect as little as 0.2 μg of MB-CK/ml (equivalent to 0.08 IU of CK activity per liter), with an upper limit of normal of 40 μg/L [55], and are precise. However, they have not achieved widespread use because they are somewhat cumbersome and necessitate use of a radionuclide.

ELISA. The enzyme-linked immunoadsorption assay, or ELISA, utilizes two antibodies, each recognizing one of the two CK subunits. Anti-M-CK antibody, bound to a solid-phase inert matrix, is exposed to the plasma sample and both MM-CK and MB-CK are bound. After washing away unbound CK, the system is flooded with a buffer containing anti-B-CK antibody linked to a "reporter molecule" (alkaline phosphatase or horseradish peroxidase). The labeled second antibody attaches to previously bound MB-CK molecules. The concentration of "sandwiched" MB isoenzyme can be determined by the intensity of a colorimetric reaction mediated by the reporter groups on the second antibody [56].

Monoclonal Antibodies. All polyclonal antibodies developed to date recognize either the M or the B polypeptide subunit and therefore react with both MB-CK and one of the two homodimers. A monoclonal antibody has been developed that recognizes an epitope unique to MB-CK and does not cross react with the MM or BB isoenzymes [57]. This antibody, linked to polystyrene beads, extracts MB-CK from serum, with subsequent assay of the bound isoenzyme using colorimetric detection [57, 58].

None of the immunoassays is currently in widespread use [43]; they tend to be cumbersome, and it has been difficult to maintain standardized antibodies [54]. The newly developed monoclonal-antibody-based system may enhance the attractiveness of immunoassays for MB-CK detection.

CK ISOENZYME TISSUE DISTRIBUTION

Skeletal Muscle
The predominance of MM-CK characteristic of mature skeletal muscle develops relatively late in fetal life. During the first 6 weeks of development only BB-CK is synthesized in fetal skeletal muscle. During the subsequent weeks, M-CK chain synthesis is induced and rapidly supplants B-CK, so that by the eighth week in utero, MB-CK is the most abundant cytosolic isoenzyme, and after the twelfth week MM-CK predominates [59, 60]. By the time of birth, MM-CK constitutes 80 percent of total cystolic CK activity in skeletal muscle [59].

Whether MB-CK is completely absent from adult skeletal muscle or present in small quantities has been the subject of some disagreement. Several investigators have found small quantities of MB-CK in normal adult skeletal muscle [61, 62], whereas others have failed to detect any cytosolic CK other than MM-CK [63, 64]. In a large study by Tsung and Tsung [61], biopsies of normal skeletal muscle were removed from 109 patients at the time of surgery; MB-CK was detected in 44 percent of all muscles tested, usually representing 1 to 3 percent of total CK activity. There was no muscle or muscle group that consistently demonstrated the presence of MB-CK.

Data from several laboratories have demonstrated that injured skeletal muscle synthesizes MB-CK at levels in excess of those reported for normal muscle. Levels of MB-CK representing 7.5 percent or more of total cytosolic CK activity have been detected in muscles affected by chronic exercise [65, 66], inflammation [67], trauma [68]; electrical current [68, 69], or genetic disease [70]. This increased skeletal muscle MB-CK synthesis is also reflected by steady-state plasma MB-CK levels exceeding normal values [67, 71]. The biologic importance of MB-CK synthesis in injured muscle is unknown. It has been postulated that the population of undifferentiated satellite cells, which can differentiate to form mature skeletal myocytes following muscle injury, repeats the developmental program of fetal skeletal muscle [72]. The potential significance of skeletal muscle MB-CK synthesis as a confounding factor in the diagnosis of AMI is discussed below.

Myocardium
Mature human myocardium contains approximately 1600 IU of CK activity/L/gm of tissue. It is the only tissue that harbors a substantial quantity of MB-CK, with 15 to 20 percent of cytosolic CK activity present as the MB isoenzyme; the remaining soluble CK is MM-CK. The adult myocardium of small mammals (rat, mouse, rabbit) contains little or no MB-CK; however, induction of MB-CK synthesis (as well as other proteins characteristic of fetal myocardium) has been observed to accompany pressure-induced hypertrophy. It has been reported that healthy cardiac tissue, like normal skeletal muscle, synthesizes only MM-CK, with MB-CK synthesis occurring only in the presence of cardiac ischemia or hypertrophy [73]. This report has not been substantiated by others and conflicts with earlier data from normal human hearts obtained at necropsy [74]. Other primates studied have approximately 15 percent of myocardial CK activity as the MB isoenzyme [75]. MB-CK in plasma has been observed to rise following catheter-directed fulgurative ablation of atrioventricular nodal bypass tracts in hearts unaffected by ischemia or hypertrophy [76]. Furthermore, we have observed a typical rise and fall of plasma MB-CK following iatrogenic

dissection of a normal right coronary artery in a young man undergoing evaluation of a cardiac murmur that was determined to be functional. Thus the weight of data supports a level of 15 percent MB-CK in nondiseased human myocardium. Whether additional accumulation of the MB isoenzyme occurs with hypertrophy remains to be determined.

Other Organs

BB-CK remains the predominant cytosolic isoenzyme in brain from development through adult life [77]. Organs other than heart, brain, and skeletal muscle, including those rich in nonstriated muscle such as the gut, uterus, and urinary bladder, contain relatively low levels of CK per gram of tissue (Fig. 6-2). More importantly from a diagnostic standpoint, none synthesizes significant quantities of MB-CK. However, the brain, gastrointestinal tract, prostate, and uterus are rich in BB-CK (Fig. 6-2); consequently, injury to these organs may result in misdiagnosis of AMI if plasma is assayed by a method that does not discriminate between MB-CK and BB-CK.

The effect of injury or disease on CK content per gram of tissue and CK isoenzyme distribution has been less well studied in tissue other than striated muscle. CK production in neoplasms, most commonly involving the lung, breast, and kidney, has been reported [78]. BB-CK is the isoenzyme most commonly detected in such tumors, but any of the cytosolic isoenzymes may occur. These tumors may cause diagnostic confusion by releasing CK into the blood. The concentration of CK per gram of tissue, predominant isoenzyme synthesized, and level of CK present in the blood do not correlate reliably with the type of tumor or its degree of differentiation.

CK Isoenzymes in AMI

Time Course

Following the onset of AMI, blood levels of total CK and MB-CK do not exceed the normal range until 6 to 10 hours after the onset of symptoms; plasma levels then rise steadily until peak values occur an average of 24 hours after the onset of symptoms. Peak CK occurs somewhat later (28 hours) with Q-wave infarctions and somewhat earlier (15 hours) with non-Q wave infarctions [79]. Peak values of

Fig. 6-2
Distribution of total CK activity and cytosolic isoenzyme activity in human tissue.

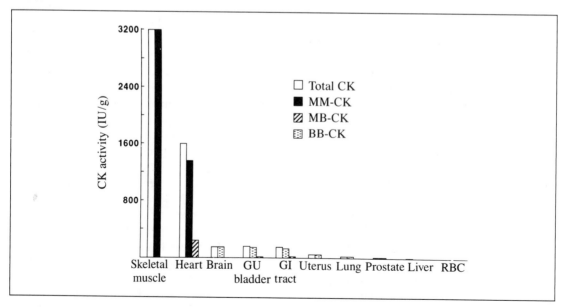

MB-CK are achieved slightly earlier for MB-CK than for MM-CK, probably because the former is cleared from the blood more rapidly. Values then gradually decline, entering the normal range by 48 to 72 hours after the onset of symptoms [19]. The MB-CK/MM-CK ratio (15:85) present in the myocardium is mirrored by a similar proportion in the blood following myocardial release after AMI. This approximate ratio is maintained throughout the CK time–activity curve.

Sensitivity and Specificity
The most important advantage of MB-CK over other biochemical markers of AMI is its great specificity for myocardium [80]. Myocardium is the only tissue that contains substantial levels of MB-CK (Fig. 6-2). The high myocardial CK activity levels, combined with the low concentration of MB-CK activity in normal plasma, which is close to the limit of detection of most assays, result in a high sensitivity of this marker for myocardial necrosis. It is generally agreed that assay of plasma MB-CK affords the most sensitive and specific, as well as cost-effective, means of diagnosing AMI. These parameters, of course, depend in part on the assay used, but for most assays the overall precision exceeds 95 percent [54, 81]. (The immunoprecipitation assays are exceptions and are substantially less reliable.) Use of the total CK assay data alone without isoenzyme study yields a similar sensitivity, but specificity is markedly lower (approximately 70 percent) [82, 83].

With the exception of the immune studies noted above, false-negative results are rare (as suggested by the high sensitivity figures) so long as blood sampling is performed within an appropriate time window. False-positive results, although also unusual, predictably occur in a variety of circumstances.

1. MB-CK may be released from tissue other than the heart. As outlined above, skeletal muscle can be induced to synthesize and release MB-CK by injury. This reaction has been documented in patients having a crush injury [68], an electrical injury [68, 69], dermatomyositis, polymyositis [67], and Du-

chenne's muscular dystrophy [84], as well as in professional athletes and marathon runners [65, 66]. Elevated levels of MB-CK have been documented not only in the blood of these patients but also directly in the skeletal muscle by analysis of extracts removed on biopsy of affected muscle. A study in our laboratory has demonstrated a late rise of MB-CK to levels above the normal range in 40 percent of individuals undergoing elective direct-current cardioversion of supraventricular arrhythmias, with peak values occurring an average of 40 hours after countershock (unpublished data). This time course corresponds to that observed following other forms of acute muscle injury and presumably reflects new synthesis and release of MB-CK by regenerating skeletal myocytes.

Release of MB-CK by skeletal muscle is suggested by: (1) An appropriate clinical setting (e.g., skeletal muscle disease or trauma). (2) An atypical time course for AMI: persistent minor degrees of MB-CK elevation in inflammatory disorders, delayed rise of MB-CK (with an immediate rise of MM-CK) following trauma. (3) A low relative percent of MB-CK. Although muscle injury may elevate the absolute plasma MB-CK level, the rise in MB-CK rarely constitutes more than 5 to 10 percent of total CK activity. Note that this figure may be in excess of the electrophoretic definition of myocardial necrosis. (4) A marked elevation of total CK activity. Myocardial infarction rarely increases total CK activity to levels in excess of 20 times the upper limit of normal (about 2500 IU/L in our laboratory); furthermore, a rise of total CK activity in excess of ten times the upper limit of normal on the basis of AMI is usually the result of substantial myocardial necrosis and therefore should be associated with diagnostic electrocardiographic (ECG) changes (usually including Q waves). Absence of these changes should raise suspicion of a nonmyocardial source of MB-CK. It should also be emphasized that certain assays, including electrophoresis and column techniques, are especially vulnerable to artifactual elevation of MB-CK values in the setting of a marked elevation of MM-CK; this situation can be avoided by sample dilution at the time of assay.

2. Apparent MB-CK plasma activity may be elevated in the absence of AMI because of artifact or laboratory error. One cause of this elevation, gel or column overload with MM-CK, has already been discussed. Hemolysis can also lead to artifactually elevated total and MB-CK values due to adenylate kinase interference. A faint band on gel electrophoresis attributable to albumin-associated fluorescence [47] is detectable slightly anodal to the expected position of the MB-CK band in most normal plasma samples. Artifactual fluorescence may also be present in patients with renal insufficiency (with or without dialysis) [85] and in those taking drugs that bind serum albumin, including diazepam, chlordiazepoxide, tricyclic antidepressants, and aspirin in high doses. Artifact should be suspected when a band migrates in an unusual position relative to MB-CK controls; such non-MB-CK bands usually also differ in color from the NADPH-generated fluorescence resulting from MB-CK activity.

3. As discussed earlier, several techniques, including ion-exchange methods and immunoassays that recognize the B-CK subunit, may yield false elevations of MB-CK activity because they fail to distinguish between MB-CK and BB-CK activity. This failure occasionally leads to misdiagnosis in patients with injury or surgery involving the prostate, uterus, gastrointestinal tract, or brain [3, 52, 86, 87] and following spontaneous or cesarean delivery [88]. Release of BB-CK is not detectable following uncomplicated ischemic stroke [89], presumably due to the integrity of the blood-brain barrier, but it may be released into the blood after trauma, infection, or diffuse hypoxic brain injury [89, 90]. Finally, tumors may rarely synthesize and release BB-CK [78]. The presence of BB-CK in the plasma is unusual outside these settings; even when detectable, it is usually present in concentrations that are insufficient to result in the

spurious elevation of MB-CK activity to levels above the reference range, and it is cleared from the blood rapidly [89].

4. Hypothyroidism has been associated with chronically elevated levels of plasma MM-CK and MB-CK. It is thought to be due to diminished plasma clearance of these isoenzymes by the reticuloendothelial system [91].

5. Macro-CK-1 may be detected as MB-CK in column assays and in immunoassays based on B-chain recognition [39, 92], resulting in a false-positive diagnosis of AMI. Macro-CK-1 is detected most commonly in the blood of elderly women and the chronically ill, with an incidence of 1.6 percent in hospitalized patients [39]. Correct diagnosis may be made by electrophoretic demonstration of band migration intermediate between control MM-CK and MB-CK bands. Macro-CK-2, when detected, is most often found in the blood of severely ill patients, possibly due to cell necrosis in the critically ill, with release of mitochondrial contents into the blood.

Current Role of MB-CK in Diagnosis of AMI

Since the introduction of enzyme markers during the late 1950s, the diagnosis of AMI has traditionally rested on the presence of "two out of three" of the triad of prolonged chest pain, ischemic ECG changes, and elevation of one of the "cardiac enzymes" [93]. However, since that time the accuracy of enzyme diagnosis has improved dramatically, whereas the sensitivity and specificity of clinical symptoms and ECG changes remain relatively poor [81]. Given the excellent sensitivity of the plasma MB-CK assay for the detection of myocardial necrosis, we believe that the diagnosis of AMI should not be made in the absence of a diagnostic rise and fall of plasma MB-CK (or LD isoenzymes) provided samples have been obtained at appropriate intervals. Conversely, a rise and fall in MB-CK and total CK in the appropriate proportion and following the typical time course, strongly suggests the diagnosis of infarction even when symptoms and ECG changes are not typical. (However, in such cases, spurious elevation of

MB-CK due to artifact, BB-CK, macro-CK, or a nonmyocardial source of MB-CK should be sought, as dictated by the clinical setting [94].)

At our institution, samples are obtained on admission and every 4 hours thereafter for 36 hours. This procedure allows for infarct size determination, as outlined below, and facilitates early transfer to stepped-down care in the approximately 70 percent of patients in whom AMI is ruled out. We utilize the glass bead assay [50], with the upper normal reference value of 14 IU/L. We consider the enzymatic data as positive for AMI if serial plasma samples separated by at least 4 hours exceed the upper reference range or if there is an increase in MB-CK of 50 percent between two samples, with at least one sample exceeding the upper reference limit. If only a single specimen is available, the diagnosis of AMI is made only if MB-CK exceeds the upper reference limit by at least 100 percent. In all cases, values should return to the normal range within 48 to 72 hours.

Between 16 and 43 percent of all CCU patients in whom plasma MB-CK activity exceeds the upper normal range have normal values for total CK activity [95, 96]. Studies suggest that these patients have myocardial necrosis as the source of their MB-CK elevation, as the incidence of typical chest pain, new ECG changes, LD_1/LD_2 "flip," and time course of the MB-CK rise and fall are similar to that seen for AMI with elevated MB-CK *and* total CK activity [96, 97]. Histologic changes of AMI have been documented in one such patient at autopsy [95]. The long-term prognosis in these patients appears to be good in the absence of superimposed severe medical illness [97, 98].

Plasma MB-CK is also useful for the diagnosis of AMI following noncardiac surgery, when MM-CK may be elevated as a result of surgical trauma. In the absence of myocardial necrosis, MB-CK remains within the normal range [99]. (It is not clear if this statement holds true after the first 1 to 2 days following surgery, when injured skeletal muscle may begin to synthesize MB-CK.) Cardiac isoenzymes are not helpful following cardiac sur-

gery, as even minimal surgical manipulation can release MB-CK.

LD Isoenzymes for the Diagnosis of AMI

BIOCHEMICAL PROPERTIES AND TISSUE DISTRIBUTION OF LD

Lactate dehydrogenase is a tetramer of MW 135,000 that catalyzes the reversible reduction of pyruvate to form lactatic acid.

$$\text{Lactate} + \text{NAD} \xrightleftharpoons{\quad LD \quad} \text{pyruvate} + \text{NADH}$$

LD thus controls an important step in carbohydrate metabolism. Under normal aerobic conditions, pyruvate, a product of glycolysis, is irreversibly converted to acetyl coenzyme A, which then enters the citric acid cycle to generate ATP. However, under the anaerobic conditions that may exist in active muscle, pyruvate accumulates at a rate too rapid for immediate oxidation and is converted to lactate by LD. The lactic acid thus formed in muscle can enter the circulation and be transported to the liver, where it is converted to glucose by gluconeogenesis. Alternatively, the liver can oxidize lactate via LD to re-form pyruvate for oxidative phosphorylation.

Two LD subunit types exist: M type, which is so designated because the homotetramer M_4 is the predominant isoenzyme in skeletal muscle; and H type, which is named for heart tissue, where H_4 is the most abundant LD isoenzyme [100]. In addition to these two homotetramers, all three heterotetramers are found: H_3M_1, H_2M_2, and H_1M_3. Dissociated polypeptide chains are inactive; only the tetramer has enzymatic activity. As is the case for CK, the two polypeptide chains differ in sequence and charge: The H chain is more negatively charged; consequently, H_4 is the fastest-migrating LD isoenzyme by gel electrophoresis, M_4 is the slowest [101], and the three heterotetramers migrate between these two based on their M and H chain content. These facts are the basis of the standard nomenclature for the LD isoenzymes: $H_4 = LD_1$, $H_3M_1 = LD_2$, . . . , $M_4 = LD_5$. The isoenzymes also differ in their biochemical characteristics: H_4 has a low K_m for pyruvate and is strongly inhibited by pyruvate; this isoenzyme favors the rapid oxidation of lactate to pyruvate in the heart; pyruvate thus formed can in turn enter the citric acid cycle. M_4 has a higher K_m for pyruvate and is not inhibited by pyruvate; it favors anaerobic metabolism in exercising muscle by converting pyruvate to lactate, which can then be transported to the liver for gluconeogenesis and resolution of the "oxygen debt." The heterotetramers have biochemical properties intermediate between the two homotetramers.

The LD molecule is stable. Enzymatic activity is maximally preserved by storage at room temperature; refrigeration results in loss of activity [102], with relatively greater loss of LD_5 and the other M-containing isoenzymes. Serum is usually assayed rather than plasma, as platelets in plasma are rich in LD activity and may result in spurious elevation. In addition, red blood cells have abundant LD activity, especially LD_1 and LD_2; therefore it is important that samples not be hemolyzed.

Assay of total LD activity may be achieved by detecting the rate of NADH production (monitored by the rate of change at ultraviolet absorbance: 340 nm) from lactate and NAD in the presence of an aliquot of serum. Isoenzyme assay is by gel electrophoresis and densitometry; no column or immune assays are in current use. The hydroxybutyrate dehydrogenase (HBD) assay gives indirect information on LD isoenzymes. This method employs 2-oxybutyrate rather than lactate as a substrate. Because 2-oxybutyrate is preferentially reduced by LD_1 and LD_2, LD release by myocardium results in substantial HBD assay elevations. This assay is less specific than electrophoresis, as LD_4 and LD_5, although lower in HBD activity than LD_1 and LD_2, do yield some signal. As a result of these drawbacks, this technique is not commonly used. Selective inactivation of LD_4 and LD_5 by heating to 56° to 65°C suffers from similar problems. Consequently, gel electrophoresis is the most widely used method for assay of LD isoenzymes.

Although LD_1 is the most abundant LD isoenzyme present in cardiac tissue, making up about one-half of the LD activity present in myocardium, other tissues are also rich in LD_1: kidney, erythrocytes, pancreas, and gastric smooth muscle contain 30 percent or more of total LD activity as the LD_1 isoenzyme. Consequently, a rise in serum LD_1 activity alone is not specific for myocardial necrosis.

SERUM LD FOR THE DIAGNOSIS OF AMI

The LD activity in the blood rises out of the normal range by 10 hours after the onset of AMI. Peak blood levels are reached between 24 and 48 hours after the onset of symptoms. Unlike CK, LD demonstrates a prolonged decline, so that serum levels do not return to the normal range until 10 to 14 days after infarction; consequently, sample collection need not be more frequent than once daily. Clearance of LD from the blood is governed by specific receptors in the surface of the cells of the reticuloendothelial system [103]. The isoenzyme profile in the blood following infarction reflects that seen in myocardium, i.e., predominance of LD_1. The LD_1/LD_2 ratio has been used to distinguish serum LD elevations due to myocardial injury from those arising from other sources. An LD_1/LD_2 ratio that is greater than or equal to 1.0 is generally regarded as the cutoff for the diagnosis of AMI. A ratio of 0.76 has also been recommended; it affords a greater sensitivity but a lower specificity than the higher cutoff [81]. Muscle or liver injury, the most common sources of elevated serum LD activity, are distinguished from cardiac necrosis by the preponderance of LD_4 and LD_5 associated with these conditions. However, injury of skeletal muscle may, in a manner analogous to CK, induce reexpression of LD_1 and LD_2 [104–106], the "fetal" isoenzymes. The effect of this response on the specificity of the LD diagnosis of AMI in the presence of skeletal injury is unclear. LD isoenzyme release patterns due to disease involving the kidney, pancreas, and stomach may be difficult to distinguish from that associated with AMI. Germ cell tumors may also give a false-positive pattern for AMI [107]. Hemolysis, either intravascular or occurring after specimen collection, also releases LD_1. Because of the widespread tissue distribution of LD and the overlap of the isoenzyme profile between tissues, no method can be entirely satisfactory for distinguishing cardiac from noncardiac sources of enzyme release. As a result, when both are available, CK isoenzyme analysis is preferable to LD isoenzyme assay for the diagnosis of AMI. However, if blood samples are not available for the first 48 hours after the suspected myocardial injury, the sustained elevation of serum LD makes assay and isoenzyme fractionation of this marker a more reliable indicator of infarction than CK.

Other Biochemical Markers of AMI

SERUM MYOGLOBIN

Myoglobin is a heme-containing protein of MW 17,800. Because of its affinity for molecular oxygen, it is believed to function as an "oxygen reservoir" in striated muscle. Myoglobin is present in high levels in both skeletal and cardiac muscle [108, 109], with no known tissue-specific isoenzymes; thus it is not a specific marker of AMI. Myoglobin functions as an oxygen carrier rather than as a catalyst; therefore its activity is measured immunologically by RIA rather than by enzymatic activity. Following AMI, myoglobin rapidly appears in the blood with detectable elevation as early as 1.5 hours after the onset of symptoms [110]. This early rise is probably a result of its low molecular weight and rapid diffusing capacity. Its relatively small molecular size also permits clearance of myoglobin through the glomerular filtration apparatus (hence the danger of myoglobin precipitation in the renal tubules and acute renal failure following massive skeletal muscle injury). Renal clearance of myoglobin is the mechanism for the rapid decline in serum levels after peak concentrations occur at 6 to 7 hours [111]; plasma myoglobin

levels often return to the normal range within 24 hours after onset of symptoms [110, 111]. Thus this marker may be falsely negative within 24 hours of AMI in patients who have sustained a small infarction. The poor specificity of myoglobin for cardiac muscle injury remains the major drawback for the use of this molecule as a diagnostic marker of AMI [112, 113].

MYOSIN LIGHT CHAINS

The myosin light chains (MLC), which are covalently linked to the myosin heavy chain together with the amino half of the myosin heavy chain make up the "head" region of the molecule. This portion of the myosin molecule is the site of ATPase activity necessary for myofilament sliding and disengagement, a critical element of the contractile apparatus. Apparently, the covalent disulfide linkages joining the two MLC molecules to each myosin heavy chain undergo breakdown following myocardial necrosis, liberating MLC into the circulation. The mechanism of this process is unknown; it has been postulated that enzymes released by inflammatory cells at the site of infarction play a role in this process [114]; acidification of the infarcted region may also be important [115]. MLC-2 appears in the serum following AMI [116], with detectable levels within 6 hours of the onset of AMI [117]. However, peak serum levels do not occur until about 5 days after AMI, presumably due to ongoing liberation of MLC from the contractile apparatus [117]. MLC-1 has also been studied as a marker of AMI [118]. Clearance of these low-molecular-weight (MW 20,000 to 27,000) markers is via the kidney. When separated from the myosin heavy chain, MLC has no enzymatic activity, and thus detection is by RIA. MLC in the diagnosis of AMI is currently under investigation but is not in routine clinical use.

AST

Aspartate transaminase, historically the first enzyme discovered to be elevated in the blood after AMI, is a less sensitive marker than CK. In addition, its presence in high levels in liver, muscle, and other tissues and the lack of myocardium-specific isoenzymes substantially limit this molecule as a diagnostic marker of AMI. It has no advantages over CK or LD and is no longer in widespread use.

A variety of other plasma markers of AMI have been employed and discarded, primarily owing to lack of specificity. During the first half of this century, prior to the observation of plasma enzyme elevations following AMI, rises in white blood cell count and erythrocyte sedimentation rate were noted 2 to 4 days after AMI. These changes were clearly nonspecific and were never taken as other than confirmatory epiphenomena.

Infarct Size Determination Using MB-CK Assay

Serial analysis of plasma MB-CK samples has been used to provide accurate estimates of infarct size. The initial impetus to assess infarct size using enzyme determinations was twofold. First, enzymatic quantitation of tissue damage would be likely to provide a better assessment of prognosis than cruder parameters such as extent of pulmonary congestion or cumulative ST-segment elevation. Second, an objective, quantitative index would be helpful in studies designed to evaluate infarct size limitation. The use of enzymatically determined infarct size as an endpoint would permit accumulation of data from each patient; far fewer patients would be required in such a study than in a comparable trial in which death or other infrequent clinical events are monitored as primary endpoints [119].

Studies during the early 1970s in the rabbit model demonstrated that CK is homogeneously distributed throughout the ventricle and that the CK activity detectable in the ventricle following AMI is diminished; furthermore, the magnitude of CK activity depletion is directly proportional to infarct size as determined histologically [120]. Studies in the dog model allowed quantitation of this relation based on plasma CK activity following a se-

ries of experimental observations: (1) A region of infarcted myocardium loses 85 percent of endogeneous CK activity; the magnitude of this CK depletion from the expected CK activity of the entire ventricle is directly proportional to infarct size. (2) Most "depleted" CK is inactivated in situ or in the cardiac lymphatic system. However, a predictable fraction (15 percent) of the depleted CK is released into the blood [121]. (3) Serial plasma CK determinations allow accurate quantitation of cumulative CK release into the blood. It is achieved by: (a) Determination of incremental CK release between each two time points as manifested by the rise in plasma CK activity corrected for concomitant CK monoexponential clearance by the reticuloendothelial system [103, 122]. (b) Summation of these values over the entire CK time–activity curve, yielding the cumulative CK release per liter of plasma. Total CK release is then obtained by correcting for the volume of distribution of CK (the plasma volume). (c) Because only a fraction of the "depleted" CK appears in the blood, cumulative CK release is converted to depleted CK activity by dividing by the "release ratio" (15 percent). (d) The quantity of depleted CK activity can be converted to infarct size in grams of tissue, as the CK content of dog (and human) myocardium is known. In humans, the monoexponential disappearance constant (K_d) for MB-CK is 0.0015 min^{-1}; the plasma volume is assumed to be 45 ml/kg of lean body mass, and myocardium contains 260 IU of MB-CK per gram of tissue. K_d has been shown to be unaffected by changes in cardiac output or by cardiac-active drugs. This method has been validated by comparing the enzymatic determination of infarct size with gross pathologic results in the animal model [123] and in humans [124]. Furthermore, enzymatic determination of infarct size in humans has been shown to be predictive of postinfarction hemodynamics [125], ejection fraction [126], prognosis [127], and incidence of ventricular arrhythmias [128].

The relations outlined above were developed and confirmed in the experimental and clinical setting of nonreperfused AMI. Reperfusion within 6 hours of the onset of AMI causes a change in the kinetics of myocardial CK release, resulting in an altered CK time–activity curve. Early reperfusion is associated with a reduction in the time from onset of infarction to peak CK, as well as an increase in the magnitude of peak CK relative to total infarct size. This is especially evident with reperfusion occurring less than 4 hours after the onset of AMI. A variety of factors may be responsible for these changes, including: (1) Augmented blood flow to the necrotic region; as a result, a greater proportion of the 85 percent of CK that is "depleted" may enter the blood rather than undergoing local denaturation. (2) Reperfusion may result in more rapid breakdown of irreversibly injured tissue, possibly due to oxidation injury.

The net effect of these changes on CK kinetics is to augment the "release ratio"; the quantity of CK depleted from the myocardium is not changed [129]. As a result, enzymatic estimates of infarct size are altered. The magnitude of change in the release ratio and whether the change is predictably dependent on the time to reperfusion are not yet clear. Therefore at the present time there is no widely accepted method for enzymatic quantitation of infarct size following successful reperfusion.

MM-CK and MB-CK Subforms

MECHANISM OF SUBFORM CONVERSION

During the late 1970s, Wevers and his colleagues showed that serum from patients who had suffered an AMI, upon prolonged electrophoresis at 90 volts, exhibited three CK bands in the MM region instead of the expected single band. On the same gels, MB-CK was resolved into two component bands [130, 131]. These multiple bands of a single isoenzyme have been designated sub-bands, and the CK molecules corresponding to each band have been termed subforms or subisoenzymes. The same group also observed a shift in relative sub-band intensity with time after AMI: The slowest migrating (most cathodal) MM-CK and MB-CK sub-bands were most intense dur-

ing the early hours after infarction; with increasing time after AMI the faster-migrating forms become dominant. Wevers et al. also showed that only the slow-migrating subforms of each isoenzyme, designated MM3 and MB2, are present in tissue. The faster migrating subforms, MB1-CK, MM2-CK, and MM1-CK, are sequentially produced by a modification of the tissue forms after release into the blood. [Like the three cytosolic CK isoenzymes, the subisoenzymes can be designated by their relative rate of electrophoretic migration toward the anode: MM3-CK and MB2-CK are the slow-migrating forms, MM1-CK and MB1-CK are the fast-migrating forms, and MM2-CK is intermediate between the MM3 and MM1 subisoenzymes (Fig. 6-3). This convention is somewhat confusing, as the numeric designation is the reverse of the sequence of appearance following AMI.] Finally, Wevers et al. reproduced the conversion of MM3-CK to MM1-CK in vitro by incubating purified tissue MM3-CK with serum [130]. This conversion can also be demonstrated in vitro with MB2-CK.

In 1981, using nondenaturing chromatofocusing chromatography, we isolated and pu-

Fig. 6-3
MM-CK and MB-CK subforms in the blood following AMI. Progressive conversion from the tissue subforms (of MM-CK and MB-CK) to the faster-migrating, modified subforms occurs with increasing time after AMI. (Courtesy of Helena Labortories.)

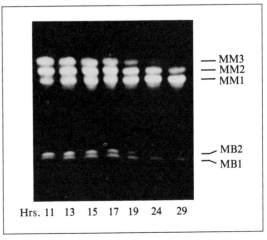

— MM3
— MM2
— MM1

— MB2
— MB1

Hrs. 11   13   15   17   19   24   29

rified the three MM subforms [132]. We subsequently demonstrated that subform conversion in the blood is mediated by the plasma enzyme carboxypeptidase-N (CP-N) and reproduced the conversion in vitro in the absence of serum by incubating purified tissue MM3-CK with CP-N [133]. Using peptide mapping and amino acid sequence analysis, the mechanism of MM3-CK modification was shown to be via cleavage of the positively charged amino acid lysine from the carboxy-terminus of the M subunit(s); the result is a polypeptide chain having a slightly greater net negative charge (by one unit) and therefore a faster rate of migration toward the positive electrode [133, 134]. The conversion reaction progresses rapidly, both in vivo and in vitro; MM3-CK is completely converted to MM1-CK in 2 hours at 37°C [133]. Thus the sequential predominance of the three MM-CK subforms can be explained as follows: Initially, release of MM3-CK from necrotic myocardium makes the tissue form the most abundant plasma MM subform; cleavage of the terminal lysine from one of the two M polypeptides of MM3-CK by CP-N then yields the heterodimer MM2-CK, which transiently becomes the predominant subform several hours after the cessation of CK release; removal of the remaining terminal lysine from the second

M-chain by CP-N produces MM1-CK (Fig. 6-4), which is the most abundant MM subform after 16 to 20 hours. Stepwise M-chain alteration has been confirmed as the mechanism of subform conversion by dissociation/reassociation experiments, in which the M chains of MM3-CK and MM1-CK were split into unpaired single chains by incubation with urea; random reassociation induced by removal of urea via dialysis produced all three subforms; similarly, dissociation and reassociation of the heterodimer MM2-CK produced all three subforms, as expected. In contrast, dissociation and reassociation of the homodimer MM1-CK alone yielded only MM1-CK; MM3-CK treated alone produced analogous results [133]. Preliminary work in our laboratory implicates a similar mechanism in the conversion of MB2-CK to MB1-CK.

CLINICAL APPLICATIONS OF SUBFORM ANALYSIS

The advent of thrombolytic therapy for AMI and the demonstration of its efficacy in reduction of mortality [135] has underlined the need for both earlier diagnosis of AMI and a noninvasive means to assess reperfusion success.

Fig. 6-4
Molecular mechanism of MM-CK subform conversion in the blood. Loss of a single positively charged lysine residue (Lys +) yields a more negatively charged molecule, resulting in faster anodal migration.

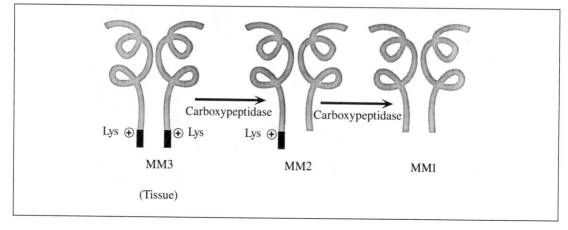

Early Diagnosis of AMI

The sensitivity of total CK and CK-MB for diagnosis of AMI is low during the early hours of AMI [136]. Myoglobin rises out of the normal range within 2 hours of AMI, but the poor specificity of this marker and the several hours required to perform the RIA assay have limited its usefulness. Consequently, no currently available biochemical marker is reliable during the first 10 hours of AMI. Because thrombolytic therapy is most efficacious only when administered within the first 3 to 4 hours of AMI, the decision to initiate treatment is, of necessity, based on symptoms and ECG findings, which are sensitive but nonspecific [136], as evidenced by the fact that only about 30 percent of patients admitted to the CCU are subsequently shown to have infarction. Because thrombolysis carries a small risk of intracranial hemorrhage and other bleeding complications, an early diagnostic marker with a low rate of false positives (i.e., high specificity) would be valuable. This problem of diagnostic uncertainty during the early hours of AMI are further compounded if the indications for thrombolysis are extended to include non-Q wave infarction, as about two-thirds of these patients present with ST-segment depression, which is nonspecific and similar to changes of transient ischemia.

CK subform analysis shows promise as an early diagnostic indicator of AMI. At steady state in a normal individual, small amounts of MM-CK from skeletal muscle, and MM-CK and MB-CK from cardiac tissue, are continuously released into the blood, converted to the modified subforms, and cleared from the blood. Because the conversion reaction is rapid, the tissue form, MM3-CK, contributes only a relatively small percent of the total MM-CK isoenzyme activity (20 to 35 percent). With the onset of AMI, the rate of myocardial MM3-CK release into the blood quickly exceeds the rate of conversion of MM3-CK to MM2-CK and MM1-CK, and MM3-CK as a percent of total MM-CK activity rises. A similar rise in the MB2-CK/MB1-CK ratio occurs. Thus rapid release of small quantities of MM3-CK is sufficient to raise the percent MM3-CK and MB2-CK before the value for total CK ac-

tivity is sufficiently increased to exceed the upper limit of normal. For example, if a patient has a baseline MM-CK activity of 60 IU/L, with the upper limit of normal at 120 IU/L, the baseline MM3-CK activity would be approximately 20 IU/L, i.e., 33 percent of MM-CK activity. An initial release of MM3-CK early in AMI might raise the MM3-CK to 60 IU/L but the total only to 100 IU/L, a value within the normal range; however, the MM3-CK now constitutes 60 percent of MM-CK activity. In effect, each patient's plasma MM-CK activity serves as its own control, with perturbations in steady-state activity readily detectable as changes in subisoenzyme distribution even when CK activity is in the normal reference range.

Initial reports using the MM-CK subform distribution for early diagnosis of AMI in animals [137] and in several studies involving human subjects [138–140] have been promising, with the MM3-CK/MM1-CK ratio rising out of the normal range 4 to 6 hours after AMI onset. However, the major drawback for the use of the MM-CK subforms is their lack of specificity. As discussed earlier, assay of total CK activity rather than MB-CK activity for the diagnosis of AMI introduces a 20 to 30 percent false-positive rate due to release of MM-CK from skeletal muscle [82, 83]. Such elevations, due to exercise [141–143] or myositis [144], have been shown to be associated with a rise in percent MM3-CK [141–144], thus reducing the specificity of this finding.

Because of the lack of specificity of MM-CK subform analysis, we have evaluated the utility of MB-CK subforms in the early diagnosis of AMI. Unlike previous systems used for subform separation, which required 1.5 hours of electrophoresis at 90 volts for adequate resolution, the prototype instrument we tested (Rep; Helena Laboratories, Beaumont, TX) performs electrophoresis at 1400 volts on a dynamically cooled gel to separate the tissue subform, MB2-CK, from the plasma-modified subform, MB1-CK, in 12 minutes. The system was validated using purified MB2-CK and MB1-CK reconstituted in heat-inactivated serum. The assay is linear for both MB-CK subforms, even at very low levels ($r = .99$ between 1.25 and 30 IU/L, N = 70; upper normal limit 14 IU/L), is highly reproducible and generates the expected MB2-CK/MB1-CK ratio when both subforms are present in serum (r = .95, N = 144). Sensitivity is 1.0 IU/L; total assay time is 20 minutes.

This MB-CK subform assay was applied to 11 patients with AMI in whom an initial plasma sample, obtained within 3 hours of the onset of symptoms, was still within the normal range for MB-CK. Results were compared with data obtained from 24 normal control subjects. The mean percent of MB2-CK was 64.1 percent among the normal individuals and 81.4 percent among the early infarct patients. Eight of eleven patients with AMI had a percent MB2-CK greater than 80 percent; samples were positive as early as 1 hour after the onset of symptoms. In contrast, among the 24 normal individuals, only one had more than 80 percent of MB-CK present as the MB2-CK subform. Thus these preliminary data suggest that MB-CK subform analysis is rapid and specific, and that it provides early diagnosis during the first 3 hours of AMI.

The role of early diagnostic methods in conjunction with thrombolysis will be defined as better methods become widely available. As currently practiced, thrombolysis is administered in the emergency room after physician evaluation. An assay with a 15-minute "turnaround time" might allow collection and reporting of objective data before initiation of therapy. Alternatively, drug therapy might be initiated in patients with a high clinical suspicion of AMI, with termination of drug infusion based on results of subform analysis available within minutes of initiating thrombolytic therapy. The latter course would maximize the potential for myocardial salvage while limiting the risk associated with a full course of therapy to a patient without AMI. A similar protocol might be employed if thrombolytic therapy were initiated by paramedics at the site of initial patient contact "in the field."

Noninvasive Diagnosis of Reperfusion

Initial studies of reperfusion therapy of AMI used intracoronary administration of drug, with coronary angiography to assess therapeutic success as well as to allow for early mechanical intervention in the event of drug failure [145]. More recently, intravenous therapy has been employed to avoid the therapeutic delay associated with acute angiography; however, early angiography was performed to evaluate reperfusion success and to permit early angioplasty in the event of drug failure [146]. Evidence is now accumulating to suggest that angioplasty performed early as an adjunct to thrombolytic therapy confers no advantage over elective angioplasty performed several days later [147]. Therefore many protocols no longer utilize early angiography; as a result, success of therapy remains obscure for several days. If thrombolytic success could be assessed noninvasively, the 30 percent of patients who fail to exhibit clot lysis would not be subjected to catheterization on day 2 or 3 for possible angioplasty, as there is no advantage in late reperfusion. Furthermore, if a noninvasive marker documented lack of success within 1 to 2 hours, mechanical reperfusion might be attempted in selected high risk patients with failure of drug-induced clot lysis.

The rationale for the use of subforms for detection of reperfusion are twofold. (1) Reperfusion is associated with rapid washout of CK from the region of infarction (see above). (2) Because MM3-CK conversion to MM2-CK and MM1-CK is rapid, prolonged MM3-CK elevation represents a marker of persistent CK release and therefore suggests failure of thrombolysis. Observations in patients undergoing thrombolytic therapy have shown that the percent MM3-CK rises to 75 percent followed by a decline (reflecting rapid MM3-CK conversion) after MM3-CK release from tissue has slowed or ceased.

In a study of 103 consecutive patients who underwent attempted reperfusion of AMI at our institutions, we compared the rate of decline of percent MM3-CK (expressed as the slope in a plot of percent MM3-CK versus time after the onset of AMI) with reperfusion success [148]. All patients underwent acute angiography to evaluate therapeutic success. Percent MM3-CK was determined by plasma electrophoresis using a commercially available system. Agarose gels from representative patients are shown in Figure 6-5. The 55 patients with successful reperfusion had an average rate of percent MM3-CK decline of 4.18 percent per hour, whereas the group of patients with angiographically proved unsuccessful reperfusion had a substantially lower rate of decline, 2.37 percent per hour; the differences between these two groups were highly statistically significant. In addition, using a cutoff value of 3.1 percent per hour, 48 of 55 successfully reperfused patients were above the cutoff, whereas 29 of 39 nonreperfused patients had a slope below the cutoff value. Thus the sensitivity for detection of reperfusion was 87 percent with a specificity of 74 percent. Among 30 patients with AMI in whom no therapy was attempted, 27 of 30 (90 percent) were below the cutoff values. In contrast, the time from onset of symptoms to peak MB-CK, which has occasionally been used as an index of reperfusion success, demonstrated marked overlap between the two groups; specificity was 49 percent.

Other investigations have reported an earlier time to peak MM3-CK/MM1-CK ratio in patients with successful reperfusion than in patients without successful reperfusion [149, 150]; because no "cutoff" times were suggested, the accuracy of this method for detecting reperfusion is not known. Work is currently in progress in our laboratory to detect reperfusion based on the MB-CK rather than the MM-CK subforms. Diagnosis with such a system would be specific, without confounding influence due to MM3-CK release from skeletal muscle injury due to cardioversion, cardiopulmonary resuscitation, or cardiac catheterization [151].

Fig. 6-5
CK-MM subforms in AMI with and without thrombolysis. *A.* Unsuccessful reperfusion is characterized by ongoing MM3-CK release and prolonged MM3-CK predominance. *B.* Successful reperfusion is characterized by cessation of CK release followed by complete conversion to the modified forms.

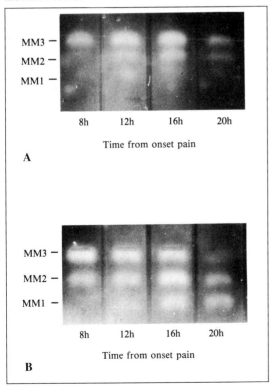

Editorial Comments

Plasma enzymes remain the "gold standard" as markers of AMI, with CK and its isoenzymes proving to be the most reliable and cost-effective markers. Several issues remain unresolved, however: Can CK release occur in sufficient amounts to measure a change above baseline in reversible ischemia? This question is probably not essential to resolve, as it depends on the definition of reversible and irreversible injury, and such a distinction is likely to represent a continuum and not a fine line. So long as we can distinguish between a definite myocardial infarction with myocardial necrosis and severe ischemia without major *myocardial necrosis, we should be able to make rational decisions about patient care. Can we develop a highly sensitive and specific enzymatic marker for myocardial necrosis that allows us to make quick decisions regarding thrombolysis? MB-CK subform analysis may provide us with a rapid and accurate "turnaround time," and we look forward to further progress in this area.* G.S.F.

References

1. Wohlgemuth, J. Unersuchungen uber die Diastasen. *Biochem. Z.* 9:10, 1908.
2. Gutman, E. B., Spraul, E. E., and Gutman, A. B. Significance of increased phosphatase activity of bone at the site of osteoblastic metastases secondary to carcinoma of the prostate gland. *Am. J. Cancer* 28:485, 1936.
3. Karmen, A., Wroblewski, F., and La Due, J. Transaminase activity in human blood. *J. Clin. Invest.* 34:126, 1954.
4. LaDue, J. S., Wroblewski, F., and Karmen, A. Serum glutamic oxaloacetic transaminase activity in human acute transmural myocardial infarction. *Science* 120:497, 1954.
5. Wroblewski, F., and LaDue, J. S. Lactic dehydrogenase activity in blood. *Proc. Soc. Exp. Biol. Med.* 90:210, 1955.
6. Sayre, F. W., and Hill, B. R. Fractionisation of serum lactic dehydrogenase by salt concentration gradient elution and paper electrophoresis. *Proc. Soc. Exp. Biol. Med.* 96:695, 1959.
7. Vesell, E. S., and Bearn, A. G. Localization of lactic acid dehydrogenase activity in serum fractions. *Proc. Soc. Exp. Biol. Med.* 94:96, 1957.
8. Wieland, T. H., and Pfleiderer, G. Nachweis der Heterogenitat von Milchsauredehydrogenase verschiedenen ursprungs durch Tragerelektrophorese. *Biochem. Z.* 329:112, 1957.
9. Markert, C. L., and Moller, F. Multiple forms of enzymes: Tissue, ontogenic, and species specific patterns. *Proc. Natl. Acad. Sci. U.S.A.* 45:753, 1959.
10. Ebashi, S., Toyakura, Y., Momoi, H., et al. High creatine phosphokinase activity of sera of progressive muscular dystrophy. *J. Biochem.* 46:103, 1959.
11. Dreyfus, V. C., Schapira, G., Resnais, J., et al. Le creatine-kinase serique dans le diagnostic de l'infarctus myocardique. *Rev. Fr. Etud. Clin. Biol.* 5:386, 1960.
12. Van der Veen, K. J., and Willebrands, A. F. Isoenzymes of creatine phosphokinase in tissue extracts and in normal and pathological sera. *Clin. Chim. Acta* 13:312, 1966.
13. Schwartz, A., Wood, J. M., Allen, J. C., et al. Biochemical and morphologic correlates of cardiac ischemia. I. Membrane systems. *Am. J. Cardiol.* 32:46, 1973.
14. Ahmed, S. A., Williamson, J. R., Roberts, R., et al. The association of increased plasma MB CPK activity and irreversible ischemic myocardial injury in the dog. *Circulation* 54:187, 1976.
15. Siegel, R. J., Said, J. W., Shell, W. E., et al. Identification and localization of creatine kinase B and M in normal, ischemic and necrotic myocardium: An immunohistochemical study.

J. Mol. Cell. Cardiol. 16:95, 1984.
16. Michael, L. H., Hunt, J. R., Weilbaecher, D., et al. Creatine kinase and phosphorylase in cardiac lymph: Coronary occlusion and reperfusion. *Am. J. Physiol.* 248(Heart Circ. Physiol. 17):H350, 1985.
17. Roberts, R. Diagnostic assessment of myocardial infarction based on lactate dehydrogenase and creatine kinase isoenzymes. *Heart Lung* 10:486, 1981.
18. Shell, W. E., DeWood, M. A., Kligerman, M., et al. Early appearance of MB-creatine kinase activity in nontransmural myocardial infarction detected by a sensitive assay for the isoenzyme. *Am. J. Med.* 71:254, 1981.
19. Roberts, R. Measurement of Enzymes in Cardiology. In R. J. Linden (ed.), *Techniques in Life Sciences.* New York: Elsevier, 1983.
20. Dawson, D. M., Eppenberger, H. M., and Kaplan, N. O. Creatine kinase: Evidence for a dimeric structure. *Biochem. Biophys. Res. Commun.* 21:346, 1965.
21. Roberts, R., and Grace, A. M. Purification of mitochondrial creatine kinase. *J. Biol. Chem.* 255:2870, 1980.
22. Basson, C. T., Grace, A. M., and Roberts, R. Enzyme kinetics of a highly purified mitochondrial creatine kinase in comparison with cytosolic forms. *Mol. Cell Biochem.* 67:151, 1985.
23. Jacobus, W. E., and Lehninger, A. L. Creatine kinase of rat heart mitochondria. *J. Biol. Chem.* 248:4803, 1973.
24. Perryman, M. B., Strauss, A. W., Buettner, T. L., et al. Molecular heterogeneity of creatine kinase isoenzymes. *Biochem. Biophys. Acta* 747:284, 1983.
25. Villareal-Levy, G., Ma, T. S., Kerner, S. A., et al. Human creatine kinase: Isolation and sequence analysis of cDNA clones for the B subunit, development of subunit specific probes and determination of gene copy number. *Biochem. Biophys. Res. Commun.* 144:1116, 1987.
26. Perryman, M. B., Kerner, S. A., Bohlmeyer, T. J., et al. Isolation and sequence analysis of a full-length cDNA for human M creatine kinase. *Biochem. Biophys. Res. Commun.* 140:981, 1986.
27. Bessman, S., and Carpenter, C. The creatine-creatine phosphate energy shuttle. *Annu. Rev. Biochem.* 54:831, 1985.
28. Mahler, M. First-order kinetics of muscle oxygen consumption, and an equivalent proportionality between QO_2 and phosphorylcreatine level. *J. Gen. Physiol.* 86:135, 1985.
29. Meyer, R. A., Sweeney, H. L., and Kushmerick, M. J. A simple analysis of the "phosphocreatine shuttle." *Am. J. Physiol.* 246(Cell Physiol. 15):C365, 1984.

30. Houk, T. W., and Putnam, S. V. Location of the creatine phosphokinase binding site of myosin. *Biochem. Biophys. Res. Commun.* 55:1271, 1973.

31. Turner, D. C., Maier, V., and Eppenberger, H. M. A protein that binds specifically to the M-line of skeletal muscle is identified as the muscle form of creatine kinase. *Proc. Natl. Acad. Sci. U.S.A.* 70:702, 1973.

32. Wallimann, T., Kuhn, H. J., Pelloni, G., et al. Localization of creatine kinase isoenzymes in myofibrils. II. Chicken heart muscle. *J. Cell. Biol.* 75:318, 1977.

33. Neumeier, D. Subcellular Distribution of Creatine Kinase Isoenzymes. In H. Lang (ed.), *Creatine Kinase Isoenzymes.* New York: Springer-Verlag, 1981.

34. Sharov, V. G., Saks, V. A., Smirnov, V. N., et al. An electron microscopic histochemical investigation of the localization of creatine phosphokinase in heart cells. *Biochim. Biophys. Acta* 468:495, 1977.

35. Saks, V. A., Lipina, N. V., Sharov, V. G., et al. The localization of the MM isozyme of creatine phosphokinase on the surface membrane of myocardial cells and its functional coupling to ouabain-inhibited (Na^+K^+)-ATPase. *Biochim. Biophys. Acta* 465:550, 1977.

36. Baskin, R. J., and Deamer, D. W. A membrane-bound creatine phosphokinase in fragmented sarcoplasmic reticulum. *J. Biol. Chem.* 245:1345, 1970.

37. Scholte, H. R., Weijers, P. J., and Wit-Peeters, E. M. The localization of mitochondrial creatine kinase, and its use for the determination of the sidedness of submitochondrial particles. *Biochim. Biophys. Acta* 291:764, 1973.

38. Morin, L. G. Creatine kinase: Stability, inactivation, reactivation. *Clin. Chem.* 23:646, 1977.

39. Urdal, P., and Landaas, S. Macro creatine kinase BB in serum, and some data on its prevalence. *Clin. Chem.* 25:461, 1979.

40. Lang, H., and Wurzburg, U. Creatine kinase, an enzyme of many forms. *Clin. Chem.* 28:1439, 1982.

41. Oliver, I. T. A spectrophotometric method for the determination of creatine phosphokinase and myokinase. *Biochem. J.* 61:116, 1955.

42. Rosalki, S. B. An improved procedure for creatine phosphokinase determination. *J. Lab. Clin. Med.* 69:696, 1967.

43. Boone, D. J., Duncan, P. H., MacNeil, M. L., et al. Results of a nationwide survey of analyses for creatine kinase and creatine kinase isoenzymes. *Clin. Chem.* 30:33, 1984.

44. Buzas, Z., and Chrambach, A. Un-supercoiled agarose with a degree of molecular sieving similar to that of crosslinked polyacrylamide. *Electrophoresis* 3:130, 1982.

45. Cook, R. B., and Witt, H. J. Agarose composition, aqueous gel, and method of making same. U.S. Patent 4,290,911, 1981.

46. Lott, J. A., and Stang, J. M. Serum enzymes and isoenzymes in the diagnosis and differential diagnosis of myocardial ischemia and necrosis. *Clin. Chem.* 26:1241, 1980.

47. Aleyassine, H., and Tonks, D. B. Albumin-bound fluorescence: A potential source of error in fluorometric assay of creatine kinase BB isoenzyme (Letter). *Clin. Chem.* 24:1849, 1978.

48. Massey, T. H., and Barta, J. S. Creatine kinase isoenzymes in neonate plasma by cellulose acetate electrophoresis: Albumin and adenylate kinase artifacts. *Clin. Chem.* 28:1174, 1982.

49. Mercer, D. W. Separation of tissue and serum creatine kinase isoenzymes by ion-exchange column chromatography. *Clin. Chem.* 20:36, 1974.

50. Henry, P. D., Roberts, R., and Sobel, B. E. Rapid separation of plasma creatine kinase isoenzymes by batch abdorption on glass beads. *Clin. Chem.* 21:844, 1975.

51. Morin, L. G. Evaluation of current methods for creatine kinase isoenzyme fractionation. *Clin. Chem.* 23:205, 1977.

52. Apple, F. S., Greenspan, N. S., and Dietzler, D. N. Elevation of creatine kinase BB CK in hospitalized patients. *Ann. Clin. Lab. Sci.* 12:398, 1982.

53. Wurzburg, U. Measurement of Creatine Kinase Isoenzyme Activity by Immunological Methods. In H. Lang (ed.), *Creatine Kinase Isoenzymes.* New York: Springer-Verlag, 1981.

54. Lott, J. A. Serum enzyme determinations in the diagnosis of acute myocardial infarction. *Hum. Pathol.* 15:706, 1984.

55. Ritter, C. S., Mumm, S. R., and Roberts, R. Improved radioimmunoassay for creatine kinase isoenzymes in plasma. *Clin. Chem.* 27:1878, 1981.

56. Chan, D. W., Taylor, E., Frye, R., et al. Immunoenzymetric assay for creatine kinase MB with subunit-specific monoclonal antibodies compared with an immunochemical method and electrophoresis. *Clin. Chem.* 31:465, 1985.

57. Vaidya, H. C., Maynard, Y., Dietzler, D. N., et al. Direct measurement of creatine kinase-MB activity in serum after extraction with a monoclonal antibody specific to the MB isoenzyme. *Clin. Chem.* 32:657, 1986.

58. Landt, Y., Vaidya, H. C., Porter, S. E., et al. Semi-automated direct colorimetric measurement of creatine kinase isoenzyme MB activity after extraction from serum by use of a CK-MB-specific monoclonal antibody. *Clin. Chem.* 34:575, 1988.

59. Foxall, C. D., and Ermery, A. E. Changes in creatine kinase and its isoenzymes in human fetal muscle during development. *J. Neurol. Sci.* 24:483, 1975.

60. Tzvetanova, E. Creatine kinase isoenzymes in muscle tissue of patients with neuromuscular diseases and human fetuses. *Enzyme* 12:279, 1971.

61. Tsung, J. S., and Tsung, S. S. Creatine kinase isoenzymes in extracts of various human skeletal muscles. *Clin. Chem.* 32:1568, 1986.

62. Wilhelm, A. H., Albers, K. M., and Todd, J. K. Creatine phosphokinase isoenzyme distribution in human skeletal and heart muscles. *I.R.C.S. Med. Sci.* 4:418, 1976.

63. Yasmineh, W. G., Ibrahim, G. A., Abbasnezhad, M. A., et al. Isoenzyme distribution of creatine kinase and lactate dehydrogenase in serum and skeletal muscle in Duchenne muscular dystrophy, collagen disease, and other muscular disorders. *Clin. Chem.* 24:1985.

64. Roberts, R., Henry, P. D., Witteveen, S. A. G. J., et al. Quantification of serum creatine phosphokinase isoenzyme activity. *Am. J. Cardiol.* 33:650, 1974.

65. Apple, F. S., Rogers, M. A., Sherman, W. M., et al. Profile of creatine kinase isoenzymes in skeletal muscles of marathon runners. *Clin. Chem.* 30:413, 1984.

66. Siegel, A. J., Silverman, L. M., and Evans, W. J. Elevated skeletal muscle creatine kinase MB isoenzyme levels in marathon runners. *JAMA* 250:2835, 1983.

67. Keshgegian, A. A., and Feinberg, N. V. Serum creatine kinase MB isoenzyme in chronic muscle disease. *Clin. Chem.* 30:575, 1984.

68. Shahanglan, S., Ash, O. W., Wahlstrom, N. O., et al. Creatine kinase and lactate dehydrogenase isoenzymes in serum of patients suffering burns, blunt trauma, or myocardial infarction. *Clin. Chem.* 30:1332, 1984.

69. McBride, J. W., Labrosse, K. R., and McCoy, H. G., et al. Is serum creatine kinase-MB in electrically injured patients predictive of myocardial injury? *JAMA* 255:764, 1986.

70. Goto, I., Nagamine, M., and Katsuki, S. Creatine phosphokinase isozymes in muscles. *Arch. Neurol.* 20:422, 1969.

71. Staubli, M., Roessler, B., Kochli, H. P., et al. Creatine kinase and creatine kinase MB in endurance runners and in patients with myocardial infarction. *Eur. J. Appl. Physiol.* 54:40, 1985.

72. Sadeh, M., Stern, L. Z., Czyzewski, K., et al. Alterations of creatine kinase, ornithine decarboxylase, and transglutaminase during muscle regeneration. *Life Sci.* 34:483, 1984.

73. Ingwall, J. S., Kramer, M. F., Fifer, M. A., et al. The creatine kinase system in normal and diseased human myocardium. *N. Engl. J. Med.* 313:1050, 1985.

74. Marmor, A., Margolis, T., and Alpan, G., et al. Regional distribution of the MB isoenzyme of creatine kinase in the human heart. *Arch. Pathol. Lab. Med.* 104:425, 1980.

75. Yasmineh, W. G., Pyle, R. B., and Nicoloff, D. M. Rate of decay and distribution volume of MB isoenzyme of creatine kinase, intravenously injected into the baboon. *Clin. Chem.* 22:1095, 1976.

76. Baraka, M., Deveaux, N., Frank, R., et al. Creatine kinase MB isoenzyme activity after endocardial catheter fulguration (Abstract). *Circulation* 76(Suppl IV):IV-174, 1987.

77. Eppenberger, H. M., Eppenberger, M. E., Richterich, R., et al. The ontogeny of creatine kinase isoenzymes. *Dev. Biol.* 10:1, 1964.

78. Tsung, S. H. Creatine kinase activity and isoenzyme pattern in various normal tissues and neoplasms. *Clin. Chem.* 29:2040, 1983.

79. Roberts, R. Recognition, pathogenesis, and management of non-Q-wave infarction. *Mod. Concepts Cardiovasc. Dis.* 56:17, 1987.

80. Roberts, R., Gowda, K. S., Ludbrook, P. A., et al. Specificity of elevated serum MB creatine phosphokinase activity in the diagnosis of acute myocardial infarction. *Am. J. Cardiol.* 36:433, 1975.

81. Lee, T. H., and Goldman, L. Serum enzyme assays in the diagnosis of acute myocardial infarction. *Ann. Intern. Med.* 105:221, 1986.

82. Grande, P., Christiansen, C., Pedersen, A., et al. Optimal diagnosis in acute myocardial infarction. *Circulation* 61:723, 1980.

83. Klein, M. S., Shell, W. E., and Sobel, B. E. Serum creatine phosphokinase (CPK) isoenzymes after intramuscular injections, surgery, and myocardial infarction. *Cardiovasc. Res.* 7:412, 1973.

84. Somer, H., Dubowitz, V., and Donner, M. Creatine kinase isoenzymes in neuromuscular diseases. *J. Neurol. Sci.* 29:129, 1976.

85. Jaffe, A. S., Ritter, C., Meltzer, V., et al. Unmasking artifactual increases in creatine kinase isoenzymes in patients with renal failure. *J. Lab. Clin. Med.* 104:193, 1984.

86. Kimler, S. C., and Sandhu, R. S. Circulating CK-MB and CK-BB isoenzymes after prostate resection. *Clin. Chem.* 26:55, 1980.

87. Tsung, S. H. Several conditions causing elevation of serum CK-MB and CK-BB. *Am. J. Clin. Pathol.* 75:711, 1981.

88. Laboda, H. M., and Britton, V. J. Creatine kinase isoenzyme activity in human placenta and in the serum of women in labor. *Clin. Chem.* 23:1329, 1977.

89. Somer, H., Kaste, M., Troupp, H., et al. Brain creatine kinase in blood after acute brain injury. *J. Neurol. Neurosurg. Psychiatry* 38:572, 1975.

90. Kaste, M., Somer, H., and Konttinen, A. Brain-type creatine kinase isoenzyme. *Arch.*

Neurol. 34:142, 1977.

91. Goldman, J., Matz, R., Montimer, R., et al. High elevations of creatine phosphokinase in hypothyroidism: An isoenzyme analysis. *JAMA* 238:325, 1977.

92. Bayer, P. M., Boehm, M., Hajdusich, P., et al. Immunoinhibition and automated column chromatography compared for assay of creatine kinase isoenzyme MB in serum. *Clin. Chem.* 28:166, 1982.

93. WHO: *Hypertension and Coronary Heart Disease: Classification and Criteria for Epidemiological Studies.* World Health Organization Technical Series 168. WHO, Geneva, 1959.

94. Roberts, R. The two out of three criteria for the diagnosis of infarction: Is it passe? (Editorial). *Chest* 86:511, 1984.

95. Dillon, M. C., Calbreath, D. F., Dixon, A. M., et al. Diagnostic problem in acute myocardial infarction: CK-MB in the absence of abnormally elevated total creatine kinase levels. *Arch. Intern. Med.* 142:33, 1982.

96. Heller, G. V., Blaustein, A. S., and Wei, J. Y. Implications of increased myocardial isoenzyme level in the presence of normal serum creatine kinase activity. *Am. J. Cardiol.* 51:24, 1983.

97. Yusuf, S., Collins, R., Lin, L., et al. Significance of elevated MB isoenzyme with normal creatine kinase in acute myocardial infarction. *Am. J. Cardiol.* 59:245, 1987.

98. White, R. D., Grande, P., Califf, L., et al. Diagnostic and prognostic significance of minimally elevated creatine kinase-MB in suspected acute myocardial infarction. *Am. J. Cardiol.* 55:1478, 1985.

99. Roberts, R., and Sobel, B. E. Elevated plasma MB creatine phosphokinase activity. *Arch. Intern. Med.* 136:421, 1976.

100. Appella, E., and Markert, C. L. Dissociation of lactate dehydrogenase into subunits with guanidine hydrochloride. *Biochim. Biophys. Acta* 6:171, 1961.

101. Wieland, T., and Pfleiderer, G. Chemical differences between multiple forms of lactic acid dehydrogenase. *Ann. N.Y. Acad. Sci.* 94:691, 1961.

102. Kreutzer, H. H., and Fennis, W. H. S. Lactic dehydrogenase isoenzymes in blood serum after storage at different temperatures. *Clin. Chim. Acta* 9:64, 1964.

103. Smit, M. J., Duursma, A. M., and Bouma, J. M. W., et al. Receptor-mediated endocytosis of lactate dehydrogenase M_4 by liver macrophages: A mechanism for elimination of enzymes from plasma. *J. Biol. Chem.* 262:13020, 1987.

104. Brody, I. A. Effect of denervation on the lactate dehydrogenase isozymes of skeletal muscle. *Nature* 205:196, 1965.

105. Emery, A. E. H. Electrophoretic pattern of lactic dehydrogenase in carriers and patients with Duchenne muscular dystrophy. *Nature* 201:1044, 1964.

106. Schapira, F., Dreyfus, J. C., and Schapira, G. Fetal-like patterns of lactic-dehydrogenase and aldolase isoenzymes in some pathological conditions. *Enzym. Biol. Clin.* 7:98, 1966.

107. McKenzie, D., Henderson, A. R., Gordesky, S. E., et al. Electrophoresis of lactate dehydrogenase isoenzymes. *Clin. Chem.* 29:189, 1983.

108. Kagen, L. J. *Myoglobin: Biochemical, Physiological and Clinical Aspects.* New York: Columbia University Press, 1972. P. 79.

109. Roberts, R. Myoglobinemia as an index to myocardial infarction. *Ann. Intern. Med.* 87:788, 1977.

110. Granadier, E., Keidar, S., Kahana, L., et al. The roles of serum myoglobin, total CPK, and CK-MB isoenzyme in the acute phase of myocardial infarction. *Am. Heart J.* 105:408, 1983.

111. Groth, T., Hakman, M., and Sylven, C. Prediction of myocardial infarct size from early serum myoglobin observations. *Scand. J. Clin. Lab. Invest.* 47:599, 1987.

112. Norregaard-Hansen, K., Petersen, P. H., Hangaard, J., et al. Early observations of S-myoglobin in the diagnosis of acute myocardial infarction: The influence of discrimination limit, analytical quality, patient's sex and prevalence of disease. *Scand. J. Clin. Lab. Invest.* 46:561, 1986.

113. Roxin, L. E., Cullhed, I., Groth, T., et al. The value of serum myoglobin determinations in the early diagnosis of acute myocardial infarction. *Acta Med. Scand.* 215:417, 1984.

114. Bird, J. W. C., Carter, J. H., Triemer, R. E., et al. Proteinases in cardiac and skeletal muscle. *Fed. Proc.* 39:20, 1980.

115. Smitherman, T. C., Dycus, D. W., and Richards, E. G. Dissociation of myosin light chains and decreased myosin ATPase activity with acidification of synthetic myosin filaments: Possible clues to the fate of myosin in myocardial ischemia and infarction. *J. Mol. Cell. Cardiol.* 12:149, 1980.

116. Nagai, R., Ueda, S., and Yazaki, Y. Radioimmunoassay of cardiac myosin light chain II in the serum following experimental myocardial infarction. *Biochem. Biophys. Res. Commun.* 86:683, 1979.

117. Katus, H. A., Diederich, K. W., Schwarz, F., et al. Influence of reperfusion on serum concentrations of cytosolic creatine kinase and structural myosin light chains in acute myocardial infarction. *Am. J. Cardiol.* 60:440, 1987.

118. Isobe, M., Nagai, R., Ueda, S., et al. Quantitative relationship between left ventricular function and serum cardiac myosin light chain

I levels after coronary reperfusion in patients with acute myocardial infarction. *Circulation* 76:1261, 1987.

119. Sobel, B. E., Roberts, R., and Larson, K. B. Estimation of infarct size from serum MB creatine phosphokinase activity: Applications and limitations. *Am. J. Cardiol.* 37:474, 1976.

120. Kjekshus, J. K., and Sobel, B. E. Depressed myocardial creatine phosphokinase activity following experimental myocardial infarction in rabbit. *Circ. Res.* 27:403, 1970.

121. Roberts, R., Henry, P. D., and Sobel, B. E. An improved basis for enzymatic estimation of infarct size. *Circulation* 52:743, 1975.

122. Sobel, B. E., Markham, J., Karlsberg, R. P., et al. The nature of disappearance of creatine kinase from the circulation and its influence on enzymatic estimation of infarct size. *Circ. Res.* 41:836, 1977.

123. Shell, W. E., Kjekshus, J. K., and Sobel, B. E. Quantitative assessment of the extent of myocardial infarction in the conscious dog by means of analysis of serial changes in serum creatine phosphokinase (CPK) activity. *J. Clin. Invest.* 50:2614, 1971.

124. Hackel, D. B., Reimer, K. A., Ideker, R. E., et al. Comparison of enzymatic and anatomic estimates of myocardial infarct size in man. *Circulation* 70:824, 1984.

125. Bleifeld, W., Mathey, D., Hanrath, P., et al. Infarct size estimated from serial serum creatine phosphokinase in relation to left ventricular hemodynamics. *Circulation* 55:303, 1977.

126. Rogers, W. J., McDaniel, H. G., Smith, L. R., et al. Correlation of CPK-MB and angiographic estimates of infarct size in man. *Circulation* 56:199, 1977.

127. Sobel, B. E., Bresnahan, G. F., Shell, W. E., et al. Estimation of infarct size in man and its relation to prognosis. *Circulation* 46:640, 1972.

128. Roberts, R., and Husain, R. Relation between infarct size and ventricular arrhythmia. *Br. Heart J.* 37:1169, 1975.

129. Roberts, R., and Ishikawa, Y. Enzymatic estimation of infarct size during reperfusion. *Circulation* 68(Suppl I):83, 1983.

130. Wevers, R. A., Delsing, M., Klein, A., et al. Post-synthetic changes in creatine kinase isoenzymes. *Clin. Chim. Acta* 86:323, 1978.

131. Wevers, R. A., Olthuis, H. P., Van Niel, J. C. C., et al. A study on the dimeric structure of creatine kinase. *Clin. Chim. Acta* 75:377, 1977.

132. Sims, H. S., Ritter, C. S., Fukuyama, T., et al. Characterization of the modification of creatine kinase following its release into plasma after infarction (Abstract). *Clin. Res.* 29:242A, 1981.

133. George, S., Ishikawa, Y., Perryman, M. B., et al. Purification and characterization of natu-

rally occurring and in vitro induced multiple forms of MM creatine kinase. *J. Biol. Chem.* 259:2667, 1984.

134. Perryman, M. B., Knell, J. D., and Roberts, R. Carboxypeptidase-catalyzed hydrolysis of C-terminal lysine: Mechanism for in vivo production of multiple forms of creatine kinase in plasma. *Clin. Chem.* 30:662, 1984.

135. Gruppo Italiano per lo Studio della Streptochinasi nell'Infarto Miocardico (GISSI): Effectiveness of intravenous thrombolytic treatment in acute myocardial infarction. *Lancet* 1:397, 1986.

136. Lee, T. H., Gregory, W. R., Weisberg, M. C., et al. Sensitivity of routine clinical criteria for diagnosing myocardial infarction within 24 hours of hospitalization. *Ann. Intern. Med.* 106:181, 1987.

137. Hashimoto, H., Abendschein, D. R., Strauss, A. W., et al. Early detection of myocardial infarction in conscious dogs by analysis of plasma MM creatine kinase isoforms. *Circulation* 71:363, 1985.

138. Jaffe, A. S., Serota, H., Grace, A., et al. Diagnostic changes in plasma creatine kinase isoforms early after the onset of acute myocardial infarction. *Circulation* 74:105, 1986.

139. Morelli, R. L., Carlson, C. J., Emilson, B., et al. Serum creatine kinase MM isoenzyme subbands after acute myocardial infarction in man. *Circulation* 67:1283, 1983.

140. Wu, A. H. B., Gornet, T. G., Wu, V. H., et al. Early diagnosis of acute myocardial infarction by rapid analysis of creatine kinase isoenzyme-3 (CK-MM) subtypes. *Clin. Chem.* 33:358, 1987.

141. Apple, F. S., Heilsten, Y., and Clarkson, P. M. Early detection of skeletal muscle injury by assay of creatine kinase MM isoforms in serum after acute exercise. *Clin. Chem.* 34:1102, 1988.

142. Apple, F. S., Rogers, M. A., and Ivy, J. L. Creatine kinase isoenzyme MM variants in skeletal muscle and plasma from marathon runners. *Clin. Chem.* 32:41, 1986.

143. Clarkson, P. M., Apple, F. S., Byrnes, W. C., et al. Creatine kinase isoforms following isometric exercise. *Muscle Nerve* 10:41, 1987.

144. Annesley, T. M., Strongwater, S. L., and Schnitzer, T. J. MM subisoenzymes of creatine kinase as an index of disease activity in polymyositis. *Clin. Chem.* 31:402, 1985.

145. Rentrop, P., Blanke, H., Kostering, K., et al. Acute myocardial infarction: Intracoronary application of nitroglycerine and streptokinase in combination with transluminal recanalization. *Clin. Cardiol.* 5:354, 1979.

146. Chesebro, J. H., Knatterud, G., Roberts, R., et al. Thrombolysis in myocardial infarction (TIMI) trial, phase I: A comparison between

intravenous tissue plasminogen activator and intravenous streptokinase. *Circulation* 76:142, 1987.

147. Califf, R. M., Topol, E. J., Kereiakes, D. J., et al. Long-term outcome in the thrombolysis and angioplasty in myocardial infarction trial (Abstract). *Circulation* 76(Suppl IV):IV-260, 1987.

148. Puleo, P. R., Perryman, M. B., Bresser, M. A., et al. Creatine kinase isoform analysis in the detection and assessment of thrombolysis in man. *Circulation* 75:1162, 1987.

149. Apple, F. S., Sharkey, S. W., Werdick, M., et al. Analyses of creatine kinase isoenzymes and isoforms in serum to detect reperfusion after acute myocardial infarction. *Clin. Chem.* 33:507, 1987.

150. Morelli, R. L., Emilson, B., and Rapaport, E. MM-CK subtypes diagnose reperfusion early after myocardial infarction. *Am. J. Med. Sci.* 293:139, 1987.

151. Roberts, R., Ludbrook, P. A., Weiss, E. S., et al. Serum CPK isoenzymes after cardiac catheterization. *Br. Heart J.* 37:1144, 1975.

7
Routine Management of Acute Myocardial Infarction

GARY S. FRANCIS

Early symptoms of ill health or prodromal chest pain are reported in 60 to 70 percent of patients ultimately diagnosed with acute myocardial infarction (AMI). *Prodromata* can be defined as a constellation of new symptoms, a sign of health deterioration, or a worsening or change in a stable pattern or symptoms or signs that occur in proximity to the myocardial infarction. Somewhat unexpectedly, a lack of college education is significantly related to the patient's recognition of prodromata [1]. In general, less educated patients tend to report a greater incidence of prodromata [1].

New or accelerated angina is one of the most common symptoms (35 percent), along with dyspnea (39 percent) and fatigue–weakness (42 percent) [1]. The most common response to prodromal symptoms is lay consultation (77 percent), with medical consultation being obtained by only 36 percent of patients prior to coming to the emergency ward [1]. Older individuals (65 years or older) are far more likely to consult a physician [1]. It is a somewhat disappointing fact that only 22 percent of patients who experience prodromata and consult their physician are evaluated within 24 hours, and only 56 percent are evaluated within 1 week [1]. The classic study of myocardial infarction prodromata by Alonzo and colleagues was conducted during the early 1970s, however, and there may be wider appreciation today by both lay people and physicians of the importance of prompt attention to the symptoms of a possible heart attack.

It is important to recognize that prodromal symptoms may be mild, intermittent, and ambiguous. The transience of the symptoms may encourage "benign" neglect. Patients who have an established relationship with a physician are more likely to seek his or her advice [1]. Public education programs do heighten awareness, despite the medical community's apprehensions, and do not appear to inundate emergency rooms and physicians' offices with false and unjustified complaints [1]. Given our current ability to deal with early myocardial infarction, we owe it to our patients to carefully and quickly evaluate complaints that might serve as prodromata for myocardial infarction. Today this process is most expeditiously done in emergency wards, which should be staffed with experienced and qualified personnel.

Classic crescendo angina seems to be clearly related on a retrospective basis to myocardial infarction [2, 3]. We now have substantial data that such patients are often undergoing a change in their coronary artery lesions [4–8], usually rupture of a plaque with intermittent thrombosis [9]. These patients should be promptly hospitalized and treated with anticoagulants and nitrates. Early coronary arteriography is necessary if pain is not easily responsive to therapy.

Of course, not all patients with prodromal symptoms go on to myocardial infarction. In fact, the Stanford group has reported that prodromata are equally reported by patients who develop myocardial infarction and those with myocardial ischemia who subsequently "rule out" [3]. The latter group, however, is well known to have a similar 18-month prognosis and should be vigorously investigated [10]. A "rule out" is not license to simply discharge the patient with a "clean bill of health." These patients, once "ruled out,"

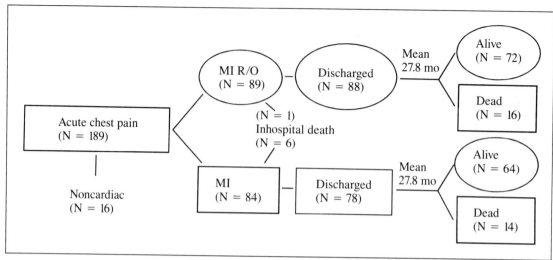

Fig. 7-1
Distribution and follow-up of 189 patients admitted with acute chest pain suspected to be a myocardial infarction. MI R/O = myocardial infarction ruled out. (From J. S. Schroeder et al. Do patients in whom myocardial infarction is ruled out have a better prognosis after hospitalization than those surviving infarction? *N. Engl. J. Med.* 303:1, 1980. Reprinted by permission.)

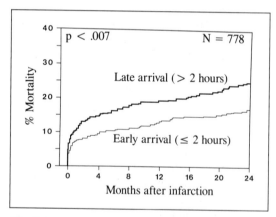

Fig. 7-2
Mortality over a 2-year period for early (within 2 hours) and late (more than 2 hours) arriving patients to the emergency ward with AMI . These data were collected prior to the thrombolysis era (August 1978 to December 1983). (From Z. G. Turi et al. Implications for acute intervention related to time of hospital arrival in acute myocardial infarction. *Am. J. Cardiol.* 58:203, 1986. With permission.)

should undergo a discharge exercise test and be considered for coronary angiography if the test is abnormal or if they continue to have evidence of myocardial ischemia at rest [10] (Fig. 7-1).

The real key to success still lies in educating the public about coming to the hospital sooner following warning symptoms of AMI. Patients who arrive early (within 2 hours of chest pain) have a significantly better prognosis during a 2-year follow-up than patients who arrive late (Fig. 7-2). Unfortunately, patients at relatively high risk of death after AMI (including those with preexisting diabetes mellitus, systemic hypertension, or congestive heart failure), along with women and older patients tend to arrive significantly later in the emergency ward than patients without these characteristics [11].

Emergency Room Strategies

The management of AMI is still rapidly evolving. There is now a growing consensus that transmural infarction is due to coronary artery thrombosis [12], after years of debate on this topic [13]. Reperfusion of an occluded artery, performed during the first few hours of evolving infarction, may reduce infarct size and improve survival [12–15]. Most of the clinical experience with reperfusion has been with streptokinase [14–17], but recombinant tissue type plasminogen activator (rt-PA), a relatively fibrin-specific agent, appears to have a superior coronary recanalization rate [18]. Several points have become clear when considering these data: (1) Time is critical—the sooner the artery is recanalized, the more striking is the improvement in survival [14]; and (2) more benefit is derived from reperfusing arteries subtending anterior myocardial infarctions than inferior infarctions. These changes in the management of AMI have profound implications for emergency care physicians [19].

To achieve beneficial results of thrombolytic therapy, a well organized and efficient emergency care system is required. Processes that ordinarily delay care, including waiting for blood tests, sending the patient for x-ray examinations, and extensive consultation, must be avoided. Instead, emphasis must be placed on the rapid and accurate diagnosis of AMI. This approach requires cardiologists to become more intimately involved with the activities of the emergency ward. In certain situations, the need for transfer of a well defined subset of patients to more specialized hospitals is necessary, but community hospitals can clearly participate [20].

Because thrombolytic therapy is not without risk, contraindications to this form of therapy must be clearly understood. The most serious complication is intracranial bleeding, which occurred with a frequency of 0.2 percent in the Grupps Italiano per lo Studio della Streptochinasi nell'Infarto Miocardico (GISSI) trial [14], 0.46 percent in the Intravenous Streptokinase in Acute Myocardial Infarction (ISAM) trial [17], and 1.6 percent in the Thrombolysis in Myocardial Infarction (TIMI) trial using 150 mg of rt-PA over 6 hours and 0.6 percent when 100 mg was given over 6 hours [21]. The frequency of cerebral hemorrhage related to streptokinase in the second

International Study of Infarct Survival (ISIS-2) trial was 0.1 percent [21a]. Patients of advanced age (75 years or older) and those with a history of stroke, transient cerebral ischemia, severe hypertension, long-standing diabetes mellitus, or other disease processes known to influence the cerebral vasculature should generally be excluded from lytic therapy. Patients who have just undergone closed chest massage should also be excluded.

It is important for each emergency care system to develop a uniform protocol for managing AMI. In general, the decision to use thrombolytic therapy for AMI and its initiation should be carried out in the emergency ward. Informed consent should be obtained. As it now stands, patients who present with electrocardiographic (ECG) evidence of anterior AMI (ST-segment elevation) under age 75 and who have no contraindications should be considered for thrombolytic therapy in the emergency ward prior to transport to the coronary care unit (CCU). The time window is narrow and not clearly defined, but our current understanding suggests that most improvement occurs when lytic therapy is begun within 4 hours of the onset of pain; this window can probably be extended to 6 hours or longer in patients who continue to have unrelenting chest pain. In fact, there is a growing body of evidence that suggests that a patent infarct-related artery may be beneficial even beyond the time that patency may salvage myocardium [21a, 21b].

In addition to the history and physical examination, the ECG remains the most useful tool in the rapid and accurate diagnosis of AMI. The sensitivity and specificity of the ECG are excellent in patients with documented anterior AMI (86.7 percent sensitive and 89.5 percent specific in one study [22]). When left bundle branch block and paced rhythm are excluded, it is the most useful early test we have for establishing the correct diagnosis [23]. Patients admitted to the hospital to "rule out myocardial infarction" despite a negative ECG often go on to infarction on follow-up (17 percent in one study [24]), so that clinical judgment remains the pivotal process. Remarkably, data by Lee and colleagues

[25] indicated that only 4 percent of patients with AMI are misdiagnosed and discharged from the emergency ward. About one-half of the missed AMIs could have been diagnosed by improved ECG reading skills [25], further emphasizing the need for cardiologists to interact with emergency care physicians.

An ECG is always performed for any patient presenting to the emergency ward with symptoms possibly due to ischemic heart disease. A completely normal ECG makes AMI unlikely [26]. Only 1 percent of such patients have AMI, and only 4 percent of this group eventually are diagnosed as having unstable angina. Most patients (60 percent) with AMI have *new* findings of ST-segment elevation or Q waves, and almost all others show *new* changes of ischemia. About 15 percent of patients with AMI present to the emergency room with an abnormal ECG but no *new* changes. One need not prove that the ECG changes are new—only that they are not known to be old. A common mistake is to assume that ECG changes are old, when in fact there is no old ECG that shows those findings. One should not rely too heavily on telephone descriptions, which are often unreliable.

The initial ECG can be helpful for determining triage options: a CCU, an intermediate care unit, or discharge [26]. Patients with ECGs that show evidence of infarction, ischemia, strain, left ventricular hypertrophy, left bundle branch block, or paced rhythm are far more likely to have a life-threatening complication (ventricular fibrillation, sustained ventricular tachycardia, or heart block) when the clinical diagnosis of AMI is suspected, and these patients should be sent to the CCU. Such complications are 23 times more likely to occur, according to one study [26]. Alternatively, a normal ECG in the face of suspected AMI portends a good prognosis (0.6 percent chance of life-threatening complication), and these patients can be admitted to an intermediate care unit. This protocol would reduce admissions to a CCU by 36 percent and thereby save considerable hospital costs without compromising patient care.

Control of Pain, Sedation, and Hypertension

The relief of pain in patients with AMI remains an important priority. Generally, two strategies are employed: (1) reduction of ischemia and (2) direct analgesia.

RELIEF OF MYOCARDIAL ISCHEMIA

Although once considered contraindicated for AMI, nitroglycerin can decrease myocardial oxygen demand by decreasing preload and afterload and decreasing left ventricular wall tension [27–29]. Nitrates may also improve collateral flow to the ischemic myocardium [30, 31]. Patients with AMI should be considered for treatment with sublingual nitroglycerin provided hypotension is not present [32]. In fact, sublingual nitroglycerin (20 to 25 mg) is comparable to intravenous morphine for pain relief and has a more favorable effect on ECG estimates of myocardial necrosis (Fig. 7-3) [32]. However, hypotension can occur with

Fig. 7-3
A patient with AMI was treated with high-dose sublingual nitroglycerin (S.L. NTG). *Arrows* denote the amount and time of administration. The effects of high-dose sublingual nitroglycerin on ST-segment change and pain are comparable to those of morphine sulfate [32]. (From Y. I. Kim and J. F. Williams, Jr. Large dose sublingual nitroglycerin in acute myocardial infarction: Relief of chest pain and reduction of Q wave evolution. *Am. J. Cardiol.* 49:842, 1982. With permission.)

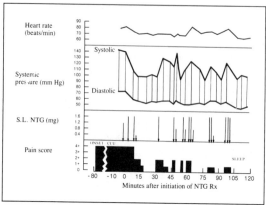

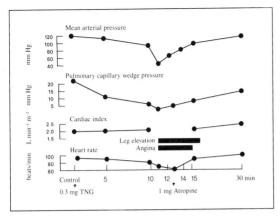

Fig. 7-4
Hemodynamic effects of 0.3 mg sublingual nitroglycerin in a patient who developed a precipitous fall in mean arterial pressure. The patient's symptoms and hypotension were relieved by raising the legs and administration of 1 mg of intravenous atropine. (From C. E. Delgado et al. Role of sublingual nitroglycerin in patients with acute myocardial infarction. *Br. Heart J.* 37:392, 1975. With permission.)

sublingual nitroglycerin (Fig. 7-4), and the patient should be observed carefully for clinical improvement or changes in hemodynamics. If the initial dose is well tolerated, intravenous nitroglycerin should be administered with careful monitoring of blood pressure [33]. The dose may vary from 10 to 200 μg/min and should be titrated so as not to allow the systolic blood pressure to fall below 90 mm Hg. Long-acting oral nitrates should be avoided during very early myocardial infarction because there is far less control over the hemodynamic response. Patients with inferior myocardial infarction are more prone to develop hypotension and bradycardia following nitroglycerin [34], so that it should be used cautiously in these patients. This complication can be reversed by raising the legs and giving intravenous atropine 0.5 to 1.0 mg (Figs. 7-5 and 7-6) [34]. Patients with presumed right

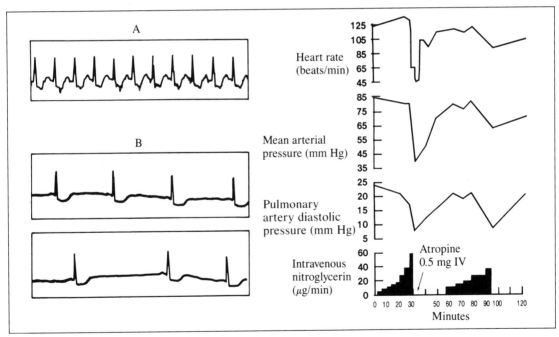

Fig. 7-5
ECG recordings (*left panel*) from a patient with acute anteroseptal myocardial infarction and sinus tachycardia (*A*). Intravenous nitroglycerin (*right panel*) caused bradycardia (*B*) and severe arterial hypotension at 20 to 40 μg/min. It was responsive to 0.5 mg of intravenous atropine but recurred following the reinstitution of intravenous nitroglycerin. (From P. C. Come and B. Pitt. Nitroglycerin induced severe myocardial infarction. *Circulation* 54:624, 1976. By permission of the American Heart Association, Inc.)

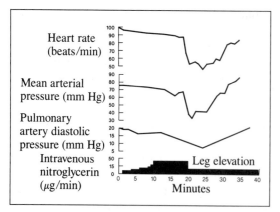

Fig. 7-6
Hemodynamic changes in a patient with acute
non-Q wave myocardial infarction given
intravenous nitroglycerin. In this case, the
hypotension responded to leg elevation.
Nitroglycerin-induced hypotension and
bradycardia can occur with the sublingual or
intravenous preparation in patients with Q-wave
or non-Q-wave infarction, or anterior or inferior
infarction, although it is more commonly observed
in patients with inferior myocardial infarction.
(From P. C. Come and B. Pitt. Nitroglycerin
induced severe myocardial infarction. *Circulation*
54:624, 1976. By permission of the American
Heart Association, Inc.)

ventricular myocardial infarction should probably not be given nitroglycerin, as they are
much more dependent on an increased preload
to maintain stroke volume [35].

Although substantial reductions in blood
pressure may be well tolerated by patients
with acute myocardial infarction given nitroglycerin [36, 37], it is prudent to achieve a reduction in mean arterial pressure of only 10
percent [38, 39]. Severe hypotension and bradycardia, which occurs in about 10 percent of
patients given nitroglycerin in the setting of
AMI, can occur even with the intravenous
preparation (Figs. 7-5 and 7-6) [34].

Nitroglycerin appears to be most useful in
patients with anterior AMI who have persistent or recurrent chest pain or heart failure. It
should be initiated at a dose of 10 μg/min and
increased by 10 μg/min every 10 minutes to
achieve a 10 percent reduction in systolic
blood pressure; heart rate should not be allowed to increase by more than 20 percent,
and systolic blood pressure should not be allowed to go below 90 mm Hg. Doses beyond
200 μg/min are rarely necessary.

Sodium nitroprusside, because of its more
balanced effect on preload and afterload,
might be considered a logical alternative to nitroglycerin. This hypothesis was tested in the
large Veterans Administration trial [40], which
required patients to have a left ventricular filling pressure of 12 mm Hg or more to enter the
protocol. In fact, early use of nitroprusside actually increased mortality compared with placebo (24 percent versus 13 percent). Patients
with pump dysfunction persistent beyond 9
hours after onset of symptoms may benefit
from nitroprusside [40], but nitroglycerin infusion is now preferred to nitroprusside early
after acute infarction.

ANALGESIA

Morphine sulfate remains the standard anal-
gesic for patients with AMI. Meperidine and
pentazocine can be substituted in patients
with well documented hypersensitivity to
morphine. Morphine is usually given in doses
of 4 to 8 mg intravenously and repeated every
5 to 15 minutes in doses of 2 to 8 mg until pain
is relieved. Occasionally, large cumulative
doses (2–3 mg/kg) are required to relieve pain.
Hypotension, bradycardia, nausea, and vomiting can occur, as well as respiratory depression. A rather pronounced peripheral venodilator effect occurs that reduces preload and is
helpful in patients with pulmonary edema [41,
42]. However, despite peripheral venous dilation, left ventricular filling pressure does not
change strikingly with morphine, and the
mechanism whereby it relieves cardiac dyspnea is not understood [43]. When combined
with other vasodilators (e.g., nitroglycerin),
the hypotensive action of morphine may be
exaggerated. This reaction can also occur in
patients who are hypovolemic, which is often
the case in patients with AMI. In the event of
morphine-induced respiratory depression, naloxone hydrochloride should be administered
in 0.4-mg increments intravenously to a total
dose of 1.4 mg. One should be prepared for
artificial ventilation in an occasional patient.

HYPERTENSION

Blood pressure elevation early during the evolution of AMI is common, occurring in 30 to 40 percent of patients, depending on the criteria used [44]. However, because an elevated blood pressure may improve perfusion to areas supplied by partially obstructed vessels, but also increases myocardial oxygen demand by increasing left ventricular wall stress, it is difficult to predict the overall effects of altering arterial pressure on myocardial oxygen supply and demand. Increasing mean arterial pressure in experimental myocardial infarction from 110 mm Hg to 145 mm Hg clearly results in extension of ischemic injury [45]. In patients with chronic coronary artery disease, at similar increases in myocardial oxygen consumption the stress of increased heart rate results in more myocardial ischemia than the stress of increased afterload [46]. In the dog with acute coronary artery occlusion, an increase in systemic arterial pressure exerts an influence on the severity of myocardial ischemic injury that is related directly to the magnitude of systemic arterial hypertension: a mild increase of pressure (diastolic pressure 95 to 115 mm Hg) reduces ischemic injury, a moderate increase (diastolic pressure 116 to 140 mm Hg) exerts no consistent effect on ischemia, and a marked increase (diastolic pressure of more than 140 mm Hg) worsens ischemic injury [47]. However, 24 hours of mildly increased aortic pressure accentuates end-diastolic wall thinning in this model and results in failure to return to control values [48]. Patients with long-standing systemic hypertension and left ventricular hypertrophy may be at particular risk during AMI. Experimental coronary occlusion in animals with hypertension and left ventricular hypertrophy is associated with reduced collateral flow to the area at risk [49]. Moreover, infarct size relative to the area at risk is increased significantly in the setting of left ventricular hypertrophy [49].

Given these experimental findings, it seems reasonable to control excessively elevated blood pressure in patients with AMI. No precise guidelines can be stated, but a persistently elevated systolic blood pressure (>150 mm Hg), diastolic blood pressure (>110 mm Hg), or both should probably be treated if it does not readily respond to analgesics and sedation. Treatment regimens vary with local policy. Nitroprusside (10–300 μg/min) usually controls blood pressure sufficiently. Intravenous labetalol (20 mg IV slowly), repeated as necessary, also is useful and usually prevents reflex tachycardia. Intravenous nitroglycerin and beta-blockers can be used to control systemic hypertension. Precipitous lowering of blood pressure by agents such as nifedipine or hydralazine should be avoided.

Routine Measures of Care

A soft or liquid diet is usually prescribed during the first 24 hours following AMI. Stable patients can be given a 1200-calorie, low-sodium, low-cholesterol diet. Caffeine and other stimulants are avoided. A stool softener is traditionally given to prevent straining at stool, and patients should be advised to use a bedside commode if possible from day 1.

Nearly all patients with AMI are hypoxemic [50, 51]. The mechanism of the hypoxemia is poorly understood but is probably related to small airway dysfunction secondary to elevated pulmonary capillary wedge pressure [52] and reduced lung volume [53]. Oxygen is routinely administered at a dose of 2 to 4 L/min for the first 3 to 4 days following AMI.

Chest Radiograph

A chest radiograph should be obtained on admission in all patients, as there is a good relation between left ventricular hemodynamics and the radiographic findings [54–56]. The heart size and extent of pulmonary vascular markings offer important prognostic information [57]. In the absence of pulmonary congestion, according to one study [54], there is a 94 percent 1-month survival and 88 percent 1-year survival. When the heart size is also normal, there is a 96 percent 1-month survival and a 91 percent 1-year survival. With diffuse alveolar edema present on the initial chest radiograph, there is an 18 percent 1-month survival and no 1-year survivals. Therefore the degree of pulmonary vascular congestion and left heart size on the initial chest radiograph after AMI are useful for defining high-risk and low-risk groups.

Drug Interactions

A careful inventory of what medications the patient already is taking at the time of the myocardial infarction must be carefully determined. Those drugs that are known to put the patient at further risk should be discontinued. For example, if the patient presents with AMI and severe congestive heart failure or complete heart block and is taking a beta-adrenergic blocker, the beta-blocker should be stopped. Contrary to widespread concern that the sudden withdrawal of beta-adrenoceptor blocking drugs may result in a rebound adrenergic hypersensitivity state, it appears not to be a major problem in patients with AMI [58]. Likewise, one would also likely discontinue other drugs known to interfere with atrioventricular (AV) nodal conduction, such as verapamil (which could also aggravate heart failure) or diltiazem, in patients with severe heart failure or heart block.

Drug interactions must be carefully assessed. For example, diltiazem, cimetidine [59], and lidocaine [60–63] can cause sinus node arrest in patients with underlying sinus node dysfunction. Any combination of these drugs, particularly if a beta-adrenergic blocker is also being used, might be expected to cause sinus node standstill. Cimetidine also increases the biologic half-life of propranolol by reducing liver blood flow [64], thereby enhancing its negative inotropic and chronotropic properties. We have been particularly impressed with the frequency of bradyarrhythmias when the combination of diltiazem and a beta-blocker are used together. The risk-benefit ratio of virtually every medication prescribed in the setting of acute myocardial infarction must be carefully weighed: How will it influence loading conditions, electrical conduction, myocardial oxygen demand, and coronary blood flow? What is the possible interaction with other agents?

Electrocardiogram

The admission ECG should always be carefully evaluated. Repeat ECGs should be routinely ordered each morning and should be obtained *during chest pain* and whenever there is a change in the patient's clinical course. Pseudoinfarct patterns may occur in healthy young athletes as well as patients with idiopathic dilated cardiomyopathy, subarachnoid hemorrhage, idiopathic hypertrophic subaortic stenosis, and preexcitation syndromes [65]. Although upright tall T waves appear simultaneously with ST-segment elevation in patients with AMI [66], the former rather than the latter is thought by some to be the earliest ECG sign of myocardial injury [67]. ST-segment elevation does not necessarily signify subsequent myocardial necrosis [68]. Marked transient giant R waves can be seen prior to or following ventricular fibrillation [69]. Lead III is most likely to have ST-segment elevation in patients with inferior AMI (94 percent), whereas lead V_2 has the highest incidence of St-segment elevation in patients with an anterior AMI [70]. Although the ECG is a good indicator of the general location of a myocardial infarction, detailed ECG classification schemes used to precisely locate infarctions are not useful [71, 72]. ECG-diagnosed anterior, posterior, and apical myocardial infarctions generally correlate with pathologic anatomy, however [73]. Circumflex coronary artery occlusion can perhaps be identified by ST-segment elevation in one or more inferior leads (II, III, aVF) with ST-segment elevation in one or more lateral leads (aVL, V_5, or V_6) without ST-segment depression in lead I [74]. ST-segment elevation (V_2) may occur when the left anterior descending coronary artery is occluded and no collateral circulation is present, whereas a similar occlusion may cause ST-segment depression when collateral function is adequate [75]. In general, however, it is treacherous to attempt to precisely define the pathologic coronary substrate based on the initial ECG.

The pathogenetic implications of precordial ST-segment depression during an acute inferior transmural myocardial infarction are controversial [76, 77]. Two hypotheses have been advanced to explain these ECG findings: (1) reciprocal changes due to the representation of the ischemic ST-segment vector in leads opposite the area of ischemia; and (2) adjacent or distant ischemia related to multiple-vessel disease. Despite the fact that this ST-segment depression may not always represent "ischemia at a distance" [78], it is now reasonably clear that *persistent* precordial lead ST-segment depression observed with a pattern of acute transmural inferior infarction predicts clinical and hemodynamic left ventricular dysfunction [79], and the prognosis is accordingly influenced [79, 80].

Non-Q Wave Myocardial Infarction

Myocardial infarction has been conventionally referred to as transmural (Q wave) and non-transmural (non-Q wave) [81]. It was not until 1944, with the introduction of the precordial leads, that the Q wave was thought to be associated with "coronary thrombosis." However, it was soon recognized that the Q wave, although rather sensitive, was lacking in specificity. Moreover, careful postmortem examinations indicated that about one-half of "subendocardial infarcts" generated pathologic Q waves, whereas one-half of the transmural infarcts did not [82]. It has been suggested that the terms Q wave and non-Q wave do not precisely relate to the previous terms transmural and nontransmural infarction [83]. In contrast to Q wave infarction, total coronary occlusion of the infarct-related vessel is unusual in the early hours of non-Q wave infarction, although it tends to increase over subsequent days [84]. Non-Q wave infarction may be related to a marginally preserved blood supply that is still sufficient to cause tissue necrosis. Although non-Q wave infarction patients may have a somewhat more benign in-hospital course compared with patients having a Q

wave myocardial infarction, their long-term prognosis is similar or even somewhat worse [81]. They are at risk for early reinfarction, angina, and bypass surgery [85, 86]. The presence of complex ventricular arrhythmias at the time of hospital discharge is an important predictor of 1-year mortality in the presence of non-Q wave infarction [87]. Because these patients are more prone to recurrent ischemic events, they frequently undergo angiography and surgery at many centers. It has been demonstrated in patients with non-Q wave infarction that diltiazem (90 mg every 6 hours) effectively prevents early reinfarction and severe angina [88].

Myocardial Infarct Extension and Expansion

The complication of myocardial infarction extension, as defined by a rise in plasma MB creatine kinase (MB-CK), occurs in 8 to 9 percent of patients [89]. Hospital mortality for these patients is increased fourfold (Fig. 7-7) but is not different for nonextension patients once they leave the hospital. Cardiogenic shock is experienced more than three times as

Fig. 7-7
Cumulative mortality in patients with and without myocardial infarct extension. There is a significant increase in early mortality in patients with extension ($p < .01$). The subsequent mortality of the two groups is not significantly different. (From J. E. Muller et al. Myocardial infarct extension: Occurrence, outcome, and risk factors in the multicenter investigation of limitation of infarct size. *Ann. Intern. Med.* 108:1, 1988. With permission.)

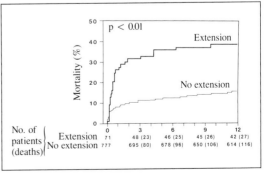

often in patients with extension, thereby contributing to the markedly increased hospital mortality. Extension can occur early, before the return of plasma MB-CK to baseline or, more often, late (days 5–7), after the return of plasma MB-CK to baseline (Fig. 7-8). Less than one-half of patients with extension have recurrent ischemic pain or ECG changes, implying that this complication is likely to be missed unless frequent sampling of enzymes is performed. Important clinical events or findings have also been shown to have predictive value with regard to myocardial extension, however. Patients with recurrent ischemic pain during the second hospital day, those with a history of previous myocardial infarction, and those with ST-segment depression on the admission ECG (non-Q wave infarction) are more likely to experience extension [89]. Such patients, known to be at risk for ex-tension, should be considered for early coronary arteriography and possible interventions to reduce the high early-hospital mortality.

Myocardial infarct expansion, a fixed, permanent, disproportionate regional thinning and dilation of the infarct zone, occurs with 35 to 40 percent of anterior transmural infarctions [90–94]. It does not occur in non-Q wave myocardial infarction. Patients with a history of systemic hypertension are at greater risk for this serious complication [95], which often leads to progressive and chronic ventricular enlargement and congestive heart failure. Antiinflammatory agents may contribute to infarct expansion [94]. There are experimental data from the rat model of myocardial infarction that captopril may reduce myocardial remodeling and thereby improve survival when given prophylactically soon after the acute injury [96]. This concept is now being applied to patients in a large, multicenter clinical trial (Survival and Myocardial Enlargement). Infarct expansion has also been shown to be reduced by administering oral nifedipine (120 mg daily) beginning on the day of infarction and continuing for 10 days [97]. Despite the severity of this complication, however, one should be cautious about applying any form of "routine" therapy. The effects of calcium channel blockers on survival after myocardial infarction have tended to favor a small excess mortality in the treated group [98]. Further study is necessary before we can know the true influence of pharmacologic and reperfusion therapy on myocardial expansion with acute infarction. Infarct expansion, extension, and reinfarction are compared in Table 7-1.

Management Beyond the First Day

Aspirin and intravenous heparin should probably be used in nearly all patients with AMI, unless contraindicated. If lytic therapy is used, it should be followed by an initial 5000 U bolus of intravenous heparin, given at the start of the rt-PA or streptokinase infusion, with a continuous infusion of heparin begun within 1 hour at a rate of 1000 U/hr. The dose of heparin should then be adjusted to maintain

Fig. 7-8
MB creatine kinase (MB-CK) time–activity curves for a patient in whom the myocardial extension occurred before return of plasma MB-CK to baseline (*top*) and a patient in whom extension occurred after return of MB-CK to baseline (*bottom*). The area below the *dashed line* represents the normal range of MB-CK values. (From J. E. Muller et al. Myocardial infarct extension: Occurrence, outcome, and risk factors in the multicenter investigation of limitation of infarct size. *Ann. Intern. Med.* 108:1, 1988. With permission.)

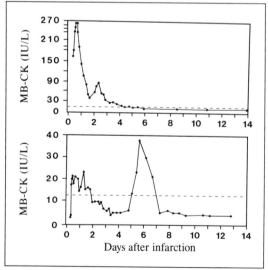

Table 7-1
Comparison of infarct expansion, extension, and reinfarction

Expansion	Extension	Reinfarction
INCIDENCE Up to 70% of all fatal infarctions About 35–45% of anterior transmural infarctions Lower incidence seen at other sites	About 15–20% of fatal infarctions Clinical incidence varies according to diagnostic criteria and patient selection, but probably is between 10% and 20% in the general population	About 10–20% in most studies; higher incidence among women
TIME COURSE Hours to several days after infarction	Arbitrarily defined as occurring between 24 hours and completion of the in-hospital postinfarction course	Arbitrarily defined as occurring after the in-hospital postinfarction course
PATHOLOGIC FEATURES Gross pathology Infarct thinning and dilatation Secondary global dilatation (possibly) Histology Myocyte slippage	Gross pathology: healing myocardial infarction with surrounding foci of more recent necrosis usually within the same vascular risk region Histology: contraction band necrosis present in the newer foci of necrosis	Gross and histologic pathology: remote healed myocardial infarction with new infarction in the same or a different vascular risk region
CONSEQUENCES Congestive heart failure Increased mortality Left ventricular dilatation (regional and global) Mural thrombus Cardiac rupture Left ventricular aneurysm Infarct extension? Postinfarction angina?	Actual increase in infarct size Congestive heart failure Cardiogenic shock Increased mortality Infarct expansion?	Increase in total infarct mass Congestive heart failure Cardiogenic shock Increased mortality

Source: From H. F. Weisman and B. Healy. Myocardial infarct expansion, infarct extension, and re-infarction: Pathophysiological concepts. *Prog. Cardiovasc. Dis.* 30:73, 1987. With permission.

the activated partial thromboplastin time between 1.5 and 2 times the control. Aspirin should be given (80 mg/day) for at least 6 days and then increased to 325 mg/day. On day 6, intravenous heparin should be replaced by subcutaneous heparin (10,000 U q12h), which should be continued until hospital discharge. There appears to be no advantage to early PTCA in terms of reduction in mortality or reinfarction over a more conservative strategy [99]. Coronary arteriography is recommended for patients who demonstrate recurrent ischemia in the hospital or during the predischarge exercise test. The results of the recently pub-

lished phase II of the National Institutes of Health-sponsored Thrombolysis in Myocardial Infarction Trial (TIMI II) demonstrate a stunning 6-week mortality rate of 4.7 percent when rt-PA in combination with aspirin and heparin is used in patients with AMI of less than 4 hours duration [99]. This stands in sharp contrast to hospital mortality rates in excess of 20 percent reported in the early days of coronary care [100, 101]. It is unknown if primary angioplasty without previous thrombolytic therapy can match this excellent clinical outcome.

Patients not on treatment with beta blockers, verapamil, or diltiazem should be considered candidates for an intravenous beta blocker. Relative contraindications to intravenous beta-blocker therapy include a ventricular rate less that 55 bpm, a systolic blood pressure less than 90 mm Hg, moist rales extending above the lower third of the lung fields, advanced AV block, or a history of asthma or severe chronic lung disease. A common practice is to use metoprolol in three 5-mg intravenous injections at 2-minute intervals, followed by oral metoprolol (50 mg bid on the first hospital day and 100 mg bid thereafter, if tolerated). Recent data from the TIMI phase II trial indicate that beta blockers given in this fashion lower the incidence of nonfatal reinfarction and recurrent ischemic events during hospitalization [99].

Patients under age 75 years who have severe resting ischemia in the hospital beyond the first 24 hours or those with a history of MI and clinical or radiographic signs of left ventricular failure in the hospital should be considered for coronary angiography [102]. The remaining patients, most of whom will perform an exercise test, should be considered for coronary arteriography if they demonstrate an ischemic response during exercise or a poor workload (less than 4 metabolic exercise equivalents [METs] where 1 MET equals the amount of oxygen used at rest). If exercise testing cannot be done, a resting radionuclide left ventriculogram is recommended, and coronary angiography should be performed if the ejection fraction lies between 0.20 and 0.44 [102]. These guidelines will identify patients at an increased 1-year risk (average mortality rate 16 percent), who make up about one-half of the postinfarction population.

Summary

It is clear to experienced physicians that there is no "routine" management of AMI in the present era. Every patient is different, and management varies accordingly. As we grow closer to understanding the mechanisms of infarction, treatments will change. We have come a great deal closer to this goal in recent years. We can now reperfuse the myocardium, abolish the residual stenosis, and limit the ischemic burden in many patients who present early in the phases of acute infarction. Most patients continue to come too late after the onset of symptoms, however. Reperfusion is not a realistic option in these patients. Nevertheless, we can still optimize left ventricular loading conditions and heart rate. We can predict which patients are likely to develop pump dysfunction and can act accordingly. The proper management of the patient with AMI requires knowledge of physiology, pathology, pharmacology, anatomy, and psychology. There is perhaps no other medical emergency that draws so completely on our role as physician and patient advocate.

Acknowledgment

The superb secretarial assistance of Sandy Thiesse is gratefully appreciated.

References

1. Alonzo, A. A., Simon, A. B., and Feinleib, M. Prodromata of myocardial infarction and sudden death. *Circulation* 52:1056, 1975.
2. Pitt, B. Natural history of myocardial infarction and its prodromal syndromes. *Circulation* 53(Suppl I):I-132, 1976.
3. Schroeder, J. S., Lamb, I. H., and Hu, M. Prodromal characteristics as indicators of cardiac events in patients hospitalized for chest pain. *Clin. Cardiol.* 2:33, 1979.
4. Ambrose, J. A., et al. Angiographic morphology and the pathogenesis of unstable angina. *J. Am. Coll. Cardiol.* 5:609, 1985.
5. Breshahan, D. R., et al. Angiographic occurrence and clinical correlates of intraluminal coronary artery thrombosis: Role of unstable angina. *J. Am. Coll. Cardiol.* 6:285, 1985.
6. Ambrose, J. A., et al. Angiographic evolution of coronary artery morphology in unstable angina. *J. Am. Coll. Cardiol.* 7:472, 1986.
7. Falk, E. Unstable angina with fatal outcome: Dynamic coronary thrombosis leading to infarction and/or sudden death. *Circulation* 71:699, 1985.
8. Wilson, R. F., Holida, M. D., and White, C. W. Quantitative angiographic morphology of coronary stenosis leading to myocardial in-

farction or unstable angina. *Circulation* 73:286, 1986.

9. Sherman, C. T., et al. Coronary angioscopy in patients with unstable angina. *N. Engl. J. Med.* 315:913, 1986.

10. Schroeder, J. S., Lamb, I. H., and Hu, M. Do patients in whom myocardial infarction is ruled out have a better prognosis after hospitalization than those surviving infarction? *N. Engl. J. Med.* 303:1, 1980.

11. Turi, Z. G., et al. Implications for acute intervention related to time of hospital arrival in acute myocardial infarction. *Am. J. Cardiol.* 58:203, 1986.

12. DeWood, M. A., et al. Prevalence of total coronary occlusion during the early hours of transmural myocardial infarction. *N. Engl. J. Med.* 303:897, 1980.

13. Chandler, A. B., et al. Coronary thrombosis in myocardial infarction. *Am. J. Cardiol.* 34:823, 1974.

14. G.I.S.S.I. Trial. Effectiveness of intravenous thrombolytic treatment in acute myocardial infarction. *Lancet* 1:397, 1986.

15. Simoons, M. L., et al. Improved survival after early thrombolysis in acute myocardial infarction. *Lancet* 2:578, 1985.

16. Kennedy, J. W., et al. Western Washington randomized trial of intracoronary streptokinase in acute myocardial infarction. *N. Engl. J. Med.* 309:1477, 1983.

17. I.S.A.M. Study Group. A prospective trial of intravenous streptokinase in acute myocardial infarction (I.S.A.M.). *N. Engl. J. Med.* 314:1465, 1986.

18. T.I.M.I. Study Group. The thrombolysis in myocardial infarction (T.I.M.I.) trial: Phase I findings. *N. Engl. J. Med.* 312:932, 1985.

19. Kennedy, J. W., et al. Recent changes in management of acute myocardial infarction: Implications for emergency care physicians. *J. Am. Coll. Cardiol.* 11:446, 1988.

20. Topol, E. J., et al. Community hospital administration of intravenous plasminogen activator in acute myocardial infarction: Improved timing, thrombolytic efficacy and ventricular function. *J. Am. Coll. Cardiol.* 10:1173, 1987.

21. The TIMI Trial (Letter). *J. Am. Coll. Cardiol.* 10:970, 1987.

21a. ISIS 2 Collaborative Group. Randomized trial of intravenous streptokinase, oral aspirin, both, or neither among 17,187 cases of suspected acute myocardial infarction: ISIS 2. *Lancet* 2:871, 1988.

21b. Braunwald, E. Myocardial reperfusion, limitation of infarct size, reduction of left ventricular dysfunction, and improved survival: Should the paradigm be expanded? *Circulation* 79:441, 1989.

22. Yasuda, T., et al. Accuracy of localization of acute myocardial infarction by 12 lead electrocardiography. *J. Electrocardiol.* 15:181, 1982.

23. McQueen, M. J., Holder, D., and El-Maraghi, N. R. H. Assessment of the accuracy of serial electrocardiograms in the diagnosis of myocardial infarction. *Am. Heart J.* 105:258, 1983.

24. Behar, S., et al. Evaluation of electrocardiogram in emergency room as a decision-making tool. *Chest* 71:486, 1977.

25. Lee, T. H., et al. Clinical characteristics and natural history of patients with acute myocardial infarction sent home from the emergency room. *Am. J. Cardiol.* 60:219, 1987.

26. Brush, J. E., et al. Use of the initial electrocardiogram to predict in-hospital complications of acute myocardial infarction. *N. Engl. J. Med.* 312:1137, 1985.

27. Smith, E. R., et al. Coronary artery occlusion in the conscious dog: Effects of alterations in arterial pressure produced by nitroglycerin, hemorrhage, and alpha adrenergic agonists on the degree of myocardial ischemia. *Circulation* 47:51, 1973.

28. Epstein, J. E., et al. Reduction of ischemic injury by nitroglycerin during acute myocardial infarction. *N. Engl. J. Med.* 292:29, 1975.

29. Gerry, J. L., Jr., et al. Effects of nitroglycerin on regional myocardial ischemia induced by atrial pacing in dogs. *Circ. Res.* 48:569, 1981.

30. Jugdutt, B. I., et al. Effect of intravenous nitroglycerin on collateral blood flow and infarct size in the conscious dog. *Circulation* 63:17, 1981.

31. Fukuyama, T., Schectman, K. B., and Roberts, R. The effects of intravenous nitroglycerin on hemodynamics, coronary blood flow and morphologically and enzymatically estimated infarct size in conscious dogs. *Circulation* 62:1227, 1980.

32. Kim, Y. I., and Williams, J. F., Jr. Large dose sublingual nitroglycerin in acute myocardial infarction: Relief of chest pain and reduction of Q wave evolution. *Am. J. Cardiol.* 49:842, 1982.

33. Mikolich, J. R., et al. Relief of refractory angina with continuous intravenous infusion of nitroglycerin. *Chest* 77:375, 1980.

34. Come, P. C., and Pitt, B. Nitroglycerin induced severe hypotension and bradycardia in patients with acute myocardial infarction. *Circulation* 54:624, 1976.

35. Ferguson, J. J., et al. Nitroglycerin induced hypotension with acute myocardial infarction: A marker of right ventricular involvement? *Circulation* 72(Suppl III):III-460, 1985.

36. Flaherty, J. T., et al. Effects of intravenous nitroglycerin on left ventricular function and ST changes in acute myocardial infarction. *Br. Heart J.* 38:612, 1976.

37. Flaherty, J. T., et al. Intravenous nitroglycerin

in acute myocardial infarction. *Circulation* 51:132, 1975.

38. Flaherty, J. T., et al. A randomized prospective trial of intravenous nitroglycerin in patients with acute myocardial infarction. *Circulation* 68:576, 1983.

39. Jugdett, B. I., et al. Persistent reduction in left ventricular asynergy in patients with acute myocardial infarction by intravenous infusion of nitroglycerin. *Circulation* 68:1264, 1983.

40. Cohn, J. N., et al. Effect of short-term infusion of sodium nitroprusside on mortality rate in acute myocardial infarction complicated by left ventricular failure: Results of a Veterans Administration Cooperative Study. *N. Engl. J. Med.* 306:1129, 1982.

41. Thomas, A. D., et al. Haemodynamic effects of morphine in patients with acute myocardial infarction. *Br. Heart J.* 27:863, 1965.

42. Timmis, A. D., et al. Haemodynamic effects of intravenous morphine in patients with acute myocardial infarction complicated by severe left ventricular failure. *Br. Med. J.* 280:980, 1980.

43. Ryan, W. F., Henning, H., and Karliner, J. S. Effect of morphine on left ventricular dimensions and function in patients with previous myocardial infarction. *Clin. Cardiol* 2:417, 1979.

44. Gibson, T. C. Blood pressure levels in acute myocardial infarction. *Am. Heart J.* 96:475, 1978.

45. Watanabe, T., et al. Effects of increased arterial pressure and positive inotropic agents on the severity of myocardial ischemia in the acutely depressed heart. *Am. J. Cardiol.* 30:371, 1972.

46. Loeb, H. S., et al. Effects of pharmacologically induced hypertension, myocardial ischemia and coronary hemodynamics in patients with fixed coronary obstruction. *Circulation* 57:41, 1978.

47. Hillis, L. D., et al. Effect of various degrees of systemic arterial hypertension on acute canine myocardial ischemia. *Am. J. Physiol.* 240:H855, 1981.

48. Roan, P. G., et al. Effects of systemic hypertension on ischemic and non-ischemic regional left ventricular function in awake, unsedated dogs after experimental coronary occlusion. *Circulation* 65:115, 1982.

49. Koyanagi, S., et al. Increased size of myocardial infarction in dogs with chronic hypertension and left ventricular hypertrophy. *Circ. Res.* 50:55, 1982.

50. Rebuck, A. S., Cade, J. F., and Campbell, E. J. M. Pulmonary aspects of myocardial infarction. *Mod. Concepts Cardiovasc. Dis.* 42:17, 1973.

51. Fillmore, S. J., et al. Blood-gas changes and pulmonary hemodynamics following acute myocardial infarction. *Circulation* 45:583, 1972.

52. Hales, C. A., and Kazemi, H. Small-airways function in myocardial infarction. *N. Engl. J. Med.* 290:761, 1974.

53. Gray, B. A., et al. Alterations in lung volume and pulmonary function in relation to hemodynamic changes in acute myocardial infarction. *Circulation* 59:551, 1979.

54. Harrison, M. O., Conte, P. J., and Heiztman, E. F. Radiological detection of clinically occult cardiac failure following myocardial infarction. *Br. Radiol.* 44:265, 1971.

55. McHugh, T. J., et al. Pulmonary vascular congestion in acute myocardial infarction: Hemodynamic and radiologic correlations. *Ann. Intern. Med.* 76:29, 1972.

56. Kostuk, W., et al. Correlations between the chest film and hemodynamics in acute myocardial infarction. *Circulation* 48:624, 1973.

57. Battler, A., et al. The initial chest x-ray in acute myocardial infarction: Prediction of early and late mortality and survival. *Circulation* 61:1004, 1980.

58. Croft, C. H., et al. Abrupt withdrawal of B-blockade therapy in patients with myocardial infarction: Effects on infarct size, left ventricular function, and hospital course. *Circulation* 73:1281, 1986.

59. Lineberger, A. S., Sprague, D. H., and Battaglini, J. W. Sinus arrest associated with cimetidine. *Anesth. Analg.* 64:554, 1985.

60. Lippestad, C. Th., and Forfang, K. Production of sinus arrest by lignocaine. *Br. Med. J.* 1:537, 1971.

61. Cheng, T. O., and Wadhwa, K. Sinus standstill following intravenous lidocaine administration. *J.A.M.A.* 223:790, 1973.

62. Dhingra, R. C., et al. Electrophysiologic effects of lidocaine on sinus node and atrium in patients with and without sinoatrial dysfunction. *Circulation* 57:448, 1978.

63. Manyari-Ortega, D. E., and Brennan, F. J. Lidocaine-induced cardiac asystole. *Chest* 74:227, 1978.

64. Feely, J., Wilkinson, G. R., and Wood, A. J. Reduction of liver blood flow and propranolol metabolism by cimetidine. *N. Engl. J. Med.* 304:723, 1981.

65. Goldberger, A. L. Recognition of ECG pseudo-infarct patterns. *Mod. Concepts Cardiovasc. Dis.* 49:13, 1980.

66. Pardee, H. E. B. An electrocardiographic sign of coronary artery obstruction. *Arch. Intern Med.* 26:244, 1920.

67. Dressler, W., and Roseler, H. High T waves in the earliest stage of myocardial infarction. *Am. Heart J.* 34:627, 1947.

68. Blumgart, H. L., et al. Experimental studies on the effect of temporary occlusion of coro-

nary arteries in producing persistent electrocardiographic changes. *Am. J. Med. Sci.* 194:493, 1937.

69. Madias, J. E., and Krikelis, E. N. Transient giant R waves in the early phase of acute myocardial infarction: Association with ventricular fibrillation. *Clin. Cardiol.* 4:339, 1981.

70. Aldrich, H. R., et al. Identification of the optimal electrocardiographic leads for detecting acute epicardial injury in acute myocardial infarction. *Am. J. Cardiol.* 59:20, 1987.

71. Sullivan, W., et al. Correlation of electrocardiographic and pathological findings in healed myocardial infarction. *Am. J. Cardiol.* 42:724, 1978.

72. Roberts, W. C., and Gardin, J. M. Location of myocardial infarcts: A confusion of terms and definitions. *Am. J. Cardiol.* 42:868, 1978.

73. Savage, R. M., et al. Correlation of post mortem anatomic findings with electrocardiographic changes in patients with myocardial infarction. *Circulation* 55:279, 1977.

74. Bairey, C. N., et al. Electrocardiographic differentiation of occlusion of the left circumflex versus the right coronary artery as a cause of acute inferior myocardial infarction. *Am. J. Cardiol.* 60:456, 1987.

75. Macdonald, R. G., Hill, J. A., and Feldman, R. L. ST segment response to acute coronary occlusion: Coronary hemodynamic and angiographic determinants of direction of ST segment shift. *Circulation* 74:973, 1986.

76. Ferguson, D. W., et al. Angiographic evidence that reciprocal ST-segment depression during acute myocardial infarction does not indicate remote ischemia: Analysis of 23 patients. *Am. J. Cardiol.* 53:55, 1984.

77. Little, W. C., Rogers, E. W., and Sodums, M. T. Mechanism of anterior ST-segment depression during acute inferior myocardial infarction: Observations during coronary thrombolysis. *Ann. Intern. Med.* 100:226, 1984.

78. Crawford, M. H., O'Rourke, R. A., and Grover F. L. Mechanism of inferior electrocardiographic ST-segment depression during acute anterior myocardial infarction in a baboon model. *Am. J. Cardiol.* 54:1114, 1984.

79. Lembo, N. J., et al. Clinical and prognostic importance of persistent precordial (V_1-V_4) electrocardiographic ST segment depression in patients with inferior transmural myocardial infarction. *Circulation* 74:56, 1986.

80. Shah, P. K., et al. Noninvasive identification of a high risk subset of patients with acute inferior myocardial infarction. *Am. J. Cardiol.* 46:915, 1980.

81. Roberts, R. Recognition, pathogenesis, and management of non-Q-wave infarction. *Mod. Concepts Cardiovasc. Dis.* 56:17, 1987.

82. Raunio, H., et al. Changes in the QRS complex and ST segment in transmural and subendocardial myocardial infarctions: A clinical pathologic study. *Am. Heart J.* 98:176, 1979.

83. Phibbs, B. "Transmural" versus "subendocardial" myocardial infarction: An electrocardiographic myth. *J. Am. Coll. Cardiol.* 1:561, 1983.

84. DeWood, M. A., et al. Coronary arteriographic findings soon after non-Q-wave myocardial infarction. *N. Engl. J. Med.* 315:417, 1986.

85. Pratt, C. M., et al. Design of a multicenter, double-blind study to assess the effects of prophylactic diltiazem on early re-infarction after a non-Q-wave acute myocardial infarction: Diltiazem re-infarction study. *Am. J. Cardiol.* 58:906, 1986.

86. Gibson, R. S., et al. The prevalence and clinical significance of residual myocardial ischemia 2 weeks after uncomplicated non-Q wave infarction: A prospective natural history study. *Circulation* 73:1186, 1986.

87. Maisel, A. S., et al. Complex ventricular arrhythmias in patients with Q wave versus non-Q wave myocardial infarction. *Circulation* 72:963, 1985.

88. Gibson, R. S., et al. Diltiazem and reinfarction in patients with non-Q-wave myocardial infarction: Results of a double-blind, randomized, multicenter trial. *N. Engl. J. Med.* 315:423, 1986.

89. Muller, J. E., et al. Myocardial infarct extension: Occurrence, outcome, and risk factors in the multicenter investigation of limitation of infarct size. *Ann. Intern. Med.* 108:1, 1988.

90. Hutchins, G. M., and Bulkley, B. H. Infarct expansion versus extension: Two different complications of acute myocardial infarction. *Am. J. Cardiol.* 41:1127, 1978.

91. Eaton, L. W., et al. Regional cardiac dilatation after acute myocardial infarction: Recognition by two-dimensional echocardiography. *N. Engl. J. Med.* 300:57, 1979.

92. Erlebacher, J. A., et al. Late effects of acute infarct dilation on heart size: A two dimensional echocardiographic study. *Am. J. Cardiol.* 49:1120, 1982.

93. McKay, R. G., et al. Left ventricular remodeling after myocardial infarction: A corollary to infarct expansion. *Circulation* 74:693, 1986.

94. Weisman, H. F., and Healy, B. Myocardial infarct expansion, infarct extension, and reinfarction: Pathophysiological concepts. *Prog. Cardiovasc. Dis.* 30:73, 1987.

95. Plerard, L. A., et al. Hemodynamic profile of patients with acute myocardial infarction at risk of infarct expansion. *Am. J. Cardiol.* 60:5, 1987.

96. Pfeffer, J. M., Pfeffer, M. A., and Braunwald, E. Hemodynamic benefits and prolonged sur

vival with long-term captopril therapy in rats with myocardial infarction and heart failure. *Circulation* 75(Suppl I):I-149, 1987.

97. Gottlieb, S. O., et al. Nifedipine reduces early infarct expansion: Results of a double blind, randomized trial (Abstract). *Circulation* 72(Suppl 3):274, 1985.

98. Yusuf, S., and Furberg, C. D. Effects of calcium channel blockers on survival after myocardial infarction. *Cardiovasc. Drugs Ther.* 1:343, 1987.

99. The TIMI Study Group. Comparison of invasive and conservative strategies after treatment with intravenous tissue plasminogen activator in acute myocardial infarction: Results of the thrombolysis in myocardial infarction (TIMI) phase II trial. *N. Engl. J. Med.* 320:618, 1989.

100. Killip, T., and Kimball, J. T. Treatment of myocardial infarction in a coronary care unit: A two-year experience with 250 patients. *Am. J. Cardiol.* 20:457, 1967.

101. Henning, H., et al. Prognosis after acute myocardial infarction: A multivariate analysis of mortality and survival. *Circulation* 59:1124, 1979.

102. Ross, J., Jr., et al. A decision scheme for coronary angiography after acute myocardial infarction. *Circulation* 79:292, 1989.

8
Hemodynamic Monitoring of Acute Myocardial Infarction

JOEL M. GORE AND PETER L. ZWERNER

The flow-directed pulmonary artery (PA) catheter introduced by Swan and associates in 1970 [1] has found widespread use in the clinical management of patients with acute myocardial infarction (AMI). Hemodynamic monitoring is a procedure that is now performed daily in most hospitals throughout the United States. The ability to measure pulmonary capillary wedge pressure and cardiac output provides hemodynamic information that can be invaluable for evaluating myocardial performance. This information may aid in classifying and treating various hemodynamic abnormalities encountered in patients with AMI.

The use of the PA catheter in AMI patients has been increasing over the years [2]. It is estimated that in 1986 500,000 PA catheters were placed, 100,000 in patients with AMI. The use of PA catheters has spawned a $2 billion industry in the United States. It is important for the clinician to remember that the catheter is not a therapy but, rather, a device to guide therapy. There is a potential to overuse the PA catheter, and this fact must be kept in perspective. The clinician should be wary not to succumb to the pressure of modern technology. The insertion of the catheter must not delay therapy nor should it replace the bedside clinical evaluation of patients.

Clinicians who employ hemodynamic monitoring should understand the fundamentals of the insertion technique, the equipment utilized, and the data that can be generated before insertion is undertaken [3]. The hemodynamic data obtained must be fully evaluated or significant information may be missed. Frequently, only two parameters are utilized— "wedge" pressure and cardiac output—whereas other parameters, including right atrial, right ventricular, and pulmonary artery pressures, are given only cursory attention. In addition, the catheter is often left in place for inappropriately long periods of time [4]. Catheters should always be removed when the the data collected are no longer being used to direct the management of the patient.

Indications

Numerous indications for insertion of the PA catheter are now accepted (Table 8-1). Critically ill patients in whom the changing function of the heart is an essential factor during treatment are candidates for hemodynamic monitoring. Hemodynamic monitoring in patients with AMI has four central objectives: (1) to assess left and/or right ventricular function; (2) to monitor changes in hemodynamic status; (3) to guide treatment with a variety of pharmacologic and nonpharmacologic agents; and (4) to provide prognostic data.

One of the most common indications for hemodynamic monitoring is the management of patients with various complications of myocardial infarction. Hypotension is common in the setting of AMI and may be secondary to a variety of conditions. Dehydration due to overly aggressive diuretic therapy, vomiting, diarrhea, or profuse diaphoresis may produce hypotension. In contrast, hypotension may be the first manifestation of cardiogenic shock. Patients with right ventricular infarction may also be hypotensive, and the diagnosis and treatment of this clinical entity can be greatly aided by hemodynamic monitoring.

Table 8-1
Indications for hemodynamic monitoring of AMI

Management of complicated AMI
  Hypovolemia vs. cardiogenic shock
  Ventricular septal rupture vs. acute mitral
    regurgitation
  Severe left ventricular failure
  Right ventricular failure
Refractory ventricular tachycardia
Differentiating severe pulmonary disease from left
  ventricular failure
Assessment of cardiac tamponade
Assessment of therapy in selected individuals
  Afterload reduction in patients with severe left
    ventricular failure
  Inotropic agents
  Beta-blockers
  Temporary pacing (ventricular vs.
    atrioventricular)
  Intra-aortic balloon counterpulsation
  Mechanical ventilation

Hemodynamic monitoring is useful for the diagnosis of individuals with severe left ventricular failure and a loud systolic murmur who may have suffered a ventricular septal rupture or acute mitral regurgitation. In other individuals, marked left ventricular failure is secondary to extensive infarction without a mechanical complication. Hemodynamic and oximetry evaluation aid in distinguishing these various entities.

Patients with refractory ventricular arrhythmias or postinfarction angina may have underlying unrecognized left ventricular failure secondary to extensive infarction or ischemia. Hemodynamic monitoring discloses the severity of left ventricular dysfunction and aids in management. In addition, cardiac arrhythmias can often cause recognizable changes in the atrial pressure tracings that can be used to both diagnose the arrhythmia and understand the hemodynamic consequences of the rhythm disturbance [5].

Coexisting pulmonary and cardiac diseases represent a difficult diagnostic and therapeutic dilemma. A confirmed pulmonary artery wedge pressure is a key hemodynamic variable. An elevated pulmonary capillary wedge pressure indicates left ventricular dysfunction, whereas a normal wedge pressure with an elevated PA diastolic pressure indicates pulmonary disease or pulmonary vasoconstriction.

Hemodynamic monitoring can be useful for assessing and maximizing therapy with various pharmacologic agents. Afterload reduction in patients with severe left ventricular failure and hypotension can be optimized with hemodynamic monitoring. In addition, the hemodynamic effects of inotropic agents and beta-blockers can be continuously monitored.

The effect of various other forms of therapy can be evaluated with hemodynamic monitoring. Therapy using various modes of temporary pacing (ventricular versus atrioventricular), the intraaortic balloon counterpulsation device, and mechanical ventilation with or without positive end-expiratory pressure can be directed utilizing hemodynamic data.

Pericardial effusion can be easily diagnosed with echocardiography, although cardiac tamponade can present with varying amounts of pericardial fluid. Hemodynamic measurements determine the physiologic significance (if any) of a specific volume of pericardial effusion. The response to therapy in these patients can be followed by means of hemodynamic monitoring.

Indications for hemodynamic monitoring in patients with AMI must be individualized. When the decision to use a PA catheter is made, one must consider the fact that it is not an innocuous procedure; the risks must be weighed against the potential benefits. Instituting hemodynamic monitoring should not delay therapy and must not replace good clinical judgment.

Hemodynamic Monitoring Equipment

PA Catheters

Pulmonary artery catheters are available in a variety of sizes and offer a range of features. The catheters are generally constructed of polyvinyl chloride, which has flexibility characteristics ideal for flow-directed catheters. Polyvinyl chloride has a high thrombogenicity, and therefore the catheters are generally coated with heparin. This heparin bonding process has been shown to be effective in reducing thrombus formation on the catheter [6, 7]. The hydrophilic properties of polyvinyl chloride have been reported to result in the absorption of certain drugs commonly utilized in the coronary care unit (CCU) setting [8, 9]. Therefore the potential for delayed drug delivery during infusion exists, and it is recommended that drug therapy always be titrated to the patient's clinical response.

The outside diameter of cardiac catheters is measured in French (Fr) gauge with 1 Fr = 0.335 mm (0.013 in.). The PA catheters utilized in the intensive care unit usually have an outside dimension of 5 to 7 Fr and are 110 cm in length. An inflatable balloon is positioned 1 to 2 cm from the tip of the catheter to allow flow direction. The balloon capacity varies according to the catheter size, and the operator must be aware of the individual balloon's maximal inflation volume, as prescribed by the manufacturer. In general, air should be used as the inflation medium. Filtered carbon dioxide may be utilized when there is a risk that balloon rupture would result in the introduction of air into the arterial system. This situation would be the case in patients with right-to-left intracardiac shunts, such as those with an atrial septal or a ventricular septal defect.

Pulmonary artery catheters are available with a number of lumens. The double-lumen catheter has a lumen for balloon inflation and a lumen for distal pressure monitoring or blood sampling. The 7 Fr triple-lumen catheter has an additional lumen 20 to 30 cm from the distal tip of the catheter that allows simultaneous measurement of central venous (right atrial) and pulmonary artery pressures. The most commonly employed PA catheter in the CCU setting is the four-lumen 7.5 Fr thermodilution catheter (Fig. 8-1). This catheter has

Fig. 8-1

Quadruple-lumen PA catheter. A = connection to thermodilution cardiac output computer; B = connection to distal lumen; C = connection to proximal lumen; D = stopcock connected to balloon at the catheter tip for balloon inflation; E = thermistor; F = balloon. Note that the catheter is marked in 10-cm increments. (From J. M. Rippe et al. *Intensive Care Medicine*. Boston: Little, Brown, 1985. P. 44. With permission.)

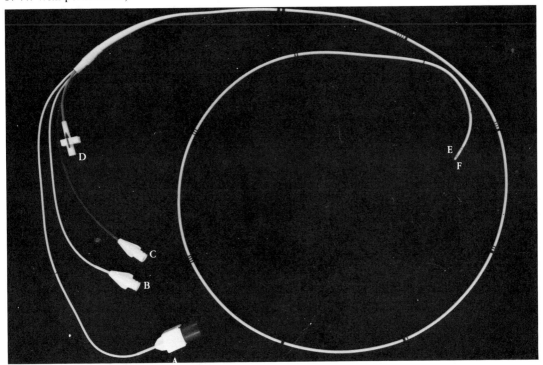

a thermister placed 4 cm proximal to the catheter tip, in addition to the three previously described lumens. The fourth lumen is utilized for placement of the electrical leads required for coupling the thermister to the cardiac output computer. This apparatus allows thermodilution cardiac output measurements.

A five-lumen catheter is also available which, in addition to the features of the four-lumen catheter, employs a fifth lumen opening 40 cm from the catheter tip. This lumen allows additional central venous access for fluid or drug infusions. This catheter is recommended when peripheral venous access is limited, volume resucitation is required, or drugs requiring infusion into a large vessel (i.e., dopamine, epinephrine) are being utilized.

Several special-purpose PA catheters are available. The "pacing PA catheter" incorporates two groups of electrodes externally on the catheter surface (six total: two ventricular, four atrial), an arrangement that enables intracardiac electrocardiographic (ECG) recording or temporary cardiac pacing. These catheters are utilized for emergency temporary cardiac pacing, although it is often difficult to position the catheter for reliable simultaneous cardiac pacing and PA pressure monitoring. The Paceport right ventricular catheter (CR Bard Inc., Billerica, MA), a five-lumen catheter, is designed with the fifth lumen located 19 cm from the distal tip. This lumen position allows passage of a specially designed pacing electrode through the catheter into the right ventricular apex (Fig. 8-2). Rapid emergency temporary intracardiac pacing can be accomplished without need for a separate central venous puncture. In addition, simultaneous PA pressure may be measured. When a pacing probe is not being used, the fifth lumen provides additional central access or the opportunity to monitor right ventricular pressure continuously.

The ability to continuously measure and record mixed venous oxygen saturation in vivo is clinically available through the use of a fiberoptic reflectance oximetry system incorporated into a five-lumen PA catheter. This catheter has an additional lumen that contains optical fibers that allow transmission of light to and from the bloodstream (Fig. 8-3). Alternating pulses of three wavelengths are emitted

from three diodes. Hemoglobin absorbs this transmitted light, which is then refracted back to a second optical detector. The amount of desaturated hemoglobin relative to oxyhemoglobin can be measured because the absorption of light by desaturated hemoglobin and oxyhemoglobin varies as a function of wavelength. The optical signal is converted to an electrical signal and transmitted to a data processor. The calculated hemoglobin oxygen saturation is averaged over a 5-second period and displayed.

PRESSURE TRANSDUCERS

Hemodynamic monitoring depends on a system that converts changes in pressure to an electrical signal suitable for interpretation. Transducers are devices that are connected through a fluid-filled tubing system to a catheter placed in an intravascular space (Fig. 8-4). The transducer has a dome that is a fluid-filled chamber directly connected to the fluid-filled catheter. Intravascular pressure changes are transmitted through the fluid-filled catheter to the fluid-filled dome. There is a diaphragm in the chamber that is connected to the pressure transducer. The diaphragm is displaced by the transmitted intravascular pressure changes, and a series of resistance wires are deformed. These wires are connected to form a Wheatstone bridge, which allows changes in resistance to induce a current. The current produced is proportional to the deformation of the diaphragm. These current changes are amplified and displayed as a waveform on a cathode ray tube and in numerical terms on a pressure meter. It allows continuous instantaneous measurement of intravascular pressure changes.

Fig. 8-2
A. Five-lumen "right ventricular Paceport" catheter; the fifth lumen, located 19 cm from the distal tip, can be used for pressure monitoring or for passage of a specially designed pacing electrode. B. Close-up view of the catheter with a pacing electrode extending out the additional lumen.

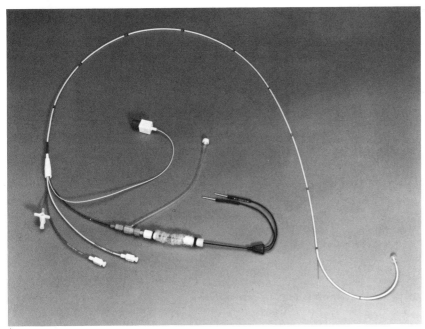

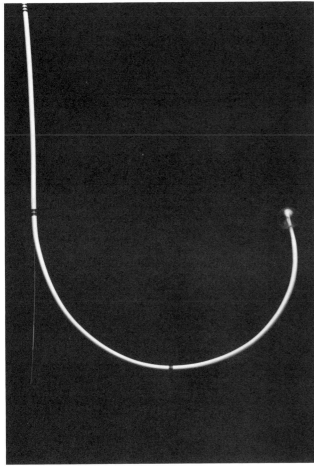

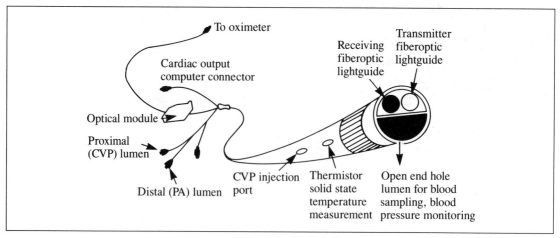

Fig. 8-3
Fiberoptic reflectance oximetry system incorporated into a five-lumen PA catheter.

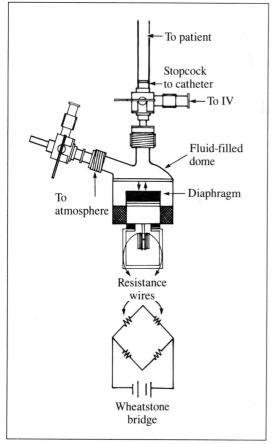

Fig. 8-4
Transducer/Wheatstone bridge.

Most systems allow either systolic, diastolic, or mean pressure numerical representation. Newer systems provide simultaneous recording of all three variables. It is recommended that the ECG be displayed simultaneous with the pressure tracing in order to time the various components of the pressure trace (i.e., A wave, V wave).

The pressure amplifier requires an integrated electronic calibration circuit and a zero control. It is essential that the pressure amplifier provide a hard-copy printout of the pressure waveform and simultaneous ECG in order to properly analyze the pressure tracing. The system should allow various recording speeds, usually 25, 50, and 100 mm/sec. Rapid speeds "expand" the recorded waveform for analysis, and slow speeds allow continuous recording.

Currently produced pressure monitors are less prone to drift, although they must be periodically calibrated and balanced. Calibration is generally accomplished against an internal electronic reference, although occasional balancing by manometry is recommended.

The ability to obtain clinically meaningful hemodynamic data depends on the fidelity of the pressure recording. *Damping* is a term referring to the property of a system to return to its resting point. Overdamping of the pressure tracing is commonly encountered in hemodynamic pressure monitoring. The usual source of overdamping is air in the pressure tubing. Reflushing the tubing system to remove air bubbles usually remedies this problem. Damping of the tracing is often caused by having the distal port of the PA catheter opposed to an intracardiac surface. Slight repositioning, inflation of the balloon, or reflushing of the catheter may correct this condition. The PA catheter has a tendency to migrate into the pulmonary vasculature periphery, leading to "overwedging" of the catheter. Caution must be exercised regarding the position of the catheter tip. Radiologic assessment of catheter position prior to balloon inflation is recommended to avoid vascular trauma due to overinflation of the balloon within the pulmonary vasculature.

Excessively exaggerated pressure waveforms may also be encountered. The length of tubing affects the damping properties. Long tubing may cause more oscillations in the pressure tubing system, resulting in underdamping of the pressure tracing. Utilizing shorter lengths of connecting tubing may ameliorate this condition.

Pressure signal quality is maximized if there is minimal distance between the transducer and the signal source. The most precise signals can be obtained with catheter tip manometers. The current generation of catheter tip micromanometers are impractical for routine CCU use owing to expense, rigidity, and drift. The expected new generations of catheter tip manometers may eliminate the problems experienced with the current devices and allow routine use of micromanometer technology.

INSERTION TECHNIQUES

Equipment Preparation

Adequate preparation is essential when performing invasive procedures, and a team approach involving the physician and nursing staff is required. The operator must be assured that the necessary equipment is present, accessible, and in operating condition prior to initiating the procedure. A careful explanation of the procedure to the patient is necessary to allay anxiety. Patients who are unable to cooperate must receive adequate sedation so invasive procedures can be performed with minimum risk. Regardless of the indications for hemodynamic monitoring, an uncooperative patient is not a candidate for introducing large-gauge intravenous devices. Once the patient has been fully informed of the procedure, he or she must be placed in as comfortable a position as possible to ensure continued cooperation. In addition, it is imperative that the person who performs the procedure assume a comfortable position in order to minimize operator fatigue.

Central Venous Access

Measurement of right heart pressures is contingent on safe and reliable access to the central venous system. Five sites are commonly utilized for insertion of PA catheters: subclavian vein, internal jugular vein, femoral vein, basilic vein, and external jugular vein. The axillary vein has also been reported to be a safe and simple alternate route for placement of PA catheters [10]. Various cannulation techniques are possible for each site. The internal jugular may be cannulated via an anterior, central, or posterior approach. The subclavian vein is reached via an intra- or supraclavicular route; the basilic vein is cannulated via a percutaneous entry or by direct visualization via a cutdown technique. It must be emphasized that no one technique is "superior," and that physicians practicing in the intensive care setting must be familiar with several approaches.

Numerous commercially prepared kits are available that contain the necessary equipment for gaining central venous access and for insertion of PA catheters (Fig. 8-5). Care should be taken to follow manufacturer's instructions regarding the specifics of the equipment utilized.

Excellent references exist for detailed explanations of various central venous catheter insertion techniques [11–13]. The internal jugular approach is the one most commonly utilized in our institution, and a detailed explanation of catheter insertion via this route follows.

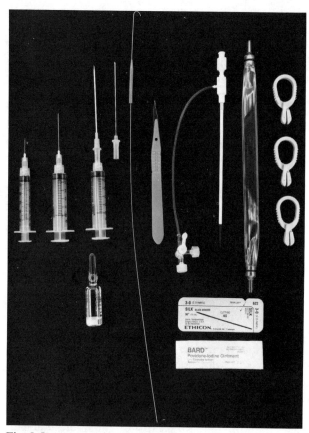

Fig. 8-5
Equipment available in a commercially supplied kit for PA
catheter introduction. Supplies shown include (clockwise
from left) 3-cc syringe with 25-gauge needle for
anesthetizing the skin; 5-cc syringe with 1.5-in., 21-gauge
needle for anesthetizing superficial tissues and locating
the vein to be cannulated; 5-cc syringe with catheter-
over-needle; 25-cm guidewire; scalpel; introducer and
sheath; sterile sheath for catheter; towel clips; 3-0 suture
for fixing catheter in place; iodine ointment; and 1%
Xylocaine. (From J. M. Rippe et al. *Intensive Care
Medicine*. Boston: Little, Brown, 1985. P. 47. With
permission.)

1. Figure 8-6 shows the surface anatomy of
   the jugular region and various approaches
   to internal jugular vein cannulation.
2. The patient and operator must be in a comfortable position with the patient placed in
   Trendelenburg position to maximize central venous pressure and venous distention. The operator should be at the head of
   the bed with the patient's head positioned
   as close to the head of the bed as possible
   and turned 30 to 45 degrees opposite the
   side of cannulation.
3. The area to be cannulated is scrubbed with
   antibacterial solution and widely draped
   with sterile barriers.
4. Local anesthesia is obtained by infiltrating
   the skin with lidocaine using a 25-gauge
   needle.
5. Deeper anesthesia is accomplished utilizing a 1.5-in. 21-gauge needle. The internal

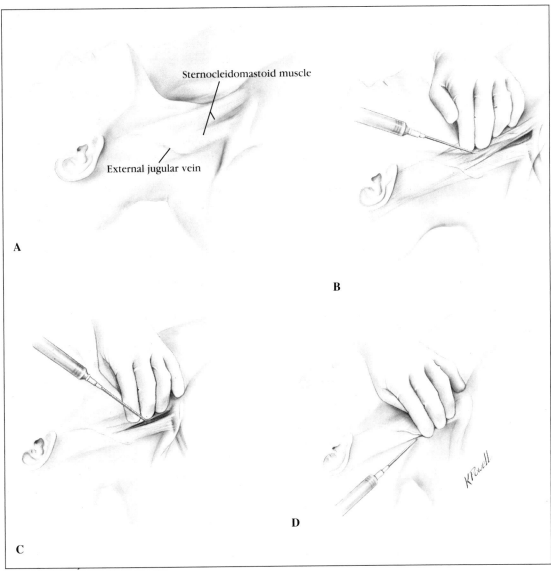

Fig. 8-6
Surface anatomy and various approaches to cannulation of the internal jugular
vein. *A*. Surface anatomy. *B*. Anterior approach. *C*. Central approach.
D. Posterior approach. (From J. M. Rippe et al. *Intensive Care Medicine*.
Boston: Little, Brown, 1985. P. 22. With permission.)

jugular vein can now be located with this needle, which is attached to a syringe. Once the vein is entered, the 21-gauge needle may be kept in place to act as a guide for vessel locations.

6. A syringe is now attached to the 18-gauge needle–cannula, which is inserted into the previously located internal jugular vein while continuously gently aspirating for free venous flow. When free flow appears, the Teflon cannula is moved over the needle into the vein using a circular motion. The needle is then removed and a syringe placed on the cannula to check for continued free venous flow. If flow is inadequate or arterial pulsations occur, the

cannula is withdrawn and pressure is applied to the area for approximately 5 minutes.

7. If free venous flow occurs, the *soft* J tip of the guidewire is advanced through the cannula. The guidewire should meet no resistance when being threaded through the cannula. Continuous ECG monitoring is necessary at this stage, as the guidewire can advance into the right ventricle and cause electrical irritability. When the guidewire is in position, the cannula can be withdrawn, leaving the guidewire in place. The guidewire must be secured (a hand on the wire) at all times to avoid loss of the guidewire into the central venous circulation.

8. A small incision in the skin is made with a scalpel at the point of the guidewire entry. This measure allows ease of placement of the vessel dilator/sheath apparatus through the skin.

9. The dilator/sheath should be placed over the guidewire and advanced through the skin into the vessel using a circular motion. Care should be taken to secure the guidewire at all times. The dilator sheath should pass smoothly into the vessel once the skin has been penetrated.

10. The dilator and guidewire are removed, leaving the introducer sheath in place. The side arm of the introducer sheath is aspirated to establish the presence of free venous blood flow. The side arm is then intermittently flushed with heparinized saline or attached to a continuous infusion to maintain patency.

PA CATHETER PREPARATION

1. Flush all lumens except the balloon lumen with sterile solution.
2. Inflate the balloon with an appropriate volume of air to check for balloon integrity and the presence of leaks.
3. Attach tubing from the transducer to all ports of the catheter and flush with saline. Turn the distal stopcock to "pressure" and check that the pressure-monitoring equipment is operational by moving the distal end of the catheter and observing for simultaneous pressure changes on the oscilloscope.

4. Place a sterile sleeve on the catheter, ensuring that the proper end is positioned to engage the introducer.

5. Gently advance the catheter into the internal jugular vein, superior vena cava, and right atrium under continuous pressure monitoring (each band mark on the catheter represents 10 cm). The right atrium is usually reached at a distance of 10 to 20 cm.

6. Right atrial oxygen saturation should be obtained.

7. Inflate the balloon, and under continuous pressure and ECG monitoring advance the catheter through the right atrium until a right ventricular pressure tracing appears. This value is recorded and the oxygen saturation obtained. Arrhythmia monitoring is critical at this stage, as the catheter may produce serious ventricular arrhythmias while in the right ventricle.

8. Advance the catheter until a PA pressure is observed. Gently continue to advance the catheter until a pulmonary capillary pressure wedge tracing is obtained. Deflate the balloon under continuous hemodynamic monitoring and record a return to a PA pressure waveform. Obtain and record the oxygen saturation. Inflation of the balloon with the prescribed amount of air should reproduce the pulmonary capillary wedge waveform, which may be recorded. Test to see that the catheter is properly positioned in the pulmonary artery by deflating the balloon completely and observing the change from a wedge pressure tracing to a PA pressure tracing.

9. The introducer and PA catheter are now sutured into place and the sterile sleeve extended to its maximum length. Sterile dressing is applied.

10. A chest radiograph in the semiupright position is obtained immediately to check for catheter position and for the presence of a pneumothorax.

SPECIAL CONSIDERATIONS

Physicians are likely to encounter several conditions in the CCU setting that require special consideration when hemodynamic monitoring is to be utilized. An individualized approach is necessary to ensure safety for any given patient. The following section discusses several situations where the approach to hemodynamic monitoring may vary from the routine.

Anticoagulated Patients

Anticoagulants are commonly prescribed for a variety of cardiac disorders. Patients in the CCU are frequently receiving either intravenous heparin or oral warfarin (Coumadin) therapy. The approach to venous access in this setting requires special attention to minimize the risk of serious hemorrhagic complications.

In general, it is recommended that patients have normal coagulation parameters prior to attempting central venous access. Anticoagulants are discontinued when possible, and sufficient time is allowed to pass prior to the procedure to allow coagulation times to return to normal. In patients receiving intravenous heparin, the drug may be discontinued 3 to 4 hours prior to the procedure to allow normalization of the partial thromboplastin time. Protamine also can acutely reverse the effect of heparin. Intravenous heparin therapy may be restarted once central venous access is obtained and the procedure is complete.

Warfarin has a protracted half-life, and discontinuance of the drug has little acute effect on the prothrombin time. The effects of this drug may be acutely reversed with infusion of fresh frozen plasma. Vitamin K also reverses the effects of warfarin, although it may take several days to normalize bleeding parameters.

In many patients it is either ill-advised or impractical to reverse the anticoagulant effects of heparin or warfarin. These patients therefore have a coagulopathy prior to PA catheter insertion. This situation represents a relative contraindication to PA monitoring, although several techniques may be utilized to minimize the risk of serious bleeding in these patients. It is recommended that the basilic vein be utilized in all patients with abnormal bleeding parameters. Visualization of the vessel via a cutdown is recommended. This approach allows direct access to the site of catheter entry and enables the operator to control sites of potential bleeding.

Central venous access via the external or internal jugular vein is a secondary choice in patients with coagulopathies. The anatomy of this region allows direct compression of potential sites of bleeding. Inadvertent puncture of the carotid artery must be avoided. If carotid artery puncture does occur, direct pressure over the vessel usually controls excessive bleeding.

The subclavian vein as a site for central venous access should be avoided in this patient population. The subclavian vessels lie under the clavicle; and in the event of uncontrolled bleeding or inadvertent puncture of the subclavian artery, the vessels would be inaccessible to direct compression.

Thrombolytic Therapy

Thrombolytic therapy has become commonplace for the treatment of AMI. Patients are frequently encountered who require invasive hemodynamic monitoring during the perithrombolytic period. Thrombolytic therapy is not an absolute contraindication for performing invasive procedures. Central venous and arterial access may be obtained with relative safety if certain guidelines are followed.

It is well established that early initiation of thrombolytic therapy is essential to have a favorable impact on AMI. It must be emphasized that it is rarely necessary to delay thrombolytic therapy in order to obtain invasive hemodynamic monitoring. Peripheral venous access for blood sampling and drug and fluid infusion should be established prior to initiating thrombolytic therapy. A peripheral arterial catheter may be placed after therapy has been initiated, in order to monitor blood pressure and aid in obtaining blood samples. At the University of Massachusetts Medical Center, peripheral arterial catheters have been placed in more than 300 patients following thrombolytic therapy with few complications. It is recommended that the use of intra-arterial catheters in general be reserved for patients who require continuous arterial blood pressure monitoring or frequent blood sampling.

Pulmonary artery catheters may be placed in patients receiving thrombolytic therapy, although caution must be exercised. When there is an indication for PA monitoring in these patients, the thrombolytic drug infusion must be immediately discontinued. Tissue plasminogen activator has a half-life of 8 to 9 minutes, which allows rapid reversal of the thrombolytic effects of this drug. Streptokinase has a longer half-life, approaching 20 minutes, and induces a fibrinolytic state that may last 24 hours following infusion due to depletion of clotting factors. Patients receiving streptokinase therapy require fresh frozen plasma in addition to discontinuation of the drug to help normalize bleeding parameters. The concomitant use of heparin may further contribute to bleeding complications following invasive procedures, and heparin should be discontinued prior to initiating invasive hemodynamic monitoring in patients receiving thrombolytic therapy.

The approach to central venous access in the setting of thrombolytic therapy should be similiar to the techniques utilized for patients receiving anticoagulants. The brachial approach via a cutdown technique is the procedure of choice; other easily compressible sites can be utilized.

Pulmonary Hypertension, Right Ventricular Dilatation, and Low Cardiac Output

In patients with severe pulmonary hypertension, dilatation of the right atrium or ventricle, or low cardiac output states, it may be difficult to place a flow-directed catheter into the right ventricle, pulmonary artery, or pulmonary capillary wedge position. Fluoroscopic guidance may be required to aid in positioning the

catheter in this setting. Occasionally, it is beneficial to stiffen the catheter by infusing 5 to 10 ml of cold sterile solution via the distal lumen. Alternately, under fluoroscopic guidance, a 0.025-cm guidewire (length 145 cm) may be placed through the distal lumen of a 7 Fr PA catheter. This maneuver makes the catheter more rigid and aids in control and placement. A guidewire should always be placed by an experienced operator under fluoroscopic guidance, as stiff catheters increase the risk of right heart perforation. In rare circumstances, it is necessary to utilize a non-flow-directed PA catheter (i.e., Cournand) because of its increased rigidity. These catheters have a potential for perforating the right heart and must always be placed via fluoroscopic guidance by a physician experienced in cardiac catheterization techniques.

Patients with right heart failure from any cause have excessively elevated central venous pressure, which places them at risk for hemorrhagic complications from central venous cannulation. It is recommended that central venous access be obtained via sites readily accessible to compression or that the brachial approach via a cutdown technique be utilized.

Mechanical Ventilation

Patients undergoing positive-pressure ventilation are at increased risk for complications of invasive hemodynamic monitoring. Hyperinflation of the lungs may predispose to pneumothorax. Ventilator-dependent patients with preexisting respiratory compromise are least likely to tolerate the consequences of a pneumothorax. A pneumothorax in this setting is under tension and requires placement of a chest tube for adequate treatment.

Central venous access via the subclavian approach is associated with the highest incidence of pneumothorax. Pneumothorax accounts for 25 percent of all complications when this route of central venous access is utilized. The internal jugular vein approach appears to have a much lower incidence of pneumothorax formation and should be util-

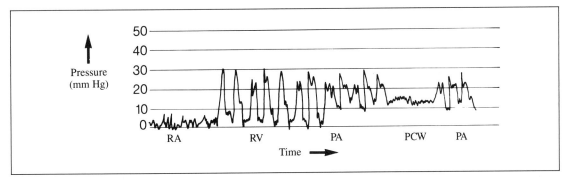

Fig. 8-7
Pressure tracing obtained from a PA catheter.

ized in patients on mechanical ventilators when practical.

Normal Physiologic Data

Hemodynamic monitoring requires careful attention to the accuracy of the data obtained. The physician must be familiar with the calibration and balancing of manometers and amplifiers, and must be able to recognize, understand, and differentiate the pressure tracings obtained from the right atrium, right ventricle, pulmonary artery, and pulmonary capillary wedge positions (Fig. 8-7).

The technical aspects of placing flow-directed catheters are not difficult to master, although the interpretation and synthesis of the data obtained require special training. The foundation of hemodynamic monitoring is built on the knowledge of normal physiologic parameters (Table 8-2). Pressure data obtained from hemodynamic monitoring are rarely specific for a particular disease, and patients may have more than one abnormality. In addition to the pressure data, analysis of the waveform is useful for recognition of certain cardiac conditions.

RIGHT ATRIUM

The normal right atrial pressure is 0 to 6 mm Hg. Two major positive atrial pressures, the A and V waves, can usually be recorded from

Table 8-2
Normal resting right heart pressures

Cardiac chamber	Pressure (mm Hg)
RIGHT ATRIUM	
Range	0–5
Mean	3
RIGHT VENTRICLE	
Systolic	17–30
Diastolic	0–6
PULMONARY ARTERY	
Systolic	15–30
Diastolic	5–13
Mean	10–18
PULMONARY CAPILLARY WEDGE	
Mean	2–12

the right atrium (Figs. 8-8 and 8-9). The A wave is due to atrial contraction and follows the P wave on the ECG. The V wave is due to venous filling of the left and right atrium during ventricular systole when the mitral and tricuspid valves are closed. The peak of the V wave occurs at the end of ventricular systole at a time when the two atria are maximally filled. The x descent, occurring after the A wave, reflects atrial relaxation and the sudden downward motion of the atrioventricular valves. The y descent is due to rapid atrial emptying following opening of the mitral and tricuspid valves. During inspiration, the mean right atrial pressures decline (owing to the decrease in intrathoracic pressure), whereas the A and V waves frequently become more prominent.

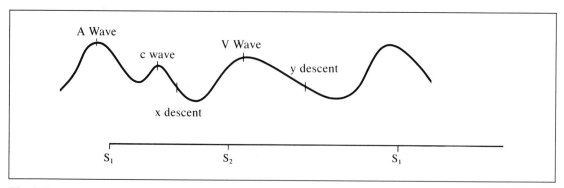

Fig. 8-8
Stylized representation of a right atrium waveform in relation to heart sounds.
(See text for discussion of A, c, and V waves and x and y descents.)

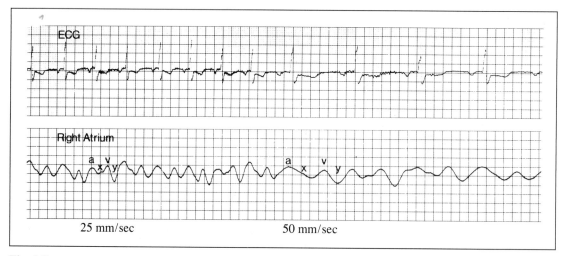

Fig. 8-9
Right atrial tracing recorded at two paper speeds.

RIGHT VENTRICLE

The right ventricular pressure and waveform are the result of both the right atrial and pulmonary arteries. The normal range is 17 to 30/0 to 6 mm Hg. The right ventricular pressure should equal the PA pressure during systole while the pulmonary valve is open. The right ventricular diastolic pressure should equal the mean right atrial pressure during diastole while the tricuspid valve is open. In the past, right ventricular hemodynamic data were not used clinically, as the catheters did not allow continuous monitoring of this chamber. The introduction of the right ventricular pacing catheter has enabled continuous observation of right ventricular hemodynamics through the port in the right ventricle. With selected disease entities, such as tricuspid regurgitation, ventricular septal rupture, cardiac tamponade, right ventricular infarction, and pulmonary embolism, monitoring the right ventricle may be beneficial.

PULMONARY ARTERY

The PA waveform is characterized by a systolic peak and diastolic trough with a dicrotic notch due to closure of the pulmonic valve.

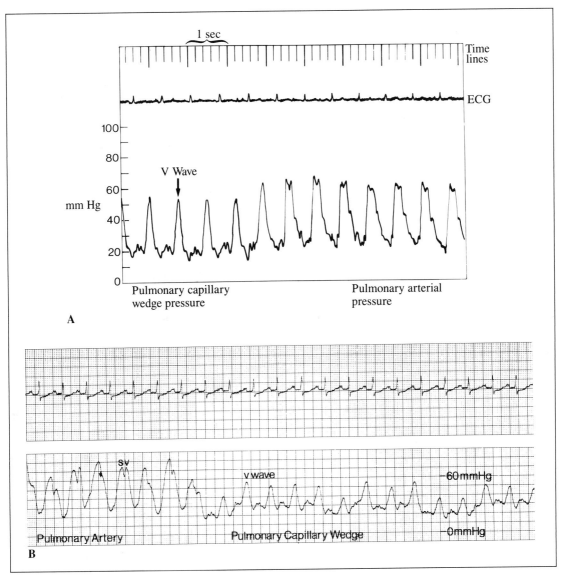

Fig. 8-10
PA and pulmonary capillary wedge pressure tracings with a giant V wave
distorting the PA pressure tracing.

The normal PA pressure is 15 to 30/5 to 13 mm Hg, with a normal mean of 10 to 18 mm Hg. A mean PA pressure of more than 20 mm Hg signifies the presence of pulmonary hypertension. The peak of the PA systolic wave occurs within the T wave of a simultaneously recorded ECG. The PA diastolic pressure is virtually equal to pulmonary capillary pressure when pulmonary vascular resistance is normal.

The morphology of the PA pressure waveform is of value for the diagnosis of conditions resulting in large volumes filling a noncompliant left atrium. In this instance, the tracing is often distorted by a V wave transmitted backward through the low-resistance pulmonary vascular bed (Fig. 8-10). The V wave may, in fact, resemble the PA waveform, and the operator may not notice that the catheter has gone from the PA position into the wedge position. This move can result in permanent wedging of the catheter.

Pulmonary Capillary Wedge

The pulmonary capillary wedge pressure is a phase-delayed and amplitude-damped version of left atrial pressure. The pressure waveform is bifid and of low magnitude. Pulmonary capillary pressure is obtained when the PA catheter is in a "PA-occluded" position. The inflated balloon prevents flow between this branch of the pulmonary artery and the left atrium, as there is no pressure drop along this vascular segment. The distal tip of the catheter is therefore monitoring left atrial pressure. The pressure obtained is more properly called the PA-occluded pressure. The mean PA-occluded pressure is normally 2 to 12 mm Hg. It should average 2 to 7 mm Hg below by the mean PA pressure.

The waveform of the PA-occluded pressure is markedly damped relative to that of the pulmonary artery. In contradistinction to the right atrial waveform, the normal PA-occluded waveform demonstrates a V wave that is slightly larger than the A wave.

Confirmation that the catheter is truly measuring PA-occluded or pulmonary capillary wedge pressure is obtained by withdrawing a sample of blood from the catheter tip and measuring oxygen saturation. Satisfactory "wedge" position is indicated by obtaining a 1- to 2-ml catheter-tip blood specimen with an oxygen saturation nearly equivalent to that of the patient's arterial blood. During procurement of the blood specimen, it is important to have the patient breathe slowly and deeply to ensure that the lung segment from which the sample is being obtained is well ventilated.

Cardiac Output

Cardiac output is an integral part of the data obtained from hemodynamic monitoring. Right-sided heart pressures should be analyzed along with the cardiac output. The thermodilution technique is the mostly commonly used bedside means of measuring cardiac output. This technique employs the principle of indicator dilution. A known quantity of cold solution is introduced into the circulation and adequately mixed by passage through two cardiac chambers (right atrium and right ventricle). A thermistor mounted on the distal tip of the PA catheter measures the temperature of PA blood, and the resulting cooling curve allows calculation of blood flow. Cardiac output is proportional to the integral of the time versus temperature curves. Cardiac output is usually calculated by a computer using a complicated formula incorporating the area under the thermodilution curve (change in temperature versus time). It can be useful to inspect the thermodilution temperature curve to ensure that the computer-derived measurement is accurate (Fig. 8-11).

The thermodilution cardiac output can be inaccurate in the presence of several clinical conditions. Thermodilution cardiac output is less accurate in low output states, tricuspid regurgitation, and atrial or ventricular septal defects. The most accurate clinical method for measuring cardiac output is the Fick technique, which employs arteriovenous (A-V) difference of blood oxygen content and total body oxygen consumption. The normal A-V oxygen content difference is 3.0 to 5.0 ml/dl. As cardiac output declines, the peripheral tissues extract more oxygen from hemoglobin and the A-V oxygen difference increases. The opposite occurs with an increase in cardiac output. Thus the A-V oxygen difference can be used to follow cardiac output. Cardiac output is defined by the following formula.

$$\text{Cardiac output} = \frac{\text{oxygen consumption}}{\substack{\text{arterial O}_2 \text{ content} - \\ \text{mixed venous O}_2 \text{ content}}}$$

If one assumes that arterial oxygen saturation and total body oxygen consumption are relatively stable over short periods of time, then, applying the Fick principle, changes in mixed venous oxygen saturation (SVO_2) reflect changes in cardiac output. The fiberoptic reflectance oximetry catheter allows continuous measurement of mixed venous oxygen

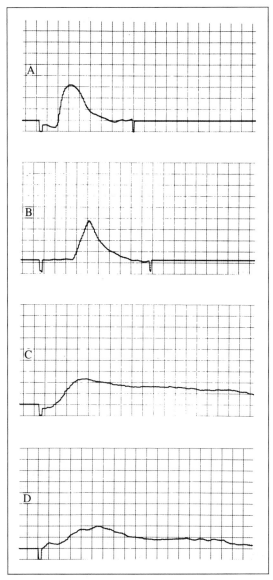

Fig. 8-11
Thermodilution temperature curves generated to determine cardiac output. *A*. Normal cardiac output. *B*. High cardiac output. *C*. Low cardiac output. *D*. Inaccurate cardiac output due to erratic injection of saline.

saturation. Changes in SVO_2 are proportional to changes in cardiac output, and this system allows continuous monitoring of this variable.

OTHER VARIABLES

The hemodynamic pressure measurements directly obtained from right heart catheterization represent only a small portion of the data that can be generated. Additional information can be obtained by making calculations based on the basic hemodynamic data that have been recorded. Tables 8-3 and 8-4 include some commonly derived variables and their normal values.

Accurate assessment of PA pressure until recently has been obtainable only with invasive right heart catheterization. In general, noninvasive techniques lack sensitivity and are limited in their ability to detect and quan-

Table 8-3
Hemodynamic formulas

Cardiac output (CO)	$HR \times SV$
Cardiac index (CI)	CO/BSA
Stroke volume (SV)	CO/HR
Stroke index (SI)	SV/BSA or CI/HR
Left ventricular stroke work index (LVSWI)	$\dfrac{1.36 \times (MAP - PCWP) \times SI}{100}$
Systemic vascular resistance (SVR)	$\dfrac{(MAP - RAP)}{CO} \times 80$
Pulmonary vascular resistance (PVR)	$\dfrac{(PAP - PCWP)}{CO} \times 80$
Mean arterial pressure (MAP)	$\dfrac{(2 \times \text{diastolic}) + \text{systolic}}{3}$
Ejection fraction (EF)	$\dfrac{SV}{\text{end-diastolic volume}} \times 100$

HR = heart rate, SV = stroke volume, BSA = body surface area, MAP = mean arterial pressure, PCWP = pulmonary capillary wedge pressure, RAP = right atrial pressure, PAP = mean pulmonary artery pressure.

Table 8-4
Selected hemodynamic values

Cardiac output	4–6 L/min
Cardiac index	2.5–4.0 L/min/m²
Stroke volume	60–90 ml
Stroke index	40 ± 7 ml/beat/m²
Left ventricular stroke work index	45–60 g-m/beat/m²
Systematic vascular resistance	800–1200 dynes/sec/cm⁻⁵
Pulmonary vascular resistance	50–150 dyne/sec/cm⁻⁵
Mean arterial pressure	70–100 mm Hg
Arteriovenous oxygen difference	4.5–6.0 vol. %

tify mild to moderate elevation of PA pressures. The introduction of Doppler echocardiography has enabled the PA pressure to be measured noninvasively. Measurement of the gradient across the tricuspid valve by quantification of the velocity of the jet of tricuspid regurgitation allows one to estimate right ventricular systolic pressure and thereby the systolic PA pressure. In addition, various indexes of pulmonary flow velocity correlate with PA pressure.

Hemodynamics in Common Clinical Situations

ACUTE MYOCARDIAL INFARCTION

It has been shown that there is a good correlation between the clinical and hemodynamic profile of patients with AMI (Table 8-5). Forester et al. [14] developed a classification method relating the clinical presentation of AMI patients to specific hemodynamic determinants of left ventricular pump performance.

> *Group I.* Patients with an uncomplicated MI, no pulmonary congestion or peripherial hypoperfusion, normal capillary wedge pressure, normal cardiac index.
> *Group II.* Patients with modest left ventricular failure as manifested by an S₃ gallop and bibasilar rales. Hemodynamics re-

veal an elevated capillary wedge pressure (>18 mm Hg), a minimally depressed cardiac index, and normal systemic blood pressure.

> *Group III.* Patients without clinical evidence of pulmonary edema but with evidence of low cardiac output and fatigue, usually in the presence of decreased renal function as evidenced by rising blood urea nitrogen (BUN) and creatinine levels. Blood pressure is usually low in these patients. Hemodynamic monitoring reveals a slightly elevated wedge pressure (12–28 mm Hg) and a reduced cardiac index (<2.2 L/min/m²). In addition, systemic vascular resistance is usually increased (>1500 dynes/sec/cm⁻⁵).
> *Group IV.* This group includes patients with cardiogenic shock that manifests clinically as hypotension, fatigue, mental obtundation, and pulmonary congestion. These patients are acidotic and hypoxic, and they have deteriorating renal function (increasing BUN and creatinine levels). Hemodynamic monitoring reveals an elevated wedge pressure (18–25 mm Hg) with evidence of pulmonary hypertension (mean PA pressure >35 mm Hg), decreased CI (<2.0 L/min/m²), and elevated systemic vascular resistance.

Appropriate therapy is guided by the hemodynamic data. In general, hemodynamic monitoring is most useful in patients in group IV in whom it is important to exclude the presence of a mechanical lesion. During the clinical course of myocardial infarction there are times when there is a discrepancy between the clinical appearance of the patient and the hemodynamic picture. It is at this time also that hemodynamic monitoring may be useful.

ACUTE MITRAL REGURGITATION

Acute mitral regurgitation (MR) can present in a variety of ways. A patient with this condition may have sudden, unexplained dyspnea with minimal cardiac auscultatory findings. The chest radiograph may reveal florid pul-

Table 8-5
Hemodynamic patterns for common clinical conditions

Cardiac condition	Chamber pressures (mm Hg)			PAOP	CI
	RA	RV	PA		
Normal	0–6	25/0–6	25/0–12	6–12	≥2.5
AMI without LVF	0–6	25/0–6	30/12–18	≤18	≥2.5
AMI with LVF	0–6	30–40/0–6	30–40/18–25	>18	>2.0
Biventricular failure	>6	50–60/>6	50–60/25	18–25	>2.0
RVMI	12–20	30/12–20	30/12	≤12	<2.0
Cardiac tamponade	12–16	25/12–16	25/12–16	12–16	<2.0
Pulmonary embolism	12–20	50–60/12–20	50–60/12	<12	<2.0

RA = right atrium, RV = right ventricle, PA = pulmonary artery, PAOP = pulmonary artery occlusion pressure, CI = cardiac index, LVF = left ventricular failure, RVMI = right ventricular myocardial infarction.

monary edema with a normal heart size. It is more common for acute MR to occur in the setting of an inferior myocardial infarction, although it can be seen with anterior AMI. In the setting of AMI, acute MR usually occurs 24 to 48 hours after the onset of infarction with sudden onset of dyspnea. The individual is usually hypotensive and tachycardic. A murmur is usually but not always present and can be nondescript.

Hemodynamic monitoring reveals a giant V wave in the wedge pressure tracing (Fig. 8-10). It results from the left ventricle ejecting blood into a normal-sized, relatively noncompliant left atrium. As mentioned, a large V wave is not definitely diagnostic of acute MR, as it can occur whenever the left atrium is distended and noncompliant, as with ventricular septal rupture or left ventricular failure of any cause [15–17]. The giant V wave of acute MR is often transmitted to the PA tracing, which yields a bifid PA waveform composed of the PA systolic wave and the V wave. As the catheter is wedged, the PA systolic wave disappears but the V wave remains. It is useful to remember that the PA systolic wave occurs earlier in relation to the QRS (between the QRS and T wave) than does the V wave (end of the T wave). Acute MR is the rare instance when the PA end-diastolic pressure may be lower than the mean pulmonary capillary wedge pressure. PA blood oxygen saturation is generally decreased owing to a reduction in cardiac output; however, in rare cases the

giant left atrial V wave is accompanied by transient reversal of pulmonary blood flow with highly oxygenated blood entering the pulmonary artery. This situation may result in overestimation of cardiac output (if one uses the Fick method) or incorrect diagnosis of a left-to-right shunt. The systemic vascular resistance is frequently elevated, and prerenal azotemia develops.

VENTRICULAR SEPTAL RUPTURE

Rupture of the ventricular septum causes acute volume overload of the right ventricle. This complication of AMI occurs 2 to 5 days after the initial event and may be found with both inferior and anterior infarction. The first clue to its appearance is the development of biventricular failure. The clinical examination usually reveals a loud holosystolic murmur along the sternum with wide radiation, an S_3 gallop, and, frequently, elevated jugular venous pressure.

The diagnosis of acute ventricular septal rupture is made by finding a significant step-up in oxygen saturation of blood between the right atrium and the pulmonary artery. The oxygen saturation value from the right atrium must be interpreted carefully, as it may be misleadingly decreased if blood is sampled near the coronary sinus. The mean right atrial, pulmonary artery, and pulmonary capillary wedge pressures are all significantly elevated.

A prominent V wave may be seen in the wedge tracing [17], but this finding is usually not as striking as that which occurs with acute mitral regurgitation.

In the setting of acute ventricular septal defect, the systemic cardiac output is less than the thermodilution-determined cardiac output. The thermodilution method measures right-sided cardiac output, i.e., pulmonary blood flow, which reflects left-to-right shunting. "Normal" thermodilution cardiac output in a patient with an acute ventricular septal defect usually reflects a severe reduction in systemic blood flow. When following Fick cardiac outputs in patients with acute ventricular septal rupture, a fall in PA blood saturation may actually represent less left-to-right shunting and an improvement in forward cardiac output. In a patient with an acute ventricular septal defect, mixed venous oxygen saturation is calculated using inferior and superior vena caval blood oxygen saturation.

CARDIAC TAMPONADE

When pericardial fluid accumulates, it may result in increased pericardial pressure, which can impair ventricular diastolic filling. Severe impairment of diastolic filling may result in cardiac tamponade. Clinically, the patient is tachycardic, hypotensive, and dyspneic. Examination reveals clear lung fields and a quiet precordium. Radiographically, the lungs are clear and the cardiac silhouette enlarged. The combination of a small, quiet heart, increased central venous pressure, and hypotension constitute *Beck's triad*.

The hemodynamic hallmarks of cardiac tamponade are elevation and equalization of the right atrial, right ventricular diastolic, PA diastolic, and mean pulmonary capillary wedge pressures. Arterial waveform analysis reveals pulsus paradoxus. Close examination of the right atrial pressure can be informative. There is a dominant x descent due to the diminished cardiac volume at this time. The y descent is frequently absent, which results in a unimodal right atrial pressure recording. Even in the presence of severe cardiac tamponade, inspiration is accompanied by a small drop in intrapericardial, and therefore right atrial, pressure, which can be detected at the bedside by an inspiratory fall in the level of the jugular venous pressure. This decline in right atrial pressure can be helpful for distinguishing cardiac tamponade from other conditions that result in elevated right-sided diastolic pressure, i.e., restriction or right ventricular infarction.

RIGHT VENTRICULAR INFARCTION

Clinically important right ventricular infarction usually occurs in the setting of inferior myocardial infarction. It is frequently accompanied by hypotension, increased jugular venous pressure, clear lung fields, and bradyarrhythmias. Right-side ECG can be useful for making the diagnosis. The hemodynamic findings are characteristic, although they may be confused with constrictive pericarditis or cardiac tamponade. The right atrial pressure is elevated (usually >10 mm Hg) with relatively low right ventricular and PA systolic pressures. The right atrial pressure is often disproportionately increased relative to the wedge pressure. With significant elevation of right atrial pressure, shunting can occur across a patent foramen ovale leading to arterial desaturation. The right atrial waveform reveals prominent x and y descents. During inspiration, the right atrial pressure usually does not decline and may actually increase (Kussmaul's sign). An increase in right atrial pressure may also be seen with compression of the liver. Right ventricular end-diastolic pressure is elevated, and the pulse pressure is narrowed in both right ventricle and pulmonary artery. Tricuspid regurgitation due to papillary muscle dysfunction and right ventricle dilatation may complicate right ventricular infarction.

Therapy is directed toward elevating the right ventricular diastolic and right atrial pressures, often to 20 mm Hg, by infusing volume in order to move blood through the right side of the heart in the face of decreased right ventricular contractility.

PULMONARY HYPERTENSION

Pulmonary hypertension is present when the mean PA pressure is more than 20 mm Hg. The cause can be either passive ("upstream" increase in pressure) or reactive (local increase in pressure). The difference between the mean PA pressure and the pulmonary capillary wedge pressures is used to make this determination. A difference of more than 12 mm Hg indicates *reactive pulmonary hypertension,* 12 mm Hg or less indicates *passive hypertension.* Pulmonary hypertension can result from a combination of passive and reactive causes.

Pulmonary hypertension is usually referred to as primary or secondary based on the underlying etiology. *Primary pulmonary hypertension* has an unknown etiology, whereas *secondary pulmonary hypertension* occurs in patients with long-standing intracardiac shunts, chronic lung disease, or chronic left ventricular failure. Pulmonary hypertension can also be classified as *passive* (upstream increase in pressure leading to increased pulmonary pressures) or *reactive* (local increase in pressure). The pulmonary capillary wedge pressure is usually normal with reactive pulmonary hypertension (primary pulmonary hypertension, pulmonary hypertension due to lung disease) and abnormal with passive pulmonary hypertension (left ventricular failure). With passive pulmonary hypertension, the PA diastolic pressure increases passively, in keeping with the elevated wedge pressure. With pulmonary hypertension of either etiology (reactive or passive), the mean PA pressure, by definition, is elevated, often exceeding 50 mm Hg. The right ventricular end-diastolic pressure is normal until late in the course of the disease. Long-standing pulmonary hypertension can lead to right ventricular dilatation with resulting tricuspid regurgitation. The right atrial pressure tracing of tricuspid regurgitation reveals accentuated V waves with steep y descents. The mean right atrial pressure is elevated. The right atrial V wave of tricuspid regurgitation is not as pronounced as the left atrial V wave of acute mitral regurgitation. With tricuspid regurgitation, Kussmaul's sign may be present, i.e., a rise in mean right atrial pressure with inspiration. Pulmonary hypertension with a dilated right ventricle and tricuspid regurgitation often presents difficulties for placement of the PA catheter. Tricuspid regurgitation interferes with the measurement of thermodilution cardiac output because of the back and forth flow of the indicator (saline) between the right atrium and right ventricle.

MASSIVE PULMONARY EMBOLISM

Massive pulmonary embolism is invariably manifested by unexplained acute dyspnea with arterial blood oxygen desaturation, low cardiac output, and elevated jugular venous pressure. The ECG usually demonstrates acute cor pulmonale. Hemodynamic monitoring reveals markedly elevated right atrial pressure (often more than 10 mm Hg). Right ventricular and PA systolic pressures are elevated but rarely exceed 40 to 50 mm Hg, as the normal right ventricle cannot generate a high PA pressure acutely. The right ventricle generally dilates and fails once right ventricular systolic pressure reaches 50 to 60 mm Hg. Higher PA pressures suggest a chronic component to the pulmonary hypertension. The pulmonary capillary wedge pressure is usually low, as is the cardiac output. The PA end-diastolic pressure remains significantly higher than the mean wedge pressure. The A and V waves of the wedge tracing are frequently absent, as the abnormal pulmonary vasculature does not allow retrograde transmission of these pressure waves from the left atrium to the distal catheter lumen. Pulmonary vascular resistance is elevated.

In patients with respiratory distress from any cause, large swings in intrathoracic pressure can occur that can be transmitted to the pulmonary capillary wedge tracing. These wide swings in intrathoracic pressure reduce the accuracy of the capillary wedge pressure as a measure of left ventricular filling pressure. It is possible for left ventricular filling pressure to be overestimated in this setting. Attempts should be made to take measurements at end expiration.

Complications of Hemodynamic Monitoring

The ability to monitor PA pressures has increased our understanding of the pathophysiology of cardiac disease. This procedure is not without risk, and the precise role in the monitoring of patients in the CCU remains controversial. Numerous case reports have described specific complications associated with the use of PA catheters, although large-scale studies are lacking. In a series of more than 500 patients, serious complications occurred in approximately 4 percent [18]. Other estimates of the incidence of significant morbidity range from 23 to 50 percent. A rate of 15.8 percent was reported when data from several series were pooled [19, 20].

Complications may be divided into three categories: (1) obtaining venous access; (2) during PA catheter insertion; and (3) catheter in situ. Most complications are avoidable when the operator is aware of the potential pitfalls and exercises careful attention to detail.

COMPLICATIONS OF CENTRAL VENOUS ACCESS

Local vascular complications can be associated with insertion of the central venous catheter. Common complications include local hematomas, inadvertent entry into the arterial system, and invasion of the pleural space with subsequent pneumothorax formation [20–26].

Hematoma formation is usually not clinically significant and can often be controlled with local pressure. Serious hematoma formation with significant bleeding or compression of mediastinal structures, with airway compromise, can occur, particularly in patients with an underlying coagulopathy [27]. Inadvertent arterial puncture is not uncommon [28]. The incidence of inadvertent carotid artery puncture with attempted internal jugular vein cannulation has been reported to be approximately 4.8 percent [29]. Reports of A-V fistula and pseudoaneurysm formation have also been described [30, 31].

Structures adjacent to vascular sites can be damaged, and there are reports of thoracic duct injury with resultant chylothorax formation [32]. Pneumothorax formation can be a serious complication of catheter insertion, although the incidence is low [29, 33]. The incidence of pneumothorax is increased utilizing the subclavian approach; hence the internal jugular approach is the preferred route in patients unlikely to tolerate a pneumothorax.

Sheared plastic catheter embolization has been reported, and caution must be exercised regarding the position of the needle and plastic cannula prior to introducer insertion [34]. Air embolism can also occur if the catheter or introducer is left open to the air and negative thoracic pressure is generated [35]. Careful attention to covering open ports in the venous system minimizes air entry into the right heart.

ARRHYTHMIAS

Insertion of PA catheters is associated with a variety of cardiac arrhythmias. Premature atrial and ventricular beats are common as the catheter passes through the right atrium and right ventricle, respectively [29, 36]. Catheter-induced atrial fibrillation and atrial flutter have been described [36]. Nonsustained ventricular tachycardia can occur as the catheter passes through the right ventricle, although the incidence of sustained ventricular tachycardia and ventricular fibrillation is low [37]. Normal electrolyte levels prior to catheter insertion minimize the potential for serious ventricular arrhythmias.

Abnormalities in electrical conduction can be encountered when right heart catheters engage the interventricular septum. Reports of transient right bundle branch block are not uncommon [38, 39], and complete heart block may also be produced [38]. Because of this potential for inducing right bundle branch block and complete heart block, it is recommended that prophylactic temporary transvenous pacing be employed prior to right heart catheterization in patients with preexisting left bundle branch block.

PULMONARY ARTERY TRAUMA

Various injuries to the pulmonary artery have been associated with the use of PA catheters. Rupture of the pulmonary artery with fatal hemorrhage has been reported [40, 41]. The onset of hemoptysis during catheter insertion signals this complication, although hemoptysis is not always present. Emergent surgical repair of the pulmonary artery or pneumonectomy may be required. PA rupture usually occurs when there is overinflation of the balloon that has migrated to a distal position. Patients with pulmonary hypertension are at increased risk for this complication. Careful consideration of catheter position prior to balloon inflation and limiting the number of balloon inflations can minimize the likelihood of PA trauma. The balloon should always be inflated with the least amount of air necessary to obtain a pulmonary capillary wedge pressure tracing.

Pulmonary artery infarction due to persistent undetected wedging of the catheter can occur [42, 43]. It may be a result of inadvertent persistent balloon inflation or, more commonly, due to distal migration of the catheter tip. These lesions are usually not clinically evident, although chest radiographs may demonstrate abnormalities in the region of the catheter tip. Careful attention to the position of the catheter tip and continuous monitoring of the pressure waveform minimize this complication.

KNOTTING

Knotting of flow-directed catheters can occur, although it is uncommon when proper technique is utilized [44]. It occurs when the catheter is advanced without the distal tip proceeding through the cardiac chambers. It is recommended that the catheter never be advanced farther than the appropriate distance for each cardiac chamber as directed by the pressure waveform. In addition, the balloon should routinely be inflated during catheter advancement to maximize flow direction of the catheter. If the catheter fails to advance

into the next heart chamber, it should be removed to the preceding chamber and re-advanced.

THROMBOTIC COMPLICATIONS

Thrombosis is a well described complication associated with the use of PA catheters. Thrombotic complications can be the result of thrombus that forms on the catheters, either proximally or distally, or within the catheter lumen with subsequent embolization to the pulmonary circulation. Thrombosis may therefore manifest clinically as either pulmonary embolism [20, 45, 46] or occlusive vascular thrombosis [45, 47]. The incidence of clinical thrombosis is uncertain; however, previously placed PA catheters have been examined at the time of open heart surgery, and the incidence of catheter thrombus formation approaches 100 percent [6, 7]. Chastre and Gilbert [48] reported a 66 percent incidence of asymptomatic thrombosis of the internal jugular vein in patients with PA catheters. Numerous cases of central venous thrombosis associated with the use of PA catheters have been reported [47, 49], as have cases of catheter-related septic central venous thrombosis [50].

Thrombosis may involve the distal tip of the PA catheter, affecting fidelity of the pressure tracing. Continuous infusion through the various catheter lumens should always be utilized to minimize this potential problem.

INFECTIONS

The use of invasive hemodynamic monitoring has been associated with both local and systemic infections [20, 22, 23, 51, 52]. The infection rate for indwelling catheters appears to be between 2 and 4 percent [24, 53, 54]. The rate may rise to 8 percent for a second catheter placed over a guidewire [53]. A large-scale prospective study of PA catheterization in patients undergoing cardiac surgery found that 18 (2.3 percent) of 794 cultured catheter tips were positive. An in situ time of more than 72 hours was associated with a significantly higher percentage (7.2 percent) of positive tip cultures [27].

Numerous factors influence the likelihood of catheter-related infection. The duration of use, care of insertion site, care of stopcocks, transducers, and infusion fluid, in addition to the patient baseline immune status, affect the rates of infection. It must be emphasized that PA catheters should be removed immediately when the hemodynamic data are no longer necessary for patient care.

Systemic Arterial Monitoring

Reliable assessment of the systemic arterial blood pressure is required in patients in the CCU setting. It is most often achieved by the use of the blood pressure cuff and auscultation of Korotkoff sounds.

Portable vital sign monitors can noninvasively and automatically measure systolic, diastolic, and mean arterial pressures. These automatic blood pressure cuff monitors operate on alternate-current line voltage or batteries and cycle automatically at operator-programmed intervals between 1 and 90 minutes. The most important consideration when obtaining indirect blood pressure measurements is use of a correctly sized cuff. A cuff that is too wide leads to underestimation of blood pressure, whereas an inappropriately narrow cuff leads to erroneously high measurements.

In most patients these indirect methods adequately assess blood pressure. There are a subset of patients in whom continuous assessment of systemic arterial pressure is required. Patients with labile blood pressure with either hyper- or hypotension constitute such a group. In these "unstable" patients, minute-by-minute assessment of blood pressure is required to determine efficacy of therapeutic interventions. Arterial cannulation and direct systemic blood pressure monitoring allow beat-to-beat monitoring of blood pressure in this critically ill population.

Multiple arterial sites are available for catheter insertion. Most common sites include the radial, dorsalis pedis, brachial, and femoral arteries. Arterial catheters may be placed either percutaneously or via a cutdown technique.

Descriptions of arterial catheter replacement are available [11, 55].

In general, it is recommended that a 2 ½ in. plastic cannula be inserted percutaneously into the radial artery. The radial artery is the preferred site because of its superficial location and the presence of collaterals with the ulnar artery via the deep and superficial volar arches (Fig. 8-12). The Allen test should always be employed prior to catheter insertion to minimize the potential for compromised arterial circulation to the hand.

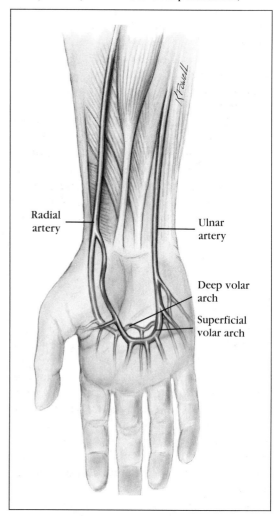

Fig. 8-12
Anatomy of the radial artery. Note the collateral circulation to the ulnar artery through the deep volar arterial arch and dorsal arch. (From J. M. Rippe et al. *Intensive Care Medicine*. Boston: Little, Brown, 1985. P. 36. With permission.)

Editorial Comments

Bedside hemodynamic monitoring has revolutionized the care of patients with AMI. Housestaff quickly become adept at utilizing invasive monitoring. Problems sometimes arise from lack of experience in interpreting hemodynamic data, which can lead to "therapeutic misadventures." One cannot learn to interpret hemodynamic data by reading a book. Experience in a laboratory or busy CCU is required. There are many pitfalls that can lead to erroneous interpretation of signals, leading in turn to incorrect therapeutic decisions. Nevertheless, hemodynamic monitoring has proved to be a valuable and powerful tool in the care of critically ill patients. If anything, it allows basic principles of physiology and pharmacology to be demonstrated at the bedside so that the clinician can experience at first hand what was previously the exclusive realm of the catheterization or experimental laboratory. G.S.F.

References

1. Swan, H. J. C., Ganz, W., Forrester, J., et al. Catheterization of the heart in man with use of a flow-directed balloon-tipped catheter. *N. Engl. J. Med.* 283:447, 1970.
2. Gore, J. M., Goldberg, T. J., Spodick, D. H., et al. A community wide assessment of the use of pulmonary artery catheters in patients with acute myocardial infarction. *Chest* 92:721, 1987.
3. Gore, J. M., Alpert, J. S., Benotti, J. R., et al. *Handbook of Hemodynamic Monitoring.* Boston: Little, Brown, 1984.
4. Robin, E. D. The cult of the Swan-Ganz catheter: Overuse and abuse of pulmonary flow catheters. *Ann. Intern. Med.* 103:445, 1985.
5. Sharkey, S. W. Beyond the wedge: Clinical physiology and the Swan-Ganz catheter. *Am. J. Med.* 83:111, 1987.
6. Hoar, P. F., Wilson, R. M., and Mangano, J. T. Heparin bonding reduces thrombogenicity of pulmonary artery catheters. *N. Engl. J. Med.* 305:993, 1981.
7. Mangano, D. T. Heparin bonding long-term protection against thrombosis. *N. Engl. J. Med.* 307:894, 1982.
8. D'Arcy, P. F. Drug interactions and reactions update. *Drug Intell. Clin. Pharm.* 17:726, 1983.
9. Jacobi, J., et al. Loss of nitroglycerin to central venous pressure catheters. *Drug. Intell. Clin. Pharm.* 16:331, 1982.
10. Martin, C., Auffray, J. P., Saux, P., et al. The axillary vein: An alternate approach to percutaneous pulmonary artery catheterization. *Chest* 90:694, 1986.
11. VanderSalm, T. J., Cutler, B. S., and Wheeler, H. B. *Atlas of Bedside Procedures.* Boston: Little, Brown, 1979.
12. Seneff, M. G., and Rippe, J. M. Central venous catheters. In: *Intensive Care Medicine.* Boston: Little, Brown, 1985. Pp. 16–33.
13. Seneff, M. G. Central venous catheterization: A comprehensive review. *J. Intensive Care Med.* 2:163, 218, 1987.
14. Forrester, J. F., Diamond, G., Chatterjee, K., and Swan, H. J. C. Medical therapy of acute myocardial infarction by application of hemodynamic subsets (Parts I & II). *N. Engl. J. Med.* 24:1356, 1404, 1976.
15. Fuchs, R. M., Heuser, R. R., Yin, F. C., and Brinker, J. A. Limitations of pulmonary wedge V waves in diagnosing mitral regurgitation. *Am. J. Cardiol.* 49:849, 1982.
16. Pichard, A. D., Kay, R., Smith, H. et al. Large V waves in the pulmonary wedge tracing in the absence of mitral regurgitation. *Am. J. Cardiol.* 50:1044, 1982.
17. Downes, T. R., Hackshaw, B. T., Kahl, F. R., et al. Frequency of large V waves in the pulmonary artery wedge pressure in ventricular septal defect of acquired (during acute myocardial infarction) or congenital origin. *Am. J. Cardiol.* 60:415, 1987.
18. Boyd, K. D., Thomas, S. J., Gold, J., and Boyd, A. D. A prospective study of complications of pulmonary artery catheterization in 500 consecutive patients. *Chest* 84:245, 1983.
19. Sprung, C. L., Jacobs, L. J., Caralis, P. V., and Karpf, M. Ventricular arrhythmias during Swan-Ganz catheterization of the critically ill. *Chest* 79:413, 1981.
20. Elliott, C. G., Zimmerman, G. A., and Clemmer, T. P. Complications of pulmonary artery catheterization in the care of critically ill patients. *Chest* 76:647, 1979.
21. Katz, J. D., Cronau, L. H., Barash, P. G., and Mandel, S. D. Pulmonary artery flow guided catheters in the perioperative period: Indications and complications. *J.A.M.A.* 237:2832, 1977.
22. Puri, V. K., Carlson, R. W., Bander, J. J., and Weil, M. H. Complications of vascular catheterization in the critically ill: A prospective study. *Crit. Care Med.* 8:495, 1980.
23. Sise, M. J., Hollingsworth, P., Brimm, J. E., et al. Complications of the flow-directed pulmonary-artery catheter: A prospective analysis in 219 patients. *Crit. Care. Med.* 9:315, 1981.
24. Davies, M. J., Cronin, K. D., and Domaingue, C. M. L. Pulmonary artery catheterization: An

assessment of risks and benefits in 220 surgical patients. *Anaesth. Intensive Care* 10:9, 1982.

25. Rao, T. L. K., Gorski, D. W., Laughlin, S., and El-Etr, A. A. Safety of pulmonary artery catheterization. *Anesthesiology* 57:A116, 1982.

26. Barash, P. G., Nardi, D., Hammon G., et al. Catheter-induced pulmonary artery perforation: Mechanisms, management and modifications. *J. Thorac. Cardiovasc. Surg.* 82:5, 1981.

27. Knoblanche, G. E. Respiratory obstruction due to hematoma following internal jugular vein cannulation. *Anaesth. Intensive Care* 7:286, 1979.

28. Silver, G. M., Bogerty, S. A., Hayashi, R. M. et al. Arterial complications of attempted Swan-Ganz insertion. *Am. J. Cardiol.* 53:340, 1984.

29. Damen, J., and Bolton, D. A prospective analysis of 1,400 pulmonary-artery catheterizations in patients undergoing cardiac surgery. *Acta Anaesthesiol. Scand.* 30:386, 1986.

30. Hansbrough, J. F., Narrod, J. A., and Rutherford, R. Arteriovenous fistulas following central venous catheterization. *Intensive Care Med.* 9:287, 1983.

31. Sheild, C. F., Richardson, J. D., Buckley, C. J., et al. Pseudoaneurysm of the brachiocephalic arteries: A complication of percutaneous internal jugular vein catheterization. *Surgery* 78:190, 1975.

32. Khalil, K. G., Parker, F. B., Jr., Mukherjee, N., et al. Thoracic duct injury: A complication of jugular vein catheterization. *J.A.M.A.* 221:908, 1972.

33. Patel, C., Laboy, V., Verus, B., et al. Acute complications of pulmonary artery catheter insertion in critically ill patients. *Crit. Care Med.* 14:195, 1986.

34. Doering, R. B., Stommer, E. A., and Connolly, J. E. Complications of indwelling venous catheters with particular reference to catheter embolism. *Am. J. Surg.* 114:259, 1967.

35. Horrow, J. C., and Laucks, S. O. Coronary air embolism during venous cannulation. *Anesthesiology* 56:212, 1982.

36. Geha, D. G., Davis, N. J., and Lappas, D. G. Persistent atrial arrhythmias associated with placement of Swan-Ganz catheter. *Anesthesiology* 39:651, 1973.

37. Cairns, J. A., and Holder, D. Ventricular fibrillation due to passage of Swan-Ganz catheter. *Am. J. Cardiol.* 35:589, 1975.

38. Thomson, I. R., Dalton, B. C., Lappas, D. G., et al. Right bundle branch block and complete heart block caused by the Swan-Ganz catheter. *Anesthesiology* 51:359, 1979.

39. Luck, J. C., and Engel T. R. Transient right bundle branch block with Swan-Ganz catheterization. *Am. Heart J.* 92:263, 1976.

40. Pape, L. A., Haffajee, C. I., Markis, J. E., et al. Fatal pulmonary hemorrhage after the use of the flow-direct balloon-tipped catheter. *Ann. Intern. Med.* 90:344, 1979.

41. Golden, M. S., Pinder, T., Anderson, W. T., et al. Fatal pulmonary hemorrhage complicating use of a flow-direct balloon-tipped catheter in a patient receiving anticoagulant therapy. *Am. J. Cardiol.* 32:865, 1973.

42. Foote, G. A., Schabel, S. I., and Hodges, M. Pulmonary complications of the flow-directed balloon tipped catheter. *N. Engl. J. Med.* 290:927, 1974.

43. Goodman, D. J., Rider, A. K., Billingham, M. E., et al. Thromboembolic complications with balloon-tipped pulmonary arterial catheter. *N. Engl. J. Med.* 291:777, 1974.

44. Lipp, H., O'Donoghue, K., and Resnekov, L. Intracardiac knotting of a flow directed balloon catheter. *N. Engl. J. Med.* 284:220, 1971.

45. Bradway, W., Bronde, R. J., Koufman, J. C., et al. Internal jugular thrombosis and pulmonary embolism. *Chest* 80:335, 1981.

46. Goldstein, M. T., Nestko, P., Olshan, A. R., et al. Superior vena cava thrombosis and pulmonary embolus. *Arch. Intern. Med.* 142:1726, 1982.

47. Yorra, F. H., Oblath, R., Jaffee, H. et al. Massive thrombosis associated with use of a Swan-Ganz catheter. *Chest* 65:682, 1974.

48. Chastre, J., and Gilbert, C. Thrombosis as complication of pulmonary artery catheterization via the internal jugular vein. *N. Engl. J. Med.* 306:1487, 1982.

49. Gore, J. M., Matsumoto, A. H., Layden, J. J., et al. Superior vena cava syndrome, its association with indwelling balloon-tipped pulmonary artery catheters. *Arch. Intern. Med.* 144:506, 1984.

50. Kaufman, J., Demas, C., Stark K., and Flancbaum, L. Catheter-related septic central venous thrombosis—current therapeutic options. *West. J. Med.* 145:200, 1986.

51. Applefield, J. J., Caruthers, T. E., and Reno, R. J. Assessment of the sterility of long-term cardiac catheterization using the thermodilution Swan-Ganz catheter. *Chest* 74:377, 1978.

52. Myers, M. L., Austin, T. W., and Silobald, W. J. Pulmonary artery catheter infections. *Ann. Surg.* 201:237, 1985.

53. Senagore, A., Waller, S. D., Bonnell, B. W., et al. Pulmonary artery catheterization: A prospective study of internal jugular and subclavian approaches. *Crit. Care. Med.* 15:35, 1987.

54. Plit, M. L., Rumbak, M. J., Lipman, J., and Eidelman, J. Invasive vascular catheterization in the critically ill. *S. Afr. Med. J.* 72:245, 1987.

55. Liebowitz, R. S., and Rippe, J. M. Arterial line placement and care. In: *Intensive Care Medicine*. Boston: Little, Brown, 1985. Pp. 33–42.

III
Electrical Complications of Acute Myocardial Infarction: Diagnosis and Treatment

9
Approach to Patients with Asymptomatic Ventricular Arrhythmias After Myocardial Infarction

ERIC N. PRYSTOWSKY

Sudden cardiac death is a major health problem, accounting for approximately 1000 deaths per day in the United States [1]. Cardiac catheterization data as well as postmortem studies demonstrate that most victims have significant coronary artery disease [2–5]. Through the efforts of Cobb et al. in association with the Seattle Fire Department, emergency care systems have been shown to decrease the mortality of cardiac arrest victims through on-the-scene cardiopulmonary resuscitation of patients who have collapsed from a malignant ventricular arrhythmia [6]. However, only a few patients with out-of-hospital ventricular fibrillation are successfully defibrillated and subsequently discharged from the hospital [6]. Clearly, a better approach would be to identify and provide prophylactic therapy for those individuals with coronary artery disease who are at high risk for future occurrences of a sustained ventricular tachyarrhythmia.

Numerous investigations demonstrated that ventricular arrhythmias, in addition to the presence and severity of coronary artery disease and left ventricular dysfunction, are risk factors for sudden cardiac death [7–19]. The presence of nonsustained ventricular tachycardia has been defined as an independent risk factor for subsequent arrhythmic death after acute myocardial infarction, and the risk appears to extend beyond the first year after myocardial infarction [19]. Califf and coworkers [20] analyzed the prognostic implications

of ventricular arrhythmias in patients who were undergoing cardiac catheterization for presumed coronary artery disease. These authors found that the severity of ventricular arrhythmias was closely associated with the extent of coronary artery disease and left ventricular dysfunction. Of patients who had nonsustained ventricular tachycardia, 71 percent had a left ventricular ejection fraction of less than 40 percent, and 16 percent of patients with an ejection fraction of less than 40 percent had nonsustained ventricular tachycardia. Although patients with more severe ventricular arrhythmias, quantitated using a modified Lown grading system, had a decreased survival rate during a 2-year follow-up period, the ventricular arrhythmia score added no additional significant prognostic information once all of the information from cardiac catheterization was included in the analysis. Thus the presence of nonsustained ventricular tachycardia has been demonstrated to be an independent risk factor for sudden cardiac death in some but not all studies.

The clinical utility of defining a high risk group for subsequent sudden cardiac death caused by a ventricular tachyarrhythmia would be to prevent the fatal arrhythmic event with appropriate antiarrhythmic therapy. Unfortunately, no data are available at the present time to document the ability of antiarrhythmic drug therapy to reduce the incidence of sudden death in these patients. The Cardiac Ar-

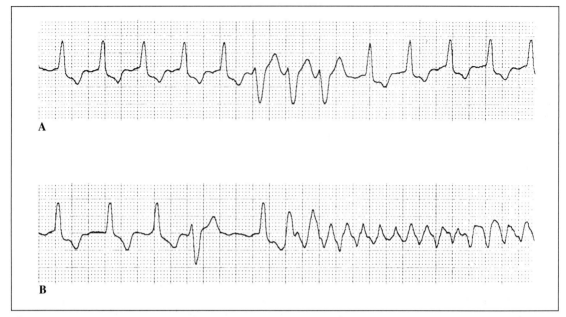

Fig. 9-1
Ambulatory ECG recording of nonsustained (*A*) and sustained (*B*) ventricular tachycardia. The patient was undergoing in-hospital evaluation of his arrhythmia at the time of the sustained ventricular arrhythmia and was cardioverted successfully.

rhythmia Pilot Study has been completed and showed that certain antiarrhythmic drugs were well tolerated by the patients for the long term without significant adverse reactions [21]; the treatment phase of this study, the Cardiac Arrhythmia Suppression Trial (CAST), is in its early stages. The study population for CAST includes patients within 2 years of a documented myocardial infarction, although patients who have nonsustained ventricular tachycardia of 15 or more complexes in duration at a rate of 120 per minute or more are excluded. The results of this study hopefully will help the clinician decide if antiarrhythmic therapy is necessary for the type of patient included in this trial; however, the results may not be applicable to subsets of patients who are excluded from this study. Importantly, the data from this investigation will not be known for several years, and the clinician is still faced with the dilemma of whether to treat these individuals at the present time.*

The prophylactic use of antiarrhythmic drugs in this situation requires an analysis of the risks and benefits of such therapy to the patient, as noted below. However, previous data regarding risk factor analysis for subsequent arrhythmic events after acute myocardial infarction have been obtained in patients undergoing traditional care during the acute myocardial infarction period. It is of note that some studies suggest that revascularization of infarcting myocardium improves survival during long-term follow-up [22–24], although the reason for the improved survival is not fully understood. Markers of electrical instability do seem to improve with reperfusion as noted by a loss of late potentials identified by signal-averaged electrocardiography [25]. Furthermore, inducibility of ventricular tachycardia at electrophysiologic study appears to occur more frequently in patients without acute reperfusion than in those who have received thrombolytic therapy [26, 27].

---

*After this chapter was written, the NHLBI removed encainide and flecainide from CAST. This action followed the recommendations from the Data and Safety Monitoring Board of this study because 56 of 730 patients assigned to encainide or flecainide died or suffered cardiac arrest compared with only 22 of 725 patients receiving placebos (NHLBI statement, April 25, 1989).

Risk Factor Analysis

NONSUSTAINED VENTRICULAR TACHYCARDIA

The relation of nonsustained ventricular tachycardia (VT-NS) to sudden cardiac death is uncertain. In some patients VT-NS triggers the onset of sustained ventricular tachycardia or ventricular fibrillation. In others, the VT-NS may become sustained at a given point. This transformation is not common in our experience, however, and the heart rate associated with VT-NS is often dissimilar from the rates seen with sustained ventricular tachycardia in a given patient (Fig. 9-1) [28]. In many patients it is also possible that VT-NS merely serves as a marker of a ventricle that is capable of supporting more serious arrhythmias. In this instance there would be no cause-and-effect relation between the nonsustained and the sustained ventricular arrhythmia.

Asymptomatic patients who have VT-NS tend to show rather characteristic features of their arrhythmia. Episodes of tachycardia are usually three to five complexes in duration, occur fewer than five times daily, and have a rate of 160 per minute or less. Several investigators have evaluated characteristics of VT-NS as predictors for the subsequent occurrence of a sustained arrhythmia, but most have failed to show any correlation. One exception was a study conducted by Meinertz et al. [29] in which there did appear to be an association between the frequency of either VT-NS or ventricular pair episodes and the subsequent clinical outcome. Other investigations have not been able to support these observations. It appears that an asymptomatic patient with three to four beats of ventricular tachycardia at a rate of 130 beats per minute (bpm) is at a risk similar to a patient who has six to eight beats of tachycardia at a rate of 180 bpm. The rate of ventricular tachycardia is often variable in these patients (Fig. 9-1). Kammerling and associates [28] showed that there was only a minimal correlation between the rate of VT-NS and the rate of sustained ventricular tachycardia in the same patient and that the more frequent the episodes of ventricular tachycardia, the more marked was the variability in tachycardia rate. Thus a lack of correlation between the rate of tachycardia and subsequent sudden cardiac death is not surprising.

SIGNAL-AVERAGED ELECTROCARDIOGRAPHY

Signal-averaged electrocardiography (ECG) is used to reduce noise, most importantly skeletal muscle activity, so that low amplitude electrical signals from the heart can be detected. The signal-averaged electrocardiogram (SAECG) usually is obtained as follows [30]: Three surface bipolar ECG leads (X, Y, Z) are acquired for 100 to 200 heart beats, and the voltage of the ECG is fed through a high-gain ($\times 1000$) amplifier. A computer averages the signal, and a high-pass filter is used to minimize the contribution of the large-amplitude low-frequency content. The high-pass filter most commonly employed is either 25 or 40 Hz. The X, Y, and Z leads are combined into a vector magnitude referred to as the filtered QRS complex (Fig. 9-2).

Three specific measurements of the filtered QRS complex are used to identify patients most likely to develop sustained ventricular tachycardia or ventricular fibrillation. These measurements are the root-mean-square voltage of the last 40 msec of the filtered QRS complex, the duration of the filtered QRS complex, and the duration of the low-amplitude signals at the end of the filtered QRS complex that are less than 40 μV [30–34]. The criteria for an abnormal SAECG vary among laboratories, but a primary goal has been to identify ventricular late potentials, which are high-frequency, low-amplitude signals that are continuous with the end of the QRS complex. These late potentials most likely represent areas of slow conduction in a damaged ventricle that may be associated with potential reentrant tachycardia circuits [35–44]. It is interesting to note that ventricular late potentials may disappear after successful ventricular tachycardia surgery [41, 43, 45–47], whereas,

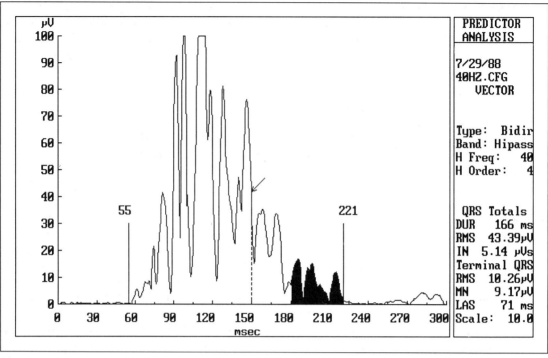

Fig. 9-2
Abnormal signal-averaged electrocardiogram. The filtered QRS duration is 166
msec, which is markedly prolonged. The root-mean-square (RMS) voltage of the
terminal 40 msec (*blackened area*) is abnormally low (10.26 μV) and constitutes a
positive late potential. Arrow = 40 μV point.

in my experience, successful antiarrhythmic
drug therapy to control ventricular tachycardia does not result in loss of late potentials.

Several studies have demonstrated that the
SAECG is a useful test to predict which patients after myocardial infarction are most
likely to develop sustained ventricular tachyarrhythmias. Kanovsky and coworkers [48]
analyzed results from the SAECG, 24-hour
ECG recording, and cardiac catheterization to
determine if the SAECG provided independent information to identify patients with a
history of sustained ventricular tachycardia.
The patient population included 76 individuals
undergoing routine cardiac catheterization who
had coronary artery disease and 98 patients
referred because of documented sustained
ventricular tachycardia. All patients had a
myocardial infarction, but the median age of
infarction differed between the patient groups;
it was 8 weeks for the control patients and 46

weeks for those with a history of sustained
ventricular tachycardia. Multivariate logistic
regression analysis identified three parameters
that were independently significant: positive
SAECG, peak premature ventricular contractions of more than 100 per hour, and the presence of a left ventricular aneurysm. Importantly, combinations of these abnormal tests
provided better predictive value than use of a
single test. If an aneurysm was excluded from
the model, a left ventricular ejection fraction
(EF) of less than 40 percent was noted to be a
significant independent variable.

A prospective study by Gomes and colleagues [34] analyzed the prognostic significance of the SAECG, left ventricular EF, and
24-hour ambulatory ECG recording in 102 patients after acute myocardial infarction. The
SAECG was obtained 10 ± 6 days after myocardial infarction, and the other tests were
performed within 72 hours of each other. The

follow-up period was 12 ± 6 months, and during this time 15 patients had either sustained ventricular tachycardia or sudden cardiac death. Arrhythmic events occurred in 29 percent of patients with an abnormal SAECG versus 3.5 percent of patients with a normal SAECG ($p< .003$); 13 of 15 patients with sustained ventricular arrhythmias were identified with this technique. Abnormal results with left ventricular EF and spontaneous ventricular arrhythmias recorded during the ambulatory ECG also presaged life-threatening arrhythmias. A high risk subset of patients was identified when all three tests were abnormal, and 8 of 16 (50 percent) of these patients had an arrhythmic event during follow-up. However, although the false-positive rate was lower, this combination of tests did not identify seven patients with a subsequent event.

In a follow-up study, Gomes and coworkers [49] investigated the relative predictive value of a 25-Hz versus a 40-Hz high-pass filter, as well as the relative predictive value of the SAECG and left ventricular EF in anterior wall versus inferior wall myocardial infarction. The sensitivity of the SAECG was slightly better at 40-Hz filtering but depended somewhat on which SAECG variable was being tested. Using 40-Hz filtering, the authors noted that patients who had inferior wall infarctions had a 100 percent sensitivity but a low (50 percent) specificity. In patients with an anterior wall myocardial infarction, the sensitivity was 75 percent and the specificity 80 percent. Thus, as has been noted in other studies of patients with chronic coronary artery disease, the SAECG has greater sensitivity in patients with an inferior versus an anterior wall myocardial infarction. It is of note that the sensitivity of an EF of less than 40 percent was high (87 percent) with a low specificity (38 percent) in patients with an anterior infarction, whereas the sensitivity was only 50 percent with a higher specificity (71 percent) in patients with an inferior wall myocardial infarction. Thus the predictive value of the SAECG was superior to that of the EF in patients with an anterior infarction, but in patients with an inferior infarction there was no difference between the two tests.

Two other investigations deserve comment. Kuchar and coworkers [50] prospectively evaluated 210 consecutive patients after acute myocardial infarction using the SAECG, 24-hour ambulatory ECG recording, and radionuclide left ventriculogram. During a median follow-up period of 14 months, seven patients had sustained ventricular tachycardia, and eight additional patients died suddenly. One patient who died suddenly had bundle branch block and did not undergo signal-averaging. Of the remaining 14 patients who had an arrhythmic event after hospital discharge, 13 had an abnormal SAECG, whereas only 1 patient (1 percent) with a normal tracing had an arrhythmic event during follow-up. Using stepwise logistic regression, an abnormal SAECG, left ventricular EF of less than 40 percent, and complex ventricular ectopy were noted to be independently significant; the EF was the most powerful variable in the model. Importantly, the combination of an abnormal SAECG and left ventricular EF was associated with a sensitivity of 80 percent and a specificity of 89 percent regarding future arrhythmic events. The combination of these variables was superior to the combination of SAECG and complex ventricular arrhythmias.

Denniss and coworkers [51] studied the prognostic significance of sustained ventricular tachycardia or ventricular fibrillation induced by programmed electrical stimulation and the presence of late potentials on SAECG in 403 patients after acute myocardial infarction. Patients who had late potentials had a higher incidence of inducible ventricular tachycardia. Patients who had inducible ventricular tachycardia had a probability of remaining free from subsequent arrhythmic events of 0.84 for the first year and 0.78 for 2 years. This rate was much worse than the event rate noted in patients in whom either no ventricular tachycardia was induced or ventricular fibrillation was initiated. Analysis of SAECG data showed that the probability of remaining free from an arrhythmic event was 0.85 at 1 year and 0.79 at 2 years with positive late potentials versus probabilities of 0.98 and 0.96, respectively, when there were no late potentials present. Multiple logistic regression analysis demonstrated that inducible ventricular tachycardia and the presence of late potentials were not independent predictors of subsequent sustained ventricular tachyarrhythmic events. However, although the positive predictive accuracy of SAECG or programmed ventricular stimulation was rather low using a single variable or a combination of variables, the negative predictive accuracy was more than 95 percent.

AUTONOMIC TESTING

Schwartz and associates [52] have investigated the relation between baroreceptor reflexes in conscious dogs and the development of ventricular fibrillation during exercise stress testing in an unique ischemic model. Results from this laboratory have now been reported on baroreflex sensitivity and subsequent cardiovascular mortality in patients after acute myocardial infarction [53]. The preliminary data suggested that patients with a markedly low baroreflex sensitivity were at risk for subsequent cardiac death. Patients with low baroreflex sensitivity scores presumably have decreased parasympathetic tone, which may in some way be related to the subsequent occurrence of sustained ventricular tachyarrhythmias, as several lines of evidence suggest that enhanced parasympathetic tone may be antiarrhythmic. Although these data are intriguing, they need to be extended and confirmed in a large prospective multicenter study.

Proposed Approach to High-Risk Patients

Prior to prescribing any specific antiarrhythmic agent to patients who appear to be at high risk for development of sustained ventricular tachyarrhythmias, it must be recognized that at the time of this writing no prospective randomized clinical trials have demonstrated the efficacy of antiarrhythmic therapy to decrease the incidence of sudden death or occurrence of sustained ventricular tachycardia in these individuals. Until data from such a trial are available, my approach is to risk-stratify patients with coronary artery disease and to treat those individuals who appear to be at highest risk for subsequent occurrence of sustained ventricular tachyarrhythmias. Data suggest that the presence of nonsustained ventricular tachycardia in patients with chronic coronary artery disease is associated with an increased mortality versus the absence of this finding (see above). Thus these patients form the primary group to which the following protocol is directed. Preliminary information regarding the use of programmed ventricular stimulation to identify a subgroup of patients at high risk for subsequent arrhythmic mortality has been published [54–58].

Patients with nonsustained ventricular tachycardia undergo SAECG and left ventricular (LV) EF determination. A "high"-risk patient is identified if the EF is less than 40 percent, an abnormal SAECG is present, or both. These patients then have programmed ventricular stimulation performed from the right ventricle using two sites, three pacing cycle lengths, and up to three extra stimuli [59]. This method appears appropriate for patients with chronic coronary artery disease, but the previously reviewed data for patients during the early postmyocardial infarction period suggest that programmed ventricular stimulation be reserved for patients with both an abnormal SAECG and an LV EF of less than 40 percent. Antiarrhythmic drug therapy is prescribed to those patients in whom sustained monomorphic ventricular tachycardia is induced by any pacing technique tried, and to patients who have ventricular fibrillation initiated with one extrastimulus, a rare event in patients without a clinical history of this arrhythmia. Drug therapy for each patient is guided by serial electrophysiologic-pharmacologic testing. Because benefit of treatment remains uncertain, "aggressive" therapy with surgery or implanted devices is not currently undertaken. In essence, we try to identify a drug(s) that prevents initiation of the sustained ventricular arrhythmia during serial electrophysiologic-pharmacologic testing. If no drug prevents inducibility, we choose the agent(s) that seemingly has provided the most benefit to the patient, as judged by the degree of spontaneous arrhythmia suppression, slowing of the rate of induced ventricular tachycardia, and change in mode of ventricular tachycardia initiation during drug therapy compared with control. The usefulness of this approach in asymptomatic patients with nonsustained ventricular tachycardia requires further investigation, and a prospective study employing a nontreatment limb is in a preliminary stage. As new data become available, a more definitive strategy for these patients can be formulated.

Editorial Comments

It is important for clinicians to remember that there is still considerable controversy regarding the treatment of patients with nonsustained ventricular tachycardia, even patients presumed to be at high risk. Until more conclusive data become available from clinical trials, this issue will remain controversial. If treatment is considered appropriate, it is now clear that drug therapy must be guided by serial electrophysiologic-pharmacologic testing or extensive Holter monitoring. Empiric therapy without rigorous testing for efficacy should be avoided. There is still uncertainty about just how to measure efficacy. G.S.F.

References

1. Lown, B. Sudden cardiac death: The major challenge confronting contemporary cardiology. *Am. J. Cardiol.* 43:313, 1979.
2. Kuller, L., Lilienfeld, A., and Fisher, R. Epidemiological study of sudden and unexpected deaths due to arteriosclerotic heart disease. *Circulation* 34:1056, 1966.
3. Liberthson, R. R., Nagel, E. L., Hirschman, J. C., et al. Pathophysiologic observations in prehospital ventricular fibrillation and sudden cardiac death. *Circulation* 49:790, 1974.
4. Reichenbach, D. D., Moss, N. S., and Meyer, E. Pathology of the heart in sudden cardiac death. *Am. J. Cardiol.* 39:865, 1977.
5. Weaver, W. D., Lorch, G. S., Alvarez, H. A., and Cobb, L. A. Angiographic findings and prognostic indicators in patients resuscitated from sudden cardiac death. *Circulation* 54:895, 1976.
6. Cobb, L. A., Werner, J. A., and Trobaugh, G. B. Sudden cardiac death. I. A decade's experience with out-of-hospital resuscitation. *Mod. Concepts Cardiovasc. Dis.* 49:31, 1980.
7. Prystowsky, E. N. Antiarrhythmic therapy for asymptomatic ventricular arrhythmias. *Am. J. Cardiol.* 61:102A, 1988.
8. Chiang, B. N., Perlman, L. V., Ostrander, L. D., Jr., and Epstein, F. H. Relationship of premature systoles to coronary heart disease and sudden death in the Tecumseh epidemiologic study. *Ann. Intern. Med.* 70:1159, 1969.
9. The Coronary Drug Project Research Group. Prognostic importance of premature beats following myocardial infarction: Experience in the Coronary Drug Project *J.A.M.A.* 223:1116, 1973.
10. Fisher, R. D., and Tyroler, H. A. Relationship between ventricular premature contractions on routine electrocardiography and subsequent death from coronary heart disease. *Circulation* 47:712, 1973.
11. Vismara, L. A., Amsterdam, E. A., and Mason, D. T. Relation of ventricular arrhythmias in the late hospital phase of acute myocardial infarction to sudden death after hospital discharge. *Am. J. Med.* 59:6, 1975.
12. Schulze, R. A., Strauss, H. W., and Pitt, B. Sudden death in the year following myocardial infarction: Relation to ventricular premature contractions in the last hospital phase and left ventricular ejection fraction. *Am. J. Med.* 62:192, 1977.
13. Ruberman, W., Weinblatt, E., Goldberg, J. D., et al: Ventricular premature beats and mortality after myocardial infarction. *N. Engl. J. Med.* 297:750, 1977.
14. Moss, A. J., David, H. T., DeCamilla, J., and Bayer, L. W. Ventricular ectopic beats and their relation to sudden and nonsudden cardiac death after myocardial infarction. *Circulation* 60:998, 1979.
15. Kotler, M. N., Tabutznik, B., Mower, M. M., and Tominaga, S. Prognostic significance of ventricular ectopic beats with respect to death in the late postinfarction period. *Circulation* 47:959, 1973.
16. Ruberman, W., Weinblatt, E., Goldberg, J. D., et al. Ventricular premature complexes in prognosis of angina. *Circulation* 61:1172, 1980.
17. Bigger, J. T., Fleiss, J. L., Kleiger, R., et al. The relationships among ventricular arrhythmias, left ventricular dysfunction, and mortality in the two years after myocardial infarction. *Circulation* 69:250, 1984.

18. Holmes, J., Kubo, S. H., Code, R. J., and Kligfield, P. Arrhythmias in ischemic and nonischemic dilated cardiomyopathy: Prediction of mortality by ambulatory electrocardiography. *Am. J. Cardiol.* 55:146, 1985.

19. Bigger, J. T., Fleiss, J. L., Orlinitzky, L. M., et al. Prevalence, characteristics and significance of ventricular tachycardia detected by 24-hour continuous electrocardiographic recordings in the late hospital phase of acute myocardial infarction. *Am. J. Cardiol.* 58:1151, 1986.

20. Califf, R. M., McKinnis, R. A., Burks, J., et al. Prognostic implications of ventricular arrhythmias during 24-hour ambulatory monitoring in patients undergoing cardiac catheterization for coronary artery disease. *Am. J. Cardiol.* 50:23, 1982.

21. The Cardiac Arrhythmia Pilot Study (CAPS) Investigators. Effects of encainide, flecainide, imipramine and moricizine on ventricular arrhythmias during the year after acute myocardial infarction: The CAPS. *Am. J. Cardiol.* 61:501, 1988.

22. Rothbaum, D. A., Linnemeier, T. J., Landin, R. J., et al. Emergency transluminal percutaneous coronary angioplasty in acute myocardial infarction: A 3 year experience. *J. Am. Coll. Cardiol.* 10:264, 1987.

23. Gruppo Italiano Per Lo Studio Della Streptochinasi Nell'Infarto Miocardico (GISSI). Effectiveness of intravenous thrombolytic treatment in acute myocardial infarction. *Lancet* 1:397, 1986.

24. Stack, R. S., Califf, R. M., Hinohara, T., et al. Survival and cardiac event rates in the first year after emergency coronary angioplasty for acute myocardial infarction. *J. Am. Coll. Cardiol.* 11:1141, 1988.

25. Irwin, J. M., Smith, P. M., Stack, R. S., et al. Successful reperfusion of infarcting myocardium is associated with reversal of electrical predictors of sudden cardiac death. *J. Am. Coll. Cardiol.* 2(II):183A, 1988.

26. Kersschot, I. E., Brugada, P., Ramentol, M., et al. Effects of early reperfusion in acute myocardial infarction on arrhythmias induced by programmed stimulation: A prospective, randomized study. *J. Am. Coll. Cardiol.* 7:1234, 1986.

27. Sager, P. T., Perlmutter, R. A., Rosenfeld, L. E., et al. Electrophysiologic effects of thrombolytic therapy in patients with a transmural anterior myocardial infarction complicated by left ventricular aneurysm formation. *J. Am. Coll. Cardiol.* 12:19, 1988.

28. Kammerling, J. M., Miles, W. M., Zipes, D. P., et al. Characteristics of spontaneous nonsustained ventricular tachycardia poorly predict rate of sustained ventricular tachycardia (Abstract). *Clin. Res.* 34:312A, 1986.

29. Meinertz, T., Hofmann, T., Kasper, W., et al. Significance of ventricular arrhythmias in idiopathic dilated cardiomyopathy. *Am. J. Cardiol.* 53:902, 1984.

30. Simson, M. B., and MacFarlane, P. W. The signal-averaged electrocardiogram. In P. W. MacFarlane and T. D. V. Lawrie (eds.), *Comprehensive Electrocardiography.* New York: Pergamon Press, 1989. Pp. 1199–1218.

31. Simson, M. B. Use of signals in the terminal QRS complex to identify patients with ventricular tachycardia after myocardial infarction. *Circulation* 64:235, 1981.

32. Breithardt, G., Borggrefe, M., Quantius, B., et al. Ventricular vulnerability assessed by programmed ventricular stimulation in patients with and without late potentials. *Circulation* 68:275, 1983.

33. Denes, P., Santarelli, P., Hauser, R. G., and Uretz, E. F. Quantitative analysis of the high-frequency components of the terminal portion of the body surface QRS in normal subjects and in patients with ventricular tachycardia. *Circulation* 67:1129, 1983.

34. Gomes, J. A., Winters, S. L., Stewart, D., et al. A new noninvasive index to predict sustained ventricular tachycardia and sudden death in the first year after myocardial infarction: Based on signal-averaged electrocardiogram, radionuclide ejection fraction and Holter monitoring. *J. Am. Coll. Cardiol.* 10(II):349, 1987.

35. Boineau, J. P., and Cox, J. L. Slow ventricular activation in acute myocardial infarction: A source of reentrant premature ventricular contraction. *Circulation* 48:702, 1973.

36. Waldo, A. L., and Kaiser, G. A. A study of ventricular arrhythmias associated with acute myocardial infarction in the canine heart. *Circulation* 47:1222, 1973.

37. El-Sherif, N., Scherlag, B. J., Lazzara, R., et al. Reentrant ventricular arrhythmias in the late myocardial infarction period. I. Conduction characteristics in the infarction zone. *Circulation* 55:686, 1977.

38. Simson, M. B., Untereker, W. J., Spielman, S. R., et al. Relation between late potentials on the body surface and directly recorded fragmented electrograms in patients with ventricular tachycardia. *Am. J. Cardiol.* 51:105, 1983.

39. Simson, M. B., Euler, D., Michelson, E. L., et al. Detection of delayed ventricular activation on the body surface in dogs. *Am. J. Physiol.* H363–H369, 1981.

40. Berbari, E. J., Scherlag, B. J., Hope, R. R., et al. Recording from the body surface of arrhythmogenic ventricular activity during the ST segment. *Am. J. Cardiol.* 41:697, 1978.

41. Rozanski, J. J., Mortara, D., Myerburg, R. J., et al. Body surface detection of delayed depo-

larization in patients with recurrent ventricular tachycardia and left ventricular aneurysm. *Circulation* 63:1172, 1981.

42. Fontaine, G., Guiraudon, G., Frank, R., et al. Stimulation studies and epicardial mapping in ventricular tachycardia: Study of mechanisms and selection for surgery. In H. Kulbertus (ed.), *Reentrant Arrhythmias*. Lancaster: MTP, 1977. Pp. 334–350.

43. Breithardt, G., Becker, R., Seipel, L., et al. Noninvasive detection of late potentials in man—a new marker for ventricular tachycardia. *Eur. Heart J.* 2:1, 1981.

44. Richards, D. A., Blake, G. J., Spear, J. F., and Moore, E. N. Electrophysiologic substrate for ventricular tachycardia: Correlation of properties in vivo and in vitro. *Circulation* 69:369, 1984.

45. Uther, J. B., Dennett, C. J., and Tan, A. The detection of delayed activation signals of low amplitude in the vectorcardiogram of patients with recurrent ventricular tachycardia by signal averaging. In E. Sandoe, D. J. Julian, and J. W. Bell (eds.), *Management of Ventricular Tachycardia—Role of Mexiletine*. Amsterdam: Excerpta Medica, 1978. Pp. 80–82.

46. Breithardt, G., Seipel, L., Ostermeyer, J., et al. Effects of antiarrhythmic surgery on late ventricular potentials recorded by precordial signal averaging in patients with ventricular tachycardia. *Am. Heart J.* 104:996, 1982.

47. Marcus, N. H., Falcone, R. A., Harken, A. H., et al. Body surface late potentials: Effects of endocardial resection in patients with ventricular tachycardia. *Circulation* 70:632, 1984.

48. Kanovsky, M. S., Falcone, R. A., Dresden, C. A., et al. Identification of patients with ventricular tachycardia after myocardial infarction: Signal-averaged electrocardiogram, Holter monitoring, and cardiac catheterization. *Circulation* 70:264, 1984.

49. Gomes, J. A., Winters, S. L., Martinson, M., et al. The prognostic significance of quantitative signal-averaged variables relative to clinical variables, site of myocardial infarction, ejection fraction and ventricular premature beats: A prospective study. *J. Am. Coll. Cardiol.* 13:377, 1989.

50. Kuchar, D. L., Thorburn, C. W., and Sammel, N. L. Prediction of serious arrhythmic events after myocardial infarction: Signal-averaged electrocardiogram, Holter monitoring and radionuclide ventriculography. *J. Am. Coll. Cardiol.* 9:531, 1987.

51. Denniss, R. A., Richards, D. A., Cody, D. V., et al. Prognostic significance of ventricular tachycardia and fibrillation induced at programmed stimulation and delayed potentials detected on the signal-averaged electrocardiograms of survivors of acute myocardial infarction. *Circulation* 74:731, 1986.

52. Schwartz, P. J., Vanoli, E., Stramba-Badiale, M., et al. Autonomic mechanisms and sudden death: New insights from analysis of baroreceptor reflexes in conscious dogs with and without a myocardial infarction. *Circulation* 78:969, 1988.

53. LaRovere, M. T., Specchia, G., Mortara, A., and Schwartz, P. J. Baroreflex sensitivity, clinical correlates, and cardiovascular mortality among patients with a first myocardial infarction: A prospective study. *Circulation* 78:816, 1988.

54. Buxton, A. E., Marchlinski, F. E., Flores, B. T., et al. Nonsustained ventricular tachycardia in patients with coronary artery disease: Role of electrophysiologic study. *Circulation* 75:1178, 1987.

55. Loughery, E. J., Miles, W. M., Fineberg, N. S., et al. Electrophysiologic testing in patients with asymptomatic nonsustained ventricular tachycardia predicts risk of sudden death or sustained ventricular tachycardia within the first year but not thereafter. *J. Am. Coll. Cardiol.* 13(II):19A, 1989.

56. Winters, S. L., Stewart, D., Targonski, A., and Gomes, J. A. Role of signal averaging of the surface QRS complex in selecting patients with nonsustained ventricular tachycardia and high grade ventricular arrhythmias for programmed ventricular stimulation. *J. Am. Coll. Cardiol.* 12:1481, 1988.

57. Kharsa, M. H., Gold, R. L., Moore, H., et al. Long-term outcome following programmed electrical stimulation in patients with high-grade ventricular ectopy. *PACE* 11:603, 1988.

58. Page, R. L., Smith, P. M., Irwin, J. M., et al. Noninvasive predictors of sustained ventricular tachycardia induction in patients with asymptomatic nonsustained ventricular tachycardia. *Circulation* 78(II):629, 1988.

59. Prystowsky, E. N., Miles, W. M., Evans, J. J., et al. Induction of ventricular tachycardia during programmed electrical stimulation: Analysis of pacing methods. *Circulation* 73 (suppl. II): 32, 1986.

10
Heart Block in Acute Myocardial Infarction

ROBERT W. PETERS

Disorders of atrioventricular (AV) and intraventricular conduction are relatively common complications of acute myocardial infarction. The pathophysiology, prognosis, and therapy of these disorders vary considerably depending on the location of the infarct and the clinical setting in which it occurs. Advances in clinical electrophysiology have provided an important means of investigating conduction system disease. In the present chapter, the functional anatomy and histopathology of the specialized conduction system are reviewed along with the clinical aspects of conduction system disease, including diagnosis and therapy, in patients with acute myocardial infarction.

Specialized Conduction System

FUNCTIONAL ANATOMY

In order to elucidate the consequences of compromised coronary blood flow, it is important to review those aspects of anatomy that are most relevant to the development conduction disorders in acute myocardial infarction (Table 10-1). More detailed descriptions of coronary anatomy and blood supply are well reviewed in other texts [1].

The AV node is a small ovoid structure formed by convergence of specialized atrial tracts within the subendocardial aspect of the right side of the interatrial septum. The proximal portion of the AV node has an abundant blood supply, primarily from the origin of the large AV nodal artery, which emanates from the posterior descending artery—a branch of the right coronary artery in 90 percent of cases

and the left circumflex coronary artery in the other 10 percent. Important collateral circulation to the proximal AV node may be provided by septal branches of the left anterior descending coronary artery. In contrast, the distal portion of the AV node receives a relatively scanty blood supply. There is extensive autonomic innervation to the AV node.

The common (His) bundle arises as a strand of Purkinje fibers that originate in the AV node and gradually converge to form a narrow tubular structure that courses through the membranous interventricular septum until it divides into the bundle branches and fascicles, usually near the crest of the muscular septum. Within the common bundle, Purkinje fibers are arranged in parallel strands divided into morphologically separate compartments by a collagenous framework. The blood supply, usually the same as that of the distal AV node, is derived from branches of the AV nodal artery or septal branches of the left anterior descending coronary artery. There is relatively little autonomic innervation of the common bundle.

There is considerable interindividual variation in the separation of the common bundle into the bundle branch system. In general, the right bundle branch tends to originate as a thin group of fibers that remains intact until it branches at the base of the anterior papillary muscle into anterior, lateral, and posterior aspects. The left bundle branch usually spreads out across the left side of the interventricular septum in a fan-like fashion which, at least in some individuals, is clearly divisible into anterior (superior), posterior (inferior), and septal portions. The bundle branch system, in

Table 10-1
Blood supply and innervation of the specialized conduction system

Area	Blood supply	Specific arteries supplying the area	Autonomic innervation
Proximal AV node	+ +	AVN, LAD	+ +
Distal AV node	+	AVN, LAD	+ +
His bundle	+	AVN, LAD	−
RBB	+ +	LAD,PDA,AVN	−
LASF	+	LAD	−
LPIF	+ +	LAD,PDA,AVN	−

AVN = AV nodal artery (a branch of the posterior descending coronary artery that comes from the right coronary artery in 90% of cases); LAD = septal perforating branches of the left anterior descending coronary artery; PDA = posterior descending coronary artery; + + = very abundant; + = less abundant; − = negligible; RBB = right bundle branch; LASF = left anterior (superior) fascicle; LPIF = left posterior (inferior) fascicle.

general, has an abundant blood supply including branches from the AV nodal artery, septal perforating branches of the left anterior descending coronary artery, Kugel's artery, septal branches of the posterior descending artery, and variable contributions from more remote branches. However, the anterior (superior) fascicle of the left bundle branch often has only a single arterial supply, rendering it the component most vulnerable to ischemic insult. The ventricular specialized conduction system has relatively little autonomic innervation.

HISTOPATHOLOGY OF ACUTE MYOCARDIAL INFARCTION

In most cases of acute inferior or inferoposterior wall myocardial infarction, the conduction system pathology is confined to the AV node, a not unexpected finding in light of the minor role that the right coronary artery plays in the blood supply to the lower aspects of the conduction system. Most clinicopathologic studies of patients with inferior wall infarction complicated by AV block report little structural damage to the AV node, even in cases of complete AV block, suggesting that reversible factors such as hypoxia are responsible.

In contrast is a study by Bilbao and coworkers. They carefully dissected the specialized conduction system in 44 patients who died from inferoposterior myocardial infarction and demonstrated that almost all patients with AV block had necrosis of the prenodal atrial myocardial fibers, whereas most patients without

AV block did not [2]. These authors noted that the supranodal atrial myocardium is supplied by a single vessel in contrast to the abundant blood supply of the AV node. It is of particular interest that patients with prenodal atrial necrosis tended to be resistant to pharmacologic therapy of AV block, whereas those without necrosis were not.

Also of note is the report of Bassan and associates that patients with inferior wall myocardial infarction and obstruction of the left anterior descending coronary artery have a sixfold greater incidence of high-grade AV block than similar patients without left anterior descending obstruction [3]. Their findings support the importance of collateral blood supply to the AV node from the left anterior descending system.

In contrast to inferior wall myocardial infarction, anterior wall infarction complicated by high-grade AV block is usually accompanied by extensive necrosis of the His bundle and bundle branches in the setting of severe left ventricular dysfunction. The AV node is usually unaffected in anterior wall infarction.

Electrocardiographic Features of Heart Block with Myocardial Infarction

AV BLOCK

The most important aspect of the electrocardiographic (ECG) evaluation of AV block with acute myocardial infarction (Table 10-2) is determining the site of block within the conduction system. When impaired AV conduction

Table 10-2
AV block in acute myocardial infarction

Severity of block	Inferior wall infarct (usually narrow QRS)	Anterior wall infarct (usually wide QRS)
First degree	PR prolongation	PR prolongation
Second degree	Type I	Usually type II
Third degree	Usually junctional escape rhythm at 50–60 bpm; may respond to pharmacologic agents	Idioventricular escape rhythm at <40 bpm; tends to be unreliable, making temporary pacing mandatory

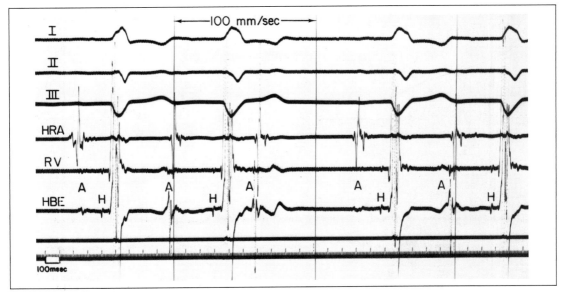

Fig. 10-1
Surface ECG leads and accompanying intracardiac recordings illustrating type I
second-degree AV block in a 54-year-old man with acute inferior wall myocardial
infarction. The arrhythmia developed abruptly 6 hours after the onset of
symptoms and was not associated with hemodynamic compromise. It
resolved spontaneously 24 hours later. I, II, III = standard ECG leads I, II, III;
HRA = high right atrial lead; RV = right ventricular lead; HBE = His
bundle electrogram; A = atrial depolarization; H = His bundle potential.

occurs during anterior wall infarction, the site
is likely to be the His-Purkinje system because
the left anterior descending coronary artery
furnishes most of the blood supply to the interventricular septum, whereas inferior/infer-
oposterior wall myocardial infarctions usually
affect the AV node. First-degree AV block
may occur with myocardial infarction of any
location, and the site of the infarction may
help localize the area of conduction delay.
Type I second-degree AV block (Wenckebach
phenomenon) (Fig. 10-1), or complete AV
block in the setting of inferior wall myocardial
infarction, is typically AV nodal in origin. In
contrast, type II second-degree AV block, or

complete AV block with a wide complex escape rhythm complicating anterior wall infarction (Fig. 10-2), is virtually always infranodal.
With 2:1 AV block, the presence of a narrow
QRS complex suggests that the block is located at the AV node, whereas a wide QRS
favors infranodal block.

Exceptions to these general rules are not
uncommon, however. For example, a preexisting intraventricular conduction defect
makes the QRS width an unreliable index of
the site of AV block. Similarly, type I second-
degree AV block complicating inferior wall
myocardial infarction has been reported within
the distal conduction system [4]. In some in-

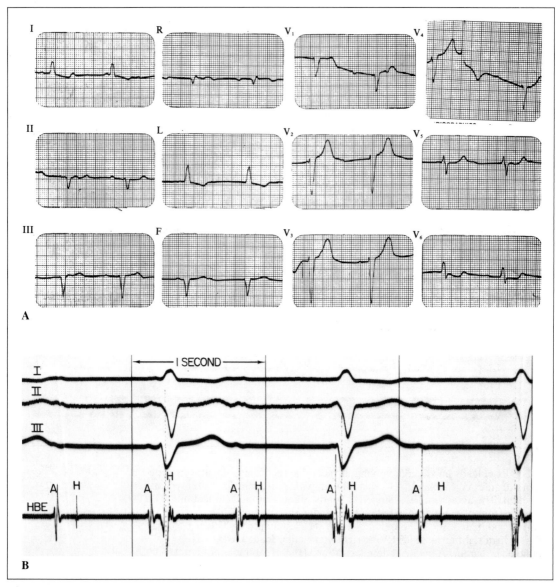

Fig. 10-2
A. Standard 12-lead ECG in a 64-year-old man with anterior wall myocardial infarction complicated by acute pulmonary edema. Complete AV block (shown here) developed 12 hours after the onset of symptoms and was preceded by left bundle branch block and first-degree AV block. Because of the slow ventricular rate and unreliability of the escape focus, immediate temporary pacemaker insertion was mandatory. B. His bundle electrogram recorded from the same patient during temporary pacemaker insertion. Block occurs below the His bundle, a pattern characteristic of anterior wall myocardial infarction.
I, II, III = standard ECG leads I, II, III; HBE = His bundle lead; A = atrial depolarization; H = His bundle potential.

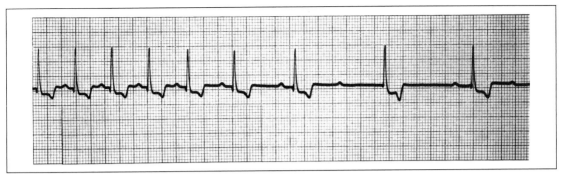

Fig. 10-3
Standard ECG lead I showing the onset of complete AV block with an
idioventricular escape rhythm in a 71-year-old woman with an otherwise
uncomplicated inferior wall myocardial infarction. The simultaneous occurrence
of sinus slowing and AV block is diagnostic of hypervagotonia. The dysrhythmia
resolved spontaneously within 30 seconds.

dividuals, the proximal portion of the right bundle branch is supplied solely by the right coronary artery, so right bundle branch block may occur in the setting of inferior wall infarction. Hypervagotonia, relatively common early in the course of inferior infarction, may mimic type II second-degree AV block (Fig. 10-3), the key to the diagnosis being simultaneous sinus slowing and nonconducted P waves [5]. In situations where the level of AV block is uncertain but clinically relevant (e.g., 2:1 AV block in the setting of anterior wall infarction) an electrophysiologic study including a recording of the His bundle electrogram can be helpful (Figs. 10-1 and 10-2).

INTRAVENTRICULAR CONDUCTION DEFECTS

ECG diagnosis of the various types of intraventricular conduction defects is well described in standard textbooks [1]. However, it is appropriate to begin with a brief review of ventricular activation as it is affected by myocardial infarction. Normal ventricular depolarization is initiated in one or more locations along the left side of the ventricular septum. Septal activation then proceeds rightward, anteriorly and inferiorly. With right bundle branch block, septal activation is normal, so the characteristic Q waves of acute myocardial infarction are often well visual-

ized (Fig. 10-4). In contrast, with left bundle branch block, the initial forces are altered (with the septum being depolarized from right to left) so the diagnosis of acute myocardial infarction is often not possible from the ECG alone. Because both left and right bundle branch block affect ventricular repolarization, the ECG diagnosis of non-Q-wave infarction is often uncertain. The fascicular blocks alter the pattern of ventricular activation and may complicate the ECG diagnosis of myocardial infarction. With left anterior (superior) fascicular block, initial forces are inferior and posterior, potentially masking inferior infarction and mimicking anterior wall infarction (Fig. 10-5). Conversely, with left posterior (inferior) fascicular block, initial forces are anterior, superior, and leftward, simulating inferior wall infarction and masking lateral wall infarction.

Clinical Aspects of AV Block in Acute Myocardial Infarction

The significance of AV block in acute myocardial infarction must be assessed in light of the clinical setting. The location of the block, the patient's hemodynamic status, the use of cardioactive medication, and other factors such as autonomic tone may be more important than the degree of the block. AV block may occur in up to 30 percent of patients with acute inferior wall infarction [6] and is especially common during the first few hours after the

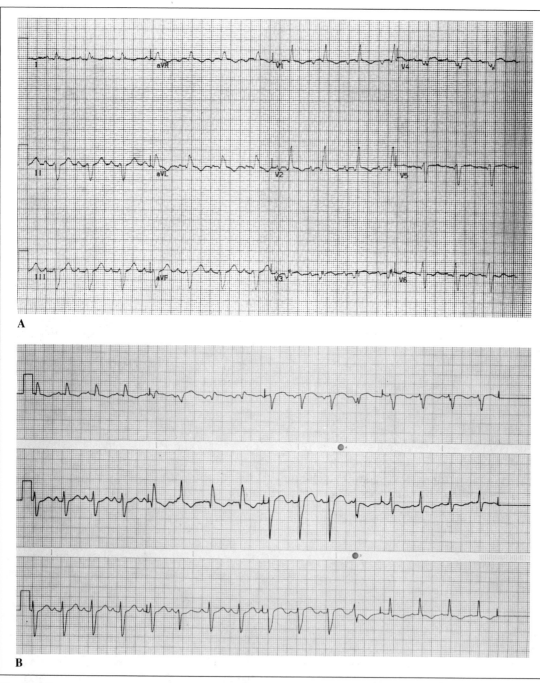

Fig. 10-4

Two ECGs from a 48-year-old man with an anteroseptal myocardial infarction complicated by left ventricular failure. *A*. Despite the presence of right bundle branch block and left anterior fascicular block, large Q waves indicative of anterior wall infarction are visible in the precordial leads. The development of new bilateral bundle branch block is an indication for temporary pacing because of the risk of high-grade AV block, but even with pacing the prognosis remains poor. *B*. Approximately 20 minutes later, the left bundle branch block developed and obscured the infarct pattern. This "alternating" bundle branch block pattern usually indicates severe infranodal disease.

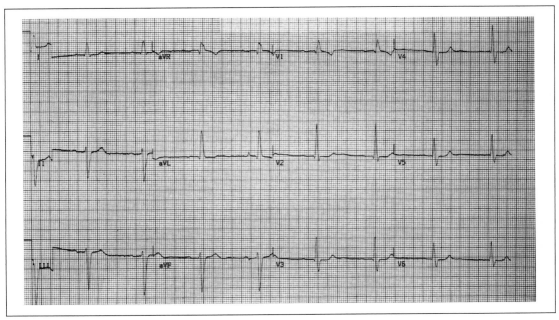

Fig. 10-5
Right bundle branch block and left anterior fascicular block in a 64-year-old
woman without coronary artery disease. The small Q waves in leads V_1–V_3 are
due to left anterior fascicular block (mimicking anteroseptal myocardial
infarction).

onset of symptoms. As would be expected from the blood supply of the inferior wall and the high degree of vagal activity accompanying inferior wall infarction, most conduction disturbances in this setting are AV nodal in origin. Accordingly, the QRS complex is usually narrow and the junctional escape rhythm stable at a reasonable rate (50–60 beats per minute [bpm]) so that even complete AV block may not require specific therapy. Although some studies have found that high-grade AV block in inferior wall infarction is associated with more extensive myocardial damage and a higher mortality rate, others have failed to confirm this finding [7–9]. Regardless of the ventricular escape rate, patients with high-grade AV block and inferior wall infarction who exhibit signs of symptoms of hypoperfusion may benefit from an increase in heart rate. (In addition to conventional findings such as hypotension or oliguria, some consider ventricular ectopy a sign of hypoperfusion.)

Pharmacologic measures include vagolytic drugs such as atropine or sympathomimetic agents such as isoproterenol. If atropine is used, intravenous therapy is preferable because of its rapid onset of action and because absorption may be erratic, especially in the presence of heart failure or hypotension. To avoid potentially deleterious tachycardia, relatively low doses of atropine (0.5 or 0.6 mg) should be used and may be repeated after several minutes if ineffective. Adverse effects of atropine include tachyarrhythmias (usually sinus tachycardia), urinary retention, central nervous system disturbances, dry mouth, and, if very low doses (0.3 mg or less) are used, paradoxical bradycardia. These adverse effects are relatively common in elderly patients and may persist for several hours, so atropine is best avoided in the presence of such conditions as prostatic enlargement and disorientation.

Intravenous isoproterenol offers the advantage of almost immediate onset of action and dissipation of effects once the infusion is discontinued. In addition, it may increase myocardial contractility in situations where this effect is desired. Isoproterenol can be initiated starting at a dose as low as 1 μg/min and titrated up to the desired increase in heart rate or hemodynamic response. Adverse effects of isoproterenol include tachyarrhythmias (potentially serious ventricular arrhythmias are not infrequent) and worsening of myocardial ischemia. Intravenous aminophylline may also improve AV conduction in at least some individuals with inferior wall myocardial infarction, but experience with this drug is limited.

If pharmacologic therapy is ineffective or undesirable, temporary transvenous pacing offers a satisfactory alternative. Pacing has the advantage of avoiding pharmacologic side effects but is invasive and has the potential for causing infection, thrombophlebitis, cardiac perforation, and arrhythmias.

Several groups have investigated the problem of AV block in the setting of inferior wall myocardial infarction with the intention of defining the mechanism and identifying subgroups who might benefit from a particular type of therapy. In a group of 144 patients with inferior wall infarction complicated by high-grade AV block, Tans and coworkers found that those with signs of low cardiac output and heart rates below 50 bpm seemed to benefit from temporary pacing, whereas patients with hypoperfusion and higher heart rates uniformly fared poorly regardless of therapy [8].

Feigl and associates, in a similar group of 34 patients, found that those who developed high-grade block suddenly (without antecedent first-degree AV block) and within 6 hours of the onset of symptoms had transient block that was responsive to atropine [10]. Individuals who developed AV block later (usually more than 24 hours after symptom onset) generally had antecedent first-degree AV block and were resistant to atropine; many required temporary pacing for block that often lasted several days. In four patients, the resolution of "early" AV block was followed by the appearance of "late" AV block with its characteristic resistance to atropine. The authors postulated the "early" AV block is due to hypervagotonia whereas "late" block is ischemically mediated and may resolve gradually as ischemia lessens.

In support of this hypothesis is a case, reported by Wesley and associates, of a 62-year-old woman with a recent inferior wall myocar-

dial infarction who developed high-grade AV block. It was resistant to atropine but dramatically responsive to aminophylline, a competitive adenosine antagonist, in doses lower than that required to release catecholamines or increase cyclic adenosine monophosphate (cAMP) [11]. Adenosine, an endogenous metabolite known to accumulate during periods of ischemia, depresses AV nodal conduction [12, 13].

Lewin and coworkers described 12 patients with alternating (multilevel) Wenckebach periods in the setting of acute inferior wall infarction [14]. They found a relatively high incidence of hemodynamic deterioration (especially during the periods of AV block) and a high mortality rate (25 percent). Atropine increased the degree of AV block, actually precipitating the multilevel Wenckebach in three patients, and isoproterenol had no effect. Thus temporary pacing was required in all.

In contrast to inferior wall infarction, high-grade AV block complicating anterior wall myocardial infarction is usually located within the His-Purkinje system (Figure 10-2). Transition from a first nonconducted sinus P wave to complete AV block is often abrupt, and the resulting idioventricular escape rhythm is slow and unreliable. Conducted beats almost always have a wide QRS complex. Interruption of the abundant septal blood supply, sufficient to cause high-grade AV block, usually causes severe left ventricular dysfunction so that mortality is high. Emergency temporary pacing (and probably permanent pacing) of these individuals is mandatory but may not improve survival appreciably.

Clinical Aspects of Intraventricular Conduction Defects with Acute Myocardial Infarction

A number of studies have examined the clinical course of patients with bundle branch block and acute myocardial infarction (Table 10-3) [15–32]. All attest to the high incidence of severe left ventricular failure and the result-

Table 10-3
Intraventricular conduction defects and progression to high-grade AV block with acute myocardial infarction

First author	No. of patients	Conduction defect	MI site	Mortality (%)	Progression to HDB (%)	Mortality of HDB patients (%)	Temporary pacing recommended
Hindman [15,16]	432	BBB	Any	28	22	47	See Table 10-4
Lamas [17]	?/698*	IVCD	Any	–	5.4	42	See Table 10-4
Dominghetti [18]	59	IVCD	Any	30	10	83	+ (BB)
Hollander [19]	49	BBB	Any	–	30	–	+ (AS MI & BB or LBBB)
Gann [20]	292	IVCD	Any	53	4.4	69	+ (Preexisting RBBB)
Waugh [21]	198	IVCD	Any	28	11.6	30	+ (BB and P–R prolongation)
Scanlon [22]	28	BB	Any	36	21	33	+
Atkins [23]	28	BB	Any	30	25	37	+
Nimetz [24]	71	BBB	Any	31	42	57	(–)
Godman [25]	68	BBB	Any	56	31	86	(–)
Godman [26]	100	BB	Any	70	47	85	(–)
Scheinman [27]	97	IVCD	Any	38	25	–	(–)
Lichstein [28]	14	BB	AS	50	21	67	(–)
Lie [29]	70	RBBB or BB	AS	74	26	–	+ (BB with prolonged H–V)
Waters [30]	27	BB	Any	44	56	–	(–)
Kubis [31]	63	BB	–	60	46	–	(–)
Hauer [32]	42	BBB	Any	57	7	0	(–)

BBB = bundle branch block; IVCD = intraventricular conduction defect; MI = myocardial infarction; HDB = high-degree block; RBBB = right bundle branch block; LBBB = left bundle branch block; LAFB = left anterior fascicular block; LPFB = left posterior fascicular block; BB = bifascicular block; AS = anteroseptal; + = temporary pacing recommended; (–) = temporary pacing not recommended; P–R = P–R interval on ECG; H–V = infranodal conduction time on intracardiac electrogram.
*Number of patients with IVCD not specified.

Table 10-4
Risk of progression to high-grade AV block with acute myocardial infarction

Multicenter retrospective study [15, 16]	
Risk factor(s)	Risk of high-grade AV block (%)
(a) 1° AV block	13
(b) New or indeterminate onset of BBB	11
(c) Bilateral BBB	10
(a) and (b)	19
(b) and (c)	31
(a) and (c)	20
(a), (b), and (c)	38

MILIS [17]		
Risk factor(s)	No. of risk factors	Risk of 3° AV block (%)
1° AV block	None	1.2
Type I 2° AV block	One	7.8
Type II 2° AV block	Two	25.0
LAFB	Three	36.4
LPFB		
RBBB		
LBBB		

BBB = bundle branch block; LAFB = left anterior fascicular block; LPFB = left posterior fascicular block; 1°, 2°, 3° = first, second, third degree AV block, respectively.

ing high mortality, although there is considerable controversy as to whether temporary or permanent pacing alters this poor prognosis.

Regarding the issue of temporary pacing, two studies are worth discussing in detail because of the large number of patients involved. The multicenter study of Hindman et al. retrospectively reviewed the clinical course of 494 patients with documented acute myocardial infarction and bundle branch block [15, 16]. Sixty-two patients developed conduction defects in the setting of cardiogenic shock and were excluded from further analysis. Hospital mortality in the remaining 432 patients (28 percent) was most closely related to severity of heart failure, although the development of high-grade AV block (22 percent of patients) was also a predictor. Specific risk factors for advanced AV block during the acute phase were bilateral bundle branch involvement, first-degree AV block, and new or indeterminate onset of the conduction defect (Table 10-4). The presence of two of these risk factors was associated with a 19 to 31 percent (depending on which two) incidence of progression to high-grade block, which certainly warrants temporary pacing (Fig. 10-4).

The Multicenter Investigation of the Limitation of Infarct Size (MILIS) study group analyzed data from 698 patients with acute myocardial infarction to determine risk factors for the development of complete heart block [17]. A total of 38 patients (5.4 percent) had documented complete heart block; and in general, this group was characterized by a high incidence of congestive heart failure and a high mortality. Specific risk factors for complete heart block (detailed in Table 10-3) each counted a single point. Patients with 3 points or more comprised a high-risk group (at least a 25 percent incidence of progression), and those with 2 points were at intermediate risk; pacing was considered (depending on the clinical situation) in these patients but was not mandatory. Their findings were then tested in two other retrospectively derived populations—one from a combination of six studies in the medical literature and the other from the

Duke data bank—with similar results. An important limitation of both the MILIS and Hindman studies is that data were analyzed regardless of infarct location (indeed, in patients with left bundle branch block the site may not have been known). Because the clinical presentation and prognosis of patients with high-grade AV block and inferior wall myocardial infarction may be different from that of anterior wall infarction, their data should be applied with caution to any individual patient.

The issue of permanent pacing for patients with intraventricular conduction defects and myocardial infarction who survive to leave the coronary care unit has also been the subject of a number of reports (Table 10-5) [15, 16, 18, 21, 23, 30–35]. The one-year follow-up provided by Hindman et al. in the multicenter retrospective study is foremost among them because of its large numbers [15, 16]. In their data, patients who experienced transient high-grade AV block during the hospitalization (regardless of whether they fulfilled the criteria for temporary pacing) had a 28 percent incidence of recurrent block, sudden cardiac death, or both over the next 12 months (compared with only 6 percent for those without high-grade block). Of particular note were a small subset of patients who experienced recurrence of high-grade block late in the hospitalization, after their temporary pacemakers had been removed, because of restoration of normal AV conduction. Thus once the decision to implant a permanent pacemaker has been made, patients should have continuous cardiac monitoring and temporary pacing until it is carried out.

Somewhat at variance with the above study is the Birmingham (England) Trial in which 50 patients who survived 2 weeks after a myocardial infarction complicated by either right bundle branch block with or without concomitant anterior fascicular block or left posterior fascicular block alone were randomized to a permanent pacemaker or a control group [35]. Specifically excluded were patients requiring permanent pacing (because of symptomatic bradycardia or persistent high-grade block). Over the follow-up period (up to 5 years), there was no difference between groups in terms of total mortality or sudden death and no observed progression of conduction system disease. Ventricular arrhythmias were an important cause of death in both groups. It is difficult to compare these data to those of Hindman et al., however, because the incidence of transient high-grade block prior to randomization is not specified. Along similar lines, Lie and associates found a high incidence of late (up to 6 weeks) in-hospital ventricular fibrillation in a large group of patients with anteroseptal myocardial infarction complicated by right or left bundle branch block [32].

The advent of intracardiac electrophysiologic studies has provided a potentially important instrument for evaluating patients with intraventricular conduction defects and myocardial infarction (Table 10-6) [28, 36–40]. It has been hypothesized that marked prolongation of infranodal conduction time (H–V interval) might be predictive of subsequent progression to high-grade AV block [41]. Initial studies, however, have been disappointing. Most have found that, although H–V prolongation may identify a group with more severe heart disease and a high mortality, most of the deaths have been due to ventricular arrhythmias and not high-grade AV block. Most of the patients studied have had only mild-to-moderate H–V prolongation, however (perhaps because patients with marked H–V prolongation do not survive), so the application of these data to patients with markedly impaired infranodal conduction may not be warranted.

From the above considerations, it seems clear that patients with acute anterior wall myocardial infarction complicated by intraventricular conduction defects have a high mortality due to left ventricular failure. However, a substantial number of these individuals do not die from heart failure alone, and it becomes imperative to avoid mortality from preventable causes such as high-grade AV block. The large studies of Hindman et al. and Lamas and associates (MILIS) have delineated high-risk groups who may benefit from temporary pacing [15–17]. Although they were compiled retrospectively, it is unlikely that a large prospective study will ever be undertaken. Similarly, the data from Hindman et al. provide

Table 10-5
Follow-up data in survivors of acute myocardial infarction complicated by intraventricular conduction defects

First author	No. of patients	Conduction defect	MI site	Follow-up (mo)	Discharged with permanent pacemaker (no.)	Mortality (%)	Sudden death (no.)	Prophylactic permanent pacing recommended
Hindman [15,16]	311	BBB	Any	2	40	28	45	+ (with transient HDB)
Atkins [23]	20	BB	Any	11 (mean)	8	50	7	+ (with transient HDB)
Dominghetti [18]	36	IVCD	Any	19 (mean)	0	25	5	+ (RBBB, LPFB)
Waugh [21]	386	IVCD	Any	12	0	9	32	+ (1° AVB and BB or LBB)
Ginks [33]	25	BBB & transient HDB	AS	49 (mean)	4	36	5	(–)
Ritter [34]	18	BB & transient HDB	Any	18 (mean)	12	28	5	+
Waters [30]	15	BB*	Any	16	3	7	0	(–)
Kubis [31]	25	BB	Any	18	11	40	4	+
Watson [35]	50	BB	Any	Up to 60	23	50	12	(–)
Hauer [32]	18	BBB	AS	13 (mean)	1	6	0	(–)

MI = myocardial infarction; BBB = bundle branch block; BB = bifascicular block; HDB = high-degree block; IVCD = intraventricular conduction defect; RBBB = right bundle branch block; LPFB = left posterior fascicular block; LBBB = left bundle branch block; 1° AVB = first-degree AV block; + = prophylactic permanent pacing recommended; (–) = not recommended.
*Six had transient high-degree block that regressed in the hospital.

Table 10-6
Studies involving intracardiac electrophysiologic studies in patients with acute myocardial infarction complicated by intraventricular conduction defects

First author	No. of patients	Conduction defects	MI site	Prolonged H–V (%)	Follow-up (mo)	Progression to HDB (%)	Predictive value of H–V	
							Mortality	HDB
Pagnoni [36]	59	IVCD	Any	24	Up to 18	2	(+)	(−)
Watson [35]	50	BB	Any	62	Up to 60	0*	(−)	(−)
Lie [37]	35	BB	AS	46	In-hospital	35	(+)	(+)
Schoenfeld [38]	14	BBB	Any	86	Up to 12	43		
Lichstein [28]	15	New BB	Any	60	Up to 6		(+)	
Gould [39]	14	BBB	Any	40	Up to 6	0	(−)	
Harper [40]	32	BBB	Any	50	Up to 3	30	(+)	

MI = myocardial infarction; H–V = infranodal conduction time; HDB = high-grade AV block; SD = sudden cardiac death; AS = anteroseptal; + = H–V has positive predictive value; (−) = H–V does not have predictive value.
*There were 23/50 patients paced prophylactically.

helpful guidelines for the use of prophylactic permanent pacing in survivors of the acute period. Although it seems clear from the work of Watson and associates, Lie and coworkers, and others that most sudden deaths following myocardial infarction are due to ventricular arrhythmias, even in patients with extensive conduction system disease, it seems prudent to implant prophylactic permanent pacemakers in individuals who have experienced transient high-degree block, especially if an intraventricular conduction defect or first-degree AV block persists. Further studies are needed to determine if intracardiac electrophysiologic studies would be of help in this population.

Therapeutic Advances: Effects on the Conduction System

No chapter would be complete without a brief discussion of some of the developments in the therapy of acute myocardial infarction and the effects of these interventions on the conduction system. Antiarrhythmic drugs, beta blockers, calcium channel blockers, and reperfusion techniques have the potential to affect intracardiac conduction in patients with acute myocardial infarction.

ANTIARRHYTHMIC DRUGS

Antiarrhythmic drugs are widely utilized during the peri- and postinfarction periods because of the prevalence and potentially malignant nature of ventricular arrhythmias. However, many of these drugs have the potential to depress AV and intraventricular conduction. Although good prospective data are not available, a large retrospectively compiled series found no adverse effects of these drugs in patients with normal AV conduction and those with first-degree AV block or type I second-degree AV block [42]. Until more definitive information is available, however, antiarrhythmic drugs, especially some of the newer

and more potent ones, should be used with caution in patients with significant conduction system disease, particularly in the setting of moderate or severe left ventricular dysfunction.

BETA BLOCKERS

Several large randomized double-blind placebo-controlled studies have demonstrated that the administration of beta blockers in therapeutic doses following acute myocardial infarction reduces mortality by 25 to 30 percent over a follow-up period of up to 2 years [43–45]. Because beta blockers may impair AV nodal conduction, patients with second- or third-degree AV block were excluded unless the block resolved within the randomization window. In all three studies there was no significant difference between treatment and placebo groups in terms of the incidence of high-grade AV block. Thus beta blockers appear generally safe to use during the peri- or postinfarction period in the absence of second- or third-degree AV block.

CALCIUM CHANNEL BLOCKERS

The Diltiazem Reinfarction Study was a randomized double-blind placebo-controlled trial of diltiazem, 360 mg daily, in patients with acute subendocardial (non-Q-wave) myocardial infarction [46]. Therapy was initiated 24 to 72 hours after the onset of symptoms and was continued for 21 days. High-grade AV block developed in 11 of 287 diltiazem-treated patients compared with 287 of 289 patients receiving placebo. Therapy needed to be discontinued in only three patients, all in the diltiazem group. Although the difference between groups did not achieve statistical significance (perhaps because the trial was relatively small), it seems advisable to administer diltiazem with caution (in a monitored setting) until more definitive information becomes available.

REPERFUSION TECHNIQUES

Heart block has been reported in association with Prinzmetal's angina [47, 48], raising the possibility that reperfusion might adversely affect AV conduction. Although there is little specific information addressing this issue, in the large GISSI study control patients actually had a slightly higher incidence of AV block (although the difference was not statistically significant) than did the thrombolysis group [49], suggesting that temporary pacing would not be of benefit.

Editorial Comments

The indications for temporary and permanent pacemakers in patients with acute myocardial infarction have remained controversial for many years, in part because a large, prospective and controlled trial has never been performed. Because the event rate of symptomatic heart block is rather small in this patient population, it is unlikely that a trial of sufficient size can be performed. Therefore clinicians must depend on the results of small studies and certain large databases (MILIS) when making decisions about heart block in the setting of acute myocardial infarction. Clearly there are selected patients who are at risk for symptomatic high-degree heart block. In such patients a prophylactic temporary intravenous pacemaker may be life-saving. We have used the external noninvasive temporary pacemaker-monitor of Paul Zoll and associates successfully in those patients at greatest risk for high-degree AV block (Zoll, P. M., et al. External noninvasive temporary cardiac pacing: Clinical trials. Circulation 71:937, 1985). G.S.F.

References

1. Schlant, R. C., and Silverman, M. E. Anatomy of the Heart. In J. W. Hurst (ed.), *The Heart* (6th ed.). New York: McGraw-Hill, 1986. Pp. 16–37.

2. Bilbao, F. J., Zabalza, I. E., Vilanova, J. R., and Froufe, J. Atrioventricular block in posterior acute myocardial infarction: A clinicopathologic correlation. *Circulation* 75:733, 1987.

3. Bassan, R., Maia, I, Dozza, A., et al. Atrioventricular block in acute inferior wall myocardial infarction: Harbinger of associated obstruction of the left anterior descending coronary artery. *J. Am. Coll. Cardiol.* 8:733, 1986.

4. Strasberg, B., Sclarovsky, S., and Agmon, J. Wenckebach block in the distal conduction system complicating a non-Q wave acute myocardial infarction. *Chest* 92:745, 1987.

5. Massie, B., Scheinman, M. M., Peters, R., et al. Clinical and electrophysiologic findings in patients with paroxysmal slowing of the sinus rate and apparent type II atrioventricular block. *Circulation* 58:305, 1978.

6. Rotman, M., Wagner, G. S., and Wallace, A. G. Bradyarrhythmias in acute myocardial infarction. *Circulation* 45:149, 1972.

7. Opolski, G., Kraska, T., Ostrzychi, A., et al. The effect of infarct size on atrioventricular and intraventricular conduction disturbance in acute myocardial infarction. *Int. J. Cardiol.* 10:141, 1986.

8. Tans, A. C., Lie, K. I., and Durrer, D. Clinical setting and prognostic significance of high degree atrioventricular block in acute inferior myocardial infarction. *Am. Heart J.* 99:4, 1980.

9. Rotman, M., Wagner, G. S., and Waugh, R. A. Significance of high degree atrioventricular block in acute posterior myocardial infarction. *Circulation* 45:257, 1973.

10. Feigl, D., Ashkenazy, J., and Kishon, Y. Early and late atrioventricular block in acute inferior myocardial infarction. *J. Am. Coll. Cardiol.* 4:35, 1984.

11. Wesley, R. C., Lerman, B. B., DiMarco, J. P., et al. Mechanism of atropine-resistant atrioventricular block during inferior myocardial infarction; possible role of adenosine. *J. Am. Coll. Cardiol.* 8:1232, 1986.

12. Belardinelli, L., Belloni, F. L., Rubio, R., and Berne, R. M. Atrioventricular conduction disturbance during hypoxia: Possible role of adenosine in rabbit and guinea pig heart. *Circ. Res.* 47:684, 1980.

13. Dimarco, J. P., Sellers, T. P., Berney, R. M., et al. Adenosine: Electrophysiologic effects and therapeutic use for terminating paroxysmal supraventricular tachycardia. *Circulation* 68:1254, 1983.

14. Lewin, R. F., Kasniec, J., Sclarovsky, S., et al. Alternating Wenckebach periods in acute inferior myocardial infarction: Clinical, electrocardiographic, and therapeutic characterization. *PACE* 9:468, 1986.

15. Hindman, M. C., Wagner, G. S., Jaro, M., et

al. The clinical significance of bundle branch block complicating acute myocardial infarction. 1. Clinical characteristics, hospital mortality, and one-year follow-up. *Circulation* 4:679, 1978.

16. Hindman, M. C., Wagner, G. S, Jaro, M., et al. The clinical significance of bundle branch block complicating acute myocardial infarction. 2. Indications for temporary and permanent pacemaker insertion. *Circulation* 4:689, 1978.

17. Lamas, G. A., Muller, J. E., Turi, Z. G., et al. A simplified method to predict occurrence of complete heart block during acute myocardial infarction. *Am. J. Cardiol.* 57:1213, 1986.

18. Dominghetti, G., and Perret, C. Intraventricular conduction disturbances in acute myocardial infarction: Short- and long-term prognosis. *Eur. J. Cardiol.* 11:51, 1980.

19. Hollander, G., Nadiminti, V., Lichstein, E., et al. Bundle branch block in acute myocardial infarction. *Am. Heart J.* 105:738, 1983.

20. Gann, D., Balachandran, P. K., El Sherif, N., and Samet, P. Prognostic significance of chronic versus acute bundle branch block in acute myocardial infarction. *Chest* 67:298, 1975.

21. Waugh, R. A., Wagner, G. S., Haney, T. L., et al. Immediate and remote prognostic significance of fascicular block during acute myocardial infarction. *Circulation* 47:765, 1973.

22. Scanlon, P. J., Pryor, R., and Blount, S. G. Right bundle branch block associated with acute myocardial infarction. *Circulation* 42:135, 1970.

23. Atkins, J. M., Leshin, S. J., Blomquist, G., and Mullins, C. B. Ventricular conduction blocks and sudden death in acute myocardial infarction: Potential indications for pacing. *N. Engl. J. Med.* 288:281, 1973.

24. Nimetz, A. A., Scubrooks, S. J., Hutter, A. M., and DeSanctis, R. W. The significance of bundle branch block during acute myocardial infarction. *Am. Heart J.* 90:439, 1975.

25. Godman, M. J., Lassers, B. W., and Julian, D. G. Complete bundle-branch block complicating acute myocardial infarction. *N. Engl. J. Med.* 282:237, 1970.

26. Godman, M. J., Alpert, B. A., and Julian, D. G. Bilateral bundle-branch block complicating acute myocardial infarction. *Lancet* 2:345, 1971.

27. Scheinman, M., and Brenman, B. Clinical and anatomic complications of intraventricular conduction blocks in acute myocardial infarction. *Circulation* 46:753, 1972.

28. Lichstein, E., Gupta, P. K., Chadda, K. D., et al. Findings of prognostic valve in patients with incomplete bilateral bundle branch block complicating acute myocardial infarction. *Am. J. Cardiol.* 32:913, 1973.

29. Lie, K. I., Wellens, H. J., and Schuilenburg, R. M. Bundle branch block and acute myocardial infarction. In H. J. J. Wellens (ed.), *The Conduction System of the Heart: Structure, Functions and Clinical Indications.* Philadelphia: Lea & Febiger, 1976.

30. Waters, D. D., and Mizgala, H. F. Long-term prognosis of patients with incomplete bilateral bundle branch block complicating acute myocardial infarction: Role of cardiac pacing. *Am. J. Cardiol.* 34:1, 1974.

31. Kubis, M., and Suejda, J. Indication of permanent pacing after acute myocardial infarction complicated by combined intraventricular block. *Cor Vasa* 24:295, 1982.

32. Hauer, R. N. W., Lie, K. I., Lier, K. L., and Durrer, P. Long-term prognosis in patients with bundle branch block complicating acute anteroseptal infarction. *Am. J. Cardiol.* 49:1581, 1982.

33. Ginks, W. R., Sutton, R., Oh, W., and Leatham, A. Long-term prognosis after acute anterior infarction with atrioventricular block. *Br. Heart J.* 39:186, 1977.

34. Ritter, W. A., Atkins, J. M., Blomquist, C. G., and Mullins, C. B. Permanent pacing in patients with transient trifascicular block during acute myocardial infarction. *Am. J. Cardiol.* 38:205, 1976.

35. Watson, R. S. D., Glover, D. R., Page, A. J. F., et al. The Birmingham trial of permanent pacing in patients with intraventricular conduction disorders after myocardial infarction. *Am. Heart J.* 108:496, 1984.

36. Pagnoni, F., Finzia, A., Valentini, R., et al. Long-term prognostic significance and electrophysiological evolution of intraventricular conduction disturbances complicating acute myocardial infarction. *PACE* 9:91, 1986.

37. Lie, K. I., Wellens, H. J., Schuilenburg, R. S., et al. Factors influencing prognosis of bundle branch block complicating acute antero-septal infarction: The value of His bundle recordings. *Circulation* 50:935, 1974.

38. Schoenfeld, C. D., Mascarenhas, E., Bhardwaj, P., et al. Clinical and electrophysiologic significance of bundle branch block in acute myocardial infarction. *PACE* 2:428, 1979.

39. Gould, L., Reddy, V. V. R., Kim, S. G., and Oh, K. C. His bundle electrogram in patients with acute myocardial infarction. *PACE* 2:428, 1979.

40. Harper, R., Hunt, D., Vohra, J., et al. His bundle electrogram in patients with acute myocardial infarction complicated by atrioventricular or intraventricular conduction disturbances. *Br. Heart J.* 37:705, 1975.

41. Aranda, J. M., Befeler, B., and Castellanos, A. His bundle recordings, bundle branch block and myocardial infarction. *Ann. Intern. Med.* 86:106, 1977.

42. Scheinman, M. M., Remedios, P., Cheitlin, M. D., et al. Effects of antiarrhythmic drugs on

atrioventricular conduction in patients with acute myocardial infarction. *Circulation* 62:20, 1980.

43. Beta-Blocker: Heart Attack Trial Research Group. A randomized trial of propranolol in patients with acute myocardial infarction. I. Mortality results. *J.A.M.A.* 247:1707, 1982.

44. Norwegian Multicenter Study Group. Timolol-induced reduction in mortality and reinfarction in patients surviving acute myocardial infarction. *N. Engl. J. Med.* 304:801, 1981.

45. Hjalmerson, A., Herlitz, J., Malek, I., et al. Effect on mortality of metoprolol in acute myocardial infarction. *Lancet* 2:823, 1981.

46. Gibson, R. S., Boden, W. E., Theroux, P., et al. Diltiazem and reinfarction in patients with non-Q-wave myocardial infarction. *N. Engl. J. Med.* 315:423, 1986.

47. Selzer, A., Langston, M., Ruggeroli, C., and Cohn, K. Clinical syndrome of variant angina with normal coronary arteriograms. *N. Engl. J. Med.* 295:1343, 1976.

48. Plotnick, G. D., Carliner, N. H., Fisher, M. L., et al. Rest angina with transient S-T segment elevation: Correlation of clinical features with coronary anatomy. *Am. J. Med.* 65:257, 1978.

49. Italian Group for the Study of Streptokinase in Myocardial Infarction (GISSI). Effectiveness of intravenous thrombolytic treatment in acute myocardial infarction. *Lancet* 1:397, 1986.

11
Treatment of Ventricular Arrhythmias in Acute Myocardial Infarction

RAYMOND L. WOOSLEY AND DAN M. RODEN

The focus of the coronary care unit (CCU) is to minimize myocardial damage during acute myocardial infarction, as well as to monitor and treat disturbances of cardiac rhythm. With the advent of intensive cardiac rhythm monitoring, the incidence and "natural history" of the various rhythm disturbances encountered during this period were defined [1–3], and the rational use of antiarrhythmic drugs is predicated on this knowledge. Our understanding of how to treat arrhythmias has advanced greatly, although there is still much to be learned. For example, there is still disagreement over the significance of "warning arrhythmias" and the risk-benefit ratio of prophylactic lidocaine therapy for patients with suspected myocardial infarction.

Many factors may underlie cardiac arrhythmias following myocardial infarction. Because these arrhythmias vary in etiology and significance, the therapeutic measures selected vary as well. For our purpose, the time frame may be broken down into three periods: during and immediately following myocardial infarction, the subsequent 3 to 10 days, and the ensuing convalescence.

The initial evaluation should include the following:

1. Several ancillary factors may underlie or provoke arrhythmias following heart attack; among them are hypoxia, electrolyte disturbance, and digitalis toxicity. Each of these possible contributors should be corrected prior to initiation of antiarrhythmic drug therapy.
2. The specific diagnosis of the arrhythmia should be made, keeping in mind that analysis of the surface electrocardiogram alone may lead to misdiagnosis, with the potential for lethal consequences.
3. The promptness with which therapy must take effect should be assessed, with the realization that the onset of action for some agents can occur within minutes, whereas others require 20 to 30 minutes or more for the safe administration of loading dosages.

In extremely urgent situations, as when patients have recurring episodes of ventricular tachycardia or fibrillation after cardioversion, lidocaine is considered the drug of first choice; it can be given safely as a bolus injection and can be active within seconds. If the patient fails to respond to adequate dosages of lidocaine and the arrhythmia still requires urgent therapy, bretylium is the next alternative. Many physicians continue the lidocaine infusion and add bretylium using a series of loading boluses and a maintenance infusion.

When more time is available, such as for treatment of a patient with sustained ventricular tachycardia who is stable hemodynamically, we prefer intravenous procainamide to convert or suppress the arrhythmia. The other antiarrhythmic agent that can be effective in this setting is lidocaine. Bretylium is not a reasonable choice in many cases not only because it does not provide an option for chronic oral therapy (true also for lidocaine) but because it is poorly tolerated, with orthostatic hypotension being an almost universal adverse effect.

Once a patient has passed the acute phase of myocardial infarction and continues to have ventricular arrhythmias, the goals of therapy are considerably different. If the arrhythmias are symptomatic, such as nonsustained or sustained ventricular tachycardia, medications that have an oral formulation and are likely to be well tolerated must be considered. Lidocaine and bretylium are no longer candidates except that they may be useful for controlling arrhythmias while one is trying to identify an orally effective regimen. Likewise, procainamide is not the optimal selection for therapy anticipated to last for years because of the high incidence of patient withdrawal due to many adverse reactions including allergy and a lupus erythematosus syndrome. Many of the newer agents are better tolerated for chronic therapy and may be considered.

The development of recurrent, sporadic, sustained ventricular tachycardia during the convalescent phase of acute myocardial infarction or afterward should prompt the physician to consider the use of programmed ventricular stimulation (PES) as the means to evaluate the effectiveness of therapy. If ventricular tachycardia recurs soon after cardioversion, PES may not be needed to evaluate therapy; however, in most cases the recurrence of tachycardia is sporadic, and for optimal drug evaluation and therapy it must be induced by PES.

The observation of asymptomatic premature ventricular beats (PVBs), by electrocardiographic monitoring or ambulatory Holter recordings after infarction, identifies individuals at high risk of sudden death. However, there is no evidence at this time to suggest that these patients benefit from antiarrhythmic therapy and there is evidence that some agents increase mortality. This subject is discussed further in the sections to follow.

Indications for Therapy

Prophylactic Therapy Less Than 12 Hours After Acute Myocardial Infarction

Lie and coworkers [4] treated 212 patients within 6 hours of the onset of acute myocardial infarction with lidocaine or placebo for 48 hours in a prospective double-blind fashion. There were 11 instances of ventricular fibrillation among the 107 patients treated with placebo, whereas none of the 105 patients treated with lidocaine developed primary ventricular fibrillation. However, patients over 65 years of age and those in shock were excluded from this study; it is possible that ventricular fibrillation may be less common in the elderly [2], and it is seen more frequently in the presence of shock or congestive heart failure. Although under these circumstances Lie and colleagues' study showed no difference in mortality due to ventricular fibrillation between those who received lidocaine and those who did not, no patients who received lidocaine developed ventricular fibrillation, whereas 11 patients receiving placebo did (two of these cases were paroxysmal ventricular fibrillation). Therefore it can be argued that treatment with lidocaine for the first 48 to 72 hours following the onset of symptoms in young patients without congestive heart failure decreases the incidence of primary ventricular fibrillation [5].

Several studies reached conflicting conclusions regarding the prophylactic effect of lidocaine (300 mg) administered intramuscularly prior to hospitalization [6, 7]. Bigger and coworkers found that lidocaine plasma levels after a similar dosage were predominantly below the range usually required for suppression of arrhythmias (mean peak 2.1 μg/ml) [1]. One study demonstrated a beneficial effect of lidocaine (400 mg) on reducing the incidence of ventricular fibrillation when administered by paramedical personnel upon reaching possible myocardial infarction victims out of hospital [8]. At 11 to 20 minutes after injection, mean plasma levels were 3 μg/ml for 369 patients, 304 of whom had levels above 2 μg/ml. Although other antiarrhythmic drugs are known to suppress "warning arrhythmias," there are few studies with sufficient numbers of patients to evaluate prophylaxis against ventricular fibrillation. As for the newer agents, a study of the effects of mexiletine compared to placebo found no statistically significant difference between the incidence of ventricular fibrillation following myocardial infarction [9] using the two treatments.

ANTIARRHYTHMIC THERAPY DURING THE FIRST 48 HOURS AFTER INFARCTION

When ventricular arrhythmias requiring therapy arise following myocardial infarction, a search must be made for the underlying exacerbating features. They include drug toxicity (digitalis, antiarrhythmic agents, bronchodilators, vasopressors, tricyclic antidepressants), low serum potassium or pH imbalance, and congestive heart failure.

Not all ventricular arrhythmias seen at this time require therapy. For instance, the accelerated idioventricular rhythms seen during the first few days following myocardial infarction are generally thought to be benign. However, there is evidence that this rhythm disturbance is associated with a high incidence of rapid ventricular tachycardia [10], and it may therefore be more ominous than previously thought. Therefore the observation of idioventricular arrhythmia should prompt the use of extensive monitoring.

Sustained ventricular arrhythmias having hemodynamic significance (ventricular tachycardia, ventricular fibrillation) require immediate direct-current (DC) cardioversion. In less urgent situations, lidocaine is the drug of choice for treatment of ventricular arrhythmias during the immediate postmyocardial infarction setting. This choice is valid following cardioversion as well. Should lidocaine prove ineffective, procainamide or bretylium are the drugs to be considered next, with bretylium being preferred in acute situations, such as recurrent ventricular fibrillation. When adequate time is thought to be available for giving loading infusions of procainamide (20–30 minutes), this agent should be administered because it is better tolerated for acute therapy than is bretylium.

Mexiletine, quinidine, aprindine, and amiodarone have been tried in patients with arrhythmias in the setting of acute infarction. However, they are no more effective than the agents already discussed and often are problematic when used in this setting.

Early intervention with beta-adrenergic blocking drugs (in patients without contraindications) may decrease subsequent mortality, although the mechanism by which it is achieved is not understood [11]. One possibility is that they lessen metabolic demand on the myocardium and thus reduce damage and preserve function. However, although therapy with beta-adrenergic receptor antagonists soon after myocardial infarction may appreciably lower the risk of subsequent sudden cardiac death, patients at the highest risk for this event generally are not candidates for beta-adrenergic blockade because of poor left ventricular function.

Polymorphic ventricular tachycardia has become increasingly recognized in the peri-infarction setting as well as in others. When this rhythm is associated with prolongation of cardiac repolarization (as in torsade de pointes) quinidine-like drugs have been implicated as causal factors, and the initiating mechanism may well be bradycardia-dependent triggered automaticity in the form of early after-depolarizations [12, 13]. Treatment with pacing, sodium bicarbonate, and isoproterenol is effective when the syndrome is recognized. On the other hand, polymorphic ventricular tachycardia that occurs in the setting of a normal Q–T interval must be distinguished because it can be treated with local anesthetic antiarrhythmic drugs. The term torsade de pointes should not be applied to all polymorphic ventricular tachycardia. The two forms described here are different, and we restrict the use of the term torsade de pointes to the syndrome that includes the arrhythmia in the presence of a markedly prolonged Q–T interval [14].

LATER ANTIARRHYTHMIC THERAPY

High-frequency ventricular ectopy and poor ventricular function have been proved to be independent predictors of increased risk of sudden cardiac death [15–17]. Because of the increased risk, many physicians choose to treat patients with frequent or complex (repetitive forms of) ventricular arrhythmias with antiarrhythmic drugs, even though these drugs have no proved benefit in patients with asymptomatic arrhythmias [18].

The development of antiarrhythmic agents

that are well tolerated and highly effective for chronic oral therapy has made it possible to conduct trials to determine if suppression of ventricular arrhythmias per se reduces the risk of sudden cardiac death in a postmyocardial infarction population [19]. The Cardiac Arrhythmia Suppression Trial (CAST) is an NIH-sponsored large-scale, double-blind study designed to address this question. Begun in 1987, CAST is evaluating the effects of antiarrhythmic drugs on mortality in patients who have had recent myocardial infarction and also have reduced myocardial function. Encainide, flecainide, and moricizine were initially chosen because of their ability to produce more than 80 percent ventricular ectopic depolarization suppression in this population. An interim report described twofold excess mortality in the group receiving encainide and flecainide. At this time the study is continuing with miricizine as the single agent being tested.

Patients who experience sudden cardiac death and are subsequently resuscitated comprise a group at high risk for recurrent sudden death [20]. Myerburg et al. [21] suggested that this subset may benefit from empiric therapy with antiarrhythmic agents (quinidine or procainamide in the absence of arrhythmia suppression), and a later report [22] suggested a beneficial effect of propanolol in these patients. These studies were performed before the development of the more recently released agents, many of which have greater antiarrhythmic potency and fewer associated adverse effects. Evaluation of antiarrhythmic drug therapy using programmed electrical stimulation has become a more acceptable approach in this group [23]. Development of the automatic implantable cardioverter/defibrillator (AICD) and surgical techniques have markedly altered therapy and reduced mortality.

A discussion of general pharmacologic principles important in the use of antiarrhythmic drugs is followed by a more detailed consideration of specific agents. Unfortunately, despite advances in elucidation of the mechanisms involved in the genesis of arrhythmias [24, 25], drug therapy remains largely empiric.

Principles of Management

PHARMACOKINETIC PRINCIPLES

The following is a brief review of pharmacokinetic principles as they apply to therapy with antiarrhythmic agents. For more extensive information, the reader is referred to a review of pharmacokinetics of antiarrhythmic drugs by Siddoway [26].

The goal is to attain myocardial drug concentrations within the range necessary for suppressing or converting an arrhythmia without reaching toxic concentrations at any site in the body. Rapid attainment of an antiarrhythmic effect is best accomplished by an intravenous loading regimen, but it has the attendant disadvantage of rapidly changing drug levels in the plasma and vital organs. Thorough understanding of drug distribution, metabolism, and elimination in both normal individuals and patients with renal, cardiac, or hepatic dysfunction provides the information necessary to arrive at initial estimates for dosage regimens, which are then individualized for the patient to be treated. The physician must be well versed in the principles of pharmacokinetics, have available the pharmacokinetic data for the drug to be administered, be familiar with the clinical condition of the patient, and understand how it pertains to the available pharmacokinetic data. Then, being prepared to adjust for any errors in predictions, the physician must monitor therapy using all of the clinical tools available, including plasma concentration monitoring.

Many antiarrhythmic drugs follow what is described as a two-compartment, open pharmacokinetic model following intravenous administration. These "compartments" are not anatomical entities; rather, they are calculated theoretical volumes. Nonetheless, these concepts are a valuable aid to designing therapy. With intravenous administration, the drug is first delivered into a central compartment, which reflects the concentration in the plasma, myocardium, and central nervous system. The drug is then distributed fairly rapidly into peripheral tissues (Fig. 11-1). Elimination, a slower process, generally takes place from the

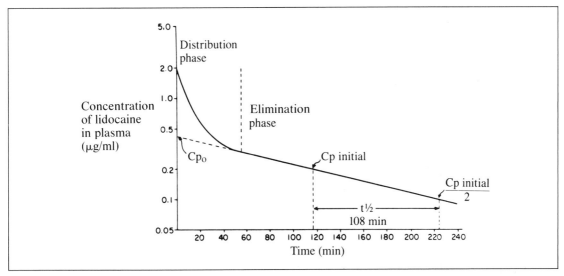

Fig. 11-1
Biexponential decay of plasma concentration of lidocaine after intravenous injection of a 50-mg dose in a normal individual. The initial rapid fall in concentration indicates distribution of lidocaine out of the central compartment into the peripheral compartment. The second phase, represented by a more gradual drop in plasma concentration, reflects elimination. C_p = plasma concentration; $t_{1/2}$ = half-life. (From R. L. Woosley. Lidocaine therapy. *Cardiac Impulse* 8:No. 2, 1987. With permission.)

central compartment. Immediately following intravenous injection, therapeutic plasma concentrations may be attained in the plasma and the myocardium; however, this effect may be short-lived because of redistribution into other tissues.

Volume of Distribution
The volume of distribution of a drug is a theoretical volume based on the original dose given and its subsequent plasma concentration. The volume of distribution (V_d) may be regarded as that theoretical volume within which a drug would be distributed in order to achieve the plasma concentration measured.

Immediately following administration of an intravenous bolus into a central compartment, the plasma concentration achieved is equal to the dose divided by the volume of distribution (of the central compartment). Volume of distribution generally does not correspond to any physiologic space and may (because of plasma levels being reduced when drug is bound to tissue) exceed the total volume of the body.

However, it provides a guide to choosing an initial dose and is one of the determinants of elimination half-life.

The volume of distribution can change in patients who develop congestive heart failure. For example, the volume of distribution for lidocaine is approximately one-half that for normal individuals.

Clearance
Clearance is a rate term describing the process of drug elimination and is expressed as milliliters per minute. For most antiarrhythmic drugs, clearance is a "first-order process," which means that the amount of drug eliminated depends on the amount of drug present in the central compartment. Dosage and clearance determine the ultimate steady-state plasma concentration (Cp_{ss}) achieved during maintenance intravenous therapy.

Cp_{ss} = infusion rate/clearance

Total clearance is the sum of renal and nonrenal clearance. An example of nonrenal

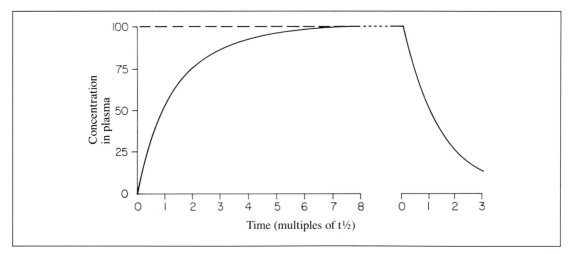

Fig. 11-2
Drug accumulation and elimination as a function of half-life ($t_{1/2}$). (From R. L. Woosley. Lidocaine therapy. *Cardiac Impulse* 8:No. 2, 1987. With permission.)

clearance for some drugs is hepatic metabolism.

Half-Life
Half-life is a convenient way to characterize processes such as elimination and distribution that proceed on a "first-order" basis. For instance, after an intravenous bolus of a rapidly distributed drug such as lidocaine is given, 50 percent of the process of distribution is complete after one distribution half-life, 75 percent after two half-lives, 87.5 percent after three half-lives, and so on (Fig. 11-2). Such processes can therefore be regarded as nearly complete after four to five half-lives. Because lidocaine's distribution half-life is usually approximately 8 minutes, distribution is complete 32 to 40 minutes after a bolus. Similarly, elimination is essentially complete after four to five elimination half-lives (8–10 hours for lidocaine in patients whose elimination half-life is 2 hours). In addition, the time required to reach steady-state conditions following initiation of chronic therapy (by any route) is four to five elimination half-lives and is dependent on the volume of distribution and clearance:

Half-life = $(0.693 \times V_d)$/clearance

Loading doses are sometimes used with the mistaken concept that they hasten the time to steady-state equilibrium. Although they may shorten the time needed to attain therapeutic plasma levels, the time required to reach steady-state equilibrium is always four to five half-lives and is unaffected by the use of loading doses.

Bioavailability
Bioavailability is the fraction of an oral dose reaching the systemic circulation when compared to the amount available (100 percent) following intravenous administration. Only a portion of an orally administered dose may be absorbed, or metabolism of a drug can take place prior to its entry into the systemic circulation. The latter can occur in the intestinal lumen, the intestinal wall, or, most commonly, the liver. Several drugs undergo such extensive "first-pass" hepatic metabolism that dosing recommendations must be considerably altered depending on the route of administration. For instance, for propranolol the respective intravenous and oral dosages are 1 to 10 mg and 40 to 80 mg.

Alterations in drug disposition due to disease states (e.g., acute myocardial infarction, congestive heart failure, hepatic or renal disease) may be conceptualized in terms of alterations of volumes of distribution, clearance, and elimination half-life. Disease states may alter volume of distribution or clearance alone (and thus alter elimination half-life) or may change both volume of distribution and clearance. Note that if clearance and volume of distribution are reduced to the same degree, elimination half-life is unaltered.

This last situation is particularly applicable to the use of lidocaine in patients with congestive heart failure. The volume of distribution for lidocaine is approximately one-half that for normal individuals, and a reduced loading dose is required. A reduced maintenance dose is also required because of reduced clearance, but the half-life may be within the usual range because both the volume of distribution and clearance have changed proportionately.

CHRONIC ORAL THERAPY

Oral therapy should start at low doses, and each dose schedule should be continued, if possible, until steady-state conditions are achieved (four to five elimination half-lives). If arrhythmia is still present and side effects are absent, a higher dosage regimen can then be tried. Plasma concentrations should be monitored to ensure the presence of adequate drug, to establish a baseline for future patient care, to warn of possible impending toxicity, and to confirm any clinical suspicion of drug toxicity. No drug can truly be declared a therapeutic failure unless arrhythmia persists in the face of side effects.

PLASMA CONCENTRATION MONITORING

The monitoring of plasma concentrations of antiarrhythmic drugs is often a valuable guide for adjusting therapy. For lidocaine, plasma concentrations parallel the effect, suggesting that the "effector" tissue site and plasma are in the same pharmacokinetic compartment. This rule does not apply to bretylium or amiodarone. Immediately following parenteral administration of the latter agents, plasma concentrations are high, although the effect may be negligible. This observation implies

that for these agents plasma and myocardium are in different compartments, and time is needed for distribution of the drug. For procainamide, long-term therapy is complicated by the production of an active metabolite in about 50 percent of the population. Nevertheless, plasma concentration monitoring can be useful for these agents once equilibrium is achieved between plasma concentration and effector site concentration.

Therapeutic ranges for plasma concentrations of antiarrhythmic drugs should be regarded as guidelines to therapy to be evaluated within the clinical setting. Although the lower limit of the published therapeutic range is the plasma concentration that is likely to produce an effect, some patients may respond to even lower concentrations. Similarly, the upper limit of the therapeutic range is the concentration beyond which an additional therapeutic benefit is unlikely to occur and the incidence of side effects rises. Again, some patients may require greater concentrations to achieve a therapeutic effect and may tolerate higher concentrations without adverse effects. Thus therapeutic ranges of plasma concentrations are no substitute for clinical judgment. Monitoring plasma concentrations during chronic therapy is useful for both verifying compliance and establishing a baseline should the patient's clinical status change (e.g., should congestive heart failure occur). It is also important to ascertain that the plasma concentration being measured is the appropriate one. Some drugs have active metabolites that may produce the dominant, or a different, pharmacologic action. Examples include procainamide, whose active metabolite N-acetylprocainamide may accumulate to antiarrhythmic concentrations in patients with renal failure [27], and encainide, converted in most patients to the O-desmethyl form, which produces arrhythmia suppression [28]. Clearly, measuring the parent drug concentrations in these settings may not be helpful and may in fact be misleading.

Drug present in plasma may exist either free or protein-bound. Because only the free drug is available to exert pharmacologic activity, a change in the free drug concentration produces a change in the effects seen. A pertinent example of these principles occurs with lidocaine. During the acute phases of myocardial infarction the plasma concentration of alpha-1-acid glycoprotein (AAG) becomes elevated. Some antiarrhythmic agents, most notably lidocaine, bind extensively to this protein, and hence their total plasma concentration is affected by changing AAG concentrations. Assays for plasma lidocaine measure both protein-bound and free lidocaine and thus do not give a true picture of the amount of free drug available. Shortly after infarction, apparent plasma lidocaine levels tend to rise, reflecting lidocaine bound to higher levels of AAG; however, the concentration of free lidocaine may change little. In this case, the lidocaine dosage should not be reduced to compensate for the higher total plasma concentration so long as the patient displays no adverse effects. Subsequent decreases in AAG concentration in the days following myocardial infarction influence measurement of the apparently available lidocaine levels as well, only in the opposite direction. Quinidine is another antiarrhythmic agent that binds to AAG, and increases in the plasma concentration of this protein explain the increase seen in total drug levels of quinidine after infarction that are not associated with excess drug effect [29, 30]. Monitoring of *free* drug levels in this setting is of unproved value but should be more reliable than measuring bound drug for guiding therapy.

REDUCING EMPIRICISM IN THERAPY

Characterization of electrophysiologic actions of drugs in in vitro or in vivo systems has provided a conceptual framework for classifying the antiarrhythmic actions of drugs [31]. Although the applicability of such a classification in the clinical setting remains limited, some conclusions and examples can be drawn. For example, patients having long Q–T interval–related arrhythmias should not receive local anesthetic-type agents that further increase the Q–T interval, i.e., those with class IA or III action. These patients are more likely to benefit from therapy with one of the lido-

caine congeners, which have little effect on the Q–T interval. A similar situation exists for those patients prone to developing hypokalemia, which can be arrhythmogenic when combined with drugs having class IA or III action [13, 32, 33].

Basic to an understanding of the mechanism of action of antiarrhythmic agents is an understanding of the cardiac sodium channel. Hodgkin and Huxley proposed that sodium channels exist in three distinct states [34]. According to the modulated receptor hypothesis of cardiac sodium channel regulation proposed by Hille [35] and Hondeghem and Katzung [36, 37], each of the three states of the sodium channel (open, closed, inactivated) has a different affinity for any given local anesthetic drug. By combining drugs such as lidocaine (which rapidly dissociate from the sodium channel and allow rapid recovery from block) with a drug such as quinidine (which dissociates from the sodium channel more slowly and requires more time for recovery from block), synergistic blockade of sodium channels (particularly during tachycardia or with premature beats) should be possible. The treatment of acute and chronic ventricular arrhythmias frequently necessitates combination therapy owing to the low efficacy of single agents. By combining drugs with differing kinetics of interaction with the sodium channel, one may produce increased sodium channel blockade and, therefore, increased drug efficacy. Additionally, drugs whose antiarrhythmic activity results from different mechanisms of action can be synergistic. A simple example is the combination of a drug that alters conduction velocity with one that prolongs repolarization and refactoriness.

Specific Antiarrhythmic Agents

LIDOCAINE

Indications
Lidocaine is often the drug of first choice for the acute suppression of ventricular arrhythmias. It also effectively decreases the incidence of primary ventricular fibrillation in

patients with documented acute myocardial infarction [4].

When a definite myocardial infarction is diagnosed, early initiation of prophylactic lidocaine therapy can be effective and safe—but only if conditions are optimal. A monitored environment is essential to permit evaluation of patient response and detection of toxicity. Based on these factors and a sound understanding of lidocaine's complex pharmacokinetics, therapy can be individualized for each patient.

An excellent example of using clinical response rather than fixed dosages or drug concentrations to evaluate therapy was reported by Alderman and coworkers [38]. Of nine patients who were apparently resistant to standard doses of lidocaine, three in fact had arrhythmias responsive at higher doses (blood levels were still within the therapeutic range), and four had arrhythmias resistant to lidocaine at usual blood levels but responsive at levels of 5 to 9 μg/ml. Only two of the nine patients were, in fact, resistant and demonstrated central nervous system side effects without an antiarrhythmic effect.

Pharmacology: In Vitro and Animal Data

In concentrations similar to those attained during clinical use, lidocaine reduces V_{max} and produces shortening or no change in action potential duration (APD) and effective refractory period of normal Purkinje fibers [39, 40]. It contrasts with quinidine and procainamide, which produce lengthening of the APD. In contrast to its actions in normal tissue, lidocaine has been shown to prolong refractoriness and slow conduction in ischemic tissue during transient coronary artery occlusion in dogs [41]. Additionally, it was found to prolong refractoriness of potential reentrant pathways within tissue 3 to 7 days following coronary artery ligation [42].

Some indications of a potential proarrhythmic action of lidocaine in certain animal models have been reported [43], and it is of interest that Adgey et al. [44] suggested that lidocaine was not a particularly effective drug for suppressing VEDs early during myocardial infarction. In contrast, both Borer et al. [45] and

Spear et al. [46] have shown that lidocaine increased ventricular fibrillation thresholds in acutely ischemic dogs. Lidocaine has little effect on atrial tissue in vitro [47], consistent with the clinical observation that it is of little use for supraventricular tachyarrhythmias.

Clinical Electrophysiology

Lidocaine has little effect on the electrophysiology of the normal conduction system. Studies on the effect of lidocaine in patients with conduction system abnormalities have produced variable results. Kunkel et al. [48] showed no change in the A–H, H–V, or QRS interval following lidocaine administration to ten patients with bundle branch block; similar results were reported by Bekheit et al. [49]. Gupta et al. [50], however, showed that lidocaine could potentiate infranodal block in patients at high risk (prolonged H–V interval or 2:1 infranodal block), and Aravindakshan et al. [51] reported abrupt slowing of the ventricular rate following lidocaine administration in 5 of 18 patients with stable AV block. In addition, the potential for advanced degrees of sinus node dysfunction has been reported in isolated instances [52, 53].

No systematically obtained data are available on the effects of lidocaine administration to patients with conduction system disturbances acquired during acute myocardial infarction. In this group, particularly in those with abnormalities involving conduction below the AV node, lidocaine (and all antiarrhythmic drugs) should be administered cautiously, if at all, unless a temporary pacemaker is inserted.

In studies carried out in patients without acute myocardial ischemia, lidocaine had inconsistent effects on atrial and AV nodal refractory periods, although it did shorten refractoriness of the His–Purkinje system [54].

Lidocaine may be useful for decreasing the ventricular response during atrial fibrillation in patients whose AV conduction follows an accessory pathway [55, 56], although some workers have reported accelerated conduction [57]; other drugs such as procainamide are probably preferred in this situation.

Absorption, Distribution, Metabolism, and Elimination

Lidocaine undergoes extensive first-pass hepatic metabolism to the deethylated forms monoethylglycinexylidide and glycinexylidide, which are excreted by the kidneys. These metabolites have less antiarrhythmic potency than the parent drug and may contribute to the production of central nervous system side effects seen with lidocaine [58, 59].

Lidocaine clearance is well approximated by measuring the liver blood flow [60, 61]. Thus although oral lidocaine is well absorbed, adequate amounts of the active parent drug cannot reach the systemic circulation without generation of toxic concentrations of the metabolites. For this reason, only intravenous lidocaine therapy is useful for arrhythmia suppression.

Following intravenous administration, lidocaine disposition is well represented by the two-compartment open model (see Fig. 11-1) [62]. The half-life of lidocaine distribution between the central compartment and peripheral tissues is approximately 8 minutes. Because antiarrhythmic activity is correlated with lidocaine's concentration in the central compartment, this activity falls rapidly following administration of a single intravenous bolus.

Little therapeutic effect is evident at lidocaine plasma concentrations below 1.5 μg/ml, whereas increasing toxicity occurs at concentrations above 5 μg/ml. In some patients, however, concentrations in the 5 to 9 μg/ml range may be required for arrhythmia suppression and can safely be achieved with cautious drug administration [38].

As discussed earlier, the prophylactic efficacy of intramuscular injections of large dosages of lidocaine by paramedical personnel has been the subject of controversy. This approach has been used for prehospital care, but resultant plasma concentrations are generally variable and at the low end of the usual therapeutic range.

Toxicity

The most frequent side effects during lidocaine administration are central nervous system symptoms. If a bolus of lidocaine is administered rapidly, seizures are likely to ensue. With more gradual attainment of excessive plasma levels, symptoms are limited to drowsiness, dysarthria, and dysesthesia; such symptoms may in fact be useful for bedside assessment of the adequacy of lidocaine dosing in the face of recurrent arrhythmia.

Excessive lidocaine can also cause coma and enters into the differential diagnosis of postcardiac arrest encephalopathy. Likewise, excessive dosages of lidocaine can depress cardiac function. A vicious cycle can occur, as depressed cardiac function decreases lidocaine clearance, thereby causing an even greater increase in the plasma concentration.

In a small subset of patients, lidocaine can also unpredictably provoke or exacerbate conduction system disturbances, as discussed above.

Dosage and Administration

Lidocaine's primary use as an antiarrhythmic agent is for the acute suppression of rhythm disturbances. In these circumstances a prompt effect is obviously desirable. Single intravenous boluses achieve therapeutic effects only transiently because the drug is rapidly distributed out of the plasma and myocardium. Increasing the size of the bolus dose is likely to produce central nervous system effects. Therefore to promptly achieve and maintain therapeutic plasma concentrations, a loading regimen of multiple doses or infusions must be used. Pharmacokinetic analyses suggest, and clinical studies confirm, that in a stable patient a total loading dose of lidocaine is approximately 3 to 4 mg/kg administered over 20 to 30 minutes. In addition, "boluses" should be administered slowly (over 2–3 minutes) while the patient is continuously observed for the presence of side effects; should side effects occur, further loading should be stopped.

One effective and well-tolerated loading regimen was outlined by Wyman et al. [63]: For a 75-kg person, an initial bolus of 75 mg is given, followed by 50 mg every 5 minutes to a total dose of 225 mg. This regimen usually achieves and maintains plasma concentrations within the usual guidelines (1.5–5.0 μg/ml). A priming dose of 75 mg followed by a loading

Table 11-1
Protocol to rapidly provide plasma lidocaine concentrations of 3 μg/ml*

Time (min)	Dose	Load by body weight (mg/kg)	
		Normal patient	Patient with heart failure
0	1st Bolus: loads central compartment	1.5	0.9
8	2nd Bolus: replaces loss in first half-life	0.8	0.4
16	3rd Bolus: replaces loss in second half-life	0.8	0.4
24	4th Bolus: replaces loss in third half-life	0.8	0.4
Total body load		3.9	2.1

*Based on: loading dose = volume of distribution × desired plasma concentration
= 1.32 L/kg × 3 μg/ml = 3.9 mg/kg
Source: From R. L. Woosley, Lidocaine therapy. *Cardiac Impulse* 8(2), 1987. With permission.

infusion of 150 mg over 18 minutes has also been used successfully [64]. Along with the loading regimen, a maintenance infusion designed to replace ongoing losses due to drug elimination should be started in the range of 20 to 60 μg/kg/min (1–4 mg/min). If symptomatic arrhythmias persist in the face of an adequate loading dosage (as assessed by plasma concentrations of more than 7 μg/ml, or the presence of side effects, or both), other agents should be used. One lidocaine dosing regimen is described in Table 11-1 [65].

Regardless of the loading regimen employed, the lidocaine concentration eventually reached at steady state is dependent only on the drug infusion rate and clearance. The time required to reach steady-state conditions is four to five elimination half-lives (approximately 8 to 10 hours in normal individuals). If the plasma concentration achieved at steady state is excessive, symptoms of lidocaine toxicity (most notably central nervous system disturbances) may occur many hours after the initiation of effective therapy and may be misinterpreted as "CCU psychosis." On the other hand, if the eventual steady-state level is too low, arrhythmia may recur many hours after the institution of seemingly effective therapy, and it may be misinterpreted as lidocaine resistance. Assuming that side effects are absent, the appropriate action in this case is the following: (1) if the patient's clinical condition permits, obtain a plasma sample for measurement of lidocaine concentration (for future reference); (2) administer a small bolus (25–50 mg); and (3) increase the maintenance infusion rate proportionately. Increasing the maintenance infusion rate without the incremental bolus may not lead to effective plasma concentrations until 8 to 10 hours later. If the arrhythmia recurs before steady state has been reached using an infusion, it might be advisable to simply administer a bolus and keep the same maintenance infusion. Again, plasma level monitoring assists in these decisions.

The practice of "tapering" lidocaine infusion rates is based on the misconception that lidocaine is eliminated rapidly. In fact, the rapid dissipation of lidocaine's effects early after an intravenous bolus is due to distribution, not elimination. Terminating a lidocaine infusion once steady-state conditions have been achieved results in a gradual decline in plasma levels over the next 8 to 10 hours as elimination occurs. Not only is there no reason to taper lidocaine infusions, if oral antiarrhythmic therapy is initiated, tapering prolongs the period during which unpredictable additive effects may occur between lidocaine and newly started oral therapy. Likewise, tapering makes it difficult to predict when lidocaine levels have fallen below the range expected to be effective.

It is possible to predict when the plasma lidocaine concentration will fall below usually therapeutic levels by determining the plasma

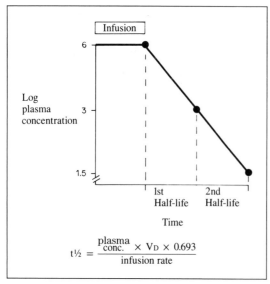

Fig. 11-3
Estimation of the half-life of lidocaine. By
determining the plasma concentration of lidocaine
at the time an infusion is terminated, one can
estimate the time needed to reach the lower limit
of the therapeutic range. V_d = volume of
distribution; $t_{1/2}$ = half-life. (From R. L. Woosley.
Lidocaine therapy. *Cardiac Impulse* 8:No. 2, 1987.
With permission.)

lidocaine concentration at the time the infusion is terminated and calculating the number
of half-lives (Fig. 11-3) needed to reach approximately 1.5 µg/ml as determined from the
following equation:

$$t_\frac{1}{} = \text{(plasma concentration)}(V_d)(0.693)/\text{(infusion rate)}$$

Modification of Dosage in Disease States
The effects of heart, liver, and renal disease
on lidocaine disposition were reported by
Thomson et al. [62]. Initial loading regimens,
dependent on volume of distribution, should
be decreased by about 50 percent in the presence of heart failure, whereas no adjustment
is necessary for renal or liver disease. Clearance is decreased by approximately 40 percent
in the presence of heart failure or liver disease; therefore intravenous maintenance infusions must be decreased in the presence of
these disease states. It is important to note
that in the presence of congestive heart failure
both the central volume of distribution and

clearance are decreased; therefore elimination
half-life is usually unchanged from that found
in normal individuals (see clearance, above).
Thus the time required to achieve steady-state
conditions following institution of a maintenance infusion is still often 8 to 10 hours even
in the presence of congestive heart failure (but
plasma concentrations will be higher due to reduced clearance and V_d). Conversely, because
clearance alone is altered in liver disease, with
little change in the volume of distribution, the
half-life of elimination is markedly prolonged
(almost 5 hours) and steady-state conditions
are not achieved until 20 to 25 hours after institution of an intravenous infusion. Despite
the fact that lidocaine metabolites are excreted by the kidneys, renal disease has not
been reported to exert any significant effect
on lidocaine dosing regimens.

In postmyocardial infarction patients receiving lidocaine infusions for more than 24
hours, plasma lidocaine levels can increase
and the elimination phase half-life can show a
marked increase (to as much as 3.2 hours)
[66]. The mechanism by which it occurs is
poorly understood: Suggestions include inhibition of lidocaine metabolism by accumulation of metabolites or changes in lidocaine
binding to plasma proteins, perhaps due to
changes in acute-phase reactants such as AAG
[67]. Monitoring lidocaine concentrations in
patients remaining on therapy for more than
24 to 48 hours may help detect those patients
with increasing drug concentrations. However, because AAG levels may be higher in
these patients, the free drug level may be unchanged and higher total lidocaine levels may
actually be required and tolerated.

Drug Interactions
An additive or synergistic depression of myocardial function or conduction may occur during combined therapy using lidocaine with
other antiarrhythmic agents [68]. A pharmacokinetic drug interaction between propranolol and lidocaine has been described in
the anesthetized dog in which beta-adrenergic
blockade caused a decrease in cardiac output
and liver blood flow. As a result, lidocaine
clearance was reduced, and lidocaine plasma

concentrations were subsequently increased [69]. A similar phenomenon has been described in man [70].

Cimetidine has been reported to decrease lidocaine's volume of distribution, decrease splanchnic (and hence liver) blood flow, and inhibit the enzymes responsible for lidocaine deethylation. All three effects serve to raise lidocaine plasma concentrations, and both loading and maintenance dosages may require downward adjustment in patients receiving cimetidine [71].

Occasionally patients are noted who have an excellent response to lidocaine but with continued therapy fail to respond. One possible explanation could be a decrease in free levels of lidocaine caused by increases in the concentration of AAG. However, another possibility has been proposed by Bennett et al. [72]. These authors found that a major metabolite of lidocaine, glycinexylidide, under certain conditions can antagonize sodium channel blockade produced by lidocaine in vitro. Such interactions call attention to the structurally specific interactions of drugs and metabolites that can occur at the receptor that regulates sodium channel function.

PROCAINAMIDE

Indications
Procainamide is effective acute parenteral therapy for ventricular arrhythmias; and, unlike lidocaine, it can be administered orally. Procainamide also has electrophysiologic characteristics that make it useful for the treatment of supraventricular tachyarrhythmias. However, as in the case of all drugs with class IA antiarrhythmic action (procainamide, quinidine, disopyramide), it should not be used in patients with a long Q-T interval syndrome, hypokalemia, or a history of torsade de pointes because of the possibility of arrhythmia aggravation.

Pharmacology
The major effects of procainamide (and quinidine or disopyramide) on atrial tissue, ventricular muscle, and Purkinje fibers are prolongation of the action potential duration and refractoriness, a decrease in phase IV depolarization (automaticity) in pacemaker cells, and a decrease in conduction velocity [73]. In patients, intravenous procainamide was found to increase the ventricular effective refractory period (VERP) as well as the ratio of VERP to the Q-T interval; it was suggested that the increase in this ratio might account for procainamide's efficacy in suppressing reentrant tachyarrhythmias [74]. Procainamide has also been suggested to prolong conduction in depressed portions of reentrant pathways, thereby creating bidirectional block and terminating tachycardia [75].

Procainamide can convert atrial flutter or fibrillation to sinus rhythm; however, patients with atrial flutter should probably receive digitalis or other AV nodal blockers prior to therapy with any of the antiarrhythmic drugs having class IA action (procainamide, quinidine, disopyramide). In the nondigitalized patient these agents may actually precipitate an increase in ventricular response. This increase is probably due to a combination of a direct drug effect, slowing of the flutter rate (which had been maintaining the ventricle in a refractory state), and an indirect anticholinergic action accelerating conduction across the AV node.

When procainamide was administered to 16 patients with intraventricular conduction delay, A–H intervals did not change, but H–V intervals increased by a mean of 18 percent. Procainamide-induced sinus node depression was noted in one of these patients [76].

Absorption, Distribution, Metabolism, and Elimination
Absorption of procainamide is rapid and almost complete (75–90 percent) following oral administration. However, because of differences in rate of absorption coupled with rapid elimination, plasma concentrations vary widely within a group of patients. Plasma concentration monitoring discussed below can help guide dosage selection [77], although it is essential to remember that plasma concentration monitoring data must be interpreted with caution, as procainamide undergoes conversion to an active metabolite.

Procainamide, like lidocaine, follows a two-compartment open kinetic model following intravenous administration. However, in this case, the concentration in plasma may not reflect the concentration in the myocardium. Galeazzi et al. [78] showed a dissociation between rate-corrected Q–T interval prolongation and plasma procainamide concentration during the first 6 hours after acute intravenous administration. Late production of N-acetylprocainamide (acecainide, NAPA) may be responsible for the change in Q–T interval.

Approximately 15 to 50 percent of a dose of procainamide is metabolized by hepatic N-acetyltransferase to NAPA. The presence of this metabolic pathway is genetically determined and is expressed in a polymorphic distribution in man [79]. Approximately 45 percent of Caucasian and 20 percent of Oriental populations have deficient N-acetyltransferase activity and are slow acetylators of procainamide. In rapid acetylators, most of a procainamide dose is converted to NAPA, and the plasma concentration of NAPA exceeds that of procainamide at steady state. NAPA is eliminated almost exclusively by the kidneys. The mean elimination half-life of procainamide is 3.5 hours in patients with normal renal and hepatic function, and the elimination half-life of NAPA is approximately 6 to 8 hours. Half-lives of both compounds are prolonged in patients with diminished creatinine clearance.

To achieve an antiarrhythmic effect, a procainamide plasma level of at least 4 μg/ml is needed for most patients [77]. An increase in both the incidence and severity of side effects, primarily gastrointestinal symptoms, is seen when plasma concentrations exceed 8 to 10 μg/ml. Plasma concentrations of NAPA are variable but are usually about equal to those of procainamide. Individuals with normal renal function and plasma NAPA-procainamide ratios of more than 1 can be defined as rapid acetylators of procainamide. NAPA has been administered to patients with arrhythmias, and its "therapeutic range" appears to be between 9 and 19 μg/ml [80]. Side effects are common during NAPA therapy, and some of the adverse effects during chronic procainamide administration are probably due to the presence of this active metabolite.

Plasma concentrations of procainamide and NAPA should be monitored under certain circumstances. In patients with renal failure, NAPA accumulates and may be the compound responsible for therapeutic effect or toxicity [27]. In rapid acetylators, excessive NAPA concentrations may be responsible for side effects, or the combined concentrations of parent drug and metabolite may produce toxicity.

Toxicity

The major dose-related side effects accompanying oral procainamide therapy are gastrointestinal symptoms. Excessively rapid intravenous administration can cause hypotension, possible due to ganglionic blockade, and depression of myocardial contractility as well as heart block.

The drug-induced lupus erythematosus syndrome is the major toxic reaction during chronic procainamide therapy. It occurs more frequently in slow acetylators of procainamide [81], and virtually any of the symptoms usually associated with systemic lupus erythematosus (e.g., rash, pericarditis, arthritis) may be present (although nephritis is rare). The syndrome resolves if procainamide therapy is stopped. One hypothesis suggests that procainamide is transformed into a reactive metabolite (other than NAPA) that then interacts with nuclear histone protein and elicits antinuclear antibody formation [82]. This theory is supported by the observation that patients who are able to rapidly acetylate the drug are relatively protected. Another line of evidence suggesting that acetylation is a "protective pathway" is that patients who have developed symptomatic drug-induced lupus erythematosus during chronic procainamide therapy can experience a remission during NAPA therapy [80]. Although virtually all patients receiving therapeutic dosages of procainamide for more than a year develop antinuclear antibodies, it alone is not an indication to stop procainamide therapy because only about 20 percent develop the lupus syndrome. Procainamide therapy has been associated with the development of agranulocytosis (0.2 percent incidence); some investigators have theorized that the sustained-release form of the drug may be particularly capable of inducing this toxicity [83], although comparative studies are not available.

Dosage and Administration

Procainamide can be administered intravenously, intramuscularly, or orally. When procainamide is used for the acute treatment of ventricular or supraventricular tachyarrhythmias, intravenous administration using a loading regimen is preferred. If the sitution is less urgent, a maintenance oral dosage can be started without a "loading dose." Intramuscular therapy appears to offer no particular advantage in either situation and makes it impossible for the physician to readjust dosage if adverse effects occur.

Loading regimens for procainamide have not been established as well as they have for lidocaine. The loading dose is 500 to 1000 mg administered either in boluses of 100 mg every 5 minutes or as a constant-rate infusion at 250 to 300 μg/kg/min. Close monitoring of the patient's electrocardiogram, blood pressure, and pulse is mandatory during loading. If no antiarrhythmic effect is seen after 1000 mg of procainamide has been administered, a further 500 mg can be given if no hypotension or excessive QRS or Q–T interval prolongation is present. Although it is unlikely that dosages of more than 1.5 gm will produce an antiarrhythmic effect when lower doses have failed, plasma concentrations should be checked to ensure that adequate drug has been given.

Depending on cardiac and renal function, the maintenance dose is 20 to 60 μg/kg/min administered as a continuous intravenous infusion. Because the elimination half-life varies from 3 to 5 hours, steady-state conditions are approached within 9 to 20 hours, regardless of the loading regimen used. Thus it is possible that many hours after the institution of effective therapy with a loading dose plasma concentrations may reach either excessive or subtherapeutic levels. In addition, 48 hours or more may be required for maximum accumulation of NAPA.

If conversion to oral procainamide therapy is desired, it should be remembered that procainamide is rapidly absorbed from the gastrointestinal tract. Adverse effects due to excessive plasma concentrations may develop if an oral dose is given as the intravenous infusion is stopped. The appropriate maneuver in this situation is to stop the intravenous infusion, wait one-half of an elimination half-life (1.5–2.0 hours), and then institute a chronic oral dosing regimen without a loading dose (because loading has already been accomplished). Because of the relatively narrow margin between therapeutic and toxic effects, and because of relatively rapid elimination, procainamide must usually be given every 3 to 4 hours. The initial dosage is 250 to 500 mg every 3 to 4 hours and is adjusted upward as necessary, guided by antiarrhythmic effects, the occurrence of side effects, and plasma concentration monitoring. Slow-release forms of procainamide allow therapy on a 6- to 8-hour basis.

Modification of Dosage in Disease States

For patients with acute myocardial infarction, procainamide loading doses should generally be lower than for normal individuals, and maintenance dosages also must be reduced to avoid accumulation to toxic levels. Although the half-life, and therefore the time to steady state, is not markedly different in these patients, total body clearance is reduced up to 40 percent, suggesting a concomitant decrease in volume of distribution [84]. Similar dosage reductions appear to be necessary in patients with heart failure.

With renal disease, there is a reduction in the elimination of both procainamide and NAPA. Maintenance dosages must be decreased, and often doses of procainamide as low as 250 mg can be administered every 8 to 12 hours with an antiarrhythmic effect in these individuals, possibly due to NAPA accumulation [27].

Drug Interactions

In an experimental setting, the combination of lidocaine and procainamide has been found to exert synergistic adverse hemodynamic effects (disproportionate hypotension) [68]. This problem has particular relevance for therapy in the CCU where patients refractory to the first drug chosen may require additional antiarrhythmic therapy before the first agent can be completely eliminated.

BRETYLIUM

Indications
Bretylium is indicated for the treatment of recurrent ventricular fibrillation, or ventricular tachycardia in an intensive care or coronary care setting [85]. Intravenous administration appears to act within minutes to suppress ventricular fibrillation, although in some patients there may be a delay of 20 minutes to 2 hours in the onset of antiarrhythmic action. This delay may be due to dosages lower than needed for antiarrhythmic effect or delayed attainment of adequate myocardial tissue levels. Of particular interest are reports that bretylium can effectively reverse ventricular tachyarrhythmias refractory to lidocaine following myocardial infarction [86, 87]. Moreover, Holder and coworkers [88] reported bretylium to be effective in 20 of 27 patients with ventricular fibrillation refractory not only to lidocaine but to DC countershock, with 12 of these 20 patients surviving to be discharged from the hospital. Rapid bretylium injection alone, in the absence of cardioversion, has been reported to restore sinus rhythm in five of seven patients with ventricular fibrillation [89].

Pharmacology
Following intravenous administration, bretylium exerts two distinct pharmacologic actions on the autonomic nervous system. It is initially sequestered into adrenergic neurons via a norepinephrine pump. This action produces release of norepinephrine, resulting in tachycardia, hypertension, and occasionally increased arrhythmias. Following this brief phase (usually less than 15 minutes but occasionally longer), further release of norepinephrine is blocked, and orthostatic hypotension is commonly present. The major electrophysiologic effect of bretylium is to prolong action potential duration and the effective refractory period, thereby decreasing dispersion of refractoriness, particularly between normal and infarcted tissue [90]. Bretylium can also hyperpolarize Purkinje fibers with low resting potentials [91] with a resultant increase in conduction velocity. There is evidence in patients that the adrenergic neuron blocking effect and the antiarrhythmic effect of bretylium can be dissociated in some patients.

Woosley and associates [92] have found that orthostatic hypotension due to bretylium can be reversed by the co-administration of protriptyline, a tricyclic antidepressant that blocks uptake of bretylium into postganglionic sympathetic neurons. Patients were able to become ambulatory without loss of bretylium's antiarrhythmic efficacy. However, one must be aware that this treatment may not be feasible in patients whose arrhythmias are controlled by the antiadrenergic actions of bretylium.

Absorption, Distribution, Metabolism, and Elimination
Bretylium is usually administered by intravenous infusion. It is eliminated by the kidneys without undergoing metabolism [93], with an elimination half-life (following intravenous dosage) calculated to be 13.6 hours. A description of the time course of myocardial drug accumulation and antifibrillatory effects following intravenous dosage in dogs demonstrated a parallel between electrophysiologic effects and myocardial drug concentrations, with peak effects occurring 3 to 6 hours after an intravenous bolus [94]. A therapeutic range of bretylium plasma concentrations (which would parallel myocardial drug concentrations once steady state was achieved) has not been established.

Toxicity
Adverse effects during bretylium administration are usually a direct consequence and extension of its pharmacologic actions. Thus transient hypertension, tachycardia, and arrhythmia worsening are occasionally seen closely following intravenous administration, and orthostatic hypotension is almost universally present a few minutes later. Bretylium did not adversely affect cardiac output or left

ventricular filling pressure in patients with recent myocardial infarction [95]. Although bretylium decreases pulmonary vascular resistance, it has been reported to increase pulmonary vascular resistance in patients with mitral valve disease following surgery [96]. Excessively rapid intravenous administration has been associated with nausea and vomiting; these effects can be reduced or prevented by decreasing the rate of administration. Postural hypotension can be most easily managed by leaving the patient in the supine position. If supine hypotension develops, the treatment of choice is volume expansion; patients receiving bretylium therapy are in a functionally denervated state and may be particularly sensitive to exogenous pressor agents such as dopamine or norepinephrine.

Dosage and Administration

Like lidocaine and procainamide, bretylium should be administered intravenously with a loading dose followed by a maintenance infusion. Bretylium's pharmacokinetics have not been intensively studied, and dose-response relations have not been clearly identified because of the difficult nature of the clinical setting in which it is used; hence exact dosing regimens have not yet been worked out. Additionally, as noted above, maximal antifibrillatory effects may not be obvious for several hours following the institution of therapy. One intravenous loading regimen involves administration of 5 to 10 mg/kg over 15 to 30 minutes followed by maintenance infusions of 2 to 4 mg/min. If rhythm control is not established, further loading doses (up to a total of 20–30 mg/kg) can be administered. The patient should be supine while bretylium is administered; hypotension is not an indication to stop therapy because, although very low dosages block autonomic neuron function, higher dosages are required for an antiarrhythmic effect.

Bretylium has also been administered intramuscularly with intermittent injections. However, this method is not recommended because absorption is uncertain and injection sites must be varied to avoid tissue necrosis.

Modifications in Disease States

Bretylium clearance is markedly reduced in the presence of renal disease [97], and the drug should be administered in the lowest effective dosage in patients with renal insufficiency. No data are available on dosage adjustments required in other conditions such as congestive heart failure or liver disease, but it is unlikely that the dosage should be adjusted for these individuals. Bretylium therapy should be avoided in patients in whom a marked drop in systemic vascular resistance may be deleterious (e.g., those with valvular aortic stenosis) and in those with pulmonary hypertension.

Drug Interactions

Because of the initial norepinephrine release induced by bretylium and the attendant risk of worsening arrhythmias, bretylium should probably be administered with caution to patients who are receiving digitalis. Once norepinephrine uptake by adrenergic neurons is blocked, a state of functional denervation hypersensitivity exists; and at this stage patients are sensitive to exogenous pressor amines. Because reversal of the antiadrenergic actions allows arrhythmic recurrence in some individuals, further evaluation of this observation in a larger patient population is needed before it is widely adopted. The interaction between bretylium and tricyclic antidepressants has already been discussed (see Pharmacology, above).

BETA-ADRENERGIC RECEPTOR BLOCKING AGENTS

One of the most significant advances in cardiovascular therapy has been the conclusion of a number of large-scale clinical trials of drugs evaluating beta-receptor antagonists in the postmyocardial infarction population. In well-conducted, double-blind, placebo-controlled trials, timolol, propranolol, metoprolol, alprenolol, and practolol have been shown to decrease the incidence of recurrent myocardial infarction and sudden cardiac death by 25 to 50 percent [11, 17]. This effect does not appear to be related to characteristics that differ among these drugs, e.g., membrane stabilization and cardioselectivity. Although some early therapeutic trials using beta-receptor antagonists showed variable effects on the recurrence of myocardial infarction and sudden cardiac death, those results most likely reflected inadequate dosages or poor study design. It is important, therefore, that the practicing physician be aware of the dosages and patient subsets that produced results in these trials. Clearly, use of any other agent or of any other dosage of these agents remains of unproved value.

Although the mechanism by which these drugs exert a protective action remains speculative, there is no question that beta-receptor antagonists can exert antiarrhythmic effects in certain settings, but it is equally possible that these agents exert their protective actions through some other mechanism. A number of trials have also studied the effects of early intervention with beta-adrenergic receptor blocking drugs in an attempt to modify infarct size. Early treatment with metoprolol (15 mg IV followed by 100 mg PO twice daily thereafter) was studied by Hjalmarson [98], who found a 36 percent reduction in mortality due to sudden cardiac death. Use of beta-receptor antagonists soon after myocardial infarction is currently accepted as being of benefit to patients who can tolerate these agents, i.e., those with good left ventricular function. The use of beta-adrenergic receptor antagonists for ventricular tachycardia during the early myocardial infarction period should be discouraged.

OTHER AGENTS

During acute myocardial infarction, most ventricular tachyarrhythmias can be controlled by lidocaine, lidocaine plus procainamide, procainamide, or bretylium. In one study examining the role of electrolytes following myocardial infarction, for the small number of patients studied there were preliminary indications that intravenous magnesium therapy could reduce the incidence of serious arrhythmias [99].

Tocainide
Studies comparing intravenous and oral tocainide regimens to lidocaine in patients with acute myocardial infarction have produced inconclusive or contradictory results. A study of 40 patients receiving 750 mg IV over 15 minutes followed by 800 mg PO found both agents to be equally effective for suppressing ventricular arrhythmias, and side effects were reported less frequently for tocainide [100]. However, another study that evaluated a lower dose of combined intravenous and oral tocainide (500 mg IV over 30 minutes followed by a 600-mg oral loading dose) on the incidence of primary ventricular fibrillation in 278 patients found it ineffective for this purpose [101]. Maintaining therapeutic plasma levels in these patients is difficult. In the latter study, tocainide plasma levels in patients with documented myocardial infarction were lower than those measured in cardiac patients who were subsequently found not to have suffered infarction. However, in the opinion of the authors, arbitrarily increasing the tocainide dosage to compensate for this low level would place individuals who had not sustained an acute infarction at risk of excessively high levels [101]. Because of significant chronic toxicity (pulmonary fibrosis and agranulocytosis) chronic oral therapy with tocainide is not recommended unless the patient is refractory to other agents.

Disopyramide
Disopyramide has been proposed as an alternate therapy for patients intolerant of lidocaine, although in a randomized study comparing it to lidocaine (33 patients receiving disopyramide), therapy with this agent was accompanied by adverse effects: supraventricular tachycardias and atrial fibrillation (21 percent), ventricular tachycardia (sustained, 3 percent; nonsustained, 18 percent), hypotension (6 percent), pulmonary congestion (6 percent), and conduction disturbances (12 percent) [102]. A major limitation of disopyramide is its ability to decrease left ventricular

function, causing new or worsened congestive heart failure [103–105]. This effect is due to a direct negative inotropic action [105] and to vasoconstriction, causing increased peripheral vascular resistance [106]. Therefore, in the opinion of the authors, there is little justification for its use in this setting.

Free disopyramide levels in plasma are known to vary because of the saturable nature of its binding to plasma proteins. During myocardial infarction, even when disopyramide is given intravenously, its serum concentration may be lower than expected. It probably reflects increased drug clearance, as suggested by Elliott and coworkers, who derived values for early and late disopyramide clearance. The former was found to be more than double the initially estimated clearance rate, although there was a range of variation among patients. They concluded that changes in disopyramide disposition that occur in the days following myocardial infarction may require measurement of free disopyramide concentrations to maintain effective therapy [107].

Propafenone
Propafenone is a new agent, still under investigation in the United States. Like procainamide, it has been given intravenously and orally. A Swedish study compared use of lidocaine and propafenone during acute myocardial infarction in 20 patients [108]. Whereas propafenone and lidocaine demonstrated equivalent antiarrhythmic efficacy, three of ten patients receiving propafenone developed increasing numbers of premature ventricular contractions and one had torsade de pointes. Although the authors concluded that propafenone was a promising agent, the possible high incidence of proarrhythmic effect requires further careful evaluation. Propafenone metabolism is polymorphic and genetically determined, and some of propafenone's metabolites possess antiarrhythmic activity.

Calcium Channel Antagonists
Clinical trials have evaluated the acute short-term use of the calcium channel blocking agents nifedipine, verapamil, and diltiazem. These agents were given within hours after the

onset of suspected myocardial infarction and demonstrated no beneficial influence on infarct size, progression to acute myocardial infarction, or mortality [109].

Initiating Chronic Therapy in the CCU

The availability of ambulatory ECG monitoring technology has enabled physicians to determine that patients with recent myocardial infarction are at higher risk for sudden death if ventricular arrhythmias are detected [110]. This risk increases in direct proportion to the log frequency of VEDs and is even higher for patients with episodes of nonsustained ventricular tachycardia. Ventricular dysfunction is an additional independent risk factor that, when coincident with ventricular arrhythmias, identifies a group at highest risk of sudden death. Patients who continue to exhibit high-grade ventricular ectopy during the convalescent phases of myocardial infarction are frequently treated with conventional antiarrhythmic therapy in the hope of reducing the risk of sudden death. However, to date there are no data to support this approach for asymptomatic patients. CAST is designed to answer this question. Patients with prior myocardial infarction, asymptomatic ventricular arrhythmias, and reduced left ventricular function whose arrhythmias are suppressed by antiarrhythmic drugs are randomized to receive placebo or drug therapy in a double-blind protocol and followed for 2 to 5 years to compare the incidence of sudden death in the two groups (see p. 198).

Patients who develop symptomatic nonsustained ventricular tachycardia either during or after the convalescent phase of infarction can be effectively treated with one of the newer antiarrhythmic agents. These drugs were frequently recommended because they effectively suppress chronic stable ventricular arrhythmias in more than 80 percent of patients and are better tolerated than either quinidine or disopyramide, particularly during long-term therapy. Of major concern are the data from CAST indicating an increased mortality with encainide and flecainide and the possibility that use of these newer agents may lead to the development of congestive heart failure, conduction disturbances, or arrhythmia aggravation. Encainide, flecainide, and propafenone markedly slow cardiac conduction (and therefore increase the P–R and QRS intervals). They have been associated with a high risk of exacerbating ventricular tachycardia in certain patient subsets (severe left ventricular dysfunction, history of sustained ventricular tachycardia). The manufacturers of encainide and flecainide recommend that they only be used in the treatment of life-threatening arrhythmias; therapy of symptomatic arrhythmias is not recommended. However, there are many patients with incapacitating arrhythmias unresponsive to other agents who can receive clinical benefit from these agents. Careful monitoring in the hospital to document both suppression of symptomatic arrhythmias by these agents and the lack of toxicity is essential. A complete assessment of the risk-benefit ratio is essential, as are discussions of this issue with patients.

The development of sustained ventricular tachycardia during this phase of recuperation is an indication for evaluation of therapy using programmed ventricular stimulation. There is less experience with the newer agents, and most physicians still choose quinidine or procainamide as the initial therapy. All of the agents with class I activity (sodium channel blockers) have been found effective but to varying extent. The lidocaine analogs (mexiletine and tocainide) and beta-receptor antagonists are not very effective, with a 10 percent or lower response rate being seen when they are used singly. Agents with class IA (quinidine, procainamide, disopyramide) or IC activity (flecainide, encainide, propafenone) have approximately 20 to 30 percent response rates. Combinations of quinidine and mexiletine may have greater potency, but the studies reported to date are relatively small. Investigational agents such as pirmenol, recainam, and lorcainide have been evaluated only in small series, and their potency does not appear to be different from that of other available agents. The investigational agent sotalol

appears to have higher potency than procainamide [111], and uncontrolled studies have reported high success rates in this population [112].

Amiodarone is being used increasingly for the acute and chronic therapy of a variety of cardiac arrhythmias. Side effects, including pulmonary fibrosis and liver damage, and the difficulty of managing arrhythmia recurrences during chronic therapy have become increasingly recognized with this drug. For these reasons most recommended it only for treatment of life-threatening arrhythmias resistant to all available agents.

The automatic implantable cardioverter-defibrillator has been approved for marketing in the United States, and ablative procedures (either surgical or catheter-directed) have been improving and are used for the management of selected arrhythmias.

It is increasingly recognized that antiarrhythmic therapy can be associated with arrhythmia exacerbation. It can range from a marked increase in the frequency of ventricular ectopic depolarizations to the new onset or increased frequency of sustained ventricular tachycardia. The latter is clearly not necessarily associated with marked Q–T prolongation, particularly with the use of drugs that markedly slow conduction velocity, e.g., encainide or flecainide. The incidence of such arrhythmia exacerbation may be as high as 20 percent in patients with severely depressed left ventricular performance, coronary artery disease, and a history of sustained ventricular tachycardia when flecainide-like agents are administered [113].

The incidence of torsade de pointes is difficult to estimate, but it is certainly seen more commonly with agents such as quinidine, procainamide, and disopyramide. It has also been seen with investigational agents that prolong the Q–T interval, e.g., sotalol and NAPA. Predisposing factors such as bradycardia and hypokalemia have been identified; and Roden et al., in a study of 24 patients, found these factors to be present in 83 percent of those who developed torsade de pointes [33]. In the population with less severe arrhythmias, the incidence of arrhythmia aggravation has been estimated to be 2 to 12 percent with currently available drugs. The Cardiac Arrhythmia Pilot Study (CAPS) was performed to determine if postinfarction ventricular arrhythmias could be satisfactorily reduced for 1 year in a large population in preparation for CAST. The overall incidence of an increase in arrhythmia frequency or severity in CAPS was 1 percent with encainide and 3 percent with flecainide—no different from that with placebo (3 percent) [114]. Therefore the increase is clearly dependent on the drug, the dose, and the clinical setting. The increased incidence of sudden death and total mortality reported in CAST may be a manifestation of the proarrhythmic potential of encainide and flecainide. However, the mechanism is unclear.

Acknowledgments

The authors thank Rosemary Hoffman for providing editorial assistance.

Editorial Comments

Physicians should be aware of an emerging sense that premature ventricular contractions (PVCs) in the setting of acute myocardial infarction need not be completely extinguished or even treated, although this subject is controversial. "Warning arrhythmias" are probably as common in patients who do not progress to ventricular fibrillation as in those who do. Moreover, ventricular fibrillation frequently occurs with no warning, except for antecedent R-on-T ventricular ectopic complexes (Campbell et al. Br. Heart J. 46:351, 1981). Ventricular tachycardia rarely is preceded by the R-on-T phenomenon. The pathogenesis and precursors of ventricular fibrillation may well be different depending on the time after the onset of infarction. It is likely that complete amelioration of PVCs with lidocaine in patients with acute myocardial infarction is cosmetic in most and prevents ventricular fibrillation in only a few. Nevertheless, this habit is etched in our therapeutic

strategy and is likely to continue to be used by most physicians. G.S.F.

The Cardiac Arrhythmia Suppression Trial has demonstrated that encainide and flecainide therapy significantly increased the risk of death and non-fatal cardiac arrest in patients with asymptomatic or mildly symptomatic ventricular arrhythmia after myocardial infarction. These data support the concept that treatment of ventricular arrhythmias in post-infarct patients should be undertaken with considerable caution (CAST Investigators, N. Engl. J. Med. 321(6):406, 1989.). J.S.A.

References

1. Bigger, J. T., Dresdale, R. J., Heissenbuttel, R. H., et al. Ventricular arrhythmias in ischemic heart disease: Mechanism, prevalence, significance, and management. *Prog. Cardiovasc. Dis.* 19:255, 1977.
2. Julian, D. G., Valentine, P. A., and Miller, G. G. Disturbances of rate, rhythm and conduction in acute myocardial infarction. *Am. J. Med.* 37:915, 1964.
3. Meltzer, L. E., and Kitchell, J. R. The incidence of arrhythmias associated with acute myocardial infarction. *Prog. Cardiovasc. Dis.* 9:50, 1966.
4. Lie, K. I., Wellens, H. J., van Capelle, F. J., and Durrer, D. Lidocaine in the prevention of primary ventricular fibrillation: A double-blind, randomized study of 212 consecutive patients. *N. Engl. J. Med.* 291:1324, 1974.
5. Harrison, D. C. Should lidocaine be administered routinely to all patients after acute myocardial infarction? (Editorial). *Circulation* 58:581, 1978.
6. Lie, K. I., Liem, K. L., Louridtz, W. J., et al. Efficacy of lidocaine in preventing primary ventricular fibrillation within 1 hour after a 300 mg intramuscular injection. *Am. J. Cardiol.* 42:486, 1978.
7. Valentine, P. A., Frew, J. L., Mashford, M. L., and Sloman, J. G. Lidocaine in the prevention of sudden death in the pre-hospital phase of acute infarction: A double-blind study. *N. Engl. J. Med.* 291:1327, 1974.
8. Koster, R. W., and Dunning, A. J. Intramuscular lidocaine for prevention of lethal arrhythmias in the prehospitalization phase of acute myocardial infarction. *N. Engl. J. Med.* 313:1105, 1985.
9. Campbell, R. W. F., Achuff, S. C., Pottage, A., et al. Mexiletine in the prophylaxis of ven-

tricular arrhythmias during acute myocardial infarction. *J. Cardiovasc. Physiol.* 1:43, 1979.

10. de Soyza, N., Bissett, J. K., Kane, J. J., et al. Association of accelerated idioventricular rhythm and paroxysmal ventricular tachycardia in acute myocardial infarction. *Am. J. Cardiol.* 34:667, 1974.

11. Hjalmarson, A., Herlitz, J., Malek, I., et al. Effect on mortality of metoprolol in acute myocardial infarction: A double-blind randomised trial. *Lancet* 2:823, 1981.

12. Brachman, J., Scherlag, B. J., Rosenshtraukh, L. V., and Lazzara, R. Bradycardia-dependent triggered activity: Relevance to drug-induced multiform ventricular tachycardia. *Circulation* 68:846, 1983.

13. Roden, D. M., and Hoffman, B. F. Action potential prolongation and induction of abnormal automaticity by low quinidine concentrations in canine Purkinje fibers: Relationship to potassium and cycle length. *Circ. Res.* 56:857, 1985.

14. Tzivoni, D., Keren, A., and Stern, S. Torsades de pointes versus polymorphous ventricular tachycardia (Editorial). *Am. J. Cardiol.* 52:639, 1983.

15. Bigger, Jr., J. T., Weld, F. M., and Rolnitzky, L. M. Prevalence, characteristics, and significance of ventricular tachycardia (three or more complexes) detected with ambulatory electrocardiographic recording in the late hospital phase of acute myocardial infarction. *Am. J. Cardiol.* 48:815, 1981.

16. Morganroth, J. Premature ventricular complexes: Diagnosis and indications for therapy. *J.A.M.A.* 252:673, 1984.

17. Mukarji, J., Rude, R. E., Poole, W. K., et al. Risk factors for sudden cardiac death following acute myocardial infarction: Two year follow-up. *Am. J. Cardiol.* 54:31, 1984.

18. Vlay, S. C. How the university cardiologist treats ventricular premature beats: A nationwide survey of 65 university medical centers. *Am. Heart J.* 110:904, 1985.

19. Woosley, R. L., Roden, D. M., Duff, H. J., and Oates, J. A. Selection of an antiarrhythmic drug for a sudden death prevention trial. *Am. Heart J.* 103:737, 1982.

20. Schaffer, W. A., and Cobb, L. A. Recurrent ventricular fibrillation and modes of death in survivors of out-of-hospital ventricular fibrillation. *N. Engl. J. Med.* 293:259, 1975.

21. Myerburg, R. J., Conde, C., Sheps, D. S., et al. Antiarrhythmic drug therapy in survivors of prehospital cardiac arrest: Comparison of effects on chronic ventricular arrhythmias and recurrent cardiac arrest. *Circulation* 59:855, 1979.

22. Cobb, L. A., Chinn, T. L., Hallstrom, A. P., et al. Effect of propranolol on long term survival in patients resuscitated from out-of-hospital ventricular fibrillation. *Circulation* 64(Suppl. IV):35, 1981.

23. Ruskin, J. N., DiMarco, J. P., and Garan, H. Out-of-hospital cardiac arrest: Electrophysiologic observations and selection of long-term antiarrhythmic therapy. *N. Engl. J. Med.* 303:607, 1980.

24. Lazzara, R., and Scherlag, B. J. Electrophysiologic basis for arrhythmias in ischemic heart disease. *Am. J. Cardiol.* 53:1B, 1984.

25. Zipes, D. P. Genesis of cardiac arrhythmias: Electrophysiological considerations. In E. Braunwald (ed.), *Heart Disease*. Philadelphia: Saunders, 1988. Pp. 581–620.

26. Siddoway, L. A., Roden, D. M., and Woosley, R. L. Clinical pharmacology of old and new antiarrhythmic drugs. *Cardiovasc. Clin.* 15:199, 1984.

27. Drayer, D. E., Lowenthal, D. T., Woosley, R. L., et al. Cumulation of N-acetylprocainamide, an active metabolite of procainamide, in patients with impaired renal function. *Clin. Pharmacol. Ther.* 22:63, 1977.

28. Roden, D. M., Reele, S. B., Higgins, S. B., et al. Total suppression of ventricular arrhythmias by encainide: Pharmacokinetic and electrocardiographic characteristics. *N. Engl. J. Med.* 302:877, 1980.

29. Edwards, D. J., Axelson, J. E. E., Slaughter, R. L., et al. Factors affecting quinidine protein binding in man. *J. Pharm. Sci.* 73:1264, 1984.

30. Garfinkel, D., Mamelok, R. D., and Blaschke, T. F. Altered therapeutic range for quinidine after myocardial infarction and cardiac surgery. *Ann. Intern. Med.* 107:48, 1987.

31. Vaughan Williams, E. M. A classification of antiarrhythmic actions reassessed after a decade of new drugs. *J. Clin. Pharmacol.* 24:129, 1984.

32. McKibbin, J. K., Pocock, W. A., Barlow, J. B., et al. Sotalol, hypokalemia, syncope, and torsade de pointes. *Br. Heart J.* 51:157, 1984.

33. Roden, D. M., Woosley, R. L., and Primm, R. K. Incidence and clinical features of the quinidine-associated long QT syndrome: Implications for patient care. *Am. Heart J.* 111:1088, 1986.

34. Hodgkin, A. L., and Huxley, A. F. A quantitative description of membrane current and its application to conduction and excitation in nerve. *J. Physiol. (Lond.)* 117:500, 1952.

35. Hille, B. Local anesthetics: Hydrophilic and hydrophobic pathways for the drug receptor reaction. *J. Gen. Physiol.* 69:497, 1977.

36. Hondeghem, L., and Katzung, B. G. Test of a model of antiarrhythmic drug action: Effects of quinidine and lidocaine on myocardial conduction. *Circulation* 61:1217, 1980.

37. Duff, H. J., Roden, D. M., Primm, R. K., et al. Mexiletine for resistant ventricular tachycardia: Comparison with lidocaine and enhancement of efficacy by combination with quinidine (Abstract). *Am. J. Cardiol.* 47:438, 1981.

38. Alderman, E. J., Kerber, R. E., and Harrison, D. C. Evaluation of lidocaine resistance in man using intermittent large-dose infusion techniques. *Am. J. Cardiol.* 34:342, 1974.

39. Bigger, Jr., J. T., and Mandel, W. J. Effect of lidocaine on the electrophysiological properties of ventricular muscle and Purkinje fibers. *J. Clin. Invest.* 49:63, 1970.

40. Davis, L. D., and Temte, J. V. Electrophysiological actions of lidocaine on canine ventricular muscle and Purkinje fibers. *Circ. Res.* 24:639, 1969.

41. Kupersmith, J. Electrophysiological and antiarrhythmic effects of lidocaine in canine acute myocardial ischemia. *Am. Heart J.* 97:360, 1979.

42. El-Sherif, N., Scherlag, B. J., Lazzara, R., and Hope, R. R. Re-entrant ventricular arrhythmias in the late myocardial infarction period. 4. Mechanism of action of lidocaine. *Circulation* 56:395, 1977.

43. Gamble, O. W., and Cohn, K. Effect of propranolol, procainamide, and lidocaine on ventricular automaticity and reentry in experimental myocardial infarction. *Circulation* 46:498, 1972.

44. Adgey, A. A. J., Allen, J. D., Geddes, J. S., et al. Acute phase of myocardial infarction. *Lancet* 2:501, 1971.

45. Borer, J. S., Harrison, L. A., Kent, K. M., et al. Beneficial effect of lidocaine on ventricular electrical stability and spontaneous ventricular fibrillation during experimental myocardial infarction. *Am. J. Cardiol.* 37:860, 1976.

46. Spear, J. F., Moore, E. N., and Gerstenblith, G. Effect of lidocaine on the ventricular fibrillation threshold in the dog during acute ischemia and premature ventricular contractions. *Circulation* 46:65, 1972.

47. Mandel, W. J., and Bigger, Jr., J. T. Electrophysiologic effects of lidocaine on isolated canine and rabbit atrial tissue. *J. Pharmacol. Exp. Ther.* 178:81, 1971.

48. Kunkel, F., Rowland, M., and Scheinman, M. M. The electrophysiologic effects of lidocaine in patients with intraventricular conduction defects. *Circulation* 49:894, 1974.

49. Bekheit, S., Murtagh, J. G., Morton, P., and Fletcher, E. Effect of lignocaine on conducting system of human heart. *Br. Heart J.* 35:305, 1973.

50. Gupta, P. K., Lichstein, E., and Chadda, K. D. Lidocaine-induced heart block in patients with bundle branch block. *Am. J. Cardiol.* 33:487, 1974.

51. Aravindakshan, V., Kuo, C-S., and Gettes, L. S. Effect of lidocaine on escape rate in patients with complete atrioventricular block. A. Distal His block. *Am. J. Cardiol.* 40:177, 1977.

52. Cheng, T. O., and Wadhwa, K. Sinus standstill following intravenous lidocaine administration. *J.A.M.A.* 223:790, 1973.

53. Marriott, H. J. L., and Phillips, K. Profound hypotension and bradycardia after a single bolus of lidocaine. *J. Electrocardiol.* 7:79, 1974.

54. Josephson, M. E., Caracta, A. R., Lau, S. H., et al. Effects of lidocaine on refractory periods in man. *Am. Heart J.* 84:778, 1972.

55. Josephson, M. E., Kastor, J. A., and Kitchen, III, J. G. Lidocaine in Wolff-Parkinson-White syndrome with atrial fibrillation. *Ann. Intern. Med.* 84:44, 1976.

56. Rosen, K. M., Barwolf, C., Ehsani, A., and Rahimtoola, S. H. Effects of lidocaine and propranolol on the normal and anomalous pathways in patients with preexcitation. *Am. J. Cardiol.* 30:801, 1972.

57. Akhtar, M., Gilbert, C. J., and Shenasa, M. Effect of lidocaine on atrioventricular response via the accessory pathway in patients with Wolff-Parkinson-White syndrome. *Circulation* 63:435, 1981.

58. Blumer, J., Strong, J. M., and Atkinson, Jr., A. J. The convulsant potency of lidocaine and its N-dealkylated metabolites. *J. Pharmacol. Exp. Ther.* 186:31, 1973.

59. Narang, P. K., Crouthamel, W. G., Carliner, N. H., and Fisher, M. L. Lidocaine and its active metabolites. *Clin. Pharmacol. Ther.* 24:654, 1978.

60. Stenson, R. E., Constantino, R. T., and Harrison, D. C. Interrelationships of hepatic blood flow, cardiac output, and blood levels of lidocaine in man. *Circulation* 43:205, 1971.

61. Zito, R. A., and Reid, P. R. Lidocaine kinetics predicted by indocyanine green clearance. *N. Engl. J. Med.* 298:1160, 1978.

62. Thomson, P. D., Melmon, K. L., Richardson, J. A., et al. Lidocaine pharmacokinetics in advanced heart failure, liver disease and renal failure in humans. *Ann. Intern. Med.* 78:499, 1973.

63. Wyman, M. G., Slaughter, R. L., Farolino, D. A., et al. Multiple bolus technique for lidocaine administration in acute ischemic heart disease. II. Treatment of refractory ventricular arrhythmias and the pharmacokinetic significance of severe left ventricular failure. *J. Am. Coll. Cardiol.* 2:764, 1983.

64. Stargel, W. W., Shand, D. G., Routledge, P. A., et al. Clinical comparison of rapid infusion and multiple injection methods for

lidocaine loading. *Am. Heart J.* 102:872, 1981.

65. Woosley, R. L. Lidocaine therapy: application of clinical pharmacokinetic principles. *Cardiac Impulse* 8:1, 1987.

66. LeLorier, J., Grenon, D., Latour, Y., et al. Pharmacokinetics of lidocaine after prolonged intravenous infusions in uncomplicated myocardial infarction. *Ann. Intern. Med.* 87:700, 1977.

67. Routledge, P. A., Shand, D. G., Barchowsky, A., et al. Relationship between alpha 1-acid glycoprotein and lidocaine disposition in myocardial infarction. *Clin. Pharmacol. Ther.* 30:154, 1981.

68. Cote, P., Harrison, D. C., Basile, J., and Schroeder, J. S. Hemodynamic interaction of procainamide and lidocaine after experimental myocardial infarction. *Am. J. Cardiol.* 32:937, 1973.

69. Branch, R. A., Shand, D. G., Wilkinson, G. R., and Nies, A. S. The reduction of lidocaine clearance by dl-propranolol: An example of hemodynamic drug interaction. *J. Pharmacol. Exp. Ther.* 184:515, 1973.

70. Ochs, H. R., Carstens, G., and Greenblatt, D. J. Reduction in lidocaine clearance during continuous infusion and by coadministration of propranolol. *N. Engl. J. Med.* 303:373, 1980.

71. Feeley, J., Wilkinson, G. R., McAllister, C. B., and Wood, A. J. J. Increased toxicity and reduced clearance of lidocaine by cimetidine. *Ann. Intern. Med.* 96:592, 1982.

72. Bennett, P. B., Woosley, R. L., and Hondeghem, L. M. Competition between lidocaine and one of its metabolites, glycylxylidide, for cardiac sodium channels. *Circulation,* 78:692, 1988.

73. Hoffman, B. F., Rosen, M. R., and Wit, A. L. Electrophysiology and pharmacology of cardiac arrhythmias. VII. Cardiac effects of quinidine and procaine amide. B. *Am. Heart J.* 90:117, 1975.

74. Kastor, J. A., Josephson, M. E., Guss, S. B., and Horowitz, L. N. Human ventricular refractoriness. II. Effects of procainamide. *Circulation* 56:462, 1977.

75. Giardina, E-G. V., and Bigger, Jr., J. T. Procaine amide against re-entrant ventricular arrhythmias. *Circulation* 48:959, 1973.

76. Scheinman, M. M., Weiss, A. N., Shafton, E., et al. Electrophysiological effects of procaine amide in patients with intraventricular conduction delay. *Circulation* 49:522, 1974.

77. Koch-Weser, J., and Klein, S. W. Procainamide dosage schedules, plasma concentrations, and clinical effects. *J.A.M.A.* 215:1454, 1971.

78. Galeazzi, R. L., Benet, L. Z., and Scheiner, L. B. Relationship between the pharmacokinetics and pharmacodynamics of procainamide. *Clin. Pharmacol. Ther.* 20:278, 1976.

79. Reidenberg, M. M., Drayer, D. E., Levy, M., and Warner, H. Polymorphic acetylation of procainamide in man. *Clin. Pharmacol. Ther.* 17:722, 1975.

80. Roden, D. M., Reele, S. B., Higgins, S. B., et al. Antiarrhythmic efficacy, pharmacokinetics and safety of N-acetylprocainamide in human subjects: Comparison with procainamide. *Am. J. Cardiol.* 46:463, 1980.

81. Woosley, R. L., Drayer, D. E., Reidenberg, M. M., et al. Effect of acetylator phenotype on the rate at which procainamide induces antinuclear antibodies and the lupus syndrome. *N. Engl. J. Med.* 298:1157, 1978.

82. Freeman, R. W., Woosley, R. L., Oates, J. A., and Harbison, R. D. Evidence for the biotransformation of procainamide to a reactive metabolite. *Toxicol. Appl. Pharmacol.* 50:9, 1979.

83. Ellrodt, A. G., Murata, G. H., Riedinger, M. S., et al. Severe neutropenia associated with sustained-release procainamide. *Ann. Intern. Med.* 100:197, 1984.

84. Lalka, D., Wyman, M. G., Goldreyer, B. N., et al. Procainamide accumulation kinetics in the immediate postmyocardial infarction period. *J. Clin. Pharmacol.* 18:397, 1978.

85. Koch-Weser, J. Drug therapy: Bretylium. *N. Engl. J. Med.* 300:473, 1979.

86. Dhurandhar, R. W., Teasdale, S. J., and Mahon, W. A. Bretylium tosylate in the management of refractory ventricular fibrillation. *Can. Med. Assoc. J.* 105:161, 1971.

87. Terry, G., Vellani, C. W., Higgins, M. R., and Doig, A. Bretylium tosylate in treatment of refractory ventricular arrhythmias complicating myocardial infarction. *Br. Heart J.* 32:21, 1970.

88. Holder, D. A., Sniderman, A. D., Frazer, G., and Fallen, E. L. Experience with bretylium tosylate by a hospital cardiac arrest team. *Circulation* 55:541, 1977.

89. Sanna, G., and Arcidiacono, R. Chemical ventricular defibrillation of the human heart with bretylium tosylate. *Am. J. Cardiol.* 32:982, 1973.

90. Cardinale, R., and Sasyniuk, B. I. Electrophysiological effects of bretylium tosylate on subendocardial Purkinje fibers from infarcted canine hearts. *J. Pharmacol. Exp. Ther.* 204:159, 1978.

91. Wit, A. L., Steiner, C., and Damato, A. N. Electrophysiologic actions of bretylium tosylate on single fibers of the canine specialized conducting system and ventricle. *J. Pharmacol. Exp. Ther.* 173:344, 1970.

92. Woosley, R. L., Reele, S. B., Roden, D. M., et al. Pharmacologic reversal of hypotensive

effect complicating antiarrhythmic therapy with bretylium. *Clin. Pharmacol. Ther.* 32:313, 1982.

93. Anderson, J. L., Patterson, E., Wagner, J. G., et al. Oral and intravenous bretylium disposition. *Clin. Pharmacol. Ther.* 28:468, 1980.

94. Anderson, J. L., Patterson, E., Conlon, M., et al. Kinetics of antifibrillatory effects of bretylium: Correlation with myocardial drug concentrations. *Am. J. Cardiol.* 46:583, 1980.

95. Chatterjee, K., Mandel, W. J., Vyden, J. K., et al. Cardiovascular effects of bretylium tosylate in acute myocardial infarction. *J.A.M.A.* 223:757, 1973.

96. Cotev, S., Merin, G., Stern, S., et al. Effect of bretylium on the pulmonary and systemic circulation in patients with mitral valve disease after cardiopulmonary bypass. *J. Clin. Pharmacol.* 11:409, 1971.

97. Adir, J., Narang, P. K., Josselson, J., and Sadler, J. H. Pharmacokinetics of bretylium in renal insufficiency (Letter). *N. Engl. J. Med.* 300:1390, 1979.

98. Hjalmarson, A. Early intervention with a beta-blocking drug after acute myocardial infarction. *Am. J. Cardiol.* 54(Suppl):11E, 1984.

99. Abraham, A. S., Rosenmann, D., Kramer, M., and Balkin, J. Magnesium in the prevention of lethal arrhythmias in acute myocardial infarction. *Arch. Intern. Med.* 147:753, 1987.

100. Rehnqvist, N., Erhardt, L., Ericsson, C-G., et al. Comparative study of tocainide and lidocaine in patients admitted for suspected acute myocardial infarction. *Acta Med. Scand.* 214:21, 1983.

101. Campbell, R. W. F., Hutton, I., Elton, R. A., et al. Prophylaxis of primary ventricular fibrillation with tocainide in acute myocardial infarction. *Br. Heart J.* 49:557, 1983.

102. Ronnevik, P. K., Gundersen, T., and Abrahamsen, A. M. Tolerability and antiarrhythmic efficacy of disopyramide compared to lignocaine in selected patients with suspected acute myocardial infarction. *Eur. Heart. J.* 8:19, 1987.

103. Podrid, P. J., Schoenberger, A., and Lown, B. Congestive heart failure caused by oral disopyramide. *N. Engl. J. Med.* 302:614, 1980.

104. Silke, B., Frais, M. A., Verma, S. P., et al. Comparative hemodynamic effects of intravenous lignocaine, disopyramide, and flecainide in uncomplicated acute myocardial infarction. *Br. J. Clin. Pharmacol.* 22:707, 1986.

105. Wilson, J. R. Use of antiarrhythmic drugs in patients with heart failure: Clinical efficacy, hemodynamic results, and relation to survival. *Circulation* 75(Suppl. IV):IV-64, 1987.

106. Kotler, V., Lindererer, T., and Schroder, R. Effects of disopyramide on systemic and coronary hemodynamics and myocardial metabolism in patients with coronary artery disease: Comparison with lidocaine. *Am. Heart J.* 46:469, 1980.

107. Elliott, H. L., Thomson, A. H., and Bryson, S. M. Disopyramide in acute myocardial infarction: Problems with changing pharmacokinetics. *Eur. J. Clin. Pharmacol.* 30:345, 1986.

108. Rehnqvist, N., Ericsson, C-G., Eriksson, S., et al. Comparative investigation of the antiarrhythmic effect of propafenone (Rytmonorm) and lidocaine in patients with ventricular arrhythmias during acute myocardial infarction. *Acta Med. Scand.* 216:525, 1984.

109. Moss, A. J. Current status of calcium channel blocking drugs after myocardial infarction. *Eur. Heart J.* 7(Suppl. A):31, 1986.

110. Multicenter Postinfarction Research Group. Risk stratification and survival after myocardial infarction. *N. Engl. J. Med.* 309:331, 1983.

111. Singh, B. N., and Nademanee, K. Sotalol: A beta-blocker with unique antiarrhythmic properties. *Am. Heart J.* 114:121, 1987.

112. Wagner, W. L., Manz, M., and Luderitz, B. Combination of sotalol with the class I B substances mexiletine or tocainide in complex ventricular extrasystole. *Z. Kardiol.* 76:296, 1987.

113. Morganroth, J., and Horowitz, L. N. Flecainide: Its proarrhythmic effect and expected changes on the surface electrocardiogram. *Am. J. Cardiol.* 53(Suppl):89B, 1984.

114. Cardiac Arrhythmia Pilot Study (CAPS) Investigators. The effect of encainide, flecainide, imipramine, and moricizine on ventricular arrhythmias occurring during the year after myocardial infarction: The CAPS. *Am. J. Cardiol.* 61:501, 1988.

12
Treatment of Supraventricular Arrhythmias in Acute Myocardial Infarction

Borys Surawicz and Simon Lee

In order to clarify the management of supraventricular arrhythmias associated with myocardial infarction, we must first recognize the general characteristics of these arrhythmias. Therefore this topic is covered first, followed by a discussion of the mechanisms of the interventions that have been found useful for treating patients with these supraventricular arrhythmias. General guidelines for such treatment are then outlined, and finally specific first-line approaches to the management of the supraventricular arrhythmias in myocardial infarction patients are proposed.

Characteristics of Supraventricular Arrhythmias in Patients with Acute Myocardial Infarction

Sinus Tachycardia

Sinus tachycardia occurs in about one-third of patients [1] and is attributed to sympathetic overactivity, particularly when associated with hypertension [2]. Persistence of sinus tachycardia for more than several days usually signifies ventricular failure and is an unfavorable prognostic sign [1]. Also, sinus tachycardia may be a precursor of primary ventricular fibrillation in the coronary care unit (CCU).

Bradycardia

Bradycardias that are secondary to atrioventricular (AV) conduction disturbances are discussed elsewhere in this book. The prevailing cause of bradyarrhythmias and accompanying hypotension in patients with myocardial infarction is vagal hyperactivity [3]. In one study, bradycardia was present in 55 percent of patients seen within 30 minutes of onset of acute myocardial infarction [2]. In several series of patients admitted to CCUs the incidence of sinus bradycardia ranged from 10 to 41 percent [1, 3].

Another cause of bradycardia is acute ischemia of the sinoatrial node, which may follow occlusion of the right coronary or left circumflex artery proximal to the takeoff of the sinus node artery [3]. However, the incidence of sinus node dysfunction precipitated by coronary occlusion is low. In one study of 431 patients admitted to the CCU, sinus node dysfunction was present in 4.6 percent [4], mostly seen in the presence of inferior wall myocardial infarction. In about two-thirds of these patients sinus bradycardia subsided following treatment with atropine or temporary pacing [4]. The remaining patients had a less benign syndrome of tachycardia-bradycardia, frequently requiring continuing treatment with antiarrhythmic drugs, pacing, or both. The most common mechanism of tachycardia-bradycardia syndrome in these patients is a combination of a slow AV junctional escape rhythm with bouts of AV nodal reentrant tachycardia, atrial flutter, or atrial fibrillation. Unlike AV block, sinus bradycardia does not appear to predispose to ventricular fibrillation [5].

ATRIAL PREMATURE COMPLEXES AND MULTIFORM ATRIAL TACHYCARDIA

Isolated atrial premature complexes occur commonly in patients with acute myocardial infarction. However, because of the high prevalence of this arrhythmia in the general population, the role of myocardial infarction in their pathogenesis is not always obvious.

Multiform atrial tachycardia, i.e., a supraventricular tachycardia with P waves of variable morphology, may be due to a multifocal ectopic activity or to unifocal impulses with variable intra-atrial conduction. This arrhythmia occurs frequently in elderly patients with chronic lung disease. In most patients with acute myocardial infarction, this arrhythmia lasts less than a few days but may be recurrent or chronic. Sometimes multiform atrial tachycardia evolves into atrial flutter or atrial fibrillation.

MONOMORPHIC ATRIAL TACHYCARDIA

Atrial tachycardia may be due to reentry, but this mechanism is rare. A more commonly postulated mechanism of this arrhythmia is nontriggered or triggered automaticity. In patients with automatic ectopic atrial tachycardia, the onset is usually precipitated by a late atrial premature complex; the P wave configuration of a tachycardia-initiating complex is identical to the P wave of succeeding complexes, and the P–R interval is not prolonged. Afterward the cycle first shortens progressively (warm-up phenomenon), but once tachycardia becomes established the P–P intervals do not vary by more than 50 msec, unless an exit block is present. However, the rate of tachycardia tends to vary appreciably from day to day, being influenced by such factors as posture and exercise.

In two studies, the reported incidence of atrial tachycardia in patients with myocardial infarction ranged from none of 400 [6] to 32 of 119 (27 percent) [7]. In three other studies the incidence of transient atrial tachycardia was 4 to 8 percent [8], 3.8 percent [9], and 2 percent [10]. The variability of these values may be due to the differences in methodology of monitoring because brief and infrequent episodes can be readily missed. Another variable is the number of patients treated with digitalis, which is the most common factor precipitating this arrhythmia. The arrhythmia is usually benign and is not associated with an increased incidence of congestive heart failure, pericarditis, or atrial infarction [7]. In one study [7] arrhythmia lasted longer than 5 minutes in only 3 of 32 patients. Because of the transient nature and short duration of this arrhythmia treatment is seldom required.

REENTRANT AV NODAL TACHYCARDIA

Tachycardias dependent on dual AV nodal conduction or a concealed AV bypass are uncommon in patients with acute myocardial infarction [3]. When present, the arrhythmias may contribute to hypotension and low cardiac output.

NONPAROXYSMAL AV JUNCTIONAL TACHYCARDIA

Nonparoxysmal AV junctional tachycardia is attributed to an abnormal automaticity or to triggered activity associated with delayed after-depolarizations, i.e., a mechanism similar to AV junctional tachycardia associated with digitalis toxicity [11]. During routine monitoring, nonparoxysmal AV junctional tachycardia was found in 3 to 16 percent of patients [12–14]. However, continuous tape-recording of patients in the CCU revealed this arrhythmia in 12 of 30 (40 percent) patients during the first 24 hours [12]. Subsequently, the incidence decreased to 13 percent at 48 hours and to 3 percent at 72 hours [12]. In this study, nonparoxysmal AV junctional tachycardia was associated with sinus arrhythmia. Although

AV junctional tachycardia rarely produces changes in the clinical status [13], the arrhythmia appears to be an independent prognostic marker for cardiogenic shock [15]. The overall mortality of patients with nonparoxysmal junctional tachycardia is higher than in the remaining patients [12, 13]. The rate of tachycardia is more rapid and mortality is higher in patients with anterior infarction than in those with inferior infarction [12, 13].

ATRIAL FLUTTER

Atrial flutter occurs as the first arrhythmia in 1 to 3 percent of patients with acute myocardial infarction [7, 9, 10]. Because of the clinical deterioration associated with the persistence of this arrhythmia, intravenous drug administration or cardioversion is frequently indicated [9] (Fig. 12-1). When diagnosis is uncertain, a right atrial electrogram may be helpful (Figs. 12-2 and 12-3).

ATRIAL FIBRILLATION

Atrial fibrillation is the most common new supraventricular arrhythmia in patients with acute myocardial infarction. The reported incidence in various studies ranged from 5 to 18 percent [10, 16–21]. The higher figures usually included individuals with preexisting atrial fibrillation. The incidence of new atrial fibrillation is closer to about 5 percent [10, 16]. Atrial fibrillation usually appears during the first 48 to 72 hours [19, 20] and in 90 percent of cases within the first 4 days [9], but it is believed to be rare during the earliest stage of infarction. In the study of Hod and coworkers [22], atrial fibrillation was present in 7 of 214 (3 percent) patients admitted within 3 hours of the onset of pain. These patients had inferior myocardial infarction, and in each case the circumflex coronary artery was occluded proximal to the left atrial circumflex branch. In five of these patients, myocardial infarction was caused by occlusion of the circumflex artery and in the

Fig. 12-1
Electrocardiogram of a 65-year-old woman with acute anteroseptal wall myocardial infarction and atrial flutter with 2:1 AV block. Intravenous verapamil (10 mg) administration failed to convert atrial flutter to sinus rhythm. DC cardioversion with 30 joules established sinus rhythm.

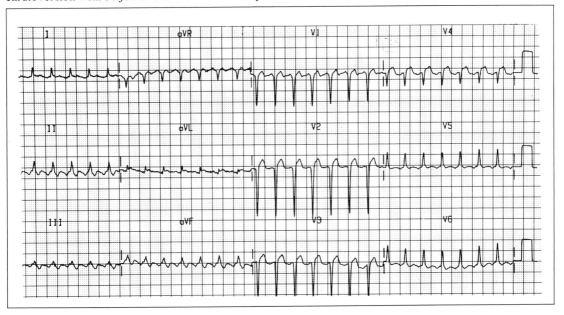

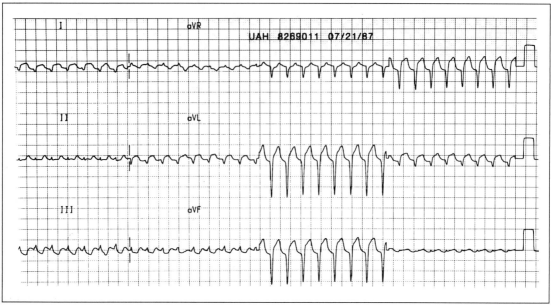

Fig. 12-2
Electrocardiogram of a 59-year-old man with acute anterolateral wall myocardial
infarction and atrial flutter with 2:1 AV block. Atrial flutter was terminated twice
by DC cardioversion but returned within a few minutes on both occasions.
Therefore pacing wire was inserted into the right atrium for rapid atrial pacing.

Fig. 12-3
Intracardiac electrogram recorded from the right
atrium in the same patient as in Figure 12-2
reveals typical flutter waves at a rate of 300/
minute. Rapid atrial pacings (400–600/min)
induced brief episodes of atrial fibrillation but
failed to establish sinus rhythm in this patient.
Sinus rhythm was established after intravenous
administration of digoxin (Lanoxin, 1 mg) and
procainamide (1 gm).

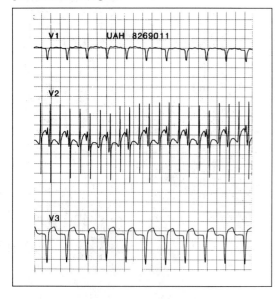

remaining two by occlusion of the right coronary artery, which supplied collaterals to the
previously occluded left circumflex artery. In
each of these seven patients, the right coronary artery was also occluded proximal to the
origin of the AV nodal artery. Thus the appearance of atrial fibrillation during the earliest stage of infarction required the combination of an occluded proximal circumflex artery
and impaired perfusion of the AV node. When
the reperfusion was successful, atrial fibrillation subsided rapidly; but in a patient in whom
reperfusion was not achieved, atrial fibrillation persisted for 16 hours [22].

In about one-half of patients with atrial fibrillation, the onset can be traced to an atrial
premature complex [10, 23] and in the other
one-half to atrial flutter [20]. Factors believed
to contribute to the appearance of atrial fibrillation in the setting of acute myocardial infarction included atrial infarction, release of catecholamines, acute pericarditis, preexisting
atrial muscle disease, chronic lung disease,
acute hypoxia, drugs, and hypokalemia [24].

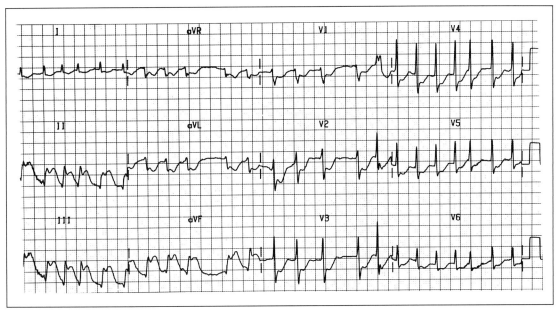

Fig. 12-4
Electrocardiogram of a 73-year-old man at the onset of acute inferior wall
myocardial infarction and atrial fibrillation with a ventricular rate of 150 per
minute. Within 30 minutes of hospital admission, sinus rhythm was established
spontaneously before infusion of tissue plasminogen activator.

In about one-half of all patients, the episodes of atrial fibrillation are single and in the other one-half multiple [17, 18]. In 50 percent of patients with single episodes, the ventricular rate was higher than 120 per minute. Multiple episodes of atrial fibrillation tend to be of shorter duration [17]. Atrial fibrillation lasted less than 2 hours in about 50 percent [17, 18], less than 4 hours in 74 percent, and less than 24 hours in 90 percent of patients [20]. An example of atrial fibrillation of brief duration is shown in Figures 12-4 and 12-5. When studied within 3 months after hospital discharge, only 6 of 77 patients still had atrial fibrillation, and in three of those patients chronic atrial fibrillation had been present before the onset of myocardial infarction [23]. The reported persistence of atrial fibrillation in as many as 33 percent of patients at the time of hospital discharge [16] may reflect the inclusion of patients with chronic atrial fibrillation predating the infarction.

In a large number of studies atrial fibrillation was associated with advanced age [10, 16–18, 21, 25], congestive heart failure, poor left ventricular function [10, 16, 21, 25–27], and extensive myocardial infarction [17, 18]. Other associated conditions included mitral regurgitation [16], pericarditis [9, 25, 26], increased incidence of ventricular tachycardia, ventricular fibrillation, right bundle branch block [17], and left bundle branch block [26]. The presence of atrial fibrillation was not related to the site of myocardial infarction [9, 16, 17] and was not linked causally to atrial infarction [17]. Transient atrial fibrillation did not contribute to an increased incidence of emboli unless the arrhythmia persisted.

Atrial fibrillation is a marker of poor prognosis. The arrhythmia is associated with an increased in-hospital [15, 17–20] and posthospital [17, 27] mortality. This increase in mortality is not attributed to the atrial fibrillation per se [9] but to a greater extent of myocardial infarction, the presence of congestive heart failure [20], more advanced age, and other complicating factors [21]. However, in patients with mild congestive heart failure,

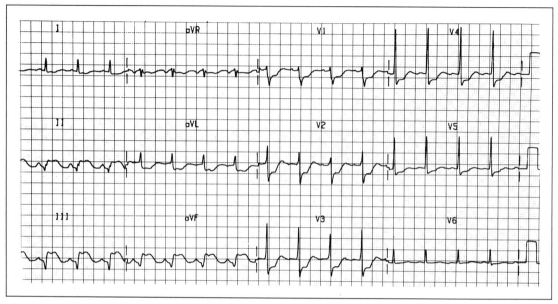

Fig. 12-5
Electrocardiogram of the same patient as in Figure 12-4 after the establishment of
sinus rhythm.

the presence of atrial fibrillation appears to worsen the prognosis [28].

PREEXCITATION

Myocardial infarction may unmask the presence of a previously nonfunctioning AV bypass tract. In one report of such an event in three patients [29], one had Wolff-Parkinson-White (WPW) pattern and two had a short P–R interval associated with supraventricular tachycardia. In the patient with the WPW pattern, autopsy revealed a bypass tract; and in one of the two patients with a short P–R interval, the interval became normal during convalescence. The authors postulated that infarction activates latent accessory pathways, possibly owing to increased sympathetic stimulation. The same mechanism was proposed in two other patients [30] in whom WPW pattern and supraventricular tachycardia appeared during the acute stage of infarction and disappeared after recovery.

Drugs and Therapeutic Procedures

DIGITALIS

In the United States digoxin is by far the most commonly used digitalis preparation, though in some regions digitoxin is the favorite drug. Digitalis may cause slowing of the ventricular rate by several mechanisms. The vagal and antiadrenergic effects of digitalis cause slowing of the ventricular rate during atrial fibrillation or flutter by blocking the conduction in the AV node. The same action may terminate AV nodal reentrant tachycardia. Administration to patients with congestive heart failure may decrease the sinus rate indirectly, owing to a decreased sympathetic tone as a result of improved ventricular function.

After oral administration of digoxin, approximately 70 to 85 percent of the drug is absorbed from the gastrointestinal tract. The half-life of digoxin is about 36 hours in the presence of normal renal function. Most laboratories have established therapeutic levels at between 0.5 to 2.2 ng/ml. In patients not treated with digitalis in the recent past, these levels can be achieved within 6 to 8 days using digoxin 0.25 mg daily by mouth. When rapid digitalization is required, the drug is given intravenously, beginning with a dose of 0.75 mg followed by 0.25 mg every 2 to 4 hours until the desired effect or the maximum dose (1.5 mg) has been reached.

It is commonly believed that patients with acute myocardial infarction exhibit increased sensitivity to digitalis, i.e., that the margin between the therapeutic and the toxic dose in these patients is reduced. This reduction may be due to an increased myocardial oxygen demand caused by the positive inotropic effect of the drug or to a loss of intracellular potassium from ischemic myocardium. Also the presence of high sympathetic tone may inhibit the vagal effects of digitalis on the AV node [31]. For these reasons many clinicians no longer consider digitalis the drug of choice for treatment of supraventricular tachyarrhythmias in patients with acute myocardial infarction.

Treatment with digitalis requires careful attention to potassium replacement. Excessive doses must be avoided if cardioversion is contemplated. Accumulation of digitalis can be prevented by using short-acting preparations, e.g., intermittent administration of ouabain intravenously [32], but this method is seldom applied in current practice.

Although administration of 1.5 mg digoxin intravenously reverses atrial fibrillation of short duration to sinus rhythm in most patients [33], this occurrence may be fortuitous because in most patients the attacks of atrial fibrillation subside spontaneously and because conversion to sinus rhythm that follows digoxin administration is seldom preceded by an appreciable slowing of ventricular rate [33].

Numerous studies have suggested that digitalis may have an adverse effect on survival during follow-up after myocardial infarction [34]. However, it has been shown that after adjusting for atrial fibrillation, left ventricular failure, and several other independent variables, the higher mortality of patients treated with digitalis was not related to digitalis per se

but to the condition of the patients treated with digitalis [34, 35].

ATROPINE

Atropine is a muscarinic receptor blocking agent that inhibits the action of endogenous acetylcholine. Atropine (0.6–2.0 mg IV) is useful for treating sinus bradycardia, especially when complicated by hypotension during the early phase of acute myocardial infarction. Administration of small doses (<0.3 mg atropine sulfate intravenously) may cause a paradoxical slowing of heart rate attributed to a stimulating effect on the central nervous system. Atropine may cause urinary retention, especially in patients with an enlarged prostate, and is contraindicated in patients with closed-angle glaucoma.

BETA-ADRENERGIC BLOCKING AGENTS

By competitive inhibition of adrenergic stimulation, beta blockers depress automaticity (phase 4 diastolic depolarization) of the sinoatrial node, AV junction, and His-Purkinje fibers [36]. Beta blockers also increase the A–H interval and prolong the effective and functional refractory periods of the AV node [37]. At concentrations 50 to 100 times higher than the therapeutic levels, certain beta blockers, e.g., propranolol, also produce sodium channel blocking effects, but they are of questionable clinical significance.

The first commercially available beta-adrenergic blocker, propranolol, is well absorbed from the gastrointestinal tract, but its systemic availability is less than 30 percent due to the first-pass effect [36]. Peak levels are reached within 1 to 2 hours after oral administration. The half-life is 2 to 4 hours but increases to 4 to 6 hours during chronic oral administration. Therapeutic blood levels range from 40 to 100 ng/ml, but several-fold differences in plasma levels may be present in patients treated with the same dose of propanolol [38].

Oral administration of propanolol (40–360 mg/day) or other beta-adrenergic blockers in

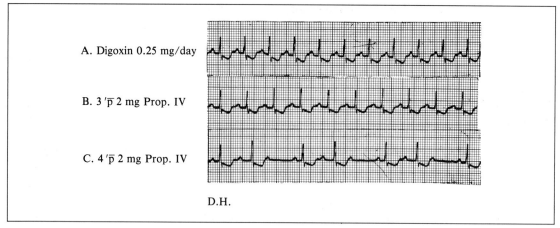

A. Digoxin 0.25 mg/day

B. 3 $'\overline{p}$ 2 mg Prop. IV

C. 4 $'\overline{p}$ 2 mg Prop. IV

D.H.

Fig. 12-6
Synergistic effect of digitalis and propranolol on AV conduction. *A.* Sinus rhythm
while receiving digoxin 0.25 mg PO daily. *B.* At 3 minutes after intravenous
propranolol (2 mg). Note the slower rate and longer P–R interval. *C.* One minute
later: Mobitz type 1 AV block.

equivalent doses helps control the ventricular
rate in patients with chronic atrial fibrillation,
especially in combination with digitalis. Side
effects include aggravation of congestive heart
failure, excessive bradycardia, fatigue, bron-
chospasm, sleep disturbance, and hypoglyce-
mia in diabetics.

Some of the newer beta-adrenergic blockers
include the nonselective beta blocker timolol
(with a half-life of 5.5 hours) and the cardioselective beta blockers metoprolol and atenolol.
The long-acting beta blockers include nadolol,
atenolol, and sustained-release preparations
of propanolol and metoprolol. Some beta-
adrenergic blockers (e.g., pindolol) possess
the properties of a partial beta agonist. The ultra-short-acting beta blockers esmolol and
flestolol with a half-life of less than 15 minutes, if used with caution, may prove to be
particularly useful in the treatment of supraventricular arrhythmias [39, 40].

The treatment of acute arrhythmias with the
beta-adrenergic blockers in patients with myocardial infarction is based on the assumption
that their negative inotropic effect is outweighed by the benefit of slowing the ventricular rate. In most cases this assumption is
valid.

The synergistic effect of beta blockers and
digitalis on the impulse transmission through

the AV node may be either advantageous or
deleterious, depending on the doses and other
circumstances (Fig. 12-6). Bradycardia that
occurs during treatment with a beta-adrenergic blocker alone or in combination with digitalis may be reversed by prompt intravenous
administration of atropine sulfate (1.0–1.5 mg)
or isoproterenol solution (0.2 mg in 250 ml of
5 percent dextrose in water) at a rate of 1 to 5
ml/min.

To slow the ventricular rate during supraventricular tachyarrhythmia, small doses
(e.g., 0.5 mg) of propanolol may be administered intravenously every 2 minutes up to an
average dose of 4.5 mg [41]. Not infrequently,
such treatment results in conversion to sinus
rhythm. Other beta-adrenergic blockers may
be administered in patients with atrial fibrillation or supraventricular tachycardia as follows.

Atenolol: 1.0 mg IV every 5 minutes up to a
    total of 5 to 15 mg [42, 43] followed by an
    oral dose of 50 to 100 mg twice daily
Metoprolol: 75 mg bolus IV followed by 4
    mg/min during the first 3 hours, subse-
    quently reduced to 2 to 3 mg/min. [44]
Alprenolol: 0.1 percent solution adminis-
    tered at a rate of 1 mg/min up to a total of
    20 mg [45]

Esmolol, an ultra-short-acting beta-adrenergic blocker with an elimination half-life of about 9 minutes, is of potential advantage because of its ultra-short action [46], but experience with the use of this drug in patients with acute myocardial infarction is still limited [40]. The drug is being titrated in doses of 50 to 300 μg/kg/min for 5 to 15 minutes and infused for up to 7 hours [40]. In several patients the infusion was terminated because of hypotension [40]. Esmolol, because of its short half-life, is rapidly gaining acceptance as the beta blocker of choice for supraventricular arrhythmias in patients with acute myocardial infarction.

CALCIUM CHANNEL BLOCKERS

Verapamil and diltiazem are the two commonly used calcium channel blockers for treatment of supraventricular arrhythmias. Both drugs depress automaticity of the sinoatrial node, slow conduction through the AV node, and terminate AV nodal reentry in a high proportion of cases. These drugs also depress slow channel-dependent depolarizations in other tissues but have little effect on the normal His-Purkinje fibers and myocardium [47]. However, they may be effective in terminating arrhythmias caused by triggered automatic activity in the atria or the AV junction. Verapamil is largely metabolized in the liver; the bioavailability is only 35 percent owing to first-pass elimination [48]. The mean half-life of verapamil after a single oral dose is 6 hours, but it increases to 12 hours during chronic therapy [49].

Verapamil consistently slows the ventricular rate in atrial fibrillation and flutter but reestablishes sinus rhythm in only about 10 percent of cases. Verapamil can precipitate ventricular tachycardia or ventricular fibrillation in patients with WPW syndrome and atrial fibrillation when the impulses are conducted anterogradely through the bypass [50].

The usual dose of verapamil is 10 mg (0.145 mg/kg body weight) administered intravenously within 1 to 2 minutes; this dose can be repeated after 30 minutes. Caution should be exercised when using a combination of verapamil and beta blockers because such combination entails the risk of AV block or significant left ventricular dysfunction [51].

Verapamil is a very useful drug for terminating paroxysmal supraventricular tachycardia [52, 53]. However, it should not be used if there is a wide QRS tachycardia. When administered at a rate of 1 mg/min up to a total dose of about 20 mg, the success rate is 80 to 90 percent. However, in about one-half of cases a dose of less than 5 mg is sufficient [54]. Verapamil also frequently converts atrial flutter to sinus rhythm but seldom restores sinus rhythm in patients with atrial fibrillation. In this condition the usual goal of therapy with verapamil is slowing the ventricular rate. The effectiveness of verapamil in slowing the ventricular rate lessens when the sympathetic tone is increased as a result of congestive heart failure, infection, or fever [31] (Fig. 12-7).

Other calcium channel blocking drugs used intravenously to terminate the supraventricular tachycardia or to slow the ventricular rate in patients with atrial fibrillation or flutter are diltiazem 0.25 mg/kg over 2 minutes [55] and tiapamil 1 mg/kg [56].

Calcium channel blocking drugs appear to be well tolerated in most patients with acute myocardial infarction, but their administration should not be continued in the presence of hypotension or increased pulmonary capillary wedge pressure [57]. Abrupt withdrawal of verapamil causes no manifestations of "withdrawal syndrome" and does not exacerbate angina pectoris [58]. Combining verapamil with digitalis to slow the ventricular rate requires caution because verapamil may increase the concentration of blood digoxin concentration [59].

In patients with adequate ventricular function, a combination of calcium channel blockers and beta blockers may be more effective than either drug alone [60]. Using a single oral dose of diltiazem (120 mg) and propranolol (160 mg), Yeh and colleagues [61] converted supraventricular tachycardia to sinus rhythm in the majority of patients within an average period of 39 ± 49 minutes. For the prevention

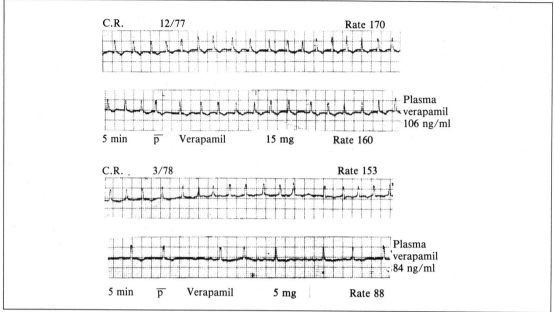

Fig. 12-7
Effectiveness of verapamil in slowing the ventricular rate depends on the patient's
sympathetic tone. Strips of electrocardiogram (lead II) before and after verapamil
in the same patient in the presence (12/77) and absence (3/78) of congestive heart
failure and fever. Note the differences in dose, plasma concentration of
verapamil, and response of ventricular rate in the presence of atrial fibrillation.
(From J. Dominic et al. Verapamil plasma levels and ventricular rate response in
patients with atrial fibrillation and flutter. *Clin. Pharmacol. Ther.* 26:710, 1979.
With permission.)

of paroxysmal supraventricular tachycardia,
the usual oral maintenance dose of verapamil
is about 120 mg, and that of diltiazem about 90
mg, administered every 8 hours [62].

In patients with ventricular preexcitation,
verapamil may increase the number of complexes conducted through the AV bypass tract
by shortening the refractory period of the bypass tract presumably as a result of reflex-
evoked hypotension [63].

Class I (Sodium Channel Blocking) Antiarrhythmic Drugs

On the basis of their effect on the electrocardiogram, sodium channel blocking drugs can
be grouped conveniently into three classes.
Class IA drugs prolong both the QRS complex

and the QT-QRS intervals. They include
quinidine, procainamide, and disopyramide.
Amiodarone, though seldom listed as a member of this class of drugs, has the same properties. Class IB drugs have no discernible effect on the duration of either the QRS or the
QT-QRS interval. The representatives of this
group are lidocaine, tocainide, mexiletine, and
phenytoin. Class IC drugs include encainide,
flecainide, and lorcainide. They prolong the
QRS duration but not the QT-QRS interval.

QUINIDINE

The three commonly used quinidine preparations are quinidine sulfate, quinidine gluconate, and quinidine polygalacturonate. Of
these agents, quinidine sulfate is most rapidly

absorbed, reaching a peak plasma level within 1 to 2 hours with a bioavailability of 60 to 100 percent. Quinidine gluconate is absorbed more slowly, reaching a peak plasma level within about 4 hours; it has a bioavailability of 40 to 90 percent [64]. Quinidine polygalacturonate is absorbed most slowly and has the lowest bioavailability. The content of quinidine base in these three preparations is 83 percent in the sulfate, 62 percent in the gluconate, and 60 percent in the polygalacturonate preparation [65]. Quinidine is used principally for the purpose of maintaining sinus rhythm after conversion to atrial fibrillation. In one study of patients treated with a long-acting quinidine sulfate preparation (0.6 gm twice daily in patients weighing less than 80 kg and 0.8 gm twice daily in patients weighing more than 80 kg), sinus rhythm was maintained in 51 percent of patients versus 28 percent in those not receiving quinidine [66]. In another study [67], 1 year after cardioversion, sinus rhythm was maintained in 50 percent of patients treated with quinidine, 30 percent of those treated with digoxin, and 23 percent of untreated patients.

The most dreaded complication of quinidine therapy is the development of polymorphic or monomorphic ventricular tachycardia. Because these arrhythmias usually occur at the beginning of therapy, monitoring the treatment during the first 5 days in the hospital is advisable. Also, a test 0.2-gm dose is usually given before the onset of therapy to detect a possible idiosyncrasy. The most common reason for discontinuing quinidine is diarrhea that can be ameliorated with aluminum-containing antacids (e.g., Amphojel).

Because of its anticholinergic action quinidine may cause acceleration of the ventricular rate during atrial flutter or atrial fibrillation. To prevent this complication, the drug is frequently administered concomitantly with digitalis or a beta-adrenergic blocker. In patients receiving digitalis, quinidine increases the plasma digoxin concentration and enhances the probability of digitalis toxicity. The reduction of digoxin dose by 30 to 40 percent has been recommended when the two drugs are administered together [68].

PROCAINAMIDE

Procainamide may be effective in the conversion of atrial fibrillation to sinus rhythm when administered intravenously at a rate of 15 to 20 mg/min up to 1000 mg. The most important determinant of the successful cardioversion is the short duration of the arrhythmia [69].

Orally administered procainamide for maintenance therapy is rapidly absorbed. Peak concentrations are reached usually within 1.0 to 1.5 hours after administration, and bioavailability is in excess of 80 percent. The half-life of procainamide is only about 3 hours, but the use of sustained-release preparations (e.g., Procan SR) enables administration of the drug every 6 to 8 hours. Procainamide is partly metabolized in the liver to N-acetyl procainamide, which has an antiarrhythmic property and is almost exclusively eliminated by the kidneys.

DISOPYRAMIDE

Disopyramide probably suppresses supraventricular arrhythmias as effectively as procainamide, but the strong anticholinergic and negative inotropic effects diminish the usefulness of disopyramide in patients with myocardial infarction.

OTHER DRUGS USED FOR TERMINATION OF SUPRAVENTRICULAR TACHYCARDIAS

Most of the information available about the drugs discussed here stems from the observations in patients with conditions other than myocardial infarction: Propafenone has been used in doses of 2 mg/kg IV [70]. Flecainide is administered in doses of 0.5 to 2.0 mg/kg IV followed by 200 to 300 mg PO per day, and encainide is given in doses of 0.3 to 2.0 mg/kg IV followed by 100 to 225 mg PO. Both flecainide and encainide depress myocardial function and should be used very cautiously in patients with acute myocardial infarction. Amiodarone can be given intravenously in a dose of 150 mg within 5 minutes, followed by 600 mg/day for 3 to 4 days [71]. Similar effects on supraventricular tachycardia can be achieved using oral amiodarone—either a single dose of 15 mg/kg [72] or 100 to 400 mg/day in divided doses. Similar to flecainide and encainide, amiodarone can depress myocardial function.

MISCELLANEOUS DRUGS

For the treatment of supraventricular tachycardia, verapamil has largely replaced the intravenous administration of two drugs commonly used in the past, i.e., edrophonium, a cholinesterase inhibitor (10 mg), and phenylephrine (1 mg/min up to 10 mg). The effectiveness of these drugs was frequently enhanced by combining the treatment with carotid sinus stimulation.

When the tachycardias are caused by AV nodal conduction or AV reentry, the AV nodal conduction can be transiently interrupted by intravenous administration of adenosine or adenosine triphosphate (ATP). This effect occurs within 15 to 30 seconds after injection. Because the antiarrhythmic effect is exerted during the first passage of the drug across the coronary circulation the bolus should be injected rapidly. The effective dose of adenosine determined by sequential increments until the arrhythmia was terminated averaged 6.6 mg and ranged from 2 to 23 mg [73]. Mild side effects of brief duration included flushing, dyspnea, and chest discomfort. Significant hemodynamic effects after a single dose were not observed, but the drug has been used seldom in patients with acute myocardial infarction.

ELECTRIC CARDIOVERSION

Synchronized direct-current (DC) cardioversion can terminate most of the arrhythmias due to reentry, but the energy required to terminate the tachycardias varies according to the type of arrhythmia. Thirty-fifty joules may be sufficient to terminate paroxysmal tachycardia and atrial flutter. However, higher energy levels (100–400 joules) are usually needed for atrial fibrillation. The delivered energy is inversely related to the square root of the resistance. The latter can be minimized by using electrode gels. The electrode paddle positions are no longer considered important modifiers of resistance, and there is no apparent advantage in using anteroposterior as opposed to anterolateral paddle placement [74].

Cardioversion should be performed after at least 6 hours of fasting. Standby cardiopulmonary resuscitation equipment such as oxygen, ventilation bag, suction tubing, and endotracheal tube should be available. Before the shock is delivered, amnesia is induced by means of intravenously administered diazepam (Valium), midazolam (Versed), or one of the short-acting barbiturates such as sodium thiopental (Pentothal) or sodium methohexital (Brevital). Diazepam is usually given 5 mg IV every minute until the patient becomes unresponsive to verbal command. The total amount of intravenously administered diazepam varies from 15 to 40 mg (0.16–0.32 mg/kg), depending on the age and body weight of the patient. Oxygen by mask is usually administered for a few minutes before and after cardioversion. Because of the drug's long half-life (30 hours), somnolence may persist for a few hours. The water-soluble benzodiazepine midazolam has pharmacologic properties similar to those of diazepam but is a more potent anesthetic with a shorter half-life (1.3–2.2 hours), allowing more rapid recovery of psychomotor functions. Methohexital, an ultrashort-acting barbiturate, is three times more potent than thiopental and has a shorter half-life.

In patients with atrial flutter, slowing the ventricular rate or conversion to sinus rhythm using digoxin or quinidine may be difficult and time-consuming. In contrast, in most cases a low-energy, i.e., 30 to 50 joules, shock can accomplish rapid cardioversion to sinus rhythm. Thus even in patients with acute myocardial infarction the electric shock is an accepted initial treatment for atrial flutter.

In the absence of digitalis toxicity or uncorrected hypokalemia, digitalis need not be discontinued for more than 1 or 2 days before cardioversion. However, DC cardioversion may precipitate ventricular arrhythmias and cause a prolonged period of sinus arrest or marked sinus bradycardia in patients with sick sinus syndrome or digitalis toxicity. In most cases, bradycardia is at least partially reversible after intravenous atropine administration (1.0–2.0 mg).

Although the risk of embolization after cardioversion is only 1 to 3 percent [75], we recommend anticoagulation whenever feasible for a period of 1 week after the procedure. If the procedure is elective, anticoagulants should be given also for 2 weeks before cardioversion.

Prophylactic pacing is recommended in patients with suspected sinus node malfunction. An alternative to cardioversion in patients with atrial flutter is rapid atrial pacing. In one study, this procedure successfully converted atrial flutter to sinus rhythm in 89 percent of trials in 46 consecutive patients [76].

General Guidelines for Treatment

Barring an emergency that may require an immediate action, a number of preliminary steps must be made before initiating antiarrhythmic therapy. We recommend in each case to: (1) establish the mechanism of arrhythmia; (2) determine whether the arrhythmia was precipitated by myocardial infarction or predated the infarction; (3) consider the role of possible precipitating or aggravating factors such as hypoxia, pulmonary insufficiency, poorly controlled diabetes, administration of sympathomimetic agent, diuretic, antiarrhythmic drugs, treatment with digitalis, presence of systemic or pulmonary emboli, anemia, hyperthyroidism, or pericarditis; (4) correct hypokalemia, even though there is no convincing evidence that it constitutes an independent cause of supraventricular arrhythmia (in contrast to well established evidence for aggravating effect on ventricular arrhythmias in patients with myocardial infarction) [77]; (5) establish possible effects of arrhythmias on hemodynamics and myocardial perfusion; (6) estimate the natural course and the expected duration of untreated arrhythmia in question; and (7) define the therapeutic goal, e.g., suppression of arrhythmia, slowing ventricular rate, increase in contribution of atrial contraction.

Specific First-Line Approaches to Management

Although therapeutic decisions should be based on the understanding of the arrhythmia mechanism and the antiarrhythmic drug action discussed above, it may be helpful to list the preferred first-line approaches recommended by the authors.

Sinus bradycardia: Atropine sulfate is given intravenously, occasionally with temporary atrial or ventricular pacing.

Sinus tachycardia: Treat the underlying cause, e.g., anxiety, fear, pain, low cardiac output, hypotension. In rare cases, intermittent intravenous administration of low doses of beta-adrenergic blockers is helpful.

Frequent premature atrial complexes: Treatment is seldom required. Occasionally one of the class I antiarrhythmic drugs (e.g., procainamide or quinidine) may be used.

Reentrant AV nodal or AV tachycardia: Interruption by verapamil or diltiazem given intravenously is accomplished. If these measures are contraindicated or ineffective, beta-adrenergic blockers are given intravenously. Beta-adrenergic blockers should not be used before the calcium channel blockers are eliminated from the body. If the arrhythmia remains refractory, amiodarone is given intravenously; and if the condition is hemodynamically unstable, electric cardioversion may be necessary.

Atrial and AV junctional tachycardia: Rule out digitalis toxicity. The general approach is the same as for AV nodal reentrant tachycardia.

Atrial flutter: If hemodynamically stable, beta-adrenergic blockers or calcium channel blockers are given intravenously. If hemodynamically unstable, electric cardioversion or rapid atrial pacing is used.

Atrial fibrillation: In previously untreated patients, digoxin is given intravenously. If arrhythmia persists and causes hemodynamic instability, electric cardioversion is applied followed by preventive therapy and anticoagulation. For prevention of recurrences, quinidine (or procainamide) is given with either digitalis or low doses of beta-adrenergic blockers. Anticoagulants are recommended in cases of recurrent, protracted, or established atrial fibrillation unless there is a bleeding tendency or other contraindication. The question of whether to use anticoagulants in the presence of pericarditis is unsettled. There is an independent association between atrial fibrillation and pericarditis both during and after the hospital course of myocardial infarction [78–80], and the continuation of anticoagulants in this condition entails a small risk of hemopericardium that may be equal to the risk of embolic complications in patients not treated with anticoagulants.

Atrial tachyarrhythmias with rapid anterograde conduction through the AV bypass tract: Digitalis and calcium channel blockers must be avoided. Intravenous administration of amiodarone or procainamide [81], electric cardioversion, or both are used for acute treatment. Oral amiodarone is given for prevention.

Acknowledgment

This study was supported in part by the Herman C. Krannert Fund; by grants HL-06308 and HL-07182 from the National Heart, Lung, and Blood Institute of the National Institutes of Health; by the American Heart Association, Indiana Affiliate; and by the Veterans Administration.

Editorial Comment

Intravenous verapamil should not be used to treat supraventricular tachycardia unless the diagnosis is secure. Numerous cases of cardiovascular collapse with ventricular fibrillation have occurred when verapamil has been mistakenly used to treat ventricular or wide QRS tachycardia.

Flecainide, as with disopyramide, the beta blockers and possibly encainide, has a distinct propensity to cause cardiodepression. When these negative inotropic properties are superimposed on an acutely infarcted myocardium, overt heart failure can be a drug-related complication. If it is elected to use a beta blocker for supraventricular tachycardia or sinus tachycardia in a patient with an acute myocardial infarction, one should consider intravenous use of the ultra-short-acting agent esmolol.

The interactions of beta blockers and diltiazem may lead to profound sinus bradycardia and heart block. It is our opinion that this drug interaction problem has been understated in the literature. Furthermore, sinus node dysfunction can be expected when an H_2 blocker such as cimetidine is combined with a beta blocker and diltiazem. These bradyarrhythmias are presumably more likely to occur if there is underlying sick-sinus node syndrome. G.S.F.

References

1. Yu, P. N. The acute phase of myocardial infarction. *Cardiovasc. Clin.* 7:45, 1975.
2. Webb, S. W., Adgey, A. A., and Pantridge, J. F. Autonomic disturbance at onset of acute myocardial infarction. *Br. Med. J.* 3:89, 1972.
3. Hindman, M. C., and Wagner, G. S. Arrhythmias during myocardial infarction: Mechanisms, significance, and therapy. *Cardiovasc. Clin.* 11:81, 1980.
4. Parameswaran, R., Ohe, T., and Goldberg, H. Sinus node dysfunction in acute myocardial infarction. *Br. Heart J.* 38:93, 1976.
5. Lie, K. I., Wellens, H. J., Downar, E., and Durrer, D. Observations on patients with primary ventricular fibrillation complicating acute myocardial infarction. *Circulation* 52:755, 1975.
6. Vazifdar, J. P., and Levine, S. A. Rarity of atrial tachycardia in acute myocardial infarction and in thyrotoxicosis. *Arch. Intern. Med.* 118:41, 1966.
7. Lesser, L. Atrial tachycardia in acute myocardial infarction. *Ann. Intern. Med.* 86:582, 1977.

8. Chung, E. K. Tachyarrhythmias associated with acute myocardial infarction: Diagnosis, frequency, and significance. *Cardiovasc. Clin.* 7:157, 1975.

9. Liberthson, R. R., Salisbury, K. W., Hutter, Jr., A. M., and DeSanctis, R. W. Atrial tachyarrhythmias in acute myocardial infarction. *Am. J. Med.* 60:956, 1976.

10. Lofmark, R., and Orinius, E. Supraventricular tachyarrhythmias in acute myocardial infarction. *Acta Med. Scand.* 203:517, 1978.

11. Rosen, M. R., Fisch, C., Hoffman, B. F., et al. Can accelerated atrio-ventricular junctional escape rhythms be explained by delayed afterdepolarizations? *Am. J. Cardiol.* 45:1272, 1980.

12. Knoebel, S. B., Rasmussen, S., Lovelace, D. E., and Anderson, G. J. Nonparoxysmal junctional tachycardia in acute myocardial infarction: Computer-assisted detection. *Am. J. Cardiol.* 35:825, 1975.

13. Fishenfeld, J., Desser, K. B., and Benchimol, A. Non-paroxysmal A-V junctional tachycardia associated with acute myocardial infarction. *Am. Heart J.* 86:754, 1973.

14. Konecke, L. L., and Knoebel, S. B. Nonparoxysmal junctional tachycardia complicating acute myocardial infarction. *Circulation* 45:367, 1972.

15. Madsen, E. B., Hougaard, P., and Gilpin, E. Dynamic evaluation of prognosis from time-dependent variables in acute myocardial infarction. *Am. J. Cardiol.* 51:1579, 1983.

16. Helmers, C., Lundman, T., Mogensen, L., et al. Atrial fibrillation in acute myocardial infarction. *Acta Med. Scand.* 193:39, 1973.

17. Hunt, D., Sloman, G., and Penington, C. Effects of atrial fibrillation on prognosis of acute myocardial infarction. *Br. Heart J.* 40:303, 1978.

18. Cristal, N., Peterburg, I., and Szwarcberg, J. Atrial fibrillation developing in the acute phase of myocardial infarction: Prognostic implication. *Chest* 70:8, 1976.

19. Sugiura, T., Iwasaka, T., Ogawa, A., et al. Atrial fibrillation in acute myocardial infarction. *Am. J. Cardiol.* 56:27, 1985.

20. Klass, M., and Haywood, L. J. Atrial fibrillation associated with acute myocardial infarction: A study of 34 cases. *Am. Heart J.* 79:752, 1970.

21. Beck, O. A., and Hochrein, H. Atrial fibrillation and flutter as a complication of acute myocardial infarction. *Dtsch. Med. Wochenschr.* 101:1148, 1976.

22. Hod, H., Lew, A. S., Keltai, M., et al. Early atrial fibrillation during evolving myocardial infarction: A consequence of impaired left atrial perfusion. *Circulation* 75:146, 1987.

23. Loewy, E. H. Effects of atrial fibrillation on prognosis of acute myocardial infarction. *Br. Heart J.* 41:255, 1979.

24. Harrison, D. C. Atrial fibrillation in acute myocardial infarction: Significance and therapeutic implications. *Chest* 70:3, 1976.

25. McLean, K. H., Bett, J. N., and Saltups, A. Tachyarrhythmias in acute myocardial infarction. *Aust. N.Z. J. Med.* 5:3, 1975.

26. Flugelman, M. Y., Hasin, Y., Shefer, A., et al. Atrial fibrillation in acute myocardial infarction. *Isr. J. Med. Sci.* 22:355, 1986.

27. Siltanen, P., Pohjola-Sintonen, S., Haapakoski, J., et al. The mortality predictive power of discharge electrocardiogram after first acute myocardial infarction. *Am. Heart J.* 109:1231, 1985.

28. Liem, K. L., Lie, K. I., Durrer, D., and Wellens, H. J. Clinical setting and prognostic significance of atrial fibrillation complicating acute myocardial infarction. *Eur. J. Cardiol.* 4:59, 1976.

29. Gavrilescu, S., Gavrilescu, M., and Luca, C. Accelerated atrio-ventricular conduction during acute myocardial infarction. *Am. Heart J.* 94:21, 1977.

30. Goel, B. J., and Han, J. Manifestation of the Wolff-Parkinson-White syndrome after myocardial infarction. *Am. Heart J.* 87:633, 1974.

31. Dominic, J., McAllister, R. G., Kuo, C. S., et al. Verapamil plasma levels and ventricular rate response in patients with atrial fibrillation and flutter. *Clin. Pharmacol. Ther.* 26:710, 1979.

32. Jewitt, D. E., Balcon, R., Raftery, E. B., and Oram, S. Incidence and management of supraventricular arrhythmias after acute myocardial infarction. *Lancet* 2:734, 1967.

33. Weiner, P., Bassan, M. M., Jarchovsky, J., et al. Clinical course of acute atrial fibrillation treated with rapid digitalization. *Am. Heart J.* 105:223, 1983.

34. Bigger, Jr., J. T., Fleiss, J. L., Rolnitzky, L. M., et al. Effect of digitalis treatment on survival after acute myocardial infarction. *Am. J. Cardiol.* 55:623, 1985.

35. Byington, R., and Goldstein, S. Association of digitalis therapy with mortality in survivors of acute myocardial infarction: Observations in the Beta-Blocker Heart Attack Trial. *J. Am. Coll. Cardiol.* 6:976, 1985.

36. Frishman, W. H. *Clinical Pharmacology of the Beta Adrenoreceptor Blocking Drugs* (2nd ed.). Norwalk: Appleton-Century-Crofts, 1984.

37. Wit, A. L., Hoffman, B. F., and Rosen, M. R. Electrophysiology and pharmacology of cardiac arrhythmias. IX. Cardiac electrophysiology effects of beta adrenergic receptor stimulation and blockade. Part C. *Am. Heart J.* 90:795, 1975.

38. Shand, D. G. Individualization of propranolol therapy. *Med. Clin. North Am.* 58:1063, 1974.

39. Swerdlow, C., Peterson, J., Liem, L. B., and Blake, K. Electropharmacology of flestolol in patients with supraventricular tachyarrhythmias. *J. Am. Coll. Cardiol.* 9:247A, 1987.

40. Kirshenbaum, J. M., Kloner, R. A., Antman, E. M., and Braunwald, E. Use of ultra-short acting beta-blocker in patients with acute myocardial ischemia. *Circulation* 72:873, 1985.
41. Lemberg, L., Castellanos, Jr., A., and Arcebal, A. G. The use of propranolol in arrhythmias complicating acute myocardial infarction. *Am. Heart J.* 80:479, 1970.
42. Ramsdale, D. R., Faragher, E. B., Bennett, D. H., et al. Ischemic pain relief in patients with acute myocardial infarction by intravenous atenolol. *Am. Heart J.* 103:459, 1982.
43. Schley, G., Beckmann, R., and Hengstebeck, W. The treatment of acute cardiac dysrhythmias with atenolol (Tenormin) particularly after myocardial infarction. *Z. Kardiol.* 67:280, 1978.
44. Miami Trial Research Group. Metoprolol in acute myocardial infarction. Arrhythmias. *Am. J. Cardiol.* 56:35G, 1985.
45. Lemberg, L., Arcebal, A. G., Castellanos, Jr., A., and Slavin, D. Use of alprenolol in acute cardiac arrhythmias. *Am. J. Cardiol.* 30:77, 1972.
46. Morganroth, J., Horowitz, L. N., Anderson, J., and Turlapaty, P. Comparative efficacy and tolerance of esmolol to propranolol for control of supraventricular tachyarrhythmia. *Am. J. Cardiol.* 56:33F, 1985.
47. Singh, B. M., Eilrodt, G., and Peter, C. T. Verapamil: A review of its pharmacological properties and therapeutic use. *Drugs* 15:169, 1978.
48. Kates, R. E., Keefe, D. L. D., Schwartz, J., et al. Verapamil dispositions: Kinetics in chronic atrial fibrillation. *J. Clin. Pharmacol. Ther.* 30:44, 1981.
49. Schwartz, J. B., Keefe, D. L., Kirsten, E., et al. Prolongation of verapamil elimination kinetics during chronic oral administration. *Am. Heart J.* 104:198, 1982.
50. McGovern, B., Garan, H., and Ruskin, J. N. Precipitation of cardiac arrest by verapamil in patients with Wolff-Parkinson-White syndrome. *Am. Intern. Med.* 104:791, 1986.
51. Packer, M., Meller, J., Medina, N., et al. Hemodynamic consequences of combined beta adrenergic and slow calcium channel blockade in man. *Circulation* 65:660, 1982.
52. Rikenberger, R. L., Prystowsky, E. N., Heger, J. J., et al. Effects of intravenous and chronic oral verapamil administration in patients with supraventricular tachycardias. *Circulation* 62:996, 1980.
53. Krikler, D. M., Verapamil in arrhythmia. *Br. J. Clin. Pharmacol.* 21(Suppl 2):183S, 1986.
54. Waxman, H. L., Myerburg, R. J., Appel, R., and Sung, R. J. Verapamil for control of ventricular rate in paroxysmal supraventricular tachycardia and atrial fibrillation or flutter. *Ann. Intern. Med.* 94:1, 1981.
55. Waleffe, A., Hastir, F., and Kulbertus, H. E.

Effects of intravenous diltiazem administration in patients with inducible tachycardia. *Eur. Heart J.* 6:882, 1985.
56. Strozzi, C., Sfrisi, C., Leutenegger, F., et al. Tiapamil in the management of supraventricular arrhythmias occurring after acute myocardial infarction. *Cardiology* 69(Suppl):187, 1982.
57. Hagemeijer, F. Verapamil in the management of supraventricular tachyarrhythmias occurring after a recent myocardial infarction. *Circulation* 57:751, 1978.
58. Danish Study Group on Verapamil in Myocardial Infarction. Abrupt withdrawal of verapamil in ischaemic heart disease. *Eur. Heart J.* 5:529, 1984.
59. Klein, H. O., and Kaplinsky, E. Verapamil and digoxin: Their respective effects on atrial fibrillation and their interaction. *Am. J. Cardiol.* 50:894, 1982.
60. Yee, R., Gulamhusein, S. S., and Klein, G. J. Combined verapamil and propranolol for supraventricular tachycardia. *Am. J. Cardiol.* 53:757, 1984.
61. Yeh, S. J., Lin, F. C., Chou, Y. Y., et al. Termination of paroxysmal supraventricular tachycardia with a single oral dose of diltiazem and propranolol. *Circulation* 71:104, 1985.
62. Yeh, S. J., Fu, M., Lin, F. C., et al. Serial electrophysiologic studies of the effects of oral diltiazem on paroxysmal supraventricular tachycardia. *Chest* 87:639, 1985.
63. Gulamhusein, S., Ko, P., Carruthers, G., and Klein, G. J. Acceleration of the ventricular response during atrial fibrillation in the Wolff-Parkinson-White syndrome after verapamil. *Circulation* 65:348, 1982.
64. Greenblatt, D. J., Pfeifer, H. J., Ochs, H. R., et al. Pharmacokinetics of quinidine in humans after intravenous, intramuscular and oral administration. *J. Pharmacol. Exp. Ther.* 202:365, 1977.
65. Woosley, R. R., and Shand, D. G. Pharmacokinetics of antiarrhythmic drugs. *Am. J. Cardiol.* 41:986, 1978.
66. Sodermark, T., Jonsson, B., Olsson, A., et al. Effect of quinidine on maintaining sinus rhythm after conversion of atrial fibrillation or flutter: A multicenter study from Stockholm. *Br. Heart J.* 37:486, 1975.
67. Grande, P., Sonne, B., and Pedersen, A. A controlled study of digoxin and quinidine in patients DC reverted from atrial fibrillation to sinus rhythm. *Circulation* 74(Suppl. II):101, 1986.
68. Doering, W. Quinidine-digoxin interactions: Pharmacokinetics, underlying mechanism, and clinical implication. *N. Engl. J. Med.* 301:400, 1979.
69. Fenster, P. E., Comess, K. A., Marsh, R., et al. Conversion of atrial fibrillation to sinus rhythm

by acute intravenous procainamide infusion. *Am. Heart J.* 106:501, 1983.

70. Shen, E. N., Keung, E., Huycke, E., et al. Intravenous propafenone for termination of reentrant supraventricular tachycardia: A placebo controlled, randomized double-blind, crossover study. *Ann. Intern. Med.* 105:655, 1986.

71. Leak, D. Intravenous amiodarone in the treatment of refractory life-threatening cardiac arrhythmias in the critically ill patient. *Am. Heart J.* 111:456, 1986.

72. Escoubet, B., Coumel, P., Poirier, J. M., et al. Suppression of arrhythmias within hours after a single oral dose of amiodarone and relation to plasma and myocardial concentration. *Am. J. Cardiol.* 55:696, 1985.

73. DiMarco, J. P., Sellers, T. D., Lerman, B. B., et al. Diagnostic and therapeutic use of adenosine in patients with supraventricular tachyarrhythmias. *J. Am. Coll. Cardiol.* 6:417, 1985.

74. Kerber, R. E., Jensen, S. R., Grayzel, J., et al. Electric cardioversion: Influence of paddle electrode location and size on success rate and energy requirement. *N. Engl. J. Med.* 305:658, 1981.

75. Mancini, G. B. J., and Goldberger, A. L. Cardioversion of atrial fibrillation: Consideration of embolization, anticoagulation, prophylactic pacemaker, and long-term success. *Am. Heart J.* 104:617, 1982.

76. Greenberg, M. L., Kelly, T. A., Lerman, B. B., and DiMarco, J. P. Atrial pacing for conversion of atrial flutter. *Am. J. Cardiol.* 58:95, 1986.

77. Nordrehaug, J. E., and von der Lippe, G. Serum potassium concentrations are inversely related to ventricular, but not to atrial, arrhythmias in acute myocardial infarction. *Eur. Heart J.* 7:204, 1986.

78. Liem, K. L., Durrer, D., Lie, K. I., and Wellens, H. J. Pericarditis in acute myocardial infarction. *Lancet* 2:1004, 1975.

79. Dubois, C., Smeets, J. P., Demoulin, J. C., et al. Frequency and clinical significance of pericardial friction rubs in the acute phase of myocardial infarction. *Eur. Heart J.* 6:766, 1985.

80. Henrard, L., and Lisin, N. Myocardial infarction and late pericarditis. *Arch. Mal. Coeur.* 72:862, 1979.

81. Cowan, J. C., Gardiner, P., Reid, D. S., et al. A comparison of amiodarone and digoxin in the treatment of atrial fibrillation complicating suspected acute myocardial infarction. *J. Cardiovasc. Pharmacol.* 8:252, 1986.

IV
Mechanical Complications of Acute Myocardial Infarction: Diagnosis and Treatment

13
Hemodynamic Profiles of Pump Disturbances in Acute Myocardial Infarction: Management Strategies

KANU CHATTERJEE

Hemodynamic disturbances following acute myocardial infarction range from little or no change to severe abnormalities. The extent, location, and rapidity of myocardial necrosis are the major determinants of the severity of hemodynamic derangements. The magnitude of left ventricular dysfunction resulting from previous myocardial infarction also contributes to the overall functional and hemodynamic impairment. Ischemic myocardium, in addition to infarcted myocardium, compromises ventricular performance and produces hemodynamic abnormalities. At the onset of myocardial infarction, the extent of ischemic but viable myocardium is relatively greater than the extent of necrosis. With prompt relief of ischemia, recovery of function of the ischemic myocardium may be associated with rapid hemodynamic improvement. In contrast, progressive deterioration in hemodynamics occurs with infarct extension and expansion.

Hyperfunctioning noninfarcted myocardial segments compensate for the loss of function of the ischemic and infarcted segments [1–3]. With adequate compensation there may be little or no hemodynamic derangement. However, profound hemodynamic disturbances may occur with inadequate, or failure of, compensations to maintain cardiac performance.

Peripheral circulatory changes in response to pump failure following myocardial infarction contributes to sustain perfusion (arterial) pressure to the vital organs and for the economic and effective distribution of decreased cardiac output. Enhanced systemic and re-gional sympathetic activity and stimulation of the renin-angiotension-aldosterone system increases systemic vascular resistance and maintains arterial pressure [4]. Increased peripheral venous tone promotes venous return to the heart and increases intracardiac volume, which enhances forward stroke volume by the Frank-Starling mechanism. Thus arterial pressure and cardiac output may remain normal despite the loss of function of ischemic and infarcted myocardium. However, these compensatory peripheral circulatory changes may also exert adverse effects on cardiac performance and hemodynamics. Marked sympathetic activation may induce tachycardia, which is associated with increased myocardial consumption. Increased systemic vascular resistance also increases left ventricular outflow resistance, which decreases stroke volume, as an inverse relation exists between left ventricular stroke volume and its outflow resistance [5]. Ventricular diastolic pressures usually increase along with increased volume, and thus pulmonary and systemic venous pressures also increase—the hemodynamic determinants of the congestive symptoms. Furthermore, myocardial oxygen consumption increases along with increased left ventricular volume. The net changes in systemic hemodynamics therefore result from a number of interacting central and peripheral adjustments accompanying acute myocardial infarction. Mechanical complications such as mitral regurgitation or ventricular septal rupture produce specific hemodynamic abnormalities. Predominant right ventricular infarction is also associated with

241

hemodynamic abnormalities different from those that result from predominant left ventricular infarction.

This chapter reviews first the general functional derangements of acute myocardial ischemia and infarction and then the hemodynamic consequences of the specific complications of acute myocardial infarction.

Systolic Dysfunction in Acute Myocardial Infarction

Total thrombotic occlusion at the site of atheromatous plaque in the infarct-related artery is the mechanism of transmural myocardial infarction in more than 90 percent of patients [6]. Within a few seconds of total interruption of coronary blood flow, systolic shortening of ischemic myocardial segments decreases; and after approximately 30 seconds of ischemia, little or no effective work is performed by the ischemic segments [7–9]. Within a few minutes, ischemic regions demonstrate bulging during isovolumic systole and akinesis during the ejection phase [7, 10]. Paradoxical shortening of the ischemic myocardium is observed during isovolumic relaxation and the early diastolic phases.

The degree of functional impairment of the ischemic myocardium is related to the magnitude of the reduction of coronary blood flow. In the presence of preexisting adequate collateral blood flow, the magnitude of reduction of effective myocardial perfusion is less despite complete occlusion of the infarct-related artery. When subtotal occlusion of the infarct-related artery is the anatomic and pathophysiologic mechanism of myocardial infarction, the degree of ischemia is also relatively less and is usually confined to the subendocardium [11]. When functionally collateral vessels are present, the extent of myocardial necrosis and the degree of functional impairment tend to be less [12–15]. The hemodynamic disturbances are likewise less pronounced.

Perfusion may be reestablished shortly after total interruption of blood flow (e.g., within 15–20 minutes), and significant recovery of

systolic function of the ischemic myocardium may occur, minimizing the hemodynamic disturbances [16–18]. If reperfusion occurs after 60 minutes of ischemia, it may require up to 4 weeks for recovery of ventricular function [19]. This prolonged impairment in myocardial function despite reestablishment of adequate coronary blood flow has been termed "stunned myocardium" [20]. The hemodynamic abnormalities resulting from nonfunctioning ischemic myocardium therefore are not immediately corrected by delayed reperfusion, although the function of the "stunned" myocardium ultimately recovers along with improvement in hemodynamics. Thus the timing of recanalization of the infarct-related artery and reperfusion of the ischemic myocardium following the onset of myocardial infarction is directly related to the severity of the hemodynamic disturbances. Although early reperfusion may avert significant hemodynamic abnormalities, delayed reperfusion may still be associated with marked hemodynamic derangements, requiring aggressive supportive and corrective therapy.

Impaired systolic function is also observed in the relatively nonischemic regions adjacent to the infarcted segments. Functional alterations can occur in the subepicardial regions with milder degrees of myocardial ischemia when subendocardial blood flow declines with little or no reduction of flow in the subepicardium [21–23]. Adjacent nonischemic subendocardial regions may also demonstrate altered function. This phenomenon probably results from mechanical "tethering" of the infarcted and nonischemic zones.

Augmented systolic function of the myocardial segments remote from the area of infarction is frequent at the early phase of infarction [1–3]. Hyperfunction of the nonischemic areas primarily result from increased utilization of the Frank-Starling mechanism, which is due to increased end-diastolic pressure, a hemodynamic consequence of acute myocardial ischemia [8, 10]. Enhanced sympathetic stimulation may also contribute to the hyperfunction of the nonischemic zones [2]. Experimental studies in animals, however, have suggested that the "compensatory" increase in shortening of the nonischemic myocardial segments primarily causes stretching of the ischemic region during isovolumic (paradoxical) systole, and there is little or no increase in the ejection phase shortening of the nonischemic zones [10]. If there is no increase in end-diastolic pressure, there is no increased utilization of the Frank-Starling mechanism; and in these circumstances there may be an actual decrease in ejection phase shortening in nonischemic regions [24]. The results of these experimental studies explain the relatively higher "optimal filling pressure" in patients with acute myocardial infarction (14–18 mm Hg pulmonary capillary wedge pressure).

Diastolic Dysfunction in Acute Myocardial Infarction

Regional and global diastolic dysfunction is as frequent as systolic dysfunction in patients with acute myocardial ischemia or infarction. Indeed, diastolic dysfunction and its hemodynamic consequences tend to precede impairment of systolic function.

During acute spontaneous or induced myocardial ischemia, the ischemic region shortens paradoxically during isovolumic relaxation and early diastolic phases, presumably due to elastic recoil of the passively stretched ischemic region or persistent late systolic active shortening [7, 25]. Nonischemic zones may demonstrate early lengthening during the isovolumic relaxation phase; the mechanism and significance of this phenomenon, however, remain unclear. Abnormalities of ventricular relaxation are also reflected in a decrease in the peak rate of left ventricular pressure fall (peak dP/dt) and an increase in the time constant of left ventricular pressure fall during isovolumic relaxation (τ or tau) [26–30].

Alterations in diastolic filling characteristics are frequent consequences of acute myocardial ischemia and infarction. Peak diastolic filling rates decrease during induced myocardial ischemia [31, 32]. In patients with ischemic heart disease, successful reperfusion by coronary angioplasty increases the peak filling rate [33]. The precise mechanism for impaired filling in patients with ischemia or infarction has not been clarified; regional abnormality of diastolic function, incomplete ventricular relaxation, and alteration in myocardial stiffness may be contributory [34]. Increased end-systolic volume and pressure resulting from impaired systolic emptying enhances inflow impedance and impairs diastolic filling [25]. Elevated left ventricular diastolic pressure also offers increased resistance to diastolic filling and decreases effective filling time [35].

Left ventricular filling pressures are elevated in many patients, particularly early during the acute phase of myocardial infarction [2, 36–39]. A number of mechanisms appear to contribute to high ventricular diastolic pressure. The left ventricular diastolic pressure-volume relation is shifted upward during induced myocardial ischemia [40–42]. Impaired ventricular relaxation [28, 29], ventricular interaction effects [43], and increased myocardial stiffness [44, 45] might be contributory. Whatever the mechanism, elevated ventricular filling pressures is a common hemodynamic consequence of abnormal diastolic function.

A mild to moderate increase in left ventricular filling pressure may augment cardiac performance because of increased utilization of the Frank-Starling mechanism by the noninfarcted, nonischemic regions. However, excessive increase in left ventricular filling pressure can produce several deleterious effects. Increased left ventricular diastolic pressure is associated with a passive increase in left atrial and pulmonary venous pressures—the hemodynamic determinant of pulmonary congestion and pulmonary edema. Compromised subendocardial perfusion resulting from decreased transmyocardial pressure gradient may enhance subendocardial ischemia and cause further deterioration of systolic and diastolic function. The therapeutic implications are that when the left ventricular filling pressure is low, it should be increased to the "optimal range" to augment stroke volume and cardiac output, if indicated. The left ventricular filling pressure should be lowered when it is excessively high in order to avoid pulmo-

Table 13-1
Subsets of acute myocardial infarction

Subset	Clinical manifestations		Hemodynamic correlates	
	Pulmonary congestion	Hypoperfusion	PCWP (mm Hg)	CI (L/min/m²)
I	Absent	Absent	≤ 18	> 2.2
II	Present	Absent	≥ 18	> 2.2
III	Absent	Present	≤ 18	< 2.2
IV	Present	Present	≥ 18	< 2.2

PCWP = pulmonary capillary wedge pressure; CI = cardiac index.
Source: Modified from J. S. Forrester et al. Medical therapy of acute myocardial infarction by application of hemodynamic subsets (first two parts). *N. Engl. J. Med.* 295:1361, 1976. Reprinted by permission.

nary congestion and to improve subendocardial perfusion.

Hemodynamic Subsets of Acute Myocardial Infarction

Based on hemodynamic derangements and their clinical manifestations, several subsets can be recognized [29, 46]. The hemodynamic subsets are based on changes in cardiac output and pulmonary capillary wedge pressure following acute myocardial infarction that reflect changes in left ventricular function. Changes in cardiac output are manifested clinically by changes in peripheral organ perfusion, and the level of pulmonary capillary wedge pressure is correlated to pulmonary congestion.

Bedside hemodynamic evaluation was performed in 200 patients with acute myocardial infarction within 72 hours of the onset of symptoms [29, 46]. Based on the initial level of pulmonary capillary wedge pressure and cardiac index, four hemodynamic subsets could be identified (Table 13-1).

In patients in subset I, the pulmonary capillary wedge pressure was 18 mm Hg or less, and the cardiac index was more than 2.2 L/min/m². Clinical evidence for pulmonary congestion or tissue hypoperfusion were absent. Hemodynamic disturbances were mild, left ventricular function was not markedly compromised, and the hospital mortality was low, only 3 percent. This hemodynamic profile occurred in approximately 25 percent of pa-

tients. No specific therapy was required until a complication supervened. As these patients could be recognized clinically, hemodynamic monitoring was also not indicated.

In patients in subset II, pulmonary capillary wedge pressure was elevated (> 18 mm Hg), but the cardiac index remained higher than 2.2 L/min/m². Clinically, these patients presented with signs and symptoms of pulmonary congestion without evidence for hypoperfusion. Approximately 25 percent of patients presented with this hemodynamic and clinical profile, and their immediate prognosis appeared to be worse than that of patients in subset I; hospital mortality was 9 percent.

The primary hemodynamic objective of treatment is to decrease pulmonary capillary wedge pressure with morphine, diuretics, and nitrates. If there is prompt relief of pulmonary edema, hemodynamic monitoring is not required in most patients. If the symptoms and signs of pulmonary congestion persist or hypotension and hypoperfusion occur, determination of pulmonary capillary wedge pressure and cardiac output aids in making further therapeutic decisions. Echocardiography-Doppler evaluation is also helpful to exclude silent, mitral regurgitation. Subsequent therapy can be tailored according to the hemodynamic abnormalities: If pulmonary capillary wedge pressure remains high, nitroglycerin and diuretics are continued. When cardiac output is also low or when pulmonary capillary wedge pressure remains elevated, the addition of sodium nitroprusside or phentolamine can produce an increase in cardiac output and further reduction of pulmonary capillary wedge pressure. Alternatively, phosphodiesterase inhibitors (amrinone, milrinone, enoximone) can be used to increase cardiac output and decrease pulmonary capillary wedge pressure. Systemic vasodilators or phosphodiesterase inhibitors, however, should be used with caution if arterial pressure is low.

The hemodynamic profile of patients in subset III was characterized by a low cardiac index (< 2.2 L/min/m^2) and low pulmonary capillary wedge pressure (< 18 mm Hg). Thus signs and symptoms of hypoperfusion rather than symptoms of pulmonary congestion were more apparent clinically. This hemodynamic profile was detected in approximately 15 percent of patients. The hospital mortality, however, was considerably higher, about 23 percent in these patients, suggesting that a decline in cardiac output is associated with worse prognosis than when only pulmonary capillary wedge pressure is elevated.

The mechanisms for the hemodynamic profile of patients in subset III are not entirely clear. Relative or absolute hypovolemia associated with decreased left and right ventricular preload can explain the low cardiac output and low ventricular filling pressures. However, the incidence of hypovolemia is low and is unlikely to be the sole or principal mechanism for these hemodynamic abnormalities. A marked decrease in left ventricular compliance, which is associated with a leftward shift of the left ventricular pressure-volume curve, may be associated with similar hemodynamic abnormalities. Decreased contractile function, increased ventricular outflow resistance, or both may produce a similar hemodynamic profile in patients with markedly reduced preload (e.g., excessive use of diuretics) prior to the onset of infarction. The hemodynamic abnormalities following right ventricular myocardial infarction (RVMI) may also be similar; however, in patients with RVMI, there is usually disproportionate elevation of right atrial pressure compared to pulmonary capillary wedge pressure. It is apparent that it is necessary to establish the mechanism of the hemodynamic profile of patients in subset III in order to select appropriate therapy. Concomitant nonin-

vasive assessment of ventricular chamber size (radionuclide ventriculography or echocardiography) along with hemodynamic determinations can potentially clarify the pathophysiologic mechanisms. Decreased right ventricular systolic function with relatively preserved left ventricular function suggests right ventricular failure, indicating RVMI in these clinical circumstances. Normal or decreased ventricular chamber size with relatively preserved systolic function indicates abnormal ventricular compliance as a mechanism for the hemodynamic changes. It is, however, appropriate to consider "volume challenge" with fairly rapid administration of intravenous fluids for the differential diagnosis and the selection of appropriate therapy. When cardiac output does not increase appreciably despite a considerable increase in pulmonary capillary wedge pressure (e.g., > 20 mm Hg) it is likely that marked impairment of left ventricular systolic function is the principal cause for the hemodynamic profile of patients in subset III [47]. In patients with true or absolute hypovolemia, a significant increase in stroke volume and cardiac output is expected along with the increase in right atrial and pulmonary capillary wedge pressures. In patients with markedly decreased left ventricular compliance, volume challenge increases left ventricular filling pressure with no substantial increase in left ventricular preload.

The hemodynamic abnormalities in patients in subset IV were characterized by an elevated pulmonary capillary wedge pressure exceeding 18 mm Hg and a low cardiac index, less than 2.2 L/min/m^2. Clinically, signs and symptoms of pulmonary congestion and hypoperfusion were present. Approximately 35 percent of the patients had this hemodynamic profile, and the hospital mortality was highest in this subset of patients, approximately 51 percent.

Marked impairment of left ventricular systolic function (reduced ejection fraction) is the principal mechanism for these hemodynamic changes. In addition to the decreased cardiac index and high pulmonary capillary wedge pressure, left ventricular stroke work index is reduced, and frequently sinus tachycardia and relative hypotension are observed. In patients with cardiogenic shock, the systolic arterial pressure is 90 mm Hg or less, and the cardiac index may be 1.5 L/min/m^2 or even less. Because of hypotension and low cardiac output, features of hypoperfusion are universally present: decreased urine output (< 20 ml/hr) and renal failure, hepatic dysfunction, pancreatic and gastrointestinal ischemia, cool and clammy skin, peripheral cyanosis, and mental obtundation. Enhanced anaerobic metabolism and metabolic acidosis frequently result and progressively worsen until a prompt increase in cardiac output can be achieved with appropriate therapeutic interventions. The cardiogenic shock syndrome occurs in approximately 10 to 15 percent of patients with acute myocardial infarction, and the immediate hospital mortality remains high, exceeding 80 percent, despite aggressive pharmacotherapy. Severe pump failure with or without clinical features of cardiogenic shock usually result from markedly impaired systolic function of large areas of ventricular myocardium. However, mechanical complications such as acute left ventricular aneurysm, papillary muscle infarction, or ventricular septal rupture may precipitate severe pump failure even in the presence of less extensive myocardial damage.

Prompt supportive therapy, based on the severity of the hemodynamic abnormalities and the hemodynamic response to therapeutic intervention, is essential. Thus hemodynamic monitoring is indicated in patients in subset IV. Preliminary uncontrolled studies suggest that early recanalization by angioplasty of the infarct-related artery with or without prior administration of thrombolytic agents may improve the prognosis of patients with cardiogenic shock [48]. Although benefits of such a therapeutic approach in the management of cardiogenic shock have not been firmly established, reperfusion therapy with angioplasty should be considered in appropriate patients, as the prognosis with supportive therapy alone remains poor. However, supportive therapy is always required, as hemodynamics and ventricular function do not improve immediately even when adequate recanalization

of the infarct-related artery is established promptly.

The major objectives of the therapy of severe pump failure with or without the clinical features of cardiogenic shock are to improve cardiac performance, correct hemodynamic abnormalities, maintain viability of ischemic myocardium, and limit the extent of myocardial damage. At present, early reperfusion therapy provides the best chance for limiting infarct size. No conclusive evidence exists to support the routine use of nitroglycerin, nitroprusside, beta blockers, calcium entry blocking agents, or intra-aortic balloon counterpulsation in patients with significant pump failure (subset IV) to decrease the extent of myocardial injury. Pharmacotherapy and intra-aortic balloon counterpulsation are employed to correct hemodynamic abnormalities and to improve cardiac performance. It is necessary to determine the hemodynamic profile, which should include, at least, arterial pressures, cardiac output, pulmonary capillary wedge pressure, and systemic vascular resistance. Prompt assessment of the hemodynamic response to an intervention is also necessary to decide "when and what" additional therapeutic interventions should be considered. The general outline for the therapy of pump failure complicating acute myocardial infarction based on hemodynamics is summarized in Figure 13-1 [49].

Fig. 13-1
Hypotension may be due to low cardiac output, low systemic vascular resistance, or both. Treatment of hypotension and pump failure is aided by hemodynamic monitoring in critically ill patients. ↑ = increase; ↓ = decrease; CO = cardiac output; SVR = systemic vascular resistance; PCWP = pulmonary capillary wedge pressure; AP = arterial pressure; RAP = right atrial pressure; IABP = intra-aortic balloon counterpulsation. (From K. Chatterjee. Bedside hemodynamic monitoring. In W. Parmley and K. Chatterjee, eds., *Cardiology*. Philadelphia: Lippincott, 1988. With permission.)

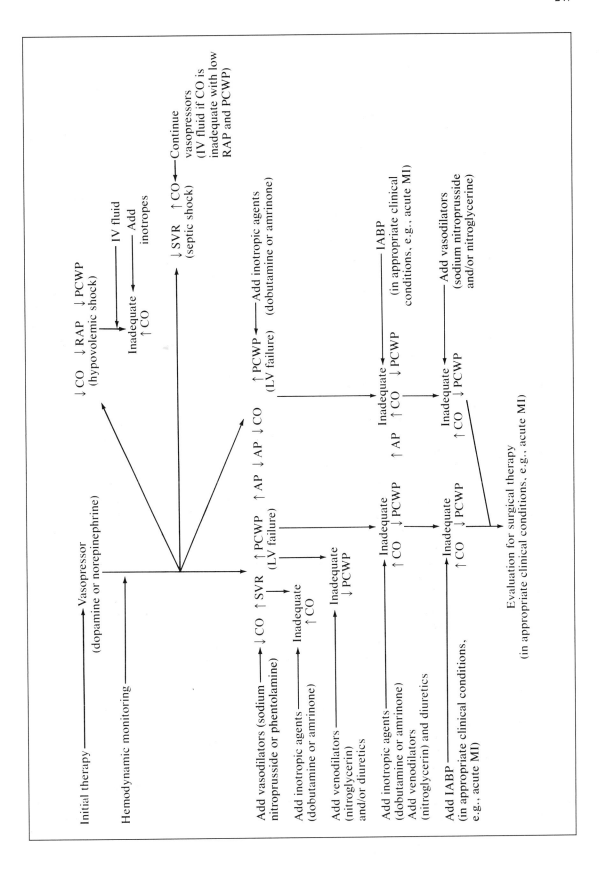

Acute Mitral Regurgitation

Mitral regurgitation can result from ischemia or necrosis of the left ventricular papillary muscles and adjacent left ventricular walls anchoring the papillary muscles, producing papillary muscle dysfunction. Rupture of the tip or trunk of the papillary muscle causes severe mitral regurgitation.

Mild mitral regurgitation is common, occurring in approximately 30 percent of patients, during the acute phase of myocardial infarction. Minor degrees of papillary muscle dysfunction resulting from ischemia of the papillary muscles or of the left ventricular walls contiguous to the papillary muscles is the likely mechanism [50]. It is likely that inefficient contraction of the papillary muscles or contraction along an abnormal axis, shifted inappropriately by dyssynergic motion of the ventricular walls anchoring papillary muscles, produces inadequate coaptation of the mitral leaflets during systole. Mitral regurgitation resulting from mild papillary muscle dysfunction does not impose any significant hemodynamic burden, and no specific hemodynamic derangements are recognized.

Papillary muscle infarction with or without rupture produces severe mitral regurgitation and is a catastrophic complication of acute myocardial infarction. The incidence is approximately 1 percent, and it accounts for about 5 percent of deaths of patients with acute myocardial infarction [51, 52]. More frequently, posteromedial papillary muscle is involved, associated with inferior or inferoposterior myocardial infarction due to occlusion of the right or left circumflex coronary artery. The extent of myocardial necrosis is relatively small in approximately 50 percent of patients and not infrequently is associated with single-vessel coronary artery disease.

Hemodynamic diagnosis of severe mitral regurgitation is usually made at the bedside by right heart catheterization with the use of balloon flotation catheters [49]. An early giant V wave in the pulmonary capillary wedge pressure tracing usually indicates acute or subacute severe mitral regurgitation. A reflected V wave, when recognized in the pulmonary artery pressure tracing, is pathognomonic of severe acute mitral regurgitation (Fig. 13-2) [49]. Giant V waves, however, may occur in the absence of mitral regurgitation, such as in patients with left-to-right shunt resulting from ventricular septal rupture. Giant V waves in the absence of mitral regurgitation are due to marked accentuation of the normal V wave because of decreased left atrial compliance or a marked increase in the venous return to the left atrium. The onset and peak of the V wave in these circumstances are delayed, in contrast to the "regurgitant wave" of mitral regurgitation, when the V waves occur at the beginning of the systole. Thus with careful attention to the details of the changes in the waveforms of pulmonary artery and pulmonary capillary wedge pressure tracings, the diagnosis of mitral regurgitation can be established at the bedside. However, clinical examination and echocardiography-Doppler evaluation are necessary and are valuable for making the correct diagnosis.

The severity of the hemodynamic derangements is related to the degree of mitral regurgitation and ischemia–infarct-related left ventricular dysfunction. In general, papillary muscle infarct produces severe mitral regurgitation and rapidly deteriorating hemodynamics. The forward stroke volume and cardiac output decline, and reflex tachycardia occurs. Systolic blood pressure falls, and the diastolic blood pressure may be maintained owing to marked peripheral vasoconstriction, and thus the pulse pressure is reduced. There is a marked increase in pulmonary venous pressure, an obligatory rise in pulmonary artery pressure, and frequently an increase in right atrial pressure, indicating right ventricular failure. Mitral regurgitation decreases left ventricular systolic impedance, elevating its ejection fraction.

Therapeutic strategies consist in rapid stabilization and early surgical intervention. Early corrective surgery may result in a significant improvement in prognosis; 60 to 70 percent of patients may survive this catastrophic complication. With conservative supportive therapy, mortality remains high, about 94 percent within 8 weeks, despite hemody-

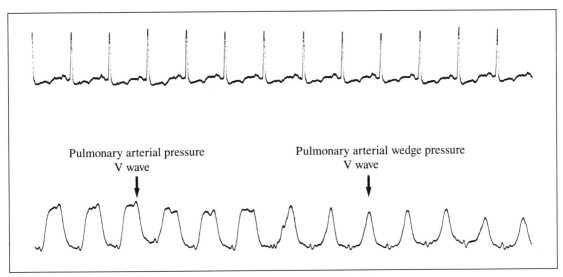

Fig. 13-2
Diagnosis of mitral regurgitation by bedside hemodynamic monitoring. A
reflected V wave in the pulmonary artery pressure tracing and a giant V wave in
the pulmonary artery wedge pressure tracing suggest severe acute or subacute
mitral regurgitation. (From K. Chatterjee. Bedside hemodynamic monitoring. In
W. Parmley and K. Chatterjee, eds., *Cardiology*. Philadelphia: Lippincott, 1988.
With permission.)

namic and clinical improvement initially in
many patients [51–53].

The objectives of supportive therapy are to
decrease regurgitant volume, increase forward
stroke volume and cardiac output, and reduce
pulmonary venous, pulmonary arterial, and
systemic venous pressures. The severity of
mitral regurgitation is related not only to the
degree of anatomic derangement of the mitral
valve apparatus but also to the aortic impedance. With increasing aortic impedance, regurgitant volume increases; with decreased
impedance, regurgitant volume declines and
forward stroke volume increases. Vasodilators
such as sodium nitroprusside or hydralazine
decrease systemic vascular resistance, reduce
regurgitant volume, and increase forward stroke
volume [54, 55]. Along with decreased regurgitant volumes, pulmonary venous pressures
fall, and right heart hemodynamics improve.
In general, with nitroglycerin there is little or
no increase in forward stroke volume, although regurgitant volume and pulmonary venous pressures decrease. Thus nitroprusside
and hydralazine are preferable to nitroglycerin
to correct the hemodynamic abnormalities of

severe mitral regurgitation. The addition of inotropic agents such as dobutamine and amrinone may cause a further improvement in
hemodynamics. Intra-aortic balloon counterpulsation is associated with decreased left
ventricular outflow resistance and an increase
in forward stroke volume and cardiac output.
Pulmonary venous pressure decreases, presumably owing to reduction of the regurgitant
volume, and the arterial diastolic pressure
(perfusion pressure) is enhanced owing to diastolic augmentation. In hypotensive patients,
intra-aortic balloon counterpulsation should
be employed prior to vasodilator therapy.
Hemodynamic monitoring is necessary to assess the response to therapy during stabilization of these patients.

Ventricular Septal Rupture

Rupture of the interventricular septum is another catastrophic complication of acute myocardial infarction. The incidence is about 0.5
to 2.0 percent and accounts for 1 to 5 percent
of all infarct-related deaths [56]. Ventricular

septal rupture produces left-to-right shunt and volume overload on both right and left ventricles. Right atrial, pulmonary artery, and pulmonary capillary wedge pressures increase. With increasing left-to-right shunt, systemic output declines with a reflex increase in systemic vascular resistance, which causes a further increase in the magnitude of left-to-right shunt.

The diagnosis can be confirmed at the bedside by demonstrating a step-up in oxygen saturation ($\geq$ 10 percent) from the right atrium to the right ventricle or proximal pulmonary artery. It can also be established by two-dimensional echocardiography, Doppler flow study, or radionuclide studies [57, 58].

The rapidity of hemodynamic deterioration is relatively slower than that in patients with papillary muscle infarction. However, the mortality associated with septal rupture remains high, 24 percent within 24 hours, 46 percent at 1 week, and 67 to 82 percent at 2 months [51–53]. Early aggressive surgical therapy with repair of the ventricular septal defect and, when necessary, coronary artery bypass surgery and aneurysmectomy have been reported to improve the short-term and long-term prognosis [59]. Conservative therapy is thus indicated to stabilize the patient prior to corrective surgery. The objectives of supportive therapy are to decrease left-to-right shunt, increase systemic output, and reduce the pulmonary capillary wedge, right atrial, and pulmonary arterial pressures.

The magnitude of the left-to-right shunt in patients with ventricular septal rupture is primarily determined by the ratio of the pulmonary and systemic vascular resistance, as the defect is usually large and offers little resistance to left-to-right shunt. A greater decrease in systemic vascular resistance than in pulmonary vascular resistance is associated with decreased left-to-right shunt and increased systemic output.

Intra-aortic balloon counterpulsation selectively decreases left ventricular outflow resistance without causing any primary change in right ventricular outflow resistance. Thus with intra-aortic balloon counterpulsation, systemic output increases along with decreased left-to-right shunt. Pulmonary and

Table 13-2
Mechanisms of decreased systemic output in right ventricular myocardial infarction

1. Decreased RV contractile function $\longrightarrow$ reduced RVSV $\longrightarrow$ decreased LV preload
2. Restricted ventricular filling due to the constraining effect of pericardium
3. Dilated RV with increased wall stress $\longrightarrow$ increased RV afterload $\longrightarrow$ reduced RNSV $\longrightarrow$ decreased LV preload
4. Increased intrapericardial pressure $\longrightarrow$ increased pulmonary venous and pulmonary arterial pressure $\longrightarrow$ increased RV ejection impedance $\longrightarrow$ decreased RNSV $\longrightarrow$ decreased LV preload
5. Interventricular septal shift toward the left ventricle $\longrightarrow$ decreased LV preload

RV = right ventricle; LV = left ventricle; RVSV = right ventricular stroke volume.

systemic venous pressures also decrease along with augmented arterial diastolic pressure.

Vasodilator drugs can improve hemodynamics, decrease left-to-right shunt, and increase systemic output. However, changes in left-to-right shunt and systemic output due to vasodilators depend on the relative changes in pulmonary and systemic vascular resistance. If the reduction in pulmonary vascular resistance is relatively greater, left-to-right shunt increases. Thus vasodilators with less pronounced effects on the pulmonary vascular bed (e.g., hydralazine) are preferable to vasodilators that cause a substantial decrease in pulmonary vascular resistance (e.g., sodium nitroprusside, nitroglycerin).

It is apparent that hemodynamic monitoring is required during supportive therapy, particularly monitoring of the oxygen saturation changes in right atrial, pulmonary, arterial, and systemic arterial blood.

Right Ventricular Infarction

Predominant right ventricular infarction occurs almost exclusively in patients with inferior or inferoposterior infarction [60, 61]. Total right coronary artery occlusion, proximal to the origins of the right ventricular branches, is the usual anatomic basis, although multivessel coronary artery disease frequently accompan-

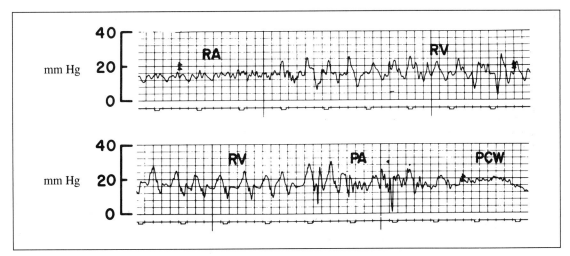

Fig. 13-3
Hemodynamic abnormalities in acute right myocardial infarction include a
disproportionate elevation of right atrial (RA) pressure compared to pulmonary
capillary wedge (PCW) pressure. In some patients the mean right atrial, right
ventricular (RV) diastolic, pulmonary artery (PA) diastolic, and mean PCW
pressure are similar. (From K. Chatterjee. Bedside hemodynamic monitoring. In
W. Parmley and K. Chatterjee, eds., *Cardiology*. Philadelphia: Lippincott, 1988.
With permission.)

ies it. A small right ventricular infarction may produce no hemodynamic abnormalities. A relatively large infarct, however, results in significant hemodynamic derangements and may be associated with decreased systemic output and hypotension. Disproportionate elevation of right atrial pressure compared to pulmonary capillary wedge pressure is the usual finding, and the ratio of the right atrial to the pulmonary capillary wedge pressure exceeds 0.86. In many patients with "low output state," equalization of right atrial and pulmonary capillary wedge pressures is observed simulating the hemodynamic abnormalities of cardiac tamponade [62]. The equalization of the "diastolic pressure" results from the increased intrapericardial pressure as the stiff pericardium does not stretch quickly enough to compensate for the increased right ventricular volume [63]. In experimental isolated right ventricular infarction in dogs, pericardiectomy prevents equalization of diastolic pressures.

There are multiple hemodynamic mechanisms that contribute to the reduction of systemic output with right ventricular infarction. Decreased right ventricular pump function reduces the venous return to the left ventricle,

reducing left ventricular preload. Increased intrapericardial pressure also restricts left ventricular filling. The interventricular septal shift toward the left ventricle also decreases left ventricular diastolic volume.

Right ventricular pump failure results not only from decreased contractility but also from augmented afterload. Right ventricular dilatation is associated with its increased wall stress. Increased left ventricular diastolic pressure resulting from increased intrapericardial pressure causes a passive increase in pulmonary arterial pressure, which also increases right ventricular outflow resistance. There is a further reduction of right ventricular stroke volume, which in turn decreases the left ventricular stroke volume. Thus a number of interacting hemodynamic mechanisms contribute to decreased left ventricular preload, which is the principal mechanism for decreased systemic output (Table 13-2).

Assessment of hemodynamics has direct relevance during the management of a "low output state" complicating right ventricular infarction (Fig. 13-3). Although intravenous fluid administration sometimes increases systemic output [64], volume expansion therapy

Table 13-3
Hemodynamic management of "low output state"
in right ventricular infarction

*Low cardiac output, right atrial pressure and
pulmonary capillary wedge pressures < 15 mm
Hg:* intravenous fluid ⟶ inadequate response
⟶ vasodilators if blood pressure is adequate
⟶ inadequate response ⟶ dobutamine.
*Low cardiac output, right atrial pressure and
pulmonary capillary wedge pressure > 15 mm
Hg:* dobutamine or nitroprusside ⟶
inadequate response ⟶ combined dobutamine
and nitroprusside.
*Low cardiac output, right atrial pressure and
pulmonary capillary wedge pressure > 15 mm
Hg, hypotension:* dopamine ⟶ inadequate
response ⟶ add dobutamine ⟶ inadequate
response but blood pressure is higher ⟶ add
nitroprusside.
In the presence of left ventricular failure: intra-
aortic balloon counterpulsation, in addition to
vasodilator therapy and inotropic agents, may
be required.

is usually ineffective when the pulmonary capillary wedge and right atrial pressures are already elevated (> 12–15 mm Hg). It is feasible that in these circumstances intravenous fluid therapy does not cause a significant increase in left ventricular preload (end-diastolic volume or transmural pressure), although right atrial and pulmonary capillary wedge pressures increase because of increased intrapericardial pressures. Inotropic drugs such as dobutamine and dopamine appear to be more effective than vasodilators or intravenous fluid therapy for increasing systemic output and improving right ventricular pump function. When vasodilators such as sodium nitroprusside or nitroglycerin are used, concomitant intravenous fluid therapy is frequently required to maintain adequate right and left ventricular preload. The therapeutic approach for the treatment of a low output state complicating right ventricular infarction based on hemodynamic abnormalities is summarized in Table 13-3.

Summary

Hemodynamic profiles are not uniform after acute myocardial infarction. They do reflect the site and extent of the infarction as well as its complications, however. Determinations of hemodynamic values are helpful in certain subsets of patients, particularly for assessing response to therapy.

References

1. Corya, B. C., Rasmussen, S., Knoebel, S. B., et al. Echocardiography in acute myocardial infarction. *Am. J. Cardiol.* 36:1, 1975.
2. Rigand, M., Rochar, P., Boschat, J., et al. Regional left ventricular function assessed by contrast angiography in acute myocardial infarction. *Circulation* 60:130, 1979.
3. Stack, R. S., Phillips, III, H. R., Grierson, D. S., et al. Functional improvement of jeopardized myocardium following intracoronary streptokinase infusion in acute myocardial infarction. *J. Clin. Invest.* 72:84, 1983.
4. Viquerat, C. E., Daly, P., Swedberg, K., et al. Endogenous catecholamines in chronic heart failure: Relation to the severity of hemodynamic abnormalities. *Am. J. Med.* 78:455, 1985.
5. Chatterjee, K., and Parmley, W. W. Role of vasodilator therapy in heart failure. *Prog. Cardiovasc. Dis.* 19:301, 1977.
6. DeWood, M. A., Spores, J., Notske, R. N., et al. Prevalence of total coronary occlusion during the early hours of transmural myocardial infarction. *N. Engl. J. Med.* 303:897, 1980.
7. Tennant, R., and Wiggins, C. J. The effect of coronary occlusion on myocardial contraction. *Am. J. Physiol.* 112:351, 1935.
8. Theroux, P., Franklin, D., Ross, Jr., J., et al. Regional myocardial function during acute coronary artery occlusion and its modification by pharmacologic agents in the dog. *Circ. Res.* 35:896, 1974.
9. Tyberg, J. V., Forrester, J. S., Wyatt, H. L., et al. An analysis of segmental ischemic dysfunction utilizing the pressure-length loop. *Circulation* 49:748, 1974.
10. Low, W. Y. W., Chen, Z., Guth, B., et al. Mechanisms of augmented segment shortening in nonischemic areas during acute ischemia of the canine left ventricle. *Circ. Res.* 56:351, 1985.
11. Gallagher, K. P., Osakada, G., Hess, O. M., et al. Subepicardial segmental function during coronary stenosis and the role of myocardial fiber orientation. *Circ. Res.* 50:352, 1982.
12. Williams, D. O., Amsterdam, E. A., Miller, R. R., et al. Functional significance of coronary collateral vessels in patients with acute myocardial infarction: Relation to pump performance, cardiogenic shock and survival. *Am. J. Cardiol.* 37:345, 1976.

13. Nohara, R., Kambara, H., Murakami, T., et al. Collateral function in early acute myocardial infarction. *Am. J Cardiol.* 52:955, 1983.

14. Bertrand, M. E., Lefebvre, J. M., Laisne, C. L., et al. Coronary arteriography in acute transmural myocardial infarction. *Am. Heart J.* 97:61, 1979.

15. Betriu, A., Castaner, A., Sanz, G. A., et al. Angiographic findings one month after myocardial infarction: A prospective study of 259 survivors. *Circulation* 65:1099, 1982.

16. Theroux, P., Ross, Jr., J., Franklin, D., et al. Regional myocardial function in the conscious dog during acute coronary occlusion and responses to morphine, propranolol, nitroglycerin and lidocaine. *Circulation* 53:302, 1976.

17. Heyndrickx, G. R., Baig, H., Nellens, P., et al. Depression of regional blood flow and wall thickening after brief coronary occlusions. *Am J. Physiol.* 234:H653, 1978.

18. Heyndrickx, G. R., Millard, R. W., McRitchie, R. J., et al. Regional myocardial functional and electrophysiologic alterations after brief coronary artery occlusion in conscious dogs. *J. Clin. Invest.* 56:978, 1975.

19. Lanakee, M., Cox, D., Pastrick, T. A., et al. Salvage of myocardial function by coronary artery reperfusion 1, 2, and 3 hours after occlusion in conscious dogs. *Circ. Res.* 53:235, 1983.

20. Braunwald, E., and Kloner, R. A. The stunned myocardium: Prolonged post-ischemic ventricular dysfunction. *Circulation* 66:1146, 1982.

21. Weintraub, W. S., Hastton, S., Agarwal, J. B., et al. The relationship between myocardial blood flow and contraction by myocardial layer in the canine left ventricle during ischemia. *Circ. Res.* 48:430, 1981.

22. Gallagher, K. P., Osakada, G., Hess, O. M., et al. Subepicardial segmental function during coronary stenosis and the role of myocardial fiber orientation. *Circ. Res.* 50:352, 1982.

23. Hattori, S., Weintraub, W. S., Agarwal, J. B., et al. Contrasting ischemic contraction patterns by zone and layer in canine myocardium. *Am. J. Physiol.* 243:H852, 1982.

24. Lew, W. Y. W., and Ban-Hayashi, E. Mechanisms of improving regional and global ventricular function by preload alterations during acute ischemia in the canine left ventricle. *Circulation* 72:1125, 1985.

25. Hess, O. M., Osakada, G., Lavelle, J. F., et al. Left ventricular geometry during partial and complete coronary occlusion in the conscious dog. *Int. J. Cardiol.* 1:387, 1982.

26. Waters, D. D., DaLuz, P., Wyatt, H. L., et al. Early changes in regional and global left ventricular function induced by graded reduction in regional coronary perfusion. *Am. J. Cardiol.* 39:537, 1977.

27. Kumada, T., Karliner, J. S., Pouleur, H., et al. Effects of coronary occlusion on early ventricular diastolic events in conscious dogs. *Am. J. Physiol.* 237:H542, 1979.

28. Mann, T., Goldberg, S., Mudge, Jr., G. H., et al. Factors contributing to altered left ventricular diastolic properties during angina pectoris. *Circulation* 59:14, 1979.

29. Carroll, J. D., Hess, O. M., Hirzel, H. O., et al. Exercise-induced ischemia: The influence of altered relaxation on early diastolic pressures. *Circulation* 67:521, 1983.

30. Sharma, B., Behrens, T. W., Erlein, D., et al. Left ventricular diastolic properties and filling characteristics during spontaneous angina pectoris at rest. *Am. J. Cardiol.* 52:704, 1983.

31. Reduto, L. A., Wickemeyer, W. J., Young, J. B., et al. Left ventricular diastolic performance at rest and during exercise in patients with coronary artery disease: Assessment with first-pass radionuclide angiography. *Circulation* 63:1228, 1981.

32. Poliner, L. R., Farber, S. H., Glaeser, D. H., et al. Alteration of diastolic filling rate during exercise radionuclide angiography: A highly sensitive technique for detection of coronary artery disease. *Circulation* 70:942, 1984.

33. Bonow, R. O., Kent, K. M., Rosing, D. R., et al. Improved left ventricular diastolic filling in patients with coronary artery disease after percutaneous transluminal coronary angioplasty. *Circulation* 66:1159, 1982.

34. Bonow, R. O., Vitale, D. F., Bacharach, S. L., et al. Asynchronous left ventricular regional function and impaired global diastolic filling in patients with coronary artery disease: Reversal after coronary angioplasty. *Circulation* 71:297, 1985.

35. Weisfeldt, M. L., Armstrong, P., Scully, H. E., et al. Incomplete relaxation between beats after myocardial hypoxia and ischemia. *J. Clin. Invest.* 53:1626, 1974.

36. Hamosh, P., and Cohn J. N. Left ventricular function in acute myocardial infarction. *J. Clin. Invest.* 50:523, 1971.

37. Rackley, C. E., and Russell, Jr., R. O. Left ventricular function in acute myocardial infarction and its clinical significance. *Circulation* 45:231, 1972.

38. Chatterjee, K., Parmley, W. W., Ganz W., et al. Hemodynamic and metabolic responses to vasodilator therapy in acute myocardial infarction. *Circulation* 48:1183, 1973.

39. Forrester, J. S., Diamond, G., Chatterjee, K., et al. Medical therapy of acute myocardial infarction by application of hemodynamic subsets. *N. Engl. J. Med.* 295:1356 (part I), 1404 (part II), 1976.

40. Diamond, G., and Forrester, J. S. Effect of coronary artery disease and acute myocardial infarction on left ventricular compliance in man. *Circulation* 45:11, 1972.

41. Barry, W. H., Brooker, J. Z., Alderman, E. L.,

et al. Changes in diastolic stiffness and tone of the left ventricle during angina pectoris. *Circulation* 49:255, 1974.

42. Mann, T., Brodie, B. R., Grossmasn, W., et al. Effect of angina on the left ventricular diastolic pressure-volume relationship. *Circulation* 55:761, 1977.

43. Hess, O. M., Osakada, G., Lavelle, J. F., et al. Diastolic myocardial wall stiffness and ventricular relaxation during partial and complete coronary occlusions in the conscious dog. *Circ. Res.* 52:387, 1983.

44. Theroux, P., Ross, Jr., J., Franklin, D., et al. Regional myocardial function in the conscious dog during acute coronary occlusion and responses to morphine, propranolol, nitroglycerin, and lidocaine. *Circulation* 53:302, 1976.

45. Edwards, II, C. H., Rankin, J. S., McHale, P. A., et al. Effects of ischemia on left ventricular regional function in the conscious dog. *Am. J. Physiol.* 240:H413, 1981.

46. Forrester, J. S., Chatterjee, K., and Jobin, G. A new conceptual approach to the therapy of acute myocardial infarction. *Adv. Cardiol.* 15:111, 1975.

47. Crexells, C., Chatterjee, K., Forrester, J. S., et al. Optimal level of left heart filling pressures in acute myocardial infarction. *N. Engl. J. Med.* 289:1263, 1973.

48. O'Neill, W. W. Management of cardiogenic shock. In J. Topol (ed.), *Acute Coronary Intervention.* New York: Alan R. Liss, 1988. Pp. 195–213.

49. Chatterjee, K. Bedside hemodynamic monitoring. In W. Parmley and K. Chatterjee (eds.), *Cardiology.* Philadelphia, Lippincott, 1988.

50. Shelburne, J. C., Rubinstein, D., and Gorlin, R. A reappraisal of papillary muscle dysfunction: Correlative clinical and angiographic study. *Am. J. Med.* 46:862, 1969.

51. Nishimura, R. A., Schaff, H. V., Shuh, C., et al. Papillary muscle rupture complicating acute myocardial infarction: Analysis of 17 patients. *Am. J. Cardiol.* 51:373, 1983.

52. Wei, J. Y., Hutchins, G. M., and Bulkley, B. H. Papillary muscle rupture in fatal acute myocardial infarction. *Ann. Intern. Med.* 90:149, 1979.

53. Clements, S. D., Story, W. E., Hurst, J. W., et al. Ruptured papillary muscle, a complication of acute myocardial infarction: Clinical presentation, diagnosis and treatment. *Clin. Cardiol.* 8:93, 1985.

54. Chatterjee, K., Parmley, W. W., Swan, H. J. C., et al. Beneficial effects of vasodilator agents in severe mitral regurgitation due to dysfunction of subvalvular apparatus. *Circulation* 48:684, 1973.

55. Greenberg, B. H., Massie, B. M., Botvinick, E. H., et al. Beneficial effects of hydralazine in severe mitral regurgitation. *Circulation* 58:273, 1978.

56. Fox, A. C., Glassman, E., and Isom, O. W. Surgically remediable complications of myocardial infarction. *Prog. Cardiovasc. Dis.* 21:461, 1979.

57. Fargot, J. C., Borsante, L., Rigaud, M., et al. Two-dimensional echocardiographic visualization of ventricular septal rupture after acute anterior myocardial infarction. *Am. J. Cardiol.* 45:370, 1980.

59. Gray, R. J., Sethna, D., and Matloff, J. M. The role of cardiac surgery in acute myocardial infarction with mechanical complications. *Am. Heart J.* 106:723, 1983.

60. Shah, P. K., Maddahi, J., Berman, D. S., et al. Scintigraphically detected predominant right ventricular dysfunction in acute myocardial infarction: Clinical, hemodynamic correlates and implications for therapy and prognosis. *J. Am. Coll. Cardiol.* 6:1264, 1985.

61. Isner, J. M., and Roberts, W. C. Right ventricular infarction complicating left ventricular infarction complicating coronary artery disease. *Am. J. Cardiol.* 42:885, 1978.

62. Lorrell, B., Leinbach, R. C., Pohost, G. M., et al. Right ventricular infarction: Clinical diagnosis and differentiation from cardiac tamponade and pericardial constriction. *Am. J. Cardiol.* 43:465, 1979.

63. Goldstein, J. A., Vlahakes, G. J., Verrier, E. D., et al. The role of right ventricular systolic dysfunction and elevated intrapericardial pressure in the genesis of low output in experimental right ventricular infarction. *Circulation* 65:513, 1982.

64. Goldstein, J. A., Vlahakes, G. J., Verrier, E. D. et al. Volume loading improves low cardiac output in experimental right ventricular infarction. *J. Am. Coll. Cardiol.* 2:270, 1983.

14
Pharmacologic Support of the Failing Circulation in Acute Myocardial Infarction

JAY N. COHN

Acute myocardial infarction is the most dramatic event that may impair ventricular performance and produce acute circulatory failure. Although the mass of the myocardium infarcted is an important determinant of pump performance and thus plays a critical role in the genesis of circulatory failure [1], a number of other factors may contribute importantly to an overall depression in ventricular pump function and the development of the shock syndrome. They include both cardiac and peripheral factors.

Factors Influencing Ventricular Function

LOCATION OF INFARCTION

The importance of the location of the infarction in the genesis of pump dysfunction is uncertain. Anterior infarcts certainly produce more hemodynamic derangement than inferior infarcts, but this difference may be largely due to the larger mass of anterior wall infarcts. Inferior infarcts often are accompanied by damage to the posterior septum and the right ventricular free wall, resulting in impairment of right ventricular function [2]. The syndrome of right ventricular infarction may precipitate circulatory failure out of proportion to the extent of the left ventricular myocardial damage. When infarcts involve valvular structures, mechanical factors may contribute to the pump dysfunction (see below).

BEHAVIOR OF INFARCTED MYOCARDIUM

Infarcts may retain some contractile function because of islands of viable myocardium within the infarcted area protected by collateral flow; infarcts may become akinetic by virtue of the loss of contractile function but with residual stiffness in the area of infarction; or infarcts may become dyskinetic because of systolic bulging in the area of the infarction [3]. The more dyskinetic the infarct area becomes, the more likely it is that it will contribute to systolic pump dysfunction and circulatory failure.

PERI-INFARCTION ISCHEMIA

Even in transmural infarctions it is likely that some tissue in the infarcted zone as well as viable myocardium at the transmural or lateral borders of the infarcted area will remain ischemic because of inadequacy of blood flow. Such ischemia, even if transient, may contribute to profound depression of overall ventricular performance. The time course of recovery of this "stunned myocardium" is controversial [4].

VENTRICULAR ARRHYTHMIAS

Premature ventricular depolarizations and runs of ventricular tachycardia are common complications of acute myocardial infarction. Although occasional premature beats have little impact on overall ventricular performance or myocardial energy requirements, frequent ventricular premature beats may have a significant adverse effect on overall myocardial function, both by impairment of systolic emptying during the premature contraction and by an increase in myocardial oxygen consumption generated by the premature beat with no appreciable external mechanical work performed by the ventricle.

ACUTE MECHANICAL DEFECTS

Rupture of the septum or ventricular free wall, or ischemia or infarction of the papillary muscles, may precipitate acute hemodynamic stress that may be corrected only by surgical repair of the physical defect. In general, surgical repairs are best postponed for several weeks until healing improves the quality of the tissue to be sutured [5].

SYSTEMIC VASOCONSTRICTION

Vasoconstriction places an added burden on the impaired left ventricle by virtue of an increase of aortic impedance and ventricular preload [6]. In the setting of acute myocardial infarction, this vasoconstriction may at least in part be contributed by activation of the sympathetic nervous system or the renin-angiotensin system. Although these systems may be activated to support blood pressure at levels compatible with life, it is likely that some of the neurohormonal response may actually be deleterious to pump function and impair it more severely than would have been the case if systemic vasoconstriction had not been stimulated by the neurohormonal mechanisms.

SODIUM AND WATER RETENTION

Impaired delivery of sodium to the distal nephron of the kidney may result from both cardiac and neurohormonal changes in the setting of acute myocardial infarction. The re-sultant sodium retention may contribute to an increase in intravascular volume that produces signs and symptoms of pulmonary and systemic congestion.

Recognition of Circulatory Failure

Some degree of ventricular pump dysfunction accompanies most acute myocardial infarctions [7]. Therefore the challenge to the physician is to recognize when pump function is so severely impaired that pharmacologic or mechanical support for the circulation is necessary. Hemodynamic monitoring is essential for this task because it becomes vital to monitor both the cardiac filling pressure and the stroke volume in order to understand the severity of the pump dysfunction and to assess its response to treatment. Arterial pressure monitoring, preferably with an intra-arterial cannula and transducer, also is essential for guiding therapy.

In the past it was considered prudent to avoid pharmacologic support of the circulation unless the shock syndrome developed with evidence of impaired perfusion to critical vascular beds [8]. The present approach is considerably more aggressive because of the recognition that intelligent use of pharmacologic and mechanical support may not only improve the performance of the ventricle acutely but may also contribute to a long-term benefit [9].

Hemodynamic monitoring of ventricular pump function usually is complemented by monitoring of urine output, blood lactate levels, and arterial blood gases for assessment of the metabolic state [10]. When metabolic acidosis begins to develop, it is clear that aggressive correction of the regional flow deficiency is mandatory. Specific deficiencies in pump function or of organ functional abnormalities may require specific therapeutic approaches.

VENTRICULAR FILLING PRESSURE

Because acute myocardial infarction usually involves the left ventricle, the pulmonary capillary pressure or left ventricular filling pressure generally is increased out of proportion to the right ventricular filling pressure [7]. The exception to this situation occurs in patients in whom the infarction involves significant portions of the free wall of the right ventricle. Under these circumstances, right ventricular filling pressure may be as high or even higher than left ventricular filling pressure, suggesting predominant right ventricular failure [2].

Correction of the elevated left ventricular filling pressure may be important for several reasons: (1) The elevated pulmonary capillary pressure may contribute to pulmonary edema, impairment of oxygenation, and increased work of breathing; (2) elevated diastolic pressure in the left ventricle during diastole may impair subendocardial blood flow owing to the compressive forces of the high ventricular chamber pressure during diastole [11] and thus contribute to aggravation of myocardial ischemia and progressive impairment of pump performance; and (3) a high ventricular diastolic pressure impairs ventricular filling and may contribute to impaired systolic pump performance.

The increase in pulmonary capillary pressure that accompanies acute myocardial infarction may result from a decrease in compliance of the left ventricle as well as from impairment of systolic emptying. The compliance abnormality associated with acute ischemia and infarction may resolve over the first 48 hours in the hospital, evidenced by a gradual fall in pulmonary capillary pressure in most patients who are monitored during this period [12]. Because this reduction of pulmonary capillary pressure is not necessarily accompanied by an improvement in left ventricular ejection fraction, it is unlikely that all of the changes in pulmonary capillary pressure can be accounted for by improvement in systolic performance.

Reduction of the elevated left ventricular filling pressure may be accomplished by contraction of intravascular volume, an increase in venous or ventricular capacitance, or improvement in systolic pump performance. In general, the latter therapeutic approach is the least effective for acutely reducing the pulmonary capillary pressure [13].

CARDIAC OUTPUT

A low cardiac output following acute myocardial infarction may be reflected by clinical signs of impaired organ perfusion. Output generally is quantitated by an indicator dilution technique, most commonly using iced dextrose solution injected into the right atrium with a thermistor probe in the pulmonary artery [14]. A low cardiac output also should be reflected in a wide arterial-pulmonary arterial oxygen difference that can be quantitated by blood gas or oximetry measurements.

The goal of therapy should be to increase a depressed cardiac output without unduly burdening the dysfunctional left ventricle. Because increases in heart rate, blood pressure, and contractility demand greater myocardial oxygen consumption [15], the ischemic ventricle may be ill-served by interventions that result in such changes. Similarly, increases in ventricular volume result in a rise in wall stress that demands more oxygen. In contrast, the cost of myocardial fiber shortening in terms of energy consumption is low. Therefore interventions that improve shortening (e.g., a reduction in aortic impedance) without altering contractility or raising blood pressure or ventricular volume would be preferred in the setting of acute myocardial infarction [16].

On the other hand, coronary perfusion depends on aortic diastolic perfusion pressure, local coronary vascular resistance, and the compressive forces that impede subendocardial flow during diastole [17]. Thus an intervention that raises arterial pressure may increase myocardial oxygen consumption but at the same time may favorably influence the myocardial metabolic balance by augmenting myocardial blood flow. The net effect of pharmacologic interventions often cannot be predicted for a given patient but, rather, must be approached empirically, with careful and frequent assessment of the overall hemodynamic response to the intervention to determine if it is favorable or unfavorable.

Pharmacologic Agents

The drug groups that may be used to support the failing circulation in acute myocardial infarction include diuretics, vasodilator drugs, positive inotropic drugs, and vasoconstrictor drugs. Antiarrhythmic drugs often are employed in this clinical situation, but they are discussed elsewhere.

DIURETICS

Administration of furosemide or potent loop diuretics in patients with acute myocardial infarction may result in a considerable diuresis that gradually reduces the elevated pulmonary capillary pressure. Caution is necessary, though, during the first 30 minutes after intravenous administration of drugs such as furosemide because a vasoconstrictor effect may be stimulated by the loop diuretics perhaps by virtue of stimulation of the renin-angiotensin system and the sympathetic nervous system [18]. This early vasoconstrictor effect of furosemide may counterbalance the beneficial volume-depleting effect of the drug and sometimes may even precipitate an acute further rise of pulmonary capillary pressure until the diuresis has become well established.

The major task of diuretic therapy for acute myocardial infarction is that a reduction in left ventricular preload may result in a further reduction in stroke volume and cardiac output. The risk of such an adverse effect can be minimized by monitoring pulmonary arterial diastolic or wedge pressure and right atrial pressure, which should be allowed to fall to below the upper limits of normal of 12 and 6 mm Hg, respectively.

An alternative strategy advocated by many experts is to utilize vasodilator drugs as concomitant therapy in all patients who require diuretics in the setting of acute myocardial infarction. The vasodilators that exert an effect on the venous capacitance vessels [19] further reduce the elevated ventricular filling pressure, and their impedance-lowering effect favorably influences cardiac output. Thus diuretics combined with vasodilators seem to provide a favorable hemodynamic and renal profile.

VASODILATOR DRUGS

Vasodilator drugs are employed in the management of circulatory failure primarily for their systemic vascular effect of reducing the loading conditions on the left ventricle. Because some of these drugs also exert an effect on the coronary circulation, the pulmonary vasculature, and certain regional vascular beds, their actions may be considerably more complicated than their effects on left ventricular loading alone.

The most popular vasodilator agents for intravenous use in circulatory failure are nitroglycerin and sodium nitroprusside. Phentolamine and trimethaphan are no longer used because of potential adverse effects. Phosphodiesterase inhibitors exert vasodilator as well as inotropic effects, but they are considered with the inotropic drugs. The converting enzyme inhibitors and hydralazine are vasodilator drugs that are generally taken orally. However, parenteral forms of these compounds are available and may find some use in the management of circulatory failure.

The most striking difference in the circulatory effects of various vasodilator drugs is their relative action on venous capacitance, arterial compliance, arteriolar resistance, and heart rate. The differing effects of some of the vasodilators are depicted in Table 14-1. Increases in venous capacitance lead to redistribution of intravascular volume so that the intrathoracic volume falls, which usually results in decreased cardiac filling pressures. Arterial compliance and arteriolar resistance are the major factors influencing impedance to left ventricular ejection. An increase in compliance or a reduction in resistance allows better left ventricular emptying in patients with left ventricular dysfunction. The result is an increase in cardiac output. The heart rate effects of various vasodilators appear to differ, perhaps because of differing effects on barorecep-

Table 14-1
Hemodynamic response to vasodilators

Vasodilator	Arterial compliance	Arteriolar resistance	Venous capacitance	Reflex response
Nitrates	+ +	+	+ +	+
Nitroprusside	+ +	+ + +	+ +	+ +
Ca²⁺ antagonists	+ +	+ +	+	+
Hydralazine	0	+ + +	0	+ + +
ACE inhibitors	+	+ +	+ +	+

tors or independent effects on baroreceptor function or sympathetic reflexes. It is also clear that there is considerable individual variation in the heart rate response to vasodilating drugs, perhaps in part because of differences in neurohormonal state or concomitant drug therapy [20].

NITROGLYCERIN

Nitroglycerin and the other nitrates have a dominant action on venous capacitance and a prominent relaxing effect on the arterial compliance vessels [21]. The net effect of infusion of this drug is a reduction in ventricular filling pressure, a fall in systolic arterial pressure, and a slight increase in cardiac output with only a modest increase in heart rate.

Because nitroglycerin relaxes conduit coronary arteries and coronary collateral vessels, the drug has also been used for acute myocardial infarction in an effort to limit infarct size [22–24]. To have such a beneficial effect it may be necessary to begin infusion within the first few hours after onset of pain.

Nitroglycerin infusion is usually begun at a dose of about 20 μg/min, with gradual increases in the infusion rate until the pulmonary arterial diastolic or wedge pressure has been reduced to the goal pressure, usually about 15 mm Hg. Side effects of headache or nausea limit increments in dosage in some patients. Although there is considerable concern expressed about the development of vascular tolerance during continuous intravenous infusion of nitroglycerin [25], some hemodynamic effect appears to persist [26].

SODIUM NITROPRUSSIDE

Sodium nitroprusside exerts a venous capacitance effect similar to that of the nitrates, but in the doses used it produces far more potent arteriolar dilation [27]. Therefore impedance is strikingly reduced, and in the patient with left ventricular failure there usually is a prominent increase in cardiac output as well as a fall in right atrial and pulmonary capillary pressures [28]. Although nitroprusside appears to exert a relaxing effect on large arteries, including the conduit coronary arteries, it has not been thought to be as effective as nitroglycerin in increasing coronary collateral flow [29]. Therefore, nitroprusside may not be the drug of choice for improving perfusion of ischemic myocardium.

A controlled double-blind trial of a 48-hour nitroprusside infusion in patients with acute myocardial infarction complicated by an elevated pulmonary wedge pressure confirmed the favorable hemodynamic effects (compared to a placebo infusion) [9]. Furthermore, the study revealed contrasting effects on survival depending on the time of institution of the infusion. Early intervention within the first 8 hours after onset of infarction appeared to increase mortality, whereas later intervention led to a long-term reduction in mortality. The best explanation for this difference is that the early-intervention group included patients whose elevated pulmonary wedge pressure was not necessarily a manifestation of severe left ventricular systolic dysfunction and would have fallen spontaneously without treatment. Hypotension induced in these patients might have a deleterious effect on the myocardium. In contrast, patients with persistent elevation of pulmonary capillary pressure probably represent a group with more severe systolic dysfunction who benefit from the preload and impedance reduction induced by nitroprusside.

The appropriate clinical implication from this study should be to reserve nitroprusside therapy for patients who manifest clear evidence of severe ventricular systolic dysfunction after acute myocardial infarction. In that group prolonged therapy may have a favorable impact on survival.

Nitroprusside is infused intravenously in increasing doses with a dual aim of reducing elevated ventricular filling pressure and increasing cardiac output and tissue perfusion. Infusions may be initiated at 15 to 20 μg/min, with increases by 20 μg/min increments at 5- to 10-minute intervals until the desired effect is achieved. Rarely is it necessary in patients with acute myocardial infarction to exceed a dose of 200 μg/min. The limiting factor in infusion increments is the fall in arterial pressure. With acute infarction, care must be taken to avoid severe hypotension, which may further aggravate flow deficiency to the ischemic myocardium.

Once a desired hemodynamic response to nitroprusside has been achieved, the effect generally is stable with a constant infusion of the drug. Continuous infusions for 2 to 5 days are usually well tolerated, although a rebound overshoot of arterial and pulmonary capillary pressures may be observed when the drug infusion is withdrawn. During long-term infusion blood thiocyanate levels should be measured occasionally to be certain that this toxic metabolic product of nitroprusside is not accumulating [30]. Levels below 10 mg/dl are well tolerated.

CALCIUM ANTAGONISTS

The dihydropyridine calcium antagonists exert potent vasodilating effects that may be beneficial in certain clinical situations. These drugs appear to have more profound arterial than venous effects, so that their major action is to reduce impedance; they have only a modest effect on preload [31]. Many of these drugs also have the potential to produce a negative inotropic effect that can directly impair myocardial contractility. An increase in coronary artery caliber in response to these drugs also may have a favorable effect on flow through stenotic coronary arteries [17].

The only calcium antagonist currently widely used for intravenous therapy is verapamil, which has considerable electrophysiologic and negative inotropic effect and is not employed for acute vasodilator action [32].

OTHER VASODILATORS

Hydralazine, a potent arteriolar dilator [33], is available in a parenteral form. However, it probably is not a drug of choice for the acutely ischemic ventricle because it is difficult to titrate accurately, and it could aggravate myocardial ischemia.

The converting enzyme inhibitors captopril and enalapril have been used in the setting of acute myocardial infarction, but drug titration is difficult because of the steep dose-response effect of these agents [34]. It seems prudent to use directly acting vasodilators for the acute phase of circulatory instability and initiate converting enzyme inhibitor therapy later, if needed, to produce a chronic reduction in preload and aortic impedance.

Phentolamine, an alpha-adrenoceptor antagonist, has been used in the past as an intravenous dilator for acute infarction. The drug, however, tends to produce a prominent reflex tachycardia, and its venous capacitance effects are less prominent than those of nitroprusside [35].

Trimethaphan is a ganglionic blocker that markedly augments venous capacitance and reduces aortic impedance. Unfortunately, however, the severe side effects (orthostatic hypotension and parasympathetic blockade) make it a relatively undesirable vasodilator drug.

INOTROPIC DRUGS

Inotropic drugs are employed in the setting of left ventricular pump failure based on the hypothesis that there is contractile reserve in the myocardium that can be called on to augment ventricular contraction and improve the depressed cardiac performance. It is assumed that the contractility increase induced by these drugs augments myocardial oxygen consumption and thus potentially aggravates a delicate balance between oxygen delivery and consumption in marginally ischemic myocardium.

Most drugs currently available as potent inotropic agents exert their effect either by stimulating myocardial beta receptors or by increasing cyclic adenosine monophosphate (cAMP) through another mechanism, usually by inhibition of phosphodiesterase. Digitalis is a less potent inotropic drug whose action to increase contractility is exerted through inhibition of Na^+, K^+-ATPase with a resultant increase in intracellular Ca^{2+}. Because of its relative lack of acute potency, its modest vasoconstrictor effect [36], and its low toxic therapeutic ratio, digitalis is not generally advocated as an agent to increase myocardial contractility in acute unstable circulatory states.

DOBUTAMINE

Dobutamine is a well-tolerated inotropic drug that exerts its effect through activation of myocardial beta-1-adrenoceptors. Because it does not release norepinephrine and has only mild direct vascular effects, the pharmacodynamic response to the drug infusion can be attributed largely to its positive inotropic properties. Furthermore, it produces less chronotropic effect than other beta agonists [37] and therefore appears to be the drug of choice when increases in contractility, without tachycardia or blood pressure effects, are sought.

Dobutamine has a fairly reproducible dose-response effect that usually reaches an optimal effect on cardiac output at a dose of 10 to 15 μg/kg/min [38]. Infusions are generally begun at a dose of 2.5 to 5.0 μg/kg/min and increased gradually until the desired hemodynamic effect is achieved. Tachycardia or ventricular arrhythmia may limit the dosing increments. Because dobutamine as well

as other sympathomimetic drugs may produce hypokalemia, serum potassium should be monitored during the infusion and potassium administered if necessary.

DOPAMINE

Dopamine is a beta-1 agonist that exerts peripheral alpha-agonistic vasoconstrictor effects as well as dopamine-mediated vasodilator effects in the renal and splanchic beds [39]. Although low doses may exhibit predominant vasodilator action, the usual clinical doses tend to raise blood pressure in part by peripheral vasoconstrictor effects. Inotropic properties augment cardiac output, but the increase in output is generally less than with dobutamine because of the increased impedance generated by peripheral vasoconstriction [40]. Tachycardia is a common complication of higher-dose dopamine administration.

When an inotropic effect is desired in a severely hypotensive patient, dopamine is the agent of choice because it probably produces less adverse effects on visceral perfusion than norepinephrine. When a selective increase in renal perfusion is described, low doses of dopamine are occasionally beneficial. However, selective vasodilation usually is a less effective means of improving renal perfusion than the increase in perfusion that accompanies inotropic-agent-mediated increases in cardiac output.

AMRINONE, MILRINONE, AND PHOSPHODIESTERASE INHIBITORS

A variety of chemical compounds that inhibit cardiac phosphodiesterase (PDE) have been demonstrated to exert in vitro and in vivo inotropic effects. These cardiac actions, which appear to be due largely to increased myocardial concentration of cAMP, are usually accompanied by vasodilation, also caused by PDE inhibition [41]. The relative cardiac and peripheral vascular effects of these drugs appear to vary from agent to agent and to depend on the dose of the drug employed. During intravenous infusion of these drugs the major side effects relate to ventricular arrhythmias and hypotension.

Because the action of these PDE inhibitors does not depend on intact beta receptors, the drugs have a theoretical advantage in individuals who may have blocked or down-regulated beta receptors. However, beta agonists rarely are ineffective when the dose is titrated upward, and the disadvantage of the PDE inhibitors is that one cannot independently titrate the inotropic and vasodilator properties as can be done with independent infusions of dobutamine and nitroprusside.

NOREPINEPHRINE

During intravenous infusion the neurotransmitter norepinephrine exerts potent beta-1 inotropic and alpha-1 and alpha-2 vasoconstrictor effects. The net effect is a dose-dependent increase in arterial pressure often at the cost of a reduction in visceral perfusion. Norepinephrine should be viewed as emergency therapy for a severely hypotensive patient whose immediate survival is threatened by impaired cerebral or coronary perfusion. More appropriate pharmacologic or mechanical attempts to increase cardiac output should be instituted as soon as the severe hypotension has been moderated.

EPINEPHRINE, ISOPROTERENOL

The catecholamines epinephrine and isoproterenol exert considerable beta-2-agonist properties that increase skeletal blood flow and myocardial contractility via beta-1-stimulating properties. Tachycardia and maldistribution of cardiac output renders these drugs less desirable for restoring disturbed hemodynamics during pump failure.

Management of the Patient

The goals of therapy are to improve tissue perfusion, control the elevated ventricular filling pressure, support arterial pressure at a level adequate to maintain renal, cerebral, and coronary perfusion, and minimize the metabolic burden on the myocardium. These goals may be only partially attainable with pharmacologic interventions, but judicious use of the available agents effectively restores hemodynamic stability to most patients with pump failure accompanying acute myocardial infarction.

The cornerstones of therapy are the manipulation of preload and impedance to left ventricular ejection. Arterial pressure represents the integration of these factors and myocardial contractility.

VENTRICULAR PRELOAD

In the past it often was recommended that left ventricular preload be "optimized" by volume manipulations intended to bring pulmonary capillary pressure to about 20 mm Hg, the "peak" of the Frank-Starling curve. In more recent years this approach has been replaced by pharmacologic efforts to reduce pulmonary capillary pressure to the *lowest level compatible with adequate tissue perfusion.* The pulmonary capillary pressure can be reduced by diuretic administration (usually high-dose furosemide) or by intravenous infusion of nitroglycerin or nitroprusside. If these interventions result in a fall in pressure below levels that maintain adequate cardiac output, volume infusion in the form of crystalloid or colloid can restore pulmonary capillary pressure to a more suitable level. It should be recognized, however, that these patients usually are sensitive to volume, and even small amounts may profoundly raise filling pressure.

Right ventricular infarcts that produce predominant right ventricular failure require a different approach to therapy. Under these circumstances high right atrial (or central venous) pressures may be necessary to produce adequate left ventricular filling, and higher volumes of fluid may be required to correct the low cardiac output.

IMPEDANCE

The acutely damaged left ventricle functions optimally when impedance to left ventricular emptying is low. Therefore vasodilator drugs should be employed whenever possible to keep impedance at the lowest level compatible with adequate arterial pressure.

In patients with pump failure accompanied by systolic arterial pressure above 120 to 130 mm Hg, vasodilator therapy should be the primary form of therapy. Titration of nitroprusside to lower the filling pressure and improve cardiac output and tissue perfusion is the most effective therapy. In patients with borderline blood pressure nitroprusside may still be the agent of choice, but careful arterial pressure monitoring is mandatory, and the need for concomitant inotropic drug support must be considered. In patients who are already severely hypotensive, vasodilator therapy should be deferred until arterial pressure can be supported by other means.

Use of agents that increase impedance in order to support arterial pressure should be discouraged unless hypotension control is the primary agenda. Vasoconstrictor agents should be employed only if they also exert an inotropic effect. Norepinephrine and dopamine may be used for this purpose.

CONTRACTILITY

Agents that increase contractility have as their major adverse effects an increase in myocardial oxygen consumption and an increase in arrhythmia risk. Consequently, preload and impedance manipulation should generally be employed when appropriate before attempts to increase contractility are initiated. Dobutamine in a dose of 5 to 15 μg/kg/min is the agent of choice when an inotropic effect is sought.

REGIONAL PERFUSION

Failure to stabilize tissue perfusion with the optimal pharmacologic support described above calls for more aggressive measures. The combination of inotropic and vasodilator drugs may exert some favorable effect, but such patients usually have a grim prognosis unless interventional or surgical procedures can be performed. Intra-aortic balloon pumping, ventricular assist devices, emergency revascularization, or correction of structural defects are rational approaches in such patients. Heart transplantation may be the only viable long-term approach if ventricular function is irretrievably impaired.

Editorial Comments

Dr. Jay Cohn has had an interest in severe pump failure since the mid-1960s. As indicated in this chapter, there is now a large array of pharmacologic agents available to help support the failing circulation. Our strategy has been to use nitroprusside as the first drug of choice when systolic blood pressure is more than 90 mm Hg. Dobutamine should be used if blood pressure falls to less than 90 mm Hg while the patient is on nitroprusside. Dopamine is primarily reserved for patients with severe hypotension, although low doses (<2 μg/ kg/min) are useful in oliguric patients. Amrinone may be useful in patients unresponsive to dobutamine and can be combined with dobutamine for augmented effects. Varying combinations of these four agents are commonly used in critically ill patients refractory to any agent used alone. G.S.F.

References

1. Page, D. L., Caulfield, J. B., Kastol, J. A., et al. Myocardial changes associated with cardiogenic shock. *N. Engl. J. Med.* 285:133, 1971.
2. Cohn, J. N., Guiha, N. H., Broder, M. I., and Limas, C. J. Right ventricular infarction: Clinical and hemodynamic features. *Am. J. Cardiol.* 33:209, 1974.
3. Weisse, A. B., Saffa, R. S., Levinson, G. E., et al. Left ventricular function during the early and late stages of scar formation following experimental myocardial infarction. *Am. Heart J.* 79:370, 1970.
4. Braunwald, E., and Kloner, R. The stunned

myocardium: Prolonged, postischemic ventricular dysfunction. *Circulation* 66:1146, 1982.

5. Cohn, L. H. Surgical management of mechanical complications of myocardial infarction. *Am. Heart J.* 102:1049, 1981.

6. Cohn, J. N. Vasodilator therapy of myocardial infarction (Editorial). *N. Engl. J. Med.* 290:1433, 1974.

7. Hamosh, P., and Cohn, J. N. Left ventricular function in acute myocardial infarction. *J. Clin. Invest.* 50:523, 1971.

8. Cohn, J. N. Treatment of shock following myocardial infarction. *Calif. Med.* 111:66, 1969.

9. Cohn, J. N., Franciosa, J. A., Francis, G. S., et al. Effect of short-term infusion of sodium nitroprusside on mortality rate in acute myocardial infarction complicated by left ventricular failure. *N. Engl. J. Med.* 306:1129, 1982.

10. Cohn, J. N. Monitoring techniques in shock. *Am. J. Cardiol.* 26:565, 1970.

11. Salisbury, P. F., Cross, E. C., and Rieban, P. A. Acute ischemia of inner layers of ventricular wall. *Am. Heart J.* 66:650, 1963.

12. Franciosa, J. A., Guiha, N. H., and Limas, C. J., et al. Arterial pressure as a determinant of left ventricular filling pressure after acute myocardial infarction. *Am. J. Cardiol.* 34:506, 1974.

13. Mikulic, E., Cohn, J. N., and Franciosa, J. A. Comparative hemodynamic effects of inotropic and vasodilator drugs in severe heart failure. *Circulation* 56:528, 1977.

14. Forrester, J. S., Ganz, W., Diamond, G., et al. Thermodilution cardiac output with a single flow-directed catheter. *Am. Heart J.* 83:306, 1978.

15. Sonnenblick, E. H., Ross, Jr., J., and Braunwald, E. Oxygen consumption of the heart: New concepts of its multifactorial determination. *Am. J. Cardiol.* 22:328, 1968.

16. Franciosa, J. A., Notargiacomo, A. V., and Cohn, J. N. Comparative haemodynamic and metabolic effects of vasodilator and inotropic agents in experimental myocardial infarction. *Cardiovasc. Res.* 12:294, 1978.

17. Cohn, J. N., Bache, R. J., and Schwartz, J. S. Calcium entry blockers in coronary artery disease. In R. P. Rubin, G. B. Weiss, and J. W. Putney (eds.), *Calcium in Biological Systems*. New York: Plenum, 1985. Pp. 471–477.

18. Francis, G. S., Siegel, R. M., Goldsmith, S. R., et al. Acute vasoconstrictor response to intravenous furosemide in patients with chronic congestive heart failure. *Ann. Intern. Med.* 103:1, 1985.

19. Cohn, J. N., and Franciosa, J. A. Vasodilator therapy of cardiac failure. *N. Engl. J. Med.* 297:27, and 254, 1977.

20. Cohn, J. N. Myocardial infarction shock revisited. *Am. Heart J.* 74:1, 1967.

21. Zobel, L. R., Finkelstein, S. M., Carlyle, P. F., and Cohn, J. N. Pressure pulse contour analysis in determining the effect of vasodilator drugs on vascular hemodynamic impedance characteristics in dogs. *Am. Heart J.* 100:81, 1980.

22. Derrida, J. P., Sal, R., and Chiche, P. Favorable effects of prolonged nitroglycerin infusion in patients with acute myocardial infarction. *Am. Heart J.* 96:833, 1978.

23. Bussmann, W. D., Passek, D., Seidel, W., and Kaltenbach, M. Reduction of CK and CK-MB indexes of infarct size by intravenous nitroglycerin. *Circulation* 63:615, 1981.

24. Flaherty, J. T., Becker, L. C., Bulkley, B. H., et al. A randomized prospective trial of intravenous nitroglycerin in patients with acute myocardial infarction. *Circulation* 68:576, 1983.

25. Abrams, J. Nitrate tolerance and dependence. *Am. Heart J.* 99:113, 1980.

26. Leier, C. V., Bambach, D., Thompson, M. J., et al. Central and regional hemodynamic effects of intravenous isosorbide dinitrate, nitroglycerin and nitroprusside in patients with congestive heart failure. *Am. J. Cardiol.* 48:1115, 1981.

27. Cohn, J. N., and Burke, L. P. Diagnosis and treatment—drugs five years later: Nitroprusside. *Ann. Intern. Med.* 91:752, 1979.

28. Franciosa, J. A., Guiha, N. H., Limas, C. J., et al. Improved left ventricular function during nitroprusside infusion in acute myocardial infarction. *Lancet* 1:650, 1972.

29. Chiariello, M., Gold, H. K., Leinbach, R. C., et al. Comparison between the effects of nitroprusside and nitroglycerin on ischemic injury during acute myocardial infarction. *Circulation* 54:766, 1976.

30. McDowall, D. G., Keaney, N. P., Turner, J. M., et al. The toxicity of sodium nitroprusside. *Br. J. Anesth.* 46:327, 1974.

31. Olivari, M. T., Levine, T. B., and Cohn, J. N. Acute hemodynamic effects of nitrendipine in chronic congestive heart failure. *J. Cardiovasc. Pharmacol.* 6:S1002, 1984.

32. Millard, R. W., Lathrop, D. A., Grupp, G., et al. Differential cardiovascular effects of calcium channel blocking agents. Potential mechanisms. *Am. J. Cardiol.* 49:499, 1982.

33. Franciosa, J. A., Pierpont, G., and Cohn, J. N. Hemodynamic improvement after oral hydralazine in left ventricular failure: A comparison with nitroprusside infusion in 16 patients. *Ann. Intern. Med.* 86:388, 1977.

34. Chaterjee, K., Rouleau, J. L., and Parmley, W. W. Hemodynamic and myocardial metabolic effects of captopril in chronic heart failure. *Br. Heart J.* 47:233, 1982.

35. Richards, D. A., Woodings, E. P., and Pritchard, B. N. C. Circulatory and alpha-adrenoceptor blocking effects of phentolamine. *Br. J. Clin. Pharm.* 5:507, 1978.

36. Cohn, J. N., Tristani, F. E., and Khatri, I. M. Cardiac and peripheral vascular effects of digitalis in clinical cardiogenic shock. *Am. Heart J.* 78:318, 1969.

37. Tuttle, R. R., and Mills, J. Dobutamine: Development of a new catecholamine to selectively increase myocardial contractility. *Circ. Res.* 36:185, 1975.

38. Akhtar, N., Mikulic, E., Cohn, J. N., and Chaudhry, M. H. Hemodynamic effect of dobutamine in patients with severe heart failure. *Am. J. Cardiol.* 36:202, 1975.

39. Goldberg, L. I. Cardiovascular and renal action of dopamine: Potential clinical applications. *Pharmacol. Rev.* 24:1, 1972.

40. Francis, G. S., Sharma, B., and Hodges, M. Comparative hemodynamic effects of dopamine and dobutamine in patients with acute cardiogenic circulatory collapse. *Am. Heart J.* 103:995, 1982.

41. Benotti, J. R., Grossman, W., Braunwald, E., et al. Hemodynamic assessment of amrinone: A new inotropic agent. *N. Engl. J. Med.* 299:373, 1978.

15
Mechanical Support of the Failing Circulation in Acute Coronary Insufficiency and Myocardial Infarction

GORDON L. PIERPONT

Pathologic studies have demonstrated that loss of function of more than 40 percent of the left ventricle leads to almost certain death [1]. If damage to the heart is extensive or large areas of myocardium are rendered functionally inadequate, a point can be reached where the heart cannot maintain adequate circulation even with the most aggressive and judicious use of supportive pharmacologic therapy. When this situation occurs, mechanical assist of left ventricular function may be the only option that can maintain survival.

This chapter reviews various methods of providing mechanical assist to the heart. After defining the physiologic goals of mechanical support, the spectrum of devices available is placed in clinical perspective. The role of circulatory assist for treatment of acute coronary insufficiency is emphasized, with only brief mention of applications to other cardiac disorders.

Physiologic Goals of Mechanical Support

There are several effects desired of mechanical support devices aimed at reversing the pathophysiologic changes that occur when acute coronary insufficiency leads to severe left ventricular dysfunction (Table 15-1). The primary goal is to improve coronary blood flow, thereby reversing the precipitating de-fect of ischemia-induced myocardial dysfunction. It can be achieved by several mechanisms. Because almost all effective coronary perfusion occurs during diastole, increasing systemic aortic pressure during diastole improves coronary perfusion pressure. Concomitant lowering of left ventricular diastolic pressure further augments coronary flow by increasing the transmyocardial perfusion gradient. Hemodynamic benefits of enhanced myocardial perfusion pressure should benefit myocardial regions perfused by both normal and stenosed coronary arteries.

A second major goal of mechanical support is to decrease cardiac work, thereby diminishing myocardial oxygen demand. It can be accomplished by decreasing both afterload and preload, with the beneficial effects of lowering afterload predominating. Decreasing afterload is accomplished by lowering systemic pressure during systole; preload is lowered indirectly by mechanical circulatory support through improved cardiac output. If the heart rate is high or significant cardiac dysrhythmias are present, promoting a slow, stable, physiologic rhythm can also have marked beneficial metabolic consequences.

At the same time that cardiac work is decreased, cardiac output needs to be maintained to improve peripheral perfusion. It requires maintaining adequate systemic perfusion pressure while lowering peripheral vascular resistance, preferably selectively in the most vital organs. A final goal in most cases

Table 15-1
Goals of mechanical support

Improve myocardial perfusion
Increase coronary perfusion pressure
Decrease diastolic wall tension
Decrease myocardial work
Decrease afterload
Decrease preload
Stabilize heart rate
Improve peripheral blood flow
Relieve pulmonary and venous congestion

of severe left ventricular dysfunction is to decrease pulmonary and venous congestion. It is basically synonymous with decreasing diastolic left ventricular filling pressure (preload). As noted above, it can be achieved by improving overall left ventricular performance and by promoting diuresis through increased blood flow to the kidneys.

It is evident that achievement of these goals requires balancing some seemingly dichotomous interactions of the hemodynamic variables involved, e.g., increasing diastolic pressure while lowering systolic pressure, or simultaneously maintaining peripheral perfusion pressure while reducing cardiac afterload. Indirect effects of mechanical support may also be important. If systemic pressure and peripheral perfusion are maintained, beneficial effects of lowering adrenergic nervous system activity, promoting diuresis, and decreasing activation of the renin-angiotensin system may be achieved. The ultimate usefulness of a mechanical support device is determined by the extent to which these therapeutic goals are attained with minimal complications, low cost, rapid application, and ease of use.

Noninvasive Devices

External circulatory assist by *mechanical compression of the chest,* either manually or mechanically, falls into the category of cardiac resuscitation rather than cardiac assist. For information on this topic, the reader is referred to Chapter 21.

Rotating tourniquets are of historical interest only. Although recommended well into the 1970s [2, 3] as a method of decreasing pulmonary congestion by diminishing venous return and thereby pooling fluid in the extremities, there was scant scientific support of the efficacy of this procedure [4, 5]. In a systematic study of ten patients with acute congestive heart failure, Bertel and Steiner [6] found no beneficial hemodynamic effects of rotating tourniquets. In view of the rapid and effective decreases in pulmonary capillary wedge pressure obtainable with currently available vasodilators, diuretics, and inotropic agents (see Chapter 14), the devices previously sold to provide rotating tourniquets for treating pulmonary congestion can be appropriately relegated to collect dust in museums of medical history.

Military antishock trousers (MAST) compress the abdomen, legs, or both. They are used primarily for hypovolemic shock in out-of-hospital settings and have no role in supporting the circulation during acute cardiac ischemia associated with left ventricular failure or shock. In one report [7] certain individuals in cardiogenic shock appeared to benefit from the MAST suit, but these patients were concomitantly volume-depleted. Rapid volume expansion would be most appropriate in such situations. Most patients in cardiogenic shock already have high preload. By further increasing preload and by aggravating dyspnea because of mechanical restraints to thoracic movement, the MAST unit is more likely to be detrimental than beneficial for acute coronary insufficiency associated with left ventricular failure [8].

The concept of supporting the circulation using synchronized *external lower body counterpulsation* (ECP) was promoted in 1963 by Dennis et al. [9]. They were able to lower peak systolic aortic pressure and raise aortic diastolic pressure using an electronically controlled external counterpulsator on the hindquarters of dogs. Further experimental support for this methodology was provided by Soroff et al. [10], who noted a decrease in systolic pressure, as well as an increase in cardiac output, in dogs provided external assist. Sil-

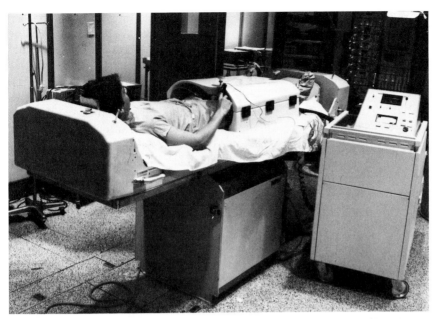

Fig. 15-1
Patient prepared for external counterpulsation of the legs. (From M. I. Kern et al. Effects of pulsed external augmentation of diastolic pressure on coronary and systemic dynamics in patients with coronary artery disease. *Am. Heart J.* 110:728, 1985. With permission.)

verstein et al. [11] demonstrated that ECP can increase diastolic perfusion pressure and improve coronary flow in experimental myocardial infarction. Their results were supported by those of Watson et al. [12], who studied dogs. After coronary artery ligation, they were able to produce increases in coronary collateral flow to ischemic myocardium with ECP equivalent to those obtained with the intra-aortic balloon pump.

Clinical application of external cardiac assist was reported by Wright to be partially responsible for survival in four patients in cardiogenic shock following cardiopulmonary bypass surgery [13]. In 17 patients with acute myocardial infarction studied by Parmley et al. [14], ECP was used in conjunction with nitroprusside to produce hemodynamic effects better than those seen with either nitroprusside or external assist alone. A patient undergoing ECP is seen in Figure 15-1.

In conjunction with reports by Kern et al. [15] of 14 patients with normal left ventricular function and by Beckman et al. [16] of 29 sur-

gical patients, it is evident that augmentation of systemic diastolic pressure can be achieved in patients using ECP, with variable increases in cardiac output. These studies provided background for a randomized cooperative trial of ECP for acute myocardial infarction that reported improved survival in patients with mild left ventricular failure treated with ECP [17]. Kuhn [18] pointed out some of the limitations of this study, and the Bethesda Conference Task Force V assessment [8] is appropriate in saying that: "Routine clinical use cannot be justified, and practical issues, in addition to efficacy, are patient discomfort and equipment cost." Although there may be a potential role of ECP in supporting the right side of the heart [19, 20], left ventricular failure is better supported by other means.

Invasive Devices

An *arterial counterpulsator* removes blood from the systemic arterial system to a reservoir chamber during ventricular systole, thereby decreasing ventricular afterload. It then empties back into the systemic circulation during diastole to augment diastolic perfusion pressure and flow to the coronary arteries and periphery. Such a device, described by Clauss et al. in 1961 [21], was used experimentally in dogs. Subsequent studies demonstrated the potential of this type of device to improve hemodynamics in experimental heart failure [22], decrease myocardial oxygen consumption [23–25], increase coronary flow [24–26], and preserve ischemic myocardium [27, 28], perhaps in part by opening dormant coronary collateral channels [29]. Despite continued evaluation of such devices [30], they have never progressed to significant clinical use, perhaps in large part because of evident superiority of the concomitantly developed intra-aortic balloon pumps and left ventricular assist devices.

The *intra-aortic balloon pump* (IABP) can be considered the circulatory assist device of choice [8]. Intra-aortic balloon counterpulsation was introduced during the early 1960s by Moulopoulos et al. [31]. It was successfully applied clinically by Kantrowitz et al. in 1967 [32] to two patients with cardiogenic shock complicating acute myocardial infarction, and one of the patients survived to leave the hospital. Early clinical use, often in preterminal patients, frequently met with relatively poor survival rates [32–39]. Nonetheless, it became clear that this technology offered improved chances of survival for some patients with a dismal prognosis. It led to progressive technologic improvement in equipment and technique, continued experimental studies evaluating physiologic effects of IABP in various animal models, and broader clinical application. A collective review by Weber and Janicki in 1974 [40] summarized the early data on IABP.

Operation of this device is conceptually illustrated in Figure 15-2. A long balloon connected to a controlling pump is positioned in

Fig. 15-2
Mechanism of circulatory support by intra-aortic balloon pumping. The balloon is collapsed during systole, allowing minimal interference with normal blood flow. Inflating the balloon during diastole increases diastolic pressure and enhances flow out of the aorta centrally and peripherally.

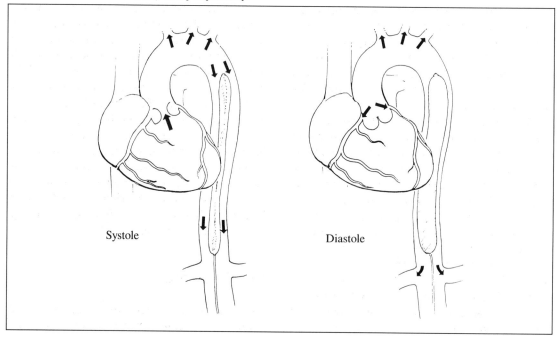

Systole

Diastole

the aorta distal to the great vessels but above the renal arteries. During systole, when blood is being ejected from the ventricle, the balloon is collapsed so as to interfere minimally with blood flow. By timing the cardiac cycle, the balloon is inflated during diastole to help force blood rapidly out of the aorta to the periphery and proximally to the heart and head. As the balloon collapses again with the next systole, blood volume in the aorta is lower, allowing easier ejection of blood from the left ventricle.

Two decades of clinical and research application of intra-aortic balloon pumping have resulted in a sound understanding of the physiologic effects of this intervention, although a few points remain controversial. The fact that peak diastolic pressure could be successfully augmented in the aorta was demonstrated early in both animals [31, 41] and man [32, 34–36, 42]. The increased peak diastolic pressure is usually associated with a lower end-diastolic aortic pressure. Augmentation of peak diastolic aortic pressure occurs independent of the status of the left ventricle so long as the

aortic valve is competent. Additional studies have supported these findings and demonstrated that systolic pressure decreases [34, 35, 42, 43] whereas mean aortic pressure changes little [42] or rises slightly [37, 44, 45] during IABP. These effects of IABP on aortic pressure are illustrated in Figures 15-3 and 15-4. Cardiac output is improved [34, 35, 37, 39, 42, 44, 46], and the pulmonary artery wedge pressure falls [37, 39, 46]. Collectively, these hemodynamic changes result in improved values for derived indices of ventricular performance. For example, the increase in cardiac output is usually greater than the increase in mean aortic pressure such that calculated peripheral vascular resistance is decreased [44, 46]. Ejection fraction [47] and stroke volume index [39] are increased. Secondarily, the heart rate is decreased [39, 42–44], and cardiac arrhythmias can sometimes be stabilized. Indeed IABP has been been used for the specific indication of treating postinfarction ventricular arrhythmias [48, 49].

Whereas the systemic hemodynamic effects

Fig. 15-3
Effect of intra-aortic balloon pump on systemic arterial pressure in a patient requiring postoperative support. With IABP treatment the peak diastolic pressure is increased, the end-diastolic pressure is decreased, the peak systolic pressure is decreased, and the mean pressure increases only slightly.

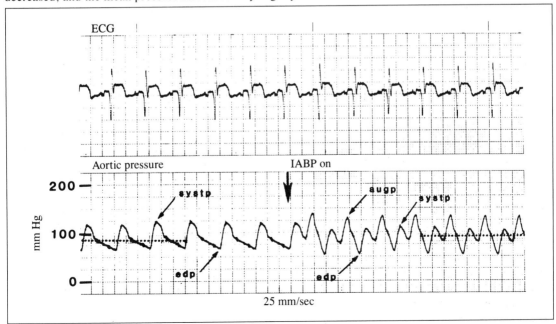

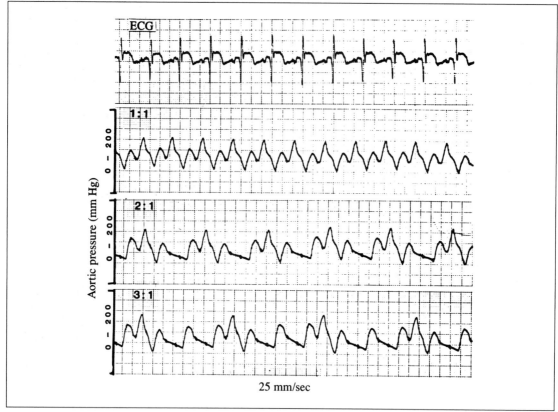

Fig. 15-4
The effects of intra-aortic balloon pumping on systemic pressure are evident as a
patient is "weaned" from support by progressing from 1:1 augmentation (balloon
inflated during every diastole) to 2:1 and then 3:1 augmentation (balloon inflated
every third diastole).

of IABP have been reproducible, changes in
myocardial blood flow have been more difficult to predict. Numerous experimental preparations in dogs have produced conflicting
results. For example, total coronary flow (coronary sinus flow) in dogs with normal hearts
was decreased during IABP in a study by
Feola et al. [50] but was essentially unchanged
in a study by Talpins et al. [51]. Talpins et al.
also found no effect of IABP on total coronary
flow if the dogs were subjected to hemorrhage
or sustained left ventricular injury by temporary left ventricular outflow occlusion. Yet
following coronary artery ligation, both Talpins et al. [51] and Feola et al. [50] noted improved total coronary flow with IABP. In right
heart bypass preparations studied by Tyberg

et al. [52], Powell et al. [53], and McDonnell
et al. [54], IABP during control conditions did
not alter coronary blood flow. However, in
this preparation coronary blood flow was improved by IABP at low cardiac output [52] and
low aortic blood pressures [53] but not following coronary artery ligation at normal systemic pressure [54].

Collectively, these results suggest that at
least in some situations (but not likely under
normal conditions) it may be possible to increase total coronary blood flow by intra-aortic balloon pumping. However, with ischemic
heart disease total coronary blood flow may
not be as important as regional flow to ischemic or peri-infarction zones. Flow to areas
fed by normal vessels would be of less impor-

tance unless left ventricular failure was severe enough to compromise total coronary flow. Using electromagnetic flowmeters, several investigators studied flow in uninvolved coronaries with or without ligation of a separate coronary artery [55–58]. Collectively, these four studies also suggest that IABP has little effect on coronary blood flow under normal conditions, but flow can be increased by intra-aortic balloon pump in normal coronaries after an adjacent coronary is ligated. Weber and Janicki [59] found similar results in calves; i.e., IABP improved coronary flow only in hypotensive animals.

Additional pertinent experimental data come from studies using alternate methods of measuring regional myocardial blood flow. Direct measurements of retrograde collateral flow distal to a coronary ligation made by Gundel et al. [60] and Feola et al. [61] in dogs demonstrated improved collateral flow during IABP. These findings were supplemented by those of Gill et al. [62], who used radioactive microspheres to demonstrate improved coronary blood flow to ischemic myocardium with IABP; in this study, however, flow to normal myocardium decreased with IABP. Shaw et al. [63] also used microspheres in dogs with ligated coronary arteries and found IABP to increase subendocardial blood flow in peri-infarction areas and normal areas but not in the infarction zone. These results were interpreted as improved collateral flow during IABP. On the other hand, using $Na^{131}I$ to measure "nutrient blood flow" to myocardium, Saini et al. [64] found that following coronary artery ligation IABP increased flow to all zones, i.e., normal, peri-infarction, and central infarction. Finally, in a study of pigs by Gewirtz et al. [65], IABP failed to alter either pressure or flow (by microspheres) distal to a coronary stenosis.

Despite the variability in the data on coronary blood flow, most studies consistently demonstrate that IABP can decrease myocardial oxygen utilization ($M\dot{V}O_2$) in experimental myocardial ischemia or infarction [53, 54, 65]. It thus remains difficult to assess whether beneficial effects of IABP on limiting infarct size [66, 67] or diminishing ischemic injury

[68] are primarily due to decreased cardiac workload and $M\dot{V}O_2$ or to improved myocardial perfusion.

Data from patients fail to provide a definitive answer to this question. Clinical studies measuring total coronary flow using coronary sinus catheterization, like the studies in animals, have been contradictory. Leinbach et al. [69] found IABP to have a variable effect on coronary flow in patients with acute myocardial infarction, with an overall surprising lack of improvement. Two reports by Mueller et al. [35, 44], on the other hand, suggested that coronary flow increases in most patients on IABP.

Similarly contradictory data evolved from studies selectively looking at flow in the great cardiac vein (which returns blood from the anterior myocardium) in patients with lesions in the left anterior descending coronary artery. Williams et al. [45] reported a decrease in selective flow from the affected area of myocardium during IABP and concluded that decreased myocardial work was more important than changes in myocardial perfusion. This conclusion was supported by the results of Port et al. [43], who used xenon ^{133} washout to measure a decrease in coronary blood flow, consistent with decreased myocardial workload, when IABP was instituted. Additionally, IABP failed to augment distal coronary perfusion pressure during percutaneous transluminal coronary angioplasty in three patients studied by MacDonald et al. [70]. By contrast, Fuchs et al. [71] found that great cardiac vein flow increased proportional to increases in systemic diastolic pressure with IABP in a similar group of patients. Whatever the mechanism (increased perfusion or decreased workload), IABP can improve myocardial lactate metabolism, i.e., increased lactate uptake and/or decreased lactate production [42], and improve regional wall motion in ischemic but not infarcted areas of the heart [72].

The inconsistencies in the results of these clinical and experimental studies are not surprising when the large number of variables that can alter coronary blood flow are considered. The effect of IABP on myocardial perfusion depends on such factors as baseline coronary and regional myocardial blood flow, the level of systemic perfusion pressure and left ventricular end-diastolic pressure, the myocardial workload, the extent to which autoregulatory mechanisms are still intact and functional, the severity of metabolic abnormalities both locally in the myocardium and systemically (e.g., pH, O_2 content), the degree of systemic and cardiac adrenergic activation and concentration of circulating neurohormones, the depth and type of anesthesia, the amount of myocardial functional reserve and extent to which pathologic changes in the myocardium are reversible, and the nature of the underlying pathologic process or processes initiating the myocardial dysfunction. Many of these factors have been discussed in the studies noted above, including some of the studies using an arterial counterpulsator, and differences in any one or more factors could easily account for variations in the results observed. It is unlikely that any single study could ever be so complete as to allow accurate prediction of the response of an individual patient with coronary insufficiency and left ventricular dysfunction to IABP. Nonetheless, independent of the mechanisms involved, it is reasonable to make two general statements.

1. IABP is not likely to be of benefit unless there is significant underlying pathology and the underlying process has some reversible component.
2. IABP can improve systemic hemodynamics and directly benefit the myocardium in appropriately selected patients.

In order to properly assess the potential benefits of IABP, the risks of this intervention must be carefully considered. Numerous studies have described myriad complications that can occur with IABP. Overall complication rates have ranged from 11 to 36 percent [73–95], with most series reporting between 10 and 20 percent. Differences between the complication rates among the reports can often be explained by factors such as whether investigators differentiated between major and minor complications, whether the series was pro-

spective or retrospective, and the percent of patients for whom extensive necropsy analysis was included. Selection criteria, insertion and maintenance techniques, and the time period over which the data were collected may also be pertinent. To gain a proper perspective, it is therefore instructive to attempt a compilation of the incidence of specific complications.

Not all attempts to insert an intra-aortic balloon are successful. Some studies on the complications of IABP fail to specifically note the number of failed attempts and if the failures were included in the series. Obviously, complications can occur even when the attempt at IABP therapy is unsuccessful. In 12 studies that reported the failure rate of attempted IABP treatment [77, 80, 82–84, 87, 95–100) the failure rate ranged from 5.7 to 21 percent, but most were approximately 10 percent.

The types of complications that can occur with IABP treatment are listed in Table 15-2 in relative order of frequency. The incidence of each type of major complication in Table 15-2 is a collective estimate based on the literature cited below.

By far the most common complication of IABP therapy is leg ischemia [73, 75–78, 82, 83, 91, 95, 97–99, 101–109). The leg is the most common site of ischemia because the femoral artery is by far the most common site of insertion for the intra-aortic balloon. Ischemia can be caused by mechanical occlusion of the ves-

Table 15-2
Complications of IABP treatment

Complication	Incidence (%)
Insertion failure	10
Leg ischemia	10
Mechanical obstruction	
Thromboembolism	
Vascular injury	5
Dissection	
Perforation	
Infection	2
Embolization/thrombosis	1
Hematologic disorder	1
Mechanical failure	1

sel from the balloon catheter or insertion sheath, by thrombosis, or by emboli that are either thrombotic or atherosclerotic in origin. The ischemia can produce necrosis requiring surgical intervention, including possible amputation. It can also lead to nerve damage resulting in footdrop or peripheral neuropathies. Residual obstruction can leave the patient who recovers with claudication.

The reported frequency of leg ischemia with IABP treatment ranges from a low of 3 percent to as high as 42 percent. However, some series reported ischemia only if subsequent permanent damage occurred, others if an additional procedure was required, and some if there was any evidence of ischemia during or following IABP insertion even if only transient. Collectively, based on the reports cited above, limb ischemia causing permanent damage or requiring intervention might be expected in 10 percent of patients undergoing treatment with the IABP.

Anticoagulation with heparin is often used to help decrease the incidence of thrombosis and embolization. Anticoagulation, of course, presents risks of bleeding, particularly in postoperative patients supported with IABP treatment. Pericardial tamponade due to anticoagulation has occurred [75], so this consideration is not trivial. The need to maintain pulsation of the balloon to decrease the incidence of thrombosis is well recognized and has been clearly demonstrated by Bernstein and Murphy [110]. It is possible that bleeding complications increase when the IABP is used subsequent to thrombolytic therapy, but pertinent data are lacking.

Vascular trauma is also reasonably common in patients on IABP treatment. Trauma to vessels is usually dissection or perforation and can lead to pseudoaneurysm formation, obstruction of branch vessels, bleeding, and hematoma formation. These complications can be expected to occur in approximately 5 percent of cases, as various reports range from 2.5 to 8.0 percent [77, 97, 102, 106, 111]. Vascular complications may well occur at the time of removal of the intra-aortic balloon [107], and careful attention to the removal technique is needed [98, 112]. Cutler et al. [113] recom-

mended surgical removal in all cases to help avoid complications.

Infection occurs in 1 to 6 percent of cases [73, 77, 82, 88, 97, 106] depending on whether local infections are included. Three studies differentiated local infection from sepsis [73, 77, 82]. In these reports sepsis ranged from 1.0 to 2.3 percent, and local infection from 3.0 to 5.7 percent. Unusual infections such as osteomyelitis of the spine have also been reported [76]. Because of the possibility of infection, many programs routinely use prophylactic antibiotics during IABP treatment.

Embolization or thrombosis of vessels other than the one used for insertion has led to a variety of complications involving multiple organ systems. Reported cases include splenic infarction [114], spinal cord infarction [115–118], mesenteric [76, 88, 99] or small bowel [119] infarction, renal artery thrombosis [42, 79], subclavian artery occlusion [120], and even cerebral vascular accident [83, 88]. The overall incidence of any one of these complications is low, but collectively a complication of this type can occur in 1 to 2 percent of cases.

Hematologic disorders, including hemolysis and thrombocytopenia, occur infrequently. Balloon malfunction, e.g., malposition, gas embolus, or balloon damage, also occur in a small percent of cases. Basically, with the widespread use of the IABP it is fair to say that almost any complication can potentially occur. For example, McCabe et al. [77] included a case of lymphocele (cystic lymphangioma) formation with lymphedema in their series, and Milgalter et al. [121] found a case in which a clot occurred in the balloon, making removal difficult. Finally, IABP treatment may have an impact on the patient's psychological status [122], particularly because it is most likely to be used in patients already under severe physical and psychological stress.

Complications are not equally likely to occur in all patients, and several factors have been identified to define patients at higher risk (Table 15-3). Peripheral vascular disease would be expected to be important and has been documented to be so by Alderman et al. [109], Goldman et al. [82], and Gottlieb et al.

Table 15-3
Risk factors for IABP complications

Peripheral vascular disease
Diabetes mellitus
Advanced age
Female gender
Shock
Hypertension
Percutaneous insertion/removal
Duration of use

---

[88]. Perhaps in part because of the high prevalence of vascular disease, diabetes mellitus is also a risk factor [99, 108, 109]. Similarly, advanced age may be important according to Weintraub and Thurer [87] and Goldberger et al. [92], although it was not in the series reported by Gottlieb et al. [88]. Women are more likely to suffer a complication of IABP treatment than men [86, 88, 93, 108, 109], perhaps because of the generally smaller size of their vessels. The importance of the status of the vasculature was further emphasized when Goldman et al. [82] noted that complications are more likely when insertion of the balloon is difficult. Aortoiliac angiography has been recommended [123] at the time of heart catheterization to assist in assessment of the pertinent vasculature for those patients likely to need IABP treatment. Not surprisingly, patients in shock may be more likely to suffer a complication than those with unstable angina but near-normal hemodynamics [82, 88, 103, 124]. Hypertension has been identified as a risk factor in one study [108], but it is not as likely to be important as the other factors noted above.

Early use of the IABP involved surgical techniques for balloon insertion. It was hoped that development of percutaneous techniques [80, 96, 105, 125, 126] would help decrease the incidence of complications. Unfortunately, it did not occur, and several studies have documented that the complication rate with percutaneous insertion is equal to or higher than that seen with surgical insertion [83–86, 88, 92–94, 113]. Complications increase the longer the balloon is in place [76, 82, 86, 88, 108,

127], and a well organized program of continuous patient monitoring is necessary to help minimize complications. Even so, the complications of IABP treatment are not trivial, in either incidence or severity, making the decision to use IABP in an individual patient a major and sometimes difficult option.

Clinical experience with the use of the IABP and knowledge of the likely outcome of its application in specific types of patient enhances the decision process when considering this intervention. Numerous institutions, encompassing thousands of patients, have reported their experience with clinical outcome following IABP treatment. The literature includes a series of specific groups with unstable angina [124, 128–131], myocardial infarction [103, 132–146], postoperative circulatory inadequacy [100, 147–154], or combinations of these and other disorders [72–75, 78, 81, 85, 87, 90, 92, 127, 155–159]. It becomes clear from an analysis of this collective experience that indications for IABP treatment cannot be easily listed in a way that will be all-inclusive. Nor is it reasonable to construct a simple decision tree that will guide us directly to the proper decision for every patient who may potentially benefit from IABP, as there are too many important factors to consider. Rather, we must carefully analyze the status of the patient along a spectrum of critical areas, then weigh the potential risks against the possible benefits of IABP treatment.

IABP therapy is useful for coronary insufficiency only when coronary lesions are critical, left ventricular function is inadequate to maintain peripheral perfusion despite optimal medical support, there are concomitant lesions such as mitral insufficiency or acquired ventricular septal defect causing inadequate cardiac output, or a combination of these situations. Moreover, because IABP treatment is supportive, not curative, the lesions must be potentially reversible. With rare exception, it means the patient with acute coronary insufficiency must be a candidate for surgery, angioplasty, or possibly cardiac transplantation [160, 161] in order for the physician to reasonably consider IABP therapy. *The first step when considering use of the IABP therefore is to establish that the patient is a candidate for further invasive procedures.*

Once it is established that a patient with acute coronary insufficiency is a candidate for aggressive, invasive therapy, subsequent management is determined by the severity of symptoms, extent of myocardial damage (and consequently the degree of hemodynamic compromise), amount of myocardium at risk, nature and severity of coronary obstruction, and presence of complications. The subsequent paragraphs provide a perspective on how IABP treatment is considered as the patient is assessed in each of these categories.

Symptoms of coronary insufficiency can range from not being present at all despite severe ischemia or infarction (silent ischemia), to severe intractable chest pain. Although the IABP has been successfully used to help alleviate the pain of unstable angina [124, 128], severe chest pain alone is not sufficient indication for its use. If the patient is hemodynamically stable, the symptoms should be treated aggressively with antianginal medication and then cardiac catheterization [162]. Olinger et al. [163] demonstrated that patients with unstable angina can be revascularized without IABP in most cases. Only when the intractable symptoms are also associated with significant cardiac dysfunction [164] or critical coronary anatomy (see below) is IABP treatment necessary. If such is the case, the IABP can be used as an adjunct to angioplasty [165] or surgery. It must also be realized that if there is ongoing myocardial necrosis, none of the available interventions may completely alleviate all pain, and narcotic analgesics are often necessary and appropriate.

The extent of myocardial damage and consequent degree of circulatory impairment are assessed with a complete hemodynamic profile as discussed in Chapter 13. *The functional status of the heart as a pump is the most critical factor determining the need for the IABP.* Pump function depends not only on the extent of myocardial dysfunction but also on the structural and functional integrity of the heart valves, interventricular septum, and electrical conduction system. Whenever there is clinical evidence of inadequate circulation, IABP

should be considered an option. However, it should be instituted only after it is evident that pharmacologic support alone (Chapter 14) is inadequate.

Assessment of the amount of myocardium at risk, as well as the nature and severity of the coronary obstruction, requires cardiac catheterization, often supplemented with data obtained by electrocardiography, echocardiography, nuclear imaging, and serum enzyme analysis. As mentioned previously, IABP is not likely to be helpful unless a reversible component to the disease is delineated with these studies. In the absence of severe pump failure, IABP may still be useful when there is a large area of myocardium at risk from a single critical coronary artery stenosis. Such is the case when there is a more than 90 percent stenosis of the left main coronary artery. This lesion carries a poor prognosis [166] and increases the risk of both cardiac catheterization [167] and coronary artery bypass surgery [168]. Perturbations in hemodynamic status that might otherwise be easily tolerated may be fatal with severe left main coronary artery disease. The experience of Cooper et al. [169] further supports use of the IABP in this situation.

Specific mention should be made of studies designed to prove the efficacy of using the IABP for acute myocardial infarction. Two randomized trials failed to detect a difference in mortality or morbidity with IABP treatment in this setting. O'Rourke et al. [133] evaluated the benefit of counterpulsation in limiting infarct size and improving survival in patients with acute myocardial infarction not considered for bypass surgery. Flaherty et al. [145] limited their study to patients in Killip class I or II at the time of entry, a group that would not likely meet the criteria for utilizing the IABP discussed above. Thus neither study examined the use of IABP therapy in the clinical setting in which we currently consider it most beneficial.

The management of acute coronary insufficiency has advanced dramatically. Interventions such as thrombolytic therapy and coronary angioplasty were not widely used over the period much of the clinical experience with the IABP cited previously was obtained. It is not likely that additional large-scale cooperative randomized trials to test the efficacy of the IABP in patients with acute coronary insufficiency will be forthcoming in the future. It would be much too difficult to limit the options available so that all patients are treated similarly and thus allow a fairly homogeneous group of patients to be randomized to IABP therapy versus conventional therapy. Moreover, "conventional therapy" is no longer easily defined and continues to evolve.

Once IABP therapy is instituted, a well structured program of patient monitoring and system maintenance by a coordinated team of well trained doctors, nurses, and technicians is necessary to ensure a good outcome and minimize complications. Routine care of patients on IABP includes use of prophylactic antibiotics, heparin anticoagulation to prevent thrombus and embolism, optimization of pump settings, treatment of complications, and careful determination of the appropriate timing and technique of balloon weaning and removal. More detailed discussion of these practical aspects of daily management of the patient on IABP treatment is contained in the books by Bolooki [170] and by Quaal [171].

Several systems have been devised to provide direct mechanical assist for the failing left ventricle. These devices are often labeled according to the degree of assist provided, whether they are designed to be temporary or permanent, and if they oxygenate the blood as well as circulate it.

Artificial hearts permanently replace the human heart and take over the total burden of maintaining circulation. None of the currently available models can maintain a person long term; and although the evolution of artificial hearts continues, they are currently limited to use at selected centers as a "bridge to cardiac transplantation." A detailed discussion of artificial heart technology and the moral and ethical considerations applicable to the use of artificial hearts is beyond the scope of this treatise.

Cardiopulmonary bypass temporarily takes over the functions of both heart and lungs and is more appropriately presented in textbooks of cardiovascular surgery. However, with current technology, there is not always a clear distinction between a cardiopulmonary bypass system and the more advanced left ventricular assist devices. When combined with an extracorporeal membrane oxygenator, some left ventricular assist systems basically become partial or even total cardiopulmonary bypass systems. We do not discuss those systems designed specifically for open heart surgery.

Skeletal muscle assistance of the left ventricle has several theoretic advantages. The energy source is intrinsic, running on mitochondrial energy derived from the food we eat, eliminating bulky power packs or lines to external power sources. In addition, using autogenous expendable muscle bundles, problems with rejection of foreign tissue or reaction to synthetic materials are avoided. Since 1958, when Kantrowitz and Mckinnon [172] first reported use of skeletal muscle to aid the heart, there have been many attempts to refine the technique. Muscle groups used have included sections of diaphragm [172–180] as well as the rectus abdominus [180–182], latissimus dorsi [182, 183], pectoralis major [182], and quadriceps femoris [184]. The muscles have been wrapped around the heart [172–174, 176, 183] or aorta [172, 182], formed into inlay or onlay grafts [173, 175, 177–180], or fashioned around chambers that could act as counterpulsation devices or valved conduits [182, 184]. In every configuration it is necessary to have a muscle-stimulating device that also senses cardiac activity and times the muscle contraction appropriately during systole or diastole.

Despite the fact that some successful augmentation has been achieved, fatigue continues to be a factor potentially limiting the technique of using skeletal muscle for left ventricular assist [176, 180, 185–187]. The structure and metabolic functions of skeletal muscle differ from those of cardiac muscle in several important ways [188]. Whereas cardiac muscle is arranged in a syncytium that contracts in unison, skeletal muscle is organized into motor units that are recruited individually. Cardiac action potentials are much longer than those of skeletal muscle, thus sustaining contraction throughout all of systole. Myocardium has more than tenfold as many mitochondria as skeletal muscle and is better suited for sustained aerobic metabolism to produce the high energy requirements of maintaining circulation. In addition, the contractile and membrane-bound proteins differ in the two types of muscle. It is not surprising that skeletal muscle cannot readily perform like cardiac muscle.

Studies have demonstrated that chronic low-frequency stimulation can condition skeletal muscle to be more fatigue-resistant [189–199]. Capillary density increases, mitochondria and enzymes of aerobic metabolism increase, and there are alterations in sarcoplasmic reticulum and contractile proteins. These changes result in transformation of "fast twitch" fibers to the slower-contracting and more fatigue-resistant "slow twitch" fibers. These phenomena have encouraged further interest in the potential use of skeletal muscle for left ventricular assist, and clinical application in two patients has been reported [200, 201]. However, because surgery is needed, followed by time for recovery and weeks of conditioning, this modality has little potential for emergency left ventricular support of acutely injured myocardium.

Electrically driven impeller pumps, roller pumps, pneumatic or electrically powered valved chamber pumps, and centrifugal pumps, have all seen service as *left ventricular assist devices* (LVADs). Impeller pumps have been limited by problems with thrombosis and hemorrhage [202] and have not progressed to clinical application. Roller pumps [203, 204], long used in cardiopulmonary bypass machines, are similarly restricted from long-term use because of blood trauma. Thus most LVADs currently in clinical use provide either pulsatile flow using chamber pumps or continuous flow using centrifugal pumps.

Chamber pumps consist of a flexible blood-filled chamber inside a rigid housing. The chamber has inlet and outlet valves to ensure unidirectional pulsatile flow as the chamber is intermittently compressed. Usually different function modes can allow pump ejection to be timed to the cardiac cycle, to run independently at set rates, or to begin ejection when complete filling is detected. One such pump, the Pierce-Donnachy [205–210], developed at Pennsylvania State University, is shown in Figure 15-5. The same group developed a similar pump (Fig. 15-6) with a pusher plate powered by a low-speed brushless DC motor [211]. Other pumps of this general type (Figs. 15-7 through 15-11) include an abdominal LVAD from the Collar Laboratory of the Texas Heart Institute [212, 213], an axisymmetric unit [214] and an electromechanical pusher-plate pump [215] developed at Children's Hospital and Harvard Medical School in Massachusetts, a microprocessor-controlled electromagnetic energy converter dual pusher-plate sac-type unit from Stanford University [216], and the hydraulic pump used at the Cleveland Clinic [217]. These units continue to evolve at a rate that often leaves a review obsolete by the time it is published.

Centrifugal pumps constitute the other ma-

Fig. 15-5
Pneumatically powered ventricular assist device is shown before chest closure as it would be used to remove blood from the left atrium and then pump it into the ascending aorta. (From W. S. Pierce et al. Ventricular-assist pumping in patients with cardiogenic shock after cardiac operations. *N. Engl. J. Med.* 305:1606, 1981. With permission.)

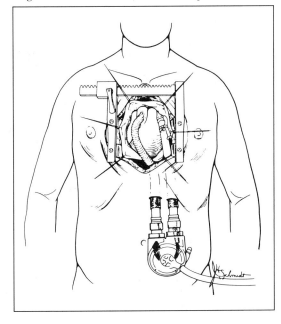

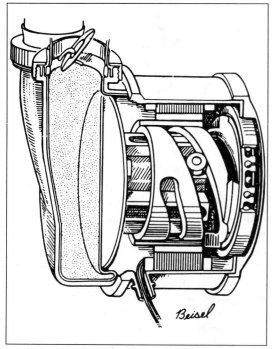

Fig. 15-6
Brushless DC electric-motor-driven cam blood pump with Bjork-Shiley inflow and outflow valves (clinical LVAD). (From W. E. Gaines et al. Development of a long-term electric motor left ventricular assist system. *Heart Transplant.* 3:323, 1984. With permission.)

jor class of devices used for left ventricular assist. These pumps move blood by centrifugal force transmitted to the blood from the rotor cones and impellar (Fig. 15-12). A pump of this type is manufactured by Biomedics, Inc. (Minneapolis, Minnesota) [207, 209, 218–223]. Although the pulsatile flow of the chamber pumps described above is more physiologic than the continuous flow provided by centrifugal pumps, centrifugal pumps do provide some advantages. Mechanically, these pumps are generally less complex than chamber pumps. Blood trauma is low, as is the propensity to develop air emboli. In conjunction with an oxygenator and heat exchanger, these pumps can provide cardiopulmonary bypass.

Most chamber pumps in general are designed for implantation, although some can be used either internally or externally. The ultimate goal of chamber pumps is an ambulatory patient with a portable power source. The centrifugal pumps are more restraining and currently are not considered for long-term ambulatory support. However, with the development of percutaneous insertion techniques [218], emergency rapid institution of ventricular support for patients with acute decomposition from ischemic heart disease is more

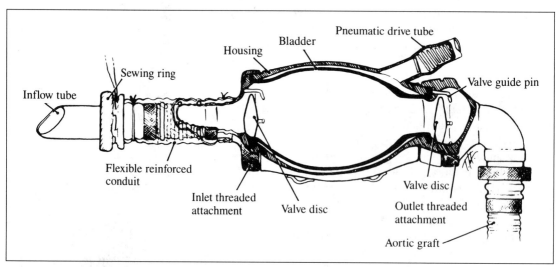

Fig. 15-7
Single-chambered balloon left ventricular assist device designed for intra-abdominal use with an external pneumatic drive console. (From D. A. Cooley. Staged cardiac transplantation: Report of three cases. *Heart Transplant.* 1:145, 1982. With permission.)

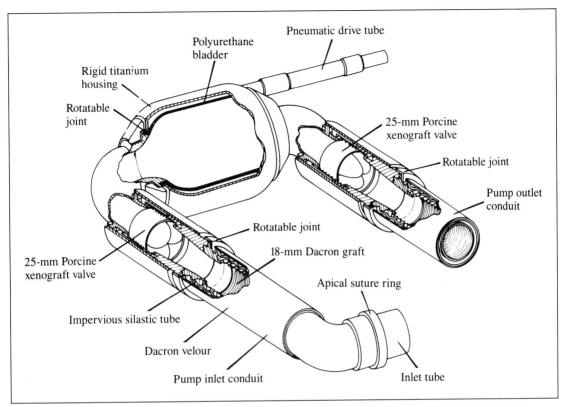

Fig. 15-8
Axisymmetric pneumatically powered ventricular assist device (clinical model 11
LVAD) fitted with porcine xenograft valves and woven Dacron grafts. (From
W. F. Bernard et al. Clinical and laboratory investigations related to temporary
and permanent ventricular bypass. *Heart Transplant.* 3:16, 1983. With
permission.)

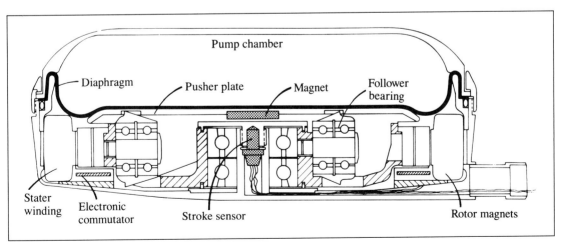

Fig. 15-9
Lateral view of an implantable pusher-plate pump powered by a 50-volt low-speed
torque motor. (From W. F. Bernhard et al. Investigations with an implantable
electrically activated ventricular assist device. *J. Thorac. Cardiovasc. Surg.*
88:11, 1984. With permission.)

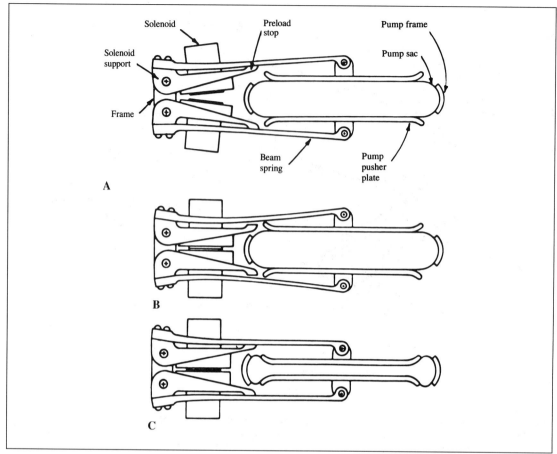

Fig. 15-10
Single-cycle spring-decoupled, pulsed solenoid electromechanical energy
converter pump. *A.* Pump filled. *B.* Solenoid closed and magnetically latched.
Start of eject stroke. *C.* End of eject stroke. (From P. M. Portner et al. An
alternative in end-stage heart disease: Long-term ventricular assistance. *Heart
Transplant.* 3:47, 1983. With permission.)

feasible. Figure 15-13 illustrates how such a pump can be hooked up for emergency left ventricular support. Percutaneous cannulation of the femoral artery and vein minimizes the time required to initiate support. By contrast, Figure 15-14 illustrates use of a pump inserted surgically, as might be done for ventricular assist following cardiovascular surgery. The latter method "unloads" the ventricle more efficiently but requires major surgery to initiate its use.

The potential use of left ventricular assistance for ischemic heart disease has been demonstrated in experiments by Pennock et al. [224] and Grossi et al. [225]. Both groups presented evidence that infarct size in dogs can be decreased using a left atrial to systemic arterial bypass. These findings were supported by those of Mickelborough et al. [223], who compared circulatory support with a centrifugal pump to that of IABP therapy combined with dopamine in dogs with myocardial depression from temporary ischemic arrest. They found less histologic evidence of necrosis in the dogs supported by left ventricular assistance. There is no similar comparison of IABP versus LVAD therapy in patients. Thus the IABP remains the first mechanical support

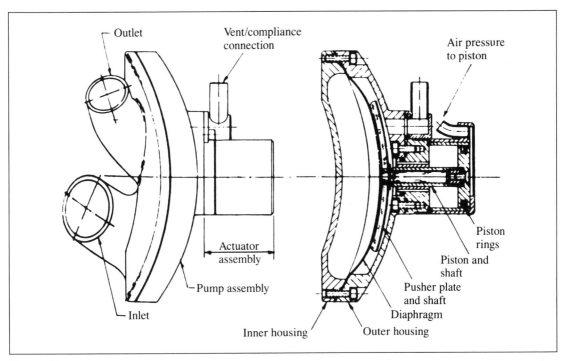

Fig. 15-11
Pneumatically powered pusher-plate left ventricular assist device. (From Y. Nose
et al. Experimental results for chronic left ventricular assist and total artificial
heart development. *Artif. Organs* 7:55, 1983. With permission.)

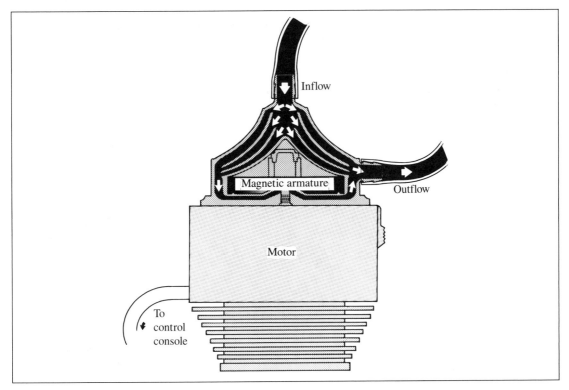

Fig. 15-12
Biomedicus centrifugal blood pump.

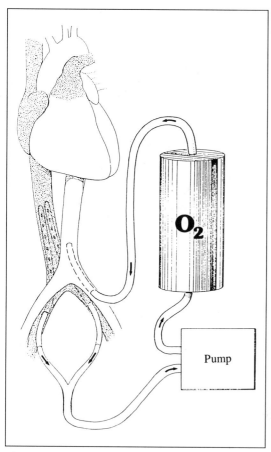

Fig. 15-13
External left ventricular assist device and extracorporeal oxygenator as it may be set up for emergency application using percutaneous arterial and venous access.

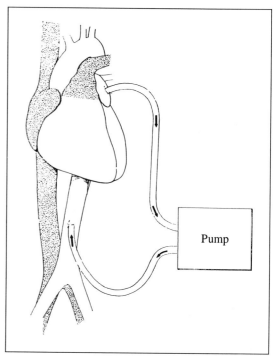

Fig. 15-14
Left ventricular assist device as it would be used to "unload" the left ventricle and sustain systemic perfusion. Surgical insertion is required.

system to be considered for acute decompensation of ischemic heart disease. An LVAD can be added (or possibly substituted) if the IABP alone is inadequate to support the circulation. The relative role of each of these devices will likely change in the future as both technology and application techniques continue to evolve.

Editorial Comments

The use of the IABP has declined at our hospital over the years, as we have learned to distinguish the patients who are not candidates for this highly invasive technique. As delineated by Dr. Pierpont, those patients not expected to be catheterized or operated should not undergo IABP placement, as there can be no certainty of effective treatment after such therapy. Patients with severe peripheral vascular disease should not be exposed to the risks of IABP placement. Interest appears to be rising for left ventricular assist devices, particularly for postoperative patients in need of cardiac transplantation. As these assist devices evolve, it is likely that our indications and needs for them will change accordingly. G.S.F.

References

1. Page, D. L., Caulfield, J. B., Kastor, J. A., et al. Myocardial changes associated with cardiogenic shock. *N. Engl. J. Med.* 285:133, 1971.
2. Robin, E. D., Cross, C. E., and Zelis, R. Pulmonary edema II. *N. Engl. J. Med.* 288:292, 1973.

3. Spann, J. F., and Hurst, J. W. Treatment of heart failure. In J. W. Hurst (ed.), *The Heart* (4th ed.). New York: McGraw-Hill, 1978.

4. Ebert, R. V., and Stead, Jr., E. A. The effect of the application of tourniquets on the hemodynamics of the circulation. *J. Clin. Invest.* 19:561, 1940.

5. Kountz, W. B., Smith, J. R., and Wright, S. T. Observations on the effect of tourniquets on acute cardiac crises, normal subjects, and chronic heart failure. *Am. Heart J.* 23:624, 1942.

6. Bertel, O., and Steiner, A. Rotating tourniquets do not work in acute congestive heart failure and pulmonary edema. *Lancet* 1:762, 1980.

7. Wayne, M. A. The MAST suit in the treatment of cardiogenic shock. *J. Am. Coll. Emerg. Physicians* 7:107, 1978.

8. Parmley, W. W., Hatcher, C. R., Ewy, G. A., et al. Task force V: Physical interventions and adjunctive therapy. *Am. J. Cardiol.* 50:409, 1982.

9. Dennis, C., Moreno, J. R., Hall, D. P., et al. Studies on external counterpulsation as a potential measure for acute left heart failure. *Trans. Am. Soc. Artif. Intern. Organs* 9:186, 1963.

10. Soroff, H. S., Birtwell, W. C., Giron, F., et al. Support of the systemic circulation and left ventricular assist by synchronous pulsation of extramural pressure. *Surg. Forum* 16:148, 1965.

11. Silverstein, D. M., Hamilton, G. W., and Hammermeister, K. E. The effect of external pressure diastolic augmentation on regional myocardial perfusion in experimental myocardial infarction. *Cardiology* 60:329, 1975.

12. Watson, J. T., Platt, M. R., Rogers, D. E., et al. Similarities in coronary flow between external counterpulsation and intra-aortic balloon pumping. *Am. J. Physiol.* 230:1616, 1976.

13. Wright, P. W. External counterpulsation for cardiogenic shock following cardiopulmonary bypass surgery. *Am. Heart J.* 90:231, 1975.

14. Parmley, W. W., Chatterjee, K., Charuzi, Y., and Swan, H. J. C. Hemodynamic effects of noninvasive systolic unloading (nitroprusside) and diastolic augmentation (external counterpulsation) in patients with acute myocardial infarction. *Am. J. Cardiol.* 33:819, 1974.

15. Kern, M. J., Henry, R. H., Lembo, N., et al. Effects of pulsed external augmentation of diastolic pressure on coronary and systemic hemodynamics in patients with coronary artery disease. *Am. Heart J.* 110:727, 1985.

16. Beckman, C. B., Dietzman, R. H., Romero, L. H., et al. Hemodynamic evaluation of external counterpulsation in surgical patients. *Surgery* 74:846, 1973.

17. Amsterdam, E. A., Banas, J., Criley, J. M., et al. Clinical assessment of external pressure circulatory assistance in acute myocardial infarction: Report of a cooperative clinical trial. *Am. J. Cardiol.* 45:349, 1980.

18. Kuhn, L. A. External pressure circulatory assistance: No light on the shadow. *Am. J. Cardiol.* 46:1069, 1980.

19. Heck, H. A., and Doty, D. B. Assisted circulation by phasic external lower body compression. *Circulation* 64(Suppl II):II-118, 1981.

20. Milliken, J. C., Laks, H., and George, B. Use of a venous assist device after repair of complex lesions of the right heart. *J. Am. Coll. Cardiol.* 8:922, 1986.

21. Clauss, R. H., Birtwell, W. C., Albertal, G., et al. Assisted circulation. I. The arterial counterpulsator. *J. Thorac. Cardiovasc. Surg.* 41:447, 1961.

22. Ellis, P. R., Lee, C., Wong, S. H., et al. Assisted circulation in treatment of experimental heart failure. *Arch. Surg.* 90:879, 1965.

23. Lefemine, A. A., Low, H. B. C., Cohen, M. L., et al. Assisted circulation. III. The effect of synchronized arterial counterpulsation on myocardial oxygen consumption and coronary flow. *Am. Heart J.* 64:789, 1962.

24. Hirsch, L. J., Lluch, S., and Katz, L. N. Counterpulsation effects of coronary blood flow and cardiac oxygen utilization. *Circ. Res.* 19:1031, 1966.

25. Spotnitz, H. M., Covell, J. W., Ross, J., and Braunwald, E. Left ventricular mechanics and oxygen consumption during arterial counterpulsation. *Am. J. Physiol.* 217:1352, 1969.

26. Goldfarb, D., Brown, B. G., Conti, C. R., and Gott, V. L. Cardiovascular responses to diastolic augmentation in the intact canine circulation and after ligation of the anterior descending coronary artery. *J. Thorac. Cardiovasc. Surg.* 55:243, 1968.

27. Goldfarb, D., Friesinger, G. C., Conti, C. R., et al. Preservation of myocardial viability by diastolic augmentation after ligation of the coronary artery in dogs. *Surgery* 63:320, 1968.

28. Sugg, W. L., Webb, W. R., and Ecker, R. R. Reduction of extent of myocardial infarction by counterpulsation. *Ann. Thorac. Surg.* 7:310, 1969.

29. Jacobey, J. A., Taylor, W. J., Smith, G. T., et al. A new therapeutic approach to acute coronary occlusion. II. Opening dormant coronary collateral channels by counterpulsation. *Am. J. Cardiol.* 11:218, 1963.

30. Nanas, J. N., Mason, J. W., Taenaka, Y., and Olsen, D. B. Comparison of an implanted abdominal aortic counterpulsation device with the intraaortic balloon pump in a heart failure model. *J. Am. Coll. Cardiol.* 7:1028, 1986.

31. Moulopoulos, S. D., Topaz, S., and Kolff,

W. J. Diastolic balloon pumping (with carbon dioxide) in the aorta—a mechanical assistance to the failing circulation. *Am. Heart J.* 63:669, 1962.

32. Kantrowitz, A., Tjonneland, S., Freed, P. S., et al. Initial clinical experience with intraaortic balloon pumping in cardiogenic shock. *J.A.M.A.* 203:135, 1968.

33. Kantrowitz, A., Krakauer, J. S., Rosenbaum, A., et al. Phase-shift balloon pumping in medically refractory cardiogenic shock. *Arch. Surg.* 99:739, 1969.

34. Buckley, M. J., Leinbach, R. C., Kastor, J. A., et al. Hemodynamic evaluation of intraaortic balloon pumping in man. *Circulation* 41,42(Suppl II):II-130, 1970.

35. Mueller, H., Ayres, S. M., Conklin, E. F., et al. The effects of intra-aortic counterpulsation on cardiac performance and metabolism in shock associated with acute myocardial infarction. *J. Clin. Invest.* 50:1885, 1971.

36. Bregman, D., and Goetz, R. H. Clinical experience with a new cardiac assist device: The dual-chambered intra-aortic balloon assist. *J. Thorac. Cardiovasc. Surg.* 62:577, 1971.

37. Dunkman, W. B., Leinbach, R. C., Buckley, M. J., et al. Clinical and hemodynamic results of intraaortic balloon pumping and surgery for cardiogenic shock. *Circulation* 46:465, 1972.

38. Leinbach, R. C., Gold, H. K., Dinsmore, R. E., et al. The role of angiography in cardiogenic shock. *Circulation* 47(Suppl III):III-95, 1973.

39. Dilley, R. B., Ross, Jr., J., and Bernstein, E. F. Serial hemodynamics during intra-aortic balloon counterpulsation for cardiogenic shock. *Circulation* 47,48(Suppl III):III-99, 1973.

40. Weber, K. T., and Janicki, J. S. Intraaortic balloon counterpulsation: A review of physiological principles, clinical results, and device safety. *Ann. Thorac. Surg.* 17:602, 1974.

41. Urschel, C. W., Eber, L., Forrester, J., et al. Alteration of mechanical performance of the ventricle by intraaortic balloon counterpulsation. *Am. J. Cardiol.* 25:546, 1970.

42. Scheidt, S., Wilner, G., Mueller, H., et al. Intra-aortic balloon counterpulsation in cardiogenic shock: Report of a co-operative clinical trial. *N. Engl. J. Med.* 288:979, 1973.

43. Port, S. C., Patel, S., and Schmidt, D. H. Effects of intraaortic balloon counterpulsation on myocardial blood flow in patients with severe coronary artery disease. *J. Am. Coll. Cardiol.* 3:1367, 1984.

44. Mueller, H., Ayres, S. M., Giannelli, Jr., S., et al. Effect of isoproterenol, l-norepinephrine, and intraaortic counterpulsation on hemodynamics and myocardial metabolism in shock following acute myocardial infarction. *Circulation* 45:335, 1972.

45. Williams, D. O., Korr, K. S., Gewirtz, H., and Most, A. S. The effect of intraaortic balloon counterpulsation on regional myocardial blood flow and oxygen consumption in the presence of coronary artery stenosis in patients with unstable angina. *Circulation* 66:593, 1982.

46. Ehrich, D. A., Biddle, T. L., Kronenberg, M. W., and Yu, P. N. The hemodynamic response to intra-aortic balloon counterpulsation in patients with cardiogenic shock complicating acute myocardial infarction. *Am. Heart J.* 93:274, 1977.

47. Steele, P., Pappas, G., Vogel, R., et al. Isosorbide dinitrate and intra-aortic balloon pumping in preinfarctional angina. *Chest* 69:712, 1976.

48. Mundth, E. D., Buckley, M. J., DeSanctis, R. W., et al. Surgical treatment of ventricular irritability. *J. Thorac. Cardiovasc. Surg.* 66:943, 1973.

49. Hanson, E. C., Levine, F. H., Kay, H. R., et al. Control of postinfarction ventricular irritability with the intraaortic balloon pump. *Circulation* 62(Suppl I):I-130, 1980.

50. Feola, M., Adachi, M., Akers, W. W., et al. Intraaortic balloon pumping in the experimental animal. *Am. J. Cardiol.* 27:129, 1971.

51. Talpins, N. L., Kripke, D. C., and Goetz, R. H. Counterpulsation and intraaortic balloon pumping in cardiogenic shock. *Arch. Surg.* 97:991, 1968.

52. Tyberg, J. V., Keon, W. J., Sonnenblick, E. H., and Urschel, C. W. Effectiveness of intra-aortic balloon counterpulsation in the experimental low output state. *Am. Heart J.* 80:89, 1970.

53. Powell, Jr., W. J., Daggett, W. M., Magro, A. E., et al. Effects of intra-aortic balloon counterpulsation on cardiac performance, oxygen consumption, and coronary blood flow in dogs. *Circ. Res.* 26:753, 1970.

54. McDonnell, M. A., Kralios, A. C., Tsagaris, T. J., and Kuida, H. Comparative effect of counterpulsation and bypass on left ventricular myocardial oxygen consumption and dynamics before and after coronary occlusion. *Am. Heart J.* 97:78, 1979.

55. Brown, B. G., Goldfarb, D., Topaz, S. R., and Gott, V. L. Diastolic augmentation by intraaortic balloon: Circulatory hemodynamics and treatment of severe, acute left ventricular failure in dogs. *J. Thorac. Cardiovasc. Surg.* 53:789, 1967.

56. Yahr, W. Z., Butner, A. N., Krakauer, J. S., et al. Cardiogenic shock: Dynamics of coronary blood flow with intra-aortic phase-shift balloon pumping. *Surg. Forum* 19:142, 1968.

57. Corday, E., Swan, H. J. C., Lang, T., et al. Physiologic principles in the application of circulatory assist for the failing heart: Intraaortic

balloon circulatory assist and venoarterial phased partial bypass. *Am. J. Cardiol.* 26:595, 1970.

58. Chatterjee, S., and Rosensweig, J. Evaluation of intra-aortic balloon counterpulsation. *J. Thorac. Cardiovasc. Surg.* 61:405, 1971.

59. Weber, K. T., and Janicki, J. S. Coronary collateral flow and intra-aortic balloon counterpulsation. *Trans. Am. Soc. Artif. Int. Organs* 19:395, 1973.

60. Gundel, W. D., Brown, B. G., and Gott, V. L. Coronary collateral flow studies during variable aortic root pressure waveforms. *J. Appl. Physiol.* 29:579, 1970.

61. Feola, M., Haiderer, O., and Kennedy, J. H. Intra-aortic balloon pumping (IABP) at different levels of experimental acute left ventricular failure. *Chest* 59:68, 1971.

62. Gill, C. C., Wechsler, A. S., Newman, G. E., and Oldham, Jr., H. N. Augmentation and redistribution of myocardial blood flow during acute ischemia by intraaortic balloon pumping. *Ann. Thorac. Surg.* 16:445, 1973.

63. Shaw, J., Taylor, D. R., and Pitt, B. Effects of intraaortic balloon counterpulsation on regional coronary blood flow in experimental myocardial infarction. *Am. J. Cardiol.* 34:552, 1974.

64. Saini, V. K., Hood, Jr., W. B., Hechtman, H. B., and Berger, R. L. Nutrient myocardial blood flow in experimental myocardial ischemia: Effects of intraaortic balloon counterpulsation and coronary reperfusion. *Circulation* 52:1086, 1975.

65. Gewirtz, H., Ohley, W., Williams, D. O., et al. Effect of intraaortic balloon counterpulsation on regional myocardial blood flow and oxygen consumption in the presence of coronary artery stenosis: Observations in an awake animal model. *Am. J. Cardiol.* 50:829, 1982.

66. Nachlas, M. M., and Siedband, M. P. The influence of diastolic augmentation on infarct size following coronary artery ligation. *J. Thorac. Cardiovasc. Surg.* 53:698, 1967.

67. Roberts, A. J., Alonso, D. R., Combes, J. R., et al. Role of delayed intraaortic balloon pumping in treatment of experimental myocardial infarction. *Am. J. Cardiol.* 41:1202, 1978.

68. Maroko, P. R., Bernstein, E. F., Libby, P., et al. Effects of intraaortic balloon counterpulsation on the severity of myocardial ischemic injury following acute coronary occlusion: Counterpulsation and myocardial injury. *Circulation* 40:1150, 1972.

69. Leinbach, R. C., Buckley, M. J., Austen, W. G., et al. Effects of intra-aortic balloon pumping on coronary flow and metabolism in man. *Circulation* 43(Suppl I):I-77, 1971.

70. MacDonald, R. G., Hill, J. A., and Feldman, R. L. Failure of intraaortic balloon counter-

pulsation to augment distal coronary perfusion pressure during percutaneous transluminal coronary angioplasty. *Am. J. Cardiol.* 59:359, 1987.

71. Fuchs, R. M., Brin, K. P., Brinker, J. A., et al. Augmentation of regional coronary blood flow by intra-aortic balloon counterpulsation in patients with unstable angina. *Circulation* 68:117, 1983.

72. Nichols, A. B., Pohost, G. M., Gold, H. K., et al. Left ventricular function during intraaortic balloon pumping assessed by multigated cardiac blood pool imaging. *Circulation* 58(Suppl I):I-176, 1978.

73. Beckman, C. B., Geha, A. S., Hammond, G. L., and Baue, A. E. Results and complications of intraaortic balloon counterpulsation. *Ann. Thorac. Surg.* 24:550, 1977.

74. Curtis, J. J., Barnhorst, D. A., Pluth, J. R., et al. Intra-aortic balloon assist: Initial Mayo Clinic experience and current concepts. *Mayo Clin. Proc.* 53:723, 1977.

75. Lefemine, A. A., Kosowsky, B., Madoff, I., et al. Results and complications of intraaortic balloon pumping in surgical and medical patients. *Am. J. Cardiol.* 40:416, 1977.

76. Pace, P. D., Tilney, N. L., Lesch, M., and Couch, N. P. Peripheral arterial complications of intra-aortic balloon counterpulsation. *Surgery* 82:685, 1977.

77. McCabe, J. C., Abel, R. M., Subramanian, V. A., and Gay, W. A. Complications of intraaortic balloon insertion and counterpulsation. *Circulation* 57:769, 1978.

78. McEnany, M. T., Kay, H. R., Buckley, M. J., et al. Clinical experience with intraaortic balloon pump support in 728 patients. *Circulation* 58:I-124, 1978.

79. Isner, J. M., Cohen, S. R., Virmani, R., et al. Complications of the intraaortic balloon counterpulsation device: Clinical and morphologic observations in 45 necropsy patients. *Am. J. Cardiol.* 45:260, 1980.

80. Subramanian, V. A., Goldstein, J. E., Sos, T. A., et al. Preliminary clinical experience with percutaneous intraaortic balloon pumping. *Circulation* 62(Suppl I):I-123, 1980.

81. Singh, J. B., Connelly, P., Kocot, S., et al. Intraaortic balloon counterpulsation in a community hospital. *Chest* 79:58, 1981.

82. Goldman, B. S., Hill, T. J., Rosenthal, G. A., et al. Complications associated with use of the intra-aortic balloon pump. *Can. J. Surg.* 25:153, 1982.

83. Hauser, A. M., Gordon, S., Gangadharan, V., et al. Percutaneous intraaortic balloon counterpulsation: Clinical effectiveness and hazards. *Chest* 82:422, 1982.

84. Alcan, K. E., Stertzer, S. H., Wallsh, E., et al. Comparison of wire-guided percutaneous

insertion and conventional surgical insertion of intra-aortic balloon pumps in 151 patients. *Am. J. Med.* 75:24, 1983.

85. Pennington, D. G., Swartz, M., Codd, J. E., et al. Intraaortic balloon pumping in cardiac surgical patients: A nine-year experience. *Ann. Thorac. Surg.* 36:125, 1983.

86. Shahian, D. M., Neptune, W. B., Ellis, F. H., and Maggs, P. R. Intraaortic balloon pump morbidity: A comparative analysis of risk factors between percutaneous and surgical techniques. *Ann. Thorac. Surg.* 36:644, 1983.

87. Weintraub, R. M., and Thurer, R. L. The intra-aortic balloon pump—a ten-year experience. *Heart Transplant.* 3:8, 1983.

88. Gottlieb, S. O., Brinker, J. A., Borkon, A. M., et al. Identification of patients at high risk for complications of intraaortic balloon counterpulsation: A multivariate risk factor analysis. *Am. J. Cardiol.* 53:1135, 1984.

89. LoCicero, J., Hartz, R. S., Sanders, Jr., J. H., et al. Interhospital transport of patients with ongoing intraaortic balloon pumping. *Am. J. Cardiol.* 56:59, 1985.

90. Vigneswaran, W. T., Reece, I. J., and Davidson, K. G. Intra-aortic balloon pumping: Seven years' experience. *Thorax* 40:858, 1985.

91. Corral, C. H. and Vaughn, C. C. Intraaortic balloon counterpulsation: An eleven-year review and analysis of determinants of survival. *Texas Heart Inst. J.* 13:39, 1986.

92. Goldberger, M., Tabak, S. W., and Shah, P. K. Clinical experience with intra-aortic balloon counterpulsation in 112 consecutive patients. *Am. Heart J.* 111:497, 1986.

93. Sanfelippo, P. M., Baker, N. H., Ewy, H. G., et al. Experience with intraaortic balloon counterpulsation. *Ann. Thorac. Surg.* 41:36, 1986.

94. Goldberg, M. J., Rubenfire, M., Kantrowitz, A., et al. Intraaortic balloon pump insertion: A randomized study comparing percutaneous and surgical techniques. *J. Am. Coll. Cardiol.* 9:515, 1987.

95. Alpert, J., Parsonnet, V., Goldenkranz, R. J., et al. Limb ischemia during intra-aortic balloon pumping: Indication of femorofemoral crossover graft. *J. Thorac. Cardiovasc. Surg.* 79:729, 1980.

96. Bregman, D., Nichols, A. B., Weiss, M. B., et al. Percutaneous intraaortic balloon insertion. *Am. J. Cardiol.* 46:261, 1980.

97. Harvey, J. C., Goldstein, J. E., McCabe, J. C., et al. Complications of percutaneous intraaortic balloon pumping. *Circulation* 64(Suppl II):II-114, 1981.

98. Vignola, P. A., Swaye, P. S., and Gosselin, A. J. Guidelines for effective and safe percutaneous intraaortic balloon pump insertion and removal. *Am. J. Cardiol.* 48:660, 1981.

99. Martin, R. S., Moncure, A. C., Buckley, M. J., et al. Complications of percutaneous intra-aortic balloon insertion. *J. Thorac. Cardiovasc. Surg.* 85:186, 1983.

100. Downing, T. P., Miller, D. C., Stofer, R., and Shumway, N. E. Use of the intra-aortic balloon pump after valve replacement: Predictive indices, correlative parameters, and patient survival. *J. Thorac. Cardiovasc. Surg.* 92:210, 1986.

101. Honet, J. C., Wajszczuk, W. J., Rubenfire, M., et al. Neurological abnormalities in the leg(s) after use of intraaortic balloon pump: Report of six cases. *Arch. Phys. Med. Rehabil.* 56:346, 1975.

102. Alpert, J., Bhaktan, E. K., Gielchinsky, I., et al. Vascular complications of intra-aortic balloon pumping. *Arch. Surg.* 111:1190, 1976.

103. O'Rourke, M. F., Sammel, N., and Chang, V. P. Arterial counterpulsation in severe refractory heart failure complicating acute myocardial infarction. *Br. Heart J.* 41:308, 1979.

104. Sutorius, D. J., Majeski, J. A., and Miller, S. F. Vascular complications as a result of intra-aortic balloon pumping. *Am. Surg.* 45:512, 1979.

105. Grayzel, J. Clinical evaluation of the percor percutaneous intraaortic balloon: Cooperative study of 722 cases. *Circulation* 66(Suppl I):I-223, 1982.

106. Perler, B. A., McCabe, C. J., Abbott, W. M., and Buckley, M. J. Vascular complications of intra-aortic balloon counterpulsation. *Arch. Surg.* 118:957, 1983.

107. Todd, G. J., Bregman, D., Voorhees, A. B., and Reemtsma, K. Vascular complications associated with percutaneous intra-aortic balloon pumping. *Arch. Surg.* 118:963, 1983.

108. Kantrowitz, A., Wasfie, T., Freed, P. S., et al. Intraaortic balloon pumping 1967 through 1982: Analysis of complications in 733 patients. *Am. J. Cardiol.* 57:976, 1986.

109. Alderman, J. D., Gabliani, G. I., McCabe, C. H., et al. Incidence and management of limb ischemia with percutaneous wire-guided intraaortic balloon catheters. *J. Am. Coll. Cardiol.* 9:524, 1987.

110. Bernstein, E. F., and Murphy, Jr., A. E. The importance of pulsation in preventing thrombosis from intra-aortic balloons. *J. Thorac. Cardiovasc. Surg.* 62:950, 1971.

111. Biddle, T. L., Stewart, S., and Stuard, I. D. Dissection of the aorta complicating intra-aortic balloon counterpulsation. *Am. Heart J.* 92:781, 1976.

112. Rodigas, P. C., and Finnegan, J. O. Technique for removal of percutaneously placed intraaortic balloons. *Ann. Thorac. Surg.* 40:80, 1985.

113. Cutler, B. S., Okike, N., and Vander Salm,

T. J. Surgical versus percutaneous removal of the intra-aortic balloon. *J. Thorac. Cardiovasc. Surg.* 86:907, 1983.

114. Busch, Jr., H. M., Cogbill, T. H., and Gundersen, A. E. Splenic infarction: Complication of intra-aortic balloon counterpulsation. *Am. Heart J.* 109:383, 1985.

115. Tyras, D. H., and Willman, V. L. Paraplegia following intraaortic balloon assistance. *Ann. Thorac. Surg.* 25:164, 1978.

116. Rose, D. M., Jacobowitz, I. J., Acinapura, A. J., and Cunningham, J. N. Paraplegia following percutaneous insertion of an intra-aortic balloon. *J. Thorac. Cardiovasc. Surg.* 87:788, 1984.

117. Harris, R. E., Reimer, K. A., Crain, B. J., Becsey, D. D., and Oldham, Jr., H. N. Spinal cord infarction following intraaortic balloon support. *Ann. Thorac. Surg.* 42:206, 1986.

118. Seifert, P. E. Late paraplegia resulting from intraaortic balloon pump. *Ann. Thorac. Surg.* 41:700, 1986.

119. Jarmolowski, C. R., and Poirier, R. L. Small bowel infarction complicating intra-aortic balloon counterpulsation via the ascending aorta. *J. Thorac. Cardiovasc. Surg.* 79:735, 1980.

120. O'Rourke, M. F., and Shepherd, K. M. Protection of the aortic arch and subclavian artery during intra-aortic balloon pumping. *J. Thorac. Cardiovasc. Surg.* 65:543, 1973.

121. Milgalter, E., Mosseri, M., Uretzky, G., and Romanoff, H. Intraaortic balloon entrapment: A complication of balloon perforation. *Ann. Thorac. Surg.* 42:697, 1986.

122. Patacky, M. G., Garvin, B. J., and Schwirian, P. M. Intra-aortic balloon pumping and stress in the coronary care unit. *Heart Lung* 14:142, 1985.

123. Bahn, C. H., Vitikainen, K. J., Anderson, C. L., and Whitney, R. B. Vascular evaluation for balloon pumping. *Ann. Thorac. Surg.* 27:474, 1979.

124. Weintraub, R. M., Voukydis, P. C., Aroesty, J. M., et al. Treatment of preinfarction angina with intraaortic balloon counterpulsation and surgery. *Am. J. Cardiol.* 34:809, 1974.

125. Wolfson, S., Karsh, D. L., Langou, R. A., et al. Modification of intraaortic balloon catheter to permit introduction by cardiac catheterization techniques. *Am. J. Cardiol.* 41:733, 1978.

126. Leinbach, R. C., Goldstein, J., Gold, H. K., et al. Percutaneous wire-guided balloon pumping. *Am. J. Cardiol.* 49:1707, 1982.

127. Macoviak, J., Stephenson, L. W., Edmunds, Jr., L. H., et al. The intraaortic balloon pump: An analysis of five years' experience. *Ann. Thorac. Surg.* 29:451, 1980.

128. Gold, H. K., Leinbach, R. C., Buckley, M. J., et al. Refractory angina pectoris: Follow-up after intraaortic balloon pumping and surgery. *Circulation* 54 (Suppl III):III-41, 1976.

129. Scully, H. E., Gunstensen, J., Williams, W. G., et al. Surgical management of complicated acute coronary insufficiency. *Surgery* 80:437, 1976.

130. Langou, R. A., Geha, A. S., Hammond, G. L., and Cohen, L. S. Surgical approach for patients with unstable angina pectoris: Role of the response to initial medical therapy and intraaortic balloon pumping in perioperative complications after aortocoronary bypass grafting. *Am. J. Cardiol.* 42:629, 1978.

131. Weintraub, R. M., Aroesty, J. M., Paulin, S., et al. Medically refractory unstable angina pectoris. I. Long-term follow-up of patients undergoing intraaortic balloon counterpulsation and operation. *Am. J. Cardiol.* 43:877, 1979.

132. O'Rourke, M. F., Chang, V. P., Windsor, H. M., et al. Acute severe cardiac failure complicating myocardial infarction: Experience with 100 patients referred for consideration of mechanical left ventricular assistance. *Br. Heart J.* 37:169, 1975.

133. O'Rourke, M. F., Norris, R. M., Campbell, T. J., et al. Randomized controlled trial of intraaortic balloon counterpulsation in early myocardial infarction with acute heart failure. *Am. J. Cardiol.* 47:815, 1981.

134. Mundth, E. D., Buckley, M. J., Gold, H. K., et al. Intraaortic balloon pumping and emergency coronary arterial revascularization for acute myocardial infarction with impending extension. *Ann. Thorac. Surg.* 16:435, 1973.

135. Baron, D. W., and O'Rourke, M. F. Long-term results of arterial counterpulsation in acute severe cardiac failure complicating myocardial infarction. *Br. Heart J.* 38:285, 1976.

136. Bardet, J., Rigaud, M., Kahn, J. C., et al. Treatment of post-myocardial infarction angina by intra-aortic balloon pumping and emergency revascularization. *J. Thorac. Cardiovasc. Surg.* 74:299, 1977.

137. Hagemeijer, F., Laird, J. D., Haalebos, M. M. P., and Hugenholtz, P. G. Effectiveness of intraaortic balloon pumping without cardiac surgery for patients with severe heart failure secondary to a recent myocardial infarction. *Am. J. Cardiol.* 40:951, 1977.

138. Johnson, S. A., Scanlon, P. J., Loeb, H. S., et al. Treatment of cardiogenic shock in myocardial infarction by intraaortic balloon counterpulsation and surgery. *Am. J. Med.* 62:687, 1977.

139. Leinbach, R. C., Gold, H. K., Harper, R. W., et al. Early intra-aorta balloon pumping for anterior myocardial infarction without shock. *Circulation* 58:204, 1978.

140. Levine, F. H., Gold, H. K., Leinbach, R. C., et al. Management of acute myocardial ischemia with intraaortic balloon pumping and coronary bypass surgery. *Circulation* 58(Suppl I):I-69, 1978.

141. Levine, F. H., Gold, H. K., Leinbach, R. C., et al. Safe early revascularization for continuing ischemia after acute myocardial infarction. *Circulation* 60(Suppl I):I-5, 1979.

142. DeWood, M. A., Notske, R. N., Hensley, G. R., et al. Intraaortic balloon counterpulsation with and without reperfusion for myocardial infarction shock. *Circulation* 61:1105, 1980.

143. Lorente, P., Gourgon, R., Beaufils, P., et al. Multivariate statistical evaluation of intraaortic counterpulsation in pump failure complicating acute myocardial infarction. *Am. J. Cardiol.* 46:124, 1980.

144. Pierri, M. K., Zema, M., Kligfield, P., et al. Exercise tolerance in late survivors of balloon pumping and surgery for cardiogenic shock. *Circulation* 62(Suppl I):I-138, 1980.

145. Flaherty, J. T., Becker, L. C., Weiss, J. L., et al. Results of a randomized prospective trial of intraaortic balloon counterpulsation and intravenous nitroglycerin in patients with acute myocardial infarction. *J. Am. Coll. Cardiol.* 6:434, 1985.

146. Laks, H., Rosenkranz, E., and Buckberg, G. D. Surgical treatment of cardiogenic shock after myocardial infarction. *Circulation* 74(Suppl III):III-11, 1986.

147. Buckley, M. J., Craver, J. M., Gold, H. K., et al. Intra-aortic balloon pump assist for cardiogenic shock after cardiopulmonary bypass. *Circulation* 47(Suppl III):III–90, 1973.

148. Bregman, D., Parodi, E. N., Edie, R. N., et al. Intraoperative unidirectional intra-aortic balloon pumping in the management of left ventricular power failure. *J. Thorac. Cardiovasc. Surg.* 70:1010, 1975.

149. Bolooki, H., Williams, W., Thurer, R. J., et al. Clinical and hemodynamic criteria for use of the intra-aortic balloon pump in patients requiring cardiac surgery. *J. Thorac. Cardiovasc. Surg.* 72:756, 1976.

150. Scanlon, P. J., O'Connell, J., Johnson, S. A., et al. Balloon counterpulsation following surgery for ischemic heart disease. *Circulation* 54(Suppl III):III-90, 1976.

151. Stewart, S., Biddle, T., and DeWeese, J. Support of the myocardium with intra-aortic balloon counterpulsation following cardiopulmonary bypass. *J. Thorac. Cardiovasc. Surg.* 72:109, 1976.

152. McGee, M. G., Zillgitt, S. L., Trono, R., et al. Retrospective analyses of the need for mechanical circulatory support (intraaortic balloon pump/abdominal left ventricular assist device or partial artificial heart) after cardiopulmonary bypass: A 44 month study of 14,168 patients. *Am. J. Cardiol.* 46:135, 1980.

153. Sturm, J. T., McGee, M. G., Fuhrman, T. M., et al. Treatment of postoperative low output syndrome with intraaortic balloon pumping: Experience with 419 patients. *Am. J. Cardiol.* 45:1033, 1980.

154. Downing, T. P., Miller, D. C., Stinson, E. B., et al. Therapeutic efficacy of intraaortic balloon pump counterpulsation: Analysis with concurrent "control" subjects. *Circulation* 64(Suppl II):II-108, 1981.

155. Foster, E. D., Subramanian, V. A., Vito, L., et al. Response to intra-aortic balloon pumping. *Am. J. Surg.* 129:464, 1975.

156. Willerson, J. T., Curry, G. C., Watson, J. T., et al. Intraaortic balloon counterpulsation in patients in cardiogenic shock, medically refractory left ventricular failure and/or recurrent ventricular tachycardia. *Am. J. Med.* 58:183, 1975.

157. Johnson, M. D., Holub, D. A., Winston, D. S., et al. Retrospective analysis of 286 patients requiring circulatory support with the intraaortic balloon pump. *Cardiovasc. Dis.* 4:428, 1977.

158. Frazier, O. H., Painvin, G. A., Urrutia, C. O., et al. Medical circulatory support: Clinical experience at the Texas Heart Institute. *Heart Transplant.* 2:299, 1983.

159. Folland, E. D., Kemper, A. J., Khuri, S. F., et al. Intraaortic balloon counterpulsation as a temporary support measure in decompensated critical aortic stenosis. *J. Am. Coll. Cardiol.* 5:711, 1985.

160. Bregman, D., Drusin, R., Lamb, J., et al. Heart transplantation in patients requiring mechanical circulatory support. *Heart Transplant.* 1:154, 1982.

161. Pennock, J. L., Pierce, W. S., Campbell, D. B., et al. Mechanical support of the circulation followed by cardiac transplantation. *J. Thorac. Cardiovasc. Surg.* 92:994, 1986.

162. Bristow, J. D., Burchell, H. B., Campbell, R. W., et al. Report of the ad hoc committee on the indications for coronary arteriography. *Circulation* 55:969A, 1977.

163. Olinger, G. N., Bonchek, L. I., Keelan, Jr., M. H., et al. Unstable angina: The case for operation. *Am. J. Cardiol.* 42:634, 1978.

164. Brundage, B. H., Ullyot, D. J., Winokur, S., et al. The role of aortic balloon pumping in postinfarction angina: A different perspective. *Circulation* 62(Suppl I):I-119, 1980.

165. Alcan, K. E., Stertzer, S. H., Wallsh, E., et al. The role of intra-aortic balloon counterpulsation in patients undergoing percutaneous transluminal coronary angioplasty. *Am. Heart J.* 105:527, 1983.

166. Takaro, T., Hultgren, H. N., Lipton, M. J., et al. The VA Cooperative Randomized Study of Surgery for Coronary Arterial Occlusive Disease. II. Subgroup with significant left main lesions. *Circulation* 54(Suppl III):III-107, 1976.

167. Davis, K., Kennedy, J. W., Kemp, Jr., H. G., et al. Complications of coronary arteriography from the collaborative study of coronary artery surgery (CASS). *Circulation* 59:1105, 1979.

168. Kennedy, J. W., Kaiser, G. C., Fisher, L. D., et al. Multivariate discriminant analysis of the clinical and angiographic predictors of operative mortality from the Collaborative Study in Coronary Artery Surgery (CASS). *J. Thorac. Cardiovasc. Surg.* 80:876, 1980.

169. Cooper, Jr., G. N., Singh, A. K., Christian, F. C., et al. Preoperative intra-aortic balloon support in surgery for left main coronary stenosis. *Ann. Surg.* 185:242, 1977.

170. Bolooki, H. *Clinical Application of Intra-aortic Balloon Pump* (2nd ed.). Mount Kisco, NY: Futura, 1984.

171. Quaal, S. J. *Comprehensive Intra-aortic Balloon Pumping*. St. Louis: Mosby, 1984.

172. Kantrowitz, A., and McKinnon, W. M. P. The experimental use of the diaphragm as an auxiliary myocardium. *Surg. Forum* 9:266, 1958.

173. Nakamura, K., and Glenn, W. W. L. Graft of the diaphragm as a functioning substitute for the myocardium. *J. Surg. Res.* 4:435, 1964.

174. Phillips, W. L., Pallin, S., and Crastnopol, P. Diaphragm transplantation: A preliminary report on an experimental form of permanent myocardial assistance. *Angiology* 20:628, 1969.

175. Shepherd, M. P. Diaphragmatic muscle and cardiac surgery. *Ann. R. Coll. Surg. Engl.* 45:212, 1969.

176. Kusaba, E., Schraut, W., Sawatoni, S., et al. A diaphragmatic graft for augmenting, left ventricular function: A feasibility study. *Trans. Am. Soc. Artif. Intern. Organs* 19:251, 1973.

177. Macoviak, J. A., Stephenson, L. W., Spielman, S. R., et al. Electrophysiologic and mechanical characteristics of diaphragmatic autograft used to enlarge right ventricle. *Surg. Forum* 31:270, 1980.

178. Macoviak, J. A., Stephenson, L. W., Spielman, S., et al. Replacement of ventricular myocardium with diaphragmatic skeletal muscle. *J. Thorac. Cardiovasc. Surg.* 81:519, 1981.

179. Macoviak, J. A., Stephenson, L. W., Alavi, A., et al. Effect of electrical stimulation on diaphragmatic muscle used to enlarge right ventricle. *Surgery* 90:271, 1981.

180. Dewar, M. L., Drinkwater, D. C., Wittnich, C., and Chu-Jeng Chiu, R. Synchronously stimulated skeletal muscle graft for myocardial repair: An experimental study. *J. Thorac. Cardiovasc. Surg.* 87:325, 1984.

181. Drinkwater, Jr., D. C., Chiu, R. C. J., Modry, D., et al. Cardiac assist and myocardial repair with synchronously stimulated skeletal muscle. *Surg. Forum* 31:271, 1980.

182. Neilson, I. R., Brister, S. J., Khalafalla, A. S., and Chiu, R. C.-J. Left ventricular assistance in dogs using a skeletal muscle powered device for diastolic augmentation. *Heart Transplant.* 4:343, 1985.

183. Termet, H., Chalencon, J.-L., Estour, E., et al. Transplantation sur le myocarde d'un muscle strie excite par pace maker. *Ann. Chir. Thorac. Cardiovasc.* 5:260, 1966.

184. Kusserow, B. K., and Clapp, J. F. A small ventricle type pump for prolonged perfusion: Construction and initial studies, including attempts to power a pump biologically with skeletal muscle. *Trans. Am. Soc. Artif. Intern. Organs* 10:74, 1964.

185. Spotnitz, H. M., Merker, C., and Malm, J. R. Applied physiology of the canine rectus abdominus: Force-length curves correlated with functional characteristics of a rectus powered "ventricle": Potential for cardiac assist. *Trans. Am. Soc. Artif. Intern. Organs* 20:747, 1974.

186. Von Recum, A., Stulc, J. P., Hamada, O., et al. Long-term stimulation of a diaphragm muscle pouch. *J. Surg. Res.* 23:422, 1977.

187. Stevens, L., and Brown, J. Can noncardiac muscle provide useful cardiac assistance? Preliminary studies of the properties of skeletal muscle. *Am. Surg.* 52:423, 1986.

188. Adams, R. J., and Schwartz, A. Comparative mechanisms for contraction of cardiac and skeletal muscle. *Chest* 78:123, 1980.

189. Salmons, S., and Sreter, F. A. Significance of impulse activity in the transformation of skeletal muscle type. *Nature* 263:30, 1976.

190. Salmons, S., and Vrbova, G. The influence of activity on some contractile characteristics of mammalian fast and slow muscles. *J. Physiol. (Lond.)* 201:535, 1969.

191. Pette, D., and Schnez, U. Coexistence of fast and slow type myosin light chains in single muscle fibres during transformation as induced by long term stimulation. *FEBS Lett.* 83:128, 1977.

192. Salmons, S., Gale, D. R., and Sreter, F. A. Ultrastructural aspects of the transformation of muscle fibre type by long term stimulation: Changes in Z discs and mitochondria. *J. Anat.* 127:17, 1978.

193. Eisenberg, B. R., and Salmons, S. The reor-

ganization of subcellular structure in muscle undergoing fast-to-slow type transformation. *Cell Tissue Res.* 220:449, 1981.

194. Salmons, S., and Henriksson, J. The adaptive response of skeletal muscle to increased use. *Muscle Nerve* 4:94, 1981.

195. Macoviak, J. A., Stephenson, L. W., Armenti, F., et al. Electrical conditioning of in situ skeletal muscle for replacement of myocardium. *J. Surg. Res.* 32:429, 1982.

196. Sreter, F. A., Pinter, K., Jolesz, F., and Mabuchi, K. Fast to slow transformation of fast muscles in response to long-term phasic stimulation. *Exp. Neurol.* 75:95, 1982.

197. Armenti, F., Bitto, T., Macoviak, J. A., et al. Transformation of canine diaphragm to fatigue-resistant muscle by phrenic nerve stimulation. *Surg. Forum* 135:258, 1984.

198. Frey, M., Thoma, H., Gruber, H., et al. The chronically stimulated muscle as an energy source for artificial organs: Preliminary results of a basic study in sheep. *Eur. Surg. Res.* 16:232, 1984.

199. Brister, S., Fradet, G., Dewar, M., et al. Transforming skeletal muscle for myocardial assist: A feasibility study. *Can. J. Surg.* 28:341, 1985.

200. Carpentier, A., and Chachques, J. C. Myocardial substitution with a stimulated skeletal muscle: First successful clinical case. *Lancet* 6:1267, 1985.

201. Magovern, G. J., Park, S. B., Magovern, Jr., G. J., et al. Latissimus dorsi as a functioning synchronously paced muscle component in the repair of a left ventricular aneurysm. *Ann. Thorac. Surg.* 41:116, 1986.

202. Unger, F., Genelin, A., Hager, J., et al. Heart replacement with biventricular assist device using nonpulsatile impeller blood pumps (Imp-BVAD). *Heart Transplant.* 2:311, 1983.

203. Litwak, R. S., Koffsky, R. M., Jurado, R. A., et al. Use of a left heart assist device after intracardiac surgery: Technique and clinical experience. *Ann. Thorac. Surg.* 21:191, 1976.

204. Rose, D. M., Colvin, S. B., Culliford, A. T., et al. Late functional and hemodynamic status of surviving patients following insertion of the left heart assist device. *J. Thorac. Cardiovasc. Surg.* 86:639, 1983.

205. Pierce, W. S., Donachy, J. H., Landis, D. L., et al. Prolonged mechanical support of the left ventricle. *Circulation* 58(Suppl I):I-133, 1978.

206. Pierce, W. S., Parr, G. V. S., Myers, J. L., et al. Ventricular-assist pumping in patients with cardiogenic shock after cardiac operations. *N. Engl. J. Med.* 305:1606, 1981.

207. Pennington, D. G., Codd, J. E., Merjavy, J. P., et al. The expanded use of ventricular bypass systems for severe cardiac failure and as a bridge to cardiac transplantation. *Heart Transplant.* 3:38, 1983.

208. Pennock, J. L., Pierce, W. S., Bull, A. P., and Waldhausen, J. A. Use of the ventricular assist pump for postcardiotomy cardiogenic shock. *Heart Transplant.* 3:26, 1983.

209. Pennington, D. G., Bernhard, W. F., Golding, L. R., et al. Long-term follow-up of postcardiotomy patients with profound cardiogenic shock treated with ventricular assist devices. *Circulation* 72(Suppl II):II-216, 1985.

210. Pae, Jr., W. E., Pierce, W. S., Pennock, J. L., et al. Long-term results of ventricular assist pumping in postcardiotomy cardiogenic shock. *J. Thorac. Cardiovasc. Surg.* 93:434, 1987.

211. Gaines, W. E., Rosenberg, G., Pennock, J. L., and Pierce, W. S. Development of a long-term electric motor left ventricular assist system. *Heart Transplant.* 3:323, 1984.

212. Norman, J. C., Duncan, J. M., Frazier, O. H., et al. Intracorporeal (abdominal) left ventricular assist devices or partial artificial hearts. *Arch. Surg.* 116:1441, 1981.

213. Cooley, D. A. Staged cardiac transplantation: Report of three cases. *Heart Transplant.* 1:145, 1982.

214. Bernhard, W. F., Clay, W., Shoen, F. J., et al. Clinical and laboratory investigations related to temporary and permanent ventricular bypass. *Heart Transplant.* 3:16, 1983.

215. Bernhard, W. F., Gernes, D. G., Clay, W. C., et al. Investigations with an implantable, electrically actuated ventricular assist device. *J. Thorac. Cardiovasc. Surg.* 88:11, 1984.

216. Portner, P. M., Oyer, P. E., Jassawalla, J. S., et al. An alternative in end-stage heart disease: Long-term ventricular assistance. *Heart Transplant.* 3:47, 1983.

217. Nose Y., Jacobs, G., Kiraly, R. J., et al. Experimental results for chronic left ventricular assist and total artificial heart development. *Artif. Organs* 7:55, 1983.

218. Phillips, S. J., Ballentine, B., Slonine, D., et al. Percutaneous initiation of cardiopulmonary bypass. *Ann. Thorac. Surg.* 36:223, 1983.

219. Eugene, J., Ott, R. A., Moore-Jeffries, E. W., and Haiduc, N. J. Left atrial-to-aortic assistance: Effect of in-line venting on myocardial oxygen consumption. *Heart Transplant.* 3:329, 1984.

220. Zumbro, Jr., G. L., Shearer, G., Kitchens, W. R., and Galloway, R. F. Mechanical assistance for biventricular failure following coronary bypass operation and heart transplantation. *Heart Transplant.* 4:348, 1985.

221. Park, S. B., Liebler, G. A., Burkholder, J. A., et al. Mechanical support of the failing heart. *Ann. Thorac. Surg.* 42:627, 1986.

222. Magovern, G. J., Park, S. B., Magovern, Jr.,

G. J., et al. Mechanical circulatory assist devices. *Texas Heart Inst. J.* 14:276, 1987.

223. Mickleborough, L. L., Rebeyka, I., Wilson, G. J., et al. Comparison of left ventricular assist and intra-aortic balloon counterpulsation during early reperfusion after ischemic arrest of the heart. *J. Thorac. Cardiovasc. Surg.* 93:597, 1987.

224. Pennock, J. L., Pierce, W. S., and Waldhausen, J. A. Quantitative evaluation of left ventricular bypass in reducing myocardial ischemia. *Surgery* 79:523, 1976.

225. Grossi, E. A., Krieger, K. H., Cunningham, Jr., J. N., et al. Time course of effective interventional left heart assist for limitation of evolving myocardial infarction. *J. Thorac. Cardiovasc. Surg.* 91:624, 1986.

16
Pump Failure, Shock, and Cardiac Rupture in Acute Myocardial Infarction

PREDIMAN K. SHAH AND GARY S. FRANCIS

Nearly 1 million patients are hospitalized in the United States each year with a diagnosis of acute myocardial infarction, and the early course (the first 2 to 4 weeks) of this disease is associated with a 5 to 15 percent mortality. Pump failure secondary to extensive myocardial loss is the leading cause of in-hospital mortality as well as a major determinant of postdischarge morbidity and mortality [1, 2]. In this chapter we discuss the pathogenesis, clinical presentation, and therapy of this important complication.

Pathogenesis of Acute Myocardial Infarction

CORONARY ARTERY

That coronary thrombosis is the culprit of evolving acute myocardial infarction in nearly all cases has now been amply confirmed by in vivo angiographic studies, careful autopsy studies, and recovery of a coronary thrombus from the artery of infarction in patients undergoing emergency coronary artery bypass surgery [3–5]. Thus the previous controversy regarding the primary versus the secondary nature of coronary thrombosis has now been laid to rest, and the primary role of coronary thrombosis in the pathogenesis of acute myocardial infarction is firmly established [4, 5].

Fissuring of an atherosclerotic plaque with subsequent exposure of the subintimal connective tissue to circulating platelets appears to initiate the process of coronary thrombosis. Coronary thrombus is totally occlusive in about 80 percent of patients studied within the early hours of evolving transmural myocardial infarction, whereas in about 20 percent of cases coronary thrombus results in subtotal or intermittent occlusion.

WAVE-FRONT PROGRESSION OF MYOCARDIAL NECROSIS

The dynamic and temporal dependence of myocardial necrosis following coronary artery occlusion has been demonstrated. After acute coronary occlusion in experimental animals, necrosis begins within 15 to 20 minutes near the subendocardium within the myocardial area at risk and progresses toward the epicardium in a wave front of cell death such that it involves about 70 to 80 percent of the risk area by 6 hours [6]. When coronary occlusion is subtotal rather than total, or when there are well developed collaterals to the area at risk, the progression of myocardial necrosis may proceed more slowly and to a smaller transmural extent.

In man, studies of myocardial perfusion, viability, and recovery of function following reperfusion suggest that the pattern and time sequence of myocardial necrosis may be similar to that in dogs and primates, with nearly complete necrosis of the area at risk within 3 to 6 hours of persistent and total occlusion of the coronary artery, although in individual patients the time required for transmural spread of necrosis may vary as a function of the magnitude of residual flow and myocardial oxygen demand. The recognition of time-dependent evolution of necrosis provides a brief "window of opportunity" during which interventions can be applied to abort the transmural speed of necrosis and to limit the eventual size of the infarction.

PUMP FAILURE

The clinical syndrome of pump failure in acute myocardial infarction (Fig. 16-1) results from one or more of the following consequences of acute myocardial infarction: (1) regional contractile dysfunction of the left or right ventricle (or both); (2) regional and global diastolic dysfunction; (3) infarct expansion and ventricular remodeling; or (4) mechanical complications such as mitral regurgitation, interventricular septal rupture, and cardiac free-wall rupture. Additional factors contributing to the pump failure syndrome include sustained or recurrent supraventricular or ventricular arrhythmias, persistent severe bradyarrhythmias including complete heart block, use of potent negative inotropic drugs, relative or absolute hypovolemia, electrolyte disturbances, acid-base disequilibrium, and abnormalities of pulmonary gas exchange.

CONTRACTILE DYSFUNCTION

Severe reduction or total cessation of coronary blood flow, the proximate cause of acute myocardial infarction, results in abnormalities of regional contractile function ranging from hypokinesis (reduction in the extent of shortening), to akinesis (loss of contraction), to dyskinesis (systolic expansion) [7] (Fig. 16-2). The extent of myocardium involved, as well as the type of regional contractile dysfunction, determines the ultimate change in global left ventricular volumes and ejection fraction (Fig.

16-2). Without compensatory mechanisms, progressive abnormalities of regional contractile function result in an increased end-systolic volume with a consequent decrease in stroke volume and ejection fraction. Similarly, an increasing extent of myocardium involved in contractile dysfunction leads to a progressively larger end-systolic volume and a lower stroke volume and ejection fraction. Reduction in stroke volume, in turn, leads to a reduction in cardiac output. When contractile dysfunction involves 10 percent of the left ventricular perimeter, the left ventricular ejection fraction declines with a minimal decrease in stroke volume, whereas fatal cardiogenic shock is usually associated with involvement of 40 percent or more. Clinical evidence of heart failure is generally observed when contractile dysfunction involves 25 to 40 percent of the left ventricular perimeter.

COMPENSATORY MECHANISMS

Several compensatory mechanisms are activated to minimize the hemodynamic consequences of contractile dysfunction in acute myocardial infarction.

1. Increased sympathoadrenal activity with increased circulating catecholamines helps to increase the heart rate, systemic vascular resistance, and inotropic state of the residual myocardium. Sympathoadrenal stimulation, however, may also increase the risk of arrhythmias, exacerbate myocardial ischemia by increasing myocardial oxygen consumption, and increase left ventricular afterload by producing systemic vasoconstriction.

Fig. 16-1
Pathogenesis of pump failure following acute myocardial infarction (AMI). VSD = ventricular septal defect; RV = right ventricular; SV = stroke volume; CO = cardiac output; BP = blood pressure; EDV = end-diastolic volume; PCW = pulmonary capillary wedge pressure; PAEDP = pulmonary arterial end-diastolic pressure; LV = left ventricular.

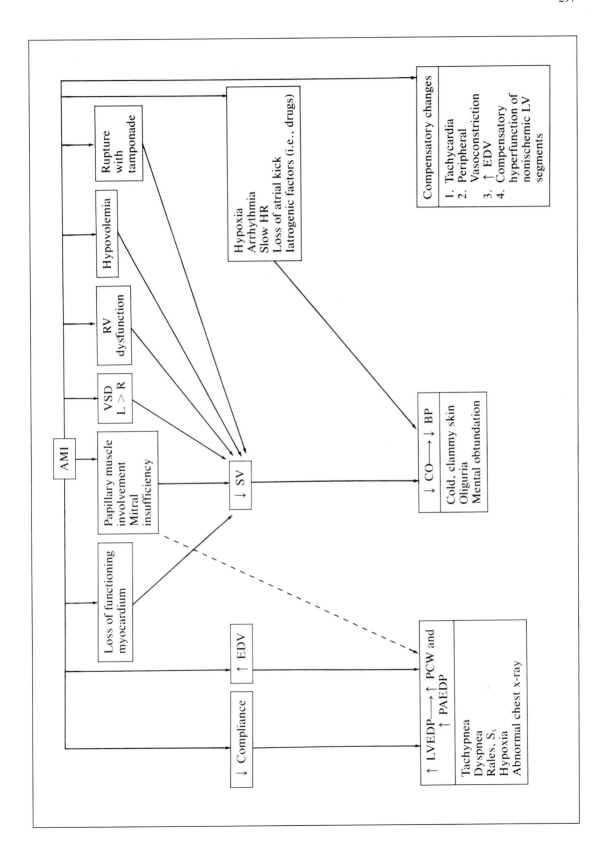

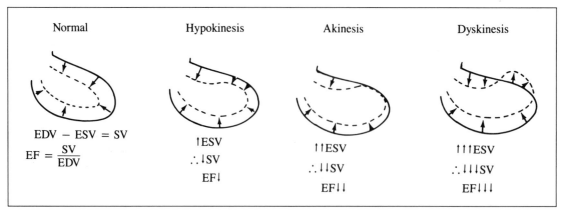

Fig. 16-2
Patterns of left ventricular regional contractile dysfunction and their influence on end-diastolic volume (EDV), end-systolic volume (ESV), stroke volume (SV), and ejection fraction (EF). Note progressive declines in EF with increasing ESV consequent to increasing gradation of contractile dysfunction.

2. Left ventricular dilatation allows the heart to utilize the Frank-Starling mechanism to minimize declines in stroke volume in the face of a depressed ejection fraction. Left ventricular dilatation, however, may produce deleterious consequences by (i) increasing wall tension and myocardial oxygen demand, (ii) leading to pulmonary venous congestion because of associated increases in left ventricular end-diastolic pressure, (iii) leading to papillary muscle dysfunction and consequent mitral regurgitation.

3. Normally perfused remote myocardial segments may hyperfunction in order to reduce the end-systolic volume, preserve the global ejection fraction, and minimize decreases in stroke volume. Such compensatory hyperfunction of remote myocardium may not be possible if remote myocardial segments become ischemic when their blood supply is jeopardized.

Diastolic Dysfunction

Diastolic function is frequently abnormal with acute myocardial infarction as reflected by changes in the ventricular diastolic pressure–volume relation or compliance. Because pulmonary capillary wedge pressure closely ap-

proximates the left ventricular mean diastolic pressure in the absence of mitral valve disease, an elevated left ventricular diastolic pressure also raises the pulmonary capillary wedge pressure. Left ventricular end-diastolic pressure may increase owing to an increased end-diastolic volume, reduced compliance, or both (Fig. 16-3). Infarct expansion appears to be an important contributor to left ventricular dilatation with acute myocardial infarction. Infarct expansion results from stretching, lengthening, and thinning of the myocardial segments with transmural necrosis, usually affecting the apical segment, which in return results in ventricular remodeling and dilatation [8, 9]. Disruption of the connective tissue framework and myofibrillar slippage may be responsible for infarct expansion.

Alteration in left ventricular diastolic compliance occurs frequently in acute myocardial infarction and may be detectable even with limited-extent infarction. Although in some instances overall compliance appears to be increased in the early phase of acute myocardial infarction, most studies suggest that the overall compliance is generally reduced, probably reflecting alterations in viscoelastic properties of the ischemic and necrotic tissue due to cellular and interstitial edema during the acute phase and healing with fibrosis during the subacute and chronic phases [10–12]. Right ven-

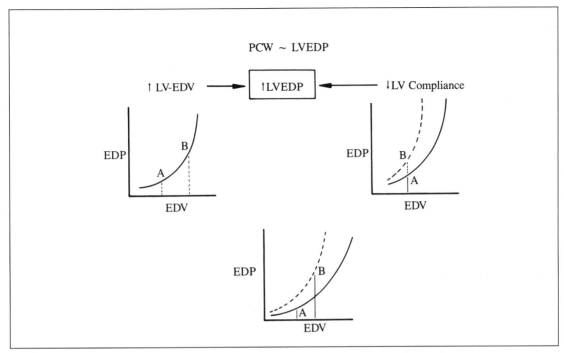

Fig. 16-3
Two mechanisms contributing to elevation of left ventricular end-diastolic
pressure (EDP)—and consequently elevation of the pulmonary capillary wedge
pressure (PCW)—are illustrated on the pressure–volume plots. *Left.* Elevation of
EDP secondary to an increase in end-diastolic volume (EDV) as the patient
moves from A to B. *Right.* Leftward and upward displacement of the pressure–
volume curve with an increase in EDP without a change in EDV, reflecting
reduced compliance, as the patient moves from A to B. *Bottom.* Composite of
increased EDV and reduced compliance as the patient moves from A to B. Note
that mitral regurgitation can raise the PCW by directly increasing the left atrial
pressure, without involving any of these mechanisms.

tricular dilatation and dysfunction accompanying ischemia or infarction of the right ventricle may produce a leftward bulging of the interventricular septum into the left ventricle as well as an increase in intrapericardial pressures contributing to abnormalities of diastolic function of the left ventricle [13].

Pump Failure

The importance of ventricular function as the chief determinant of short-term as well as long-term survival following acute myocardial infarction has been well established [1, 13–17]. Infarct size, in turn, is a major determinant of ventricular function, although alterations in

compliance, contractile function of noninfarcted remote myocardium, and mechanical disruption of infarcted structures may modify this relation. Investigators have attempted to characterize the severity of ventricular dysfunction and pump failure using clinical, invasive hemodynamic, and noninvasive techniques, not only to assist in prognostic assessment but also to provide rational guidelines for therapeutic interventions [15–18].

CLINICAL SUBSETS

In 1967 Killip and Kimbal [15] characterized patients with acute myocardial infarction into four classes based on physical findings on ad-

Table 16-1
Clinical and hemodynamic subsets in acute myocardial infarction

Subset	Clinical features	Approximate % of patients with AMI	Hospital mortality (%)
Killip class			
1	No signs of CHF	40–50	6
2	S_3 gallop, bibasilar rales	30–40	17
3	Acute pulmonary edema	10–15	38
4	Cardiogenic shock	5–10	81
Cedars-Sinai clinical subsets			
1	No pulmonary congestion or tissue hypoperfusion	25	1
2	Pulmonary congestion only	25	11
3	Tissue hypoperfusion only	15	18
4	Pulmonary congestion and tissue hypoperfusion	35	60
Cedars-Sinai hemodynamic subsets	Hemodynamic features		
1	PCW $\leq$ 18; CI > 2.2	25	3
2	PCW > 18; CI > 2.2	25	9
3	PCW $\leq$ 18; CI $\leq$ 2.2	15	23
4	PCW > 18; CI $\leq$ 2.2	35	51

AMI = acute myocardial infarction; PCW = pulmonary capillary wedge pressure (mm Hg); CI = cardiac index (L/min/m^2).

mission: class I (no signs of left ventricular failure), class II (S_3 gallop and/or pulmonary congestion limited to basal lung segments), class III (acute pulmonary edema), and class IV (shock syndrome) (Table 16-1). Subsequently, Forrester and colleagues stratified patients with acute myocardial infarction into four subsets: subset I (no evidence of pulmonary congestion or systemic hypoperfusion), subset II (evidence of pulmonary congestion without evidence of systemic hypoperfusion), subset III (evidence of systemic hypoperfusion without evidence of pulmonary congestion), and subset IV (evidence of pulmonary congestion and systemic hypoperfusion) [16, 17].

More recently, patients with acute myocardial infarction have also been characterized into prognostic subsets based on left and right ventricular ejection fractions determined by radionuclide ventriculography (Fig. 16-4) [18]. Such categorization is particularly relevent in patients who do not have clinical signs of severe pump failure on admission. The severity of ventricular dysfunction determined by more objective invasive or noninvasive means often shows considerable overlap between various clinical classes and subsets of patients. Such discrepancies arise because patients exhibit clinical "phase lags" as pulmonary congestion develops or resolves, when symptoms and signs secondary to coexistent chronic obstructive lung disease are mistakenly interpreted as pulmonary congestion, or when patients pass from one subset to another with or without therapy or due to confounding effects of changes in ventricular compliance or loading conditions that occur with mechanical complications such as mitral regurgitation and cardiac rupture.

HEMODYNAMIC ASSESSMENT OF PUMP DYSFUNCTION

Introduction of the balloon-flotation pulmonary artery thermodilution catheter by Swan,

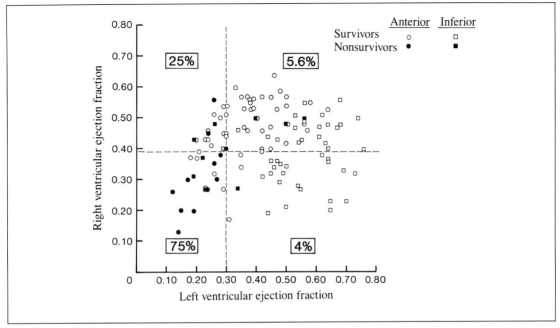

Fig. 16-4
Relation of mortality to left and right ventricular ejection fractions during acute myocardial infarction in 112 Killip class 1 or 2 patients. Note that mortality is high when LVEF is ≤0.30 and RVEF is ≤0.38, whereas mortality is low in the presence of LVEF >0.30 regardless of RVEF.

Ganz, and colleagues during the early 1970s made it feasible to objectively assess left ventricular function in acute myocardial infarction [19]. Based on invasive hemodynamic evaluation of pulmonary capillary wedge pressure and cardiac index in 200 patients with acute myocardial infarction, Forrester et al. described four subsets of patients (Table 15-1) [16, 17]. This stratification was suggested for predicting mortality, and it can be used as well as a guide for selecting appropriate therapy.

In acutely ill patients with myocardial infarction, clinical evidence of pulmonary congestion is often present when the pulmonary capillary wedge pressure is 18 to 20 mm Hg or higher, whereas evidence of systemic hypoperfusion is frequently present when the cardiac index is less than 2.0 to 2.2 L/min/m². However, in 20 to 30 percent of cases, discrepancies between clinical findings and hemodynamic variables may be found for reasons described earlier.

Hemodynamic Monitoring of Acute Myocardial Infarction

There is little evidence to support the practice of routine hemodynamic monitoring in patients with a clinically uncomplicated acute myocardial infarction. Such patients can be well assessed by carefully and meticulously performed clinical observation, which takes into account the overall appearance of the patient, heart rate and rhythm, systemic blood pressure, careful repeated cardiac examination for gallops or murmurs, careful pulmonary auscultation for rales, assessment of pulmonary vasculature on a chest radiograph, and assessment of the adequacy of vital organ perfusion (i.e., urine output, mental status).

On the other hand, hemodynamic monitoring may be useful in selected subsets of patients with hemodynamic complications following an acute myocardial infarction in order to: (1) clarify the role of hypovolemia, left ventricular failure, valvular regurgitation, septal rupture, right ventricular infarction, and cardiac tamponade in producing a state of hypotension, low-output syndrome, or pulmonary congestion and edema; and (2) assist in the selection of appropriate therapeutic intervention and follow the response to the intervention (Table 16-2). Thus hemodynamic monitoring should be considered only in those patients with acute myocardial infarction who demonstrate clinical evidence of severe low-output state, persistent hypotension and shock unrelated to correctable bradycardia, persistent unexplained sinus tachycardia, or appearance of a new systolic murmur.

In recent years, noninvasive studies such as two-dimensional echocardiography, Doppler flow studies, and radionuclide scintigraphy have proved useful for fully characterizing abnormalities of regional and global left and right ventricular function and detection of complications of myocardial infarction (Table 16-3). Thus in recent years the role of invasive hemodynamic monitoring for diagnosing complications of acute myocardial infarction has assumed a secondary rather than a primary role.

CLINICAL SUBSETS

It is useful to categorize patients with pump failure following acute myocardial infarction into subsets that are clinically meaningful and that provide guidelines for appropriate diagnostic and therapeutic strategies (Table 16-4).

Pulmonary Congestion Without a Low-Output State

Some degree of pulmonary congestion (pulmonary capillary wedge pressure 18 to 25 mm Hg) is common in patients with acute myocardial infarction. The increased pulmonary capillary wedge pressure results from an elevated left ventricular end-diastolic pressure due to decreased diastolic compliance, increased end-diastolic volume, or both, although it may also be due to mitral regurgitation. The patient may be asymptomatic or may complain of dyspnea and orthopnea. Findings on physical ex-

Table 16-2
Invasive hemodynamic monitoring of acute myocardial infarction

Uses
1. Clarifying role of hypovolemia, left ventricular failure, mitral regurgitation, interventricular septal rupture, right ventricular infarction and cardiac tamponade in the genesis of pump failure
2. Selection of appropriate therapy for pump failure, i.e., inotropes, vasodilators, volume
3. Rapid assessment of response to therapy
4. Prognostic assessment (see Table 16-1)

Indications
1. Persistent low-output state, hypotension, or shock
2. Recurrent or refractory pulmonary congestion or edema
3. Appearance of a new systolic murmur
4. During the use of intravenous vasoactive drugs or intra-aortic balloon counterpulsation
5. Unexplained persistent sinus tachycardia

amination may include tachypnea, bibasilar pulmonary rales, mild to moderate hypoxemia, and radiologic evidence of mild to moderate pulmonary venous congestion.

Therapy in such patients is aimed at ensuring adequate arterial oxygenation and relieving pulmonary venous congestion. These goals can usually be accomplished by supplemental oxygen and judicious use of small doses of intravenous diuretics. Reduction of left ventricular filling pressure not only relieves pulmonary congestion but may also reduce left ventricular volume, wall tension, and myocardial oxygen demand while facilitating subendocardial coronary perfusion. Measurements of venous capacitance in patients with acute myocardial infarction have suggested that the diuretic effect of intravenous furosemide may be preceded by a venodilator action, contributing to its preload reducing effect [20], although a transient vasoconstrictor effect preceding a diuretic effect has been noted in patients with chronic congestive heart failure [21]. Excessive diuresis should be avoided to prevent electrolyte depletion (notably hypokalemia) and hypotension secondary to hypovolemia.

Vasodilators such as nitrates or sodium ni-

Table 16-3
Role of noninvasive techniques for assessing complications of acute myocardial infarction
with pump dysfunction

Technique	Useful for diagnosis
Echocardiography	Papillary muscle rupture
	Ventricular septal rupture
	Pseudoaneurysm
	True aneurysm and mural thrombus
	Infarct expansion
	Right ventricular infarction
	Pericardial effusion and tamponade
Doppler echocardiography	Acute mitral regurgitation
	Ventricular septal rupture
Radionuclide techniques	
Radionuclide ventriculography	Ventriculopenic state
	Right ventricular infarction
	Ventricular septal rupture (first-pass method)
	Pseudoaneurysm and true aneurysm
	Mural thrombus
	Subacute cardiac rupture with intrapericardial bleeding
Rest and redistribution thallium 201 scintigraphy	Differentiation of ischemia and viable tissue from infarcted myocardium
Technetium 99m pyrophosphate scintigraphy	Diagnosis of right ventricular infarction

troprusside may also be used, particularly when pulmonary congestion is accompanied by evidence of mitral regurgitation or systemic hypertension. Vasodilators produce their beneficial effects in pulmonary congestion by producing (1) venodilation, (2) improved ventricular compliance directly or by unloading the right ventricle, (3) decreased ventricular afterload through arteriolar dilator effects resulting in improvement in left ventricular function, and (4) reduction in mitral regurgitation or the degree of left-to-right shunt across a ventricular septal rupture. Nitrates, such as sublingual isosorbide dinitrate (in doses of 2.5–10.0 mg) every 3 to 4 hours or 2% nitroglycerin ointment (0.5–1.0 inch) applied cutaneously every 6 to 8 hours may provide mild to moderate vasodilator effects. Although hemodynamic monitoring is not generally necessary in patients with pulmonary congestion and adequate perfusion, objective documentation of effects of vasodilators, if they are used, may be appropriate when clinical assessment of efficacy is ambiguous. Continuous exposure to nitrates may lead to tolerance, and nitrate therapy should be used in such a way as to allow a 6- to 12-hour nitrate-free interval during each 24-hour period of therapy.

Acute Pulmonary Edema Without Shock

Acute pulmonary edema without shock is characterized by severe, dramatic manifestations of acute pulmonary congestion, i.e., severe respiratory distress, sometimes accompanied by expectoration of pink, frothy sputum and frequently accompanied by cool, clammy, diaphoretic skin, an increased heart rate, and elevated blood pressure indicative of a reactive sympathoadrenal response. Pulmonary edema may be precipitated by (1) extensive left ventricular contractile failure due to massive acute myocardial infarction or cumulative effects of old and new myocardial infarction, (2) primary decrease of diastolic function with only modest systolic contractile dysfunction (stiff heart), (3) acute, persistent or intermittent mitral regurgitation resulting from papillary muscle dysfunction or rupture, or (4) profound global myocardial ischemia in association with a relatively small or modest degree of myocardial necrosis (ischemic paralysis).

Table 16-4
Categories of pump dysfunction in acute myocardial infarction

Clinical category	Pathophysiologic basis	Equivalent clinical subsets		Equivalent Cedars-Sinai hemodynamic subset
		Killip	Cedars-Sinai	
Subclinical	Compensated ventricular dysfunction or normal or near-normal ventricular function	I	I	I
Clinically overt				
Pulmonary congestion	Systolic and/or diastolic LV dysfunction Mitral regurgitation Ventricular septal rupture	II	II	II
Acute pulmonary edema	As above but more severe	III	II	II
Low-output state, hypotension, and shock				
With pulmonary congestion and edema				
Ventriculopenic state	Severe systolic and diastolic LV dysfunction	IV	IV	IV
Mechanical lesions	Acute mitral regurgitation Septal rupture	IV	IV	IV
Without pulmonary congestion or edema	Hypovolemia Dominant RV dysfunction Cardiac rupture Cardiac tamponade Electromechanical dissociation Severe bradyarrhythmias	IV	III	III

LV = left ventricular; RV = right ventricular.

Patients with pulmonary edema usually exhibit severe hypoxemia and may demonstrate respiratory alkalosis or metabolic acidosis depending on the degree and duration of the problem. Physical examination generally reveals tachypnea, cyanosis, tachycardia, elevated blood pressure, cool and moist skin, and extensive bilateral pulmonary rales, occasionally accompanied by wheezing (cardiac asthma) or even diminished breath sounds due to poor respiratory efforts. Acute pulmonary edema in myocardial infarction is invariably due to a rapid, marked elevation of pulmonary capillary wedge pressure (exceeding 25 mm Hg), although in some patients decreased capillary colloid oncotic pressure has been thought to play a contributory role. A hypooncotic state has been implicated when pulmonary edema is precipitated by rapid infusion of crystalloid volume that results in dilution of serum proteins and a fall in intravascular oncotic pressure. Acute pulmonary edema complicating myocardial infarction is associated with 30 to 50 percent mortality.

The salient principles of therapy of acute pulmonary edema involve maintenance of adequate gas exchange, a stable rhythm and blood pressure, and rapid reduction of pulmonary capillary wedge pressure.

MAINTENANCE OF ADEQUATE GAS EXCHANGE

Maintenance of adequate gas exchange requires immediate assessment with analysis of arterial blood gases and administration of high concentrations (50–100%) of oxygen via a face mask. Endotracheal intubation should be considered when patients are moribund, unable to maintain an arterial PO_2 of at least 60 mm Hg on a face mask, or develop a rising PCO_2 or falling arterial pH. Following endotracheal intubation, mechanical ventilation may need to be supplemented with positive end-expiratory pressure (PEEP) in order to maintain adequate systemic oxygenation and allow the use of relatively safer concentrations of oxygen, i.e., $FiO_2 \leq 60$ percent. PEEP should be used judiciously to avoid lung barotrauma and to minimize declines in cardiac output secondary to reduced left ventricular preload and increased right ventricular afterload. Hemodynamic and arterial blood gas monitoring is useful for determining the effects of PEEP on tissue oxygen delivery (a product of cardiac output and arterial oxygen content) and for selecting optimal amounts of PEEP.

RAPID REDUCTION OF PULMONARY CAPILLARY WEDGE PRESSURE

Nitrates are useful for rapidly lowering an elevated pulmonary capillary wedge pressure in the presence of acute pulmonary edema [22, 23]. Nitrates produce a pharmacologic phlebotomy by their peripheral venodilator effects, shifting blood volume away from the intrathoracic compartment to the extrathoracic compartment, thereby rapidly lowering pulmonary venous and capillary pressures. A direct vasodilator effect of nitrates on pulmonary vasculature may contribute in some patients to unloading of the right ventricle, resulting in improved left ventricular compliance. Improvement in left ventricular function resulting from a reduction in afterload and improved function of ischemic segments, as well as a decrease or elimination of mitral regurgitation consequent to reduction of afterload, may be additional important acute effects of nitrates. The effects of nitrates may be supplemented by small intravenous doses of morphine sulfate, which helps calm the agitated patient and contributes to venodilator and arteriolar dilator actions.

Diuretics, especially intravenous furosemide, are frequently used as the primary treatment; however, their effect is slower and their use should generally be considered as secondary and adjunctive to nitrates. In severely hypertensive patients or in those with significant mitral regurgitation, continuous infusion of sodium nitroprusside may be useful. Acute digitalization, intermittent positive-pressure ventilation, and routine use of aminophylline are generally not beneficial for acute pulmonary edema. In some patients, use of rotating tourniquets or phlebotomy is recommended, but in our experience it is rarely necessary. The role of inotropic-vasopressor therapy and intra-aortic balloon pumping for acute pulmonary edema in selected patients is discussed later in this chapter.

After successful emergency therapy of acute pulmonary edema, patients should be assessed for the presence of (1) intermittent or persistent severe mitral regurgitation, (2) ventricular septal rupture, and (3) intermittent ischemia. Recognition of these complications is important, as surgical intervention may be highly desirable for such patients.

Shock

Shock can be defined as a clinical syndrome characterized by evidence of acute, severe, prolonged tissue hypoperfusion, usually associated with a low arterial blood pressure (≤ 90 mm Hg systolic) and a markedly reduced cardiac output. In addition to hypotension and tachycardia, patients generally have cool, clammy skin, diaphoresis, mental obtundation, and oliguria. Depending on the dominant pathophysiologic event precipitating shock, additional clinical findings may also be present. Similarly, hemodynamic findings of shock may also vary depending on the pathophysiologic state resulting in the shock syndrome. Shock syndrome can be considered under two main categories: shock with pulmonary congestion or edema and shock without pulmonary congestion or edema.

SHOCK WITH PULMONARY CONGESTION OR EDEMA

Shock syndrome that includes pulmonary congestion or edema may result from extensive left ventricular dysfunction (ventriculopenic state) or mechanical complications, i.e., acute mitral regurgitation and ventricular septal rupture.

Ventriculopenic Shock
Ventriculopenic shock syndrome occurs in 10 to 15 percent of patients with acute myocardial infarction. However, in recent years the incidence of cardiogenic shock appears to have declined, perhaps related to the common use of infarct-size-limiting strategies, i.e., reperfusion with thrombolytic therapy and coronary angioplasty during evolving myocardial infarction. Shock generally results from severe left ventricular contractile dysfunction due to: (1) extensive acute myocardial infarction, (2) acute myocardial infarction of less severe nature in patients with prior loss of myocardial function from old infarction; and (3) less commonly, large areas of ischemic nonfunctioning but viable myocardium along with only modest areas of myocardial infarction (ischemic paralysis). It may be the predominant mechanism of shock that occurs within the first few hours of onset of acute myocardial infarction. Aggressive strategies aimed at reperfusion during early evolving myocardial infarction may be most useful for salvaging ischemic but viable myocardium in this subset of patients with cardiogenic shock.

Several pathologic studies have indicated that patients succumbing to this type of shock invariably demonstrate a cumulative involvement of at least 35 to 40 percent of the total left ventricular mass [24, 25]. In addition, patients frequently demonstrate marginal extension of recent areas of necrosis and focal necrotic areas remote from the major location of recent infarction. Profound impairment of ventricular function perpetuates ischemia and necrosis secondary to hypotension and the coronary artery underperfusion. This vicious cycle is responsible for the progressive nature of myocardial damage found in this syndrome, reflected by stuttering and progressive elevation of plasma levels of myocardium-specific enzymes [26]. Nearly 70 percent of patients succumbing to this type of shock demonstrate extensive, severe multivessel coronary obstructive disease with a high prevalence of left anterior descending coronary artery involvement [27]. It has been suggested that early thinning, lengthening, and stretching of transmurally necrotic myocardium (infarct expansion) may contribute to acute ventricular dilatation and precipitation of pump failure in patients with acute myocardial infarction [8, 28, 29].

CONSEQUENCES OF SHOCK

Severe hypoperfusion of various body organs due to low cardiac output and hypotension results in impairment of organ function, e.g., renal failure, hepatic dysfunction, pancreatic and gastrointestinal ischemia, enhanced anaerobic metabolism, and lactic acidosis. Pulmonary congestion and edema produce hypoxemia, atelectasis, and in rare cases acute respiratory distress syndrome. Supraventricular and ventricular arrhythmias are common, and complications such as systemic or pulmonary sepsis, renal failure, and gastrointestinal hemorrhage further contribute to the poor overall outlook of the patient. Older patients, those with diabetes, patients with prior infarction, and those with anterior myocardial infarction are most likely to develop cardiogenic shock.

Patients in shock are generally cool and clammy with peripheral cyanosis, oliguria, and impaired mentation [30]. The systolic blood pressure is generally less than 90 mm Hg, or 60 mm Hg below the previous basal level, and the pulse is rapid with a narrow pulse pressure. Lactic acidosis may be present in advanced cases. Indirect cuff pressures may be 10 to 20 mm Hg lower in the presence of intense peripheral vasoconstriction, arguing in favor of direct intra-arterial measurements. Some patients have recurrent episodes of ischemic cardiac pain, whereas others remain moribund. Depending on the severity of the pulmonary congestion, patients demonstrate varying degrees of respiratory distress, hypoxemia, and hyperpnea. Cerebral underperfusion and use of narcotic analgesics, particularly in elderly patients, may result in Cheyne-Stokes respirations. Other clinical features of organ dysfunction may also be evident as the shock syndrome progresses. Cardiac examination generally demonstrates diminished intensity of heart sounds, atrial or ventricular gallop (or both), pericardial friction rub, and dyskinetic apical impulse; the pulmonary examination reveals rales of varying distribution.

Hemodynamic findings demonstrate a low arterial pressure, severely depressed cardiac and stroke work indices, and elevated pulmonary arterial and capillary wedge pressures. Systemic vascular resistance and arteriovenous oxygen differences are also increased. The left ventricle is generally dilated with severe and extensive regional contractile dysfunction, and the global ejection fraction is frequently less than 0.20 to 0.30.

The prognosis of this type of "cardiogenic shock" is poor, with 80 to 100 percent in-hospital mortality. The small number of hospital survivors often live with continued heart failure and dysrhythmias, and they are faced with a low probability of long-term survival. Prognosis appears to be more favorable in relatively young patients, in those with single-vessel coronary disease, and in that subgroup of patients in whom early reperfusion with or without subsequent coronary artery revascularization salvages substantial amounts of jeopardized nonfunctioning but viable myocardium [31–34].

TREATMENT STRATEGIES

The main goals of management of ventriculopenic cardiogenic shock are to: (1) improve ventricular performance and cardiac output and maintain adequate systemic arterial pressure in order to sustain perfusion to vital organs and reduce pulmonary congestion; and (2) preserve the viability and function of ischemic and jeopardized myocardium and limit the ultimate infarct size.

General Supportive Measures
General supportive measures are essential, such as relief of pain and discomfort with judicious use of small doses of analgesics such as morphine, maintenance of adequate oxygenation and ventilation (which requires endotrachael intubation in some patients), prompt correction of electrolyte and acid-base abnormalities, control of fever, treatment of nausea and vomiting, control of cardiac dysrhythmias, and maintenance of an adequate heart rate with atrioventricular synchrony. An ischemic ventricle is more susceptible to negative inotropic effects of drugs, particularly the antiarrhythmic agents, which are frequently misused in such patients. The need for the use of such drugs and their dosage must be carefully reviewed and monitored in order to avoid deleterious consequences.

Specific Therapeutic Modalities

Until a few years ago specific therapy of "cardiogenic shock" not only required careful clinical assessment but, in addition, virtually mandated the use of bedside hemodynamic monitoring using a Swan-Ganz thermodilution catheter as well as an indwelling intra-arterial cannula. Such invasive monitoring has been useful for excluding the presence of other complications that could produce pump failure or shock, i.e., mitral regurgitation, septal or free-wall rupture, hypovolemia, and right ventricular infarction (Table 16-5). Moreover, it has helped in the selection of specific drugs and other therapeutic interventions, as well as monitoring the response to such therapy. Refinements in noninvasive techniques such as two-dimensional echocardiography, Doppler flow techniques, and radionuclide scintigraphy have made it possible to expand and refine the information obtained by clinical means. In most modern cardiac intensive care units, bedside assessment of critically ill patients can now be made with a combination of clinical and noninvasive techniques that considerably facilitate diagnosis and treatment.

Specific therapeutic interventions used in patients with shock are pharmacologic agents (inotropic and vasopressor drugs, vasodilators, diuretics), mechanical circulatory assist devices (intra-aortic balloon pumping, left heart assist device), reperfusion (thrombolysis, percutaneous transluminal angioplasty, coronary artery bypass graft surgery), and surgery for correction of mechanical complications (Table 16-6).

INOTROPIC AND VASOPRESSOR AGENTS

Inotropic and vasopressor agents are necessary in many patients to maintain peripheral tissue perfusion by improving cardiac output and maintaining an adequate systemic blood pressure (usually in the range of at least 90 to 100 mm Hg systolic).

CARDIAC GLYCOSIDES

Cardiac glycosides are relatively ineffective or only marginally effective in patients with severe pump failure following acute myocardial infarction. Ischemic myocardium appears to be more susceptible to arrhythmogenic effects of digitalis, and the coronary as well as peripheral vasoconstrictor effects of rapid intravenous administration of digitalis have produced deleterious consequences [35]. However, digitalis may be indicated for atrial arrhythmias (i.e., fibrillation, flutter) complicating myocardial infarction and pump failure.

SYMPATHOMIMETIC AGENTS

Sympathomimetic drugs are the most commonly used inotropic-vasopressor drugs for cardiogenic shock (Table 16-7). Dopamine and dobutamine are the most frequently used agents, whereas norepinephrine is used infrequently.

Dopamine. Dopamine exerts its cardiovascular effects by directly stimulating dopaminergic-specific receptors as well as releasing endogenous norepinephrine from sympathetic nerve endings [36, 37]. At low doses (2–5 μg/kg/min), most patients increase their stroke volume and cardiac output; their renal blood flow is also increased, with redistribution toward the inner one-third of the renal cortex, an effect mediated by interaction with dopaminergic-specific receptors. At this low dosage chronotropic and peripheral vasoconstrictor effects are minimal, and deleterious effects on myocardial ischemia are not generally observed. With increasing doses, there is a dose-dependent increase in chronotropic, arrhythmogenic, and alpha-adrenergically mediated vasoconstrictor and vasopressor effects that may result in decreased tissue perfusion and increased pulmonary arterial and left ventricular filling pressures secondary to elevated afterload. At large doses (>15–20 μg/kg/min), inotropic, chronotropic, and vasopressor effects may provoke or exacerbate myocardial ischemia.

The dose of dopamine infusion in "cardiogenic shock" requires careful individual titration beginning with a low dose (2–5 μg/kg/min). The object of therapy is to improve cardiac output, increase renal and other organ perfusion, and maintain a systolic blood pressure of 90 to 100 mm Hg without permitting excessive increases in heart rate (>110–115 beats per minute), arrhythmias, or excessive peripheral vasoconstriction to occur. Because of marked individual variations in dose response, it is crucial to use the lowest dose that produces optimal hemodynamic and clinical improvement with the fewest adverse effects. Adverse effects include sinus tachycardia, atrial and ventricular arrhythmias, excessive peripheral vasoconstriction and compromise of tissue blood flow, precipitation or worsening of myocardial ischemia, gangrene at the infusion site especially when extravascular extravasation occurs, nausea and vomiting, and increased heart rate in the presence of supraventricular arrhythmias resulting from facilitation of atrioventricular conduction.

Dobutamine. Dobutamine, a synthetic catecholamine, differs from dopamine in that it has predominantly beta-adrenergic agonist actions (accounting for its positive inotropic and chronotropic effects) with only minimal alpha-adrenergic agonist effects (accounting for its lack of appreciable vasoconstrictor effects even at large doses) [38]. Furthermore, dobutamine does not release endogenous norepinephrine and has no direct renal vasodilator effects. Dobutamine produces dose-dependent increases in stroke volume and cardiac output, and a modest reduction in pulmonary capillary wedge pressure. Excessive increases in heart rate are uncommon at infusion rates under 15 to 20 µg/kg/min, and vasoconstriction does not occur.

Because dobutamine tends to produce equivalent increases in cardiac output but with lesser increments in heart rate, a lower risk of arrhythmias, no vasoconstrictor effects, and more consistent reduction in left ventricular filling pressures than dopamine, it is generally preferred as a starting drug. However, lack of direct renal vasodilator effects and only a modest pressor effect compared to dopamine make dobutamine less desirable when arterial pressure is low, i.e., less than 80 mm Hg. The optimal use of dobutamine for cardiogenic shock requires that guidelines similar to those for dopamine be followed.

Norepinephrine. Norepinephrine produces potent arteriolar and venous constrictor effects through stimulation of alpha-adrenergic receptors. It has relatively modest beta-1-adrenergically mediated myocardial inotropic and chronotropic effects. The peripheral vasoconstrictor effects of norepinephrine make it a potent pressor agent with much fewer overall positive chronotropic or arrhythmogenic effects than dopamine or dobutamine. Although such effects may temporarily maintain adequate arterial pressure in severely hypotensive patients, little increase or an actual decrease in cardiac output and compromise of peripheral organ blood flow may result in later deterioration [39]. However, in patients with cardiogenic shock with a low systemic arterial pressure ($\leqslant$70 mm Hg) and a normal or reduced systemic vascular resistance in whom pressor doses of dopamine produce serious adverse effects (tachyarrhythmias), small doses of norepinephrine may be used to maintain systemic arterial pressure around 90 mm Hg systolic with improvement in cardiac output in some patients. Combined use of norepinephrine with an alpha-adrenergic blocking drug, e.g., phentolamine, or direct vasodilators, e.g., nitroglycerin or sodium nitroprusside, is preferred, as such therapy minimizes peripheral vasoconstrictor effects and helps unmask the positive inotropic effects of norepinephrine [40]. As with dopamine and dobutamine, norepinephrine is generally begun at a low dose (1–4 µg/min) and increased to an optimal clinical and hemodynamic effect before excessive peripheral vasoconstriction or arrhythmias occur. Adverse effects are mostly related to excessive vasoconstriction and compromise of organ blood flow, worsening of ventricular function due to increased afterload, tissue necrosis and sloughing if extravascular extravasation occurs, increased heart rate, and cardiac arrhythmias. In some patients, an excessive increase in blood pressure may produce reflex slowing of the heart rate.

VASODILATORS

The rationale for using vasodilators in patients with shock is predicated on their ability to (1) reduce ventricular afterload by dilating the systemic arteriolar bed and (2) reduce ventricular preload by dilating the peripheral venous or capacitance bed. Reduction in ventricular afterload results in decreased outflow imped-

Table 16-5
Low-output state and shock following acute myocardial infarction

Underlying abnormality	Recognition			Guide to management
	Clinical	Hemodynamic	Others	
Ventriculopenic shock	Shock syndrome Rales, S_3 Abnormal chest x-ray	Elevated PCW Depressed CI High SVR Low BP	Markedly depressed LVEF (i.e., ≤0.30)	Inotropes-pressors to maintain systolic BP ~90 mm Hg and CI of >2 L/m² Vasodilators added to keep PCW 12–15 mm Hg IABP if no response to above + General supportive care Consider acute reperfusion with PICA and/or thrombolysis
Acute severe mitral regurgitation	Shock syndrome Rales, S_3, abnormal x-ray Holosystolic murmur; occasionally murmur not heard or soft and brief	Elevated PCW with tall V waves Depressed CI High SVR Low BP	LVEF may be normal, elevated, or variably depressed depending on extent of necrosis of LV Echo shows flail leaflet Doppler shows regurgitation	Vasodilators + inotropes to maintain systolic BP ~90, PCW 12–15 mm Hg, and CI >2 L/m² IABP followed by early catheterization and surgery + General supportive care
Acute VSD	Shock syndrome Rales, S_3 Holosystolic murmur with precordial thrill in 50%	O_2 stepup from RA to RV or PA Thermodilution curve shows evidence of L→R shunt	First-pass radionuclide study shows L→R shunt LV and RVEF are variable as in mitral regurgitation and depend on extent of necrosis 2D echo visualizes defect Shunt seen on Doppler	Same as above + General supportive care

	Clinical features	Hemodynamic findings	2D echocardiographic findings	Treatment
Hypovolemia	Shock syndrome Lungs and x-rays do not show signs of LV failure (but in some patients may show persistent signs of LV failure if hypovolemia is superimposed on a patient with prior LV failure, generally from overdiuresis) Orthostatic ↑ in HR and/or ↓ in BP	PCW generally <12–15 mm Hg CI depressed SVR may be high BP may be low Some patients with this profile have RV infarction		If patient has clinical evidence for hypoperfusion, then rapid but careful volume expansion until PCW is ~15 mm Hg but no higher than 18 mm Hg
Predominant acute right ventricular infarction	Shock syndrome in a patient with inferior infarction JVD or HJR in 70% of cases Lungs and x-rays generally clear with minimal or no signs of LV failure Occasionally pulsus paradoxus and Kussmaul sign Rarely severe hypoxia from R→L shunt across a PFO	RA pressure ≥PCW Reduced PA and RV pulse pressure Depressed CI 30% May have normal RA pressure (Volume challenge may bring out occult findings)	Dilated RV with ↓RVEF (<0.39) LVEF generally >0.45 Some patients have severely depressed LV and such patients should be categorized differently	Increase volume if PCW <15 mm Hg PCW is ~15 mm Hg If no improvement add inotropic agent and/or vasodilator depending on BP

PCW = pulmonary capillary wedge pressure; CI = cardiac index; SVR = systemic vascular resistance; BP = blood pressure; LVEF = left ventricular ejection fraction; IABP = intra-aortic balloon pumping; PTCA = percutaneous transluminal coronary angioplasty; LV = left ventricle; VSD = ventricular septal defect; RA = right atrium; RV = right ventricle; PA = pulmonary artery; L→R = left to right; RVEF = right ventricular ejection fraction; 2D = two-dimensional; HR = heart rate; JVD = jugular venous distension; HJR = hepatojugular reflux; PFO = patent foramen ovale.

Table 16-6
Beneficial and adverse effects of therapeutic interventions for postinfarction pump dysfunction

Intervention	Potential effects	
	Beneficial	Adverse
↑ Heart rate	May ↑ depressed CO and BP if HR is slow	↑ MVO$_2$ and possible increase in ischemia, loss of atrial contribution if ventricular pacing is performed
Diuretics	Decrease PCW, improve pulmonary congestion	Hypovolemia, low CO and BP, azotemia, hypokalemia
Volume loading	May ↑ depressed CO and BP in presence of hypovolemia or RV infarction	↑ MVO$_2$ by increasing preload, and possible ↑ in ischemia, pulmonary edema if PCW is not carefully monitored
Inotropic agents Digitalis Dopamine Norepinephrine Dobutamine	May ↑ depressed CO and BP in presence of LV failure	May ↑ MVO$_2$ by ↑ HR (dopamine, dobutamine, norepinephrine), ↑ contractility (all agents), ↑ SVR (norepinephrine, digitalis, dopamine), may worsen LV failure and produce tissue hypoperfusion if SVR increased markedly or tachyarrhythmias occur
Vasodilators Nitroprusside Nitroglycerin	May decrease elevated PCW and SVR, reduce MR, L→R shunt, and elevate depressed cardiac output	May ↑ BP and compromise myocardial and other organ perfusion; may produce hypoxia; may produce toxic effects
IABP	Similar to above with maintenance and/or augmentation of diastolic coronary perfusion pressure	Complications related to IABP insertion and stay in the vascular compartment, i.e., vascular insufficiency, infection
Early reperfusion (thrombolysis, anticoagulants, PTCA)	May stop ischemia, limit infarction, improve LV function, restore inotropic responsiveness, prevent ischemia-related arrhythmias, reverse conduction abnormalities, prevent mural thrombus formation	Bleeding complications, hypotension, allergy, etc. (with thrombolytic anticoagulant drugs)

CO = cardiac output; BP = blood pressure; HR = heart rate; LV = left ventricular; PCW = pulmonary capillary wedge pressure; SVR = systemic vascular resistance; MR = mitral regurgitation; L→R = left to right; MVO$_2$ = myocardial O$_2$ demand; HR = heart rate; IABP = intra-aortic balloon pumping; PTCA = percutaneous transluminal angioplasty.

Table 16-7
Guidelines for use of intravenous catecholamines and vasodilators in pump failure
following myocardial infarction

Catecholamines
   Begin with a low dose and titrate every 10–15 minutes to a therapeutic endpoint without provoking
      unacceptable adverse effects.
   Dopamine: Begin with 1–3 μg/kg/min and increase as needed to increase blood pressure.
   Dobutamine: Begin with 2–5 μg/kg/min and increase as needed to improve cardiac output;
      dobutamine is not effective as sole therapy to increase blood pressure and should be used only
      when BP has been adequately restored.
   Norepinephrine: Begin with 1–3 μg/min and increase by 0.5–2.0 μg increments. Preferably use in
      combination with alpha blocker, i.e., phentolamine.
   Use acidic solutions as diluents.
   Observe for adverse effects.
      Sinus tachycardia (rarely bradycardia may occur with norepinephrine-induced hypertension)
      Accelerated AV conduction and increased ventricular response in supraventricular arrhythmias
      Atrial and ventricular premature beats and tachyarrhythmias
      Worsening or provocation of ischemia or ventricular dysfunction
      Tissue hypoperfusion from excessive vasoconstriction; necrosis (from extravascular extravasation)
         from dopamine or norepinephrine
      Nausea and vomiting
Vasodilators
   Begin with low doses and titrate every 10–15 minutes to a therapeutic endpoint without provoking
      adverse effects.
   Sodium nitroprusside: Begin with 10–20 μg/min and increase by 10–20 μg/min increments.
   Intravenous nitroglycerin: Begin with 10–20 μg/min and increase by 10–20 μg/min increments.
   Intravenous phentolamine: Begin with 0.5 mg/min and increase by 0.25 mg/min increments.
   Use freshly prepared solutions of nitroprusside (<6–8 hours old) and shield the reservoir from light.
   Preferably use nonabsorbent plastic tubings when giving intravenous nitroglycerin to avoid adherence
      of nitroglycerin to plastic tubing.
   Observe for adverse effects.
      Flushing, headaches, hypotension
      Reflex tachycardia; rarely reflex bradycardia
      Worsening or precipitation of ischemia due to excessive hypotension and tachycardia and, possibly,
         maldistribution of coronary nutrient flow
      Arterial desaturation from intrapulmonary shunting
      Methemoglobinemia (nitroglycerin and nitroprusside)
      Thiocyanate and cyanide intoxication (nitroprusside)
      Precipitation of increased intracranial and intraocular pressure (nitrates)
      Ethanol intoxication during prolonged high-dose infusions of intravenous nitroglycerin containing
         ethanol as a vehicle
Miscellaneous
   Infuse these potent drugs through free-flowing non-posture-dependent large-bore intravenous,
      preferably central, lines using well-calibrated constant-infusion pumps.
   Avoid abrupt cessation of infusion (unless serious adverse effects occur); preferably, wean gradually.
   Avoid flushing infusion lines through which catecholamines or vasodilators are infusing without first
      clearing the infusion line by withdrawing blood through it.
   If cardiac outputs are being performed using a Swan-Ganz catheter, avoid infusing drugs through the
      right atrial port of the Swan-Ganz catheter.

ence to left ventricular ejection, thereby increasing forward stroke volume and cardiac output. In the presence of mitral regurgitation and ventricular septal rupture, decreased impedance to ejection into the aorta reduces the degree of regurgitation and left-to-right shunt while increasing forward output into aorta. Preload reduction contributes to the reduction of ventricular filling pressures, thereby reducing pulmonary capillary wedge pressure, pulmonary arterial pressure, and right atrial pressure. Although favorably influencing ventricular function, the afterload and preload reducing effects also tend to decrease myocardial oxygen demand and may favor subendocardial perfusion during diastole. Vasodilators may also influence the left ventricular diastolic pressure–volume relation, shifting it down and to the right owing to right ventricular unloading and reduction in the degree of pericardial restraint.

The use of vasodilators in this clinical setting is limited by their potential to produce excessive hypotension. Blood flow through coronary arteries with severe flow-limiting stenosis is highly dependent on perfusion pressure because of loss of autoregulatory reserve. Thus vasodilator-induced hypotension may decrease coronary blood flow and increase oxygen demand when hypotension provokes a reflex tachycardia. Hypotension may also compromise perfusion to other organs, i.e., brain, kidney, splanchnic bed. Excessive reduction of left ventricular filling pressures or use of vasodilators in patients with low or normal filling pressures predisposes to hypotension and tachycardia. Because of these considerations, caution is necessary when using vasodilators in critically ill patients with a precarious hemodynamic state.

The effects of vasodilator therapy on the outcome of patients with cardiogenic shock have never been examined in properly controlled studies. Chatterjee and colleagues reported an apparent improvement in short-term survival of close to 50 percent in a small group of patients with severe pump failure complicating acute myocardial infarction treated with vasodilators; the 1-year survival, however, was 20 percent, and most survivors continued to have severe heart failure [41].

Currently the most commonly used vasodilators in patients with severe heart failure and shock are intravenous sodium nitroprusside and nitrates. Intravenous agents are preferred because they have a rapid onset of action (1–2 minutes) and a short half-life (2–4 minutes), and their effects rapidly dissipate within 10 to 15 minutes after cessation of the infusion. *Sodium Nitroprusside.* Sodium nitroprusside infusion has a prompt peripheral vasodilator effect on both arterial and venous circulations. It produces hemodynamic and short-term clinical improvement in patients with severe heart failure with or without shock accompanying acute myocardial infarction [42]. The beneficial effects tend to be greater in patients with a markedly elevated pulmonary capillary wedge pressure and in those with mitral regurgitation or septal rupture. Therapy is generally begun with a low dose (10–20 µg/min) followed by rapid increases every 15 to 20 minutes until the pulmonary capillary wedge pressure is lowered to 15 to 20 mm Hg without permitting systolic arterial pressure to drop below 90 mm Hg (Table 16-7). In many patients with cardiogenic shock, vasodilator therapy alone may produce unacceptable degrees of arterial hypotension unless combined with an inotropic drug (dopamine or dobutamine) or intra-aortic balloon counterpulsation.

Adverse effects of nitroprusside therapy include excessive hypotension reflex tachycardia, potential for worsening of myocardial ischemia, accumulation of thiocyanate (particularly in the presence of renal insufficiency and prolonged infusions) with thiocyanate toxicity, accumulation of cyanide and cyanide toxicity, worsening of arterial hypoxemia due to an increasing intrapulmonary ventilation–perfusion mismatch, and rarely methemoglobinemia and vitamin B_{12} deficiency. Limiting the dose and duration of therapy, frequent monitoring of serum thiocyanate levels to avoid exceeding levels of 6 mg/dl, and prophylactic use of the cyanide chelating agent hydroxycobalamin have been recommended to avoid cyanide intoxication [43].
Intravenous Nitroglycerin. Intravenous nitroglycerin is a rapidly acting vasodilator that tends to reduce the pulmonary capillary wedge pressure with more variable increases

in stroke volume and cardiac output in patients with severe left ventricular failure [44]. These differential effects have been attributed to preferential venodilation particularly at lower doses, but significant arteriolar dilation is also observed with increasing doses. Nitroglycerin may have a more favorable effect on the distribution of coronary blood flow to ischemic myocardium than nitroprusside, but there have been no careful comparative studies of cardiogenic shock to confirm or refute the superiority of one agent over the other.

The adverse effects of nitroglycerin, like those of nitroprusside, include hypotension with reflex tachycardia, headaches due to cerebral vasodilation and possibly increased intracranial pressure, increasing intraocular pressure in patients with glaucoma, methemoglobinemia, Wernicke's encephalopathy, and ethanol intoxication (ethanol is the vehicle for many intravenous nitroglycerin preparations). Hypotension and paradoxical profound bradycardia are rare but generally respond to atropine administration and cessation of nitroglycerin therapy [45]. As with nitroprusside therapy, the use of intravenous nitroglycerin for cardiogenic shock frequently requires concomitant use of an inotropic drug (dopamine or dobutamine) or intra-aortic balloon counterpulsation to maintain or elevate a low systemic arterial pressure.

Phentolamine. Phentolamine was one of the earliest agents to be used as a vasodilator. It is a nonselective alpha-adrenergic blocking agent with direct smooth muscle relaxant and mild direct inotropic and chronotropic effects. In comparison to nitroprusside and nitroglycerin, phentolamine produces a relatively greater increase in heart rate (and cardiac output) and a lesser decrease in filling pressures; it is considerably more expensive. It is mainly used to minimize vasoconstrictor effects of norepinephrine infusion and the deleterious effects of extravascular extravasation of norepinephrine or dopamine.

COMBINED VASODILATOR AND
SYMPATHOMIMETIC DRUGS
Afterload and preload reducing effects of vasodilators improve cardiac output and lower ventricular filling pressures, but systemic arterial hypotension remains a potential drawback. Inotropic drugs may improve ventricular function and cardiac output, but it may have inconsistent effects on ventricular filling pressures and potentially deleterious excessive peripheral vasoconstrictor effects. Thus by using lower doses of more than one agent, combined therapy may offset each other's adverse effects while augmenting overall ventricular function. Vasodilators frequently used for this purpose include alpha-adrenergic blockers such as phentolamine and direct vasodilators such as nitroglycerin and sodium nitroprusside. The principal advantage of adding a vasodilator to dopamine or dobutamine is that increments in cardiac output are achieved at much lower left ventricular filling pressures and systemic vascular resistance. Combined use of dopamine and dobutamine has also been suggested for treatment of cardiogenic shock as a means of achieving better acute hemodynamic response at lower doses.

INTRA-AORTIC BALLOON PUMPING
Intra-aortic balloon counterpulsation (see Chapter 15) is a mechanical circulatory assist device commonly used for management of shock syndrome. The development of a percutaneous insertion technique has made it easier to initiate balloon counterpulsation, although rarely insertion through a surgical femoral arteriotomy is needed. Intra-aortic balloon pumping reduces left ventricular oxygen demand by its afterload reducing effect while the increased diastolic aortic pressure helps to maintain or improve coronary perfusion pressure and subendocardial blood flow. The combined systolic unloading and diastolic augmentation tend to reduce myocardial ischemia, left ventricular filling pressures, mitral regurgitation, and left-to-right shunt across a ventricular septal rupture, whereas the forward stroke volume and cardiac output tend to increase. Electrocardiographic synchronization is used to begin balloon inflation at the time of aortic valve closure to produce diastolic pressure augmentation and to initiate deflation just prior to the onset of systole, thereby causing systolic unloading (Fig. 16-5). Hemodynamic effects of balloon counterpul-

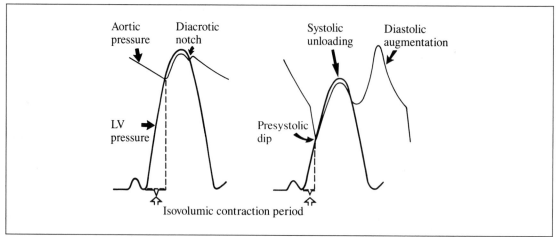

Fig. 16-5
Principle of intra-aortic balloon counterpulsation. Initiation of balloon inflation is timed to the arterial dicrotic notch producing diastolic augmentation in arterial pressure, whereas deflation of the balloon prior to the next ventricular systole contributes to systolic unloading.

sation may be further augmented by concomitant use of vasodilator or inotropic drugs.

Although patients with cardiogenic shock frequently demonstrate temporary clinical and hemodynamic improvement during intra-aortic balloon pumping, short- and long-term mortality remain high unless intra-aortic balloon pumping is used for short-term stabilization of the patient; it is done in preparation for salvage of jeopardized nonfunctioning (but still viable) ischemic myocardium with coronary revascularization or for correction of severe mechanical complications, i.e., mitral regurgitation and ventricular septal rupture. The patients least likely to benefit from intra-aortic balloon pumping are those with multiple previous infarctions, large areas of myocardial scarring with massive irreversible necrosis, or late and advanced stages of cardiogenic shock; elderly patients with peripheral vascular disease who are most at risk of morbidity from insertion of the device also belong in this group [46, 47]. For patients with evidence of large areas of ischemic but viable myocardium or in whom there are mechanical complications (both amenable to definitive surgical therapy), balloon counterpulsation begun within a few hours after development of shock offers the best prospect of benefit when

subsequent definitive surgical intervention is combined with it [48, 49].

From a pragmatic standpoint, balloon counterpulsation should be considered for relatively young patients, who are free of severe aortoiliac disease or aortic regurgitation, who have developed cardiogenic shock after their first infarction, and who have failed to improve with a trial of pharmacologic therapy given for 30 to 60 minutes. Every attempt should be made to determine the presence of surgically remediable lesions as described earlier using noninvasive and invasive techniques. Early cardiac catheterization, usually within 48 to 96 hours of the onset of balloon counterpulsation, should be performed and surgical intervention instituted for suitable patients. Those patients who are unsuitable for surgery or in whom surgery must be delayed because of intercurrent complications should undergo weaning from balloon counterpulsation after a stabilization period of 2 to 4 days. The prognosis in such patients is generally unfavorable.

Complications occur in up to 30 percent of patients subjected to intra-aortic balloon counterpulsation and tend to be more frequent with the use of percutaneous methods [46, 47]. The complications are mostly vascular (i.e., vascular compromise of extremities and abdominal viscera, damage to femoral artery, aortic dissection,) but also include infection, hemolysis, thrombocytopenia, gas leak, and embolism. In the authors' experience, complications are particularly likely in older individuals (>70 years), especially older women, and in those with aortoiliac vascular disease [46]. We generally recommend the use of small-caliber balloon catheters for the elderly and women whose native vessels tend to be smaller.

EARLY REPERFUSION

Because ventriculopenic shock results from large areas of nonfunctioning left ventricular myocardium, early restoration of myocardial blood flow during the evolutionary phase of myocardial infarction (phases of ischemia and mixed pathology), when substantial amounts of nonfunctioning myocardium are still viable, may be the most rational and effective therapy for preventing death and morbidity. Early reperfusion can relieve ischemia of jeopardized myocardium, restore its contractile function immediately or over time, render reperfused, salvaged but nonfunctioning myocardium more responsive to inotropic agents, limit the eventual degree of necrosis, preserve ventricular function, and dramatically improve the outlook of these patients. Preliminary reports of reperfusion using early percutaneous transluminal coronary angioplasty with or without prior thrombolytic therapy in selected patients with cardiogenic shock have been encouraging, with reports of 40 to 60 percent survival [31–34]. Furthermore, randomized trials of thrombolytic therapy for evolving myocardial infarction have demonstrated a reduction in the frequency with which acute myocardial infarction progresses to cardiogenic shock.

A report from a multicenter registry documented 59 percent in-hospital survival among 69 patients with cardiogenic shock after an acute myocardial infarction, using coronary balloon angioplasty [34]. When angioplasty was successful, short-term survival was 69 percent compared to a 20 percent survival

when angioplasty failed to accomplish reperfusion. At a mean of 32 months' follow-up, 55 percent of successfully reperfused patients were surviving compared to only 20 percent of those in whom angioplasty had failed [34]. In another study involving 53 patients, survival was 40 percent among patients who were successfully reperfused with angioplasty, thrombolytic therapy, or both within 6 hours of the onset of symptoms, whereas nonreperfused patients had only a 19 percent survival rate [34].

Combining angioplasty with thrombolytic therapy, rather than thrombolytic therapy alone, appears to be more successful in reversing shock and improving survival. Thus from these preliminary reports, the modern approach to management of cardiogenic shock within the first 6 hours of the onset of acute myocardial infarction appears to be moving toward aggressive attempts at reperfusion rather than the palliative use of cardioactive-vasoactive drugs and mechanical assist devices alone. It is important, however, to recognize that, despite reperfusion, short-term circulatory support with drugs or devices may still be necessary to tide the patient through the early phase of shock.

CARDIAC SURGERY

Cardiac surgery may improve the long-term survival of selected patients with shock following acute myocardial infarction. These patients may benefit from coronary revascularization or corrective repair of a potentially lethal mechanical complication, i.e., severe mitral regurgitation or ventricular septal or subacute free-wall rupture [50]. The potential value of myocardial revascularization in the absence of mechanical complications depends on the existence of ischemic but viable myocardium with impaired function, which would gain sufficient function from revascularization to sustain global ventricular function. After stabilization of the patient with general supportive, specific pharmacologic, and in many cases balloon counterpulsation therapy, prompt cardiac catheterization is recommended to define the presence and feasibility of cardiac surgery. Survival rates of 50 to 75 percent may be accomplished with this approach in properly selected cases.

SHOCK SYNDROME WITHOUT PULMONARY CONGESTION OR PULMONARY EDEMA

A clinical syndrome of low-output hypotensive state following myocardial infarction may occur without signs of left ventricular failure. Such a clinical syndrome may result from bradyarrhythmias, hypovolemia, right ventricular infarction, and superimposed complications such as pulmonary embolism or sepsis.

Invasive hemodynamic studies of acute myocardial infarction have demonstrated that in some patients with shock the left ventricular filling pressure is normal, low, or only minimally elevated; and in some of these patients the clinical and hemodynamic state may improve with rapid volume loading. The precise reasons for this hypovolemic state are not clear, but overdiuresis, excessive use of vasodilators, possible reflexly mediated inappropriate peripheral vasodilation, and in some cases diaphoresis and vomiting resulting in dehydration may contribute to volume depletion. These patients can be recognized when low-output state or shock is associated with collapsed neck veins without signs of pulmonary congestion on physical examination and chest radiograph and without an S_3 gallop. In other patients the diagnosis can be made with certainty only using invasive hemodynamic monitoring. The hemodynamic profile of these patients is typified by the Cedars-Sinai subset III, i.e., a cardiac index of 2.2 or less with a pulmonary capillary wedge pressure of, at most, 18 mm Hg but usually considerably lower. It is also important to recognize that some patients with predominant right ventricular dysfunction complicating an acute inferior infarction may have a similar hemodynamic profile.

The treatment of hypovolemic shock requires rapid volume infusion using aliquots of 50 to 100 ml of fluid (colloid or crystalloid) under close clinical and hemodynamic observation until the pulmonary capillary wedge pressure is elevated to a maximum of 15 to 18 mm Hg. Further volume infusion may precipitate pulmonary congestion or edema and should be avoided. In some patients, particularly those receiving crystalloid infusions, pulmonary congestion and edema may even occur at lower pulmonary wedge pressures possibly owing to a reduction in intracapillary oncotic pressure resulting from dilutional hypoalbuminemia. Thus careful clinical assessment in addition to hemodynamic monitoring is essential while volume loading is under way. Some patients fail to improve their pump function despite restoration of pulmonary capillary wedge pressure to seemingly adequate levels. Such patients generally have a severely reduced left ventricular systolic function (ejection fraction) with the ventricle operating along a flat Starling curve. Alternatively, volume loading may elevate pulmonary capillary wedge pressure without a real increase in left ventricular preload or end-diastolic volume when left ventricular compliance is abnormal.

Right Ventricular Infarction

Ischemia and infarction of the right ventricle may occur in as many as 30 to 40 percent of patients with acute inferior or posterior myocardial infarction and rarely with anterior infarction [51, 52]. Associated infarction of the posterior part of the interventricular septum and variable degrees of inferoposterior left ventricular infarction are common, as these territories share a common blood supply from the right coronary artery [51]. Right ventricular dysfunction due to ischemia or infarction is clinically silent in many patients, but in 30 to 40 percent of cases it is associated with a low-output, hypotensive syndrome often simulating true cardiogenic shock. Diagnosis of hemodynamically significant predominant right ventricular dysfunction in acute myocardial infarction (Fig. 16-6) should be considered in any patient with acute inferior or posterior myocardial infarction complicated by a low-output or hypotensive syndrome; it is especially considered when accompanied by ele-

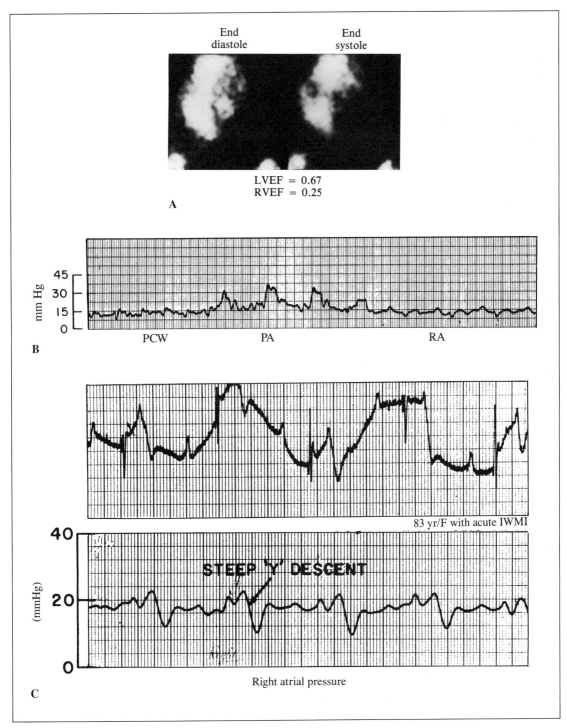

Fig. 16-6
A. Radionuclide ventriculogram in a 45-degree left anterior oblique projection demonstrating predominant right ventricular dysfunction in a patient with acute inferior infarction. LV = left ventricle; RV = right ventricle; EF = ejection fraction. *B.* Hemodynamic findings of equalization of right atrial and pulmonary capillary wedge pressures in a patient with postinfarction predominant right ventricular dysfunction. *C.* Abnormal right atrial pressure waveform showing a steep y descent in a patient with postinfarction predominant right ventricular dysfunction.

vated jugular venous pressure or increased jugular venous pressure during inspiration (Kussmaul sign) or during abdominal compression (abdominojugular reflux) with little evidence of pulmonary congestion. In about 30 percent of patients, however, the jugular venous pressure may be within normal limits. Rarely, a murmur of tricuspid regurgitation secondary to right ventricular papillary muscle dysfunction may be heard. The presence of pulsus paradoxus in some patients leads to an erroneous diagnosis of cardiac tamponade [53].

The electrocardiogram, in addition to the changes of acute inferior infarction, frequently shows ST segment elevation in right-sided precordial leads (V_{3R} or V_{4R}) or, less commonly, over V_1–V_5. Such precordial ST elevations may create confusing electrocardiographic patterns simulating concomitant left anterior descending coronary occlusion [54].

A wide spectrum of hemodynamic abnormalities may be observed, with elevation of right atrial and right ventricular end-diastolic pressure equal to or above the pulmonary capillary wedge pressure, which may be low, normal, or only modestly elevated. Other hemodynamic findings may include a steep right atrial y descent (Fig. 6-6C) with a paradoxical increase in the right atrial pressure during inspiration (Kussmaul sign), a dip and plateau during diastole in the right ventricular pressure tracing, pulmonary arterial and right ventricular pulsus alternans, and diminished pulse pressures in the right ventricle and pulmonary artery. Many of these hemodynamic findings overlap with those of cardiac tamponade, constrictive pericarditis, or restrictive myocardial disease [53]. In nearly 30 percent of patients, however, abnormalities of right atrial pressure are not evident initially but appear only later in the course of illness or following volume infusion. Severe arterial desaturation secondary to a right-to-left shunt through a stretched patent foramen ovale has rarely been observed [55]. Echocardiography and radionuclide ventriculography demonstrate disproportionate right ventricular dilation, dyssynergy, and a depressed ejection fraction (<0.39) compared

to the left ventricle, which generally demonstrates an ejection fraction of 0.45 or more. Technetium 99m pyrophosphate imaging may show uptake in the right ventricle. However, severe left ventricular global and regional dysfunction coexist in some cases of right ventricular infarction, and such patients with severe biventricular dysfunction may behave differently from patients with predominant right ventricular dysfunction [18].

The low-output hypotensive syndrome results predominantly from reduced left ventricular filling and low left ventricular end-diastolic volume [52]. However, bradyarrhythmias, which are frequently observed with this syndrome (particularly when associated with loss of appropriately timed atrial contraction), may aggravate or even precipitate the low-output syndrome. The reduction in left ventricular volume results from reduced right ventricular systolic function with a consequent decrease in pulmonary blood flow and left ventricular inflow, as well as an increase in intrapericardial pressure secondary to right ventricular dilation, producing in effect a tamponade of the left ventricle [52, 53, 56]. In addition, diastolic septal bulge into the left ventricle (reverse Bernheim effect) may contribute to decreased left ventricular volume.

It is important to recognize that volume infusion alone is rarely successful in improving the hemodynamic or clinical state in patients with right ventricular infarction and that concomitant use of inotropic or vasoactive drug therapy is necessary in most patients [52]. The overall survival is generally favorable in this subset of patients owing probably to spontaneous improvement that occurs in right ventricular function over time [52]. However, when severe left ventricular dysfunction (hemodynamic evidence of which may remain masked) coexists or if papillary muscle, free-wall, or ventricular septal rupture occurs, the outlook becomes grave [18, 52]. Rarely, tricuspid valve replacement has been necessary to treat shock and severe tricuspid regurgitation; and closure of a patent foramen ovale has been necessary for refractory right-to-left shunt and life-threatening hypoxemia.

Mechanical Complications

Mechanical complications following myocardial infarction include acute mitral regurgitation (papillary muscle dysfunction and rupture) or septal or free-wall rupture. Cardiac rupture contributes to 15 to 30 percent of all deaths related to acute myocardial infarction. Papillary muscle rupture accounts for 5 percent of all cardiac ruptures, ventricular septal rupture for 10 percent, and free-wall rupture for 85 percent.

ACUTE MITRAL REGURGITATION

Acute mitral regurgitation following myocardial infarction can result from: (1) ischemia or necrosis of the left ventricular papillary muscles and the contiguous portion of the left ventricular wall from where the papillary muscles originate (papillary muscle dysfunction); (2) rupture of the tip or, less commonly, the trunk of papillary muscle; and (3) rarely, from rupture of the chordae tendineae.

PAPILLARY MUSCLE DYSFUNCTION

An intricate balance of geometry and function of components of the mitral valve complex is necessary for normal competent function of the mitral valve, failure of which can result in varying degrees of malfunction and regurgitation. The mitral valve complex consists of the annulus, mitral leaflets (anterior and posterior), papillary muscles (anterolateral and posteromedial), 120 chordae tendineae, the left ventricular wall where the two papillary muscles are attached, and the left atrial wall. The posteromedial papillary muscle receives blood supply predominantly from the posterior descending branch of the angiographically dominant coronary artery [commonly the right (90 percent) but occasionally the left (10 percent) circumflex] with few twigs from the nondominant artery. The anterolateral papillary muscle receives its blood supply from the left anterior descending coronary artery or its diagonal branches and from the marginal termination of the left circumflex coronary artery. The anterolateral papillary muscle originates from the midportion of the anterolateral left ventricular wall and receives chordal attachment from both mitral leaflets. The bulkier posteromedial papillary muscle originates from the junction of the lower or middle one-third of the ventricular septum and the posterior left ventricular wall, and it receives chordal attachment from the medial one-half of both mitral leaflets. The high propensity of papillary muscle for ischemia and infarction in coronary disease is related partly to its disadvantaged blood supply from inconstant and tenuous sources and its innermost cardiac location at the terminus of cardiac arterial circulation; it is also subject to exiguous perfusion and a relatively high degree of tension development during systole. Its attendant high metabolic oxygen cost is similar to that of subendocardial myocardium. Posteromedial papillary muscle ischemia, infarction, or rupture is five to ten times more common than that of anterolateral papillary muscle, possibly because of its more tenuous blood supply, which comes predominantly from a single artery.

Papillary muscle ischemia or infarction is rarely sufficient to result in severe mitral regurgitation unless there is deranged contractile function of the left ventricular myocardium contiguous to the base of the papillary muscle [57]. It is likely that in many cases mitral regurgitation resulting from papillary muscle dysfunction occurs when papillary muscle contraction fails to occur or occurs along an abnormal axis, shifted inappropriately by coexistent ventricular dilatation and dyssynergy, resulting in an inability of the mitral leaflets to coapt appropriately during systole.

Recognition of papillary muscle dysfunction complicating acute myocardial infarction is based on the appearance of intermittent or persistent mitral regurgitation. Mitral regurgitation is suspected in patients with a new systolic apical murmur of variable intensity, duration, pitch, and radiation who demonstrate disproportionately large V waves on pulmonary capillary wedge pressure or severe mitral regurgitation on left ventricular angiography. However, the systolic murmur may be ephemeral and lingering, soft or loud, high- or low-pitched, holosystolic or midsystolic, or even completely absent despite severe mitral regurgitation [58, 59]. Depending on the concomitant severity of left ventricular dysfunction and the degree of acute mitral regurgitation, the patient may develop clinical manifestations of persistent or intermittent pulmonary congestion, pulmonary edema, hypotension, or shock.

Recognition of severe mitral regurgitation, persistent or intermittent, requires a high index of clinical suspicion. Advances in echocardiography and Doppler techniques have made it possible to detect mitral regurgitation and assess its severity at the bedside. Such patients should be subjected to prompt cardiac catheterization followed by surgery that may include mitral valve repair or replacement as well as coronary artery bypass.

In preparation for cardiac catheterization and surgery, the condition of a severely symptomatic patient may require stabilization using pharmacologic support (intravenous vasodilators and inotropic agents) and mechanical circulatory assist (intra-aortic balloon pumping). A report of three patients with acute myocardial infarction complicated by mitral regurgitation and pulmonary edema or shock treated successfully with coronary angioplasty is provocative, as prompt resolution of hemodynamic instability and resolution of mitral regurgitation was documented [60].

PAPILLARY MUSCLE RUPTURE

Rupture of the left ventricular papillary muscle, a serious complication of acute myocardial infarction, occurs in approximately 1 percent of cases and accounts for up to 5 percent of infarcts resulting in death [61, 62]. Papillary muscle rupture tends to occur 2 to 7 days after infarction, but up to 20 percent of cases may occur within 24 hours of the onset of infarction. Most of the ruptures involve the posteromedial papillary muscle, a complication of inferior or posterior infarction resulting from occlusive disease of the circumflex or the right coronary artery for reasons described earlier. The degree of left ventricular myocardial ne-

crosis is variable, with nearly 50 percent of patients demonstrating relatively small or subendocardial infarction [62]. Likewise, the extent of coronary artery disease is variable, with nearly 50 percent of patients having single-vessel disease [61]. The most frequent form of papillary muscle rupture involves one of the smaller heads of the papillary muscle, whereas rupture of the main trunk of the papillary muscle is less common and generally incompatible with more than brief survival [61].

The clinical presentation is dominated by the sudden development of severe pulmonary congestion and pulmonary edema, with many patients rapidly progressing to shock. A loud holosystolic apical murmur with widespread radiation may be detected. However, the systolic murmur may be brief (owing to rapid equilibration of left atrial and left ventricular pressures during late systole), nondescript, or even completely absent (silent mitral regurgitation) in some patients. The severe respiratory distress and adventitious pulmonary sounds caused by pulmonary edema may make it difficult to hear a murmur even when it is present. A palpable thrill is distinctly rare with papillary muscle rupture. The electrocardiogram often shows evidence of inferior or posterior infarction, which in many cases may be limited to seemingly minor ST–T changes, a deceptively benign appearance despite the catastrophic clinical deterioration. The chest radiograph shows pulmonary congestion or edema, which may be preferentially distributed to upper lung lobes particularly on the right side, simulating pulmonary infiltrates. This preferential location may be the outcome of the mitral regurgitant jet being directed toward the orifice of the right upper lobe pulmonary veins. The left ventricular ejection fraction may be normal or supernormal because of the relatively limited degree of myocardial necrosis coupled with the unloading effect of severe mitral regurgitation depressed when infarction is extensive. However, the right ventricular ejection fraction may be depressed owing to associated acute pulmonary arterial hypertension or coexistent right ventricular infarction.

The diagnosis can be made noninvasively in the presence of the appropriate clinical con-

Table 16-8
Papillary muscle rupture with acute mitral regurgitation versus ventricular septal rupture

Papillary muscle rupture with acute mitral regurgitation	Ventricular septal rupture
Characteristics	
Occurs in 1% of all infarcts	Occurs in 1–2% of all infarcts
Peak incidence 3–5 days after infarct	Peak incidence 3–5 days after infarct
More frequent in inferoposterior infarcts (posterior papillary more frequently involved)	Equally frequent in anterior and inferior infarcts
Murmur usually loud and holosystolic but may be soft and nonholosystolic or completely absent	Murmur loud and holosystolic with widespread radiation
Palpable precordial thrill, rarely	Palpable precordial thrill in 50%
Diagnostic techniques	
Two-dimensional echocardiography: flail or prolapsing leaflet	Visualization of defect in septum (with or without contrast echocardiography)
Doppler: systolic regurgitant jet into left atrium	Detection of transseptal left-to-right shunt
Radionuclide ventriculography: normal, increased, or reduced LV ejection fraction with abnormal stroke/count ratio	Normal, increased, or reduced LV ejection fraction with abnormal stroke/count ratio; left-to-right shunt on a first-pass study
Pulmonary artery catheterization	
Prominent V waves on PCW tracing, reflected V waves on PA tracing	Oxygen saturation in RV and PA shows a step-up compared to RA (PA>RA by $\geq$ 10% saturation)
Left ventricular angiography: mitral regurgitation visualized	Ventricular septal defect visualized

text. Echocardiography may show a flail mitral leaflet as well as hyperdynamic left ventricular wall motion. When a Doppler flow study is performed, the presence and severity of mitral regurgitation can be gauged at the bedside. Even when a characteristic mitral valve echo of papillary muscle rupture is not observed on echocardiography, hyperdynamic left ventricular wall motion in a postinfarction patient with pulmonary edema and shock suggests the diagnosis. Hemodynamic evaluation shows elevated pulmonary capillary wedge pressure with tall V waves, which are sometimes reflected in the pulmonary arterial tracing as well. Papillary muscle rupture can be differentiated from ventricular septal rupture by several features (Table 16-8).

Patients with papillary muscle rupture experience 50 percent mortality within 24 hours and 94 percent mortality within 8 weeks [61–63]. Although some patients appear to stabilize and improve with supportive medical therapy, such improvement is transitory and is usually followed by deterioration. Early surgical correction by valve replacement or repair can salvage up to 60 to 70 percent of patients.

The catastrophic clinical course, the frequent evidence of relatively limited extent of myocardial necrosis and obstructive coronary artery disease, and a better outcome with surgery provide an impetus and rationale for early recognition of and early surgery for papillary muscle rupture [61, 62]. In preparation for urgent cardiac catheterization and subsequent surgery, patients frequently require intra-aortic balloon pumping and additional diuretic, vasodilator, or inotropic therapy for temporary stabilization. Papillary muscle rupture is one of the few causes of pulmonary edema or shock complicating myocardial infarction whereby aggressive and early surgical correction can result in improved short- and long-term survival rates compared to the natural history of this complication when untreated.

VENTRICULAR SEPTAL RUPTURE

Rupture of the interventricular septum is a catastrophic and serious complication of acute myocardial infarction that occurs in 0.5 to 2.0 percent of infarction cases and is responsible for 1 to 5 percent of all infarct-related deaths [64]. Septal rupture occurs with both anterior and inferior or posterior infarction and is associated with infarction of the interventricular septum as well as a variable extent of the left or right ventricular myocardium. Although multivessel obstructive coronary artery disease is common, septal rupture may complicate single-vessel disease. Rupture of the septum may occur as early as within the first 24 hours of the onset of infarction or as late as 2 weeks hence; however, most cases tend to occur 3 to 7 days after infarction. Rupture of the septum results in a left-to-right interventricular shunt producing right ventricular volume overload, increased pulmonary blood flow, and reduced systemic blood flow. Reduction in systemic blood flow results in a low-output hypotensive syndrome that rapidly progresses to shock. The left ventricular ejection fraction is usually normal or supernormal but may be variably depressed depending on the magnitude of the ventricular infarction. The unloading effect of the left-to-right shunt may result in a higher left ventricular ejection fraction relative to the extent of myocardial necrosis. The right ventricular ejection fraction may be depressed secondary to right ventricular volume overload and increased pulmonary arterial pressure, particularly in patients with concomitant ischemic damage or infarction of the right ventricle.

Ventricular septal rupture is associated with the development of a new harsh, loud holosystolic precordial murmur with widespread radiation. It is accompanied by a palpable thrill in about 50 percent of the cases. Clinically, the patient may have recurrence of chest pain and dyspnea followed by signs and symptoms of a low-output state, hypotension, or shock. Right ventricular volume overload secondary to the shunt, concomitant right ventricular ischemic damage, and tricuspid regurgitation may produce signs of systemic venous congestion out of proportion to those of pulmonary venous congestion. The diagnosis can be confirmed rapidly at the bedside using two-dimensional echocardiography, which demonstrates the site and approximate size of the septal rupture [65, 66]. The diagnosis can be further refined by using echo-bubble contrast or Doppler echocardiography. First-pass radionuclide ventriculography may also demonstrate an intracardiac left-to-right shunt. Bedside right heart catheterization is useful for confirming the diagnosis and permits an approximate calculation of the degree of left-to-right shunt. An increase in oxygen saturation (≥ 10 percent) from right atrium to right ventricle or proximal pulmonary artery in the appropriate clinical setting is virtually diagnostic of ventricular septal rupture.

The clinical course of septal rupture is ominous, with a 24 percent mortality within 24 hours, 46 percent mortality at 1 week, 67 to 82 percent mortality at 2 months, and only 5 to 7 percent survival at 1 year [50, 64]. Conservative medical therapy of septal rupture is generally ineffective. Afterload reduction by vasodilators may decrease left ventricular systolic pressure and reduce the degree of left-to-right shunt, but more pulmonary than systemic vasodilation could actually increase the shunt. Severe systemic hypotension frequently precludes the aggressive use of vasodilators. Inotropic and vasopressor drug therapy may be necessary to sustain arterial blood pressure, but it could produce tachyarrhythmias, systemic vasoconstriction with increasing left-to-right shunt, and myocardial ischemia. Transient stabilization can be achieved with intra-aortic balloon counterpulsation alone or in conjunction with vasodilator and inotropic drug therapy, but such stabilization is often temporary and should be used only in preparation for urgent cardiac catheterization to confirm the diagnosis, define the coronary anatomy, or determine mitral valve competence and left ventricular function.

It should be followed by prompt cardiac surgery involving repair of the defect and, when necessary, coronary bypass surgery and aneurysmectomy. Such an aggressive surgical approach results in 48 to 75 percent short-term survival [50]. Follow-up over 17 to 91 months has shown a late mortality of 5 to 14 percent in some series [50]. Cardiogenic shock, right ventricular infarction, and evidence of end-organ failure (pulmonary, renal) appear to portend a higher perioperative mortality [58]. The results of surgery appear more favorable for anteriorly located septal ruptures compared to posteriorly located defects possibly because of technical problems encountered during repair of posteriorly located defects, coexistent mitral regurgitation, and ischemic right ventricular dysfunction.

FREE-WALL RUPTURE

Free-wall rupture contributes to 8 to 24 percent of deaths related to acute myocardial infarction and occurs in 1.5 to 8.0 percent of all acute myocardial infarcts [67]. The peak incidence of rupture appears to be around the second to eighth day after infarction, although about 30 percent of ruptures occur within 24 hours of the onset of infarction. Rupture occurs through an area of transmural necrosis and expansion; the infarct-related coronary artery is invariably totally occluded with a thrombus, and the collateral circulation is sparse or absent [67, 68]. The rupture occurs mainly in the left ventricle. Free-wall rupture may occur with anterior and inferior infarcts. Rarely, right ventricular rupture occurs as a complication of right ventricular infarction. Free-wall rupture occurs most frequently after a first infarction, during and after the seventh decade of life, in women, and in those with a history of systemic hypertension or hypertension complicating myocardial infarction [68]. Early ambulation, short-term use of anti-inflammatory drugs (steroids, indomethacin), and anticoagulants have been implicated in predisposing to cardiac rupture, although firm evidence is lacking.

Early thrombolytic-anticoagulant therapy initiated before transmural infarction is complete does not appear to increase the risk of cardiac rupture. Early reperfusion therapy may in fact halt transmural spread of myocardial infarction and thereby reduce the risk of free-wall rupture by preserving a viable shell of epicardial tissue. This theory is supported by published data on the incidence of cardiac rupture among patients receiving thrombolytic therapy when compared to conventionally treated patients with acute myocardial infarction. It is possible, however, that thrombolytic anticoagulant therapy, when administered after completion of transmural necrosis and occurrence of pericarditis, may actually increase the risk of cardiac rupture or hemopericardium.

Free-wall rupture generally presents as a catastrophic clinical syndrome characterized by sudden severe and often tearing pain that is rapidly followed by hypotension, jugular venous distention, and electromechanical dissociation. Frequently there is a vagally mediated junctional or sinus bradycardia associated with the hypotension. In some patients this clinical scenario may be preceded or accompanied by intense agitation and mental confusion, whereas in other patients intermittent chest pain may precede the full-blown catastrophic syndrome. In most such patients, death from hemopericardium and tamponade ensues rapidly, and few cases with this mode of presentation can be salvaged by anything short of heroic measures, i.e., immediate pericardiocentesis, emergency thoracotomy, and surgical repair.

A more subacute form of free-wall rupture with progressively increasing signs of cardiac tamponade over hours or days occurs in some patients. Only a high index of suspicion can lead to proper investigation, diagnosis, and appropriate surgery [69]. It is important to recognize this subacute form of rupture, as surgery can lead to gratifying long-term results [50, 69].

Rarely, free-wall rupture of the left ventricle leads to pseudoaneurysm formation, which is a consequence of containment of the resulting hemopericardium by circumferential adhesions between the pericardium and the epicardium (Fig. 16-7). Most pseudoaneurysms reported in the literature, however, have resulted from complications of cardiac surgery, chest trauma, and bacterial endocarditis [70]. In one retrospective review, a pseudoaneurysm was detected in 0.5 percent of 1050 patients referred for cardiac catheterization [71]. The pseudoaneurysm frequently contains a thrombus and communicates with the body of

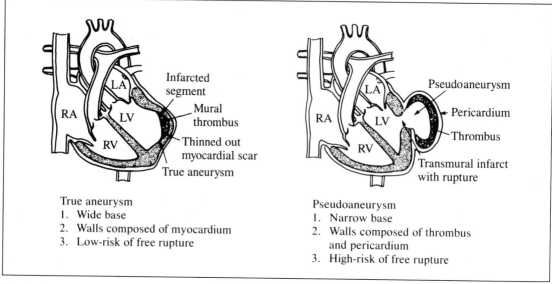

Fig. 16-7
Differences between a pseudoaneurysm and a true aneurysm.

the left ventricle through a narrow isthmus. It may remain small or enlarge progressively, eventually becoming larger than the main left ventricle in some cases. In contrast to a true aneurysm, the walls of the pseudoaneurysm are composed of pericardium and adhesions and are devoid of myocardial tissue and coronary arteries. Pseudoaneurysm may remain clinically silent and be discovered only during routine investigation. In some patients it leads to progressively worsening congestive heart failure, recurrent ventricular arrhythmias, cardiomegaly with an abnormal bulge on the cardiac border, and persistent elevation of the ST segment overlying an area of infarction on the electrocardiogram, thereby simulating a true aneurysm. Systolic and diastolic murmurs, presumably related to back-and-forth movement of blood across the narrow isthmus of the aneurysm, may occur, simulating valvular heart disease [72]. The pseudoaneurysm is prone to free rupture with an invariably fatal outcome, whereas such a complication is rare with chronic true aneurysm [70]. Two-dimensional echocardiography, radionuclide ventriculography, or invasive left ventriculography, cine-computed tomography, and magnetic resonance imaging can be used to make a diagnosis of pseudoaneurysm. Surgical resection

is strongly recommended in symptomatic as well as asymptomatic patients, irrespective of the size of the pseudoaneurysm, to prevent a catastrophic outcome from rupture.

Acknowledgments

The authors gratefully acknowledge the secretarial work of Beverly Yoshioka and Sharon Hulse-Adler, and the artwork of the Audiovisual Department (Cedars-Sinai Medical Center, Los Angeles).

Figures 16-1 to 16-3, 16-5 to 16-7, Tables 16-1 to 16-5, 16-7 and 16-8 were reprinted with permission from K. Chatterjee, Complications of Acute Myocardial Infarction. In W. Parmley and K. Chatterjee (eds.), *Cardiology*. Philadelphia: Lippincott, 1987.

References

1. Multicenter Post Infarction Research Group: Risk stratification and survival after myocardial infarction. *N. Engl. J. Med.* 309:331, 1983.
2. May, G. S., Furberg, C. D., Eberlein, K. A., et al. Secondary prevention after myocardial infarction: A review of short term acute phase trials. *Prog. Cardiovasc. Dis.* 25:335, 1983.

3. Herrick, J. B. Clinical features of sudden obstruction of the coronary arteries. *J.A.M.A.* 59:2015, 1912.

4. Roberts, W. C. Coronary arteries in fatal acute myocardial infarction. *Circulation* 45:215, 1972.

5. DeWood, M. A., Spores, J., Notske, R., et al. Prevalence of total coronary occlusion during the early hours of transmural myocardial infarction. *N. Engl. J. Med.* 303:897, 1981.

6. Reimer, K. A., Lowe, J. E. Rasmussen, M. M., et al. The wave-front phenomenon of ischemic cell death. *Circulation* 56:786, 1977.

7. Herman, M. V., Heinle, R. A., Klein, M. D., et al. Localized disorders in myocardial contraction. *N. Engl. J. Med.* 227:222, 1967.

8. Eaton, L. W., and Bulkley, B. H. Expansion of acute myocardial infarction: Its relationship to infarct morphology in a canine model. *Circ. Res.* 49:80, 1981.

9. Erlebacher, J. A., Weiss, J. L., Eaton, L. W., et al. Late effects of acute infarct dilation on heart size: A two dimensional echocardiographic study. *Am. J. Cardiol.* 49:1120, 1982.

10. Bertrand, M., Rousseau, M. F., LaBlanche, J. M., et al. Cineangiographic assessment of left ventricular function in the acute phase of transmural myocardial infarction. *Am. J. Cardiol.* 43:472, 1979.

11. Bardet, J., Rocha, P., Rigaud, M., et al. Left ventricular compliance in acute myocardial infarction in man. *Cardiovasc. Res.* 11:122, 1977.

12. Swan, H. J. C., Forrester, J. S., Diamond, G., et al. Hemodynamic spectrum of myocardial infarction and cardiogenic shock. *Circulation* 45:1097, 1972.

13. Shah, P. K., Pichler, M., Berman, D. S., et al. Left ventricular ejection fraction determined by radionuclide ventriculography in early stages of first transmural myocardial infarction: Relation to short term prognosis. *Am. J. Cardiol.* 45:542, 1980.

14. Bigger, J. T., Fleiss, J. L., Kleiger, R., et al. The relationship among ventricular arrhythmias, left ventricular dysfunction, and mortality in the 2 years after myocardial infarction. *Circulation* 69:250, 1984.

15. Killip, T., and Kimbal, J. T. Treatment of myocardial infarction in a coronary care unit: A two year experience with 250 patients. *Am. J. Cardiol.* 20:457, 1967.

16. Forrester, J. S., Diamond, G. A., Chatterjee, K., et al. Medical therapy of acute myocardial infarction by application of hemodynamic subsets (first of two parts). *N. Engl. J. Med.* 295:1356, 1976.

17. Forrester, J. S., Diamond, G. A., Chatterjee, K., et al. Medical therapy of acute myocardial infarction by application of hemodynamic subsets (second of two parts). *N. Engl. J. Med.* 295:1404, 1976.

18. Shah, P. K., Maddahi, J., Staniloff, H. M., et al. The variable spectrum and prognostic implications of left and right ventricular ejection fractions determined early in the course of acute myocardial infarction associated with clinical evidence of no or mild heart failure. *Am. J. Cardiol.*, in press.

19. Swan, H. J. C., Ganz, W., Forrester, J., et al. Catheterization of the heart in man with use of a flow-directed balloon-tipped catheter. *N. Engl. J. Med.* 283:447, 1970.

20. Dikshit, K., Vyden, J. K., Forrester, J. S., et al. Renal and extrarenal hemodynamic effects of furosemide in congestive heart failure after acute myocardial infarction. *N. Engl. J. Med.* 288:1087, 1973.

21. Francis, G. S., Siegel, R. M., Goldsmith, S. R., et al. Acute vasoconstrictor response to intravenous furosemide in patients with chronic congestive heart failure. *Ann. Intern. Med.* 103:1, 1985.

22. Bussman, W. D., and Kaltenbach, M. Sublingual nitroglycerin in the treatment of left ventricular failure and pulmonary edema. *Eur. J. Cardiol.* 4:327, 1976.

23. Shah, P. K. Buccal nitroglycerin ointment in acute cardiac pulmonary edema. *Ann. Intern. Med.* 103:153, 1985.

24. Page, D. L., Caulfield, J. B., Kastor, J. A., et al. Myocardial changes associated with cardiogenic shock. *N. Engl. J. Med.* 285:133, 1971.

25. Alonso, D. R., Scheidt, S., Post, M., et al. Pathophysiology of cardiogenic shock: Quantification of myocardial necrosis: Clinical, pathologic and electrocardiographic correlation. *Circulation* 48:588, 1973.

26. Gutovitz, A. L., Sobel, B. E., and Roberts, R. Progressive nature of myocardial injury in selected patients with cardiogenic shock. *Am. J. Cardiol.* 41:469, 1978.

27. Wackers, F. J., Lie, K. I., and Becker, A. E. Coronary artery disease in patients dying from cardiogenic shock or congestive heart failure in the setting of acute myocardial infarction. *Br. Heart J.* 38:906, 1976.

28. Eaton, L. W., Weiss, J. L., Bulkley, B. H., et al. Regional cardiac dilatation after acute myocardial infarction: Recognition by 2-D echocardiography. *N. Engl. J. Med.* 300:57, 1979.

29. Meizlish, J. L., Berger, H. J., Plankey, M., et al. Functional left ventricular aneurysm formation after acute anterior transmural myocardial infarction: Incidence, natural history and prognostic implications. *N. Engl. J. Med.* 311:1001, 1984.

30. Doherty, N. E., Ades, A., Shah, P. K., et al. Hypothermia as a consequence of acute myocardial infarction: Reversal with intra-aortic balloon counterpulsation. *Ann. Intern. Med.* 101:863, 1984.

31. Lew, A. S., Weiss, A. T., Shah, P. K., et al. Extensive myocardial salvage and reversal of cardiogenic shock after reperfusion of the left main coronary artery by intravenous streptokinase. *Am. J. Cardiol.* 54:450, 1984.

32. Mathey, D. G., Kuck, K. H., Tilsner, V., et al. Nonsurgical coronary artery recanalization in acute transmural myocardial infarction. *Circulation* 63:489, 1981.

33. Meyer, J., Merx, W., Dorr, R., et al. Successful treatment of acute myocardial infarction shock by combined percutaneous transluminal coronary artery recanalization and angioplasty. *Am. Heart J.* 103:132, 1982.

34. Ramos, R. G., et al. The effect of coronary reperfusion on the survival of patients with cardiogenic shock due to acute myocardial infarction (Abstract). *J. A. M. Coll. Cardiol.* 9:233A, 1987.

35. Cohn, J. N., Tristani, F. E., and Khatri, I. M. Cardiac peripheral vascular effects of digitalis in clinical cardiogenic shock. *Am. Heart J.* 78:318, 1969.

36. Goldberg, L. O. Cardiovascular and renal actions of dopamine. I. Potential clinical applications. *Pharmcol. Rev.* 21:1, 1972.

37. Mueller, H. S., Evans, R., and Ayres, S. M. Effects of dopamine on hemodynamics and myocardial metabolism in shock following acute myocardial infarction in man. *Circulation* 57:361, 1978.

38. Sonnenblilck, E. H., Frishman, W. H., and Lejemtel, T. H. Dobutamine: A new synthetic cardioactive sympathetic amine. *N. Engl. J. Med.* 300:17, 1979.

39. Mueller, H., Ayres, S., Giarinelli, Jr., S., et al. Effect of isoproterenol, l-norepinephrine and intraaortic counterpulsation on hemodynamics and myocardial metabolism in shock following myocardial infarction. *Circulation* 55:325, 1972.

40. Gray, R. J., Shah, P. K., Singh, B. N., et al. Low cardiac-output states following open heart surgery: Comparative hemodynamic effects of dobutamine, dopamine and norepinephrine plus phentolamine. *Chest* 80:16, 1981.

41. Chatterjee, K., Swan, H. J. C., Kaushik, V. S., et al. Effects of vasodilator therapy for severe pump failure in acute myocardial infarction on short term and late prognosis. *Circulation* 53:797, 1976.

42. Franciosa, J. B., Buiha, N. M., Limas, C. J., et al. Improved left ventricular function during nitroprusside infusion in acute myocardial infarction. *Lancet* 1:650, 1972.

43. Cottrell, J. E., Casthely, P., Brodie, J. D., et al. Prevention of nitroprusside induced cyanide toxicity with hydroxycobalamin. *N. Engl. J. Med.* 298:809, 1978.

44. Jaffe, A. S., and Roberts R. The use of intravenous nitroglycerin in cardiovascular disease. *Pharmacotherapy* 2:273, 1982.

45. Nemerowski, M., and Shah, P. K. Syndrome of severe bradycardia and hypotension following sublingual nitroglycerin administration. *Cardiology* 67:180, 1981.

46. Goldberger, M., Tabak, S. W., and Shah, P. K. Clinical experience with intra-aortic balloon counterpulsation in 112 consecutive patients. *Am. Heart J.* (in press).

47. Isner, J. M., Cohen, S. R., Vermani, R., et al. Complications of intra-aortic balloon counterpulsation device, clinical and morphological observations in 45 necropsy patients. *Am. J. Cardiol.* 45:260, 1980.

48. Dewood, M. A., Notske, R. N., Hensley, G. R., et al. Intra-aortic balloon counterpulsation with or without reperfusion for myocardial infarction shock. *Circulation* 61:1105, 1980.

49. Leinbach, R. C., and Gold, H. K. Intra-aortic Balloon Pumping: Use in Treatment of Cardiogenic Shock and Acute Myocardial Ischemia. In J. S. Karliner and G. Gregoratos (eds.), *Coronary Care.* New York: Churchill Livingstone, 1981.

50. Gray, R. J., Sethna, D., and Matloff, J. M. The role of cardiac surgery in acute myocardial infarction with mechanical complications. *Am. Heart J.* 106:723, 1983.

51. Isner, J. M., and Roberts, W. C. Right ventricular infarction complicating left ventricular infarction complicating coronary artery disease. *Am. J. Cardiol.* 42:885, 1978.

52. Shah, P. K., Maddahi, J., Berman, D. S., et al. Scintigraphically detected predominant right ventricular dysfunction in acute myocardial infarction: Clinical, hemodynamic correlates and implications for therapy and prognosis. *J. Am. Coll. Cardiol.* 6:1264, 1985.

53. Lorrell, B., Leinbach, R. C., Pohost, G. M., et al. Right ventricular infarction: Clinical diagnosis and differentiation from cardiac tamponade and pericardial constriction. *Am. J. Cardiol.* 43:465, 1979.

54. Geft, I. L., Shah, P. K., Rodriguez, et al. ST elevations in leads V_1 to V_5 may be caused by right coronary occlusion and acute right ventricular infarction. *Am. J. Cardiol.* 53:991, 1984.

55. Morris, A. L., and Donen, N. Hypoxia and intracardiac right to left shunt complicating inferior myocardial infarction with right ventricular extension. *Arch. Intern. Med.* 138:1405, 1978.

56. Goldstein, J. H., Blahaker, G. J., Verriez, E. D., et al. The role of right ventricular systolic dysfunction and elevated intrapericardial pressure in the genesis of low cardiac output in experimental right ventricular infarction. *Circulation* 65:513, 1981.

57. Shelburne, J. C., Rubinstein, D., and Gorlin, R. A reappraisal of papillary muscle dysfunction: Correlative clinical and angiographic study. *Am. J. Med.* 46:862, 1969.

58. Heikkila, J. Mitral incompetence complicating acute myocardial infarction. *Acta Med. Scand.* 176:287, 1967.

59. Forrester, J. S., Diamond, G., Freedman, S., et al. Silent mitral insufficiency in acute myocardial infarction. *Circulation* 44:877, 1971.

60. Heuser, R. R., Maddoux, G. L., Gross, J. E., et al. Coronary angioplasty for acute mitral regurgitation due to myocardial infarction. *Ann. Intern. Med.* 107:852, 1987.

61. Nishimura, R. A., Schaff, H. V., Shuh, C., et al. Papillary muscle rupture complicating acute myocardial infarction: Analysis of 17 patients. *Am. J. Cardiol.* 51:373, 1983.

62. Wei, J. Y., Hutchins, G. M., and Bulkley, B. H. Papillary muscle rupture in fatal acute myocardial infarction. *Ann. Intern. Med.* 90:149, 1979.

63. Clements, S. D., Story, W. E., Hurst, J. W., et al. Ruptured papillary muscle, a complication of acute myocardial infarction: Clinical presentation, diagnosis and treatment. *Clin. Cardiol.* 8:93, 1985.

64. Fox, A. C., Glassman, E., and Isom, O. W. Surgically remediable complications of myocardial infarction. *Prog. Cardiovasc. Dis.* 21:461, 1979.

65. Farcot, J. C., Borsante, L., Rigaud, M., et al. Two dimensional echocardiographic visualization of ventricular septal rupture after acute anterior myocardial infarction. *Am. J. Cardiol.* 45:370, 1980.

66. Richards, K. L., Hoekenga, D. E., Leach, J. K., et al. Doppler cardiographic diagnosis of interventricular septal rupture. *Chest* 76:101, 1979.

67. Rasmussen, S., Leth, A., Kjoller, E., et al. Cardiac rupture in acute myocardial infarction: A review of 72 consecutive cases. *Acta Med. Scand.* 205:11, 1979.

68. Bates, R. J., Beutler, S., Resnekov, L., et al. Cardiac rupture—challenge in diagnosis and management. *Am. J. Cardiol.* 40:1231, 1977.

69. O'Rourke, M. F. Subacute heart rupture following myocardial infarction—clinical features of a correctable condition. *Lancet* 2:124, 1973.

70. Knowlton, A. A., Grauer, J., Plehn, J. F., et al. Ventricular pseudoaneurysm: A rare but ominous condition. *Cardiovasc. Rev. Rep.* 6:508, 1985.

71. Catherwood, E., Mintz, G. S., Kotler, M. N., et al. Two dimensional echocardiographic recognition of left ventricular pseudoaneurysm. *Circulation* 62:294, 1980.

72. Lopez-Martinez, J. I. Pulsatory and auscultatory phenomena in pseudoaneurysm of the heart. *Am. J. Cardiol.* 15:422, 1965.

17
Pericardial Complications of Myocardial Infarction

DAVID H. SPODICK

As the nearest neighbor of the heart, the pericardium is increasingly shown to participate directly or indirectly in many cardiac lesions and cardiac responses to physiologic, pharmacologic, and metabolic challenges [1] (Table 17-1). They are due in part to the immediate proximity of the pericardial sac, to direct anatomic involvement, or to pericardial constraint of the heart [2]. The latter is a function of the parietal pericardium, which begins to act after anything more than minimal cardiac dilation or individual chamber enlargement due to injury or to circulatory volume overload [3]. Thus there is an increasingly recognized pericardial role in ventricular failure, acute valvular regurgitation, and rapid chamber enlargement, as in acute right ventricular myocardial infarction [4]. These entities sometimes raise problems in the differential diagnosis from primarily pericardial disease.

The pericardial tissue responses to all the foregoing include irritative, inflammatory, transudative, and immunopathic reactions and healing, i.e., pericardial scarring [5], individually and in combinations. It must be emphasized that, as with most disease, data obtained at necropsy differ from clinical and laboratory (e.g., imaging) results obtained during life, and that the differences are exaggerated as these types of data are temporally separated.

Acute Fibrinous "Pericarditis" (*Pericarditis Epistenocardiaca*)

Forty percent of patients who die during acute myocardial infarction show fibrinous exudation into the pericardial sac [6]. Although it is classically known as epistenocardiac pericarditis [7] this response appears to be irritative rather than inflammatory, as no separate leukocytic response necessarily accompanies it—hence the term "pericarditis" [8]. In line with common usage, the quotation marks are eliminated hereafter. An important datum here is that every patient with fresh infarct-associated pericarditis [9] has an anatomically transmural infarct [6]. (Anatomically is stressed here because the electrocardiogram has been shown to be incapable of detecting infarct transmurality with certainty [10].) Thus although transmural infarction need not be a homogeneously necrotic block of tissue, at least the apex of the infarcted "pyramid" must extend into the epicardial muscle layers and involve the visceral pericardium to account for the production of fibrin at that point, which is also the site of any future pericardial scarring or adhesion. Smaller amounts of fibrinous exudate remain localized, whereas larger amounts are spread throughout the pericardial cavity by the action of the heart. Heart size appears to be unrelated to the occurrence of epistenocardiac pericarditis [11].

CLINICAL CHARACTERISTICS

Epistenocardiac pericarditis appears most often to be clinically silent—without subjective or objective manifestations. Pain is probably the most frequent manifestation, but unfortunately can be firmly ascribed to pericardial involvement only if a pericardial rub is discovered [9]. However, the characteristics of the pain are such that the inference of peri-

Table 17-1
Pericardial complications of myocardial infarction

Fibrinous "pericarditis" (pericarditis
    epistenocardiaca)
Intrapericardial bleeding
Pericardial effusion
    Noncompressing
        Acute: transudative or exudative
        Chronic
    Compressing: cardiac tamponade
Recurrent acute pericarditis (postmyocardial
    infarction syndrome)
    Clinically "dry"
    Effusive pericarditis
    Constrictive pericarditis
Pericardial scarring
    Epistenocardiac adhesions
    Constrictive pericarditis
    Effusive-constrictive pericarditis
Pseudoaneurysm

cardial involvement can be strong. The most common pain is precordial or substernal and is pleuritic, i.e., increased by breathing, body movement, and usually recumbency, all of which tend to distinguish it from renewed ischemic pain.

The only pain quasi-pathognomonic of pericardial injury is that which is perceived in one (usually the left) or both trapezius ridges, either in association with chest pain or by itself [7]. It is important to have the patient point to the area of involvement because he or she (or the physician) usually describes it as "shoulder" pain. Shoulder pain also occurs with pericarditis, which indeed can have all the areas of reference and radiation of anginal pain [7]; anginal pain, however, is not referred to the trapezius ridge.

On a scale of one to ten, the pain of epistenocardiac pericarditis is commonly rated between one and five, though occasionally it can be as much as ten; and in some patients it is more distressing than the pain of their myocardial infarction. The mildest pain may not evoke spontaneous complaints from the patient and may be transient, though often fluctuating in presence and intensity. Persistence for more than 2 to 3 days is unusual. It is im-

portant to distinguish it from extending or renewed infarction, as pericardial involvement does not appear to worsen the in-hospital prognosis.

Because of the rarity of characteristic electrocardiographic changes (see below), virtually the only objective manifestation of pericardial involvement in acute myocardial infarction is the appearance of a pericardial rub. More than perhaps most other types of pericarditis, the rub here not only fluctuates rapidly but is especially likely to be evanescent and therefore largely undiscovered. Indeed, its discovery may be strongly linked to the frequency of auscultation, not only because of transience but also because many patients with possible or probable pericardial pain do not appear to have rubs, whereas occasional pain-free patients have them. This situation is responsible for the wide discrepancy in the proportion of patients with acute myocardial infarction reported to have pericarditis: roughly between 6 and 30 percent [9]. In large series of consecutive patients with acute myocardial infarction in which patients with pericarditis were carefully compared with either the other patients with infarcts as a control group or selected control patients, the incidence of infarction-associated pericarditis ranged from 6.3 to 10.1 percent [12].

Pericardial rubs are an early phenomenon, most appearing within the first 4 days after admission, with more than one-half of them on day 1 or day 2 [9]. In the absence of the postmyocardial infarction syndrome of recurrent pericarditis (never a secure exclusion), rubs may first appear as late as the twelfth day and, exceptionally, may disappear only to reappear from the first to the third week after onset.

Pericardial rubs may be typical, i.e., three-component [13], in patients with sinus rhythm; but often they are biphasic, and some are confined to ventricular systole. In each case, differentiation from a murmur is essential, although usually easy, unless a murmur coexists with a rub. Rubs, like pain, are likely to vary more with posture and respiration than most murmurs associated with infarction, and they nearly always sound "more superficial," as if they are just under the diaphragm of the stethoscope (which is preferred for auscultation because nearly every rub is of high frequency).

The most important differential diagnoses are from papillary muscle dysfunction, which may be perceived as a murmur anywhere from the apex to the left lower sternal border, ventricular septal perforation (which may be heard in the same areas), and tricuspid regurgitation (detected at the right lower sternal border). The pericardial lesion is distinguished from these entities (again, so long as they do not coexist) by the absence of expected hemodynamic abnormalities and of characteristic pharmacologic and physiologic responses to challenges such as respiratory and postural maneuvers as well as administration of nitrates.

ELECTROCARDIOGRAPHY

Although there is some evidence that special techniques can show increased total ST segment elevation (Σ ST) in patients with infarct-associated pericarditis, the electrocardiogram is of virtually no help, probably because the pericardial involvement is local and because there is not usually an element of true pericardial inflammation. Thus the quasi-diagnostic stage I electrocardiographic changes of pericarditis [7, 14] were found in only 1 of 31 consecutively diagnosed patients [9]. Experience shows that in these rare cases the J points are displaced from the baseline in accordance with the criteria for stage I ST changes, obliterating any preexisting ST depressions, reciprocal or otherwise, but usually not interfering with any T-wave evolution of the infarct that has already commenced. In contrast to the approximately 43 percent of atypical electrocardiograms in patients with acute pericarditis of mixed causes [15], the rarity of this finding among patients with acute myocardial infarction raises strong questions of either an intercurrent true pericarditis of other etiology or myopericarditis masquerading from the outset as myocardial infarction [16].

OTHER CHARACTERISTICS

Careful observations failed to show any increase in the incidence of arrhythmias in patients with pericarditis of myocardial infarction [9, 12], which is not surprising because even generalized, truly inflammatory pericarditis does not by itself provoke arrhythmias [17] and because pericardial involvement is strictly localized to the infarct itself [6]. This is of additional interest because most patients with pericarditis have Q-wave infarcts [9, 12], and an increased number of patients are in Killip classes II, III, and IV [9]. Yet in prospectively observed series the in-hospital mortality of patients with pericarditis versus patients without pericarditis is no different [9, 12]. Finally, it is not surprising that pericarditis is discovered equally among anterior and inferior infarcts, as the exudate is free to slosh throughout the pericardial sac. The sporadic identification of a more generalized pericardial involvement may well be related to the unusually early appearance of the postmyocardial infarction (Dressler's) syndrome (see below), which could also be a cause of the rare stage I electrocardiographic changes. Finally, in company with most forms of pericardial disease [15] there is a male-to-female ratio of about 4:1, far in excess of the male dominance ($<$ 2:1) among patients with acute myocardial infarction [9].

Treatment for infarct-associated pericarditis is primarily for relief of pain. Nonsteroidal anti-inflammatory drugs, usually aspirin or ibuprofen, are preferred. Indomethacin should be avoided.

Intrapericardial Bleeding

Although many, if not most, forms of pericardial inflammation are accompanied by some escape of red blood cells into the pericardial cavity, this entity is associated with either direct injury of the pericardium by the inciting agent or disease or the capillary-rich granulation tissue that appears with early healing [7]. With infarction-associated pericardial involvement, this problem should be minimal to absent because of the common absence of true inflammation and the restriction of the lesion to the smallest part of any transmural infarct, i.e., its epicardial apex. (An unusually early postmyocardial infarction syndrome could be an exception owing to presumed widespread pericardial involvement.) Thus the source of any significant intrapericardial bleeding could be smaller or larger amounts of myocardial perforation (rupture) into the sac [18–20]. This explanation, of course, raises the question as to the effect of antithrombotic—including anticoagulant, "antiplatelet," and thrombolytic—therapy, which would either promote hemorrhage or impede its cessation. Overall experience indicates that any of these treatments, even after recognition of pericarditis, does not in fact produce catastrophic bleeding (including patients who were put in a thrombolytic state by treatment when acute pericarditis was mistaken for acute myocardial infarction). Evidence, on the other hand, exists for individuals given anticoagulants and thrombolytics with significant pericardial bleeding, i.e., hemopericardium, sometimes causing cardiac tamponade that was not always recognized before death. Some of the latter reports come from an era when anticoagulant control was not at the present standards, and indeed the level of anticoagulation was higher than the currently accepted levels [20]. Moreover, experience now is more with heparin than coumarin derivatives. Finally, the major, if not the sole, cause of frank hemopericardium appears to be ventricular rupture.

The danger of hemopericardium from anticoagulant therapy appears to be remote in patients with infarct-associated pericardial lesions, particularly with appropriate, careful control of the level of anticoagulation and of thrombolysis, and therefore these forms of therapy should be applied if there is an appropriate indication. Of course, it is prudent on such occasions to increase further the already high level of patient observation following the appearance or persistence of pericardial rubs or effusion (see below), particularly when they appear later than the first week after onset of infarction. Cardiac tamponade (also discussed under Pericardial Effusion, below) is a

major, though rare, emergency with or without an underlying infarct and indeed may be difficult to diagnose from other consequences of infarction.

Pericardial Effusion

Despite the 40 percent incidence of pericardial effusion in necropsied patients with infarct-associated pericardial involvement, only about 18 percent were found to have excess pericardial fluid content (although despite a careful necropsy-clinical correlation it was unclear how many of them were the same patients [11]). Clinical experience and laboratory evaluation (principally by echocardiography) indicate that very different individuals may be involved because pericardial effusion can be inflammatory or irritative (an exudate) or noninflammatory (a transudate). An exudative effusion could be further complicated by intrapericardial bleeding of the types mentioned above. Transudates accumulate because of either metabolic abnormalities, including fluid and electrolyte imbalances, or high intracapillary pressures due to heart failure or even venous and lymphatic obstruction. Such transudates are probably much more common.

Careful echocardiography of consecutive patients with acute myocardial infarction by Galve and colleagues [21] and Pierard and colleagues [22] detected 28 percent and 26 percent, respectively, with pericardial effusion and compared them with acute myocardial infarction patients who did not develop pericardial effusions. In both reports there were no significant differences for the following factors: sex, initial acute infarction, Q-wave versus non-Q-wave infarction, in-hospital mortality, and major supraventricular arrhythmias. In both studies pericardial effusion was more often associated with anterior infarction and with heart failure. In Galve et al.'s study [21] there was no difference in peak creatine kinase MB (CK-MB); in Pierard and associates' study [22] peak CK was higher with pericardial effusion, as was peak lactate dehydrogenase. In the latter study late mortality (15 days to 1 year) was greater in those with pericardial effusion, whereas in Galve et al.'s study the 6-month mortality was no different. Moreover, Galve et al. found no difference among those requiring resuscitation maneuvers, cardioversion, or both and no statistical difference for atrioventricular block, ventricular arrhythmias, and non-Q-wave infarction [21]; Pierard et al. found no difference among those with lateral infarcts and no difference between the groups for heparin therapy; but for those with pericardial effusion, there were a higher average Killip class, more ventricular arrhythmias, and much more aneurysm formation with their first acute infarction, along with an equally heavy preponderance of wall motion abnormalities [22]. These careful reports clearly supersede earlier investigations utilizing only M-mode echograms.

Finally, pericardial effusion may rarely be localized in patients with acute infarction [23] and is probably related to new or preexisting pericardial adhesions. Series such as that of Wunderink [24] can be discounted because they are M-mode studies and especially because the echocardiographic incidence (5.6 percent) is equivalent to the prevalance of posterior echo-free spaces (5 percent) found in the Framingham Study for individuals of the same age and sex [25] and for the same control group by Galve et al [21]—which by itself can be accounted for by pericardial fat [26]. (Several differences between the carefully studied series of Galve et al. [21] and Pierard et al. [22] may be ascribed largely to group differences and perhaps in part to study protocol.)

It is important that the presence of excess pericardial fluid does not correlate with the presence of pericardial rubs or inflammatory signs but, rather, with the clinical extent of the infarction, cardiac dilation, and particularly aneurysm formation (an expected feature of anterior infarctions especially). It also correlates with both heart failure and admission Killip class, as well as late mortality [21, 22]. The absence of correlation with heparin therapy is also significant. Indeed, there were no differences in the incidence of pericardial effusion in patients at either full- or low-dose heparin and no case with severe effusion or tamponade [21].

Pericardial effusion is thus common during acute myocardial infarction and is usually small, although slowly reabsorbed. It is probably rarely, if ever, related to a fibrinous pericardial reaction to localized injury but, rather, to heart failure with the attendant hemodynamic and fluid–electrolyte effects that can produce effusions in other serous cavities as well. It is not clear if aneurysm formation produces irritative effects of its own. The poor late prognosis probably reflects only the larger size of acute damage and generally poor prognosis for patients with myocardial infarction who have developed congestive heart failure.

Occasional patients show persistence (i.e., poor reabsorption) of pericardial fluid, which may be related to persistent cardiac failure and attendant fluid–electrolyte abnormalities. It has been shown that even a small amount of fluid has detectable physiologic, if not pathologic, effects [27]. This finding suggests that rapid cardiac dilation in the presence of otherwise clinically insignificant amounts of fluid may raise the pressure in the pericardial sac to some degree of cardiac compression (tamponade).

CARDIAC TAMPONADE

Following acute myocardial infarction, cardiac tamponade is virtually always due to bleeding into the percardial sac with or without concomitant pericardial effusion. Any demonstrable association with anticoagulant and antithrombotic therapy is not clear (see above), but the situation is rare, as is atrial rupture [28], whereas ventricular rupture is a relatively common mode of death during early infarction because it causes overwhelming cardiac tamponade, usually before treatment is available, and with the characteristic sign of electromechanical dissociation. It may be preceded by a somewhat lesser degree of tamponade, resembling (and extremely difficult to differentiate from) cardiogenic shock. Especially because of extremely low blood pressures, the characteristic sign, pulsus paradoxus, may be imperceptible (and it does not occur in hypertrophied hearts). Because bedside pressure curves and portable radiographs may be difficult to interpret, the situation calls for emergency echocardiography. In patients with either a minute myocardial perforation or myocardial hemorrhage of other cause, an increase in cardiopericardial silhouette with pulsus paradoxus, particularly with clear lung fields, should prompt a hemodynamic study (for diastolic pressure equilibration and absence of the y descent in venous and atrial curves); emergency echocardiography is also performed if necessary.

There is but one effective treatment for cardiac tamponade: evacuation of the pericardial contents. Little proof exists that the medical measures to support the hemodynamic state or intravascular fluid volume (which is dangerous in some patients with heart disease) have more than evanescent, temporizing effects on cardiac tamponade. Therefore needle pericardiocentesis or subxiphoid surgical drainage (which can be done under local anesthesia if necessary) should be instituted as soon as there is a firm diagnosis or on reasonable suspicion if the patient is sinking rapidly. Needless to say, should bloody fluid be encountered, all anticoagulant and antithrombotic therapy should be discontinued.

Postmyocardial Infarction (Dressler's) Syndrome

Between 1 week and 2 months after an acute myocardial infarction (rarely earlier [29, 30] and rarely later) patients may develop constitutional symptoms such as malaise and fever along with pericardial and pleuritic pain (sometimes severe and nearly always more intense than that of epistenocardiac pericarditis). Also present are leukocytosis, rapid erythrocyte sedimentation rate, sinus tachycardia, and sometimes pulmonary infiltrates and effusion. The latter are seen on chest films; and at the bedside pericardial and pleural rubs are frequent.

Examination of the patient may also reveal signs of the acute infarction if it is an early postmyocardial infarction syndrome (PMIS);

such signs may be disconcerting, particularly in patients recovering from a painless or minimally symptomatic infarction. The rub is more likely to be loud and to have two or three components than is the usual rub of infarct pericarditis. Cardiac tamponade is rare [31], although it is probably always indicative of a generalized pericarditis (in contrast to the infarct lesion, which is localized). Individual attacks are also more protracted, even with therapy, and may last as long as 6 weeks.

Chest films usually show some increase in the cardiopericardial silhouette. Pleural effusion may be bilateral; but as with other forms of pericarditis, it is usually on the left, irrespective of whether there is pericardial effusion [32]. There are no cardiac enzyme changes unless there is also extension of the infarct. Echocardiography should show pericardial effusion when it is present as well as the expected wall motion and other changes due to infarction. The electrocardiogram is sometimes unchanged, although J–ST changes may occur and are more often typical of pericarditis (i.e., stage I) than of epistenocardiac pericarditis [30]. PR segments may or may not be depressed.

Recurrences are common and may go on indefinitely after the index attack, although 2 years is a common cutoff point. Recurrence is thus one of the characteristics that point to an immunopathic basis for the PMIS, i.e., an immune response to products of myocardial damage, including antimyocardial antibodies [33], like the postmyocardial and pericardial injury syndromes. The other characteristics pointing to an immune basis include the time interval from the tissue damage, frequent evidence of generalized pericardial involvement as well as systemic involvement, and response to anti-inflammatory treatment. On the other hand, the question has been raised of activation of a latent virus [34] producing what is clinically idiopathic or viral pericarditis complicating infarction. This situation is more likely in patients with a lesion confined to the pericardium; but although these forms of pericarditis recur, one rarely sees associated lesions.

The incidence of the PMIS appears to be declining; and in Dressler's hospital among 229 consecutive patients there were no cases [35]. Elsewhere three cases were found among 779 patients [36]. It is unclear why the PMIS may be disappearing. Perhaps there is some element of the management of infarct patients—e.g., no longer is there prolonged strict bed rest, and the anticoagulant dicumarol is not used—but this remains speculative.

Differential diagnosis includes epistenocardiac pericarditis, usually distinguished by the differences noted above, its earlier onset in nearly every case, and a much milder course. Recurrent or extending acute infarction should be recognizable by enzyme increases, and its pain should be different. Cardiac tamponade is rare [31] but may mimic right ventricular infarction by producing increased jugular venous pressure with essentially clear lungs and pulsus paradoxus [3]. Moreover, a pericardial rub was found in 11 of 12 patients with right ventricular infarction [4]. The differential diagnosis should be made by pulmonary artery catheterization for the characteristic features of right ventricular infarction (a right ventricular pressure curve resembling pericardial constriction and right atrial pressure equal to or greater than left atrial pressure versus left ventricular infarction with left atrial pressure exceeding right atrial pressure); right precordial leads may show ST elevation but without stage I electrocardiographic changes of pericarditis (unless they coexist); pericardial effusion is usually absent by echocardiography. Differentiation from pulmonary embolism is important, as anticoagulants are needed for that condition but are relatively, if not absolutely, contraindicated by the presence of PMIS. Exclusion of pericarditis by bedside and laboratory techniques is the most dependable differential approach. Should the picture resemble pneumonia, appropriate sputum and blood cultures (negative in PMIS) as well as careful radiography, are needed.

Patients who have been discharged should be readmitted to the hospital for their initial episode of PMIS because of the remote possibility of cardiac tamponade and especially for the differential diagnosis of the conditions noted above. For recurrent episodes, admission is not needed so long as they are recognizable and so long as the patient is not seriously uncomfortable or threatened by any of the changes.

Treatment is primarily with nonsteroidal anti-inflammatory agents, including aspirin as tolerated. Perhaps the first drug to use is ibuprofen because it has the widest dose range and the lowest side effect profile. Indomethacin should be avoided because, at least in experimental animals, it has been shown to reduce coronary flow, raise blood pressure, and increase infarct size. If nonsteroidal agents are of no avail after trying several, corticosteroid therapy may be attempted. It is likely to work but may predispose to recurrences and, in some patients, to steroid side effects and dependence. Standard doses of prednisone (e.g., 60 mg/day in divided doses) may be given until symptoms and signs have decreased (usually rapidly). This agent should be tapered over approximately 2 weeks while introducing a nonsteroidal agent, which can then be tapered after the last dose of prednisone.

Pericardial Scarring

Adhesions and scarring of the pericardium, usually minor and localized, are the rule after epistenocardiac pericarditis [5]. They are localized to the area of the infarct and are of little or no clinical significance. Rare patients develop constrictive pericarditis [37] or effusive-constrictive pericarditis [38]. It is so uncommon as to raise a question of intercurrent infectious pericarditis or PMIS masquerading as epistenocardiac pericarditis, as PMIS rarely proceeds to constriction.

Pseudoaneurysm

Occasionally, ventricular rupture is minor and not fatal, occurring in such a form and at such a tempo that the pericardium contains the bleeding. Thus an aneurysmal bulge is formed that may resemble a true ventricular aneurysm. However, the wall is formed by pericardium, usually with a narrow neck connecting the aneurysm cavity to the ventricular cavity, in contrast to a true ventricular aneurysm, which has a wide communication with the ventricle and a wall of myocardium in various states of damage and fibrosis [39]. Because pseudoaneurysms are more likely to rupture than aneurysms, the diagnosis should lead to surgical intervention when possible.

Editorial Comments

The clinical incidence of infarction-associated pericarditis is in the range of 6 to 10 percent. Pericarditis following myocardial infarction implies transmural myocardial infarction. The presence of a pericardial rub is diagnostic of pericarditis in this setting. Echocardiography is not routinely necessary, as cardiac tamponade is rare. Aspirin or ibuprofen is effective therapy for most patients. G.S.F.

References

1. Spodick, D. H. The normal and diseased pericardium: Current concepts of pericardial physiology, diagnosis and treatment. *J. Am. Coll. Cardiol.* 1:240, 1983.
2. Spodick, D. H. Threshold of pericardial constraint: The pericardial reserve volume and auxiliary pericardial functions. *J. Am. Coll. Cardiol.* 6:296, 1985.
3. Shirato, K., Shabetai, R., Bhargava, V., et al. Alteration of left ventricular diastolic pressure-segment length relation produced by the pericardium: Effects of cardiac distension and afterload reduction in conscious dogs. *Circulation* 57:1191, 1978.
4. Lorell, B., Leinbach, R. C., Pohost, G. M., et al. Right ventricular infarction: Clinical diagnosis and differentiation from cardiac tamponade and pericardial constriction. *Am. J. Cardiol.* 43:465, 1979.
5. Spodick, D. H. *Chronic and Constrictive Pericarditis.* New York: Grune & Stratton, 1964.
6. Erhardt, L. R. Clinical and pathological observations in different types of acute myocardial infarction: A study of 84 patients deceased after treatment in a coronary care unit. *Acta Med Scand [Suppl]* 560:1, 1974.
7. Spodick, D. H. *Acute Pericarditis.* New York: Grune & Stratton, 1959.
8. Roberts, W. C., Spray, T. L. Pericardial Heart Disease: A Study of Its Causes, Consequences, and Morphologic Features. In D. H. Spodick, (ed.), *Pericardial Diseases.* Philadelphia: Davis, 1976. Pp. 11–65.
9. Krainin, F. M., Flessas, A. P., and Spodick, D. H. Infarction-associated pericarditis: Rarity of diagnostic electrocardiogram. *N. Engl. J. Med.* 311:1211, 1984.
10. Spodick, D. H. Q-wave infarction versus ST-infarction: Nonspecificity of ECG criteria for differentiating transmural and nontransmural lesions. *Am. J. Cardiol.* 51:913, 1983.
11. Roeske, W. R., Savage, R. M., O'Rourke, R. A., and Bloor, C. M. Clinicopathologic correlations in patients after myocardial infarction. *Circulation* 63:36, 1981.
12. Lichstein, E., Liu, H. M., and Gupta, P. Fundamentals of clinical cardiology: Pericarditis complicating acute myocardial infarction: incidence of complications and significance of electrocardiogram on admission. *Am. Heart. J.* 87:246, 1974.
13. Spodick, D. H. The pericardial rub: A prospective, multiple observer investigation of pericardial friction in 100 patients. *Am. J. Cardiol.* 35:357, 1975.
14. Spodick, D. H. The electrocardiogram in acute pericarditis: Distributions of morphologic and axial changes by stages. *Am. J. Cardiol.* 33:470, 1974.
15. Bruce, M. A., and Spodick, D. H. Atypical electrocardiogram in acute pericarditis: Characteristics and prevalence. *J. Electrocardiol.* 13:61, 1980.
16. Spodick, D. H. Infection and infarction: Acute viral (and other) infection in the onset, pathogenesis and mimicry of acute myocardial infarction. *Am. J. Med.* 81:661, 1986.
17. Spodick, D. H. Frequency of arrhythmias in acute pericarditis determined by Holter monitoring. *Am. J. Cardiol.* 53:843, 1984.
18. Miller, R. L. Hemopericardium with use of oral anticoagulant therapy. *J.A.M.A.* 209:1362, 1969.
19. Anderson, M. W., Christensen, N. A., and Edwards, J. E. Hemopericardium complicating myocardial infarction in the absence of cardiac rupture. *Arch. Intern. Med.* 90:634, 1952.
20. Goldstein, R., and Wolff, L. Hemorrhagic pericarditis in acute myocardial infarction treated with bishydroxycoumarin. *J.A.M.A.* 146:616, 1951.
21. Galve, E., Garcia-Del-Castillo, H., Evangelista, A., et al. Pericardial effusion in the course of myocardial infarction: Incidence, natural history, and clinical relevance. *Circulation* 73:294, 1986.
22. Peirard, L. A., Albert, A., Henrard, L., et al. Incidence and significance of pericardial effusion in acute myocardial infarction as deter-

mined by two-dimensional echocardiography. *J. Am. Coll. Cardiol.* 8:517, 1986.

23. Gore, J. M., Haffagee, C. I., Love, J. C., and Dalen, J. E. Isolated right ventricular tamponade after pericarditis from acute myocardial infarction. *Am. J. Cardiol.* 53:372, 1984.

24. Wunderink, R. G. Incidence of pericardial effusion in acute myocardial infarctions. *Chest* 85:494, 1984.

25. Savage, D. D., Garrison, R. J., Anderson, B. F., et al. Prevalence and correlates of posterior extra echocardiographic spaces in a free-living population based sample (the Framingham Study). *Am. J. Cardiol.* 51:1207, 1983.

26. Rifkin, R. D., Isner, J. M., Carter, B. L., and Bankoff, M. S. Combined posteroanterior subepicardial fat simulating the echocardiographic diagnosis of pericardial effusion. *J. Am. Coll. Cardiol.* 3:1333, 1984.

27. Spodick, D. H., Paladino, D., and Flessas, A. P. Respiratory effects on systolic time intervals during pericardial effusion. *Am. J. Cardiol.* 51:1033, 1983.

28. Bishop, Jr., L. H., Estes, Jr., E. H., and McIntosh, H. D. The electrocardiogram as a safeguard in pericardiocentesis. *J.A.M.A.* 162:264, 1956.

29. Kossowsky, W. A., Epstein, P. J., and Levine, R. S. Post-myocardial-infarction syndrome: An early complication of acute myocardial infarction. *Chest* 63:35, 1973.

30. Berman, J., Haffajee, C. I., and Alpert, J. S. Therapy of symptomatic pericarditis after myocardial infarction: Retrospective and prospec-

tive studies of aspirin, indomethacin, prednisone, and spontaneous resolution. *Am. Heart J.* 101:750, 1981.

31. Tew, F. T., Mantle, J. A., Russell, R. O., and Rackley, C. E. Cardiac tamponade with nonhemorrhagic pericardial fluid complicating Dressler's syndrome. *Chest* 72:93, 1977.

32. Weiss, J. M., Spodick, D. H. Association of left pleural effusion with pericardial disease. *N. Engl. J. Med.* 308:696, 1983.

33. Fowler, N.O. Autoimmune heart disease. *Circulation* 44:159, 1971.

34. Burch, G. E., and Colcolough, H. L. Postcardiotomy and postinfarction syndrome—a theory. *Am. Heart J.* 80:290, 1970.

35. Lichstein, E., Arsura, E., Hollander, G., et al. Current incidence of postmyocardial infarction (Dressler's) syndrome. *Am. J. Cardiol.* 50:1269, 1982.

36. Thadani, U., Chopra, M. P., Aber, C. P., et al. Pericarditis after acute myocardial infarction. *Br. Med. J.* 2:135, 1971.

37. Haiat, R. Post-myocardial infarction constrictive pericarditis (Letter). *Am. Heart J.* 101:358, 1981.

38. Friedman, B. J., and Segal, B. L. Chronic effusive pericarditis associated with healed myocardial infarction: Report of a case. *Dis. Chest* 49:217, 1966.

39. Wang, R., DeSantola, J. R., Reichek, N., and Edie, R. An unusual case of postoperative pseudoaneurysm of the left ventricle: Doppler echocardiographic findings. *J. Am. Coll. Cardiol.* 8:699, 1986.

18
Diastolic Abnormalities of Acute Myocardial Infarction

J. A. BIANCO

In 1970 Hood and colleagues [1] first demonstrated that left ventricular (LV) compliance, as measured by pressure–volume or pressure–segment length curves, was reduced (i.e., there was an upward and leftward shift of the curves) in canine myocardial infarction during the 3- to 5-day postinfarct period. This observation has held unchallenged since that time, providing an expected functional abnormality of the postinfarcted heart.

During the 1970s, LV diastole was investigated in terms of relaxation, i.e., the rate of diastolic LV pressure decline, and its characterization by the time constant T. However, these measurements as well as the study of pressure–volume relations of the left ventricle were invasive and complex. There was a pressing need to offer the clinician a simpler diagnostic assessment of diastolic parameters. Radionuclide and Doppler determination of diastolic events have been explored, and much data from these investigations have become available.

A review of diastolic function by Harizi and coworkers [2] described (1) the current physiologic understanding of LV diastole, (2) indexes of diastolic function (especially radionuclide and Doppler studies), (3) the role of pericardium and ventricular interdependence in influencing diastolic phenomena, and (4) diastolic abnormalities in patients with myocardial ischemia and myocardial infarction. Another timely review by Labovitz and Pearson [3] addressed concepts on LV diastolic function with highlights on Doppler echocardiographic methodology.

To describe diastolic abnormalities in patients with myocardial infarction, it is useful to relate Doppler and radionuclide data to hemodynamic events (Fig. 18-1). The top panel of Figure 18-1 shows the lower portion of a tracing of LV pressure obtained in the catheter laboratory. The second panel exhibits a typical Doppler signal with the two waveforms of mitral inflow: the early velocity (E), which is greater than the velocity during atrial systole (A). MVO indicates the time of opening of the mitral valve and the beginning of diastolic filling. The third panel is the radionuclide LV time–activity curve (counts/time, which are proportional to LV volume). The radionuclide maximum rate of diastolic filling (Max dC/dt or peak filling rate = PFR) corresponds to the peak E on the Doppler waveform. T-PFR is the time interval from end-systole to PFR. The bottom panel in Figure 18-1 is the electrocardiogram (ECG).

It is important to remember that the diastolic filling rates (specifically the PFR) are a function of ejection fraction, heart rate, age, and ventricular volume [2]. PFR is also determined by the left atrial pressure and the LV relaxation rate [4]. All of these factors, singly and in combination, must be considered when assessing diastolic properties in patients with myocardial infarction. It is critical that when Doppler or radionuclide studies are performed the investigator or clinician determines the interobserver, intraobserver, and interstudy variabilities of the method used to evaluate LV diastole.

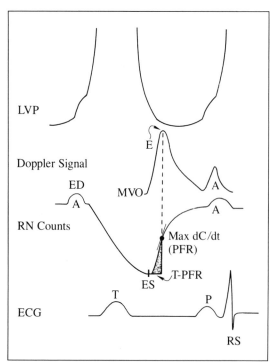

Fig. 18-1
Relation between LV filling parameters and hemodynamics. The figure is structured to portray four physiologic recordings. *Top to bottom:* Bottom part of LV pressure tracing, Doppler signal, radionuclide counts as a function of time, and electrocardiogram.

The pressure tracing is shown as a reference to highlight the diastolic phase of the cardiac cycle. With the Doppler signal, transmitral flow occurs mainly as early diastolic (E) and late diastolic (A = atrial contraction-related) components. The areas under the velocity signals reflect the amount of diastolic inflow.

The radionuclide time–activity curve is closely equivalent to the Doppler signal. It is expressed as counts (C) as a function of time, i.e., C(t). The maximum rate of filling, dC/dt_{max} = PFR, defines the maximal derivative of early rapid diastolic filling, which corresponds to the peak of the velocity signal on the Doppler recording (E). The second flow signal in the radioisotopic C(t) curve is the atrial kick (A), which corresponds to the A signal on the Doppler signal. The time interval between end-systole (ES) and PFR is designated as time to peak filling rate (T-PFR). The shaded area under the diastolic time activity curve corresponds to the maximal fraction of diastolic filling.

Diastolic Function in Patients with Myocardial Infarction

PRESSURE–VOLUME CHARACTERISTICS

In our original investigation, as discussed above [1], we found increased LV passive diastolic stiffness during the healing phase of acute canine myocardial infarction. This concept is illustrated in Figure 18-2. However, before the necrotic cardiac tissue is replaced by fibrosis (i.e., during the first days in the course of an evolving acute cardiac infarct), LV diastolic function typically demonstrates an increase in distensibility (lower LV volumes per any given LV pressure), which is thought to minimize the rise in filling pressure [5].

Investigators have designed studies to evaluate the changes in ventricular volumes associated with myocardial infarction. McKay et al. [6] investigated LV geometric changes by LV angiography and echocardiography on admission and 2 weeks after thrombolytic therapy in 30 patients presenting with acute myocardial infarction. At 2 weeks after thrombolysis, there was an increase in LV end-diastolic and end-systolic volumes. The increase in LV end-diastolic volume correlated directly with the percentage at the left ventricle that was akinetic or dyskinetic on initial catheterization. In a model for LV remodeling after infarction proposed by these workers, it is postulated that LV pressure also tends to increase at the time ventricular volume increases. Incidentally, the postinfarct increase in LV volume was by far more common in patients with anterior infarcts.

In a related study, Lamas and Pfeffer [7] found that in patients with left anterior descending artery–related remote myocardial infarction, there were substantial increases in systolic and diastolic LV volumes. The increase in these volumes was inversely related to the patient's computed ejection fraction but directly related to the severity of wall motion abnormality. The increase in ventricular volumes in this study was accompanied by milder increases in LV end-diastolic pressures.

Similarly, in the clinical study of Seals et al.

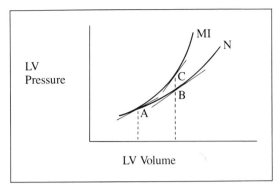

Fig. 18-2
Passive LV pressure–volume characteristics. N is the normal curve. The stiffness of the left ventricle is given by the tangents to the curves at points A and B. MI is the curve of the heart with acute myocardial infarction in the healing phase [1]. At point A, the stiffness of both the normal and the infarcted left ventricles are similar. However, at point B the distensibility of the infarcted heart (C) is decreased. (Adapted from D. Gibson. Ventricular Function. In R. H. Anderson, F. J. MaCartney, E. A. Shinebourne, and M. Tynan, eds., *Pediatric Cardiology* (Vol. 1). New York: Churchill Livingstone, 1987. P. 174.)

[8], documented by radioisotopic ventriculography, substantial LV dilatation during the initial 24 hours of acute myocardial infarction occurred. Such increases in end-diastolic and end-systolic volumes were even more significant in a repeat study 10 days after acute myocardial infarction. Volume augmentation was again more prominent in those patients with anterior infarcts. Also, the increase of LV volume in these patients was inversely correlated to the global ejection fraction. No pressure data were reported in this investigation.

From the foregoing, the following can be concluded.

1. In patients with acute myocardial infarction, LV end-diastolic pressure may be variable depending on: (1) the age of the infarct, (2) the degree of global LV dysfunction, (3) the extent of the wall motion abnormalities, and (4) possibly, medical therapy.
2. LV end-diastolic and end-systolic volumes increase in patients with acute cardiac necrosis in relation to: (1) age of the infarction, (2) location of the infarction (anterior versus than inferior), and (3) severity of global and regional LV function.
3. It is useful to consider pressure–volume characteristics (when available) in these patients, as such data may offer prognostic and treatment clues. The caveat here is that preload manipulation (i.e., by medication) can and does influence measured volumes and pressures.

ABNORMALITIES IN LV DIASTOLIC FILLING

Because the radionuclide ventriculogram displays systolic and diastolic information, it was reasonable to analyze the radioisotopic time–activity curve (which is proportional to LV volume) to record important systolic and diastolic events in a manner similar to that used by Hammermeister and Warbasse [9]. Bonow et al. [10] and Reduto et al. [11], using radionuclide angiography, found that most patients with remote myocardial infarction (or with wall motion abnormalities likely due to cardiac infarction) had a decreased peak filling rate (PFR) (this index is discussed in Figure 18-1) and decreased early diastolic fractional diastolic filling.

In these patients with remote myocardial infarction, the decrease in the speed of diastolic filling as well as the decrease in the fraction of filling during the first one-third of diastole could be related to chronic ischemia, or it could be a manifestation of altered mechanical properties (e.g., viscosity, elasticity, stretchability) of the LV wall.

Masuyama et al. [12] investigated the effects of changes in coronary stenosis on LV diastolic filling. Fifty patients with stable angina (note that 16 of these patients had prior myocardial infarction) were studied before and after coronary angioplasty. Patients with severe coronary stenosis (> 90 percent reduction of coronary arterial lumen) had postangioplasty improvement in LV diastolic filling that was greater than in patients with milder degrees of coronary stenosis. This research thus indicated that chronic ischemia may be responsible for the existence of preangioplasty diastolic abnormalities that may be apparent in the radionuclide or Doppler investigations and that respond to restoration of blood flow.

Normal mitral inflow is biphasic with early (E) and late (A) filling phases, as indicated in Figure 18-1. There is reason to believe that the information on early and late diastolic filling can be useful for assessing patients with myocardial infarction. In the presence of myocardial infarction, chronic ischemia, or any other causes of reduced compliance (e.g., hypertension and hypertrophic cardiomyopathy) there is a shift in the velocity waveform profile (or in the temporal occurrence of PFR) such that higher diastolic velocity and functional diastolic filling occur later and later during diastole.

This temporal shift in diastolic filling can be seen after coronary arterial occlusion in the dog [13]. At the University of Massachusetts Medical Center, an institution participating in the TIMI protocol, we (J. A. Bianco, J. S. Alpert, and J. Gore) noted prominent late diastolic filling (larger A waves and decreased PFR) in patients after acute myocardial infarction before and after tissue plasminogen activator (tPA) therapy. However, these observations (unpublished) remain preliminary.

The magnitude of the shift in early diastolic filling in myocardial infarction may be related to the change in LV end-diastolic pressure in patients with myocardial infarction [1, 5].

Discussion

It is now appreciated that abnormalities of diastolic function are potentially important for the practice of cardiology [2]. Therapeutic decisions are frequently made and directed to a specific cardiac pathophysiologic mechanism, such as altered diastolic compliance. In such instances, calcium channel blockers are given because it is believed that calcium plays an important role in cardiac relaxation [2].

This chapter emphasizes that shifts in pressure–volume characteristics of the left ventricle do occur in patients with myocardial infarction. However, pressure and volume LV measurements are not practical. Furthermore, as both pressure and volume are pathologically increased in myocardial infarction, it is impossible to determine where in the pressure–volume curve an individual patient's left ventricle operates.

Radionuclide or Doppler measurements of diastolic speed of filling and of the time integral of diastolic filling have become widely available. They appear to be related in some way to pressure–volume relations. After proper standardization of measurements of diastolic filling, a physician using these parameters is in a position to assess ventricular diastolic function, which may be of practical diagnostic, prognostic, or therapeutic importance when evaluating a patient with acute myocardial infarction.

Study of indexes of the diastolic properties of the heart has added data that have increased our understanding of the biologic features of acute myocardial infarction. The difficulties have not been unexpected: To correlate intricate ultrastructural phenomena such as calcium intracellular transients (relaxation) with overall LV pump performance is equivalent to equating electronic behavior in the atom to the earth's motion in the planetary system.

Editorial Comments

Now that Doppler echocardiography is readily available, there is seemingly more interest in diastolic properties of the heart. Acute myocardial infarction undoubtedly alters LV chamber stiffness, which has important clinical implications. The increase in pulmonary capillary wedge pressure so characteristic of acute infarction is often related in part to a change in diastolic heart function. Even a small change in LV volume may substantially raise pulmonary capillary wedge pressure. In some cases the diastolic compliance changes are transient (days), whereas in others there may be long-term abnormalities of chamber stiffness and relaxation following acute myocardial infarction.

Left ventricular diastolic filling is a complex phenomenon determined by multiple factors, including LV relaxation, intrinsic myocardial muscle properties, and loading conditions of the left ventricle. It cannot be adequately characterized by a single measurement. Peak filling rate may be independent of ventricular compliance or its reciprocal, chamber stiffness. LV relaxation and compliance are both elements of diastolic function, but the terms are not synonymous. Noninvasive imaging methods such as Doppler echocardiography are simple to perform, but they must be rigorously validated before they can be accepted as routine tests of diastolic function.
G. S. F.

References

1. Hood, W. B., Bianco, J. A., Kumar, R., and Whiting, R. B. Experimental myocardial infarction. IV. Reduction of left ventricular compliance in the healing phase. *J. Clin. Invest.* 49:1316, 1970.
2. Harizi, R. C., Bianco, J. A., and Alpert, J. S. Diastolic function of the heart in clinical cardiology. *Arch. Intern. Med.* 148:99, 1988.
3. Labovitz, A. J., and Pearson, A. C. Evaluation of left ventricular diastolic function: Clinical relevance and recent Doppler echocardiographic insights. *Am. Heart J.* 114:836, 1987.
4. Ishida, Y., Meisner, J. S., Tsujioka, K. et al. Left ventricular filling dynamics: Influence of left ventricular relaxation and left atrial pressure. *Circulation* 74:187, 1986.
5. Forrester, J. S., Diamond, G., Parmley, W. W., and Swann, H. J. C. Early increase in LV compliance after myocardial infarction. *J. Clin. Invest.* 51:598, 1972.
6. McKay, R. G., Pfeffer, M. A., Pasternak, R. C., et al. Left ventricular remodeling after myocardial infarction: A corollary to infarct expansion. *Circulation* 74:693, 1986.
7. Lamas, G. A., and Pfeffer, M. A. Increased left ventricular volume following myocardial infarction in men. *Am. Heart J.* 111:30, 1986.
8. Seals, A. A., Pratt, G. M., Mahmarian, J. H., et al. Relation of left ventricular dilatation during acute myocardial infarction to systolic performance, diastolic dysfunction, infarct size and location. *Am. J. Cardiol.* 61:224, 1988.
9. Hammermeister, K. E., and Warbasse, J. R. The rate of change of left ventricular volume in man. II. Diastolic events in health and disease. *Circulation* 49:739, 1974.
10. Bonow, R. O., Bacharach, S. L., Green, M. V., et al. Impaired left ventricular diastolic filling in patients with coronary artery disease: Assessment with radionuclide angiography. *Circulation* 64:315, 1981.
11. Reduto, L. A., Wickemeyer, W. J., Young, J. B., et al. Left ventricular diastolic performance at rest and during exercise in patients with coronary artery disease. *Circulation* 63:1228, 1981.
12. Masuyama, T., Kodama, K., Nakatani, S., et al. Effects of changes in coronary stenosis on left ventricular diastolic filling assessed with pulsed Doppler echocardiography. *J. Am. Coll. Cardiol.* 11:744, 1988.
13. Armstrong, W. F. Echocardiography in coronary artery disease. *Prog. Cardiovasc. Dis.* 30:267, 1988.

V
Miscellaneous Complications of Acute Myocardial Infarction

19
Unstable Angina Pectoris

GARY S. FRANCIS

There is no general agreement about the precise definition of unstable angina. The condition is said to present when there is recurrent rest angina that is more prolonged, intense, and more frequent than usual. There are often ST–T changes observed on the electrocardiogram (ECG) during pain and no significant rise in serum enzymes. It may be defined as the new onset of angina pectoris or previously "stable" angina that is now brought on by minimal activity. Unstable angina may also be a change from previously predictable, exertional angina to rest angina.

Although most patients with acute myocardial infarction have a prodrome of discomfort (60–70 percent) (see Chapter 5), only 7 to 22 percent of patients with unstable angina go on to develop acute myocardial infarction [1–3]. On the other hand, the 1-year mortality is high following the onset of unstable angina [4] and can approach 20 percent [3]. Patients with unstable angina whose symptoms do not promptly respond to medical therapy (<48 hours) are a particularly high-risk group [5], as are patients who develop frequent episodes of ECG changes without chest pain (silent ischemia) [6].

Pathophysiology

There are now compelling angiographic [7–13], angioscopic [14], and autopsy [15, 16] data to indicate that unstable angina is due to a change in the coronary endothelial surface. For reasons that are still unclear, an atherosclerotic plaque ruptures, platelets are activated, and thrombus formation ensues. Vasospasm, progression of underlying disease, and an increased myocardial demand for oxygen under certain conditions can also play some role. The pathogenesis of unstable angina has been extensively discussed in several reviews [17–22] as well as in Chapter 1.

It is now recognized that plaque disruption is the major underlying event that seems to precede most acute coronary syndromes [15, 20, 23]. It is often superimposed on the progression of underlying coronary stenosis [24]. Complex arteriographic lesions including eccentric stenosis, scalloping, and overhanging edges are observed angiographically and at autopsy in patients with unstable angina [7, 25]. A plaque may rupture within a relatively minor preexisting lesion. Thrombosis may be intermittent in unstable angina, in contrast to a Q-wave or non-Q-wave infarction in which the thrombosis may be more firmly fixed. Aggregated platelets may contribute to local vasoconstriction by releasing thromboxane [26]. Fibrinopeptide A, a sensitive marker of in vivo thrombin generation, is increased in patients with unstable angina [27], as is the concentration of fibrin and fibrinogen-related antigens [28]. Taken together, these observations strongly support a role for endothelial change (plaque fissure/rupture, platelet adhesion and activation, vasoconstriction, thrombosis, spontaneous lysis) in the pathogenesis of unstable angina).

Diagnosis

The diagnosis of unstable angina depends on the definition and is therefore subjective. A characteristic history accompanied by ECG changes during pain is conventionally used to make the diagnosis. Enzymes are usually negative, although some investigators have allowed the presence of a "slight enzyme leak." We have stressed the importance of obtaining a 12-lead ECG *during pain* to confirm the diagnosis; we also accept for diagnosis a change from a previous ECG in the absence of enzyme changes. This strategy, however, does not take into account that more than 90 percent of ECG changes are asymptomatic in the setting of unstable angina when calibrated amplitude-modulated Holter monitoring recordings are used [6].

Management

MEDICAL MANAGEMENT

Most if not all patients should be admitted to the coronary care or intensive care unit, where appropriate surveillance and intensive nursing care are available. Although invasive monitoring is usually not necessary, it should be available if the patient becomes hemodynamically unstable. Supplemental oxygen by nasal prongs and sedation with benzodiazepam is standard care. Pharmacologic therapy for unstable angina has improved substantially, and our experience is that roughly 80 percent of patients respond to medical treatment. Urgent cardiac catheterization is reserved for a subset of patients who continue to have angina despite aggressive medical therapy (Table 19-1).

Intravenous nitroglycerin is used for nearly all patients because it is easier to titrate than oral nitrates and may offer additional benefit [29, 30]. The dose is highly variable, but 10 to 200 μg/min usually relieves or prevents angina.

Aspirin has been extensively studied in patients with unstable angina, where it has proved to be exceptionally beneficial [31, 32]. In the Veterans Administration Cooperative Study [31] 1266 men were treated with aspirin or placebo for 12 weeks following admission to the hospital for unstable angina. The authors observed a 51 percent reduction in mortality and acute myocardial infarction in the

aspirin group ($p < .0005$). The Canadian Multicenter Trial [32] randomized 555 patients with unstable angina to aspirin, sulfinpyrazone, both drugs, or placebo; the investigators then followed these patients for up to 2 years. The incidence of cardiac death or nonfatal myocardial infarction was reduced by 51 percent in patients treated with aspirin ($p = .008$), once again establishing the utility of aspirin for treatment of unstable angina. Taken together, these two well controlled studies offer strong support for the role of platelet activation in the syndrome of unstable angina.

Intravenous heparin has been shown in one small, controlled study to significantly reduce progression to transmural infarction when compared to atenolol in patients with unstable angina [33]. Although not systematically studied, a small dose of aspirin (325 mg/day or less) used with full-dose heparin may prevent progression to infarction while minimizing bleeding complications. It has been our strategy to use both small-dose aspirin and full-dose heparin in patients with unstable angina unless contraindicated. However, a contrary view might be that, unless heparin can be demonstrated to be of direct benefit in unstable angina syndromes, it may be wise to withhold it when anticipating the use of systemic lytic agents in order to hold bleeding complications to a minimum. This strategy is under continual reevaluation.

Numerous studies have demonstrated improved control of rest angina by adding calcium channel blockers to nitrates or beta blockers. One well controlled study demonstrated that adding nifedipine to nitrates and propranolol significantly reduced sudden death, myocardial infarction, or persistent angina requiring surgery [34]. Similar controlled studies have demonstrated the usefulness of verapamil in patients with unstable angina [35, 36]. The precise reasons whereby calcium channel blockers improve unstable angina are not clear, but multiple mechanisms are likely operative. Coronary blood flow may improve, spasm may be prevented, and verapamil and diltiazem are well known to reduce the heart rate. Moreover, all three commonly used calcium channel blockers (nifedipine, verapamil,

Table 19-1
Treatment of unstable angina

Mechanism	Treatment	Dose	Comments
Plaque rupture	Aspirin	40–325 mg/day	
Platelet adhesion and aggregation			
Spasm?	Nifedipine	10–30 mg tid	Should be combined with a beta blocker
	Verapamil	400 mg/day	Contraindicated for overt CHF or symptomatic bradyarrhythmias
	Diltiazem	60–120 mg qid	
	Nitroglycerin	10–200 μg/min IV	
	Heparin	50 units/kg IV followed by 10–25 units/kg/hr IV according to PTT	
Thrombosis	Streptokinase, urokinase, tPA	Variable; see refs. 47–51	Still under investigation
Stenosis	Angioplasty surgery		Culprit lesion only
↑MV̇O₂	Esmolol	500 μg/kg/min IV loading dose followed by 25–300 μg/kg/min	Should be used to achieve resting pulse of 50–60 bpm
	Propranolol	1–10 mg IV; 10–100 mg bid PO	
	Metoprolol	5–15 mg IV; 50–100 mg bid PO	
	Nitroglycerin	10–200 μg/min IV	
	IABC		

CHF = congestive heart failure; PTT = partial thromboplastin time; tPA = tissue plasminogen activator; IABC = intra-aortic balloon counterpulsation; MV̇O₂ = myocardial oxygen consumption.

and diltiazem) are known to have some anti-platelet activity [37].

The use of beta blockers for unstable angina is more controversial. Although introduced during the early 1970s as treatment for unstable angina [4], there has been only one controlled trial demonstrating their usefulness [38]. Another controlled trial failed to show the effectiveness of propranolol [39], and some experts have questioned the drug's use for unstable angina [40]. It appears that benefit is best derived when propranolol is combined with nifedipine [38].

Our own experience with beta blockers for treating unstable angina is that they are generally beneficial. In fact, use of the ultra-short-acting agent esmolol may help to control severe angina when used in selected patients who are refractory to more conventional therapy.

INVASIVE SUPPORTIVE MEASURES

Some patients continue to have rest angina despite maximal medical therapy. Intra-aortic balloon counterpulsation (IABC) has been demonstrated to control refractory symptoms [41]. However, there is a substantial risk when using IABC, especially in older patients, women, diabetics, and those with severe peripheral vascular disease [42]. Patients who remain refractory to medical therapy are likely to undergo urgent cardiac catheterization and possibly angioplasty or surgery. The IABC device now serves primarily as a temporary support system prior to urgent catheterization, angioplasty, or surgery (see Chapter 15).

Coronary sinus retroperfusion is a technique that allows delivery of arterial blood and medications to the coronary veins during diastole. Venous drainage occurs during systole through a synchronized coronary sinus balloon catheter and pump system. Animal studies have documented beneficial effects with coronary sinus retroperfusion [43–45], and preliminary experience in patients appears promising [46]. More experience is necessary with this device and with the newer catheter-based systems, including laser, intracoronary

stents, and atherectomy techniques, before their role in unstable angina is secured.

THROMBOLYTIC THERAPY

The well recognized role of intracoronary thrombus in unstable angina has generated much interest in thrombolytic therapy for this syndrome. Intravenous [47] and intracoronary [48, 49] streptokinase have been used with expected success. Gold and colleagues [50, 51] have used recombinant tissue-type plasminogen activator (tPA) in patients with unstable angina. In a placebo-controlled trial, tPA in doses of 1.75 mg/kg IV over 12 hours was given at a rate of 0.75 mg/kg over 1 hour and 0.5 mg/kg over 11 hours; it ameliorated angina in 11 of 12 patients, whereas placebo was effective in only 6 of 11 patients. Oozing at puncture sites was not observed in patients treated with placebo but occurred in 8 of 12 patients treated with tPA. In three patients tPA was terminated before the 12-hour infusion was completed because of bleeding complications. Subsequent coronary arteriography demonstrated subocclusive thrombus in 8 of 11 patients receiving placebo but in none of the patients treated with tPA. Although the numbers are small, this preliminary study suggested that tPA may be beneficial in selected patients with unstable angina. A large, randomized, controlled trial of thrombolytic therapy for unstable angina seems clearly warranted.

INTERVENTIONAL MANAGEMENT

The timing and even the necessity of coronary arteriography for patients with unstable angina has been controversial and even somewhat cyclical. The early 1970s was an era of emergency arteriography and surgery [52, 53], soon followed by a general consensus that if patients can be medically controlled arteriography and catheterization can be delayed [54, 55]. This change was in part predicated on the large National Cooperative Study Group Report on Unstable Angina, which concluded that patients with unstable angina can be managed acutely with intensive medical therapy, followed by elective surgery performed if the patient fails to respond to medical therapy [56]. In this study 36 percent of medically treated patients crossed over to surgery because of refractory symptoms during follow-up. The Veterans Administration Cooperative Study on Unstable Angina [57] found a similar survival at 2 years' follow-up in patients treated medically or surgically; but once again 34 percent of patients assigned to chronic medical therapy became refractory with recurrent symptoms and crossed over to surgery. Interesting, the Veterans Administration study found that patients with a modestly low ejection fraction (30–59 percent) demonstrated significantly greater improvement in survival when treated surgically [57]. This improvement in survival in surgically treated patients with unstable angina who showed some reduction in ejection fraction is similar to observations made in patients with stable angina [58, 59].

It is probably fair to say that many centers, at least until recently, treated most patients with unstable angina medically in the coronary care unit, performed coronary arteriography electively within 2 to 3 days when patients were pain-free, and operated on a substantial proportion of patients depending on the individual circumstances. Indeed, coronary bypass surgery has proved to be a safe, effective treatment for medically refractory or medically responsive unstable angina pectoris when performed in an elective manner in a stable, quiescent patient. Our approach is to obtain coronary arteriography data early in the patient's hospital course because knowledge of the anatomy helps the physician make judgments regarding therapy and sometimes helps to avoid later emergency catheterization in patients who subsequently become unstable.

Percutaneous transluminal coronary angioplasty (PTCA) has more recently been used to treat patients with unstable angina [60, 61] and those with evolving acute myocardial infarction [62–64] (see Chapter 23). Reports of angioplasty in patients with unstable angina have

generally been favorable [65–73], with primary success rates of 61 to 93 percent and complication rates of 2.0 to 12.5 percent. Interpretation of these studies is difficult because many were conducted with the older, stiff, fixed guidewire catheter systems. Today the primary success rate is probably much greater in high-volume centers using steerable guidewires and low-profile angioplasty catheters. As in patients with stable angina, the restenosis rate approximates 30 percent.

There has been interest in "culprit lesion angioplasty," in which PTCA is performed on a single lesion in patients with unstable angina and multivessel disease. The culprit lesion is identified by observing ECG changes during ischemia or by regional thallium redistribution. Angiography, exercise-induced wall motion abnormalities during exercise gated blood pool scan, dipyridamole thallium perfusion scintigraphy, and positron emission tomography can also be used to identify culprit lesions. The good symptomatic response to culprit lesion angioplasty in patients with unstable angina suggests that the single-site dilation strategy should be the rule unless there is a substantial amount of myocardium in jeopardy from other lesions.

Summary

The past few years have witnessed a remarkable transition in therapeutic approaches to the acutely ischemic myocardium. Reduction in myocardial oxygen demand, a strategy shown to be beneficial in the laboratory setting for reducing infarct size, has not proved to reduce infarct size in patients [74]. Instead, a realization that unstable angina may be caused by a reversible change in the endothelial surface of the coronary artery has emerged. This new concept of how stable coronary disease becomes unstable is still incompletely understood, but it has nevertheless fostered new approaches to therapy.

Antiplatelet drugs, usually in the form of low-dose aspirin, are now routinely given to patients unless there is a contraindication. A strong case can also be made for administering intravenous heparin to patients with unstable angina. Beta-adrenergic blocking drugs may be useful in selected patients with unstable angina who have excessive myocardial oxygen demands. Intravenous nitroglycerin followed by long-acting oral nitrates are time-proved remedies for unstable angina. Calcium channel blocking agents may be useful. If nifedipine is used, it should be combined with a beta blocker. Lytic therapy with streptokinase or tPA might be considered, but experience with these agents to date is primarily in patients with evolving acute transmural (Q-wave) infarction and not unstable angina.

Early cardiac catheterization is usually indicated in patients once they respond to treatment and have stabilized. Patients who fail to stabilize should have urgent cardiac catheterization with consideration toward angioplasty of the culprit lesion. Rarely, IABC and emergency catheterization are necessary. Operative therapy is preferred for many patients, especially those with multivessel disease and modest left ventricular dysfunction.

References

1. Fulton, M., Lutz, W., Donald, R. W., et al. Natural history of unstable angina. *Lancet* 1:860, 1972.
2. Gazes, P. C., Mobley, E. M., Jr., Faris, H. M., Jr., et al. Preinfarction (stable) angina—a prospective study: Ten year follow-up prognostic significance of eletrocardiographic changes. *Circulation* 48:331, 1973.
3. Mulcahy, R., Awahdi, A. H. L., de Buitleor, M., et al. Natural history and prognosis of unstable angina. *Am. Heart J.* 109:753, 1985.
4. Fischl, S. J., Herman, M. V., and Gorlin, R. The intermediate coronary syndrome: Clinical angiographic and therapeutic aspects. *N. Engl. J. Med.* 288:1193, 1973.
5. Roberts, K. B., Califf, Harrell, F. E., Jr., et al. The prognosis for patients with new-onset angina who have undergone cardiac catheterization. *Circulation* 68:970, 1983.
6. Gottleib, S. O., Weisfeldt, M. L., Ouyang, P., et al. Silent ischemia as a marker for early unfavorable outcomes in patients with unstable angina. *N. Engl. J. Med.* 314:1214, 1986.
7. Ambrose, J. A., Winters, S. L., Stern, A., et al. Angiographic morphology and the pathogenesis of unstable angina. *J. Am. Coll. Cardiol.* 5:609, 1985.
8. Alpert, J. S., Coronary vasomotion, coronary thrombosis, myocardial infarction and the camel's back (Editorial). *J. Am. Coll. Cardiol.* 5:617, 1985.
9. Bresnahan, D. R., Davis, J. L., Holmes, D. R., Jr., et al. Angiographic occurrence and clinical correlates of intraluminal coronary artery thrombus: Role of unstable angina. *J. Am. Coll. Cardiol.* 6:285, 1985.
10. Ambrose, J. A., Winters, S. L., Arora, R. R., et al. Angiographic evolution of coronary artery morphology in unstable angina. *J. Am. Coll. Cardiol.* 7:472, 1986.
11. Gotoh, K., Minamino, T., Katoh, O., et al. The role of intracoronary thrombus in unstable angina: Angiographic assessment and thrombolytic therapy during ongoing anginal attacks. *Circulation* 77:526, 1988.
12. Wilson, R. F., Holida, M. D., and White, C. W. Quantitative angiographic morphology of coronary stenoses leading to myocardial infarction or unstable angina. *Circulation* 73:286, 1986.
13. Ambrose, J. A., and Hjemdalh-Monsen, C. E. Arteriographic anatomy and mechanisms of myocardial ischemia in unstable angina (Editorial). *J. Am. Coll. Cardiol.* 9:1397, 1987.
14. Sherman, C. T., Litvack, F., Grundfest, W., et al. Coronary angioscopy in patients with unstable angina pectoris. *N. Engl. J. Med.* 315:913, 1986.
15. Falk, E. Unstable angina with fatal outcome: Dynamic coronary thrombosis leading to infarction and/or sudden death. *Circulation* 71:699, 1985.
16. Davies, M. J., Thomas, A. C., Knapman, P. A., et al. Intramyocardial platelet aggregation in patients with unstable angina suffering sudden ischemic cardiac death. *Circulation* 73:418, 1986.
17. Epstein, S. E., and Palmeri, S. T. Mechanisms contributing to precipitation of unstable angina and acute myocardial infarction: Implications regarding therapy. *Am. J. Cardiol.* 54:1245, 1984.
18. Fuster V., and Chesebro. J. W. Mechanism of unstable angina. *N. Engl. J. Med.* 315:1023, 1986.
19. Willerson, J. T., Hillis, L. D., Winniford, M., et al. Speculation regarding mechanisms responsible for acute ischemic heart disease syndromes (Editorial). *J. Am. Coll. Cardiol.* 8:245, 1986.
20. Gorlin, R., Fuster, V., and Ambrose, J. A. Anatomic-physiologic links between acute coronary syndromes (Editorial). *Circulation* 74:6, 1986.
21. Forrester, J. S., Litvack, F., and Grundfest, W.

A perspective of coronary disease seen through the arteries of living man. *Circulation* 75:505, 1987.

22. Fuster, V., Badiman, L., Cohen, M., et al. Insights into the pathogenesis of acute ischemic syndromes. *Circulation* 77:1213, 1988.

23. Davies, M. J., and Thomas, A. C. Plaque fissuring: The cause of acute myocardial infarction, sudden ischemic death, and crescendo angina. *Br. Heart J.* 53:363, 1985.

24. Moise, A., Théroux, P., Taymans, Y., et al. Unstable angina and progression of coronary atherosclerosis. *N. Engl. J. Med.* 309:685, 1983.

25. Levin, D. C., and Fallon, J. T. Significance of the angiographic morphology of localized coronary stenosis: Histopathological correlates. *Circulation* 66:316, 1982.

26. Fitzgerald, D. J., Roy, L., Catella, F., et al. Platelet activation in unstable coronary disease. *N. Engl. J. Med.* 315:983, 1986.

27. Théroux, P., Latour, J-G, Léger-Gauthier, C., et al. Fibrinopeptide A and platelet factor levels in unstable angina pectoris. *Circulation* 75:156, 1987.

28. Kruskal, J. B., Commerford, P. J., Franks, J. J., et al. Fibrin and fibrinogen-related antigens in patients with stable and unstable coronary artery disease. *N. Engl. J. Med.* 317:1361, 1987.

29. Kaplan, K., Davison, R., Parker, M., et al. Intravenous nitroglycerin for the treatment of angina at rest unresponsive to standard nitrate therapy. *Am. J. Cardiol.* 51:694, 1983.

30. Curfman, G. D., Heinsimer, J. A., Lozner, E. C., et al. Intravenous nitroglycerin in the treatment of spontaneous angina pectoris. *Circulation* 67:276, 1983.

31. Lewis, H. D., Jr., Davis, J. W., Archibald, D. G., et al. Protective effects of aspirin against acute myocardial infarction and death in men with unstable angina. *N. Engl. J. Med.* 309:396, 1983.

32. Cairns, J. A., Gent, M., Singer, J., et al. Aspirin, sulfinpyrazone, or both in unstable angina: Results of a Canadian multicenter trial. *N. Engl. J. Med.* 313:1369, 1985.

33. Telford, A. M., and Wilson, C. Trial of heparin versus atenolol in prevention of myocardial infarction in intermediate coronary syndrome. *Lancet* 1:1225, 1981.

34. Gerstenblith, G., Ouyang, P., Achuff, S. C., et al. Nifedipine in unstable angina: A double-blind, randomized trial. *N. Engl. J. Med.* 306:885, 1982.

35. Mehta, J., Pepine, C. J., Day, M., et al. Short-term efficacy of oral verapamil in rest angina—a double-blind, placebo-controlled trial in CCU patients. *Am. J. Med.* 71:977, 1981.

36. Parodi, O., Maseri, A., and Simonetti, I. Management of unstable angina at rest by verapamil: A double-blind, cross-over study in the coronary care unit. *Br. Heart J.* 41:167, 1979.

37. Johnson, G. J., Leis, L. A., and Francis, G. S. The calcium channel blockers, nifedipine and verapamil, have different effects on alpha$_2$ adrenergic receptors and thromboxane-induced aggregation of human platelets. *Circulation* 73:847, 1986.

38. Gottlieb, S. O., Weisfeldt, M. L., Ouyang, P., et al. Effect of the addition of propranolol to therapy with nifedipine for unstable angina pectoris: A randomized, double-blind, placebo-controlled trial. *Circulation* 73:331, 1986.

39. Parodi, O., Simonetti, I., Michelassi, C., et al. Comparison of verapamil and propranolol therapy for angina pectoris at rest: A randomized, multiple-crossover, controlled trial in the coronary care unit. *Am. J. Cardiol.* 57:899, 1986.

40. Singh, B. H., and Nademanee, K. Beta-adrenergic blockade in unstable angina pectoris. *Am. J. Cardiol.* 57:992, 1986.

41. Gold, H. K., Leinbach, R. C., Sanders, C. A., et al. Intraaortic balloon pumping for control of recurrent myocardial ischemia. *Circulation* 47:1197, 1973.

42. Alderman, J. D., Gablioni, G. I., McCabe, C. H., et al. Incidence and management of limb ischemia with percutaneous wire-guided intraaortic balloon catheters. *J. Am. Coll. Cardiol.* 9:524, 1987.

43. Meerbaum, S., Lang, T., Osher, J. V., et al. Diastolic retroperfusion of acutely ischemic myocardium. *Am. J. Cardiol.* 37:588, 1976.

44. Drury, J. K., Yamazaki, S., Fishbein, M. C., et al. Synchronized diastolic coronary venous retroperfusion: Results of a pre-clinical safety and efficacy study. *J. Am. Coll. Cardiol.* 6:328, 1985.

45. Chang, B-L., Drury, J. K., Meerbaum, S., et al. Enhanced myocardial washout and retrograde blood delivery with synchronized retroperfusion during acute myocardial ischemia. *J. Am. Coll. Cardiol.* 9:1091, 1987.

46. Gore, J. M., Weiner, B. H., Benotti, J. R., et al. Preliminary experience with synchronized coronary sinus retroperfusion in humans. *Circulation* 74:381, 1986.

47. Lawrence, J. R., Shephard, J. T., Bone, I., et al. Fibrinolytic therapy in unstable angina: A controlled clinical trial. *Thromb. Res.* 17:767, 1980.

48. Vetrovec, G. W., Leinbach, R. C., Gold, H. K., et al. Intracoronary thrombolysis in syndromes of unstable ischemia: Angiographic and clinical results. *Am Heart J.* 104:946, 1982.

49. Shapiro, E. P., Brinker, J. A., Gottleib, S. O., et al. Intracoronary thrombolysis 3 to 13 days after acute myocardial infarction for postinfarc-

tion angina pectoris. *Am. J. Cardiol.* 55:1453, 1985.

50. Gold, H. K., Johns, J. A., Leinbach, R. C., et al. A randomized, blinded, placebo-controlled trial of recombinant human tissue-type plasminogen activator in patients with unstable angina pectoris. *Circulation* 75:1192, 1987.

51. Gold, H. K., Johns, J. A., Leinbach, R. C., et al. Thrombolytic therapy for unstable angina pectoris: Rationale and results. *J. Am. Coll. Cardiol.* 10:91B, 1987.

52. Bonchek, L. I., Rahimtoola, S. H., Anderson, R. B., et al. Late results following emergency saphenous vein bypass grafting for unstable angina. *Circulation* 50:972, 1974.

53. Matloff, J. M., Sustaita, H., Chatterjee, K., et al. The rationale for surgery in preinfarction angina. *J. Thorac. Cardiovasc. Surg.* 69:73, 1975.

54. Golding, L. A. R., Loop, F. D., Sheldon, W. C., et al. Emergency revascularization for unstable angina. *Circulation* 58:1163, 1978.

55. Cohn, L. H., Alpert, J., Koster, J. K., et al. Changing indications for the surgical treatment of unstable angina. *Arch. Surg.* 113:1312, 1978.

56. Russell, R. O., Jr., Moraski, R. E., Kouchoukos, N., et al. Unstable angina pectoris: National cooperative study group to compare surgical and medical therapy. *Am. J. Cardiol.* 42:839, 1978.

57. Luchi, R. J., Scott, S. M., Deupree, R. H., et al. Comparison of medical and surgical treatment for unstable angina pectoris. *N. Engl. J. Med.* 316:977, 1987.

58. Passamani, E., Davis, K. B., Gillespie, M. J., et al. A randomized trial of coronary artery bypass surgery: Survival of patients with a low ejection fraction. *N. Engl. J. Med.* 312:1665, 1985.

59. Veterans Administration Coronary Artery Bypass Surgery Cooperative Study Group. Eleven-year survival in Veterans Administration randomized trial of coronary bypass surgery for stable angina. *N. Engl. J. Med.* 311:1333, 1984.

60. Meltzer, R. S., van den Brand, M., Serruys, P. W., et al. Sequential intracoronary streptokinase and transluminal angioplasty in unstable angina with evolving myocardial infarction. *Am. Heart J.* 104:1109, 1982.

61. De Feyter, P. J., Serruys, P. W., van den Brand, M., et al. Emergency coronary angioplasty in refractory unstable angina. *N. Engl. J. Med.* 313:342, 1985.

62. Goldberg, S., Urban, P. L., Greenspon, A., et al. Combination therapy for evolving myocardial infarction: Intracoronary thrombolysis and percutaneous transluminal angioplasty. *Am. J.*

Med. 72:994, 1982.

63. Myer, J., Merx, W., Schmitz, H., et al. Percutaneous transluminal coronary angioplasty immediately after intracoronary streptolysis of transmural myocardial infarction. *Circulation* 66:905, 1982.

64. Yasuno, M., Saito, Y., Ishida, M., et al. Effects of percutaneous transluminal coronary angioplasty: Intracoronary thrombolysis with urokinase in acute myocardial infarction. *Am. J. Cardiol.* 53:1217, 1984.

65. Williams, D. O., Riley, R. S., Singh, A. K., et al. Evaluation of the role of coronary angioplasty in patients with unstable angina pectoris. *Am. Heart J.* 102:1, 1981.

66. Meyer, J., Schmitz, H., Erbel, R., et al. Treatment of unstable angina pectoris with percutaneous transluminal coronary angioplasty (PTCA). *Cathet. Cardiovasc. Diagn.* 7:361, 1981.

67. Erbel, R., Moyer, J., Schmitz, H., et al. Percutaneous transluminal coronary angioplasty in patients with unstable angina. *Postgrad. Med. J.* 59(Suppl 3):22, 1983.

68. Faxon, D. P., Detre, K. M., McCabe, C. H., et al. Role of percutaneous transluminal coronary angioplasty in the treatment of unstable angina: Report from the National Heart, Lung and Blood Institute percutaneous transluminal coronary angioplasty and coronary artery surgery study registries. *Am. J. Cardiol.* 53:131C, 1984.

69. Quigley, P. J., Erwin, J., Maurer, B. J., et al. Percutaneous transluminal coronary angioplasty in unstable angina: Comparison with stable angina. *Br. Heart J.* 55:227, 1986.

70. Timmis, A. D., Griffen, B., Crick, J. C. P., et al. Early percutaneous transluminal coronary angioplasty in the management of unstable angina. *Int. J. Cardiol.* 14:25, 1987.

71. De Feyter, P. J., Serruys, P. W., Soward, A., et al. Coronary angioplasty for early postinfarction unstable angina. *Circulation* 74:1365, 1986.

72. Gottlieb, S. O., Walford, G. D., Ouyang, P., et al. Initial and late results of coronary angioplasty for early postinfarction unstable angina. *Cathet. Cardiovasc. Diagn.* 13:93, 1987.

73. Safian, R. D., Snyder, L. D., Snyder, B. A., et al. Usefulness of percutaneous transluminal coronary angioplasty for unstable angina pectoris after non-Q-wave acute myocardial infarction. *Am. J. Cardiol.* 59:263, 1987.

74. Roberts, R., Croft, C., Gold, H. K., et al. Effect of propranolol on myocardial infarct size in a randomized blinded multicenter trial. *N. Engl. J. Med.* 311:218, 1984.

20
Pulmonary Embolism and Systemic Embolism in Patients with Acute Myocardial Infarction

JAMES E. DALEN

The incidence of venous thromboembolism (VTE) in patients with acute myocardial infarction has decreased dramatically. The primary factors predisposing to VTE in patients with acute myocardial infarction are immobility and congestive heart failure. In the past patients with acute myocardial infarction were kept at bed rest for 6 weeks, whereas at the present time patients with uncomplicated myocardial infarction rarely remain in bed for more than a few days and the total hospital stay is usually less than 7 to 10 days. The clinical incidence of pulmonary embolism in patients with uncomplicated myocardial infarction is approximately 1 to 8 percent [1].

Venous thromboembolism is most likely to occur in myocardial infarction patients who are at prolonged bed rest due to complications, particularly those associated with congestive heart failure. The myocardial infarction patients who are at greatest risk are those who have additional risk factors for VTE (Table 20-1). A history of VTE is an important risk factor.

Prevention of Venous Thromboembolism

In patients with an uncomplicated myocardial infarction who do not have additional risk factors for VTE, low-dose heparin (5000 units SC q12h) and early mobilization are adequate to prevent VTE [2]. The risks of low-dose heparin are minimal. It is our policy to begin low-dose heparin in all patients who are admitted with suspected acute myocardial infarction. When the infarction is excluded and the patient is ambulatory, heparin is discontinued. If the diagnosis of myocardial infarction is confirmed, we continue low-dose heparin until the patient is out of the coronary care unit and is ambulating actively.

In patients with myocardial infarction complicated by congestive heart failure or prolonged bed rest, and in those with additional risk factors for VTE (Table 20-1), low-dose heparin is inadequate to prevent VTE. In this circumstance, intravenous heparin is indicated. After a 5000-unit bolus, intravenous heparin at a rate of 1000 units/hr is begun. The hourly dose is adjusted to prolong the partial thromboplastin time (PTT) to 1.5 to 2.0 times the control value. Heparin should be continued until the patient is ambulatory.

If heparin is contraindicated, external compression devices can effectively prevent deep vein thrombosis [3]. They should be utilized until the patient is ambulatory. In patients at very high risk, e.g., a patient with recent VTE whose myocardial infarction is complicated and in whom heparin is contraindicated, it may be appropriate to place a filter in the inferior vena cava [4].

Detection of Deep Vein Thrombosis

Pulmonary embolism nearly always originates as venous thrombosis in the lower extremities. Unfortunately, this process is usually clini-

Table 20-1
Risk factors for venous thromboembolism in patients with acute myocardial infarction

Prolonged bed rest, especially when due to congestive heart failure
History of venous thromboembolism
Cancer
Advanced age
Obesity
Malignancy

cally silent. The most specific sign of proximal deep vein thrombosis is unilateral leg swelling; however, this finding is not sensitive in that it occurs in only a few patients with deep vein thrombosis.

The most useful diagnostic test for deep vein thrombosis is impedance plethysmography, which is noninvasive and is easily performed at the bedside [5]. A unilaterally positive test is essentially diagnostic of proximal deep vein thrombosis, and this finding is sufficient to begin full-dose heparin therapy [6]. If the impedance plethysmography is bilaterally positive, it may reflect bilateral acute or bilateral old deep vein thrombosis, or it may be a false-positive result [7]. In this circumstance, venography is indicated for definitive diagnosis. Bilaterally normal impedance plethysmography essentially excludes proximal deep vein thrombosis.

If proximal deep vein thrombosis is documented by impedance plethysmography or venography, full-dose intravenous heparin is indicated to prevent pulmonary embolism. If heparin is contraindicated, an inferior vena cava filter should be placed.

Detection of Pulmonary Embolism

If deep vein thrombosis is not prevented, and if it is not detected and treated, pulmonary embolism may occur and cause one of three syndromes: acute cor pulmonale, pulmonary infarction, or acute unexplained dyspnea.

Acute Cor Pulmonale

Acute cor pulmonale due to massive pulmonary embolism obstructing more than 60 percent of the pulmonary circulation is the most dramatic but the least frequent manifestation of acute pulmonary embolism. When more than 60 percent of the pulmonary circulation is acutely obstructed by emboli, the right ventricle dilates and fails. The central venous pressure increases and the stroke volume and cardiac output decrease, with resultant hypotension, syncope, or cardiac arrest [8].

The principal symptoms of acute cor pulmonale are dyspnea, anxiety, and possible syncope. On physical examination, one notes tachypnea (>20/min), tachycardia, and hypotension in most cases. The signs of acute right ventricular failure include distended neck veins, an S_3 gallop, and a parasternal heave. The lungs are usually clear. The most important diagnostic tests are the electrocardiogram (ECG), which demonstrates a new S_1 Q_3 T_3 pattern or new incomplete right bundle branch block in most cases [9]. Arterial blood gases demonstrate significant hypoxemia, hypocapnia, and respiratory alkalosis. The diagnosis may be confirmed by a V/Q lung scan or pulmonary angiography.

Pulmonary Infarction

Pulmonary infarction occurs when pulmonary embolism causes complete obstruction of a distal branch of the pulmonary circulation [10]. Because patients with pulmonary infarction have submassive pulmonary embolism, there are no signs or symptoms of acute cor pulmonale. The dominant symptom of pulmonary infarction is pleuritic chest pain, which may be accompanied by dyspnea, cough, and hemoptysis. The pleuritic pain may be confused with the pain of pericarditis, or it may be attributed to a pulmonary infection.

On physical examination the principal findings are in the lungs, which may include rales, wheezes, or a pleural friction rub. In addition to tachypnea, tachycardia may be present. The cardiac examination remains unchanged.

The ECG is of little benefit other than helping to exclude pericarditis. The chest radiograph is usually abnormal, demonstrating an infiltrate (which is rarely wedge-shaped) or a small unilateral pleural effusion [9].

Arterial blood gases may demonstrate hypoxemia, or the PO_2 may remain in the low-normal range, as a small portion of the pulmonary circulation is compromised. Hypocapnia and respiratory alkalosis are usually present.

Because the principal differential diagnosis (once pericarditis is excluded) is pulmonary infection, viral or bacterial, the white blood cell count, temperature, and sputum analysis are important. The diagnosis can usually be determined by V/Q scan and impedance plethysmography. If the lung scan is nonspecific and impedance plethysmography is bilaterally normal, pulmonary embolism is unlikely. If the findings are inconclusive, a selective pulmonary angiogram to evaluate the findings of the perfusion scan may be indicated.

Acute, Unexplained Dyspnea

If pulmonary embolism is submassive, and if pulmonary infarction does not occur, the only symptoms may be dyspnea and possibly anxiety. Pulmonary embolism is often overlooked in this setting. The physical examination is unchanged except for tachypnea and possibly tachycardia. The ECG and chest radiograph are unchanged. The dyspnea is often attributed to left ventricular (LV) failure secondary to acute myocardial infarction. Examination of the lungs and a chest radiograph help to exclude LV failure. If a pulmonary artery catheter is in place, the wedge pressure is normal in the absence of LV failure, but the pulmonary artery pressure is elevated owing to precapillary pulmonary hypertension secondary to the pulmonary embolism [11]. Assay of arterial blood gases is helpful in this setting. If dyspnea is due to acute pulmonary embolism, the arterial PO_2 (breathing room air) demonstrates obvious hypoxemia. A V/Q scan and impedance plethysmography should lead to the correct diagnosis.

Treatment of Acute Pulmonary Embolism

The cornerstone of treatment for acute pulmonary embolism in patients with acute myocardial infarction is heparin given by intravenous infusion at a rate sufficient to prolong the PTT to 1.5 to 2.0 times control. Heparin should be continued for 7 to 10 days [12]. Studies are currently under way to determine if a shorter course of heparin is sufficient.

Warfarin should be begun early in the treatment course, perhaps on day 1 or 2 of heparin therapy. The dose of warfarin should be adjusted to prolong the prothrombin time to 1.2 to 1.5 times control using North American rabbit brain thromboplastin. This result corresponds to a value of 2.0 to 3.0 using the more sensitive human brain thromboplastin widely used in Europe [13]. The duration of warfarin therapy depends on the factors that predisposed to VTE. If these factors are ongoing, e.g., a patient immobilized by severe congestive heart failure, warfarin therapy should be continued indefinitely. In patients in whom the predisposition to VTE is chronic, inferior vena caval interruption with a filter may be considered. Anticoagulant therapy with heparin followed by warfarin is effective in patients with pulmonary embolism uncomplicated by hypotension. The major threat to life in these patients is recurrent, potentially lethal episodes of pulmonary embolism.

In patients with massive pulmonary embolism complicated by acute cor pulmonale and hypotension, prophylactic therapy with anticoagulation may be insufficient. In this circumstance, definitive therapy may be indicated. Pulmonary embolectomy is rarely, if ever, feasible in patients with acute myocardial infarction. However, in some centers transvenous pulmonary embolectomy may be feasible [14].

As an alternative to embolectomy in patients with massive pulmonary embolism complicated by shock, fibrinolytic therapy may be appropriate. The most extensive experience is with urokinase and streptokinase. Treatment with these agents has been shown to increase the early resolution rate of pulmonary embolism, but they have not been shown to decrease the mortality associated with acute pulmonary embolism [15]. The primary complication of fibrinolytic therapy is bleeding, especially from the sites of arterial or venous procedures. Preliminary reports indicate that treatment of pulmonary embolism with tissue plasminogen activator (tPA) may be more effective than with urokinase and streptokinase [16]. However, further studies are required to determine the efficacy and the hemorrhagic complication rate of tPA.

It should be stressed that only a few patients with pulmonary embolism require definitive therapy with embolectomy or fibrinolytic agents. Most of these patients do well if further episodes are prevented with appropriate prophylactic therapy.

Systemic Embolism

Systemic emboli in patients with acute myocardial infarction may arise from two sources: the left ventricle and the left atrium. Left atrial thrombi leading to systemic embolism may occur in patients with atrial fibrillation [17] or other arrhythmias characterized by a lack of effective atrial contraction [18] and in patients with coexistent mitral valve disease [19].

The most common source of systemic embolism in patients with acute myocardial infarction is from left ventricular thrombi. It is now clear from studies utilizing two-dimensional echocardiography, that LV thrombi are most frequently associated with transmural anterior wall infarction, where the incidence of thrombi may be as high as 30 to 40 percent [20]. The incidence in patients with inferior wall infarction is much lower. It should be noted that two-dimensional echocardiography fails to detect up to 20 percent of LV thrombi [21] and that only a few LV thrombi result in systemic embolism.

The exact incidence of systemic embolism in patients with acute myocardial infarction is uncertain because many systemic emboli are not detected clinically. In postmortem studies the incidence has been reported to be 5 percent [22]. Most (70 percent) systemic emboli result in cerebral embolism. Embolic stroke occurs in approximately 3 percent of patients with acute myocardial infarction [23].

Prevention

At least three clinical trials have demonstrated that full-dose heparin followed by oral anticoagulation decreases the incidence of stroke in patients with acute myocardial infarction [24–26]. In these three studies, the incidence of stroke was decreased from 2 to 3 percent in control patients to approximately 1 percent in patients who were anticoagulated. Given the hemorrhagic complications of anticoagulant therapy, full-dose anticoagulation is not appropriate in all patients with acute myocardial infarction.

The high incidence of LV thrombi in patients with transmural anterior myocardial infarction indicates that they are the acute myocardial infarction patients at greatest risk of systemic embolism. Several small case–control studies have shown that anticoagulation decreases the incidence of LV thrombi in patients with transmural anterior myocardial infarction as detected by two-dimensional echocardiography [27, 28]. To date, no large randomized trial has demonstrated that anticoagulation decreases the incidence of systemic embolism in patients with transmural anterior myocardial infarction.

Given the available incomplete data, it was recommended by the ACCP-NHLBI National Conference of Antithrombotic Therapy [29] that, in the absence of contraindications, patients with transmural anterior myocardial infarction should receive full-dose anticoagulation. They recommended heparin sufficient to prolong the PTT to 1.5 to 2.0 times control, followed by low-intensity warfarin therapy (prothrombin time 1.2 to 1.5 times control using rabbit brain thromboplastin) for 3 months.

It must be noted that there is no evidence that low-dose heparin, aspirin, or other platelet-active agents decrease the incidence of systemic embolism in patients with acute myocardial infarction.

Treatment

The treatment of systemic embolism in patients with acute myocardial infarction depends on the site of the embolism. Emboli to the upper or lower extremities may be removed by the use of the Fogarty catheter [30], with follow-up anticoagulation with heparin and warfarin to prevent recurrent embolism. When emboli affect the viscera, thrombolytic therapy may be appropriate in addition to anticoagulation.

Treatment of the most common form of systemic embolism—cerebral embolism—is somewhat controversial. Some clinicians are reluctant to anticoagulate because of the fear of brain hemorrhage due to hemorrhagic transformation of a bland infarct. The Cerebral Embolism Study Group addressed this problem, utilizing serial computed tomography (CT) scans [31]. They found that the incidence of hemorrhagic transformation was greatest in patients with large infarcts and in those in whom anticoagulation was initiated less than 12 hours after the onset of symptoms [31]. The recommendation of the ACCP/NHLBI Task Force on Antithrombotic Therapy [32] was that patients with small to moderate-sized embolic strokes should have a CT scan 24 hours or more after stroke onset. If the CT scan documents the absence of spontaneous hemorrhage and there are no contraindications, intravenous heparin treatment sufficient to prolong the PTT to 1.5 to 2.0 times control should be initiated. Heparin therapy should be followed by warfarin therapy at a dose that prolongs the prothrombin time to 1.5 to 2.0 times control using rabbit brain thromboplastin. Warfarin therapy should be continued for 3 months.

Editorial Comments

The clinical incidence of venous and arterial thromboembolism in patients with acute myocardial infarction seems to be on the decline, perhaps in part due to the more aggressive use of heparin and thrombolytic therapy. Nevertheless, pulmonary embolism and systemic embolism are devastating complications and must be prevented if possible. Despite incomplete data, full anticoagulation should at least be considered for most patients with acute anterior myocardial infarction. The role of tPA in the face of established pulmonary or left ventricular thrombi is still evolving, but we can expect more research activity in this area.
G.S.F.

References

1. Salzman, E. W., and Hirsch, J. Prevention of Venous Thromboembolism. In R. W. Colman et al. (eds.), *Hemostasis and Thrombosis: Basic Principles and Clinical Practice* (2nd ed.). Philadelphia: Lippincott, 1987.
2. Hull, R. D., and Hirsch, J. Preventing venous thromboembolism. *J. Cardiovasc. Med.* 63, 1984.
3. Moser, G., Krahenbuhl, B., Barroussel, R., et al. Mechanical versus pharmacologic prevention of deep venous thrombosis. *Surgery* 152:448, 1981.
4. Kanter, B., and Moser, K. M. The Greenfield vena cava filter. *Chest* 93:170, 1988.
5. Wheeler, H. B. Diagnosis of deep vein thrombosis. *Am. J. Surg.* 150:7, 1985.
6. Hull, R. D., Hirsch, J., Carter, C. J., et al. Diagnostic efficacy of impedance plethysmography for clinically suspected deep-vein thrombosis. *Ann. Intern. Med.* 102:21, 1985.
7. Curley, F. J., Pratter, M. R., Irwin, R. S., et al. The clinical implications of bilaterally abnormal impedance plethysmography. *Arch. Intern. Med.* 147:125, 1986.
8. Thames, M. D., Alpert, J. S., and Dalen, J. E. Syncope in patients with pulmonary embolism. *J.A.M.A.* 238:2509, 1977.
9. Szucs, Jr., M., Brooks, H. L., Johnson, L. W., et al. Diagnostic sensitivity of laboratory findings in acute pulmonary embolism. *Arch. Intern. Med.* 74:161, 1971.
10. Dalen, J. E., Haffajee, C. I., Alpert, J. S., et al. Pulmonary embolism, pulmonary hemorrhage, pulmonary infarction. *N. Engl. J. Med.* 296:1431, 1977.
11. Dalen, J. E., Dexter, L., Ockene, I. S., and Carlson, J. Precapillary pulmonary hypertension; Its relationship to pulmonary venous hypertension. *Trans. Am. Clin. Climatol. Assoc.* 86:207, 1974.
12. Hyers, T. M., Hull, R. D., and Weg, J. G. Antithrombotic therapy for venous thromboembolic disease. *Chest* 89:26S, 1986.

13. Hirsh, J., Deykin, D., and Poller, L. "Therapeutic range" for oral anticoagulant therapy. *Chest* 89:26S, 1986.

14. Greenfield, L. J., and Zocco, J. J. Intraluminal management of acute massive pulmonary thromboembolism. *J. Thorac. Cardiovasc. Surg.* 77:402, 1979.

15. Dalen, J. E. The case against fibrinolytic therapy. *J. Cardiovasc. Med.* 5:799, 1980.

16. Goldhaber, S. Z., Markis, J. E., Meyerovitz, M. F., et al. Acute pulmonary embolism treated with tissue plasminogen activator. *Lancet* I:886, 1986.

17. Abbott, W. M., Maloney, R. D., McCabe, C. C., et al. Arterial embolism: A 44 year perspective. *Am. J. Surg.* 1243:460, 1982.

18. Fairfax, A. J., Lambert, C. D., and Leatham, A. Systemic embolism in chronic sinoatrial disorder. *N. Engl. J. Med.* 295:190, 1976.

19. Coulshed, N., Epstein, E. J., McKendrick, C. S., et al. Systemic embolism in mitral valve disease. *Br. Heart J.* 32:26, 1970.

20. Asinger, R. W., Mikell, F. L., Elsperger, J., et al. Incidence of left ventricular thrombosis after acute transmural myocardial infarction. *N. Engl. J. Med.* 305:297, 1981.

21. Ezekowitz, M. D., Wilson, D. A., Smith, E. O., et al. Comparison of indium-111 platelet scintigraphy and two-dimensional echocardiography in the diagnosis of left ventricular thrombi. *N. Engl. J. Med.* 306:1509, 1982.

22. Hilden, T., Iversen, K., Raaschou, F., et al. Anticoagulants in acute myocardial infarction. *Lancet* 2:327, 1961.

23. Drapkin, A., and Merskey, C. Anticoagulant therapy after acute myocardial infarction: Relation of therapeutic benefit to patient's age, sex and severity of infarction. *J.A.M.A.* 222:541, 1972.

24. United States Veterans Administration: Long-term anticoagulant therapy after myocardial infarction. *J.A.M.A.* 193:157, 1965.

25. Second Report of the Working Party on Anticoagulant Therapy in Coronary Thrombosis to the Medical Research Council: An assessment of long-term anticoagulant administration after cardiac infarction. *Br. Med. J.* 2:837, 1964.

26. Veterans Administration Cooperative Trial on Anticoagulation. Anticoagulants in acute myocardial infarction: Results of a cooperative clinical trial. *J.A.M.A.* 225:724, 1973.

27. Weinreich, D. J., Burke, J. F., and Pauletto, F. J. Left ventricular mural thrombi complicating acute myocardial infarction: Long-term follow-up with serial echocardiography. *Ann. Intern. Med.* 100:789, 1984.

28. Keating, E. C., Gross, S. A., Schlamowitz, R. A., et al. Mural thrombi in myocardial infarctions: Prospective evaluation of two-dimensional echocardiography. *Am. J. Med.* 74:989, 1983.

29. Resnekov, L., Chediak, J., Hirsch, J., and Lewis, D. Antithrombotic agents in coronary artery disease. *Chest* 89:54S, 1986.

30. Sheiner, N. M., Zeltzer, J., and MacIntosh, E. Arterial embolectomy in the modern era. *Can. J. Surg.* 25:373, 1982.

31. Cerebral Embolism Study Group: Cardioembolic stroke, early anticoagulation, and brain hemorrhage. *Arch. Intern. Med.* 147:636, 1987.

32. Sherman, D. G., Dyken, M. L., Fisher, M., et al. Cerebral embolism. *Chest* 89:82S, 1986.

21
Cardiopulmonary Resuscitation in Patients with Acute Myocardial Infarction

KARL B. KERN AND GORDON A. EWY

Cardiopulmonary resuscitation is intended to revive individuals who have experienced an unexpected cardiac arrest [1–3]. Thus not all patients with myocardial infarction are candidates for resuscitation. Although clinical death occurs when the patient's heart stops beating, cellular metabolism continues for a limited period of time. Unless effective cardiopulmonary resuscitation is promptly instituted, cellular ischemia and death quickly follow. The probability of successful cardiopulmonary resuscitation depends on the duration of the arrest prior to initiating therapy, the age of the patient, and the degree of cardiac damage sustained prior to the cessation of circulation [4–6]. Early recognition is an essential initial step. For this reason, all patients with acute or suspected myocardial infarctions should be monitored electrocardiographically.

Defibrillation is the most important single event of successful resuscitation. Accordingly, the new standards for cardiopulmonary resuscitation and emergency cardiac care have been changed [7].

In the intensive care setting, respiratory arrest can precede cardiac arrest, but prompt assisted ventilation prevents the problem. Because this sequence is rare in the patient with acute myocardial infarction, respiratory arrest is not addressed.

Mechanism of Blood Flow with External Chest Compression

In 1960 Kouwenhouven and associates [1] described a noninvasive technique for cardiopulmonary resuscitation (CPR). Over the ensuing two decades there was little change in what was known as conventional or standard CPR. By the mid-1970s, one of the few remaining questions concerning CPR was the rate at which external chest compression should be applied. In 1977 Taylor and others indicated that over a range of 40 to 80 compressions per minute the *duration* of chest compression was more important than the *rate* of chest compression [8, 9]. At 50 percent chest compression and 50 percent relaxation, duty cycle at a rate of 60 compressions per minute was thought to be optimal [7]. However, work from Duke University indicated that a faster chest compression rate produces better blood flow during closed-chest CPR [10, 11]. Some of these data were available at the time of the last National Conference on CPR [7]. Consequently, this information played a role in the present recommendations for a chest compression rate of 80 to 100 per minute [7].

Physiologists and physicians have assumed that external chest compression in the arrested patient created artificial circulation by compressing the heart in much the same manner as open-chest internal cardiac massage. It was assumed that during sternal compression there was cardiac compression and that blood moved from the left ventricle into the aorta as closure of the mitral valve prevented retrograde blood flow. This widely held concept was challenged during the late 1970s by Weisfeldt and associates [12–16]. These physicians from Johns Hopkins University thought that this concept was inconsistent with a number of observations. The first was that when sternal compression was performed in a patient with a flail chest no radial arterial blood pressure was recorded until the remainder of the chest was bound to prevent paradoxical expansion [12, 14]. The second clinical observation was that patients with chronic obstructive lung disease and a marked increase in anterior-posterior chest diameter and a relatively small heart could be resuscitated by sternal compression [12, 14]. The third observation was that during conventional CPR the compression cycle that followed ventilation often resulted in increased blood pressure and blood flow [12, 14]. Weisfeldt's group extended these observations by maintaining airway pressure with a bag–mask device and noted that this method also increased radial artery pressure during external chest compression [12]. These findings suggested that forward blood flow was related to an increase in intrathoracic pressure. This theory was supported by the studies of Criley and associates on "cough CPR" (see below).

Another important observation was the rediscovery that the pressures in the aorta and right atrium were often similar during external sternal compression. This observation had been reported by Weale and Rothwell-Jackson in 1962 but had received little attention [17]. Weisfeldt and associates found that during chest compression not only were the central venous and aortic pressures similar but the pressures in all cardiac chambers as well as in all the intrathoracic structures were nearly equal. In a fluid-filled system with a resistance, there must be a pressure gradient across the resistance to allow fluid to flow. When the heart is pumping normally, there is a large pressure gradient between the aorta and the right atrium and central veins. The lack of a gradient during external chest compression in their arrested subjects suggested to these investigators that the heart was not functioning as a pump [12, 14]. They concluded that the entire thorax was the "pump" during CPR.

In contrast to the similar pressures inside the thorax, Weisfeldt and associates found a significant pressure difference between the extrathoracic carotid artery and jugular veins.

This pressure gradient was thought to be sufficient to produce cerebral blood flow. The reason for the pressure difference between the intrathoracic and extrathoracic veins was initially not clear [14]. At the same time, Criley and coworkers demonstrated that jugular venous valves were operative during coughing [18]. This observation led to a renewed appreciation of the internal jugular valves that were well described by early anatomists [19]. Figure 21-1 illustrates how the thorax, in conjunction with these jugular venous valves, acts as a "pump."

Further support for the theory that increasing intrathoracic pressure is the driving force for the forward blood flow during external chest compression came from early echocardiographic studies [20, 21]. These two-dimensional echocardiographic studies during cardiopulmonary resuscitation in man showed that the mitral valve did not close and that the left ventricular internal diameter was little changed. These findings supported the observation that in some patients increased intrathoracic pressure and not cardiac compression accounted for the forward blood flow during external chest compression.

Cardiac compression does occur in humans [12]. In a few of the patients studied by the Johns Hopkins group, simultaneous central venous pressures were lower than arterial pressures during external chest compression, indicating cardiac compression [12]. It is of interest that in patients in whom cardiac compression is present the arterial pressure generated is generally higher than that found in patients without cardiac compression [9]. Weisfeldt et al. emphasized that "in these patients in whom direct cardiac compression can be applied effectively, a particularly attractive feature of the maneuver is that the aortic diastolic pressure seems to rise significantly more than it does when the blood is moved solely by manipulating intrathoracic pressure; this means coronary perfusion is probably improved. For this reason, we strongly recommend that chest compression be included in any new CPR system designed to take advantage of the potentially useful effects of manipulating generalized intrathoracic pres-

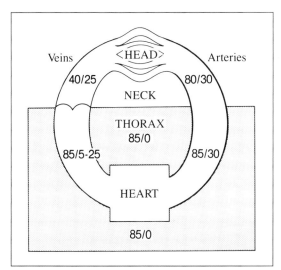

Fig. 21-1
Thoracic "pump" wherein pressures produced in the thorax are equally transmitted to an intrathoracic vascular structure. Note the reflection of that transmitted pressure by the extrathoracic venous jugular valve, which allows a pressure gradient across the central nervous system vascular bed resulting in antegrade flow to the head.

sure" [12]. The importance of this statement has been underscored by more recent studies (see below).

If in most patients blood flow during external chest compression depends on increased intrathoracic pressure, the question that logically follows is if altering techniques of conventional CPR could enhance blood flow during external chest compression. Accordingly, the group from Johns Hopkins explored two basic strategies: direct increases in intrathoracic pressure and abdominal binding [14]. Although increased intrathoracic pressure could be obtained by clamping the endotracheal tube during chest compression, the initial increase in pressure and flow dissipated rapidly, undoubtedly because venous return is inhibited by the continuous high intrathoracic pressure [12]. The Johns Hopkins group [14] then reported that maintaining inflated lungs during external chest compression resulted in a significant increase in arterial pressure and carotid flow when compared to conventional CPR (Table 21-1). These results have been

confirmed by other investigators using simultaneous high-pressure ventilation and chest compression in large [22] but not small [22, 23] dogs. In small dogs, true cardiac compression evidently occurs with relatively good blood pressure and flow, and the addition of simultaneous high-pressure ventilation does not appear to improve these hemodynamics [22]. In large animals, where cardiac compression plays a small role, the addition of simultaneous ventilation improves peripheral circulation [22].

The second approach to augment blood flow during CPR was abdominal binding (Table 21-1). Redding was the first to show that abdominal binding during CPR improves survival as well as hemodynamics [24]. However, further investigation of this technique was interrupted by studies that reported a high incidence of liver laceration secondary to abdominal binding [25]. Studies that applied abdominal binding during CPR using military antishock trousers (MAST) also revealed a high incidence of liver laceration and exsanguination [26]. The technique advocated by the group at Johns Hopkins utilized a device similar to an enlarged blood pressure cuff that distributes pressure over the abdomen in a broader fashion. They then reported the use of such a device in humans [16].

The ultimate utility of simultaneous high-pressure ventilation or abdominal binding would be determined by whether these interventions resulted in an increase in survival. In an effort to answer this question, an experimental form of CPR that utilized high-pressure (60 torr) ventilation, chest compression with a broad flat surface, and abdominal binding (60 torr) was compared to standard CPR in our laboratory. Standard or experimental CPR was performed during ventricular fibrillation [27]. Five of the six animals that underwent standard CPR had a return of blood pressure and survived, whereas none of the six animals that underwent simultaneous high-pressure ventilation, diffuse chest compression, and abdominal pressure had a return of blood pressure following defibrillation, and none could be resuscitated despite intensive efforts [27]. Nevertheless, a National Heart, Lung, and

Table 21-1
Effects of maintaining lungs inflated and binding the abdomen during chest compression

Treatment	Aortic systolic blood pressure (mm Hg)	Carotid flow (ml/min)
Chest compression plus lung inflated	27	9
	58	29
Chest compression plus abdominal binding	29	15
	58	32

Source: After M. T. Rudikoff et al. Mechanisms of blood flow during cardiopulmonary resuscitation. *Circulation* 61:345, 1980.

Blood Institute (NHLBI) funded study in humans that was performed in Dade County, Florida by Chandra, Nagel, and associates. To our knowledge, the results of these studies were never formally published, but simultaneous chest compression and ventilation did not improve survival and is therefore not recommended [28]. The hemodynamic reasons for the deleterious effect of simultaneous chest compression and ventilation are discussed below.

In contrast to the "thoracic pump" mechanism of blood flow during CPR, Rankin and associates were convinced from their clinical experience that faster chest compression rates were more effective and that cardiac compression was the mechanism of blood flow during CPR. Maier, Rankin, and associates from Duke University studied the effects of varying the manual compression rate, force, and duration in large dogs [10, 11]. They reported that the relative contributions of the thoracic pump and direct cardiac compression mechanisms to blood flow varied with the method of CPR being performed [10, 11]. Direct cardiac compression seemed to be more significant during high-impulse (increased frequency) CPR, and the thoracic pump mechanism was predominant during low-momentum compression techniques. Echocardiographic studies by Deshmukh et al. [29, 30] in anesthetized minipigs demonstrated cardiac valve motion and a change in left ventricular dimensions during the early phases of closed-chest CPR, adding further support for direct cardiac compression as a mechanism of blood flow during CPR.

As with most disagreements, there is probably truth on both sides. It is our conclusion that the mechanism of blood flow during closed-chest compression is a spectrum varying from a purely thoracic pump mechanism (cough or vest CPR) on one end of the spectrum and cardiac compression (open-chest CPR) on the other; with still others, e.g., standard, mechanical thumper, or high-impulse CPR, there are varying combinations of thoracic pump and cardiac pump depending on the anatomic attributes of the subject and the duration of CPR. This conclusion is based on the following observations. Patients in sinus rhythm and subjects in cardiac arrest undergoing open-chest cardiac compression display a large difference between the aortic and right atrial systolic pressures. In contrast, there appear to be little or no systolic pressure difference between the aorta and right atrium in those subjects in whom blood moves by the thoracic pump mechanism during CPR. Because of this observation we evaluated the absolute difference between aortic and right atrial systolic pressure (which we called the systolic pressure gradient, or SPG) in 63 adult mongrel dogs undergoing five methods of CPR [31]. After 3 minutes of "down time," during which no CPR was performed, the animals were ventilated and one of five methods of CPR was initiated. Systolic pressure gradients were measured at 1, 7, and 17 minutes of CPR. The systolic pressure gradient was greatest during open-chest cardiac massage (true cardiac compression), intermediate with external mechanical (Thumper) and standard CPR, and lowest with CPR performed with a combined

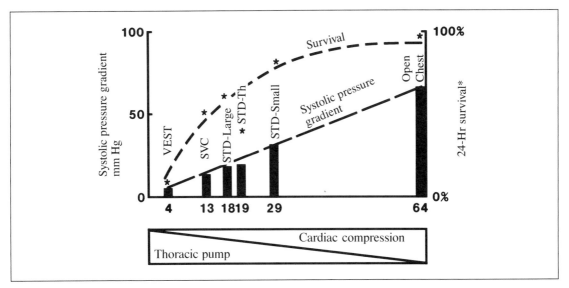

Fig. 21-2
Systolic pressure gradient as a potential indicator of the mechanism of CPR-generated blood flow. Of note is the relation between increased survival and CPR blood flow resulting from cardiac compression.

thoracic and abdominal vest apparatus (predominantly thoracic pump) [31]. The findings are shown in Figure 21-2.

It was also noted that 24-hour survival was greatest in the groups with cardiac compression and least in those with the thoracic pump mechanism (Fig. 21-2) [31]. This latter observation is of interest in light of the report by Deshmukh and associates concerning a two-dimensional echocardiographic study of eight minipigs [29, 30]. The aortic and mitral valves demonstrated appropriate systolic and diastolic behavior for the first 5 minutes in all animals but for 12 minutes in the three minipigs successfully resuscitated [29, 30].

We concluded that the mechanism of blood flow during closed-chest CPR varies according to *technique;* it is greatest with the open-chest technique (see below) and high-impulse CPR and lowest with vest CPR. The mechanism also varies with *duration* of CPR, with cardiac compression being the mechanism early and thoracic pump later. The fact is that the patients reported by the Johns Hopkins group were studied only after the house staff had "given up" and turned the patient over to the CPR research team, who then had to instrument the patients prior to their studies. The average *systolic* arterial pressure generated by these investigators with standard CPR was less than 30 mm Hg (Table 21-1). Thus by the time these measurements were made, the thoracic pump mechanism was predominant. The third determinant of blood flow during closed-chest CPR is the *anatomic makeup* of the subject. Patients with narrow anterior-posterior chest diameters and a large heart have more cardiac compression than does the emphysematous patient with a large anterior posterior chest diameter and a small heart. In summary, the mechanism of blood flow during closed-chest CPR depends on the anatomy and pathology of the patient, the duration of CPR, and the technique used. We recommend a compression rate of at least 100 per minute with a 50 percent compression/50 percent relaxation ratio.

Cough Resuscitation

Criley and associates introduced cough CPR, accomplished by having the patient with recent-onset asystole or ventricular fibrillation

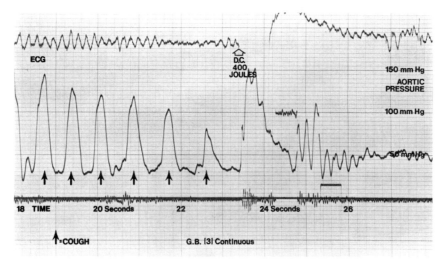

Fig. 21-3
Marked aortic pressure spikes seen with simple rhythmic coughing during
ventricular fibrillation. Aortic peak pressure ranges from 80 to 145 mm Hg. No
compressions of any type were performed during this tracing. (From G. A. Ewy
and R. Bressler, eds., *Cardiovascular Drugs and Management of Heart Disease.*
New York: Raven Press, 1982. P. 365.

cough forcefully every 1 to 2 seconds [32, 33].
The obvious disadvantage of this technique is
that it must be initiated before the patient
loses consciousness. Forceful cough results in
an abrupt increase in intrathoracic pressures,
which can result in striking aortic systolic
pressures (Fig. 21-3). By employing cough
CPR in the cardiac catheterization laboratory,
Criley et al. have 'had patients sustain consciousness for 24 and 39 seconds after the onset of ventricular fibrillation [32, 33]. Cough
CPR has several advantages: It enables laboratory personnel to turn their full attention to
preparing for and using the defibrillator rather
than performing cardiac massage; it can be
performed by a patient in any position and on
any surface, including the lateral position of
the angiographic cradle; and, finally, not only
are the hazards of fracture avoided, but ventilation also occurs spontaneously [32, 33].
The potential for using cough CPR in areas
other than the cardiac catheterization laboratory needs further exploration. Cough has
been used not only for resuscitation but for
termination of ventricular tachycardia [34].

Open-Chest Cardiac Massage

Open-chest cardiac massage sounds primitive
in the present era but may well be indicated in
selected situations. Conventional CPR, which
produces only 6 to 30 percent of normal blood
flow, cannot sustain tissue viability—it only
slows the process of dying. The question is
whether open-chest cardiac massage provides
sufficient increase in blood flow over standard
noninvasive resuscitation methods to justify
its use.

There have been few published studies in
humans comparing closed- and open-chest
CPR. Del Guercio and associates recorded
hemodynamics of patients undergoing CPR
with closed-chest compression and repeated
these measurements with open-chest cardiac
massage [35]. The cardiac output and circulation times were significantly improved by the
open-chest technique. However, this study
has been criticized because the green dye dilution techniques used are inaccurate at low
flow states [36].

There are indications for open-chest cardiac

massage in clinical medicine. Patients with cardiac arrest and major chest trauma or penetrating chest wounds should be treated with open-chest massage once they arrive at the hospital. Patients undergoing thoracic surgery should also undergo open-chest massage should they arrest. The major question concerns the use of open-chest massage when standard closed-chest compression is not effective. This issue is further complicated by another major deficit in the field of CPR, namely the inability to determine the effectiveness of closed-chest compression. If an arterial pulse is not perceptible, one can be sure that external chest compression alone is inadequate. If a pulse is palpable, the question remains whether this pulse is only a transmitted pressure wave or is a true arterial pulse. Even if it is a true arterial pulse, if the diastolic pressure is not adequate the subject is not likely to survive.

If a pulse cannot be generated after a reasonable trial of external chest compression, the patient may be hypovolemic or have cardiac tamponade—conditions that are difficult to diagnose during cardiac arrest. Likewise, the patient might simply be inadequately perfused with closed-chest compression CPR. How long should efforts with ineffective closed-chest compression persist before more drastic therapy such as open-chest cardiac massage be instituted? In an experimental model of cardiac arrest, we found open-chest massage effective if instituted after 15 minutes of ineffective closed-chest resuscitation [37]. However, if internal massage was delayed for 20 minutes of closed-chest efforts, successful resuscitation with open-chest massage was less likely; and if 25 minutes elapsed before open-chest cardiac compressions were performed, none of the experimental subjects could be resuscitated. It appears that though open-chest massage can effectively produce excellent myocardial perfusion pressures, if a lengthy period of poor myocardial perfusion precedes the use of internal resuscitation techniques no improvement in resuscitation outcome results.

Open-chest cardiac massage has clearly been shown to improve hemodynamics, car-

diac output, and short-term resuscitation success. However, the long-term effects of internal resuscitation, with its inherent morbidity, was less clear. Could open-chest cardiac massage, when instituted after 15 minutes of closed-chest compressions, improve long-term survival as well as initial resuscitation outcome? In an experiment designed to evaluate this question, we found that open-chest massage begun after 15 minutes of ventricular fibrillation and closed-chest compression was strikingly superior for producing 7-day survival compared to continued closed-chest efforts [38] (Fig. 21-4).

Geehr and associates performed a limited trial of open-chest cardiac massage in victims of out-of-hospital cardiac arrest. They found no difference in open-chest massage versus continued closed-chest compressions in 50 patients. Both groups had three initial resuscitated survivors, but no patient lived long term [39]. Careful evaluation of the details of this study revealed that all patients had a minimum of 20 to 30 minutes of cardiac arrest and closed-chest compression prior to randomization to continue closed-chest efforts versus open-chest massage. Hence their results were similar to the findings of our experimental work showing that open-chest cardiac massage does not improve survival when instituted after a lengthy period of closed-chest efforts. In both experimental models and limited clinical trials it appears that open-chest cardiac massage is unlikely to improve survival from cardiac arrest if used only as a last ditch effort. Nonetheless, it is also apparent that, with proper timing, open-chest cardiac massage is clearly the superior resuscitation technique at present.

Open-Chest Cardiac Massage During Acute Myocardial Infarction

Open-chest massage is one resuscitation technique that has been experimentally evaluated in the setting of myocardial infarction and cardiac arrest. Weiser and associates studied the hemodynamic effects of closed- and open-chest

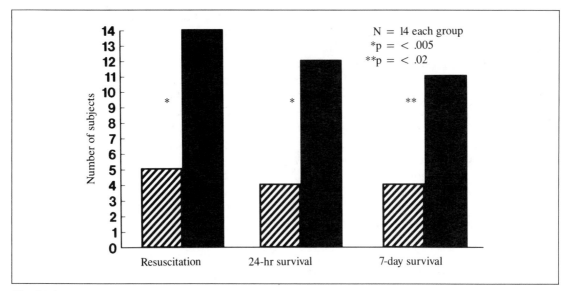

Fig. 21-4
Open-chest cardiac massage (*closed bars*) improves initial resuscitation results,
24-hour survival, and 7-day survival when instituted after 15 minutes of standard
closed-chest compression CPR (*hatched bars*) and failed external defibrillation.

cardiac resuscitation in both normal dogs and those with myocardial infarction [40]. Experimental myocardial infarctions were attempted by injecting plastic microspheres into the ascending aorta and allowing random entry into the coronary circulation, though no documentation of actual infarction was provided. The authors comment on the superiority of open-chest massage for producing higher aortic pressures and cardiac outputs, but no analysis compared the effect of the bead-induced myocardial infarction on hemodynamics, cardiac output, or outcome. Another study of external versus internal cardiac massage in normal and chronically ischemic dogs was reported in 1980 by Byrne and associates [41]. These investigators measured myocardial blood flow using radioactive microspheres in normal animals and in those with complete circumflex coronary artery occlusions produced by a surgically placed ameroid constrictor. Myocardium supplied by the occluded circumflex artery, presumably then perfused by canine epicardial collaterals, had significantly less blood flow than any other area during external cardiac massage. The authors speculated that similar hypoperfused areas of myocardium are

likely to exist in many patients who developed cardiac arrest and that such areas may be more adequately perfused by internal massage. No data were given concerning the relation of CPR-produced intravascular pressures, the amount of blood flow to the normal and ischemic myocardium, or the success of the resuscitation effort.

We have completed preliminary work of adapting a nonsurgical method for the production of a coronary stenosis in closed-chest animals for CPR research. The model, originally described by Gewirtz and Most [42], involves percutaneous transcatheter placement of a plastic cylinder in a coronary artery of the pig. We modified this procedure for the production of a discrete anterior myocardial infarction by occluding the mid-portion of the left anterior descending coronary artery. We found that allowing thrombotic occlusion of the stenosis in the mid left anterior coronary artery resulted in an anteroseptal infarction involving 28 ± 3 percent of the left ventricle [43] Subsequently, we produced both discreet patent stenoses and complete coronary occlusions in the pig through the judicious use of anticoagulation therapy.

We have begun to apply this model of coronary obstructive disease in preliminary studies of coronary blood flow during CPR. Nine pigs have been studied with nonradioactive, colored microspheres for regional blood flow during normal sinus rhythm and ventricular fibrillation treated with CPR [44]. All animals have one or more Teflon cylinders successfully placed in the left anterior coronary artery during the study. An advantage of this method for creating an "abnormal" heart model for CPR research is avoidance of a thoracotomy. External chest compressions can be performed without concern for nonphysiologic changes within the thorax or chest wall.

We found that prior to coronary manipulations left ventricular myocardial blood flow was 124 ± 56 ml/min/100 gm during sinus rhythm. These data correspond well to published levels of myocardial blood flow in pigs [45–51]. Comparisons of left ventricular blood flow during sinus rhythm showed no difference between the anterior and lateral locations or between blood flows to the epicardium and endocardium.

Blood flow to the left ventricular anterior wall supplied by the left anterior descending coronary artery was studied above and below the location of the experimentally placed intracoronary cylinder. Preliminary data showed that in pigs in which the cylinder is occluded no distal left anterior decending flow occurred. Hence regardless of the coronary perfusion pressure generated by CPR, no blood flow occurred to the myocardium below the level of the obstruction. This initial finding, if confirmed, is important to understanding the distribution of CPR-produced blood flow during acute myocardial infarctions complicated by cardiac arrest. Evidence indicates that most myocardial infarctions indeed result from acute thrombotic occlusions [52]. Hence if a person arrests during an acute coronary occlusion and myocardial infarction, CPR does not produce the same regional myocardial blood flow as in patients without such coronary disease.

The most important finding, though, again from a small number of animals, is that CPR performed in an arrest victim with a left anterior descending coronary artery stenosis pro-duces markedly different regional myocardial blood flows above and below that lesion. We found that, for any given coronary perfusion pressure, blood flow below a patent stenosis was only one-half of that above the coronary lesion. The consequences of diminished myocardial blood flow in the presence of coronary stenosis and occlusion is of obvious importance, as greater CPR-produced perfusion pressure may be needed to produce enough blood flow for successful resuscitation.

Drug Therapy During Cardiac Arrest

Proper drug therapy generally increases the effectiveness of CPR. The objectives of drug therapy during cardiac arrest are, first, to increase peripheral vascular constriction and, second, to minimize the adverse effects of metabolic acidosis.

The value of epinephrine in cardiac resuscitation has long been known. Because the drug has both inotropic and chronotropic (beta-adrenergic) effects on the beating heart and also produces peripheral vasoconstriction (alpha-adrenergic effects), there has been confusion regarding which of these effects is the most important to restarting an arrested heart. As early as 1906, Crile and Dolley [53] noted the importance of securing an adequate aortic diastolic perfusion pressure during cardiac resuscitation. They stated that it usually was not possible to achieve an adequate aortic diastolic pressure via cardiac massage without the addition of epinephrine. Since that time, it has been repeatedly demonstrated that the value of epinephrine does not lie in its direct action on the heart. Instead, epinephrine increases peripheral vascular resistance, transiently decreasing perfusion of most of the body and, in the process, increasing aortic diastolic pressure [54, 55]. The increased peripheral vascular constriction increases aortic diastolic blood pressure, which improves the coronary perfusion pressure. Because coronary artery blood flow occurs during diastole in either the spontaneously beating or arrested heart, the result is increased coronary blood flow.

Table 21-2
Successful drug therapy for cardiac arrest

Cardiac arrest	Survival
Asphyxial arrest	
Epinephrine	10/10
Isoproterenol	0/10
Methoxamine	9/10
VF arrest	
Epinephrine	9/10
Phenylephrine	10/10
Saline	1/10
Epinephrine	10/10
Phenylephrine plus propranolol	10/10
Isoproterenol plus phenoxybenzamine	3/11

The now classic studies of Redding and Pearson, in which asphyxial cardiac arrest was produced, are worth emphasizing [56]. Standard CPR and drug administration resulted in survival of all of ten animals that received epinephrine, none of ten animals that received isoproterenol, and nine of ten animals that received methoxamine [56]. In a similar study of cardiac arrest produced by ventricular fibrillation, one of ten animals survived without drugs, nine of ten with epinephrine, and ten of ten with phenylephrine. In a reexamination of this phenomenon, it was found that alpha-adrenergic blockade administered with epinephrine prevented resuscitation in animals with cardiac arrest. Resuscitation of animals with beta-adrenergic blocking drugs administered with epinephrine was uniformly successful [57]. Table 21-2 summarizes these data.

Drugs that have their principal effect by cardiac stimulation, such as isoproterenol, dobutamine, or calcium salts, may be useful for supporting the circulation after the heart has restarted but have not been shown to be helpful during the period of cardiac arrest. Drugs that do not have epinephrine's cardiac stimulating effect but are potent peripheral vasoconstrictors, such as phenylephrine, methoxamine, or dopamine, are as effective as epinephrine during CPR [54–60]. However, because none of these medications has been shown to be superior to epinephrine, epinephrine remains the drug of choice. There should

be no delay in using an appropriate dose of epinephrine during resuscitation from either cardiac standstill or ventricular fibrillation. Because the useful action of the drug is on the peripheral circulation, intracardiac injection has no advantage over intravenous injection. In fact, when an endotracheal tube is in place and intravenous access is not available, drugs may be diluted and administered via the endotracheal tube (see below). Intracardiac injections, although relatively safe [60], should be reserved for the rare situation where intravenous and endotracheal routes are not available.

Two drugs, sodium bicarbonate and calcium chloride, are often used in excess during CPR. In the absence of adequate tissue perfusion, anaerobic metabolism results in the production of lactic acid and other metabolites that cause metabolic acidosis. Following the widespread adoption of CPR, there were many advocates of the early use of sodium bicarbonate to correct the acidosis on the assumption that it would promote early restoration of cardiac function. For several years it was common to observe the administration of large amounts of sodium bicarbonate while drugs of established value were neglected. This attitude was based on observations that the administration of bicarbonate to the animals before the induction of cardiac arrest made the animals easier to resuscitate, that acidotic animals had a diminished response to catecholamines, and that calves made hypotensive by infusion of hydrochloric acid could be restored by infusion of sodium bicarbonate [61–63].

Subsequent investigation showed that sodium bicarbonate alone given during CPR did not promote return of cardiac contractility [64]. In fact, accurate correction of metabolic acidosis was not feasible until cardiac resuscitation had been successful and improved tissue perfusion mobilized acid metabolites sequestered in the tissues. Administration of bicarbonate did not potentiate the effect of suboptimal doses of epinephrine, whereas 1 mg of epinephrine was found to be effective even in the presence of severe metabolic acidosis [64]. Other experiments demonstrated that the susceptibility of the heart to the development of ventricular fibrillation was increased in the presence of metabolic acidosis, and that it could be corrected by administration of bicarbonate. However, respiratory acidosis or alkalosis had no such effect [65]. Hyperosmolar states considered incompatible with life have been found in a series of patients given bicarbonate during resuscitation efforts. The hyperosmolar state was attributed directly to the injection of hypertonic sodium bicarbonate [66, 67]. Sodium bicarbonate infusion results in a significant rise in arterial carbon dioxide tension that parallels the rise in pH [68].

These facts indicate that caution should be used in the administration of sodium bicarbonate. Observations by Bishop and Weisfeldt indicated that cardiac arrest can be managed for a "considerable period of time" by adequate ventilation in patients not previously acidotic [68]. Animals fibrillated and immediately begun on CPR with adequate ventilation become progressively alkalotic during the first 5 minutes. After 20 minutes of standard CPR, metabolic acidosis is present. Thus if a patient develops primary ventricular fibrillation, sodium bicarbonate is probably not needed unless CPR is excessively long. In this situation, the need for sodium bicarbonate should be determined by blood gas analysis. In some patients, cardiac arrest is secondary to acidosis. In these patients, sodium bicarbonate 1 mg/kg should be administered initially with subsequent doses based on blood gas determinations. If blood gases are not available, one-half of the initial dose can be given empirically every 10 to 15 minutes during arrest [2].

The second drug that is probably used in excess during cardiac arrest is calcium. Calcium ions have long been known to increase the force of myocardial contraction [69–71]. Because of their integral role in myocardial excitation-contraction coupling, calcium ions have been postulated to be useful during profound cardiovascular collapse when accompanied by electrical mechanical dissociation, and for restoring electrical rhythm in some instances of electrical standstill. Not only are there few experimental data to support this postulate [56, 72], but intravenous injections

in the quantities usually given result in potentially dangerous high serum calcium levels in the arrested patient [73, 74]. After 5 mg of 10% calcium chloride administration as an intravenous bolus to arrested victims, serum calcium levels were found to vary from 12.9 to 18.2 ml/dl [74]. The mean serum calcium level was 15.3 ml/dl at 5 minutes and 11.2 ml/dl at 10 minutes. Calcium has the potential of being particularly dangerous in patients receiving digitalis.

Calcium may be needed in a rare patient, as in a cardiac arrest victim who has had considerable blood loss and citrated blood replacement or the hyperkalemic patient who arrests. The near routine use of calcium chloride in victims of cardiac arrest and during asystole or idioventricular rhythm has little support in the medical literature and is no longer recommended [7].

Endotracheal Administration of Drugs

Epinephrine is rapidly absorbed when given via the endotracheal tube (Table 21-3); epinephrine peak blood levels occur within 15 seconds, but the effects last much longer than with intravenous administration [75–78]. Because metabolism of the drug is the same following intravenous or endotracheal administration, the endotracheal route must provide a depot for continued delayed release [75–79]. Other drugs that have been shown to be well absorbed via the endotracheal route are atropine and lidocaine for dysrhythmias, naloxone for morphine overdose, and diazepam for therapy of status epilepticus [80] (Table 21-3).

All endotracheally administered drugs have

Table 21-3
Endotracheal administration of
cardiac arrest drugs

Acceptable	Not acceptable
Epinephrine	Calcium
Atropine	Norepinephrine
Lidocaine	
Naloxone	
Diazepam	

a two to five times longer duration of action than when given by the intravenous route [81, 82]. Repeated doses by the endotracheal route should be administered with this extended period in mind. The volume of endotracheal drug should not be excessive.

Sterile normal saline is probably the diluent of choice for endotracheal drug administration because this solution should result in less deleterious effects than distilled water. However, Pearson and Redding have shown that endotracheal epinephrine has a faster effect when diluted in distilled water than when diluted in saline. Endotracheal drugs should be administered deep into the lungs, preferably with a catheter as long as the endotracheal tube. Forceful administration with nebulization of the solution enhances its absorption. Its delivery should be followed by a short period of hyperventilation (about five inflations with a breathing bag).

Because absorption is nearly complete, drugs administered endotracheally have the same toxicity as those administered intravenously. Drugs that should not be administered via the endotracheal tube are calcium chloride and norepinephrine. Sodium bicarbonate has not been studied but will probably not be practical if for no other reason than because of the large volume of fluid necessary for an effective dose.

The endotracheal route of administration of drugs may be especially valuable in the prehospital CPR setting where paramedics have the skills for endotracheal intubation but where field conditions or patient factors might preclude efficient intravenous access.

Bradydysrhythmias During Cardiac Arrest

Asystole and idioventricular rhythm are the dominant bradydysrhythmias seen during cardiac arrest and resuscitation. Yet during cardiac arrest these disorders of impulse formation and conduction are almost invariably the result of myocardial ischemia and do not respond to pacing. Even when pacing results in electrical depolarization of the myocardium, there is seldom an associated myocardial contraction. Thus during CPR one must resist the temptation to focus only on the electrocardiogram. The therapy of choice is to improve myocardial perfusion by appropriate CPR techniques and drugs. Pacing is seldom indicated.

On rare occasions, sinus arrest, profound sinus bradycardia, and advanced heart block with long periods of ventricular asystole occur because of isolated conduction defects. In these patients, emergency pacing is indicated. In such acute emergencies, temporizing measures may be necessary before pacing can be initiated. These temporizing measures include cough CPR, rhythmic chest thumps, standard CPR, and intravenous drugs.

Cough CPR may be effective if initiated before the patient loses consciousness. A sharp blow to the precordium (chest thump) may initiate cardiac contraction. Continued rhythmic chest thumps are indicated only if each blow produces a palpable pulse or the series maintains consciousness [83].

If the patient is unconscious and chest thumps are ineffective, standard external chest compression and assisted ventilation should be initiated while an intravenous access is being obtained. Drugs that might be beneficial in patients with severe bradycardia or recent-onset asystole include anticholinergic drugs such as atropine and beta-adrenergic stimulants such as isoproterenol. Some patients who have sustained trauma or have an acute illness may develop a marked vasovagal reaction that results in profound bradycardia or asystole. In these patients, intravenous atropine 0.5 to 1.0 mg or even more may be effective. The potential for adverse reactions to a single dose of atropine in the setting of asystole or severe bradycardia is so minimal that its use is to be encouraged. Isoproterenol infusion may also be helpful in patients with high-grade heart block or severe symptomatic bradycardia, but as noted (see Drug Therapy During Cardiac Arrest, above) isoproterenol is contraindicated in the patient with true cardiac arrest. In such patients, epinephrine is the drug of choice.

There are three basic approaches to pacing: transvenous, transthoracic, and external. External pacing is the oldest and simplest technique and is another temporizing approach to stabilizing patients with profound bradydysrhythmias [84]. The major virtue of external pacing is its ease of application. Zoll et al. modified the external electrodes and the pacing waveform to effect external cardiac pacing without excessive pain or skeletal-muscle stimulation [85]. This device is now available for clinical use [86].

Ventricular Fibrillation

Cardiac arrest may result from a variety of dysrhythmias including ventricular fibrillation, ventricular tachycardia, ventricular asystole, electromechanical dissociation, and high-grade heart block. Ventricular fibrillation, the most common cause of cardiac arrest, almost invariably requires defibrillation for definitive therapy. Ventricular tachycardia may respond to pharmacologic therapy but frequently requires electrical intervention. The remaining ventricular dysrhythmias often require some form of electrical intervention as definitive or adjunctive therapy. Fifty to seventy percent of the annual deaths from coronary artery disease occur suddenly and are the result of ventricular fibrillation [87]. Fortunately, primary ventricular fibrillation is usually responsive to immediate defibrillation [88]. Patients with witnessed, exertion-related cardiac arrest in well established cardiac rehabilitation units have been reported to respond uniformly to prompt defibrillation [89]. Similarly, nearly 40 percent of patients treated for out-of-hospital cardiac arrest are discharged alive following prompt application of CPR and early defibrillation [90, 91]. Because rapidity of delivery of defibrillation continues to be the major determinant in survival from cardiac arrest secondary to ventricular fibrillation, therapy that can be administered by bystanders or emergency medical technicians trained in defibrillation is assuming increasing importance [92–94].

A sharp blow to the chest with the fist 8 to 12 inches above the precordium, the chest thump, is effective in only 2 percent of patients with ventricular fibrillation [95] but has the distinct advantages of ready availability and ease and speed of application. These features have resulted in the recommendation that the chest thump be the initial therapy for witnessed unmonitored cardiac arrest [7].

RECOMMENDED MANAGEMENT

1. In a witnessed arrest due to ventricular fibrillation the initial step is prompt defibrillation, providing a defibrillator is available.
2. If a defibrillator is not available, initiate external sternal compression and assisted ventilation (basic cardiac life support [BCLS]) and call for defibrillation equipment and assistance. If the patient is monitored and has ventricular fibrillation or has witnessed nonasphyxial unmonitored collapse, give a precordial thump.
3. The following steps should be followed while interrupting chest compressions for as brief a time as possible.
   a. Apply conductive, low-resistance interface to metal defibrillator paddles or apply self-adhesive electrodes.
   b. Place electrode paddles so that the delivered current traverses the left ventricle.
   c. Select the appropriate energy level (joules) and charge the defibrillator capacitor. In adults the initial attempt at defibrillation is made using approximately 200 joules of delivered energy. If defibrillation is successful at 200 joules but the patient later has recurrent ventricular fibrillation, higher energies are not necessary for subsequent shocks.
   d. If the first shock is unsuccessful, the second shock is 200 to 300 joules.
   e. If unsuccessful, a third shock of up to 360 joules is administered as soon as possible.
   f. If the patient does not defibrillate following the third shock, look for factors producing high impedance.
   g. Administer epinephrine, continue chest compression and assisted ventilation, and administer an additional one or two

shocks at 360 joules. Follow American Heart Association recommendations for advanced cardiac life support (ACLS).

4. After delivery of electrical current, the electrocardiogram and arterial pulse are assessed to determine effectiveness of therapy.

Successful defibrillation of patients in ventricular fibrillation depends on many factors, including the duration of the ventricular fibrillation, the environment and condition of the myocardium, and if an adequate electrical current traverses a critical mass of the ventricles [96, 97]. Current delivery through the ventricles depends on the energy delivered from the defibrillator, the resistance (impedance) between the defibrillator capacitor and the heart, and the electrode size and position.

Energy Requirements for Defibrillation

The amount of energy desirable for direct-current external defibrillation is controversial [98]. It is clear that a defibrillation threshold exists, i.e., shocks of inadequate strength do not defibrillate [99–103]. Yet excessively strong defibrillation shocks are known to produce dysrhythmias and myocardial damage [99]. Animals varying markedly in size require a wide range of energy for defibrillation [99]. However, observations in human adults indicate that body weight is not a major determinant of the energy levels necessary for defibrillation [103–106]. It is now generally agreed that although there is a relation between body size and the energy needed for defibrillation (infants and small children require less energy than large adults) over the range of weights in most adults, size does not appear to be a clinically important variable [107].

Previous ACLS guidelines have advised that "the initial attempt at defibrillation should be made using 200 to 300 joules of delivered energy" [2]. Since this recommendation was made, two clinical studies have suggested that an initial shock energy of no more than 200 joules should be used. In a prospective out-of-hospital study, Weaver et al. compared the effects of low and high energy shocks in 249 patients with ventricular fibrillation [108].

"Low-energy" shocks (two 175-joule shocks; if ineffective, an additional 320-joule shock) were compared on alternate days with "high-energy" shocks (three 320-joule shocks). Defibrillation rates were virtually identical with either shock energy, as was the proportion of patients resuscitated and subsequently discharged from the hospital [108]. Kerber and associates conducted a prospective in-hospital study of 183 patients who received direct-current shocks for ventricular fibrillation [109]. Patients received initial shocks of either 200 joules or 300 to 400 joules. This study also showed no difference in the first-shock or cumulative success rates of these two energy levels. Neither study therefore showed any benefit from initial shocks above 200 joules. Moreover, using a lower energy may be safer. Weaver and associates found a higher incidence of atrioventricular block in patients receiving 320-joule shocks compared to the lower-energy shocks; it was particularly evident in patients who received several shocks at the higher energy level [108].

The appropriate energy level for the second shock is still somewhat controversial. The previous ACLS guidelines suggested that the initial and second shock should be of similar energies [2]. This recommendation was based on three points. First, defibrillation appears to be a probability function; that is, at any given energy there is a specific probability that defibrillation can be achieved [110]. Thus if the first shock fails, there is a possibility that a second shock of the same energy will succeed. The rationale for a second shock is that transthoracic impedance declines with repeated shocks [111, 112]. Such a decline results in greater current flow for any given energy, and this increase in current flow should improve the chances of achieving defibrillation with a second shock using the same energy. However, Kerber and associates have shown that, although the transthoracic impedance in humans does fall with repeated shocks, the change is modest [113]. They concluded that a greater and more predictable increase in current flow occurs if the shock energy is raised. Another argument against increasing the energy for the second shock is the result of a study by Weaver et al. [108]. Because of the conflicting evidence, the present recommendation for the strength of the second shock remains at 200 to 300 joules [2]. Should the first two shocks fail to defibrillate, a third shock not to exceed 360 joules should be delivered immediately. This method is another change incorporated in the 1986 guidelines for ACLS [2].

Because defibrillation success is significantly decreased by a delay of minutes, the present guidelines suggest three consecutive shocks [2, 114]. Again, because early defibrillation is so important, the guidelines are written so that it is acceptable to deliver three successive 200-joule shocks (the maximum output of the presently available automatic external defibrillators is less than 360 joules).

For recurrent ventricular fibrillation, it may not be necessary to increase the defibrillation energy on successive shocks. If ventricular fibrillation recurs frequently, it may be desirable to reduce the energy of subsequent defibrillatory shocks. This approach has the theoretical advantage of minimizing electrical injury to the heart. Appropriate external chest compression and assisted ventilation should be performed until a defibrillator is available and between shocks while the defibrillator capacitor is charging, *except* with automatic or semiautomatic external defibrillators. These devices require a period of time for diagnosis and capacitor charging. During this time, external chest compression interferes with the diagnostic process and delays or aborts discharge. Therefore because the most important aspect of survival in out-of-hospital fibrillation is prompt defibrillation, a period of up to 1.5 minutes for diagnosing and delivering three shocks by automatic or semiautomatic external defibrillators without chest compression is, by consensus, acceptable [115].

Defibrillation is accomplished by passage through the heart of an electrical current of sufficient energy to depolarize a critical mass of the myocardium. Although the operator selects the energy (joules), it is the current flow (amperes) that is responsible for defibrillation. Current flow is determined by the shock strength and the transthoracic resis-

tance (impedance). Many of the factors determining transthoracic impedance to direct-current defibrillator discharge are known. They include the energy level [116], electrode size [117–120], interface between the skin and the electrode [119, 121, 122], number and time interval of previous shocks [111, 112], phase of ventilation [123], distance between electrodes [113], and paddle electrode pressure [113]. Human transthoracic impedance to cardioversion or defibrillator shock ranges between 14 and 143 ohms [124]. If the impedance is high, low-energy shocks fail to defibrillate [125]. Factors affecting transthoracic impedance are less important at high-energy defibrillations. However, if all three defibrillation attempts fail, one should evaluate factors that may contribute to a high transthoracic impedance or resistance to defibrillation. These factors include pneumothorax, inadequate electrode chest wall interface, inadequate electrode position or skin contact, excessive distance between electrodes, and inadequate electrode pressure.

Because defibrillation depends on an adequate current traversing the myocardium, *paddle electrode placement* is critical. The electrodes should be placed in a position that maximizes current flow through the ventricular myocardium. There are two accepted locations for paddle placement. The standard placement is one electrode with its edge just to the right of the upper sternum and below the clavicle, with the other paddle placed to the left of the nipple with the center of the electrode in the mid-axillary line. An alternative approach is to place one paddle anteriorly over the left precordium and the other posteriorly behind the heart. The paddle should be applied to the chest wall with firm pressure (about 25 lb).

On occasion, external cardioversion of defibrillation is necessary in patients with a permanent pacemaker. The external defibrillation electrodes should not be placed too near (not closer than 5 inches) the subcutaneous pacemaker generator, as defibrillation shocks may cause pacemaker malfunction by raising the pacing threshold [126]. It has been suggested that patients with permanent pacemakers who have been defibrillated or cardioverted should have the pacing thresholds checked at frequent intervals for 6 weeks after the shock [126].

Conclusions

Cardiopulmonary resuscitation and defibrillation can be life-saving. The time to defibrillation is the most important aspect for successful resuscitation and survival. Hence major emphasis should continue to be on early defibrillation. Effective CPR can improve defibrillation success, providing myocardial blood flow during cardiac arrest. Systemic blood flow appears to result from at least two distinct mechanisms: the "cardiac compression mechanism" and the "thoracic pump mechanism." Both mechanisms may play a role in blood flow production in individual patients depending on the circumstances surrounding the resuscitation efforts. Regardless of the mechanism of CPR-generated blood flow, acute and chronic coronary disease has a profound effect on myocardial perfusion. The effect on CPR of acute coronary occlusion, as is often seen with acute myocardial infarction, and coronary stenosis, which is present in 95 percent of all victims of cardiac arrest, requires further study.

Editorial Comments

Cardiopulmonary resuscitation is currently undergoing continuing evaluation in hopes of fine-tuning its effectiveness. Drs. Kern and Ewy have been at the forefront of this movement, primarily in the experimental laboratory. Resuscitation in the patient with acute myocardial infarction usually means electrical defibrillation. The initial shock should be 200 joules, which is successful in up to 90 percent of cases. A second shock of 200 to 360 joules may be used if the first defibrillation attempt is unsuccessful. Until the new technique of simultaneous compression-ventilation is established, conventional CPR at a cycle of 80 to 100 per minute, with lung inflation being performed separately, is recommended. G.S.F.

References

1. Kouwenhoven, W. B., Jude, J. R., and Knickerbocker, G. C. Closed chest cardiac massage. *J.A.M.A.* 137:1064, 1960.
2. Standards and guidelines for cardiopulmonary resuscitation (CPR) and emergency cardiac care (ECC). *J.A.M.A.* 244:453, 1980.
3. McIntyre, K. M., and Lewis, A. J. *Textbook of Advanced Cardiac Support.* Dallas: American Heart Association, 1981.
4. Cole, S. L., and Corday, E. Four minute limit for cardiac resuscitation. *J.A.M.A.* 161:1454, 1956.
5. Cobb, L. A., Baum, R. S., Alvarez, J., et al. Resuscitation from out-of-hospital ventricular fibrillation. *Circulation* 51,52(Suppl 3):223, 1975.
6. Eisenberg, M. S., Bergner, L., and Hallstrom, A. Cardiac resuscitation in the community: Importance of rapid provision and implications of program planning. *J.A.M.A.* 241:1905, 1979.
7. Standards and guidelines for cardiopulmonary resuscitation (CPR) and emergency cardiac care (ECC) *J.A.M.A.* 255:2905, 1986.
8. Taylor, G. J., Tucker, W. M., Green, H. L., et al. Importance of prolonged compression duration during cardiopulmonary resuscitation in man. *N. Engl. J. Med.* 296:1515, 1977.
9. Fitzgerald, K. R., Babbs, C. F., Frissors, H. A., et al. Prediction of cardiac output during cardiopulmonary resuscitation at various compression rates and duration. *Am. J. Physiol.* (submitted).
10. Maier, G. W., Tyson, G. S., Olsen, C. O., et al. The physiology of external cardiac massage: High impulse cardiopulmonary resuscitation. *Circulation* 70:86, 1984.
11. Maier, G. W., Tyson, G. S., Olsen, C. O., et al. Optimal techniques of external cardiac massage. *Surg. Forum* 33:282, 1982.
12. Weisfeldt, M. I., Chandra, N., Tsitlik, J. E., et al. New Attempts to Improve Blood Flow During CPR. In J. Schluger and A. F. Lyon (eds.), *CPR and Emergency Cardiac Care. Looking to the Future.* New York: EM Books, 1980. Pp. 29–45.
13. Chandra, N., Rudikoss, M., Tsitlik, J., et al. Augmentation of carotid flow during cardiopulmonary resuscitation (CPR) in the dog by simultaneous compression and ventilation with high airway pressure. *Am. J. Cardiol.* 43:422, 1979.

14. Rudikoff, M. T., Maughan, W. L., Effron, M., et al. Mechanisms of blood flow during cardiopulmonary resuscitation. *Circulation* 61:345, 1980.

15. Chandra, N., Rudikoff, M., and Weisfeldt, M. L. Simultaneous chest compression and ventilation at high airway pressure during cardiopulmonary resuscitation. *Lancet* 1:175, 1980.

16. Chandra, N., Snyder, L. D., and Weisfeldt, M. L. Abdominal binding during cardiopulmonary resuscitation in man. *J.A.M.A.* 246:351, 1981.

17. Weale, F. E., and Rothwell-Jackson, R. L. The efficiency of cardiac massage. *Lancet* 1:1990, 1962.

18. Niemann, J. T., Garner, D., Rosborough, D. S., et al. The mechanism of blood flow in closed chest cardiopulmonary resuscitation (Abstract). *Circulation* 59(Suppl II):74, 1979.

19. Weathersby, H. T. The valves of the axillary, subclavian, and internal jugular vein (Abstract). *Anat. Rec.* 124:379, 1956.

20. Werner, J. A., Greene, H. L., Janko, C., et al. Visualization of cardiac valve motion in man during external chest compression using two-dimensional echocardiography: Implications regarding the mechanism of blood flow. *Circulation* 63:1417, 1981.

21. Rich, S., Wix, H. L., and Shapiro, E. Two-dimensional echocardiography resuscitation in man. *Am. J. Cardiol.* 47:398, 1981.

22. Babbs, C. F., Tacker, W. A., Paris, R. J., et al. Cardiopulmonary resuscitation with simultaneous compression and ventilation at high airway pressure in four animal models. In: Abstracts of the Fourth Purdue Conference on Cardiac Defibrillation and Cardiopulmonary Resuscitation. Purdue University, September 15–17, 1981. P. 5.

23. Redding, J. S., Haynes, R. R., and Thomas, J. D. "Old" and "new" CPR manually performed in dogs. *Crit. Care Med.* 9:386, 1981.

24. Redding, J. S. Abdominal compression in cardiopulmonary resuscitation. *Anesth. Analg.* 50:668, 1971.

25. Harris, L. C., Kirimli, B., and Safar, P. Augmentation of artificial circulation during cardiopulmonary resuscitation. *Anesthesia* 28:730, 1967.

26. Alifimoff, J. K., Barnett, W. M., Safar, P., et al. Comparisons of standard cardiopulmonary resuscitation, new CPR, abdominal restraint—augmented CPR and open-chested CPR. In: Abstracts of the Fourth Purdue Conference on Cardiac Defibrillation and Cardiopulmonary Resuscitation. Purdue University, September 15–17, 1981. P. 2.

27. Sanders, A., Ewy, G. A., Alferness, C., et al. Failure of one method of simultaneous chest compression, ventilation, and abdominal binding during cardiopulmonary resuscitation. *Crit. Care Med.* 10:509, 1982.

28. Weisfeldt, M. Personal communication.

29. Deshmukh, H. G., Weil, M. H., Gudipati, C. V., et al. Blood flow during CPR is maintained by direct cardiac compression (Abstract). *Clin. Res.* 34:88A, 1986.

30. Deshmukh, H. G., Weil, M. H., Rackow, E. C., et al. Echocardiographic observations during cardiopulmonary resuscitation: A preliminary report. *Crit. Care Med.* 13:904, 1985.

31. Raessler, K. L., Kern, K. B., Sanders, A. B., et al. Aortic and right atrial systolic pressures as an indicator of the mechanism of blood flow during CPR. *Am. Heart J.* 115:1021, 1988.

32. Criley, J. M., Blaufuss, A. H., and Kissel, G. L. Cough-induced cardiac compression. *J.A.M.A.* 236:1246, 1976.

33. Criley, J. M. Cough CPR. In J. Schluger and A. F. Lyon (eds.), *CPR and Emergency Cardiac Care: Looking to the Future.* New York: EM Books, 1980. P. 47.

34. Wei, J. Y., Greene, H. L., and Weisfeldt, M. L. Cough facilitated conversion of ventricular tachycardia. *Am. J. Cardiol.* 45:174, 1980.

35. Del Guercio, L. R. M., Feins, N. R., Cohn, J. D., et al. Comparison of blood flow during external and internal cardiac massage in man. *Circulation* 31 and 32(Suppl 1):171, 1965.

36. Jacobson, S. Current Status of Open Chest Procedures. In J. Schluger and A. F. Lyon (eds.), *CPR and Emergency Cardiac Care: Looking to the Future.* New York: EM Books, 1980. P. 127.

37. Sanders, A. B., Kern, K. B., Atlas, M., et al. Importance of the duration of inadequate coronary perfusion pressure on resuscitation from cardiac arrest. *J. Am. Coll. Cardiol.* 6:113, 1986.

38. Kern, K. B., Sanders, A. B., Badylak, S. F., et al. Long-term survival with open chest cardiac massage after ineffective closed chest compression in a canine preparation. *Circulation* 75:498, 1987.

39. Geehr, E. C., Lewis, F. R., and Auerbach, P. S. Failure of open heart massage to improve survival after pre-hospital non-traumatic cardiac arrest. *N. Engl. J. Med.* 314:1189, 1986.

40. Weiser, F. M., Adler, L. N., and Kuhn, L. A. Hemodynamic effects of closed and open chest cardiac resuscitation in normal dogs and those with acute myocardial infarction. *Am. J. Cardiol.* 10:555, 1962.

41. Byrne, D., Pass, H. I., Neely, W. A., et al. External versus internal cardiac massage in normal and chronically ischemic dogs. *Am. Surg.* 46:657, 1980.

42. Gewirtz, H., and Most, A. S. Production of a critical coronary stenosis in closed chest laboratory animals. *Am. J. Cardiol.* 47:589, 1981.

43. Lancaster, L. D., Kern, K. B., Morrison, D., et al. Right ventricular dysfunction during acute anteroseptal myocardial infarction in pigs (Abstract). *Clin. Res.* 35:179A, 1987.

44. Kern, K. B., Lancaster, L. D., Perrault, P., et al. Myocardial blood flow during CPR in pigs with obstructive coronary lesions. *Clin. Res.* 36:109A, 1988.

45. White, F. C., Roth, D. M., and Bloor, C. M. The pig as model for myocardial ischemia and exercise. *Lab. Anim. Sci.* 36:351, 1986.

46. Bellamy, R. F., DeGuzman, L. R., and Pedersen, D. C. Coronary blood flow during cardiopulmonary resuscitation in swine. *Circulation* 69:174, 1984.

47. Guth, B. D., White, F. C., Gallagher, K. P., and Bloor, C. M. Decreased systolic wall thickening in myocardium adjacent to ischemic zones in conscious swine during brief coronary artery occlusion. *Am. Heart J.* 107:458, 1984.

48. Fedor, J. M., McIntosh, D. M., Rembert, J. C., and Greenfield, Jr., J. Coronary and transmural myocardial blood flow responses in awake domestic pigs. *Am. J. Physiol.* 255:H435, 1978.

49. Tranquilli, W. J., Manohar, M., Parks, C. M., et al. Systemic and regional blood flow distribution in unanesthetized swine and swine anesthetized with halothane and nitrous oxide, halothane, or enflurane. *Anesthesiology* 56:369, 1982.

50. Manohar, M., and Parks, C. M. Porcine systemic and regional organ flow during 1.0 and 1.5 minimum alveolar concentrations of sevoflurane anesthesia without and with 50 percent nitrous oxide. *J. Pharmacol. Exp. Ther.* 231:640, 1984.

51. Brown, C. G. Regional blood flow measurements during cardiopulmonary resuscitation following prolonged ventricular fibrillation in a swine model. *Resuscitation* 16:107, 1988.

52. DeWood, M. A., Spores, J., Motske, R., et al. Prevalence of total occlusion during the early hours of transmural myocardial infarction. *N. Engl. J. Med.* 303:897, 1980.

53. Crile, G., and Dolley, D. H. Experimental research into resuscitation of dogs killed by anesthetics and asphyxia. *J. Exp. Med.* 8:713, 1906.

54. Pearson, J. W., and Redding, J. S. Epinephrine in cardiac resuscitation. *Am. Heart J.* 66:210, 1963.

55. Pearson, J. W., and Redding, J. S. Influence of peripheral vascular tone on cardiac resuscitation. *Anesth. Analg.* 46:253, 1967.

56. Redding, J. S., and Pearson, J. W. Evaluation of drugs for cardiac resuscitation. *Anesthesiology* 24:203, 1963.

57. Yakaitis, R. W., Otto, C. W., and Blitt, C. D. Relative importance of alpha- and beta-adrenergic receptors during resuscitation. *Crit. Care Med.* 7:293, 1979.

58. Otto, C. W., Yakaitis, R. W., and Blitt, C. D. Mechanism of action of epinephrine in resuscitation from asphyxial arrest. *Crit. Care Med.* 9:364, 1981.

59. Otto, C. W., Yakaitis, R. W., Redding, J. S., et al. Comparison of dopamine, dobutamine, and epinephrine in CPR. *Crit. Care Med.* 9:366, 1981.

60. Davison, R., Barresi, V., Parker, M., et al. Intracardiac injections during cardiopulmonary resuscitation: A low-risk procedure. *J.A.M.A.* 244:1110, 1980.

61. Ledingham, I. M. A., and Norman, J. N. Acid-base studies in experimental circulatory arrest. *Lancet* 2:967, 1962.

62. Thrower, W. B., Darby T. D., and Aldinger, E. E. Acid-base derangements and myocardial contractibility. *Arch. Surg.* 82:56, 1961.

63. Stewart, J. S. S. Management of cardiac arrest. *Lancet* 1:106, 1964.

64. Redding, J. S., and Pearson, J. W. Metabolic acidosis: A factor in cardiac resuscitation. *South. Med. J.* 60:926, 1967.

65. Gerst, P. H., Fleming, W. H., and Malm, J. R. Increased susceptibility of the heart to ventricular fibrillation during metabolic acidosis. *Circ. Res.* 19:63, 1966.

66. Mattar, J. A., Weil, M. H., Shubin, H., et al. Cardiac arrest in the critically ill. II. Hyperosmolar states following cardiac arrest. *Am. J. Med.* 56:162, 1974.

67. Cohn, J. D., and Del Guercio, L. R. M. Cardiorespiratory analysis of cardiac arrest and resuscitation. *Surg. Gynecol. Obstet.* 123:1066, 1966.

68. Bishop, R. L., and Weisfeldt, M. L. Sodium bicarbonate administration during cardiac arrest: Effect on arterial pH, PCO_2, and osmolality. *J.A.M.A.* 235:506, 1976.

69. Niedergerke, R. The rate of action of calcium ions on the contraction of the heart. *J. Physiol. (Lond.)* 138:506, 1957.

70. Weber, A., Herz, R., and Reiss, I. Role of calcium in contraction and relaxation of muscle. *Fed. Proc.* 28:896, 1964.

71. Borle, A. B. Calcium metabolism of the cellular level. *Fed. Proc.* 32:1944, 1973.

72. White, B. C., Petinga, T. J., Hoehner, P. J., et al. Incidence, etiology and outcome of pulseless idioventricular rhythm treated with dexamethasone during advanced CPR. *J. Am. Coll. Emerg. Physicians* 8:188, 1979.

73. Carlon, G. C., Howland, W. S., Kahn, R. C.,

et al. Calcium chloride administration in nor-mocalcemic critically ill patients. *Crit. Care Med.* 8:209, 1980.

74. Dembo, D. H. Calcium in advanced life sup-port. *Crit. Care Med.* 9:358, 1981.

75. Redding, J. S., Asuncion, J. S., and Pearson, J. W. Effective routes of drug administration during cardiac arrest. *Anesth. Analg.* 46:253, 1967.

76. Roberts, J. R., Greenberg, M. I., Kanub, M. A., et al. Blood levels following intrave-nous and endotracheal epinephrine adminis-tration. *J. Am. Coll. Emerg. Physicians* 8:53, 1979.

77. Roberts, J. R., Greenberg, M. I., and Baskin, S. I. Endotracheal epinephrine in cardiorespi-ratory collapse. *J. Am. Coll. Emerg. Physi-cians* 8:515, 1979.

78. Greenberg, M. I., Roberts, J. R., and Baskin, S. I. Endotracheal naloxone reversal of mor-phine-induced respiratory depression in rab-bits. *Ann. Emerg. Med.* 9:289, 1980.

79. Greenberg, M. I., Roberts, J. R., and Krusz, J. C. Endotracheal epinephrine in a canine anaphy-lactic shock model. *J. Am. Coll. Emerg. Physi-cians* 8:500, 1979.

80. Greenberg, M. I. Endotracheal medication in cardiac emergencies. In: Abstracts of the Fourth Purdue Conference on Cardiac Defi-brillation and Cardiopulmonary Resuscitation. Purdue University, September 15–17, 1981. P. 9.

81. Roberts, J. R., Greenberg, M. I., Knaub, M., et al. Comparison of the pharmacological ef-fects of epinephrine administered by the intra-venous and endotracheal routes. *J. Am. Coll. Emerg. Physicians* 7:260, 1978.

82. Elam, J. O. The Interpulmonary Route for CPR Drugs. In P. Safar and J. O. Elam (eds.), *Advances in Cardiopulmonary Resuscitation.* New York: Springer-Verlag, 1977.

83. Zoll, P. M., Belgard, A. H., Weintraub, M. J., and Frank, H. A. External mechanical cardiac stimulation. *N. Engl. J. Med.* 294:1274, 1976.

84. Zoll, P. M. Resuscitation of the heart in ven-tricular standstill by external electrical stimu-lation. *N. Engl. J. Med.* 247:768, 1952.

85. Zoll, R. H., Zoll, P. M., and Belgard, A. H. Non-invasive cardiac stimulation. In: Ab-stracts of the Fourth Purdue Conference on Cardiac Defibrillation and Cardiopulmonary Resuscitation. Purdue University, September 15–17, 1981. P. 20.

86. Zoll, P. M., Zoll, R. H., Falk, R. H., et al. External noninvasive temporary cardiac pac-ing: Clinical trial. *Circulation* 71:937, 1985.

87. Julian, D. G. Toward preventing coronary death from ventricular fibrillation. *Circulation* 54:360, 1976.

88. Eisenberg, M. S., Copass, M. K., Hallstrom, A. P., et al. Treatment of out-of-hospital car-diac arrests with rapid defibrillation by emer-gency medical technicians. *N. Engl. J. Med.* 302:1379, 1980.

89. Hossck, K. F., and Hartwig, R. Cardiac arrest associated with supervised cardiac rehabilita-tion. *J. Cardiac Rehabil.* 2:402, 1982.

90. Cobb, L. A., and Hallstrom, A. P. Community-based cardiopulmonary resuscitation: What have we learned? *Ann. N.Y. Acad. Sci.* 382:330, 1982.

91. Eisenberg, M. S., Bergner, L., and Hallstrom, A. P. Cardiac resuscitation in the community: Importance of rapid provision and implications for program planning. *J.A.M.A.* 241:1905, 1979.

92. Stults, K. R., Brown, D. D., Schug, V. L., and Bean, J. A. Pre-hospital defibrillation per-formed by emergency medical technicians in rural communities. *N. Engl. J. Med.* 310:219, 1984.

93. Rozkovec, A., Crossley, J., Walesby, R., et al. Safety and effectiveness of a portable external automatic defibrillator-pacemaker. *Clin. Car-diol.* 6:527, 1983.

94. Weaver, W. D., Copass, M. K., Cobb, L. A., et al. A new, compact, automatic external de-fibrillator designed for layperson use (Ab-stract). *J. Am. Coll. Cardiol.* 5:457, 1985.

95. Caldwell, G., Millor, G., Quinn, E., et al. Sim-ple mechanical method of cardioversion: De-fense of the precordial thump and cough ver-sion. *Br. Med. J.* 291:627, 1985.

96. Garrey, W. E. The nature of fibrillatory con-tractions of the heart and its relation to tissue mass and form. *Am. J. Physiol.* 33:397, 1914.

97. Zipes, D. P., Fisher, J., King, R. M., et al. Ter-mination of ventricular fibrillation in dogs by depolarizing a critical amount of myocardium. *Am. J. Cardiol.* 36:37, 1975.

98. Ewy, G. A., Tacker, Jr., W. A. Transchest electrical ventricular defibrillation. *Am. Heart J.* 91:403, 1976.

99. Geddes, L. A., Tacker, W. A., Rosborough, J. P., et al. Electrical dose for ventricular de-fibrillation of large and small animals using precordial electrodes. *J. Clin. Invest.* 53:310, 1974.

100. Gutgesell, H. P., Tacker, W. A., Geddes, L. A., et al. Energy dose for defibrillation in children. *Pediatrics* 58:898, 1976.

101. Dahl, C. F., Ewy, G. A., Warner, E. D., et al. Myocardial necrosis from direct current coun-tershock. *Circulation* 50:956, 1974.

102. Warner, E. D., Dahl, C., and Ewy, G. A. Myo-cardial injury from transthoracic defibrillator countershock. *Arch. Pathol.* 99:55, 1975.

103. Pantridge, J. R., Adgey, A. A. J., Webb,

S. W., et al. Electrical requirements for ventricular defibrillation. *Br. Med. J.* 2:313, 1975.

104. Adgey, A. A. Electrical energy requirements for ventricular defibrillation. *Br. Heart J.* 40:1197, 1978.

105. Crampton, J. A., Crampton, R. S., Sipes, J. N., et al. Energy levels and patient weight in ventricular defibrillation. *J.A.M.A.* 242:1380, 1984.

106. Gascho, J. A., Crampton, R. S., Cherwek, M. L., et al. Determinants of ventricular defibrillation in adults. *Circulation* 60:231, 1979.

107. Lown, B., Crampton, R. S., DeSilva, R. A., and Gascho, J. The energy for ventricular fibrillation—too little or too much? *N. Engl. J. Med.* 298:1252, 1978.

108. Weaver, W. D., Cobb, L. A., Copass, M. K., and Hallstrom, A. P. Ventricular defibrillation—a comparative trial using 175 J and 320 J shocks. *N. Engl. J. Med.* 307:1101, 1982.

109. Kerber, R. E., Jensen, S. R., Gascho, J. A., et al. Determinants of defibrillation: Prospective analysis of 183 patients. *Am. J. Cardiol.* 52:739, 1985.

110. Tacker, W. A., and Geddes, L. A. *Electrical Defibrillation.* Boca Raton, FL: CRC Press, 1980. P. 141.

111. Geddes, L. A., Tacker, W. A., Cabler, D. P., et al. Decrease in transthoracic resistance during successive ventricular defibrillation trials. *Med. Instrum.* 9:179, 1975.

112. Dahl, C. F., Ewy, G. A., Ewy, M. D., and Thomas, E. D. Transthoracic impedance to direct current discharge: Effect of repeated countershocks. *Med. Instrum.* 10:151, 1976.

113. Kerber, R. E., Grayzel, J., Hoyt, R., et al. Transthoracic resistance of human defibrillation: Influence of body weight, chest size, serial shocks, paddle size and paddle contact pressure. *Circulation* 63:676, 1981.

114. Yakaitis, R. W., Ewy, G. A., Oho, C. W., et al. Influence of time and therapy on ventricular defibrillation in dogs. *Crit. Care Med.* 8:157, 1980.

115. Ewy, G. A. Electrical therapy for cardiovascular emergencies. *Circulation* 74(Suppl IV):111, 1986.

116. Ewy, G. A., Ewy, M. D., Nuttall, A. J., and Nuttall, A. W. Canine transthoracic resistance. *J. Appl. Physiol.* 32:91, 1972.

117. Thomas, E. D., Ewy, G. A., Dahl, C. F., and Ewy, M. D. Effectiveness of direct current defibrillation: Role of paddle electrode size. *Am. Heart J.* 93:463, 1977.

118. Patel, A. S., and Galysh, F. T. Experimental studies to design safe external pediatric paddles for DC defibrillation. *IEEE Trans. Biomed. Eng.* 19:228, 1972.

119. Connell, P. N., Ewy, G. A., Dahl, C. F., et al. Transthoracic impedance to defibrillation discharge: Effect of electrode size and electrode chest wall interface. *J. Electrocardiol.* 6:313, 1973.

120. Ewy, G. A., and Horan, W. J. Effectiveness of direct current defibrillations. II. Role of paddle electrode size. *Am. Heart J.* 93:674, 1977.

121. Ewy, G. A., Horan, W. J., and Ewy, M. D. Disposable defibrillator electrodes. *Heart Lung* 6:127, 1977.

122. Ewy, G. A., and Taren, D. Comparison of paddle electrode pastes used for defibrillation. *Heart Lung* 6:847, 1977.

123. Ewy, G. A., Hellman, D. A., McClung, S., et al. Influence of ventilation phase on transthoracic impedance and defibrillation effectiveness. *Crit. Care Med.* 3:164, 1980.

124. Ewy, G. A., Ewy, M. K., and Silverman, J. Determinants of human transthoracic resistance to direct current discharge. *Circulation* 46(Suppl II):II–150, 1972.

125. Kerber, R. E., Kouba, C., Martins, J., et al. Advanced prediction of transthoracic impedance in human defibrillation and cardioversion: Importance of impedance in determining the success of low energy shocks. *Circulation* 70:303, 1984.

126. Levine, P. A., Barold, S. S., Fletcher, R. D., and Talbot, P. Adverse acute and chronic effects of electrical defibrillation and cardioversion on implanted unipolar cardiac pacing systems. *J. Am. Coll. Cardiol.* 1:1413, 1983.

VI
Special Procedures in Acute Myocardial Infarction

22
Coronary Arteriography in Acute Myocardial Infarction

Marcus A. DeWood, William F. Stifter, A. Henry Reisig, Donald B. Canaday, Terrance P. Judge, and J. Paul Shields

During the early years after the development of coronary arteriography, investigation of the coronary tree was confined to patients with chronic stable angina pectoris. Increasing experience demonstrated that coronary arteriography could be used to define the nature and extent of coronary obstruction in acute ischemic syndromes and their most profound expression, acute myocardial infarction [1–4]. Furthermore, advancing interest in the pathophysiology of acute myocardial infarction shifted attention from animal models and pathology studies of acute myocardial infarction to clinical studies of acute ischemia in patients. This situation occurred because animal models or autopsy studies frequently do not mimic the clinical situation. In addition, therapeutic interventions are usually based on careful definition of coronary anatomy.

The coronary vasculature in the various acute ischemic syndromes is different and probably reflects a broad spectrum of acute manifestations of chronic coronary disease. Thus precise categorization of arteriographic findings is difficult because the biology of the coronary lesion for each type of clinical event is variable. For example, although it is known that coronary thrombosis occurs frequently with Q-wave infarction (i.e., transmural) [5], there are variable amounts of interaction between underlying atherosclerotic plaque, coronary arterial spasm, and platelet aggregates. The contribution of each is not well defined, even though the clinical manifestation of Q-wave infarction is similar from patient to patient. In contrast, non-Q-wave (formerly nontransmural or subendocardial) myocardial infarction presents a confusing and variable clinical picture [6, 7]. Associated with this clinical picture are the findings of less coronary thrombosis and coronary occlusion. Furthermore, the two types of infarction have different angiographic features depending largely on the time that elapses between the onset of symptoms and when arteriography is performed during the evolution of the infarction [1, 6].

The status of the coronary tree soon after sudden cardiac death due to myocardial infarction has been unexplored. Accordingly, the mechanisms of ventricular arrhythmias associated with sudden cardiac death are mostly unknown. In the setting of acute myocardial infarction, vulnerability to ventricular tachycardia, fibrillation, or both may occur secondary to complete coronary occlusion or may be associated with reperfusion rhythm disturbances. Rhythm disturbances associated with coronary occlusion are usually termed *ischemic arrhythmias*, whereas the category associated with antegrade blood flow is termed *reperfusion arrhythmias*. The mechanisms of each differ significantly and have been defined in the laboratory setting [8–12].

Because little prospective investigation has been done in this area, the patient who undergoes sudden cardiac death is usually perceived as unstable, and the clinician is reluctant to perform arteriography or thrombolytic therapy soon after cardiopulmonary arrest or resuscitation, especially if the cerebral status is not immediately clear. Furthermore, because therapeutic options are limited following cardiopulmonary arrest, the nature and extent of coronary obstruction following sudden death have been undetermined.

Even though coronary arteriography was previously reserved for chronic stable angina, clearly there has been exceptional interest in determining the coronary arteriographic findings in a variety of disease dates. The goal of this chapter is to present the angiographic findings of the early stages of Q-wave myocardial infarction as well as those arteriographic findings associated with non-Q-wave myocardial infarction. Furthermore, preliminary data regarding the angiographic findings in patients evaluated soon after sudden cardiac death are discussed. Finally, some of the complications associated with arteriography during bouts of each type of acute ischemic syndrome are explored.

Q-Wave Myocardial Infarction

Until the past few years, there has been a general reluctance to subject patients to coronary arteriography during acute myocardial infarction. Because interest has shifted to the pathophysiology of acute myocardial infarction in patients, therapies directed toward thrombolysis, restoration of myocardial perfusion, and limitation of the extent of acute myocardial infarction have evolved. Despite early reticence to perform arteriography during early acute infarction, the procedure has been performed in our center since 1970. Early Q-wave myocardial infarction is defined as chest pain in conjunction with persistent ST segment elevation on the electrocardiogram with evolution of pathologic Q waves and typical cardiac enzyme elevations.

Multiple clinical studies [1, 5, 13–16] have demonstrated that the prevalence of coronary occlusion is high in patients hospitalized within the first few hours after the onset of symptoms of Q-wave myocardial infarction. Results reported from most centers suggest that coronary thrombosis is present in the involved coronary artery in approximately 80 percent of cases seen early. We attempted to address the arteriographic findings with and without coronary thrombosis during Q-wave

myocardial infarction in a 10-year study that began in 1971 [5].

PATIENT POPULATION

During the 10-year period from 1971 to 1981, more than 500 patients underwent coronary arteriography and left ventriculography within 24 hours of symptom onset of Q-wave myocardial infarction. Overall average age for the groups was 54 years (range 32 to 76 years). Seventy-nine percent were male. Seventy-two patients (13.9 percent) had suffered previous myocardial infarction.

Coronary arteriography was performed in the 517 patients within 24 hours of symptom onset. Because earlier data [1] demonstrated that the prevalence of coronary occlusion in Q-wave myocardial infarction changed over a period of hours, the 517 patients were divided into three subsets reflecting the intervals from symptom onset to performance of coronary arteriography. This step was taken to define the frequency of coronary occlusion and to investigate the prevalence of coronary thrombosis in each patient group. The population characteristics of each subset are presented in Table 22-1. The clinical classification of each group is described according to average age, gender, area of infarction defined by the electrocardiogram on study entry, and clinical class [17]. As is demonstrated, 368 patients underwent coronary arteriography within 0 to 6 hours of symptom onset, and 85 patients and 64 patients underwent investigation in the 6- to 12-hour and the 12- to 24-hour periods, respectively. Anterior wall infarction included anterior, anteroseptal, and lateral infarcts. Inferior infarction included inferior, inferoposterior, and inferolateral infarction, that is, infarcts likely caused by occlusion of the right or circumflex system.

RESULTS OF ARTERIOGRAPHIC STUDIES

Eighty-one percent of the patients in the overall population (419 of 517) demonstrated total coronary occlusion. The patient group evalu-

Table 22-1
Clinical characteristics of subsets on study entry

Characteristics	At 0–6 hours	At 6–12 hours	At 12–24 hours
No. of patients	368	85	64
Age (years)	52.5 ± 7.2	53.7 ± 8.2	55.1 ± 8.2
Sex (% male)	79.4	82.3	76.8
Area of infarction by ECG			
Anterior	199 (51.9%)	46 (54.1%)	32 (50.0%)
Inferior	177 (48.1%)	39 (45.8%)	32 (50.0%)
Clinical class*			
I	227 (61.7%)	47 (55.3%)	39 (61.0%)
II	99 (26.9%)	23 (27.0%)	15 (23.4%)
III	18 (4.9%)	4 (4.7%)	2 (3.2%)
IV	24 (6.5%)	11 (12.9%)	8 (12.5%)

Values are mean ± SD.
*Criteria of Killip and Kimball [17].

ated within 6 hours of symptom onset demonstrated an 85 percent (320 of 368) frequency of complete coronary occlusion (Fig. 22-1). The frequency fell to 68 percent (58 of 85) in the 6- to 12-hour group and to 64 percent (41 of 64) in the 12- to 24-hour study group. This trend was statistically significant.

ARTERIOGRAPHIC FEATURES OF CORONARY THROMBOSIS

The angiographic features that best define "fresh" intracoronary thrombus include (1) staining of intraluminal material at the distal end of the column of injected contrast agent (Figs. 22-2 and 22-3); (2) local retention of the contrast agent in the involved coronary artery (Figs. 22-2B and 22-3B); and (3) an intracoronary filling defect usually best seen in patients with subtotal coronary obstruction (Fig. 22-4).

PREVALENCE OF CORONARY THROMBOSIS

In the *overall* population, angiographic features suggestive of coronary thrombosis were observed in 73 percent (379 of 517). As with complete coronary occlusion, the frequency of coronary thrombus declined in each patient group (Fig. 22-5). Of the patients evaluated

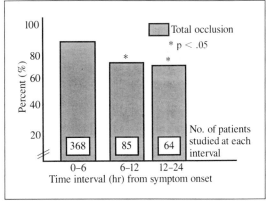

Fig. 22-1
Frequency of total occlusion in patient groups evaluated during time intervals over 24 hours after the onset of symptoms in Q-wave myocardial infarction. There is less complete occlusion in the 6- to 12-hour and the 12- to 24-hour groups than in the patients studied over 0–6 hours. (From M. A. DeWood et al. Coronary arteriographic findings in acute transmural myocardial infarction. *Circulation* 68[Suppl I]:I-39, 1983. By permission of the American Heart Association, Inc.)

within 6 hours of symptom onset, one or more angiographic features consistent with thrombus were present in 80 percent (294 of 368), whereas the frequency of coronary thrombosis fell to 59 percent (50 of 85) and 54 percent (35 of 64) in the 6- to 12-hour and 12- to 24-hour groups, respectively. The decline in the fre-

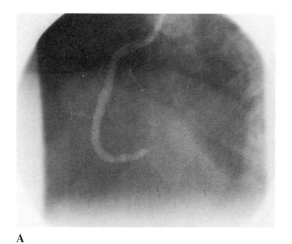

A

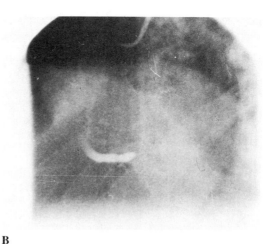

B

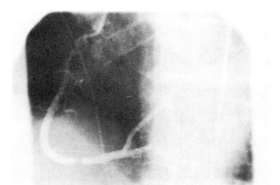

C

Fig. 22-2
A. Total coronary occlusion of the right coronary artery in a patient seen within 3 hours of acute myocardia infarction. B. Retention of dye in the involved vessel. C. After intracoronary streptokinase perfusion of the distal right coronary artery. (From M. A. DeWood et al. Coronary arteriographic findings in acute transmural myocardial infarction. *Circulation* 68[Suppl I]:I-39, 1983. By permission of the American Heart Association, Inc.)

quency of coronary thrombosis by angiography was a statistically significant trend.

When comparing Figures 22-1 and 22-5, it becomes apparent that the decline in arteriographic features favoring coronary thrombus parallels the fall in the prevalence of total coronary occlusion. Also demonstrated in Figures 22-1 and 22-5 is that the frequencies of total coronary occlusion and of coronary thrombosis are slightly different even though most patients are completely occluded by coronary thrombus. Likewise, the presence of total coronary occlusion and coronary thrombus declined in patient groups in the 6- to 12-hour and 12- to 24-hour periods. This difference between occlusion and thrombosis (approximately 10 percent) was systematic and suggests that the two phenomena differ somewhat in terms of selected patients. Other factors that may affect the coronary tree at the point of occlusion and coronary thrombus may not be present in these instances. For example, rupture of a softened plaque with progressive occlusion of the coronary lumen (Fig. 22-6), coronary spasm (Fig. 22-7), or gradual reduction of blood flow due to multiple stenoses (Fig. 22-8) may be causative of myocardial infarction. The angiographic findings detailed in Figure 22-9 suggest that the pathophysiology of myocardial infarction in a selected group might not involve coronary thrombus even though complete occlusion is usual. This difference between occlusion and thrombus may partly explain failure of thrombolytic agents to restore antegrade blood flow in selected patients [13–16].

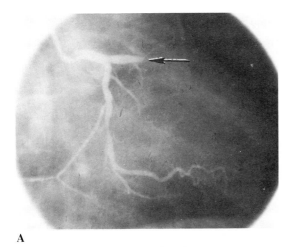

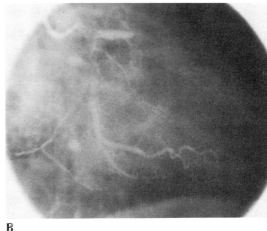

A

B

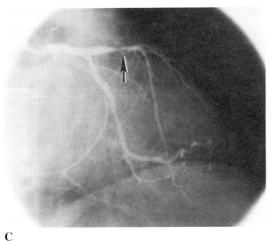

C

Fig. 22-3
A. Complete occlusion of the left anterior descending coronary artery. B. Retention of dye with staining of the intraluminal material in the same vessel while contrast is disappearing from the circumflex system. C. Restoration of blood flow to the left anterior descending artery after guidewire recanalization. Thrombus is noted after reinjection of the vessel at the point of the arrow. (From M. A. DeWood et al. Coronary arteriographic findings in acute transmural myocardial infarction. *Circulation* 68[Suppl I]:I-39, 1983. By permission of the American Heart Association, Inc.)

CORRELATION OF SURGICAL AND PATHOLOGIC FINDINGS

To assess the accuracy of coronary arteriography in determining the presence or absence of coronary thrombus, we reviewed the surgical findings in 96 patients who underwent emergency bypass surgery for Q-wave myocardial infarction. This procedure has been described elsewhere [1]. Briefly, at surgery a Fogarty catheter was passed into the coronary tree in an attempt to retrieve thrombus. Of the 96 patients, 71, 14, and 11 were in the 0- to 6-hour group, the 6- to 12-hour group, and the 12- to 24-hour group, respectively. The coronary obstruction observed during arteriography was graded as positive or negative for the presence of thrombus depending on cri-

teria agreed on prospectively and outlined above. Seventy-three patients (76 percent) had angiographic features of thrombus, and clot was recovered from the coronary artery of 65 (89 percent). These thrombi were situated at or near a critical stenosis. In contrast, coronary thrombus was incorrectly judged to be present in 11 percent of the patients with features of coronary thrombosis. Possibly the absence of coronary thrombus occurred because of spontaneous thrombolysis that may have occurred in the interval between arteriography and surgery. This interval was usually 1 hour or less.

It is especially noteworthy that a 26 percent false-negative rate was observed because, even though thrombus was judged absent, thrombus was recovered in 6 of 23 cases. Fig-

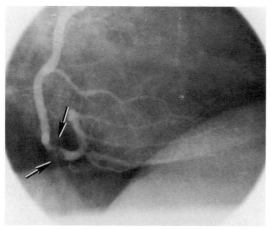

Fig. 22-4
Subtotal occlusion of the right coronary artery demonstrating an intraluminal filling defect (arrow). Thrombus was recovered at surgery. (From M. A. DeWood et al. Coronary arteriographic findings in acute transmural myocardial infarction. *Circulation* 68[Suppl I]:I-39, 1983. By permission of the American Heart Association, Inc.)

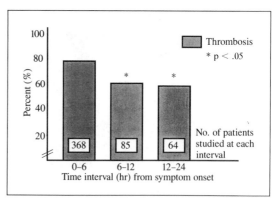

Fig. 22-5
Frequency of coronary thrombosis detected by coronary arteriography in patients evaluated during discrete time intervals after symptom onset. There was a significant decrease ($p < .05$) in the prevalence of coronary thrombosis that paralleled the decrease in total coronary occlusion. (From DeWood et al. Coronary arteriographic findings in acute transmural myocardial infarction. *Circulation* 68[Suppl I]:I-39, 1983. By permission of the American Heart Association, Inc.)

ure 22-6 is an example of this situation. This finding suggests that in selected patients the presence of thrombus is not detected by the resolution of the coronary angiogram. Nevertheless, coronary arteriography appears to be very sensitive in the detection of coronary thrombus during the early hours of Q-wave infarction. It does lack some specificity, especially in patients evaluated after 6 hours from symptom onset.

COMPLICATIONS ASSOCIATED WITH CORONARY ARTERIOGRAPHY

Of the 517 patients, 51 (10 percent) had major complications during the procedure. Most (44 of 51) complications were due to ventricular fibrillation. Overall, this represented an 85 percent (44 of 517) prevalence of ventricular fibrillation. None of these instances was fatal. More than half of the 44 patients had experienced recurrent bouts of paired or multiple premature ventricular contractions, ventricular tachycardia, or fibrillation prior to the procedure. Thus we usually institute intravenous lidocaine therapy if ventricular irritability is demonstrated prior to the cardiac catheterization. Other complications included intramyocardial injection of contrast agent, which occurred twice (0–4 percent), and plaque was raised in a vessel not involved with the acute infarct in two other patients (0.4 percent). Four patients (0.7 percent) did not survive the procedure. Three had been suffering from cardiogenic shock prior to the procedure. Hypotension was occasionally observed. Importantly, however, no deaths occurred secondary to hypotension associated with cardiac catheterization. Thus in experienced hands cardiac catheterization during early acute Q-wave myocardial infarction is relatively safe and is associated with low morbidity and mortality.

Non-Q-Wave (Nontransmural) Myocardial Infarction

Whereas "early Q-wave myocardial infarction" is usually diagnosed by ST segment elevation with pathologic Q waves on the elec-

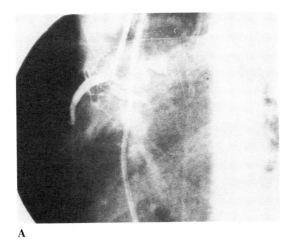

A

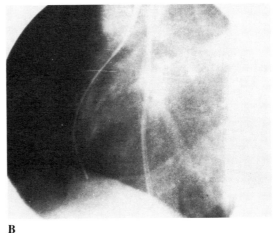

B

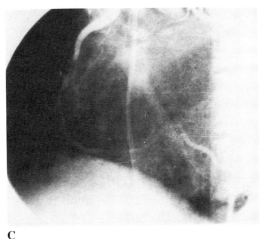

C

Fig. 22-6
A. Abrupt cutoff of forward flow in the right coronary artery with retention of dye. There was no staining, however. B. Passage of a guidewire through the lumen of the right coronary artery demonstrates that reperfusion of the distal vessel is possible. C. Perfusion of the distal right coronary artery is present. Beyond the previous occlusion, a channel through the thrombus has been generated by the guidewire. (From M. A. DeWood et al. Coronary arteriographic findings in acute transmural myocardial infarction. *Circulation* 68[Suppl I]:I-39, 1983. By permission of the American Heart Association, Inc.)

trocardiogram, non-Q-wave (nontransmural) myocardial infarction is not associated with a distinctive electrocardiographic marker. Frequently, these patients present with chest pain and nondiagnostic ST and T-wave abnormalities, but they do not develop Q waves.

The clinical distinction between Q-wave and non-Q-wave myocardial infarction relies heavily on electrocardiographic criteria, but autopsy studies have shown that these criteria are relatively nonspecific [18–22]. Furthermore, patients with ST and T-wave abnormalities on the electrocardiogram with only minor abnormalities of cardiac enzymes have been perceived as having unstable angina pectoris or a less important form of coronary disease. Because of this perception, few prospective clinical studies aimed at defining the arterio-

graphic features associated with non-Q-wave infarction have been performed in the past. Because the arteriographic features of Q-wave infarction have been well defined, however, investigation of the acute ischemic syndrome has shifted to non-Q-wave myocardial infarction. It is especially so because the clinical behavior of non-Q-wave infarction indicates that the initial mortality is lower, but most reports indicate the overall mortality equals or surpasses mortality associated with Q-wave infarction in long-term observations [23–27].

Because clinical observations have indicated that non-Q-wave myocardial infarction is associated with unexpectedly high long-term mortality, we assumed that it reflected unstable pathophysiologic events in the coronary arteries. Accordingly, we performed an-

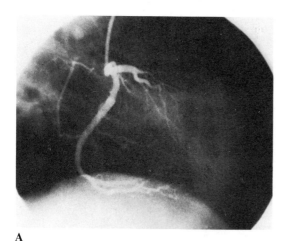

A

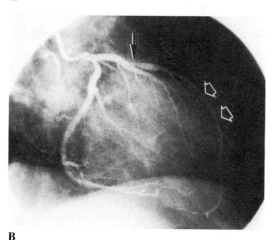

B

Fig. 22-7
A. Right anterior oblique projection of the left anterior descending coronary artery showing "beaking" appearance. *B*. After injection of intracoronary nitroglycerin, the distal left anterior descending coronary artery is injected as resolution of coronary spasm has occurred. (From M. A. DeWood et al. Coronary arteriographic findings in acute transmural myocardial infarction. *Circulation* 68[Suppl I]:I-39, 1983. By permission of the American Heart Association, Inc.)

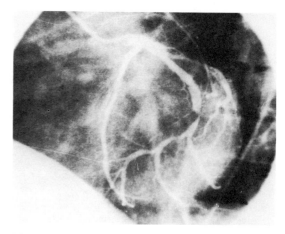

Fig. 22-8
Multiple severe stenosis of the circumflex vessels causative of Q-wave myocardial infarction. Several stenoses were observed in multiple eccentric lesions. No thrombus was seen. (From M. A. DeWood et al. Coronary arteriographic findings in acute transmural myocardial infarction. *Circulation* 68[Suppl I]:I-39, 1983. By permission of the American Heart Association, Inc.)

PATIENT POPULATION

During the 10-year period from 1974 through 1984, 341 patients underwent left heart studies within 1 week of the peak symptoms of non-Q-wave infarction. This group represented 75 percent of the patients (341 of 451) who were hospitalized within 1 week of peak symptoms during the period of study. The clinical characteristics of the patients are summarized in Table 22-2. Because earlier studies with Q-wave myocardial infarction demonstrated that coronary arteriographic findings were associated with the duration from symptom onset to performance of arteriography, the total population with non-Q-wave myocardial infarction was divided into three large groups.

One group of 192 patients underwent left heart catheterization within 24 hours of peak symptoms, another of 94 patients underwent evaluation within the 24- to 72-hour period, and 55 patients underwent left heart catheterization 3 to 7 days after peak symptoms. Table 22-2 demonstrates that the age, gender, incidence of previous myocardial infarction, creatine kinase characteristics, number of vessels

giography in patients suffering early non-Q-wave infarction. The goals of the study were (1) to define the frequency of complete coronary occlusion in patients hospitalized within 1 week of non-Q-wave myocardial infarction and (2) to correlate the arteriographic and clinical findings associated with non-Q-wave myocardial infarction.

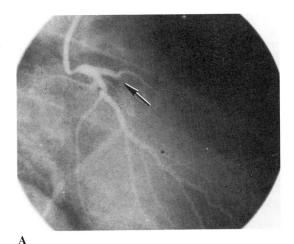

A

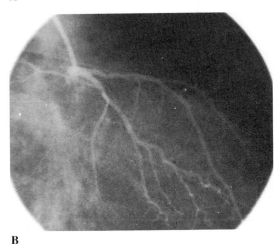

B

Fig. 22-9
A. Total occlusion of the left anterior descending coronary artery in the right anterior blight projection. There was no staining or retention of dye on the left anterior descending vessel. Contrast agent perfused the circumflex system, which is well defined. B. Successful reperfusion of the distal left anterior descending coronary artery after thrombolytic therapy. There was a minor irregularity noted. (From M. A. DeWood et al. Coronary arteriographic findings in acute transmural myocardial infarction. *Circulation* 68[Suppl I]:I-39, 1983. By permission of the American Heart Association, Inc.)

diseased, and the area of infarction seen by electrocardiogram were similar among the three groups. As with the Q-wave myocardial infarction group, anterior infarction included patients with anterior, anteroseptal, anterolateral, and lateral infarctions, whereas inferior

wall infarction encompassed inferior, infero-posterior, posterior, and inferolateral infarctions.

RESULTS OF CORONARY ARTERIOGRAPHIC STUDIES

In contrast to the Q-wave myocardial infarction group (see Fig. 22-1), only 32 percent (107 of 341) of the entire population demonstrated complete coronary occlusion. Figure 22-10 shows that total coronary occlusion occurred in 26 percent (49 of 192) in the 0- to 24-hour group, 37 percent (35 of 94) of the 24- to 72-hour group, and 42 percent (23 of 55) of the 3- to 7-day group ($p<.05$). Thus a significant increase in the frequency of complete coronary occlusion in the infarct-related vessel was observed over time.

Importantly, in the same groups, stenosis of more than 90 percent (i.e., subtotal occlusion) occurred in 34 percent (65 of 192), 26 percent (24 of 94), and 18 percent (10 of 55), respectively ($p<.05$). As is demonstrated in Figure 22-10, stenosis of 70 to 90 percent occurred in similar proportions across the patient populations studied. Stenosis of less than 70 percent was seen in 3 percent, 1 percent, and 0 percent in the three groups, respectively. Thus a clear trend toward higher prevalence of total coronary occlusion and a decline in the frequency of subtotal occlusion occurred over time. As is shown in Figure 22-10, the prevalence of collaterals beyond the infarct-related vessel was also defined. Overall, collateral vessels that opacified the distal infarct-related vessel almost universally occurred with patients who had complete coronary occlusion and in 32 percent of the entire population (107 of 341). As is shown in Figure 22-10, collateral vessels occurred in 27 percent (52 of 192) in the 0- to 24-hour group, 34 percent (32 of 94) in the 24- to 72-hour group, and 42 percent (23 of 55) of the patients in the 3- to 7-day group ($p<.05$). Thus there was parallel increase in visible collateral vessels that was associated with the progression to total coronary occlusion among the three groups. Furthermore, collateral ves-

Table 22-2
Clinical characteristics of the three subsets of patients on entry into the study*

Characteristic	Time after peak symptoms		
	<24 hours	24–72 hours	72 hours to 7 days
No. of patients	192	94	55
Age (yr), mean ± SD	59 ± 10	58 ± 9	60 ± 9
Men (No. and % of total)	166 (86%)	83 (88%)	45 (82%)
Previous MI (No.)	42 (22%)	28 (30%)	10 (18%)
Mean initial CK (IU)	200	198	218
Mean peak CK (IU)	547	465	358
No. of diseased vessels			
1	53 (28%)	25 (27%)	11 (20%)
2	77 (40%)	28 (30%)	21 (38%)
3 or more	62 (32%)	41 (44%)	23 (42%)
Area of infarct by ECG			
Anterior	96 (50%)	51 (54%)	32 (58%)
Inferior	45 (23%)	26 (28%)	11 (20%)
Indeterminate	28 (15%)	7 (7%)	5 (9%)
Both	23 (12%)	10 (11%)	7 (13%)

*The three groups did not differ significantly in any of the characteristics on entry into the study.
MI = myocardial infarction; CK = total creatine kinase activity (>90 IU = abnormal); ECG = electrocardiogram.

sels were almost never seen in the absence of complete coronary occlusion.

COMPLICATIONS ASSOCIATED WITH CORONARY ARTERIOGRAPHY

Although the complications rate was 10.8 percent in the Q-wave myocardial infarction group, we observed a much lower complication rate in patients with non-Q-wave myocardial infarction: 2 percent (8 of 342). Major complications included ventricular fibrillation (N = 3), allergic dye response (N = 1), and severe hypotension (N = 3) that required extensive volume expansion and vasopressor therapy. One patient needed transvenous pacing. No deaths were attributable to cardiac catheterization.

ANGIOGRAPHIC FEATURES

Most patients demonstrated high grade stenosis, as shown in Figure 22-11. When complete coronary occlusion was present (Fig. 22-12), usually the distal vessel was completely opa-

cified by collaterals from a noninfarct-related vessel. Occasionally, there were intraluminal filling defects consistent with intracoronary thrombus. Because they were rarely associated with complete coronary occlusion, there was neither local retention of contrast agent nor staining of intraluminal material. An example of these filling defects is seen in Figures 22-13 and 22-14. More recent studies using intraoperative angioscopy have confirmed that intraluminal filling defects observed by angiographic methods are microthrombi [28].

SUDDEN CARDIAC DEATH DUE TO MYOCARDIAL INFARCTION: PRELIMINARY ARTERIOGRAPHIC FINDINGS

The mechanisms of ventricular rhythm disturbances in cardiac death are generally unknown. In the setting of acute myocardial infarction, vulnerability to ventricular tachycardia or fibrillation may be secondary to complete occlusion, or it may be due to reperfusion rhythm disorders. Rhythm disturbances associated with complete coronary

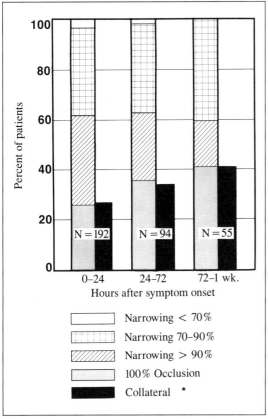

Fig. 22-10
Extent of occlusion in the three groups suffering non-Q-wave myocardial infarction. Percentage of stenosis applies to the infarct-related vessel. There was a significant increase in the frequency of coronary occlusion with time in the three groups and an inverse decrease (90 percent or more) in the percentage of patients with stenosis. There is no significant change in patients with 70–90 percent narrowing. (From M. A. DeWood et al. Coronary angiographic findings soon after non-Q-wave myocardial infarction. *N. Engl. J. Med.* 315:417, 1986. With permission.)

occlusion are usually termed *ischemic arrhythmias,* whereas the other category is designated *reperfusion arrhythmias.* The mechanisms for each differ in the experimental setting [8–12, 29–34].

In patients successfully resuscitated after sudden cardiac death, coronary arteriography suggests extensive coronary atherosclerosis, but only 20 percent of these patients evolved Q waves consistent with myocardial infarc-

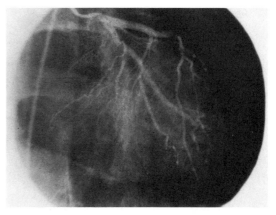

Fig. 22-11
Subtotal stenosis demonstrated in non-Q-wave myocardial infarction. This 90 percent stenosis was typical of patients studied within 24 hours of symptom onset. (From DeWood et al. Coronary angiographic findings soon after non-Q-wave myocardial infarction. *N. Engl. J. Med.* 315:417, 1986. With permission.)

tion. Thus study of patients without evolution of Q waves results in two groups of patients: (1) those who have primary electrocardiographic disturbances but no evidence of acute myocardial necrosis, and (2) those with non-Q-wave infarction. Although cardiac enzyme studies confirm myocardial infarction in 40 percent [35], most patients who undergo successful resuscitation usually undergo coronary angiography several weeks after the acute event. Accordingly, little is known about the arteriographic findings associated with disturbances soon after the onset of myocardial infarction. Along those same lines, little is known about whether coronary thrombus or aggregates are partially responsible for either ischemic or reperfusion rhythm disturbances.

Laboratory investigation [36] indicated that coronary blood flow is phasic. In these preparations, a 70 percent reduction in luminal diameter of coronary arteries was generated by placement of a snare. It resulted in periodic and phasic decreases in coronary blood flow in more than half of the animals. Usually, there was a gradual decrease in flow followed by a return to control levels. Nevertheless, some animals spontaneously occluded, which resulted in ventricular fibrillation and sudden cardiac death.

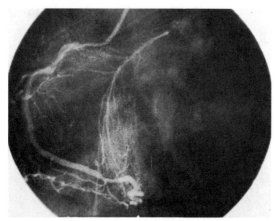

Fig. 22-12
Complete filling of the left anterior descending coronary artery in a patient with an anterior non-Q-wave myocardial infarction. The right coronary artery completely fills the distal left anterior descending coronary artery.

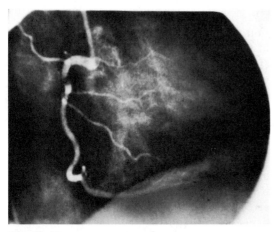

Fig. 22-13
Subtotal occlusion with a large thrombus in the right coronary artery causative of non-Q-wave inferior wall myocardial necrosis.

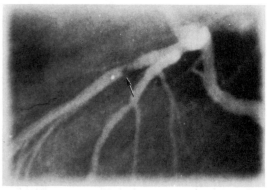

Fig. 22-14
Small thrombus in the left anterior descending coronary artery in the lateral projection vessel in a patient soon after symptom onset of non-Q-wave myocardial infarction. The patient has recurrent bouts of severe ischemia and required coronary bypass surgery. Thrombus was retrieved at surgery.

Table 22-3
Overall group characteristics

Characteristic	Nonsudden death	Sudden death
No. of patients	78	78
Age ($\pm$ SD)	54 $\pm$ 10	54 $\pm$ 10
Gender (% male)	78%	75%
Area of MI		
Anterior	39	39
Inferior	39	39
Previous MI	12/78 (15%)	11/78 (14%)
No. vessels diseased		
1	36/78 (46%)	35/78 (45%)
2	28/78 (36%)	32/78 (41%)
3 or 3 +	14/78 (18%)	11/78 (14%)
Global EF	51 $\pm$ 10	47 $\pm$ 13 (N = 71)
LVFP (mm Hg)	21 $\pm$ 9	20 $\pm$ 9
$\bar{A}_0$ (mm Hg)	101 $\pm$ 15	98 $\pm$ 18

EF = ejection fraction; LVFP = left ventricular filling pressure; $\bar{A}_0$ = mean aortic pressure

Equally as important, abrupt restoration of blood flow may also result in ventricular fibrillation. The duration of preceding ischemia has been shown to influence the incidence of malignant arrhythmias associated with reperfusion [34]. Importantly, the cyclic changes in coronary blood flow can be inhibited by antiplatelet agents, suggesting that thrombus formation at the site of the narrowing is important in some instances.

In patients, little is known about the status of the coronary arteries except for pathology data. These data usually demonstrate that almost all cases of sudden cardiac death are accompanied by some abnormality, although none is pathognomonic of sudden death. Some studies have shown microthrombi, whereas others [37] described platelet aggregates in the microcirculation of young patients who had no other abnormalities of the coronary arteries.

Because the arteriographic features of the patients dying suddenly following myocardial infarction are not known, we performed a series of studies. The goals of these investigations were (1) to define the prevalence of coronary occlusion in patients with sudden cardiac death associated with myocardial infarction, and (2) to determine if coronary anatomy is different from that in patients who sustain myocardial infarction but not sudden cardiac death. We attempted to determine whether most rhythm disturbances are caused by ischemic arrhythmias or reperfusion rhythm disturbances [38].

The clinical characteristics, coronary arteriographic features, and left ventriculographic findings in 78 patients with documented ventricular fibrillation, tachycardia, or asystole leading to sudden cardiac death after the symptoms of myocardial infarction were in-

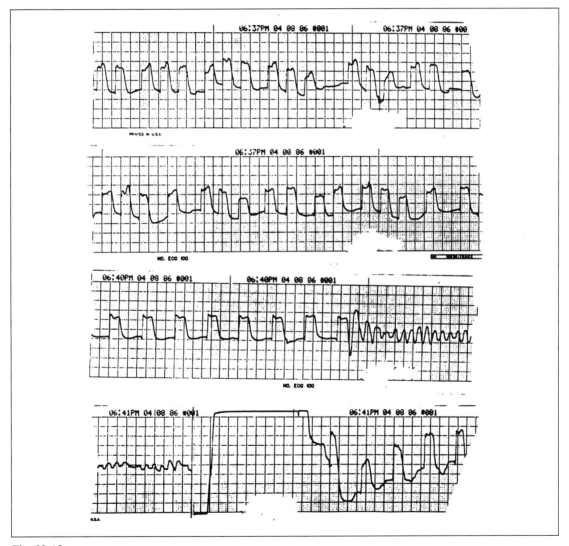

Fig. 22-15
Supraventricular arrhythmia with acute inferior wall myocardial infarction. The arrhythmia deteriorates into ventricular tachycardia and fibrillation. Electrical countershock is applied, and normal sinus rhythm resumes. Note the significant ST segment elevation in lead II.

vestigated. In each case sudden death was witnessed and rhythm disturbances were documented by a cardiac monitor, either by paramedics in the field or by hospital personnel.

The sudden cardiac death group was compared to a nonsudden cardiac death group with myocardial infarction who also underwent left heart catheterization, left ventriculography, and coronary arteriography within 6 hours of symptom onset. The groups were matched for age, area of infarction (determined by the electrocardiogram), and the vessels believed to be responsible for the infarct. Other variables included number of vessels diseased, prevalence of complete coronary occlusion, incidence of previous myocardial infarction, left ventricular filling pressure, central aortic blood pres-

sure, and left ventricular function (estimated by global ejection fraction determinations).

As shown in Table 22-3, 78 patients were studied an average of 2.3 hours after cardiopulmonary resuscitation. These patients were compared to the group that did not have rhythm disturbances but also underwent left heart catheterization for interventions in acute myocardial infarction.

An example of this type of patient is shown in Figure 22-15. This patient presented to the emergency room with chest discomfort. He experienced ventricular fibrillation following a bout of ventricular tachycardia. After the patient became pulseless he was defibrillated. Regular rhythm was immediately restored, as was the blood pressure. Coronary arteriography was performed within the hour of this

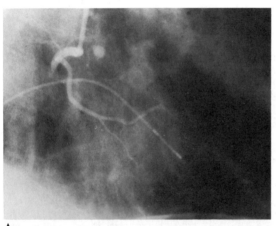

A

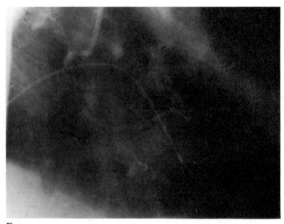

B

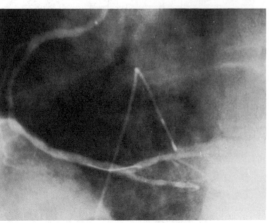

C

Fig. 22-16
A. Left anterior oblique projection of the right coronary artery, which was causative of the Q-wave myocardial infarction, in sudden death patients (characterized in Figure 22-15). B. Staining of the thrombus in the right coronary artery is seen in the same patient. C. The patient underwent coronary angioplasty and was discharged uneventfully in 3 days. The floppy guidewire is seen in the distal right coronary artery. Good perfusion of the distal vasculature was observed.

instance of sudden death. The results are demonstrated in Figure 22-16. Evidence favoring coronary thrombus was present because of intracoronary retention of the contrast agent.

There was a significant difference in the prevalence of coronary occlusion in the non-sudden death group (Fig. 22-16). Even though this information is preliminary, the study suggests that total coronary occlusion is frequent in sudden cardiac death associated with myocardial infarction and supports the concept that most rhythm disturbances are due to ischemic arrhythmias. Within this group, however, there is an unexpectedly but significantly lower frequency of complete coronary occlusion when compared to a matched group not sustaining sudden death in this clinical situation. In these patients, it may be that sudden cardiac death is secondary to spontaneous thrombolysis and reperfusion rhythm disturbances. Further ongoing investigation must be designed to define the frequency of each type of arrhythmia and its clinical significance.

Summary

The role of coronary thrombosis in Q-wave myocardial infarction is the final common pathway converting chronic coronary disease to acute ischemia in the presence of Q-wave myocardial infarction. It occurs in approximately 80 percent of such patients within 6 hours of symptom onset. This finding has been confirmed with multiple studies. There is less certainty when dealing with non-Q-wave myocardial infarction because few systematic prospective studies have been done. Certain features are suggestive of coronary thrombus.

Coronary arteriographic findings in sudden death patients are currently an area of investigation. Among patients who evolve acute myocardial infarction, coronary thrombus is present in many, as is total coronary occlusion with thrombosis. However, less coronary occlusion is demonstrated in those patients who do not have ventricular fibrillation or tachycardia (Fig. 22-17). In selective cases this finding may reflect spontaneous thrombolysis.

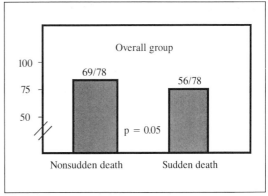

Fig. 22-17
Frequency of coronary occlusion in sudden-death versus non-sudden-death patients suffering Q-wave myocardial infarction. There was significantly less coronary occlusion in patients who suffered sudden cardiac death following myocardial infarction than in patients who did not.

Acknowledgments

The authors thank Cynthia Brandt for her wonderful organizational and secretarial support. We hope she understands how much we appreciate her dynamic on and off screen performances.

Supported in part by the Deaconess Medical Center Foundation, the Sacred Heart Medical Center Foundation, the Max Bayer Heart Fund of the Fraternal Order of Eagles, and the Inland Northwest Heart Research Foundation.

Editorial Comments

We owe DeWood and colleagues major tribute for providing the seminal observations that proved the role of coronary thrombosis in patients with acute transmural myocardial infarction. This work has forever changed the management of acute myocardial infarction, setting the stage for the "thrombolytic era" currently in vogue. It appears as though the coronary arteries can be safely cannulated, probed, dilated, and subjected to various injurious procedures to a far greater extent than was imagined even 15 years ago. However, we are reminded by DeWood et al. that compli-

cations still occur, even in the most experienced hands. Although the role of thrombosis is secure in acute transmural myocardial infarction, ongoing work by these investigators should provide us with more information regarding the mechanisms of non-Q-wave infarction and sudden death. G.S.F.

References

1. DeWood, M. A., Spores, J., Notske, R., et al. Prevalence of total coronary occlusion during the early hours of transmural myocardial infarction. *N. Engl. J. Med.* 303:897, 1980.
2. Oliva, P. B., and Breckenridge, J. C. Arteriographic evidence of coronary arterial spasm in acute myocardial infarction. *Circulation* 56:366, 1977.
3. Neill, W. A., Wharton, T. P., Jr., Fluri-Lundeen, J., and Cohen, I. S. Acute coronary insufficiency—coronary occlusion after intermittent ischemic attacks. *N. Engl. J. Med.* 302:1157, 1980.
4. Alison, H. W., Russell, R. O., Jr., Mantle, J. A., et al. Coronary anatomy and arteriography in patients with unstable angina pectoris. *Am. J. Cardiol.* 41:204, 1978.
5. DeWood, M. A., Spores, J., Hensley, G. R., et al. Coronary arteriographic findings in acute transmural myocardial infarction. *Circulation* 68(Suppl I):1-39, 1983.
6. DeWood, M. A., Stifter, W. F., Simpson, C. S., et al. Coronary angiographic findings soon after non-Q-wave myocardial infarction. *N. Engl. J. Med.* 315:417, 1986.
7. Gibson, R. S., Beller, G. A., Gheorghiade, M., et al. The prevalence and clinical significance of residual myocardial ischemia 2 weeks after uncomplicated non-Q-wave infarction: A prospective natural history study. *Circulation* 73:1186, 1986.
8. Axelrod, P. J., Verrier, R. L., and Lown, B. Vulnerability to ventricular fibrillation during acute coronary arterial occlusion and release. *Am. J. Cardiol.* 36:776, 1975.
9. Corbalan, D., Verrier, R. L., and Lown, B. Differing mechanisms for ventricular vulnerability during coronary artery occlusion and release. *Am. Heart J.* 92:223, 1976.
10. Levite, R., Banka, V. S., and Helfant, R. H. Electro-physiologic effects of coronary occlusion and reperfusion, observation of dispersion of refractoriness and ventricular automaticity. *Circulation* 52:760, 1975.
11. Ramanathan, K. B., Bodenheimer, M. M., Banka, V. S., et al. Electrophysiological effects of partial coronary occlusion and reperfusion. *Am. J. Cardiol.* 40:50, 1977.
12. Battle, W. E., Naimi, S., Avitall, B., et al. Distinction time course of ventricular vulnerability of fibrillation during and after release of coronary ligation. *Am. J. Cardiol.* 34:42, 1974.
13. Raisner, A. E., Tortoledo, F. A., Verani, M. S., et al. Intracoronary thrombolytic therapy in acute myocardial infarction: A prospective, randomized, controlled trial. *Am. J. Cardiol.* 55:301, 1985.
14. Stadius, M. L., Maynard, C., Fritz, J. K., et al. Coronary anatomy and left ventricular function in the first 12 hours of acute myocardial infarction: The Western Washington randomized intracoronary streptokinase trial. *Circulation* 72:292, 1985.
15. Simoons, M. L., Serruys, P. W., Van den Brand, M., et al. Improved survival after early thrombolysis in acute myocardial infarction: A randomized trial by the Interuniversity Cardiology Institute in The Netherlands. *Lancet* 2:578, 1985.
16. Rentrop, K. P., Feit, F., Blanke, H., et al. Effects of intracoronary streptokinase and intracoronary nitroglycerin infusion on coronary angiographic patterns and mortality in patients with acute myocardial infarction. *N. Engl. J. Med.* 311:1457, 1984.
17. Killip, T., III, and Kimball, J. T. Treatment of myocardial infarction in a coronary care unit: A two year experience with 250 patients. *Am. J. Cardiol.* 20:457, 1967.
18. Abbott, J. A., and Scheinman, M. M. Nondiagnostic electrocardiogram in patients with acute myocardial infarction: Clinical and anatomic correlations. *Am. J. Med.* 55:608, 1973.
19. Sullivan, W., Voldaver, Z., Tuna, N., et al. Correlation of electrocardiographic and pathologic findings in healed myocardial infarction. *Am. J. Cardiol.* 42:724, 1978.
20. Savage, R. M., Wagner, G. S., Ideker, R. E., et al. Correlation of postmortem anatomic findings with electrocardiographic changes in patients with myocardial infarction: Retrospective study of patients with typical anterior and posterior infarcts. *Circulation* 55:279, 1977.
21. Cook, R. W., Edwards, J. E., and Pruitt, R. D. Electrocardiographic changes in acute subendocardial infarction. I. Large subendocardial and large nontransmural infarcts. *Circulation* 18:603, 1958.
22. Horan, L. G., Flowers, N. C., and Johnson, J. C. Significance of the diagnostic Q-wave of myocardial infarction. *Circulation* 43:428, 1971.
23. Thanavaro, S., Krone, R. J., Kleiger, R. E., et al. In-hospital prognosis of patients with first nontransmural and transmural infarctions. *Circulation* 61:29, 1980.
24. Fabricius-Bjerre, N., Munkvad, M., and Knud-

sen, J. B. Subendocardial and transmural myocardial infarction: A five year survival study. *Am. J. Med.* 66:986, 1979.

25. Szklo, M., Goldberg, R., Kennedy, H. L., and Tonascia, J. A. Survival of patients with nontransmural myocardial infarction: A population-based study. *Am. J. Cardiol.* 42:648, 1978.

26. Cannom, D. S., Levy, W., and Cohen, L. S. The short- and long-term prognosis of patients with transmural and nontransmural myocardial infarction. *Am. J. Med.* 61:452, 1976.

27. Hutter, A. M., Jr., DeSanctis, R. W., Flynn, T., and Yeatman, L. A. Nontransmural myocardial infarction: A comparison of hospital and late clinical course of patients with that of matched patients with transmural anterior and transmural inferior myocardial infarction. *Am. J. Cardiol.* 48:595, 1981.

28. Sherman, C. T., Litvack, F., Grundfest, W., et al. Coronary angioscopy in patients with unstable angina pectoris. *N. Engl. J. Med.* 315:913, 1986.

29. Penkoske, P.A., Sobel, B.E., and Corr, P. B. Disparate electrophysiological alterations accompanying dysrhythmia due to coronary occlusion and reperfusion in the cat. *Circulation* 58:1023, 1978.

30. Murdock, D. K., Loeb, J. M., Euler, D. E., and Randall, W. C. Electrophysiology of coronary reperfusion, a mechanism for reperfusion arrhythmias. *Circulation* 61:175, 1980.

31. Kaplinsky, E., Ogawa, S., Michelson, E. L., and Dreifus, L. S. Instantaneous and delayed ventricular arrhythmias after reperfusion of acutely ischemic myocardium: Evidence for multiple mechanisms. *Circulation* 63:333, 1981.

32. Sewell, W. H., Koth, D. R., and Huggins, C. E. Ventricular fibrillation in dogs after sudden return of flow to the coronary artery. *Surgery* 38:1050, 1955.

33. Scherlag, B. J., El-Sherif, N., Hope, R., and Lazzara, R. Characterization and location of ventricular arrhythmias resulting from myocardial ischemia and infarction. *Circ. Res.* 33:372, 1974.

34. Balke, C. W., Kaplinsky, E., Michelson, E. L., et al. Reperfusion tachyarrhythmias: Correlation with antecedent coronary artery occlusion tachyarrythmias and duration of myocardial ischemia. *Am. Heart J.* 101:449, 1981.

35. Cobb, L. A., Werner, J. A., and Trobaugh, G. B. Sudden cardiac death. 1. A decade's experience with out-of-hospital resuscitation. *Mod. Concepts Cardiovasc. Dis.* 49:31, 1980.

36. Folts, J. D., Gallagher, K., and Rowe, G. G. Blood flow reductions in stenosed canine coronary arteries: Vasospasm or platelet aggregation. *Circulation* 65:248, 1982.

37. Frink, R. J., Trowbridge, J. O., and Rooney P. A., Jr. Nonobstructive coronary thrombosis in sudden cardiac death. *Am. J. Cardiol.* 42:48, 1978.

38. DeWood, M. A., Spores, J., Notske, R. N., et al. Coronary artery occlusion determined early after sudden cardiac death due to myocardial infarction. *J. Am. Coll. Cardiol.* 5:401, 1985.

23
Percutaneous Transluminal Coronary Angioplasty in Acute Myocardial Infarction

BERTRAM PITT

Thrombolytic therapy with intravenous strep-tokinase, recombinant tissue plasminogen activator (rt-PA), and anisoylated plasminogen streptokinase activator complex (APSAC) has been shown to improve ventricular function and survival in patients with acute myocardial infarction. The GISSI trial [1], demonstrating a marked reduction in mortality in patients seen within the first few hours of onset of symptoms of infarction, marked the beginning of the modern "reperfusion era." The ISIS-II trial [2] extended these observations and demonstrated a significant reduction in mortality in patients receiving aspirin, streptokinase, or combination of aspirin and streptokinase seen within 24 hours from onset of symptoms. Similar reductions in mortality have been seen with rt-PA [3] and APSAC [4], at least within the early hours of acute infarction.

Despite the beneficial effects of intravenous thrombolytic agents, animal and clinical data suggest that intravenous thrombolysis alone may not provide optimal results. For example, Tomada [5] compared the effects of coronary artery thrombotic occlusion without intervention, coronary occlusion with thrombolysis, and coronary occlusion with PTCA in an animal model. He found that the animals who underwent PTCA had a significantly smaller infarct size/area at risk than the animals treated with thrombolysis alone. Studies at the University of Michigan by Grines et al. [6] in patients with acute myocardial infarction undergoing reperfusion show that patients with more than a 50 percent residual stenosis of their infarct-related artery had a significantly increased incidence of postinfarction angina, exercise-induced ischemia prior to hospital discharge, and mortality compared to patients with less than 50 percent stenosis. These observations in animals and man suggest that a residual stenosis of the infarct-related artery may limit the beneficial effects of reperfusion. The residual stenosis of the infarct-related artery after reperfusion with thrombolytic agents is in part due to the underlying atherosclerotic lesion that led to the acute thrombosis and in part to partially lysed thrombus.

Although currently available intravenous agents may achieve reperfusion in 60 to 75 percent of patients [7–9], this reperfusion may not be optimal, at least during the first few hours of thrombolysis. Serial angiographic studies in patients receiving intravenous streptokinase in the Western Washington trial [10] have shown that clot lysis is not complete at 90 minutes and may not be complete for several days. Studies at the University of Michigan by Nicklas et al. [11] have shown that restoration of coronary blood flow after thrombolysis is suboptimal. The failure to completely restore flow after thrombolysis is likely due to the residual stenosis of the infarct-related artery and active vasoconstriction due to continued platelet deposition on to the unlysed residual thrombus, with release of thromboxane A_2 and serotonin as well as other vasoconstrictive agents.

Direct PTCA

PTCA of patients with acute myocardial infarction in an attempt to achieve more complete reperfusion was first attempted by Meyer et al. in West Germany [12] and Hartzler et al. in the United States [13]. Hartzler et al. [14] have performed more than 400 direct PTCAs without concomitant thrombolytic therapy in patients with acute myocardial infarction. They have achieved a greater than 90 percent primary success rate with a relatively low in-hospital mortality and excellent long-term follow-up.

The only random trial of direct PTCA without thrombolytic agents to date was performed by O'Neill et al. at the University of Michigan and William Beaumont Hospital [15]. In this study patients with acute myocardial infarction seen within the first 6 hours of onset of symptoms of infarction were randomized to a strategy of PTCA without prior thrombolytic therapy or to thrombolytic therapy alone with intracoronary streptokinase. Approximately 85 percent of patients were successfully reperfused with either PTCA or intracoronary streptokinase. Although the reperfusion rates were similar, the patients randomized to PTCA had significantly less residual stenosis of their infarct-related artery, better improvement in global and regional left ventricular function, less postinfarction angina, less exercise-induced ischemia on prehospital discharge submaximal thallium 201 stress testing, and a tendency toward less reocclusion. Bleeding rates, however, as evidenced by the need for blood transfusion, were similar in the two groups. Although it was postulated that an advantage of direct PTCA might be a reduction in bleeding compared to that seen with thrombolytic agents, it is likely that the concomitant use of intravenous heparin negated this potential advantage. The number of patients in this trial was unfortunately too small to give any insight into the relative effect of these two strategies on survival. Although relatively small (56 patients), this trial provided encouragement for the use of direct (primary) PTCA.

We remain enthusiastic about the potential of direct PTCA, but it is obvious that this strategy is unlikely to be broadly applicable. The advantages of direct PTCA include a high success rate of reperfusion (85–95 percent), a low incidence of residual stenosis of the infarct-related artery, significantly better global and regional left ventricular function, less postinfarction angina, and less exercise-induced ischemia prior to hospital discharge compared to patients receiving thrombolysis alone. A major disadvantage of this strategy, however, is the time necessary to get the patient to the cardiac catheterization laboratory and to perform PTCA compared to the administration of an intravenous thrombolytic agent alone. Second, most patients with acute myocardial infarction are seen in community hospitals without facilities for acute angiography or PTCA. Even in institutions with adequate facilities for PTCA, adoption of a strategy of direct PTCA would result in performance of PTCA in individuals who might not need it if they have received intravenous thrombolytic therapy. Approximately 15 percent of patients who receive an intravenous thrombolytic agent are shown to have a less than 50 percent residual stenosis of their infarct-related artery on follow-up coronary angiography prior to hospital discharge. If seen within the early hours of infarction, these patients may have a more than 50 percent residual stenosis of their infarct-related artery, which might lyse over time and may not be hemodynamically significant (*minimal lesion syndrome*). Until prospective controlled trials are available comparing direct PTCA to intravenous thrombolysis in regard to ventricular function and survival it is difficult to justify the use of direct PTCA in light of the significant improvement in ventricular function and survival when intravenous thrombolytic agents are administered alone.

In view of animal studies by Reimer et al. [16] demonstrating the importance of the time to reperfusion, a delay in time to achieve reperfusion by PTCA cannot be justified unless, as mentioned above, further studies demonstrate that the better reperfusion afforded by PTCA outweighs the delay in achieving reperfusion. Although regionalized care for the patient with acute infarction using helicopter transport has been shown to be safe and feasible [17], the transport necessarily results in a potential delay in establishing reperfusion compared to administration of an intravenous thrombolytic agent in the community hospital. In consideration of the costs and risks associated with direct angioplasty, this strategy can be recommended only for patients in whom there is a contraindication to intravenous thrombolytic therapy, such as those with hypertension or a history of a cerebral vascular accident—for whom transport to a regional center appears justified, especially the high-risk patient. Direct PTCA may also be of value in the patient who has an episode of infarction while in a regional hospital with facilities for PTCA in whom the PTCA could be performed expeditiously within an hour or so.

Urgent PTCA

In view of the limitations of the strategy of direct PTCA, we and others have explored the strategy of urgent PTCA after intravenous thrombolysis. With this strategy patients are given an intravenous thrombolytic agent when initially seen in the early hours of acute infarction and then immediately transported to a regional center where PTCA and coronary bypass graft surgery are available on a 24-hour basis.

In a pilot study at the University of Michigan [18], patients with acute myocardial infarction were administered intravenous streptokinase when seen in their community hospitals and transported by helicopter to the university hospital, where angiography was performed within 90 minutes of administering intravenous streptokinase. In this study a reperfusion rate of approximately 95 percent could be achieved with an improvement in left ventricular function.

With these encouraging data, a relatively large-scale prospective randomized study was begun to compare the strategy of urgent PTCA in patients with successful reperfusion after

intravenous thrombolysis with rt-PA to an elective or noninvasive strategy in which patients with successful reperfusion would undergo PTCA only if they had postinfarction angina pectoris or exercise-induced ischemia by thallium 201 myocardial imaging on submaximal exercise stress testing prior to hospital discharge [9]. This trial, The Thrombolysis and Angioplasty in Acute Myocardial Infarction (TAMI) trial [9], failed to show any significant advantage of urgent PTCA, compared to the elective or noninvasive strategy, in regard to global or regional left ventricular function when evaluated 7 to 10 days after infarction prior to hospital discharge. In addition, there appeared to be increased risk and mortality in performing PTCA within the early hours of infarction compared to performing it electively. This study has subsequently been confirmed by the European Cooperative Study group [19] and the TIMI-IIA investigators [20]. The data from the three trials failed to demonstrate any improvement in left ventricular function when the urgent PTCA strategy was compared to an elective (TAMI) [9], delayed (TIMI-IIA) [20], or no PTCA (European Cooperative Study Group) [19] strategy and a significant increase in risk. Thus despite the initial promise, urgent PTCA could not be demonstrated to significantly improve left ventricular function and was associated with an increased risk.

Salvage PTCA

Another potential strategy is that of salvage or rescue PTCA in patients who fail to achieve reperfusion after administration of an intravenous thrombolytic agent. Although success could be demonstrated in an initial pilot study [18], the TAMI trial [9], which had an obligatory shunt to PTCA if the initial angiogram after intravenous rt-PA demonstrated an occluded infarct-related artery, found that there was a high early reclosure rate (29 percent) when PTCA was performed under these circumstances. The procedure was associated with a high in-hospital mortality rate (10 percent) and failure, on an attempt to treat basis, of an improvement in left ventricular function.

The TIMI-II investigators [21] in a small study comparing patients undergoing PTCA for failed intravenous thrombolysis to patients with failed intravenous thrombolysis not undergoing PTCA, also failed to demonstrate any improvement in left ventricular function in the group undergoing PTCA. Thus the strategy of rescue or salvage PTCA, at least with intravenous rt-PA alone, has not been demonstrated to be of benefit.

One situation where urgent PTCA or rescue PTCA after successful thrombolysis may have a role is in the patient with cardiogenic shock. Studies in Worcester, Massachusetts [22] over the last three decades have failed to show any improvement in survival from cardiogenic shock despite introduction of the coronary care unit, hemodynamic monitoring, and the availability of intra-aortic balloon pumping and inotropic agents. Intravenous thrombolytic therapy has resulted in a significant reduction in mortality in patients with acute myocardial infarction and improved ventricular function with a resultant reduction in the incidence of cardiogenic shock. Once cardiogenic shock is manifest, intravenous thrombolytic agents may have a beneficial effect on survival, but the mortality rate in these patients remains high. Although there have as yet been no prospective randomized studies, the experience summarized by Lee et al. [23] has suggested that direct PTCA or PTCA after intravenous thrombolytic therapy may improve survival from approximately 20 to 50 percent, at least in those with anterior infarction and a proximal single left anterior descending coronary artery obstruction. The patients in cardiogenic shock with multivessel disease do not appear to have been improved by PTCA of the infarct-related artery. If mortality is to be reduced in these patients, multivessel PTCA with aortofemoral bypass in the catheterization laboratory or coronary bypass graft surgery may be required. Further carefully controlled studies are, however, necessary before any definitive conclusions can be reached concerning the role of PTCA in cardiogenic shock.

Delayed PTCA

Another potential strategy for PTCA in acute infarction is the delayed strategy. With this strategy patients receiving an intravenous thrombolytic agent undergo routine coronary arteriography 18 to 72 hours after infarction and PTCA of the infarct-related vessel if there is a residual stenosis and acceptable coronary artery anatomy.

In the Johns Hopkins Hospital randomized trial of intravenous rt-PA [24], patients were randomized to PTCA or no PTCA after 3 days and then studied by rest and exercise radionuclide ventriculography at 7 to 10 days prior to hospital discharge. This study showed that delayed PTCA could be accomplished safely and that those patients who underwent delayed PTCA had a significantly better improvement in exercise left ventricular function and significantly fewer ischemic events than patients who did not undergo delayed PTCA.

This strategy of delayed coronary angiography and PTCA has been studied in a larger number of patients by the TIMI-IIB investigators [25]. In this trial patients were randomized to an invasive strategy of delayed PTCA, including administration of intravenous rt-PA followed by angiography at 18 to 72 hours and PTCA in vessels with a significant residual stenosis of the infarct-related artery or to a "noninvasive strategy" in which patients who received intravenous rt-PA underwent PTCA only if they had postinfarction angina pectoris or developed evidence of myocardial ischemia on stress testing prior to hospital discharge. In this trial of several thousand patients, no benefit in regard to resting left ventricular ejection fraction or survival could be demonstrated in the group randomized to the invasive versus the noninvasive strategy. There was, however, a significant improvement in exercise left ventricular ejection fraction in patients undergoing delayed PTCA [25], similar to that reported by the Johns Hopkins Hospital group [24].

In view of the significant reduction in acute and long-term mortality in the GISSI [1], ISIS-II [2], AIMS [4], and ASSET [3] trials of intravenous thrombolytic therapy where PTCA was only rarely used, and in conjunction with the TAMI [9] and TIMI-IIB data [25] in which there was no apparent major benefit of PTCA, an urgent or delayed PTCA strategy cannot be recommended at this time.

Elective Strategy

An elective, or "noninvasive," strategy has the advantage of early administration of intravenous thrombolytic agents with a demonstrated improvement in left ventricular function and survival and avoids the need for early coronary angiography and PTCA and therefore does not require a regional approach. Disadvantages of this strategy include a lack of early angiographic definition, with a consequent inability to detect high risk anatomic subsets such as those with left main coronary artery disease, and failure to detect and reperfuse patients with failed intravenous thrombolysis. In view of the currently available data, an elective or "noninvasive" strategy appears to be advantageous. It should be emphasized, however, that in the TAMI [9] and TIMI-IIB [25] trials the elective (noninvasive) strategy included PTCA for those with postinfarction angina pectoris or exercise-induced myocardial ischemia prior to hospital discharge. The hospitals in which these trials were conducted had facilities for PTCA and skilled angioplasty operators available on a 24-hour basis. The situation in community hospitals may not be identical to these referral centers. There may be a longer delay in detecting and transferring those patients who have recent ischemia to a regional center and having them undergo PTCA. Nevertheless, as emphasized above, the burden of proof is now with those who advocate an invasive strategy of urgent or delayed PTCA.

Comments

In view of the preclinical and clinical data suggesting that a residual stenosis of the infarct-related artery limits the benefits of reperfusion, why has the strategy of sequential urgent or delayed PTCA failed to be beneficial? One possibility is that prior administration of a thrombolytic agent predisposes the patient undergoing PTCA to a greater risk of hemorrhage into the area of infarction.

Studies by Waller et al. have shown extensive hemorrhagic infarction in patients who died subsequent to PTCA after receiving an intravenous thrombolytic agent [26]. Another possible explanation relates to the finding that rt-PA and streptokinase activate platelets [27, 28]. With "successful" intravenous thrombolysis, clot lysis is, as mentioned above, often incomplete [10]. The clot surface serves as a nidus for further platelet deposition. Injury of the arterial wall as a result of PTCA in conjunction with activated platelets and a residual thrombus predisposes to rethrombosis. The potential benefits of successful PTCA are lost by reocclusion. Given the high rate of early reocclusion in patients undergoing PTCA who have received intravenous rt-PA, it is not surprising that this strategy has failed to show any benefit. If this later hypothesis is correct, interventions that reduce the tendency to platelet aggregation and the incidence of reocclusion should result in an improved benefit of PTCA. One piece of evidence supporting this hypothesis comes from a pilot trial of rt-PA and urokinase carried out by the TAMI investigators [29]. Collen and Van de Werf [30] have shown in animal studies that there is a synergistic effect of rt-PA and either urokinase or prourokinase on clot lysis. In the TAMI-II trial [29] reported by Topol et al. this strategy was tested by administering increasing doses of intravenous rt-PA and urokinase in successive groups of patients until at the highest dose patients received 100 mg of intravenous rt-PA and 2 million units of urokinase. In this pilot trial a synergistic effect on thrombolysis could not be confirmed. The patency rate with full doses of rt-PA (100 mg) and urokinase (2 million units) was not significantly better than that found in the TAMI-I study with rt-PA alone [9]. This combination did, however, result in a significant reduction in angiographically determined reocclusion while in the hospital. The reocclusion rate of 15 percent seen in the TAMI-I study with rt-PA alone was reduced to 9 percent with rt-PA plus urokinase [29]. It was accomplished without any increase in bleeding rate.

The mechanism responsible for the reduction in reocclusion is uncertain but may be related to the systemic fibrinolytic effect induced by urokinase, a direct effect of urokinase, or an effect of the combination of urokinase plus rt-PA. To explore these possibilities further the TAMI group has begun a larger prospective trial in which patients with acute myocardial infarction are randomized to rt-PA, urokinase, or the combination of rt-PA plus urokinase (TAMI-V). These patients are then further randomized to undergo coronary angiography and PTCA for failed thrombolysis or to a noninvasive strategy. The potential importance of the study can be seen in the subset of patients with failed thrombolysis who underwent salvage or rescue PTCA in the TAMI-II pilot trial or rt-PA plus urokinase [29]. As mentioned above, salvage PTCA in the TAMI-I trial [9] with rt-PA alone was associated with a 29 percent reocclusion rate and a 10 percent in-hospital mortality without any significant benefit on left ventricular ejection fraction. In the TAMI-II trial [29] with rt-PA plus urokinase, patients who underwent salvage PTCA had a significantly lower reocclusion rate (approximately 4 percent), no in-hospital mortality, and a significant increase in left ventricular ejection fraction. Thus if reocclusion can be prevented, it appears that the safety and benefits of PTCA can be demonstrated. It should be pointed out, however, that this conclusion is based on only a relatively small number of patients and requires confirmation in the ongoing TAMI-V trial or other studies.

Other strategies to block rethrombosis are currently being explored in several centers. At the University of Michigan initial studies with the antibody to the platelet glycoprotein IIb/IIIa receptor have been carried out in a model of acute angioplasty by Bates et al. [31]. This animal model of acute PTCA is associated with a relatively high incidence of acute thrombotic occlusion. Pretreatment with aspirin reduces the rate of reocclusion to approximately 15 percent. Pretreatment with the 7E3 antibody to the glycoprotein IIb/IIIa re-

ceptor completely blocks the tendency toward acute thrombotic reocclusion. Studies by Gold et al. at the Massachusetts General Hospital [32] have also shown the 7E3 platelet antibody to be effective in preventing reocclusion after thrombolysis with rt-PA in an animal model of thrombotic coronary artery occlusion. If this antibody or one of the other antithrombotic strategies being pursued proves successful, the prospects for performing PTCA in patients with acute myocardial infarction will be enhanced and the full potential of the strategy possibly realized. Other advances in angioplasty and interventional angiography, such as the use of stents, are also likely to alter the current results with PTCA and improve its safety and efficacy. However, until it can be convincingly demonstrated that PTCA can be performed safely in patients with acute myocardial infarction, an elective (noninvasive) strategy, as suggested by the TAMI-I [9], European Cooperative Study Group [19], and TIMI-II trials [20, 25], must be recommended for clinical use. The available data should not, however, preclude further clinical investigation. In fact, the encouraging data from the TAMI-II trial [29] with salvage or rescue PTCA and the exciting advances in antithrombotic strategies should be a stimulus for further carefully controlled clinical trials in this area.

Editorial Comments

Dr. Pitt's group at the University of Michigan has been instrumental in providing insight into therapeutic strategies for acute myocardial infarction. Although scientific data favor a conservative strategy regarding PTCA, there continues to be much debate regarding this issue. It appears to be a case of what seems intuitively correct (lytic therapy followed by immediate PTCA) versus what is supported by scientific data (lytic therapy followed by PTCA only in patients with spontaneous or exercise-induced ischemia). We now know that the conservative strategy has much to commend it, but debate will likely continue. G.S.F.

References

1. Gruppo Italiano Per Lo Studio Della Streptochinasi Nell'Infarcto Miocardio (GISSI). Effectiveness of intravenous thrombolytic treatment in acute myocardial infarction. *Lancet* 1:397, 1986.
2. ISIS-2 Collaborative Group. Randomized trial of intravenous streptokinase, oral aspirin, both or neither among 17187 cases of suspected acute myocardial infarction: ISIS-2. *Lancet* 2:349, 1988.
3. Wilcox R. G., Olsson, C. G., Skene, A. M., et al. Trial of tissue plasminogen activator for mortality reduction in acute myocardial infarction: Anglo-Scandinavian Study of Early Thrombolysis (ASSET). *Lancet* 2:525, 1988.
4. AIMS Trial Study Group. Effect of intravenous APSAC on mortality after acute myocardial infarction: Preliminary report of a placebo-controlled clinical trial. *Lancet* 1:545, 1988.
5. Tomada, H. Experimental study on myocardial salvage by coronary thrombolysis and mechanical recanalization. *Am. Heart J.* 116:687, 1988.
6. Grines, C. L., Topol, E. J., Bates, E. R., et al. Infarct vessel status after intravenous tissue plasminogen activator and acute coronary angioplasty: Prediction of clinical outcome. *Am. Heart J.* 115:1, 1988.
7. Chesebro, J. H., Knatterud, G., Roberts, R., et al. Thrombolysis in Myocardial Infarction (TIMI) Trial, Phase I: A comparison between intravenous tissue plasminogen activator and intravenous streptokinase. *Circulation* 76:142, 1987.
8. Verstraete, M., Brower, R. W., Collen, D., et al. Double-blind randomised trial of intravenous tissue-type plasminogen activator versus placebo in acute myocardial infarction. *Lancet* 2:965, 1985.
9. Topol, E. J., Califf, R. M., George, B. S., et al. A randomized trial of immediate versus delayed elective angioplasty after intravenous tissue plasminogen activator in acute myocardial infarction. *N. Engl. J. Med.* 317:581, 1987.
10. Stadius, M. L., Maynard, C., Fitz, J. K., et al. Coronary anatomy and left ventricular function in the first 12 hours of acute myocardial infarction: The Western Washington Randomized Intracoronary Streptokinase Trial. *Circulation* 72:292, 1985.
11. Nicklas, J. M., Diltz, E. A., O'Neill, W. W., et al. Quantitative measurement of coronary flow during medical revascularization (thrombolysis or angioplasty) in patients with acute infarction. *J. Am. Coll. Cardiol.* 10:284, 1987.
12. Meyer, J., Merx, W., Schmitz, H., et al. Percutaneous transluminal coronary angioplasty after streptolysis of transmural myocardial infarction. *Circulation* 66:905, 1982.
13. Hartzler, G. O., Rutherford, B. D., McConahay, D. R., et al. Percutaneous transluminal coronary angioplasty with and without thrombolytic therapy for treatment of acute myocardial infarction. *Am. Heart J.* 106:965, 1987.
14. Giorgi, L. V., Rutherford, B. D., Hartzler, G. O., et al. Direct PTCA for acute myocardial infarction in patients commonly excluded from thrombolytic trials. *Circulation* 78 (Suppl II):377, 1988.
15. O'Neill, W., Timmis, G., Bourdillon, P., et al. A prospective randomized clinical trial of intracoronary streptokinase versus coronary angioplasty therapy of acute myocardial infarction. *N. Engl. J. Med.* 314:812, 1986.
16. Reimer, K. A., Lowe, J. E., Rasmussen, M. M., and Jennings, R. B. The wavefront phenomenon of ischemic cell death. I. Myocardial infarct size vs. duration of coronary occlusion in dogs. *Circulation* 56:786, 1977.
17. Topol, E. J., Fung, A. Y., Kline, E., et al. Safety of helicopter transport and out-of-hospital intravenous fibrinolytic therapy in patients with evolving myocardial infarction. *Cathet. Cardiovasc. Diagn.* 13:151, 1986.
18. Fung, A. Y., Lai, P., Topol, E. J., et al. Value of percutaneous transluminal coronary angioplasty after unsuccessful intravenous streptokinase therapy in acute myocardial infarction. *Am. J. Cardiol.* 58:686, 1986.
19. Simoons, M. L., Arnold, A. E. R., Betriu, A., et al. Thrombolysis with rt-PA in acute myocardial infarction: No beneficial effects of immediate PTCA. *Lancet* 1:197, 1988.
20. TIMI Study Group. Immediate vs. delayed catheterization and angioplasty following thrombolytic therapy for acute myocardial infarction: TIMI-IIA results. *JAMA* (in press).
21. Baim, D. S., Diver, D. J., Knatterud, and the TIMI-IIA Investigators. PTCA "salvage" for thrombolytic failures—implications from TIMI-IIA (Abstract). *Circulation* 78(Suppl II):112, 1988.
22. Frid, D. J., Gore, J. M., Goldberg, R. J., et al. Cardiogenic shock in acute myocardial infarction: inhospital and long-term survival: A community-wide perspective (Abstract). *Circulation* 76 (Suppl IV):546, 1987.
23. Lee, L., Bates, E. R., Pitt, B., et al. Percutaneous transluminal coronary angioplasty improves survival in acute myocardial infarction complicated by cardiogenic shock. *Circulation* 78:1345, 1988.
24. Guerci, A. D., Gerstenblith, G., Brinker, J. A., et al. A randomized trial of intravenous tissue plasminogen activator for acute myocardial infarction with subsequent randomization to elective angiography. *N. Engl. J. Med.* 317:613, 1987.

25. The TIMI Study Group. Comparison of invasive and conservative strategies after treatment with intravenous tissue plasminogen activator in acute myocardial infarction. *N. Engl. J. Med.* 320:618, 1989.

26. Waller, B. F., Rothbaum, D. A., Pinkerton, C. A., et al. Status of the myocardium and infarct-related coronary artery in 19 necropsy patients with acute recanalization using pharmacologic (streptokinase, r-tissue plasminogen activator), mechanical (percutaneous transluminal coronary angioplasty) or combined types of reperfusion therapy. *J. Am. Coll. Cardiol.* 9:785, 1987.

27. Fitzgerald, D. J., Catella, F., Roy, L., et al. Marked platelet activation in vivo after intravenous streptokinase in patients with acute myocardial infarction. *Circulation* 77:142, 1988.

28. Ohlstein, E. H., and Shebuski, R. J. Tissue-type plasminogen activator (rt-PA) increases plasma thromboxane levels which is associated with platelet aggregation (Abstract). *Circulation* 76 (Suppl IV):100, 1987.

29. Topol, E. J., Califf, R. M., George, B. S., and the TAMI Study Group. Coronary arterial thrombolysis with combined recombinant tissue-type plasminogen activator and urokinase in patients with acute myocardial infarction. *Circulation* 77:1100, 1988.

30. Collen, D., and Van de Werf, F. Coronary thrombolysis with low dose synergistic combinations of recombinant tissue-type plasminogen activator (rt-PA) and recombinant single chain urokinase-type plasminogen activator (scu-PA) in man. *Am. J. Cardiol.* 60:431, 1987.

31. Bates, E. R., McGillem, M. J., Mickelson, J. K., et al. A monoclonal antibody to the platelet receptor GPIIb/IIIa (7E3) prevents acute thrombosis in a canine model of coronary angioplasty. *Circulation* 78 (Suppl II):289, 1988.

32. Gold, H. K., Coller, B. S., Yasuda, T., et al. Rapid and sustained coronary artery recanalization with combined bolus injection of recombinant tissue-type plasminogen activator and monoclonal antiplatelet GPIIb/IIIa antibody in a canine preparation. *Circulation* 77:670, 1988.

24
Streptokinase in Acute Myocardial Infarction

ALLAN S. LEW, K. NAGENDRA NATH REDDY, AND WILLIAM GANZ

Experimental models of acute myocardial infarction indicate that reperfusion of reversibly ischemic myocardium limits myocardial necrosis [1–6]. Clinical studies have confirmed that the implications of these experimental studies are applicable to patients with acute myocardial infarction and that reperfusion can "salvage" ischemic myocardium [7–9] and hence preserve ventricular function [10–12] and improve survival [13–15]. Implicit in this therapeutic strategy of reperfusion is the concept that myocardial necrosis occurs in a progressive sequence that can be arrested prior to its completion [16, 17]. Consequently, the amount of myocardium that can potentially be salvaged by reperfusion is a function of the size of the ischemic zone at risk of undergoing necrosis [18, 19] as well as the duration of myocardial ischemia prior to reperfusion [20–22] and the rapidity of its progression from reversible injury to irreversible necrosis [5, 16].

In current clinical practice, the only one of these variables that has been shown to be amenable to modification is the duration of ischemia, which can be shortened by early initiation of treatment. Accordingly, reperfusion within about 2 to 4 hours of the onset of symptoms of a heart attack has been shown to reduce infarction size [23–25], thereby improving ventricular function [10, 12, 26] and survival [14, 15, 26]; later reperfusion generally does not achieve significant myocardial salvage. However, because the rate of progression of necrosis is directly related to the severity of myocardial ischemia (or inversely related to residual myocardial perfusion) [27], patients with severe ischemia usually have a narrower "therapeutic window of opportunity" and may complete their infarction rapidly, whereas patients in whom some perfusion to the ischemic myocardium is preserved because of coronary occlusion is intermittent or not total or because there are well developed collaterals may still benefit from later reperfusion [28].

Because the final common pathway of coronary artery occlusion that leads to acute myocardial infarction is thrombus formation at the site of an ulcerated or fissured atheromatous plaque [29, 30], thrombolysis of the occlusive coronary artery thrombus should be an effective intervention. During the 1960s and 1970s, several large randomized studies addressed the question of the value of intravenous thrombolytic therapy for acute myocardial infarction and reached negative conclusions [31]. The reason for these unfavorable findings was probably the failure to appreciate the brevity of the time period during which the ischemic myocardium within the infarction zone remains reversible, and consequently treatment was usually initiated far too late to achieve any myocardial salvage (up to 72 hours after the onset of symptoms). The lack of clinical impact in these studies together with a growing belief that thrombotic coronary artery occlusion was not the primary pathogenetic mechanism of acute myocardial infarction [32] led to the abandonment of thrombolytic therapy. Early reperfusion was resurrected during the latter part of the 1970s following the realization that complete or nontotal thrombotic occlusion of the infarcted artery is almost always the cause of acute myocardial infarction [33] and that restoration of perfusion to the zone of infarction resulted in clinical improvement [34, 35].

An early approach to achieve reperfusion of the infarcting myocardium was emergency coronary artery bypass surgery (CABG) [36–38], but its widespread application was not feasible; even in the relatively few centers where it could be performed, it usually involved long time delays so that the need for nonsurgical reperfusion was obvious. When it was shown that intracoronary administration of fibrinolytic agents was an effective means for coronary recanalization and myocardial reperfusion, the era of thrombolytic therapy was ushered in [39–41]. It was soon followed by application of acute percutaneous coronary angioplasty (PTCA) [42–44], but both of these intracoronary techniques for reperfusion were restricted in application and had inherent delays in the initiation of treatment. Therefore the utility of intravenous administration of fibrinolytic agents for the treatment of acute myocardial infarction was readdressed, but in contrast to the studies two decades earlier treatment was started early and high-dose protocols were employed [45–48]. It is now accepted that intravenous thrombolysis is currently the most rapidly implementable and most widely applicable method of achieving reperfusion during acute myocardial infarction.

Streptokinase: Mechanism of Action

Thrombolysis is a complex physiologic process that is controlled by an interplay of enzyme precursors, their activators, and enzyme inhibitors. The enzyme responsible for fibrin digestion is plasmin, a nonspecific serine protease that is present in the circulation as the inactive proenzyme precursor plasminogen. Plasminogen is synthesized by the liver and is a 90-kilodalton (kD) glycoprotein containing 20 percent carbohydrate [49]. The protein molecule is composed of a single polypeptide chain containing 791 amino acids [49]. The native form of plasminogen is known as Glu-plasminogen with glutamic acid in the N-terminus position. Another form of plasmino-

gen, Lys-plasminogen, with amino-terminal lysine arises when plasmin cleaves off a 77 amino acid residue peptide from the amino-terminal portion of Glu-plasminogen [50]. The biologic properties of Glu- and Lys-plasminogens are significantly different. The plasminogen content of plasma is approximately 180 mg/L, and the protein has a half-life of 2.2 days. Plasmin degrades fibrin (thrombolysis) and other peptides, including fibrinogen, clotting factors V, VIII, and XII, and some hormones [51]. Both endogenous (intrinsic and extrinsic) and exogenous activators of plasmin are recognized. The intrinsic activators, which include factor XII, kallikrein, and kinins, circulate in the plasma in a precursor state, whereas the extrinsic plasminogen activators are of tissue or cellular origin (kidney, endothelial cells) and appear to be released and act locally. The exogenous activators are those used for the pharmacologic activation of plasminogen to plasmin. Currently, there are three groups of pharmacologic activators of plasmin: (1) streptokinase and its related agents, (2) urokinase and its related agents, and (3) tissue plasminogen activator. In this report, only streptokinase is discussed.

Streptokinase (SK) is an extracellular bacterial protein produced by several strains of hemolytic streptococci [52]. It is composed of a single polypeptide chain with a molecular weight of 47 to 50 kD. SK is not an enzyme; it cannot cleave peptide bonds in proteins, has no esterase or amidase activities against synthetic substrates, and is not inhibited by any of the inhibitors specific for proteolyic enzymes [53]. The activation of plasminogen is an enzymatic reaction in which a single peptide bond is cleaved to give rise to plasmin. Although not an enzyme, SK activates plasminogen to plasmin. How this nonenzymatic protein catalyzes an enzyme reaction was discovered by Reddy and Markus [54] and is summarized in Table 24-1.

Streptokinase reacts rapidly with plasminogen and forms a stoichiometric complex with it (reaction 1). As a result of this complex formation, a conformational change occurs in the plasminogen moiety of the complex, and the complex acquires the properties of an "en-

Table 24-1
Mechanism of action of streptokinase

Reaction sequence	Reaction	
1	Plasminogen + SK $\longrightarrow$	SK–plasminogen complex
2	Plasminogen + SK–plasminogen $\longrightarrow$	plasmin
3	SK–plasminogen + SK–plasminogen $\longrightarrow$	SK–plasmin
4	Plasminogen + SK–plasmin $\longrightarrow$	plasmin

zyme." Thus the mere association of two in-active proteins, SK and plasminogen, by non-covalent bonds leads to the formation of a new protein complex with enzyme activity. The complex catalyzes the conversion of plasmin-ogen to plasmin (reaction 2). The SK–plasmin-ogen complex is also transformed into the SK–plasmin complex by the newly formed en-zyme active site (reaction 3). SK–plasmin is the relatively stable final product formed by the reaction of SK with plasminogen and is an activator of plasminogen (reaction 4). An im-portant consequence of complex formation between SK and plasminogen is that when SK enters the circulation it makes use of an equi-molar amount of plasminogen for activator formation and thus decreases the amount of "substrate" plasminogen available for conver-sion to plasmin.

STREPTOKINASE–PLASMINOGEN COMPLEX

The SK–plasminogen complex is an enzyme formed by the noncovalent association of one molecule of SK with one molecule of plasmin-ogen. Thus SK–Glu-plasminogen and SK–Lys-plasminogen complexes are formed from the respective plasminogens. Plasminogen is the only natural substrate known for the SK–plasminogen enzyme. The complex shows cat-alytic activity toward lysine methyl ester, ace-tyl lysine methyl ester, and tosyl arginine methyl ester at rates approximately one-half that of the SK–plasmin complex [55]. The en-zyme also exhibits amidase activity against H-D-Val-Leu-Lys-pNA and Tos-Gly-Pro-Lys-pNA [56, 57]. The SK–Glu-plasminogen com-plex activates Lys-plasminogen at a higher

rate (sixfold) than Glu-plasminogen [58]. The plasminogen activator activity of the SK–plas-minogen complex is two- to threefold greater than the activity of the SK–plasmin com-plex [55]. However, the SK–plasmin complex shows higher activity (2.5-fold) toward Lys-plasminogen as the substrate compared to Glu-plasminogen. Thus during thrombolytic therapy with SK, if plasmin generated in the circulation is not inactivated rapidly, the cas-cade of reactions amplifies the rate of plasmin-ogen activation to plasmin.

Although the SK–plasminogen complex can be prepared by mixing stoichiometric amounts of the two components, its existence is short-lived. It is continuously transformed into the SK–plasmin complex, and this conversion is completed within 5 minutes at room tempera-ture [54]. Reddy and Markus were able to pre-pare a stable derivative of the SK–plasmino-gen complex by blocking the enzyme active site with a guanidinobenzoyl group [54]. Similarly, acylated anisolylated plasminogen streptokinase activator complex (APSAC) (see below) was prepared by blocking the ac-tive site with acyl or anisoyl groups, respec-tively [59].

STREPTOKINASE–PLASMIN COMPLEX

The SK–plasmin complex is the relatively stable form of plasminogen activator en-zyme formed from the reaction between SK and plasminogen. The same complex is also formed by reaction of SK with plasmin; it has a dissociation constant of 5×10^{-11} for the complex [60, 61]. The formation of the SK–plasmin complex involves cleavage of two peptide bonds in the plasminogen molecule, between Arg_{560}–Val_{561} and Lys_{77}–Lys_{78}, giving rise to the two-chain structure of plasmin. The SK molecule also undergoes proteolytic cleavages, giving rise to a modified SK [53].

The enzyme properties of the SK–plasmin complex are similar to many of the properties exhibited by plasmin. A significant difference between the two enzymes is their reaction with plasminogen. Plasmin cannot activate plasminogen, whereas the complex is an efficient activator of plasminogen. The SK–plasmin complex activates both Glu and Lys plasminogens to give Lys-plasmin. One important difference between plasmin and SK–plasmin complex is that whereas plasmin is rapidly and efficiently inhibited by alpha-2-antiplasmin [62] the inhibitor has no effect on the complex [61]. The interaction of plasmin with the inhibitor is practically instantaneous, and a 2×10^7-fold reduction is seen in its interaction with the SK–plasmin complex [60, 61]. This difference in the reaction of the physiologically important inhibitor has important consequences for the in vivo activity of SK: Because of the inability of the alpha-2-antiplasmin to inhibit the SK–plasmin complex, plasminogen activation in the circulation proceeds until both plasminogen and the inhibitor are depleted.

Mechanism of Clot Lysis

In man, both the circulating plasminogen and the thrombus-bound plasminogen are converted to plasmin, but the thrombus-bound plasmin appears to be more important in thrombolysis [62–64]. Most of the circulating plasmin is either rapidly inactivated by circulating antiplasmins and then cleared from the circulation [65], or it hydrolyzes circulating fibrinogen and other clotting factors, producing the "lytic state" characterized by hypofibrinogenemia, elevated serum fibrin(ogen) degradation products, a shortened euglobulin lysis time, a prolonged thrombin time, and a prolonged partial thromboplastin time [66, 67]. These changes in clotting function are dose-dependent and contribute to the bleeding tendency produced by streptokinase administration. The half-life of streptokinase is approximately 20 minutes, whereas the half-life of the plasminogen activator complex appears to be considerably longer, about 80 minutes. Similarly, the systemic lytic effects last longer than either the circulating streptokinase or its activator complex and plasma fibrinogen is depressed for 24 to 72 hours with recovery to levels of more than 100 mg/dl (minimum for adequate coagulation) within about 24 hours [68].

Species Specificity of Streptokinase

Plasminogen from various mammalian species show variation in their interaction with SK [53] and can be divided into three groups.

1. Plasminogens that can be activated with a small amount of SK (human and monkey)
2. Plasminogens that require large amounts of SK (dog and rabbit)
3. Plasminogens that are resistant to activation by SK (cow, sheep, mouse)

As described above, the mechanism of plasminogen activation by SK involves several steps, and any block in these steps affects the activation process. For example, cow, sheep, and mouse plasminogens do not form the respective SK–plasminogen complexes, and no activation can take place. In the dog and rabbit, high concentrations of SK are needed for complete activation, as the added SK was rapidly degraded to give inactive SK species. When native SK of 47 kD was added to dog plasminogen, the final product of the reaction was a SK–dog plasmin complex in which the SK was found to be degraded to a fragment of approximately 25 kD [69]. Moreover, the SK–dog plasmin complex had no plasminogen activator activity. In contrast to the very high activator activity of the SK–human plasmin complex is the fact that alpha-2-antiplasmin inhibited the former completely and had no effect on the latter [70]. Lack of activator activity in the SK–dog plasmin complex and its rapid inhibition by alpha-2-antiplasmin explains why SK infusion in the dog does not result in efficient thrombolysis. Although purified rabbit plasminogen requires a large excess of SK for activation, significant thrombolysis is achieved in vivo with low doses of SK due to enhancement of activation by rabbit fibrin [71]. In cats, SK infusion results in depletion of plasminogen and fibrinogen in the circulation similar to changes seen in humans [72].

EFFECT OF FIBRIN ON SK ACTIVITY

The plasminogen activator activity of SK is enhanced in the presence of fibrinogen, fibrin, and fibrinogen fragment D. Fibrinogen was found to stimulate the rate of complex formation between SK and plasminogen as well as the activator activity of the complex [73–75]. Fibrin was found to stimulate Glu-plasminogen activation at a higher rate (6.5-fold) than fibrinogen (2.0-fold). The amidolytic activity of the SK–plasminogen complex against the synthetic substrate S-2251 is also enhanced by the stimulators [18].

ANTIGENICITY OF STREPTOKINASE

Because exposure to the streptococcus is almost ubiquitous in man, after administration of streptokinase an amnestic immunologic response usually substantially increases the titer of circulating antistreptokinase antibodies [76–78]. This response is variable, but antibody titers are usually elevated within about 5 days after treatment and persist for up to 6 months [79]. During this time, infusion of standard doses of streptokinase may be ineffective [80], and the dosage required to overcome these antibodies can be determined only after determination of the antistreptokinase titer. Because this assay requires several hours to perform, alternative thrombolytic agents are recommended for patients requiring urgent thrombolytic therapy between 5 days and 6 months after a previous treatment with streptokinase. Notwithstanding the inhibitory role of antistreptokinase antibodies, allergy following streptokinase is rarely a problem in clinical practice.

NEW FORMS OF STREPTOKINASE

New forms of streptokinase have been developed by molecular engineering technologies that covalently bind streptokinase–plasminogen activator complex to compounds such as acyl or anisoyl groups, which render the complex inactive. The new product, acylated plasminogen streptokinase activator complex (APSAC), becomes a functioning plasminogen activator only after removal of the acyl group or deacylation exposes the active site on the complex [81, 82]. Because deacylation proceeds much more rapidly in the presence of fibrin than in the circulation, APSAC is relatively inert following intravenous injection until it reaches the thrombus interface. However, the compound slowly deacylates in the circulation, and the ultimate systemic effects of APSAC are usually similar in degree to those of streptokinase [83–85]. One advantage of APSAC over streptokinase is that it may be given as a bolus [83] because the systemic activation of plasmin is slow and the drug does not cause a hypotensive effect when given rapidly [86, 87]. Otherwise, the thrombolytic effects of APSAC are similar to that of streptokinase, and it is both antigenic to man and inactivated by antistreptokinase antibodies.

Thrombolysis During Acute Myocardial Infarction

PATIENT INCLUSION CRITERIA

Because all patients in whom an acute myocardial infarction is still evolving may benefit from limitation of the extent of necrosis by reperfusion, there are only two considerations for patient selection for intravenous thrombolytic therapy: (1) the presence of reversibly ischemic myocardium in the zone of infarction and (2) the risk of complications, primarily hemorrhagic, from the thrombolytic and anticoagulant therapy.

The clinical assessment of reversibility is based on an estimate of the stage of evolution of the infarction and is probably best gauged by consideration of the duration of chest pain, the persistence or intermittence of the chest pain, and the "acuteness" of the electrocardiographic changes. The experimental and clinical data indicate that reperfusion probably benefits all patients with infarction of less than 2 hours' duration, most patients with infarction of 2 to 4 hours' duration in whom there is still chest pain and acute electrocardiogram changes, and some patients with infarction of more than 4 hours' duration in whom the chest pain has been intermittent or there are acute electrocardiogram changes [20, 23–25, 88]. A fully evolved electrocardiographic pattern of infarction probably precludes a significant benefit with respect to myocardial salvage from reperfusion, but QR complexes per se that accompany acute electrocardiographic changes do not necessarily imply completion of infarction [89–91], whereas QS complexes probably do. This remains an area of uncertainty.

Who Should Be Excluded?

An understanding of the risks of thrombolytic therapy is essential for its safe utilization [92, 93]. Most patients at risk of hemorrhagic complications can be recognized clinically (Table 24-2). The risk increases with age, especially beyond 75 years, and appears to be higher in women, patients with hypertension, and patients with diabetes mellitus [94].

The most serious complication of thrombolytic therapy is intracranial hemorrhage, which fortunately occurs infrequently with an overall incidence of about 0.3 to 0.9 percent [93, 95]. However, this low incidence of intracranial bleeding also makes its prediction difficult, and there are no systematic studies on how to best avoid this complication so that the clinician must rely on several empiric recommendations based on the accumulated clinical experience. The risk of intracranial bleeding is higher in patients with chronic hypertension, but what level or what duration of hypertension constitutes a contraindication is not known. As guidelines, we have generally recommended alternative methods of reperfusion, such as PTCA, for patients with hyper-

Table 24-2
Contraindications for streptokinase use

Risk of intracranial hemorrhage
Poorly controlled chronic hypertension
Acute hypertension: >180 mm Hg systolic or >115 mm Hg diastolic
Hypertensive or diabetic hemorrhagic retinopathy
Any known cerebrovascular pathology
CNS surgery within 6 months
Risk of hemorrhage
Active bleeding or potentially hemorrhagic disease
Surgery, trauma, or organ biopsy/aspiration within 6 weeks
Puncture of a noncompressible vessel or traumatic CPR
Age 75 years or older
Bleeding diathesis
Severe liver or kidney disease or malignancy
Pregnancy or the postpartum state
Risk of systemic embolization
Known or strongly suspected chronic left heart thrombus
Infective endocarditis

tension of more than 10 years' duration and diastolic pressures of more than 110 mm Hg, but we have generally accepted for thrombolytic therapy patients with less than 5 years of well controlled hypertension and no evidence of end-organ damage. We have also excluded patients with hypertension of lesser severity in whom there was coexistent diabetes mellitus and all patients with hemorrhagic retinopathy of any cause, as these patients almost certainly have abnormal cerebral microvasculature. Patients who fall between these extremes must be evaluated on an individual basis with consideration of the likely risk of extensive myocardial necrosis or death from the infarction.

Severe acute hypertension may also pose an increased risk of intracranial bleeding from thrombolytic therapy but fortunately can almost invariably be controlled by pharmacologic means, after which thrombolytic therapy can proceed.

Thrombolytic therapy is absolutely contraindicated in patients with any evidence of parenchymal or vascular cerebral pathology.

Specifically, a history of cerebrovascular accident, no matter how remote, is an absolute contraindication because it is unlikely that the underlying cerebrovascular disease would have regressed with the passage of time; rather, it would be expected to have progressed. The only exception may be the patient in whom a cerebrovascular accident had been known to be due to a nonrecurrent embolic event.

Puncture of a noncompressible vessel such as the subclavian or the jugular vein may lead to uncontrollable bleeding and should be avoided in patients who could potentially receive thrombolytic therapy. Although cardiopulmonary resuscitation and traumatic endotracheal intubation also predispose to severe bleeding, these procedures may be unavoidable in some critically ill patients, and therefore it is sometimes necessary to weigh the potential benefits of reperfusion against the risks of hemorrhage. In general, reperfusion in patients at risk of serious bleeding should be accomplished by alternative means, such as PTCA; but if thrombolytic therapy is deemed essential in such patients, there should be early discontinuation of heparin. Implicit in this strategy of thrombolysis without anticoagulation for high risk patients is the early performance of coronary angiography and, if possible, early PTCA or coronary bypass surgery in order to reduce the risk of reocclusion.

Although the use of "thrombus-selective" agents such as rt-PA may reduce the severity of hemorrhagic complications [96], these agents do not decrease the list of contraindications to thrombolytic therapy, as they still cause fibrinolysis at the site of hemostatic plugs [97, 98] and post-treatment heparinization is still required.

Classically, thrombolytic therapy is contraindicated in the presence of a known or strongly suspected chronic left heart thrombus and in patients with infective endocarditis because of the potential for systemic embolization. However, fresh mural left ventricular thrombus in the setting of acute myocardial infarction may be effectively lysed by thrombolytic therapy with a low risk of embolization [99], as can a thrombus that forms on a left-sided heart valve and compromises its function.

Should Patients with Inferior Infarction Receive Thrombolytic Therapy?

The available data suggest that the group of patients with inferior acute myocardial infarction derive less benefit from early thrombolytic therapy than those with anterior acute myocardial infarction because inferior infarctions are generally small and consequently associated with a good prognosis, whereas anterior infarctions tend to be larger and carry a worse prognosis [15, 100, 101]. Accordingly, it has been proposed that patients with inferior infarction do not warrant treatment with thrombolytic therapy. However, large inferior infarctions that are not clinically benign do occur, and these patients derive benefit from early reperfusion with respect to infarction size and prognosis [19, 25, 102, 103]. Because size of infarction is not necessarily reliably represented by clinical or electrocardiographic criteria during its first few hours, it has been our policy to offer thrombolytic therapy to patients with inferior infarction who are not at high risk of bleeding. Furthermore, initially stable patients with inferior infarction may destabilize due to: (1) the development of high grade atrioventricular block [104] or (2) lethal tachyarrhythmias, which may be prevented by early reperfusion and termination of ischemia [105–107]; (3) myocardial rupture, which may be avoided by preventing transmural necrosis and thereby preserving at least a "rim" of viable subepicardial myocardium [108, 109]; and (4) infarction extension caused by progression of a nontotal coronary occlusion (clinically a "small" infarction) to total occlusion, which may be prevented by lysis of the coronary clot [110, 111].

Even when reperfusion does not influence short-term prognosis, it may improve the patient's chance of surviving a subsequent infarction. Physiologic considerations indicate that, in the event that another coronary artery becomes acutely occluded, a patent right or circumflex coronary artery may be a source of collateral perfusion, which reduces the severity of the acute ischemia and the rapidity of its progression to myocardial necrosis [112]. These collaterals may therefore facilitate greater myocardial salvage by reperfusion of the second infarction.

RECOGNITION OF REPERFUSION

Angiographic Signs

Angiographic patency is the "gold standard" of successful reperfusion (Fig. 24-1). The first angiographic sign of reperfusion is frequently establishment of a sluggish flow of contrast through the thrombus. In both experimental and clinical studies, the lumen and coronary flow generally increase as thrombolysis continues, although sometimes a cyclic pattern of reperfusion and reocclusion may occur before definitive reperfusion is achieved [113, 114]. In our experience, once there is evidence of reperfusion, the artery remains open if thrombolytic therapy is continued, even when the patency is initially intermittent. Neither nitroglycerin nor calcium channel blocking drugs have proved effective in relieving this intermittent occlusion.

For the purposes of description of the adequacy of antegrade perfusion of the artery of infarction, the following four-point scoring code has been proposed by the investigators of the Thrombolysis in Myocardial Infarction (TIMI) study: TIMI 0 = no antegrade perfusion; TIMI 1 = contrast penetrates beyond the occlusive thrombus but does not fill the entire distal artery; TIMI 2 = the entire distal artery fills sluggishly at a rate much slower than that in the normal coronary arteries; and TIMI 3 = normal antegrade perfusion [115].

NONANGIOGRAPHIC CLINICAL SIGNS
The therapeutic advantage of intravenous thrombolytic therapy is that it does not require pretreatment coronary angiography and therefore can be initiated earlier than intracoronary thrombolysis. Implicit in this approach is the need for nonangiographic recognition of the end-point of treatment, i.e., reperfusion.

The nonangiographic assessment of reperfusion is based on: (1) clinical evidence of termination of ischemia (Fig. 24-2); (2) the occurrence of arrhythmias that have been reported to occur following recanalization of an occluded artery of infarction (reperfusion arrhythmias); and (3) an abrupt rise in plasma cardiac enzyme kinase activity that results from their accelerated washout by reperfusion from the necrotic portion of the infarcting myocardium [116].

Termination of ischemia results in the close temporal occurrence of abatement of chest pain and resolution of ST segment elevation (Fig. 24-2A) as well as the resolution of recent, ischemia-mediated atrioventricular or bundle branch block, if present.

Relief of chest pain following reperfusion is readily apparent to both the patient and the

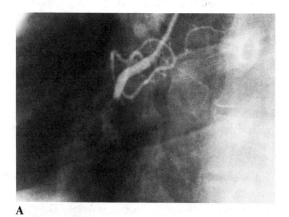

A

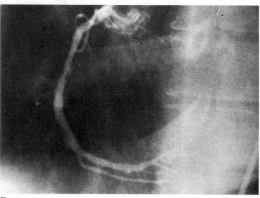

B

Fig. 24-1
Serial selective right coronary angiograms from a patient with inferior acute myocardial infarction showing (A) complete proximal occlusion and (B) restoration of patency following intracoronary streptokinase.

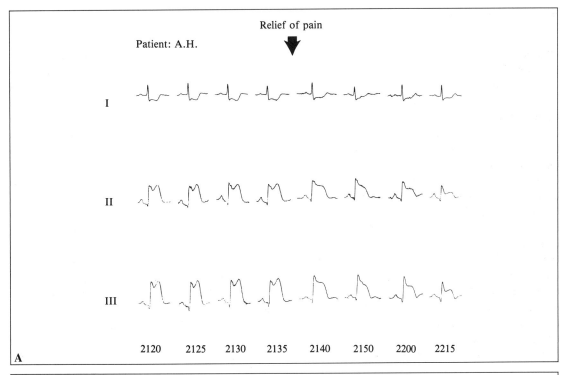

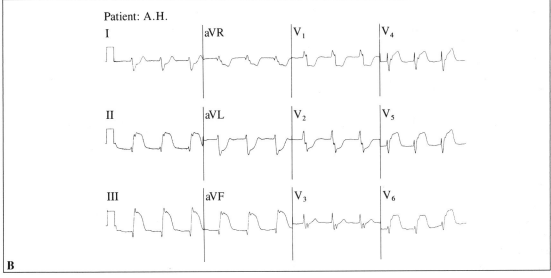

Fig. 24-2
"Simultaneous" appearance of the nonangiographic signs of reperfusion in a patient with inferior acute myocardial infarction who received intravenous streptokinase commencing at 2120. Note (*A*) the onset of resolution of chest pain and ST segment elevation between 2135 and 2140; (*B*) the occurrence of accelerated idioventricular rhythm at 2142; and (*C*) the onset of an abrupt rise in plasma creatine kinase between 2130 and 2200 followed by early peaking of the time–activity curve within 4 hours of the commencement of its rise.

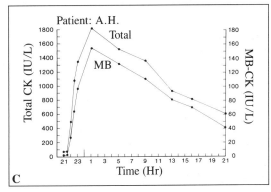

physician and easy to recognize, even after treatment with narcotic analgesics. The patient usually reports a feeling of well-being and also appears well, becoming more conversive and attentive to his or her environment. Occasionally, the abatement of chest pain is preceded by a period of fluctuation of chest pain [117] consistent with the intermittency of patency observed angiographically. Similarly, reperfusion usually results in rapid resolution of the electrocardiographic manifestations of ischemia, e.g., ST segment elevation. Some patients also manifest a cyclic pattern of oscillating ST segment changes that is probably the electrocardiographic counterpart of this phenomenon. Many patients manifest a sudden but transient worsening of both the chest pain and the ST segment elevation at the moment of reperfusion, but neither the pathogenesis nor the significance of these findings is known [118].

Importantly, however, these findings have not been universal in clinical studies of thrombolysis [119–121]. One possible explanation for the discrepant observations is that both the symptomatic and electrocardiographic signs of reperfusion are based on evidence of termination of ischemia. Therefore they are observed only in patients in whom some part of the myocardium is still ischemic at the time of reperfusion; conversely, they are not likely to be observed following reperfusion of a fully evolved infarction. This fact may explain why the studies that have not found the clinical signs of reperfusion to be reliable have generally been those in which patients were treated late, probably following completion of their infarction, and why these same studies often found the clinical signs to be "paradoxically" useful only in the subset of patients with nontotal occlusion [121, 122], that is, those in whom there was most likely to be an element of reversible ischemia [123]. Reperfusion usually produces a rapid resolution of ischemic ST–T wave changes [124–127] followed by rapid evolution of the electrocardiographic signs of infarction commensurate with the extent of necrosis that had evolved prior to termination of the ischemia by reperfusion [90, 121, 128]. Although patients who have sus-

tained no or minimal necrosis may not develop pathologic Q waves, reperfusion is usually not early enough to completely prevent myocardial necrosis; thus in clinical practice, evolution of pathologic Q waves is the norm. However, the appearance of Q waves immediately after reperfusion does not imply transmural necrosis [91], and in experimental studies pathologic Q waves appear following necrosis of as little as 25 percent of the transmural thickness of the wall [129]. Furthermore, Q waves that appear early after reperfusion may disappear, and "lost" R waves may recover within a few days to weeks [10, 89, 121, 126]. This finding contrasts with the evolution of the electrocardiogram following infarction in the absence of reperfusion in which there is typically a gradual but permanent loss of R waves [125, 126].

When atrioventricular or intraventricular conduction block is present at the outset, it often disappears shortly after reperfusion; it has also been reported to resolve following delayed reperfusion [104]. This resolution of conduction block should not be confused with the vagally mediated sinoatrial or atrioventricular block that may transiently appear at the time of reperfusion in some patients with inferior wall infarction and that is frequently associated with nausea, vomiting, and hypotension. This reaction is probably due to triggering of the Bezold-Jarisch reflex by restoration of perfusion to the inferior and posterior wall of the left ventricle [130, 131]; importantly, it responds readily to intravenous atropine.

Reperfusion arrhythmias are ventricular arrhythmias that occur at the time of reperfusion or shortly thereafter and have been reported in about 90 percent of patients with proved reperfusion [105, 106, 132–134]. Although experimental studies indicate that the electrophysiologic basis of reperfusion arrhythmias is probably increased automaticity [135, 136], in clinical practice almost any ventricular arrhythmia may accompany reperfusion. The commonest reperfusion arrhythmias are accelerated idioventricular rhythm (AIVR) (Fig. 24-2B) and ventricular ectopic beats that occur late during diastole and appear either as isolated ectopic or fusion beats or as part of a bigeminal or trigeminal pattern [106, 134]. Although AIVR occurs at the time of reperfusion in only about 50 percent of patients, Holter monitor studies indicate that about 90 percent of patients have self-terminating runs of AIVR or slow ventricular tachycardia at about 70 to 90 beats per minute (bpm) during the 12 hours following reperfusion [106] (Fig. 24-3). This relative slowness of the rate of AIVR may delay its appearance until the sinus rate slows and may be the reason why some patients manifest only delayed AIVR. Although reperfusion arrhythmias are generally transient and benign, and therefore do not usually require any treatment, sustained or rapid ventricular tachycardia occasionally occurs and responds to the usual antiarrhythmic agents. Ventricu-

lar fibrillation is a rare reperfusion arrhythmia following intravenous thrombolysis.

"Washout" of creatine kinase (CK) and other cardiac enzymes into the circulation occurs following reperfusion [137–140] owing to the abrupt and marked increase in antegrade coronary blood flow to the myocardium compared with the collateral blood flow that existed prior to reperfusion. Therefore immediately following reperfusion there is a rapid increase in serum CK activity; in most cases, the CK time-activity curve peaks earlier (See Fig. 24-2C) than with nonreperfused infarctions [141]. Reperfusion also results in a more complete "washout" of CK from the myocardium, with considerably less CK inactivation [142, 143] such that the peak serum CK activity as well as the total amount of CK released

Fig. 24-3
Time course of the prevalence of ventricular arrhythmias during the first 24 hours after reperfusion with intravenous streptokinase. R = hour during which reperfusion occurred; VPB = ventricular premature beat; AIVR = accelerated idioventricular rhythm; VT = ventricular tachycardia. (From B. Cercek et al. Time course and characteristics of ventricular arrhythmias following reperfusion in acute myocardial infarction. *Am. J. Cardiol.* 60:214, 1987. With permission.)

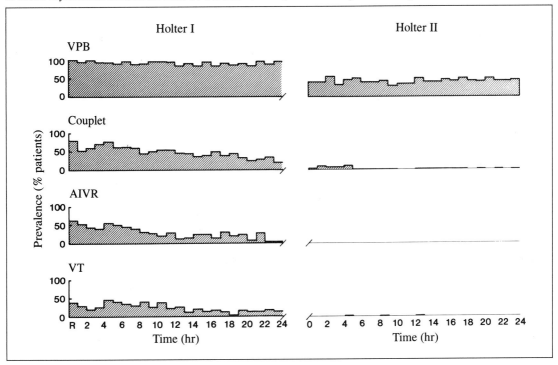

are considerably higher following reperfusion (two to three times higher in canine models) than for an equivalent sized nonreperfused myocardial infarction [144].

Similar findings of more rapid enzyme washout have also been reported for beta-hydroxydehydrogenase [145], myoglobin [146], and isoforms of creatine kinase [147, 148].

In our experience, the simultaneous occurrence of (1) relief of chest pain, (2) resolution of ST segment elevation, and (3) abrupt CK "washout" following thrombolytic therapy reliably indicated coronary artery reperfusion in patients treated by thrombolysis [149, 150]. Furthermore, consistent with the sound physiologic basis of the nonangiographic signs of reperfusion, there was an excellent concordance between these signs and angiographically recognized reperfusion in several intracoronary streptokinase studies [116].

In order to facilitate the recognition of reperfusion at the bedside, we ask the patient to grade his or her chest pain on a scale of 0 to 10 immediately before treatment and subsequently at 5- to 10-minute intervals. Reperfusion is accompanied by a rapid, progressive decrease in pain intensity to a score of 0 or 1 within 30 minutes of the onset of its abatement. Resolution of ST segment elevation is assessed by both continuous monitoring of the ST segment elevation and by recording a 12-lead electrocardiogram prior to treatment and whenever a change in pain, monitored ST segment elevation, or cardiac rhythm suggesting reperfusion occurs. We defined resolution of ST segment elevation as its progressive decrease to less than 50 percent of its baseline elevated value within 30 minutes of the onset of its decline. The time of onset of the rise in CK is determined by sampling blood at 30-minute intervals until the time of reperfusion and then every 2 to 4 hours for another 12 hours. An abrupt rise in serum CK temporarily related to the bedside signs of reperfusion was defined as a first hour rise of 15 percent or more of the peak value commencing during the same 30-minute period as the other signs of reperfusion. It is important to remember, however, that none of the noninvasive signs of reperfusion is completely reliable.

INTRACORONARY STREPTOKINASE

Most studies using intracoronary thrombolytic therapy for acute myocardial infarction have used streptokinase, but similar results have been reported following intracoronary administration of urokinase [151], rt-PA [152], and acylated streptokinase–plasminogen activator complex [85]. In these studies reperfusion occurred in 60 to 95 percent of completely occluded arteries of infarction, but few of the studies observed patients for longer than 90 minutes. The reperfusion rate averaged about 75 percent for 1453 patients enrolled in three large registries of intracoronary streptokinase [153–155] with a mean time interval from commencement of streptokinase to reperfusion of about 40 minutes for the successfully treated patients. In these studies the dosage, infusion rate, and technique of infusion varied, but in general a streptokinase loading dose of 10,000 to 20,000 units was followed by a constant infusion of 2000 to 4000 units/min until coronary artery patency was restored and then for a further 30 to 60 minutes in order to "clean up" the thrombus. The total dose varied from less than 100,000 units to more than 500,000 units and was usually greater than 250,000 units. In most studies streptokinase was infused into the ostium of the coronary artery via the coronary angiography catheter, but in a few it was administered subselectively within a few millimeters of the thrombus following advancement of a special 2.5 Fr infusion catheter via the coronary angiography catheter [156]. Pooled data suggest that administration of larger doses of streptokinase and the use of a subselective technique each resulted in a higher rate of reperfusion, whereas intracoronary nitroglycerin or perforation of the thrombus with a guidewire was of no added benefit and only rarely achieved reperfusion alone [6, 40, 156].

Despite these encouraging results, intracoronary thrombolysis is limited in application to medical centers with angiographic facilities; even when these facilities exist, they may not be immediately available when a patient is admitted during the working hours and in many centers are not available at all during the night. Because in patients with an evolving acute myocardial infarction who are eligible for thrombolytic therapy "time is myocardium," the inherent delay of preliminary coronary angiography decreases the impact of the intracoronary approach in terms of myocardial salvage. These constraints fostered renewed interest in intravenous administration of thrombolytic agents.

INTRAVENOUS STREPTOKINASE

Intravenous administration of streptokinase is an effective and widely applicable means of achieving reperfusion, and several studies comparing intravenous to intracoronary streptokinase have found similar rates of reperfusion with either approach [19, 157–161]. Although the reported reperfusion rates following intravenous streptokinase have varied widely, from as low as 10 to 30 percent [162, 163] to more than 90 percent [164], the studies in which treatment was initiated early have generally reported higher reperfusion rates of more than about 85 percent [157, 164–167]. These differences probably reflect differences in several aspects of study design, including the dosage, time of treatment, patient inclusion criteria, method of assessing reperfusion, and pretreatment with heparin.

Dosage

The rate at which clot lysis proceeds with any thrombolytic agent is a function of its plasma concentration [65, 98, 168]; therefore intravenous studies have given higher doses at faster infusion rates than were administered in the intracoronary studies. Streptokinase doses of 0.5 to 1.5 million units were infused over 30 to 60 minutes. Although the "optimal" dose for intravenous streptokinase has not been determined, some investigators have found a direct relation between dosage and reperfusion rates with doses up to about 1.5 million units [160, 162]. In our experience, about 30 percent of the patients treated with 750,000 IU received an inadequate dose and required a second dose of streptokinase to achieve reperfusion [169]. Although these patients tended to be heavy (>75 kg) or had a high titer of anti-SK antibodies, they could not be reliably recog-

nized before treatment. However, because the larger dose did not cause an increased incidence of bleeding, we currently recommend a routine intravenous streptokinase dose of 1.5 million IU.

Consistent with the relation between the plasma level of streptokinase and its efficacy, reperfusion by intravenous streptokinase occurs more rapidly during fast infusion rates, whereas it may take considerably longer with slow infusion rates (Fig. 24-4); thus slow administration may be relatively ineffective [170]. This effect of infusion rate was also noted in intracoronary streptokinase studies [156]. Therefore it may seem logical to give intravenous streptokinase rapidly or as a bolus. However, rapid infusion of streptokinase may cause sudden and sometimes severe transient hypotension [171] (Fig. 24-4). In our experience, limiting the rate of infusion of streptokinase to about 400 to 500 IU/kg/min together with frequent monitoring of the blood pressure during the infusion (e.g., every 1–2 minutes using a Dinamap) can minimize this potential complication. A practical, easy formula for es-

Fig. 24-4
Reciprocal effects of the rate of infusion of streptokinase on the time interval to reperfusion (*bottom*) and the fall in systolic blood pressure (*top*). Slow infusion rates of streptokinase have a small effect on blood pressure but achieve reperfusion slowly, whereas rapid infusion rates of streptokinase achieve prompt reperfusion but may cause considerable hypotension.

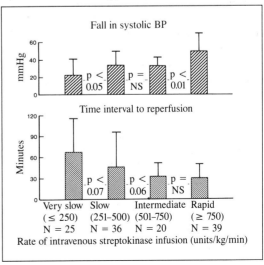

tablishing an infusion of 500 IU/kg/min is given in Table 24-3.

Mild hypotension responds promptly to temporary interruption of the infusion, but more severe hypotension may require placing the patient in the Trendelenburg position or even giving a low dose infusion of a vasopressor, such as norepinephrine. Note that for hemodynamically compromised patients and those with baseline hypotension, slower infusion rates of streptokinase (about 200–250 IU/kg/min) should be used, and preparation of a "standby infusion" of norepinephrine may be in order. This hypotensive effect of intravenous streptokinase may pose an important limitation for its use in out-of-hospital settings.

Time of Treatment
Consistent with experimental studies showing that older thrombi are more resistant to lysis [4, 172], several clinical studies have found that the delay between onset of infarction and treatment was a determinant of both the rate of successful reperfusion and the time required to achieve reperfusion [21, 153, 155, 170, 172]. The probable reason for these observations is that the interval between onset of symptoms and treatment is related to the thrombus age or at least the age of its final occlusive component. Because older thrombi tend to be larger, have a lower plasminogen content due to retraction, and have a higher degree of fibrin cross-linking than fresher thrombi [173, 174], they become more resistant to lysis and require a longer exposure to increased amounts of thrombolytic agents to be lysed than do smaller and fresher clots [175, 176]. Anderson et al. [10] reported reperfusion rates of 87 and 85 percent for the intra-

Table 24-3
Setting up a streptokinase infusion
of 500 IU/kg/min

Because: 500 IU/kg/min = 30,000 IU/kg/hr
1. Reconstitute 1.5 million units of streptokinase in 50 ml = 30,000 IU/ml.
2. Set infusion rate in *milliliters per hour* = patient's body weight in kilograms.

---

coronary and intravenous routes, respectively in patients who were admitted within 4 hours of the onset of chest pain, whereas the rate of successful reperfusion tended to be about 60 to 70 percent in studies that delayed treatment for more than 6 hours after the onset of chest pain [157–159, 162, 163]. However, it is still probable that some patients will derive benefit when streptokinase is given between 6 and 24 hours.

Patient Inclusion Criteria
Some studies have required pretreatment coronary angiography and included only patients with total occlusion of the artery of infarction, whereas others have included patients according to the clinical criteria of acute myocardial infarction. In general, the latter studies, in which treatment was not delayed by 1 to 2 hours for preliminary angiography and patient inclusion was limited to 3 to 4 hours, have reported high rates of reperfusion (80–90 percent) following intravenous thrombolysis [164–167], whereas when patient inclusion was extended for 6 hours or longer and treatment was delayed for angiography the reperfusion rate was considerably lower (40–70 percent) [46–48, 159–163]. The greater clinical efficacy of the studies that did not delay treatment for angiography may reflect two factors: (1) higher reperfusion following earlier treatment because of the direct relation between clot age and the efficacy of most thrombolytic agents; and (2) inclusion of patients in whom acute infarction was due to a nontotal, rather than a total, coronary occlusion, as these patients generally show a good clinical response to thrombolytic therapy because the clot is not only smaller but presents a relatively larger surface area to the thrombolytic agent. However, only 15 to 25 percent of patients with acute infarction have a nontotal occlusion from the outset, and therefore [33, 177] the inclusion of these patients could not entirely account for the higher reperfusion rate of patients not undergoing pretreatment angiography.

The effect of preliminary coronary angiography is illustrated by studies of intravenous streptokinase reported by Schroder et al. [46]

and Rogers et al. [162, 165]. Schroder et al. treated two groups of patients, only one of which underwent pretreatment angiography. In this group, reperfusion of a totally occluded coronary artery occurred within 3 hours in 71 percent of patients, whereas the group without pretreatment angiography had a reperfusion rate of 94 percent. Rogers et al. reported two studies. In their initial postangiography study [162] they reported a 40 percent reperfusion rate in patients with total coronary occlusion treated within 12 hours of the onset of pain, but in a subsequent study performed without preliminary angiography [165] they reported an 86 percent reperfusion rate in patients treated within 6 hours of the onset of pain.

Method for Recognizing Reperfusion

Perhaps the most controversial aspect of intravenous thrombolysis for acute myocardial infarction is the method of assessing reperfusion. Some studies have done so by immediate post-treatment angiography, whereas others (including our own) have relied primarily on nonangiographic recognition of reperfusion confirmed by early, but not immediate, angiography. Most studies relying on angiographic patency have also required pretreatment angiography, and the lower reperfusion rate in these studies may reflect the delay to treatment. However, even studies that performed only post-treatment angiography may have underestimated the reperfusion rate, as the period of observation was usually limited to 60 to 90 minutes, and about 20 percent of patients may show signs of reperfusion more than 90 minutes after the initiation of therapy [178], especially if treated with a slow infusion rate.

The study by Schroder et al. [46] also illustrated the impact of the time of assessment, as angiographically determined reperfusion was 52 percent at 1 hour, 71 percent at 3 hours, and 81 percent by 24 hours. It is of note that reperfusion in the TIMI studies may have been underestimated, as it was assessed angiographically at 90 minutes after commencement of treatment even though rt-PA was given as a 3-hour infusion.

In our studies, reperfusion assessed nonan-

giographically occurred in about 90 percent of patients treated by either intravenous streptokinase [164] or rt-PA [179]. The mean time interval to reperfusion was about 45 minutes, which is similar to that following intracoronary thrombolysis.

Role of Anticoagulation

Pretreatment with a bolus of heparin is recommended because of both experimental and clinical evidence that it potentiates the efficacy of thrombolytic agents by inhibiting ongoing fibrin incorporation by the thrombus during thrombolysis [180–182]. This step appears to be especially important when circulating fibrinogen is preserved, as may occur with clot-selective agents such as rt-PA. The risk of rethrombosis and reocclusion at the reexposed site of arterial pathology that initially precipitated thrombosis is lessened by post-treatment anticoagulation [183, 184], and the most critical period appears to be the first 3 days. The protocol recommended in Table 24-4 is designed to maintain the partial thromboplastin time (PTT) at about 70 to 80 seconds, but individual responses are highly variable and therefore frequent monitoring of the PTT is critical until its level is stable. For several hours after the bolus, anticoagulation can usually be maintained with about 10 IU/kg/hr; but as the effects of the bolus dissipate (4–6 hours) and as clotting factors recover and fibrin(ogen) degradation products are cleared from the circulation, the heparin requirements usually increase to about 12 to 15 IU/kg/hr. Because reperfusion may be delayed, heparin should not be withheld on the basis of pre-

Table 24-4
Anticoagulation

1. Pretreatment bolus of heparin 40 U/kg IV.
2. Post-treatment heparin infusion at 10–15 U/kg/hr IV to maintain PTT at 70–80 seconds.
3. Heparin requirements may increase during inital 24–48 hours.
4. Heparin is not discontinued prior to coronary angiography, PTCA, or CABG.
5. Patients not undergoing CABG or PTCA receive coumadin.

sumed failure until it is verified by angiography, and heparin should not be interrupted prior to angiography, PTCA, or CABG. Patients in whom no procedure is contemplated are commenced on coumadin after at least 3 days of heparin, and continued coumadin is recommended for at least 2 months. The role of anti-platelet agents such as aspirin as a substitute for coumadin is unclear, but some preliminary data suggest that these agents may afford adequate protection against reocclusion [26, 185–187]. This point may be especially pertinent in patients in whom the residual stenosis is not severe.

Complications

Hemorrhagic complications are the only significant cause of morbidity attributable to thrombolytic therapy [68, 92, 153–155, 188, 189]. Bleeding results from either (1) lysis of hemostatic fibrin–platelet thrombi at the site of previous trauma or tissue injury or (2) prevention of adequate clot formation by heparin and fibrinogen degradation products at sites of traumatic procedures. Although some degree of bleeding has been reported in up to 50 percent of patients following either intracoronary or intravenous thrombolytic therapy and heparin, severe bleeding occurs in fewer than 15 percent of patients and in some series in fewer than 5 percent [15, 26]. In our experience, most instances of bleeding can be attributed to either invasive procedures or inappropriate patient selection, and most patients at high risk of a hemorrhagic complication can be identified by a careful history and examination. If these high risk patients are excluded and if invasive procedures can be avoided, the incidence of bleeding is low.

The commonest site of severe bleeding is the femoral artery puncture site performed for coronary angiography, and the factors that predispose to bleeding from this site include repeated attempts at vascular access, puncture of the posterior wall of the femoral artery, and inadequate attention to postprocedure hemostasis, which, following thrombolytic therapy, may require prolonged groin pressure or clamping for up to 4 to 6 hours. Repeated veni-

puncture is another common cause of minor and sometimes severe bleeding that can be prevented by placement of one or more venous cannulas in each arm prior to therapy for later drug infusions and blood sampling. Whenever possible, vascular access lines are maintained until recovery of coagulation factors if they are depleted (approximately 24 hours) and until the dissipation of fibrinolytic effects (about 12 to 24 hours for streptokinase or urokinase but less than an hour for rt-PA).

A guide to the management of bleeding complications is presented in Table 24-5. The use of topical thrombin and cryoprecipitate can assist in hemostasis [190], but, as with all blood products, their use should be restricted to refractory bleeding. Discontinuation of heparin should prompt consideration of early PTCA in suitable patients with a tight residual coronary stenosis that may predispose to reocclusion. It is of note that, even for severe bleeding, anti-fibrinolytic agents such as epsilonaminocaproic acid are usually not indicated if bleeding occurs after the fibrinolytic effects of the drug have dissipated [191]. For early and severe bleeding, currently available antifibrinolytic agents may be useful but should be considered a second line approach as they are only partially effective and the

Table 24-5
Management of hemorrhagic complications

Minor complications
1. Secure local hemostasis; apply pressure dressings; apply topical thrombin powder or topical cryoprecipitate/thrombin glue.*
2. Discontinue anticoagulation if bleeding cannot be controlled.

Moderate complications
1. As above.
2. Discontinue anticoagulation.
3. Reverse anticoagulation if bleeding not controlled. Give protamine sulfate for heparin or fresh frozen plasma for coumadin.

Severe complications
1–3. As above.
4. If fibrinogen <100 mg/dl, administer 5–10 units of cryoprecipitate.
5. Transfuse blood as required.
6. Consider epsilonaminocaproic acid.*
7. Consider surgical control of bleeding site.

*See Complications section in text.

bleeding is more likely to respond to withdrawal of anticoagulant therapy and repletion of coagulation factors. The development of monoclonal antibodies that specifically inhibit the circulating plasminogen activators may potentially provide a tool for controlling severe hemorrhage.

Streptokinase is now highly purified, and allergic reactions following its use are rare. Despite almost a decade of routine pretreatment with steroids or antihistamines prior to streptokinase, there is no proof that these agents are necessary or effective. Because there were no allergic reactions in any of 70 consecutive patients in whom we omitted pretreatment with anti-allergy medications, we believe such routine pretreatment is not justified.

Management of the Residual Coronary Artery Stenosis

Early reocclusion occurs in about 10 to 15 percent of patients treated with thrombolytic therapy and has been reported in up to 40 percent of patients in some studies [192–195]. Therefore coronary thrombolysis in acute myocardial infarction begets the question of how to manage the residual stenosis at the site of reperfusion, which is often severe with superimposed residual unlysed thrombus [155, 196–200]. Because a tight residual stenosis is associated with a high risk of reocclusion or recurrent ischemic manifestations [201, 202] some investigators have advocated PTCA of severe stenoses [203–207]. However, others have not found post-thrombolysis PTCA to reliably prevent reocclusion; furthermore, PTCA in the presence of residual thrombus may precipitate sudden reocclusion, which may then mandate urgent CABG [208, 209]. This fact was highlighted by a report from Topol et al. [210], who found that immediate post-thrombolysis PTCA was (1) associated with a higher incidence of abrupt reocclusion than elective PTCA deferred until 1 week after reperfusion and (2) frequently unnecessary because the residual stenosis tended to improve spontaneously during this interval. Indeed, if early reocclusion can be prevented and/or if only those patients with clinical evidence of reocclusion or recurrent ischemia are selected for PTCA, the residual stenosis in the remaining (most) patients tends to improve spontaneously over a few days to weeks due to ongoing (endogenous) thrombolysis (Fig. 24-5) and during the ensuing weeks to months due to plaque healing and remodeling [196, 197, 200, 201, 211]. This "natural history" of the conservatively managed residual stenosis

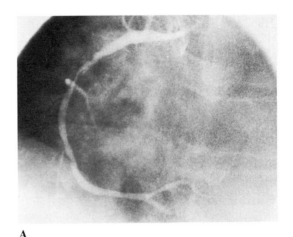

A

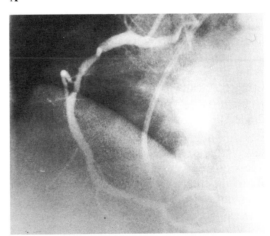

B

Fig. 24-5
Serial selective right coronary angiograms from a patient with inferior acute myocardial infarction at (A) 2 hours and (B) 24 hours after treatment with intravenous tissue plasminogen activator. Note the early post-reperfusion tight residual stenosis of the right coronary artery proximal to the right ventricular branch with a superimposed intraluminal thrombus (A) that has markedly improved by 24 hours following additional intravenous rt-PA and anticoagulation with heparin (B).

contrasts markedly with the 30 percent or more restenosis rate induced by PTCA [212].

Therefore at present the role of post-thrombolysis PTCA is unclear, although current evidence suggests that the decision for its application should not be based solely on an anatomic determination of the severity of the residual stenosis. Perhaps some functional assessment of both the viability and the adequacy of perfusion to the reperfused myocardium is a better guide for this selection [213, 214]. Currently, our indications for early PTCA after thrombolytic therapy are (1) failure to recanalize the artery of infarction, (2) severe heart failure or shock, (3) recurrent resting ischemia or reocclusion (which may be retreated by thrombolysis prior to PTCA), (4) the need to discontinue anticoagulation, and (5) exercise-induced ischemia. With respect to the latter, the tendency for improvement in the caliber of the stenosis during the weeks to months following thrombolysis implies that a mild to moderate positive response on a predischarge exercise test in an asymptomatic patient may bear observation and subsequent retesting 6 to 12 weeks later.

In accordance with a growing trend toward more conservative management of the residual stenosis, Gold et al. [215, 216] have reported that reocclusion of tight stenoses following rt-PA may be prevented by prolonging the duration of thrombolytic therapy with a 4-hour low-dose "maintenance" infusion, thereby achieving more complete clot lysis. However, it is not clear whether the beneficial effects of such a protocol are due to protraction of the treatment period or the ultimately larger dose of rt-PA that is given. In our experience, a 150-mg dose of rt-PA given over a relatively brief 2-hour infusion period was associated with only a 10 percent incidence of reocclusion—a rate similar to that reported for Gold et al.'s protocol [179]. Furthermore, the relevance of this approach for streptokinase and other thrombolytic agents is not known.

Patients with surgically amenable severe multivessel coronary artery disease should be considered for elective CABG prior to discharge, as the risk of early CABG is not significantly increased by thrombolytic therapy

[217–219], especially with short-acting clot-selective agents such as rt-PA; however, surgery performed during the first 24 hours after streptokinase administration may be associated with an increased requirement for blood and blood products [220, 221].

Myocardial Salvage and Patient Survival

Early reperfusion results in a reduction in the extent of myocardial necrosis as assessed by electrocardiographic [10, 121, 125, 126, 128], enzymatic [9, 20, 222], scintigraphic [7–9, 222–229], functional [10–12, 23, 24, 230–233], and metabolic [234–237] criteria, whereas reperfusion that is delayed for more than about 4 hours after the onset of infarction usually does not achieve significant measurable myocardial salvage [20, 23, 25, 238–240] (Fig. 24-6). The importance of early initiation of therapy is highlighted by a study from Israel [24]

Fig. 24-6

Electrocardiographic (A), thallium-201 scintigraphic (B), and radionuclide ventricular functional (C) evidence of myocardial salvage following reperfusion of the left main coronary artery by intravenous streptokinase. A. Serial 12-lead electrocardiograms demonstrating rapid resolution of marked anterior ST segment elevations and right bundle branch block without evolution of pathologic Q waves. B. Serial thallium-201 scintigrams showing an extensive perfusion defect involving the anterior (ANT), apical (AP), septal (SEPT), and posterolateral (PL) walls of the left ventricle on day 1. Only posterolateral and apical perfusion defects are present by day 10, with marked improvement of anterior and septal isotope uptake. C. Serial technetium 99m radionuclide wall motion studies in the left anterior oblique 45° projection showing a dilated and poorly functioning left ventricle with regional ventricular septal, inferoapical, and posterolateral wall motion abnormalities on day 1 that significantly improved by day 10. (From A. S. Lew et al. Extensive myocardial salvage and reversal of cardiogenic shock following reperfusion of the left main coronary artery by intravenous streptokinase. Am. J. Cardiol. 54:451, 1984. With permission.)

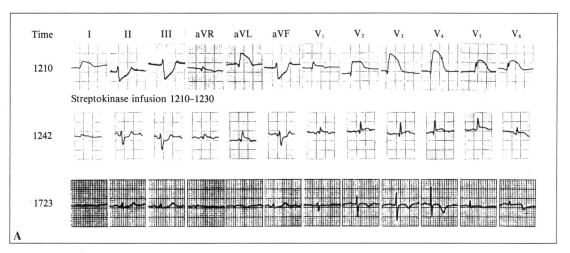

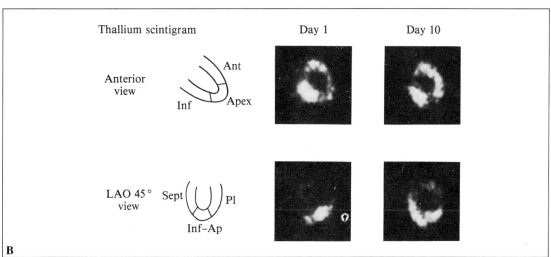

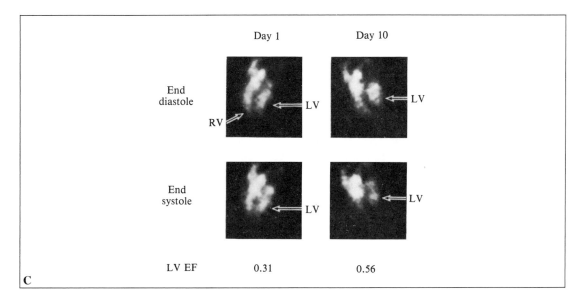

in which intravenous streptokinase was either given by ambulance officers at the patient's home or delayed until arrival at the hospital emergency room. All parameters of infarction size were markedly reduced in the group treated by the ambulance officers compared with those treated in the emergency room.

When assessing the impact of reperfusion on ventricular function, it is important to appreciate the distinction between global ventricular function and regional function in the reperfused zone [101–231]. Because global ventricular function or ejection fraction reflects the additive contribution to the function of both the nonischemic and ischemic zones of the myocardium, its recovery may be an insensitive index of myocardial salvage. This point is especially true if prior to reperfusion the hypofunction of the ischemic zone was compensated by hyperkinesia in the nonischemic myocardium, which, following functional recovery of the salvaged myocardium, subsequently regresses to normal function and thereby "neutralizes" or offsets any measurable gain in global function. This phenomenon may also explain why improvement in global function following reperfusion is more apparent in patients with extensive initial involvement [241–243] as in these patients the nonischemic zone is relatively small, and hence the impact of the early compensatory hyperkinesis and its subsequent regression is small compared to the impact of the changes in the large ischemic zone. In contrast, with a small infarction the compensatory hyperkinesia of a large nonischemic zone may be sufficient to preserve initially normal global function.

Furthermore, because the contractile function of the salvaged and viable but "stunned" myocardium may remain depressed for several days or even weeks following reperfusion, an improvement in ventricular function may not be apparent during the relatively short period during which the patient is hospitalized. It is of importance, however, that this viable but stunned reperfused myocardium is responsive to inotropic stimulation immediately after reperfusion [244–246], which may explain why hemodynamically compromised patients who are refractory to inotropic agents before reperfusion frequently become responsive to them after reperfusion. This property has important implications for the effective management of patients with cardiac failure or cardiogenic shock [247, 248].

Several investigators have suggested that the amount of myocardium salvaged by reperfusion may be augmented by adjuvant pharmacologic therapy designed to decrease the rate of progression of myocardial necrosis prior to reperfusion or to inhibit the potentially toxic effects of increased delivery of calcium ions, superoxide radicals, and other metabolic products to the reperfused myocardium [249–251].

Although limiting the rate of progression of necrosis by administration of beta blockers [252–255], calcium channel antagonists [255–258], glucose–insulin–potassium infusion [259–261], or nitroglycerin [262] is theoretically sound and based on their salutory effects in experimental studies, the ability of these agents to augment the myocardial salvage achieved by reperfusion in clinical practice is unknown. Beta-blocker given in conjunction with rt-PA appeared to afford benefit according to the recent TIMI-IIB trial, but in the clinical study of White et al. [26] there was no potentiation of salvage by pretreatment with beta blockers. These agents may be relatively ineffective in clinical practice, not due to an intrinsic inefficacy at reducing myocardial ischemia but because—in contrast to experimental studies in which they are given prior to or at the commencement of the infarction—in clinical studies they have a limited opportunity to act (only during the relatively short time interval between initiation of treatment and reperfusion). Naylor and colleagues [263] have provided data that seem to support this view by demonstrating that experimental reperfusion injury could be prevented by calcium antagonists only if they had been administered before the onset of ischemic injury rather than only prior to reperfusion. It is conceivable that these agents may be beneficial in circumstances in which there is an anticipated delay until reperfusion, such as when a patient in whom thrombolysis is contraindicated must be transferred for PTCA.

The role of pharmacologic adjuvant therapy in preventing the potentially deleterious consequences of reperfusion is much more tenuous, as there is no firm evidence that reperfusion injury exists [264]. In experimental studies the results of prereperfusion administration of oxygen free-radical scavengers such as catalase and superoxide dismutase have been conflicting [265], and the findings may be model-dependent. A deleterious role for calcium influx into the reperfused myocardium is also controversial, and postreperfusion cellular calcium overload may be a secondary event confined to cells that are already irreversibly damaged at the time of reperfusion [264, 266]. Although it is conceivable that there is a subgroup of patients (yet to be defined) in whom clinically important reperfusion injury does occur, it is likely that in most clinical circumstances reperfusion injury either does not occur or is small and unimportant relative to the extent of salvage achieved by reperfusion.

That myocardial salvage following reperfusion translates into improved survival has been demonstrated by several randomized [13–15, 26, 93, 267, 268] and nonrandomized [232, 269] studies of thrombolysis in acute myocardial infarction. The importance of the early initiation of therapy for survival is highlighted by the Italian (GISSI) study [15, 268], which randomized nearly 12,000 patients to receive either a 1-hour intravenous infusion of 1.5 million units streptokinase or no thrombolytic therapy. There was an overall 18 percent reduction in 21-day mortality in the group who received streptokinase, but the beneficial effect was limited to patients treated within 6 hours of the onset of symptoms. It is of note that the improved survival was proportionately greater with earlier treatment to the extent that the mortality reduction was 47 percent in the subgroup of patients who were treated within 1 hour of the onset of their symptoms. This survival benefit of streptokinase was still apparent at the 12-month follow-up [268]. More recently, White et al. [26] reported an 80 percent reduction in hospital mortality by early treatment with streptokinase. It is likely that similar data will soon be available for the newer thrombolytic agents such as rt-PA.

Summary and Perspective

The available evidence suggests that thrombolytic therapy in patients with evolving acute myocardial infarction can lyse coronary artery thrombus, restore antegrade coronary blood flow, preserve myocardial viability and function, and improve survival. Because the clinical impact of reperfusion is critically dependent on how early it is achieved, future innovative protocols that permit earlier initiation of treatment or treatment in the patient's home or in the ambulance together with the introduction of safer and more effective agents that can achieve a more rapid rate of clot lysis should enhance the potential benefits of thrombolytic therapy.

Editorial Comments

Streptokinase and urokinase are now being widely used as lytic agents for patients with acute myocardial infarction. Until there is a head-to-head comparison of streptokinase with rt-PA, urokinase, and APSAC, debate will continue regarding the various advantages and disadvantages of these agents. A large clinical trial including streptokinase, rt-PA, and possibly APSAC is currently in the planning stages, and a prospective randomized trial comparing streptokinase with rt-PA has begun (GISSI-II). These large clinical trials, although expensive and time-consuming, are our best hope for establishing which lytic agents are most effective. Moreover, such trials provide information on important ancillary issues, such as the concomitant use of heparin, aspirin, and beta blockers. Large trials also more accurately define the "therapeutic window," which currently stands at 0 to 6 hours but may be much larger for certain subsets of patients. The recent ISIS-II trial demonstrated a 25 percent reduction in 5-week mortality with 160 mg of aspirin daily for 1 month. Streptokinase reduced mortality by 35 percent. The benefits of streptokinase and aspirin were highly additive in this study, with the largest reduction in mortality (40–60 percent) observed when the two agents were given together very early. Even the late institution of aspirin and streptokinase had a favorable influence on mortality. G.S.F.

References

1. Maroko, P. R., Libby, P., Gings, W. R., et al. Coronary artery reperfusion 1. Early effects on local myocardial function and the extent of myocardial necrosis. *J. Clin. Invest.* 51:2710, 1972.
2. Ginks, W. R., Sybers, H. D., Maroko, P. R., et al. Coronary artery reperfusion. II. Reduction of myocardial infarct size at 1 week after the coronary occlusion. *J. Clin. Invest.* 51:2717, 1972.
3. Geary, G. G., Smith, G. T., and McNamara, J. J. Defining the anatomic perfusion bed of an occluded coronary artery and the region at risk to infarction: A comparative study in the baboon, pig and dog. *Am. J. Cardiol.* 47:1240, 1981.
4. Karsch, K. R., Hofmann, M., Rentrop, K. P., et al. Thrombolysis in acute experimental myocardial infarction. *J. Am. Coll. Cardiol.* 1:427, 1983.
5. Jennings, R. B., and Reimer, K. A. Factors involved in salvaging ischemic myocardium: Effect of reperfusion of arterial blood. *Circulation* 68(Suppl I):25, 1983.
6. Ganz, W., Ninomya K., Hashida, J., et al. Intracoronary thrombolysis in acute myocardial infarction: Experimental background and clinical experience. *Am. Heart J.* 102:1145, 1981.
7. Markis, J. E., Malagold, M., Parker A., et al. Myocardial salvage after intracoronary thrombolysis with streptokinase in acute myocardial infarction: Assessment by intracoronary thallium-201. *N. Engl. J. Med.* 305:777, 1981.
8. Maddahi, J., Ganz, W., Ninomiya, K., et al. Myocardial salvage by intracoronary thrombolysis in evolving acute myocardial infarction: Evaluation using intracoronary injection of thallium-201. *Am. Heart J.* 102:664, 1981.
9. Schwarz, F., Schuler, G., Katus, H., et al. Intracoronary thrombolysis in acute myocardial infarction: Correlations among serum enzymes, scintigraphic and hemodynamic findings. *Am. J. Cardiol.* 50:32, 1982.
10. Anderson, J. L., Marshall, H. W., Askins, J. C., et al. A randomized trial of intravenous and intracoronary streptokinase in patients with acute myocardial infarction. *Circulation* 70:606, 1984.
11. Charuzi, Y., Beder, C., Marshall, L. A., et al. Improvement in regional and global left ventricular function after intracoronary thrombolysis: Assessment with two-dimensional endocardiography. *Am. J. Cardiol.* 53:662, 1984.
12. Serruys, P. W., Simoons, M. L., Suryapranata, H., et al. Preservation of global and regional left ventricular function after early thrombolysis in acute myocardial infarction. *J. Am. Coll. Cardiol.* 7:729, 1986.
13. Kennedy, J. W., Ritchie, J. L., Davis, K. B., and Fritz, J. K. Western Washington randomized trial of intracoronary streptokinase in acute myocardial infarction. *N. Engl. J. Med.* 309:1477, 1983.
14. Simoons, M. L., van der Brand, M., de Zwaan, C., et al. Improved survival after early thrombolysis in acute myocardial infarction. *Lancet* 2:578, 1985.
15. Gruppo Italiano per lo Studio della Streptochinasi Nell'Infarto Miocardico (GISSI): Effectiveness of intravenous streptokinase thrombolytic treatment in acute myocardial infarction. *Lancet* 1:397, 1986.
16. Reimer, K. A., Lowe, J. E., Rasmussen, M. M., and Jennings, R. B. The wave-front phenomenon of ischemic cell death. I. Myocardial infarct size vs duration of coronary occlusion in dogs. *Circulation* 56:786, 1977.
17. Reimer, K. A., and Jennings, R. B. The wave-front phenomenon of myocardial ischemic cell death. II. Transmural progression of necrosis within the framework of ischemic bed size. *Lab. Invest.* 40:633, 1979.
18. Lee, J. T., Ideker, R. E., and Reimer, K. A. Myocardial infarct size and location in relation to the coronary vascular bed at risk in man. *Circulation* 64:526, 1981.
19. Timmis, G. C., Westveer, D. C., Hauser, A. M., et al. The influence of infarction site and size on the ventricular response to coronary reperfusion. *Arch. Intern. Med.* 145:2188, 1985.
20. Schwarz, F., Schuler, G., Katus, H., et al. Intracoronary thrombolysis in acute myocardial infarction: Duration of ischemia as a major determinant of late results after recanalization. *Am. J. Cardiol.* 50:933, 1982.
21. Lee, G., Joye, J. A., Amsterdam, E. A., et al. Determinants of beneficial coronary streptokinase therapy in acute myocardial infarction: Success and rapidity of thrombolysis depends on minimal time from symptom onset to treatment (Abstract). *Am. J. Cardiol.* 49:973, 1982.
22. Lavallee, M., Cox, D., Patrick, T. A., and Vatner, S. F. Salvage of myocardial function by coronary artery reperfusion 1, 2 and 3

hours after occlusion in conscious dogs. *Circ. Res.* 53:235, 1983.

23. Mathey, D. G., Sheehan, F. H., Schofer, J., and Dodge, H. T. Time from onset of symptoms to thrombolytic therapy: A major determinant of myocardial salvage in patients with acute transmural acute myocardial infarction. *J. Am. Coll. Cardiol.* 6:518, 1985.

24. Koren, G., Weiss, A. T., Hasin, Y., et al. Prevention of myocardial damage in acute myocardial ischemia by early treatment with intravenous streptokinase. *N. Engl. J. Med.* 313:1384, 1985.

25. Vermeer, F., Simoons, M. L., Bar, F. W., et al. Which patients benefit most from early thrombolytic therapy with intracoronary streptokinase. *Circulation* 6:1379, 1986.

26. White, H. D., Norris, R. M., Brown, M. A., et al. Effect of intravenous streptokinase on left ventricular function and early survival after acute myocardial infarction. *N. Engl. J. Med.* 317:850, 1987.

27. Schaper, W., and Pasyk, S. Influence of collateral flow on the ischemic tolerance of the heart following acute and subacute coronary occlusion. *Circulation* 53(Suppl I):57, 1976.

28. Rogers, W. J., Hood, W. P., Jr., Mantle, J. A., et al. Return of left ventricular function after reperfusion in patients with myocardial infarction: Importance of subtotal stenoses or intact collaterals. *Circulation* 69:338, 1984.

29. Friedman, M. The coronary thrombus: Its origin and fate. *Hum. Pathol.* 2:81, 1971.

30. Chandler, A. B., Chapman, I., Erhardt, L. R., et al. Coronary thrombosis in myocardial infarction: Report of a workshop on the role of coronary thrombosis in the pathogenesis of acute myocardial infarction. *Am. J. Cardiol.* 34:823, 1974.

31. Stampfer, M. J., Goldhaber, S. Z., Yusup, S., et al. Effect of intravenous streptokinase on acute myocardial infarction: Pooled results from randomized trials. *N. Engl. J. Med.* 307:1180, 1982.

32. Roberts, W. C., and Buja, L. M. The frequency and significance of coronary arterial thrombi and other observations in fatal acute myocardial infarction: A study of 107 necropsy patients. *Am. J. Med.* 52:425, 1972.

33. DeWood, M. A., Spores, J., Notske, R., et al. Prevalence of total coronary occlusion during the early hours of transmural myocardial infarction. *N. Engl. J. Med.* 303:897, 1981.

34. Rentrop, K. P., Blanke, H., Karsch, K. R., et al. Acute myocardial infarction: Intracoronary application of nitroglycerin and streptokinase. *Clin. Cardiol.* 2:354, 1979.

35. Kanmatsuse K., Lando, U., Mercier, J. F., et al. Rapid lysis of coronary thrombi by local application of fibrinolysin (Abstract). *Circulation* 60(Suppl II):216, 1979.

36. Phillips, S. J., Kongtahworn, C., Skinner, J. R., and Zeff, R. H. Emergency coronary artery reperfusion; a choice therapy for evolving myocardial infarction: Results in 339 patients. *J. Thorac. Cardiovasc. Surg.* 86:679, 1983.

37. Spencer, F. C. Emergency coronary bypass for acute myocardial infarction: An unproved clinical experiment. *Circulation* 68(Suppl II):17, 1983.

38. DeWood, M. A., Spores, J., Berg, R., et al. Acute myocardial infarction: A decade of experience with surgical reperfusion in 701 patients. *Circulation* 68(Suppl II):8, 1983.

39. Rentrop, P., Blanke, H., Karsch, K. R., et al. Selective intracoronary thrombolysis in acute myocardial infarction and unstable angina pectoris. *Circulation* 63:307, 1981.

40. Ganz, W., Buchbinder, N., Marcus, H., et al. Intracoronary thrombolysis in evolving myocardial infarction. *Am. Heart J.* 101:4, 1981.

41. Mathey, D. G., Kuck, K. H., Tilsner, V., et al. Nonsurgical coronary artery recanalization in acute transmural myocardial infarction. *Circulation* 63:489, 1981.

42. Hartzler, G. O., Rutherford, B. D., McConahay, D. R., et al. Percutaneous transluminal coronary angioplasty with and without thrombolytic therapy for treatment of acute myocardial infarction. *Am. Heart J.* 106:965, 1983.

43. O'Neill, W., Timmis, G. C., Bourdillion, P. D., et al. A prospective randomized clinical trial of intracoronary streptokinase versus coronary angioplasty for acute myocardial infarction. *N. Engl. J. Med.* 314:812, 1986.

44. Rothbaum, D. A., Linnemeier, T. J., Landin, R. J., et al. Emergency percutaneous transluminal coronary angioplasty in acute myocardial infarction: A 3 year experience. *J. Am. Coll. Cardiol.* 10:264, 1987.

45. Ganz, W., Geft, I., Maddahi, J., et al. Nonsurgical reperfusion in evolving myocardial infarction. *J. Am. Coll. Cardiol.* 1:1247, 1983.

46. Schroder, R., Biamino, G., Leitner, E. R., et al. Intravenous short-term infusion of streptokinase in acute myocardial infarction. *Circulation* 67:536, 1983.

47. Neuhaus, K. L., Tebbe, U., Sauer, G., et al. High dose intravenous streptokinase in acute myocardial infarction. *Clin. Cardiol.* 6:426, 1983.

48. Spann, J. F., Sherry, S., Carabello, B. A., et al. Coronary thrombolysis by intravenous streptokinase in acute myocardial infarction: Acute and follow up studies. *Am. J. Cardiol.* 53:655, 1984.

49. Sottrup-Sensen, L., Claeys, H., Zasdel, M., et al. The primary structure of human plasmino-

gen: Isolation of two lysine binding fragments and one miniplasminogen (MW 38,000) by elastase-catalyzed-specific limited proteolysis. In J. F. Davidson, R. M. Rowan, M. M. Samama, and P. C. Desnoyers (eds.), *Progress in Chemical Fibrinolysis and Thrombolysis* (Vol. 3). New York: Raven Press, 1978. Pp. 191–209.

50. Claeys, H., Molla, A., and Verstraete, M. Conversion of NH_2-terminal glutamic acid to NH_2-terminal lysine human plasminogen by plasmin. *Thromb. Res.* 3:515, 1973.

51. Sherry, S., Alkjaersig, N., and Fletcher, A. P. Fibrinolysis and fibrinolytic activity in man. *Physiol. Rev.* 39:343, 1959.

52. Tillet, W. S., Edwards, L. B., and Garner, R. L. Fibrinolytic activity of hemolytic streptococci: The development of resistance to fibrinolysis following acute hemolytic streptococcus infections. *J. Clin. Invest.* 13:47, 1934.

53. Reddy, K. N. N. Mechanism of activation of human plasminogen by streptokinase. In Kline and K. N. N. Reddy (eds.), *Fibrinolysis*. Boca Raton: CRC Press, 1980. Pp. 71–94.

54. Reddy, K. N. N., and Markus, G. Mechanism of activation of human plasminogen by streptokinase: Presence of an active center in the streptokinase-plasminogen complex. *J. Biol. Chem.* 247:1683, 1972.

55. Reddy, K. N. N., and Markus, G. Esterase activities in the zymogen moiety of the streptokinase-plasminogen complex. *J. Biol. Chem.* 249:4851, 1974.

56. Claeson, G., Aurell, L., Karlsson, G., and Friberger, P. Substrate structure and activity relationships. In J. F. Davidson, R. M. Rowan, M. M. Samama, and P. C. Desnoyers (eds.), *Progress in Chemical Fibrinolysis and Thrombolysis* (Vol. 3). New York: Raven Press, 1978. Pp. 299–304.

57. Robbins, K. C., Summaria, L., and Wohl, R. C. Human plasmin. *Methods Enzymol.* 80:379, 1981.

58. Wohl, R. C., Arzadon, L., Summaria, L., and Robbins, K. C. Kinetics of activation of human plasminogen by different activation species at pH 7.4 and 37°C. *J. Biol. Chem.* 255:2005, 1980.

59. Smith, R. A. G., Dupe, R. J., English, P. D., and Green, J. Fibrinolysis with acyl-enzymes: A new approach to thrombolytic therapy. *Nature* 290:505, 1981.

60. Cederholm-Williams, S. A., De Cock, F., Lijnen, H. R., and Collen, D. Kinetics of the reaction between streptokinase, plasmin and $alpha_2$-antiplasmin. *Eur. J. Biochem.* 100:125, 1979.

61. Wilman, B. On the reaction of plasmin or plasmin-streptokinase complex with aprotinin or $alpha_2$-antiplasmin. *Thromb. Res.* 17:143, 1980.

62. Fletcher, A. P., Alkjaersig, N., and Sherry, S. The maintenance of a sustained thrombolytic state in man. I. Induction and effects. *J. Clin. Invest.* 38:1096, 1959.

63. Fletcher, A. P., Sherry, S., Alkjaersig, N., et al. The maintenance of a sustained thrombolytic state in man. II. Clinical observations on patients with myocardial infarction and other thromboembolic disorders. *J. Clin. Invest.* 38:1111, 1959.

64. Alkjaersig, N., Fletcher, A. P., and Sherry, S. The mechanism of clot dissolution by plasmin. *J. Clin. Invest.* 38:1086, 1959.

65. Spottl, F., and Holzknecht, F. The influence of inhibitors of plasmin and plasminogen activation on the streptokinase-induced fibrinolytic state. *Thromb. Diath. Haemorrh* 24:101, 1970.

66. Alkjaersig, N., Fletcher, A. P., and Sherry, S. Pathogenesis of the coagulation defect developing during pathological plasma proteolytic ("fibrinolytic") states. I. The significance of fibrinogen proteolysis and circulating fibrinogen breakdown products. *J. Clin. Invest.* 41:896, 1962.

67. Alkjaersig, N., Fletcher, A. P., and Sherry, S. Pathogenesis of the coagulation defect developing during pathological plasma proteolytic ("fibrinolytic") states. II. The significance of, mechanism and consequences of defective fibrin polymerization. *J. Clin. Invest.* 41:917, 1962.

68. Timmis, G. C., Gangadharan, V., Ramos, R. G., et al. Hemorrhage and the products of fibrinogen digestion after intracoronary administration of streptokinase. *Circulation* 69:1146, 1984.

69. Reddy, K. N. N. Kinetics of active center formation in dog plasminogen by streptokinase and activity of a modified streptokinase. *J. Biol. Chem.* 251:6626, 1976.

70. Reddy, K. N. N., Cercek, B., Lew, A. S., and Ganz, W. Interaction of SK-human plasmin, SK-dog plasmin complexes with α_2-antiplasmin and $alpha_2$-macroglobulin. *Thromb. Res.* 41:671, 1986.

71. English, P. D., Smith, R. A. G., Dupe, R. J., et al. The thrombolytic activity of streptokinase in the rabbit. *Thromb. Haemost.* 46:525, 1981.

72. Einarsson, M., Mattson, C., and Nilsson, S. Effect on haemostasis of intravenous injection of $alpha_2$-antiplasmin in cats treated with streptokinase. *Thromb. Res.* 30:205, 1983.

73. Fears, R., Hibbs, M. J., and Smith, R. A. G. Kinetic studies in the interaction of streptokinase and other plasminogen activators with

plasminogen and fibrin. *Biochem. J.* 229:555, 1985.

74. Takada, A., and Takada, Y. Kinetic analysis of potentiation of plasminogen activation by streptokinase in the presence of fibrin or its degradation products. *Haemostasis* 17:1, 1987.

75. Takada, A., Takada, Y., and Sugawara, Y. The activation of Glu- and Lys-plasminogens by streptokinase: Effects of fibrin, fibrinogen and their degradation products. *Thromb. Res.* 37:465, 1985.

76. Spottl, F., and Kaiser, R. Rapid detection and quantitation of precipitating streptokinase antibodies. *Thromb. Diathes. Haemorrh.* 32:608, 1974.

77. James, D. C. O. Anti-streptokinase levels in various hospital patient groups. *Postgrad. Med. J.* 49(Suppl):26, 1973.

78. Hirsh, J., O'Sullivan, E. F., and Martin, M. Evaluation of a standard dosage schedule with streptokinase. *Blood* 35:341, 1970.

79. Moran, D. M., Standring, R., Lavender, E. A., and Harris, G. S. Assessment of anti-streptokinase antibody levels in human sera using a microradioimmunoassay procedure. *Thromb. Haemost.* 52:281, 1984.

80. Lew, A. S., Neer, T., Rodriguez, L., et al. Clinical failure of streptokinase due to an unsuspected high titer of antistreptokinase antibody. *J. Am. Coll. Cardiol.* 4:183, 1984.

81. Prowse, C. V., Hornsey, V., Ruckley, C. V., and Boulton, F. E. A comparison of acylated streptokinase-plasminogen complex in healthy volunteers. *Thromb. Haemost.* 47:132, 1982.

82. Staniforth, D. H., Smith, R. A. G., and Hibbs, M. Streptokinase and anisoylated streptokinase-plasminogen complex: Their action on haemostasis in human volunteers. *Eur. J. Clin. Pharmacol.* 24:751, 1983.

83. Marder, V. J., Rothbard, R. L., Fitzpatrick, P. G., and Francis, C. W. Rapid lysis of coronary artery thrombi with anisoylated plasminogen:streptokinase activator complex: Treatment by bolus injection. *Ann. Intern. Med.* 104:304, 1986.

84. Been, M., De Bono, D. P., Muir, A. L., et al. Coronary thrombolysis with intravenous anisoylated streptokinase-plasminogen complex BRL 26921. *Br. Heart J.* 53:253, 1985.

85. Kasper, W., Erbel, R., Meinhertz, T., et al. Intracoronary thrombolysis with an acylated streptokinase-plasminogen activator (BRL 26921) in patients with acute myocardial infarction. *J. Am. Coll. Cardiol.* 4:357, 1984.

86. Timmis, A. D., Griffin, B., Crick, J. C. P., and Sowton, E. Anisoylated plasminogen streptokinase activator in acute myocardial infarction: A placebo-controlled arteriographic coronary recanalization study. *J. Am. Coll. Cardiol.* 10:205, 1987.

87. Hillis, W. S., and Hornung, R. S. The use of BRL 26921 (APSAC) as fibrinolytic therapy in acute myocardial infarction. *Eur. Heart J.* 6:909, 1985.

88. Fine, D. G., Weiss, A. T., Sapoznikov, D., et al. Importance of early initiation of intravenous streptokinase therapy for acute myocardial infarction. *Am. J. Cardiol.* 58:411, 1986.

89. Bateman, T. M., Czer, L. S. C., Gray, R. J., et al. Transient pathological Q waves during acute ischemic events: An electrocardiographic correlate of the stunned but viable myocardium. *Am. Heart J.* 106:1421, 1983.

90. Mikell, F. L., Petrovich, J., Snyder, M. C., et al. Reliability of Q-wave formation and QRS score in predicting regional and global left ventricular performance in acute myocardial infarction with successful reperfusion. *Am. J. Cardiol.* 57:923, 1986.

91. Lew, A. S., Cercek, B., Lee, M., et al. The relation of the evolution of pathological Q waves following reperfusion in acute myocardial infarction to transmural necrosis: Findings at surgical inspection. *Clin. Res.* 35:110A, 1987.

92. Verheugt, F. W. A., van Eenige, M. J., Res, J. C. J., et al. Bleeding complications of intracoronary fibrinolytic therapy in acute myocardial infarction: Assessment of risk in a randomized trial. *Br. Heart J.* 54:455, 1985.

93. Yusuf, S., Collins, R., Peto, R., et al. Intravenous and intracoronary fibrinolytic therapy in acute myocardial infarction: Overview of results on mortality, reinfarction and side-effects from 33 randomized controlled trials. *Eur. Heart J.* 6:556, 1985.

94. Lew, A. S., Hod, H., Cercek, B., et al. Mortality and morbidity of patients older and younger than 75 years with acute myocardial infarction treated with intravenous streptokinase. *Am. J. Cardiol.* 59:1, 1987.

95. TIMI Operations Committee. Announcement of protocol change in thrombolysis and myocardial infarction change. *J. Am. Coll. Cardiol.* 9:467, 1987.

96. Collen, D. Human tissue-type plasminogen activator: From the laboratory to the bedside. *Circulation* 72:18, 1985.

97. Sobel, B. E., Gross, R. W., and Robison, A. K. Thrombolysis, clot selectivity, and kinetics. *Circulation* 70:160, 1984.

98. Garabedian, H. D., Gold, H. K., Leinbach, R. C., et al. Dose-dependent thrombolysis, pharmacokinetics and hemostatic effects of recombinant human tissue-type plasminogen activator for coronary thrombosis. *Am. J. Cardiol.* 58:673, 1986.

99. Kremer, P., Fiebig, R., Tilsner, V., et al. Lysis

of left ventricular thrombi with urokinase. *Circulation* 72:112, 1985.

100. Stadius, M. L., Davis, K., Maynard, C., et al. Risk stratification for 1 year survival based on characteristics identified in the early hours of acute myocardial infarction: The Western Washington Intracoronary Streptokinase Trial. *Circulation* 74:703, 1986.

101. Ritchie, J. L., Davis, K. B., Williams, D. L., et al. Global and regional left ventricular function and tomographic radionuclide perfusion: The Western Washington Intracoronary Streptokinase in Myocardial Infarction Trial. *Circulation* 70:867, 1984.

102. Simoons, M. L., Serruys, P. W., van der Brand, M., et al. Early thrombolysis in acute myocardial infarction: Limitation of infarct size and improved survival. *J. Am. Coll. Cardiol.* 7:717, 1986.

103. Bates, E. R., Topol, E. J., Kline, E. M., et al. Early reperfusion therapy improves left ventricular function after acute inferior myocardial infarction associated with right coronary artery disease. *Am. Heart J.* 114:261, 1987.

104. Wilber, D., Walton, J., O'Neill, W., et al. Effects of reperfusion on complete heart block complicating anterior myocardial infarction. *J. Am. Coll. Cardiol.* 4:1315, 1984.

105. Kersschot, I. E., Brugada, P., Ramentol, M., et al. Effects of early reperfusion in acute myocardial infarction on arrhythmias induced by programmed stimulation: A prospective, randomized study. *J. Am. Coll. Cardiol.* 7:1234, 1986.

106. Cercek, B., Lew, A. S., Laramee, P., et al. Time course and characteristics of ventricular arrhythmias following reperfusion in acute myocardial infarction. *Am. J. Cardiol.* 60:214, 1987.

107. Gang, E., Hong, M., Wang, F., et al. Does reperfusion influence the incidence of ventricular late potentials in acute myocardial infarction. *Circulation* 76(Supp IV):217, 1987.

108. Nobuyoshi, M., Nosaka, H., and Yasumoto, H. Can intracoronary thrombolysis prevent free wall rupture of acute myocardial infarction? *J. Am. Coll. Cardiol.* 7:107A, 1986.

109. Hochman, J. S., and Choo, H. Limitation of myocardial infarct expansion by reperfusion independent of myocardial salvage. *Circulation* 75:299, 1987.

110. Hutchins, G. M., and Bulkley, B. H. Infarct extension versus extension: Two different complications of acute myocardial infarction. *Am. J. Cardiol.* 41:1127, 1978.

111. Shapiro, E. P., Brinker, J. A., Gottlieb, S. O., et al. Intracoronary thrombolysis 3 to 13 days after acute myocardial infarction for postinfarction angina pectoris. *Am. J. Cardiol.* 55:1453, 1985.

112. Schaper, W. *The Collateral Circulation of the Heart.* Amsterdam: North Holland, 1971.

113. Davis, G. J., Chierchia, S., and Maseri, A. Prevention of myocardial infarction by very early treatment with intracoronary streptokinase. *N. Engl. J. Med.* 311:1488, 1984.

114. Schumacher, W. A., Buda, A. J., and Lucchesi, B. R. Streptokinase thrombolysis in experimental coronary artery thrombosis: Pattern of reflow and effect of a stenosis. *Int. J. Cardiol.* 6:615, 1984.

115. TIMI Study Group. The thrombolysis in myocardial infarction (TIMI) trial: Phase I findings. *N. Engl. J. Med.* 312:932, 1985.

116. Udall, J. A. Noninvasive markers of intravenous streptokinase coronary thrombolysis. *Clin. Cardiol.* 6:86, 1983.

117. Monassier, J. P., Valeix, B., Bory, M., et al. Intracoronary thrombolysis: "Paradoxical" increasing of chest and pain ST elevation during reperfusion (cooperative study) (Abstract). *Eur. Heart J.* 5:25, 1984.

118. Sato, H., Kodama, K., Nanto, S., et al. Abrupt augmentation of ST segment evaluation as a marker of successful coronary thrombolysis in acute myocardial infarction. *Circulation* 74(Suppl II):367, 1986.

119. Kircher, B. J., Topol, E. J., O'Neill, W. W., and Pitt, B. Prediction of infarct artery recanalization after intravenous thrombolytic therapy. *Am. J. Cardiol.* 49:513, 1987.

120. Timmis, G. C., Gangadharan, V., Huaser, A. M., et al. Intracoronary streptokinase in clinical practice. *Am. Heart J.* 104:925, 1982.

121. Bren, G. B., Wasserman, A. G., and Ross, A. M. The electrocardiogram in patients undergoing thrombolysis for myocardial infarction. *Circulation* 76(Suppl II):18, 1987.

122. Ross, A. M., for the TIMI investigators. Electrocardiographic and angiographic correlations in myocardial infarction patients treated with thrombolytic agents: A report from the NHLBI Thrombolysis in Myocardial Infarction (TIMI) trial (Abstract). *J. Am. Coll. Cardiol.* 5:495, 1985.

123. Schwartz, H., Leiboff, R. L., Katz, R. J., et al. Arteriographic predictors of spontaneous improvement in left ventricular function after myocardial infarction. *Circulation* 71:466, 1985.

124. Beller, G. A., Hood, W. B., Jr., and Smith, T. W. Effects of ischaemia and coronary reperfusion on regional myocardial blood flow and on the epicardial electrogram. *Cardiovasc. Res.* 11:489, 1977.

125. Blanke, H., Scherff, F., Karsch, K. R., et al. Electrocardiographic changes after streptokinase-induced recanalization in patients with acute left anterior descending artery obstruction. *Circulation* 68:406, 1983.

126. Von Essen, R., Schmidt, W., Uebis, R., et al. Myocardial infarction and thrombolysis: Electrocardiographic short term and long term results using precordial mapping. *Br. Heart J.* 54:6, 1985.

127. Krucoff, M. W., Green, C. E., Satler, L. F., et al. Noninvasive detection of coronary artery patency using continuous ST-segment monitoring. *Am. J. Cardiol.* 57:916, 1986.

128. Goldberg, S., Urban, P., Greenspon, A., et al. Limitation of infarct size with thrombolytic agents—electrocardiographic indexes. *Circulation* 68(Supp I):77, 1983.

129. Durrer, D., Van Lier, A. A. W., and Buller, J. Epicardial and intramural excitation in chronic myocardial infarction. *Am. Heart J.* 68:765, 1964.

130. Wei, J. Y., Markis, J. E., Malagold, M., and Braunwald, E. Cardiovascular reflexes stimulated by reperfusion of ischemic myocardium in acute myocardial infarction. *Circulation* 67:796, 1983.

131. Esente, P., Giambartolomei, A., Gensini, G. G., and Dator, C. Coronary reperfusion and Bezold-Jarisch reflex (bradycardia and hypotension). *Am. J. Cardiol.* 52:221, 1983.

132. Goldberg, S., Greenspon, A. J., Urban, P. L., et al. Reperfusion arrhythmia: A marker of restoration of antegrade flow during intracoronary thrombolysis for acute myocardial infarction. *Am. Heart J.* 105:26, 1983.

133. Westveer, D. G., Stewart, J., Hauser, A. M., et al. The significance of reperfusion arrhythmias with thrombolytic coronary recanalization (Abstract). *Circulation* 68(Suppl III):410, 1983.

134. Gorgels, A. P., Letsch, I. S., Bar, F. W., et al. Accelerated idioventricular rhythm in persistent ischemic chest pain indicates necrosis and reperfusion (Abstract). *Circulation* 74(Suppl II):11, 1986.

135. Corr, P. B., and Witkowski, F. X. Potential electrophysiologic mechanisms responsible for dysrhythmias associated with reperfusion of ischemic myocardium. *Circulation* 68(Suppl I):16, 1983.

136. Fujimoto, T., Peter, T., Hamamoto, H., and Mandel, W. J. Electrophysiological observations on ventricular tachyarrhythmias following reperfusion. *Am. Heart J.* 105:201, 1983.

137. Blumenthal, M. R., Wang, H. H., and Liu, L. M. P. Experimental coronary artery occlusion and release: Effect on enzymes, electrocardiograms, myocardial contractility and reactive hyperemia. *Am. J. Cardiol.* 36:225, 1975.

138. Vatner, S. F., Baig, H., Manders, W. T., and Maroko, P. R. Effects of coronary artery reperfusion on myocardial infarct size calculated

139. Shell, W., Mickle, D. K., and Swan, H. J. C. Effects of nonsurgical myocardial reperfusion of plasma creatine kinase kinetics in man. *Am. Heart J.* 106:665, 1983.

140. Blanke, H., von Hardenberg, D., Cohen, M., et al. Patterns of creatine kinase release during acute myocardial infarction after nonsurgical reperfusion: Comparison with conventional treatment and correlation with infarct size. *J. Am. Coll. Cardiol.* 3:675, 1984.

141. Herlitz, J., Hjalmarson, A., and Waldenstrom, J. Time lapse from estimated onset of acute myocardial infarction to peak serum enzyme activity. *Clin. Cardiol.* 7:433, 1984.

142. Sato, Y., Degawa, T., Geft, I., et al. Reperfusion makes the relationship of creatine kinase release to infarct size linear and allows accurate measurement of infarct size (Abstract). *Circulation* 68(Suppl III):196, 1983.

143. Sato, Y., Degawa, T., Isojima, K., et al. Following early reperfusion, all the creatine kinase depleted from the necrotic myocardium appears in the blood (Abstract). *J. Am. Coll. Cardiol.* 3:22, 1984.

144. Roberts, R., and Ishikawa, Y. Enzymatic estimation of infarct size during reperfusion. *Circulation* 68(Suppl I):83, 1983.

145. Van der Laarse, A., Vermeer, F., Hermens, W. T., et al. Effects of early intracoronary streptokinase on infarct size estimated from cumulative enzyme release and on enzyme release rate: A randomized trial of 533 patients with acute myocardial infarction. *Am. Heart J.* 112:672, 1986.

146. Drexel, H., and Dienstl, F. Myoglobinemia and reperfusion in myocardial infarction. *N. Engl. J. Med.* 309:1457, 1983.

147. Devries, S. R., Sobel, B. E., and Abendschein, D. R. Early detection of myocardial reperfusion by assay of plasma MM-creatine kinase isoforms in dogs. *Circulation* 74:567, 1986.

148. Puleo, P. R., Perryman, M. B., Bresser, M. A., et al. Creatine kinase isoform analysis in the detection and assessment of thrombolysis in man. *Circulation* 6:1162, 1987.

149. Laramee, P., Lew, A. S., Cercek, B., et al. Evidence that abrupt acceleration of creatine kinase release (washout) and rapid resolution of ST-T elevation are signs of coronary reperfusion. *Circulation* 72(Suppl III):418, 1985.

150. Lewis, B. S., Lew, A. S., and Ganz, W. Bedside recognition of coronary artery reperfusion during thrombolytic therapy. In R. M. Califf, D. B. Mark, and G. S. Wagner (eds.), *Acute Coronary Care in the Thrombolytic Era.* Chicago: Year Book Medical Publishers, 1988 Pp. 260–272.

from creatine kinase. *J. Clin. Invest.* 61:2048, 1978.

151. Tennant, S. N., Dixon, J., Venable, T. C., et al. Intracoronary thrombolysis in patients with acute myocardial infarction: Comparison of the efficacy of urokinase and with streptokinase. *Circulation* 69:756, 1984.

152. Van de Werf, F., Ludbrook, P. A., Bergmann, S. R., et al. Coronary thrombolysis with tissue-type plasminogen activator in patients with evolving myocardial infarction. *N. Engl. J. Med.* 310:609, 1984.

153. Weinstein, J. Treatment of myocardial infarction with intracoronary streptokinase: Efficacy and safety data from 209 United States cases in the Hoechst-Roussel registry. *Am. Heart J.* 104:894, 1982.

154. Weinstein, J. The international registry to support approval of intracoronary streptokinase thrombolysis in the treatment of myocardial infarction. *Circulation* 68(Suppl I):61, 1983.

155. Kennedy, J. W., Gensini, G. G., Timmis, G. C., and Maynard, C. Acute myocardial infarction treated with intracoronary streptokinase: A report of the Society for Cardiac Angiography. *Am. J. Cardiol.* 55:871, 1985.

156. Cowley, M. J. Methodologic aspects of intracoronary thrombolysis: Drugs, dosage and duration. *Circulation* 68(Suppl I):90, 1983.

157. Taylor, G. J., Mikell, F. L., Moses, H. W., et al. Intravenous versus intracoronary streptokinase therapy for acute myocardial infarction in community hospitals. *Am. J. Cardiol.* 54:256, 1984.

158. Valentine, R. P., Pitts, D. E., Brooks-Brunn, J. A., et al. Intravenous versus intracoronary streptokinase in acute myocardial infarction. *Am. J. Cardiol.* 55:309, 1985.

159. Alderman, E. L., Jutzy, K. R., Berte, L. E., et al. Randomized comparison of intravenous versus intracoronary streptokinase for acute myocardial infarction. *Am. J. Cardiol.* 54:14, 1984.

160. Woollard, K. V., Mews, G. C., Cope, G. D., et al. A comparison of intravenous and intracoronary streptokinase in acute myocardial infarction. *Aust. N.Z. J. Med.* 14:475, 1984.

161. Blunda, M., Meister, S. G., Shechter, J. A., et al. Intravenous versus intracoronary streptokinase for acute transmural myocardial infarction. *Cathet. Cardiovasc. Diagn.* 10:319, 1984.

162. Rogers, W. J., Mantle, J. A., Hood, W. P., et al. Prospective randomized trial of intravenous and intracoronary streptokinase in acute myocardial infarction. *Circulation* 68:1051, 1983.

163. Hillis, L. D., Borer, J., Braunwald, E., et al. High dose intravenous streptokinase for acute myocardial infarction: Preliminary results of multicenter trial. *J. Am. Coll. Cardiol.* 6:957, 1985.

164. Ganz, W., Geft, I., Shah, P. K., et al. Intra-venous streptokinase in evolving acute myocardial infarction. *Am. J. Cardiol.* 53:1209, 1984.

165. Rogers, W. J., Hood, W. P., Jr., Reeves, R. C., and Whitlow, P. L. Randomized trial of intracoronary versus intravenous streptokinase in acute myocardial infarction (Abstract). *J. Am. Coll. Cardiol.* 3:525, 1984.

166. Mayer, G., Story, W. E., Seco, J. E., et al. Intravenous streptokinase in acute myocardial infarction. *Ann. Emerg. Med.* 14:410, 1985.

167. Chopra, K. L., Chopra, H. K., Aggarwal, K. K., and Parashar, S. K. Intravenous streptokinase and oral nifedipine in evolving myocardial infarction—a pilot study. *Indian Heart J.* 36:347, 1984.

168. Collen, D. On the regulation and control of fibrinolysis. *Thromb. Haemost.* 73:77, 1980.

169. Lew, A. S., Cercek, B., Hod, H., et al. A high residual plasma fibrinogen following intravenous streptokinase predicts delay or failure of reperfusion in acute myocardial infarction. *Am. J. Cardiol.* 58:680, 1986.

170. Lew, A. S., Laramee, P., Cercek, B., et al. The effects of the rate of intravenous infusion of streptokinase and the duration of symptoms on the time interval to reperfusion in acute myocardial infarction. *Circulation* 72:1053, 1985.

171. Lew, A. S., Laramee, P., Cercek, B., et al. The hypotensive effect of intravenous streptokinase in patients with acute myocardial infarction. *Circulation* 72:1321, 1985.

172. Rutsch, W., Schartl, M., Mathey, D., et al. Percutaneous transluminal coronary recanalization: Procedure, results, and acute complications. *Am. Heart J.* 102:1178, 1981.

173. Gottlob, R., Blumel, G., Piza, F., et al. Studies on thrombolysis with streptokinase. II. The influence of changes due to age in thrombi and whole blood clots. *Thromb. Diath. Haemorrh.* 19:516, 1968.

174. McDonagh, J. Structure and function of factor XIII. In R. W. Colman, J. Hirsch, V. J. Marder, and E. W. Salzman (eds.), *Hemostasis and Thrombosis: Basic Principles and Clinical Practice.* Philadelphia: Lippincott, 1982. Pp. 168–169.

175. Cercek, B., Hod, H., Lew, A. S., et al. 4-Hr old thrombi are bigger and more resistant to lysis than 1-hr old thrombi (Abstract). *Clin. Res.* 34:5A, 1986.

176. Korninger, C., and Collen, D. Studies on the specific fibrinolytic effect of human extrinsic (tissue-type) plasminogen activator in human blood and in various animal species. *Thromb. Haemost.* 46:561, 1981.

177. Stadius, M. L., Maynard, C., Fritz, J. K., et al. Coronary anatomy and left ventricular function in the first 12 hours of acute myocar-

dial infarction: The Western Washington Randomized Intracoronary Streptokinase Trial. *Circulation* 72:292, 1985.

178. Verstraete, M., Bory, M., Collen, D., et al. Randomized trial of intravenous recombinant tissue-type plasminogen activator versus intravenous streptokinase in acute myocardial infarction: Report from the European Cooperative Study Group for recombinant tissue-type plasminogen activator. *Lancet* 1:842, 1985.

179. Lew, A. S., Cercek, B., Lewis, B. S., et al. Efficacy of a 2-hour infusion of 150 mg tissue plasminogen activator in acute myocardial infarction. *Am. J. Cardiol.* 60:1228, 1987.

180. Cercek, B., Lew, A. S., Sato, Y., et al. Heparin enhances experimental thrombolysis by preventing new fibrin deposition. *Circulation* 72(Suppl III):194, 1985.

181. Cercek, B., Lew, A. S., Hod, H., et al. Ancrod enhances the thrombolytic effect of streptokinase and urokinase. *Thromb. Res.* 47:417, 1987.

182. Cercek, B., Lew, A. S., Hod, H., et al. Pretreatment with heparin enhances thrombolysis by tissue type plasminogen activator. *Circulation* 74:683, 1986.

183. Chandler, J. W., Nath, H. P., and Rogers, W. J. Heparin and antiplatelet drugs following streptokinase in acute myocardial infarction (Abstract). *J. Am. Coll. Cardiol.* 3:600, 1984.

184. Kaplan, K., Davison, R., Parker, M., et al. Role of heparin after intravenous thrombolytic therapy for acute myocardial infarction. *Am. J. Cardiol.* 59:241, 1987.

185. Merx, W., Dorr, R., Rentrop, P., et al. Evaluation of the effectiveness of intracoronary streptokinase infusion in acute myocardial infarction: Postprocedure management and hospital course in 204 patients. *Am. Heart J.* 102:1181, 1981.

186. Raizner, A. E., Tortoledo, F. A., Verani, M. S., et al. Intracoronary thrombolytic therapy in acute myocardial infarction: A prospective, randomized, controlled trial. *Am. J. Cardiol.* 55:301, 1985.

187. Urban, P. L., Cowley, M. J., Hastillo, A., et al. Clinical course after myocardial reperfusion during myocardial infarction (Abstract). *Circulation* 68(Suppl III):210, 1983.

188. Bell, W. R., Duckert, H., Fletcher, A. P., et al. Thrombolytic therapy in thrombosis: A National Institutes of Heart consensus development conference. *Ann. Intern. Med.* 93:141, 1980.

189. Sharma, G. V. R. K., Cella, G., Parisi, A. F., and Sasahara, A. A. Thrombolytic therapy. *N. Engl. J. Med.* 306:1268, 1982.

190. Lupinetti, F. M., Stoney, W. S., Alford, W. C., Jr., et al. Cryoprecipitate-topical thrombin glue: Initial experience in patients undergoing cardiac operations. *J. Thorac. Cardiovasc. Surg.* 90:502, 1985.

191. Mentzer, R. L., Budzynski, A. Z., and Sherry, S. High-dose, brief-duration infusion of streptokinase in acute myocardial infarction: Description of effects in the circulation. *Am. J. Cardiol.* 57:1220, 1986.

192. Gold, H. K., Leinbach, R. C., Palacios, I. F., et al. Coronary reocclusion after selective administration of streptokinase. *Circulation* 68(Suppl I):50, 1983.

193. Schroder, R., Vohringer, H., Linderer, T., et al. Follow-up after coronary arterial reperfusion with intravenous streptokinase in relation to residual myocardial infarct artery narrowings. *Am. J. Cardiol.* 55:313, 1985.

194. Schaer, D. H., Ross, A. M., and Wasserman, A. G. Reinfarction, recurrent angina, and reocclusion after thrombolytic therapy. *Circulation* 76(Suppl II):57, 1987.

195. Williams, D. O., Borer, J., Braunwald, E., et al. Intravenous recombinant tissue-type plasminogen activator in patients with acute myocardial infarction: A report from NHLBI thrombolysis in myocardial infarction trial. *Circulation* 73:338, 1986.

196. Karsch, K., Blanke, H., Pichard, A., et al. Changes in the degree of stenosis of the infarct vessel following intracoronary streptokinase (Abstract). *Circulation* 64(Suppl IV):107, 1981.

197. Terrosu, P., Ibba, G. V., Contini, G. M., and Franceschino, V. Angiographic features of the coronary arteries during intracoronary thrombolysis. *Br. Heart J.* 52:154, 1984.

198. Fallon, J. T., Aretz, H. T., and Gold, H. K. Coronary arterial pathology following thrombolytic therapy for acute myocardial infarction (Abstract). *Circulation* 66(Suppl II):336, 1982.

199. Ambrose, J. A., Haft, J. I., Winters, S. L., et al. Coronary morphology in myocardial infarction—response to streptokinase (Abstract). *Clin. Res.* 32:667A, 1984.

200. Brown, B. G., Gallery, C. A., Badger, R. S., et al. Incomplete lysis of thrombus in the moderate underlying atherosclerotic lesion during intracoronary infusion of streptokinase for acute myocardial infarction: Quantitative angiographic observations. *Circulation* 73:653, 1986.

201. Harrison, D. G., Ferguson, D. W., Collins, S. M., et al. Rethrombosis after reperfusion with streptokinase: Importance of geometry of residual lesions. *Circulation* 69:991, 1984.

202. Gash, A. K., Spann, J. F., Sherry, S., et al. Factors influencing reocclusion after coronary thrombolysis for acute myocardial infarction. *Am. J. Cardiol.* 57:175, 1986.

203. Meyer, J., Merx, W., Schmitz, H., et al. Percutaneous transluminal coronary angioplasty

immediately after intracoronary streptolysis of transmural myocardial infarction. *Circulation* 66:905, 1982.

204. Serruys, P. W., Wijns, W., Van Den Brand, M., et al. Is transluminal coronary angioplasty mandatory after successful thrombolysis? Quantitative coronary angiographic study. *Br. Heart J.* 50:257, 1983.

205. Gold, H. K., Cowley, M. J., Palacios, I. F., et al. Combined intracoronary streptokinase infusion and coronary angioplasty during acute myocardial infarction. *Am. J. Cardiol.* 53:122C, 1984.

206. Papapietro, S. E., MacLean, W. A. H., Stanley, A. W. H., et al. Percutaneous transluminal coronary angioplasty after intracoronary streptokinase in evolving acute myocardial infarction. *Am. J. Cardiol.* 55:48, 1985.

207. Holmes, D. R., Jr., Smith, H. C., Vliestra, R. E., et al. Percutaneous transluminal coronary angioplasty, alone or in combination with streptokinase therapy during acute myocardial infarction. *Mayo Clin. Proc.* 60:449, 1985.

208. Mabin, T. A., Holmes, D. R., Smith, H. C., et al. Intracoronary thrombus: Role in coronary occlusion complicating percutaneous transluminal coronary angioplasty (PTCA) (Abstract). *J. Am. Coll. Cardiol.* 3:506, 1984.

209. Sugrue, D. D., Holmes, D. R., Smith, H. C., et al. Coronary artery thrombus as a risk factor for acute vessel occlusion during percutaneous transluminal coronary angioplasty: Improving results. *Br. Heart J.* 56:62, 1986.

210. Topol, E. J., Califf, R. M., George, B. S., et al. A randomized trial of immediate versus delayed elective angioplasty after intravenous tissue plasminogen activator in acute myocardial infarction. *N. Engl. J. Med.* 317:585, 1987.

211. Terrosu, P., Ibba, G. V., Franceschino, V., and Contini, G. M. Late improvement of residual stenosis and LV function after intracoronary thrombolysis (Abstract). *Circulation* 68(Suppl III):413, 1983.

212. Satler, L. F., Green, C. E., McNamara, N. M., et al. Late angiographic follow-up after successful coronary arterial thrombolysis and angioplasty during acute myocardial infarction. *Am. J. Cardiol.* 60:210, 1987.

213. Lew, A. S., Maddahi, J., Hod, H., et al. Utility of early post-reperfusion Tl-201 scintigraphy to assess myocardial viability: Implications for early coronary angioplasty. *Circulation* 74(Suppl II):211, 1986.

214. Nicklas, J. M., Diltz, E. A., O'Neill, W. W., et al. Quantitative measurement of coronary flow during medical revascularization (thrombolysis or angioplasty) in patients with acute infarction. *J. Am. Coll. Cardiol.* 10:284, 1987.

215. Gold, H. K., Leinbach, R. C., Garabedian, H. D., et al. Acute coronary reocclusion after thrombolysis with recombinant human tissue-type plasminogen activator: Prevention by a maintenance infusion. *Circulation* 73:347, 1986.

216. Gold, H. K., Leinbach, R. C., Johns, J. A., et al. Prevention of coronary reocclusion and reduction in late coronary stenosis by maintenance recombinant tissue-type plasminogen activator (rt-PA) infusion (Abstract). *Circulation* 74(Suppl II):368, 1986.

217. Sterling, R. P., Walker, W., Weiland, A. P., et al. Early bypass grafting following intracoronary thrombolysis with streptokinase. *J. Thorac. Cardiovasc. Surg.* 87:487, 1984.

218. Kay, P., Ahmad, A., Floten, S., and Starr, A. Emergency coronary artery bypass surgery after intracoronary thrombolysis for evolving myocardial infarction. *Br. Heart J.* 53:260, 1985.

219. Wellon, H. A., Schneider, J. A., Mikell, F. L., et al. Early operative intervention after thrombolytic therapy for acute myocardial infarction. *J. Vasc. Surg.* 2:186, 1985.

220. Skinner, J. R., Phillips, S. J., Zeff, R. H., and Kongtahworn, C. Immediate coronary bypass following failed streptokinase infusion in evolving myocardial infarction. *J. Thorac. Cardiovasc. Surg.* 87:567, 1984.

221. Becher, H., Schroder, Ch., Mathey, D. G., et al. Coronary artery bypass grafting within 24 hours after intracoronary thrombolysis-risk of bleeding (Abstract). *Eur. Heart J.* 5:177, 1984.

222. Tamaki, S., Murakami, T., Kadota, K., et al. Effects of coronary artery reperfusion on relation between creatine kinase-MB release and infarct size estimated by myocardial emission tomography with thalliun-201 in man. *J. Am. Coll. Cardiol.* 2:1031, 1983.

223. Simoons, M. L., Wijns, W., Balakumaran, K., et al. The effect of intracoronary thrombolysis with streptokinase on myocardial thallium distribution and left ventricular function assessed by blood-pool scintigraphy. *Eur. Heart J.* 3:433, 1982.

224. Maddahi, J., Weiss, A. T., Garcia, E. V., et al. Split-dose thallium-201 quantitative imaging for immediate post-reperfusion assessment of intravenous coronary thrombolysis. *Eur. Heart J.* 6(Suppl E):127, 1985.

225. Maddahi, J., Weiss, I., Geft, I., et al. Coronary thrombolysis with intravenous streptokinase salvages jeopardized myocardium in evolving myocardial infarction: Assessment by quantitative Tl-201 imaging (Abstract). *Circulation* 68(Suppl III):120, 1983.

226. Schuler, G., Schwarz, F., Hofmann, M., et al. Thrombolysis in acute myocardial infarction using intracoronary streptokinase: Assessment by thallium-201 scintigraphy. *Circulation* 66:658, 1982.

227. Maddahi, G., Geft, I., Berman, D., et al. Intracoronary technetium-99m pyrophosphate immediately demonstrates necrosis in reperfused myocardium and complements post-reperfusion intracoronary thallium-201 imaging (Abstract). *Circulation* 66(Suppl II):86, 1982.

228. Schofer, J., Mathey, D. G., Montz, R., et al. Use of dual intracoronary scintigraphy with thallium-201 and technetium-99m pyrophosphate to predict improvement in left ventricular wall motion immediately after intracoronary thrombolysis in acute myocardial infarction. *J. Am. Coll. Cardiol.* 2:737, 1983.

229. De Coster, P. M., Melin, J. A., Detry, J. M. R., et al. Coronary artery reperfusion in acute myocardial infarction: Assessment by pre- and postintervention thallium-201 myocardial perfusion imaging. *Am. J. Cardiol.* 55:889, 1985.

230. Rentrop, P., Blanke, H., Karsch, K. R., et al. Changes in left ventricular function after intracoronary streptokinase infusion in clinically evolving myocardial infarction. *Am. Heart J.* 102:1188, 1981.

231. Sheehan, F. H., Mathey, D. G., Schofer, J., et al. Effect of interventions in salvaging left ventricular function in acute myocardial infarction: A study of intracoronary streptokinase. *Am. J. Cardiol.* 52:431, 1983.

232. Smalling, R. W., Fuentes, F., Mathews, M. W., et al. Sustained improvement in left ventricular function and mortality by intracoronary streptokinase administration during evolving myocardial infarction. *Circulation* 68:131, 1983.

233. Stack, R. S., Phillips, H. R., III, Grierson, D. S., et al. Functional improvement of jeopardized myocardium following intracoronary streptokinase infusion in acute myocardial infarction. *J. Clin. Invest.* 72:84, 1983.

234. Bergmann, S. R., Lerch, R. A., Fox, K. A., et al. Temporal dependence of beneficial effects of coronary thrombolysis characterized by positron tomography. *Am. J. Med.* 73:573, 1982.

235. Sobel, B. E., Geltman, E. M., Tiefenbrunn, A. J., et al. Improvement of regional myocardial metabolism after coronary thrombolysis induced with tissue-type plasminogen activator or streptokinase. *Circulation* 69:983, 1984.

236. Schwaiger, M., Schelbert, H. R., Keen, R., et al. Retention and clearance of C-11 palmitic acid in ischemic and reperfused canine myocardium. *J. Am. Coll. Cardiol.* 6:311, 1985.

237. Guth, B. D., Martin, J. F., Heusch, G., and Ross, J. Regional myocardial blood flow, function and metabolism using phosphorus-31 nuclear magnetic resonance spectroscopy during ischemia and reperfusion. *J. Am. Coll. Cardiol.* 10:673, 1987.

238. Khaja, F., Walton, J. A., Brymer, J. F., et al. Intracoronary fibrinolytic therapy in acute myocardial infarction: Report of a prospective randomized trial. *N. Engl. J. Med.* 308:1305, 1983.

239. Verani, M. S., and Roberts, R. Preservation of cardiac function by coronary thrombolysis during acute myocardial infarction. *J. Am. Coll. Cardiol.* 10:470, 1987.

240. Sheehan, F. H., Braunwald, E., Canner, P., et al. The effect of intravenous thrombolytic therapy on left ventricular function: A report on tissue-type plasminogen activator and streptokinase from the Thrombolysis in Myocardial Infarction (TIMI phase I) trial. *Circulation* 75:817, 1987.

241. Ferguson, D. W., White, C. W., Schwartz, J. L., et al. Influence of baseline ejection fraction and success of thrombolysis on mortality and ventricular function after acute myocardial infarction. *Am. J. Cardiol.* 54:705, 1984.

242. Rentrop, P., Smith, H., Painter, L., and Holt, J. Changes in left ventricular ejection fraction after intracoronary thrombolytic therapy: Results of the Registry of the European Society of Cardiology. *Circulation* 68(Suppl I):55, 1983.

243. Sheehan, F. H., Mathey, D. G., Schofer, J., et al. Factors that determine recovery of left ventricular function after thrombolysis in patients with acute myocardial infarction. *Circulation* 71:1121, 1985.

244. Mercier, J. C., Lando, U., Kanmatsuse, K., et al. Divergent effects of inotropic stimulation on the ischemic and severely depressed reperfused myocardium. *Circulation* 66:397, 1982.

245. Ellis, S. G., Wynne, J., Braunwald, E., et al. Response of reperfusion-salvaged, stunned myocardium to inotropic stimulation. *Am. Heart J.* 107:13, 1984.

246. Arnold, J. M. O., Braunwald, E., Sandor, T., and Kloner, R. A. Inotropic stimulation of reperfused myocardium with dopamine: Effects on infarct size and myocardial function. *J. Am. Cardiol.* 6:1026, 1985.

247. Lewis, B. S., Eigler, N. L., Lew, A. S., and Litvack, F. Salvage of patients in cardiogenic shock by flexible interventional strategies. *Circulation* 76(Suppl IV):261, 1987.

248. Lew, A. S., Weiss, A. T., Shah, P. K., et al. Extensive myocardial salvage and reversal of cardiogenic shock following reperfusion of the left main coronary artery by intravenous streptokinase. *Am. J. Cardiol.* 54:451, 1984.

249. McCord, J. M. Oxygen-derived free radicals in postischemic tissue injury. *N. Engl. J. Med.* 312:159, 1985.

250. Hammond, B., and Hess, M. L. The oxygen free radical system: Potential mediator of myocardial injury. *J. Am. Coll. Cardiol.* 6:215, 1985.

251. Cheung, J. Y., Bonventre, J. V., Malis, C. D., and Leaf, A. Calcium and ischemic injury. *N. Engl. J. Med.* 314:1670, 1986.

252. Reimer, K. A., Rasmussen, M. M., and Jennings, R. B. On the nature of protection by propranolol against myocardial necrosis after temporary coronary occlusion in dogs. *Am. J. Cardiol.* 37:520, 1976.

253. Hammerman, H., Kloner, R. A., Briggs, L. L., and Braunwald, E. Enhancement of salvage of reperfused myocardium by early beta-adrenergic blockade (Timolol). *J. Am. Coll. Cardiol.* 3:1438, 1984.

254. Van de Werf, F., Vanhaecke, J., Jang, I-K., et al. Reduction in infarct size and enhanced recovery of systolic function after coronary thrombolysis with tissue-type plasminogen activator combined with β-adrenergic blockade with metoprolol. *Circulation* 75:830, 1987.

255. Naylor, W. G., Ferrari, R., and Williams, A. Protective effect of pretreatment with verapamil, nifedipine and propranolol on mitochondrial function in the ischemic and reperfused myocardium. *Am. J. Cardiol.* 46:242, 1980.

256. Lange, R., Ingwall, J., Hale, S. L., et al. Preservation of high-energy phosphates by verapamil in reperfused myocardium. *Circulation* 70:734, 1984.

257. McDonagh, P. F., and Roberts, D. J. Prevention of transcoronary macromolecular leakage after ischemia-reperfusion by the calcium entry blocker nisoldipine. *Circ. Res.* 58:127, 1986.

258. Knabb, R. M., Rosamond, T. L., Fox, K. A. A., et al. Enhancement of salvage of reperfused ischemic myocardium by diltiazem. *J. Am. Coll. Cardiol.* 8:861, 1986.

259. Maroko, P. R., Libby, P., Sobel, B. E., et al. Effect of glucose-insulin-potassium infusion on myocardial infarction following experimental coronary artery occlusion. *Circulation* 45:1160, 1972.

260. Rackley, C. E., Russell, R. O., Rogers, W. J., et al. Glucose-insulin-potassium administration in acute myocardial infarction. *Annu. Rev. Med.* 33:375, 1982.

261. Satler, L. F., Green, C. E., Pearle, D. L., et al. The coadministration of streptokinase and glucose-insulin-potassium during acute myocardial infarctions: Effects on left ventricular function (Abstract). *Clin. Res.* 32:832A, 1984.

262. Flaherty, J. T., Becker, L. C., Bulkley, B. H., et al. A randomized prospective trial of intravenous nitroglycerin in patients with acute myocardial infarction. *Circulation* 68:576, 1983.

263. Naylor, W. G., Panagiotopoulos, S., Elz, J. S., and Sturrock, W. J. Fundamental mechanisms of action of calcium antagonists in myocardial ischemia. *Am. J. Cardiol.* 59:75B, 1987.

264. Naylor, W. G., and Elz, J. S. Reperfusion injury: Laboratory artifact or clinical dilemma? *Circulation* 74:215, 1986.

265. Przyklenk, K., and Kloner, R. A. Free radicals: Role in ischemia and infarction. *Cardiology* November, 55, 1986.

266. Murphy, J. G., Marsh, J. D., and Smith, T. W. The role of calcium in ischemic myocardial injury. *Circulation* 75(Suppl V):15, 1987.

267. Kennedy, J. W., Ritchie, J. L., Davis, K. B., et al. The Western Washington randomized trial of intracoronary streptokinase in acute myocardial infarction: A 12 month follow-up report. *N. Engl. J. Med.* 312:1073, 1985.

268. Franzocsi, M. G., Mauri, F., Pampallona, S., et al. The GISSI study: further analysis: Gruppo Italiano per lo Studio della Streptochinasi Nell'Infarto Miocardico. *Circulation* 76(Suppl II):52, 1987.

269. Lew, A. S., Geft, I. L., Shah, P. K., et al. Intracoronary and intravenous streptokinase in acute myocardial infarction—a comparative report. *Eur. Heart J.* 6(Suppl E):223, 1985.

25
Recombinant Tissue Plasminogen Activator in Acute Myocardial Infarction

Eugene R. Passamani

Tissue plasminogen activator is a serine protease found in small concentration (several nanograms per milliliter) in circulating blood; it originates, at least in part, in vascular endothelium [1]. This activator, like all thrombolytic agents, acts by converting plasminogen to plasmin. Streptokinase and urokinase, first-generation thrombolytic agents, are nonspecific plasminogen activators, converting plasminogen to plasmin in circulating blood as well as at the surface of a clot. The second-generation thrombolytic agents, of which tissue plasminogen activator is perhaps the most extensively studied, preferentially activate plasminogen on the surface of thrombus, which considerably increases clot-dissolving efficacy and reduces plasmin-driven consumption of clotting factors. In the absence of fibrin, tissue plasminogen activator is an ineffective activator because of poor plasminogen affinity [2].

Tissue plasminogen activator has been produced in clinically useful amounts by means of recombinant DNA techniques [3]. The U.S. Food and Drug Administration approved a recombinant DNA produced tissue plasminogen activator for use in selected patients with acute myocardial infarction in November 1987.

Thrombosis and Thrombolysis

Intravascular thrombus formation and dissolution are finely balanced processes; pathophysiologic accentuation of either can result in either hemorrhage or vascular closure. Each competing process requires the activation of a key protease from an inert precursor, which in the case of clot formation is thrombin and in the case of thrombolysis is plasmin. A number of circulating inhibitors of these two proteases limit activity to the vicinity of vascular breach or thrombus surface. Appreciable circulating quantities of either thrombin or plasmin cause serious distortion of normal function of both clotting and clot-dissolving systems.

Tissue plasminogen activator (rt-PA) is composed of 527 amino acids. The primary structure of the protein is displayed in Figure 25-1. The molecule has several functional domains [4, 5]. The amino terminus is the location of fibrin-avid structures that draw this protein to fibrin; the carboxy portion contains the active site, which converts plasminogen to plasmin by cleavage of the 560-561 arginine/valine bond. Plasminogen conversion in the absence of fibrin requires large concentrations of rt-PA [2]. Thus the fibrin specificity of rt-PA is lost with large doses given over lengthy periods. Fortunately, the intravenous dose (100 mg) required to produce 80 percent coronary patency rates in acute infarction patients is below the threshold of substantial loss of fibrin specificity in most patients as evidenced by maintenance of fibrinogen levels [6].

Thrombolytic therapy with fibrin-specific agents results in generation of plasmin on the surface of thrombus. As demonstrated in Figure 25-2, the plasmin so generated is immune from inactivation by blood inhibitors and is

443

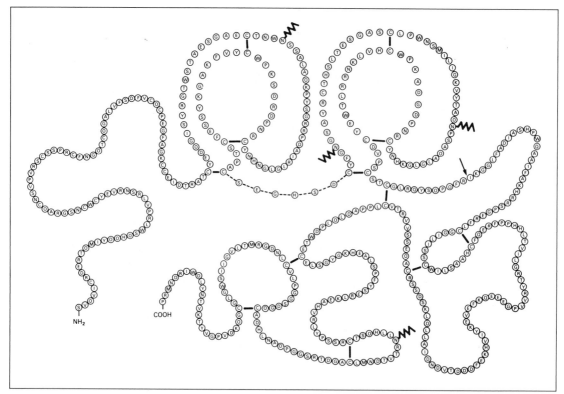

Fig. 25-1
Potential structure of human tissue-type plasminogen activator. Each amino acid is represented by a one-letter code in the open circles. Cysteine residues are shaded, and solid black bars indicate potential disulfide bridges. The two-chain molecule is created from the one-chain form by cleavage at the arrow between arginine and isoleucine. The zigzag lines indicate potential glycosylation sites, and the broken line connects the six amino acids between the two kringles. (From D. Pennica et al. Cloning and expression of human tissue-type plasminogen activated cDNA in *E. coli. Nature* 301:214, 1983. With permission.)

concentrated at the point of action. Commonly used doses of first-generation thrombolytic agents (streptokinase and urokinase) and high doses of rt-PA result in widespread indiscriminate plasminogen activation [7, 8]. Rapid plasmin generation exhausts plasmin inhibitors, resulting in circulating plasmin and consumption of fibrinogen, factor V, and factor VIII. Uncontrolled production of plasmin produces the twin evils of exhaustion of plasminogen supply, wasting plasmin bound by inhibitors, and consumption of clotting reserve with concomitant increased risk of bleeding.

Coronary Thrombosis

Clinicians and pathologists of the nineteenth century recognized coronary thrombosis at necropsy and believed it to be instantaneously fatal. Herrick, in an important paper in 1912, asserted that coronary closure with thrombus was not always fatal and thus described the syndrome of nonfatal myocardial infarction secondary to coronary thrombosis [9]. However, myocardial necrosis can occur in the absence of occlusive coronary thrombus, and the primacy of thrombotic coronary closure in the pathophysiology of myocardial infarction was vigorously debated for 70 years [10, 11].

During the late 1970s, application of coronary arteriography to patients in the early hours of myocardial infarction permitted a direct test of this hypothesis. It quickly became apparent that 80 percent of patients with ischemic chest pain of 30 minutes' duration as-

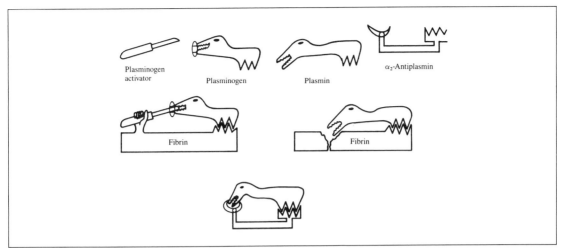

Fig. 25-2
Molecular scheme of fibrin-specific thrombolysis. The fibrin surface provides a platform for efficient plasminogen activation and protects plasmin from inactivation by α_2-antiplasmin. (From M. Verstraete and J. Vermylen. *Thrombosis*. London: Pergamon, 1984. P. 43. With permission.)

sociated with ST segment elevation had closed coronary arteries subtending ischemic myocardium; intracoronary infusion of thrombolytic drugs opened these arteries in 60 to 90 percent of patients [12, 13].

Clinical Trial Findings

Investigative attention was quickly drawn to the use of intravenous thrombolytic drugs in the hope of avoiding the delay, discomfort, risk, and expense of immediate coronary arteriography and intracoronary delivery by catheter. An international clinical trial effort has produced important data from a number of randomized trials on which therapeutic decisions can be based. In general, the form of these trials tended to fall into one of two categories: (1) simple protocols involving thousands of patients utilizing mortality as the primary endpoint; (2) smaller, more complex protocols designed either to compare coronary thrombolytic potential of various intravenously administered clot-dissolving drugs or to make drug–placebo comparisons using the left ventricular ejection fraction determined several weeks later as the primary endpoint.

Two large trials designed to assess the effect of large-dose intravenous streptokinase (SK) have revealed modest but important reductions in hospital mortality. The first trial,

GISSI, involved nearly 12,000 patients admitted to the trial within 12 hours of onset of chest pain [14, 15]. These patients were randomly assigned to intravenous SK (1.5 million units over 1 hour) or to no SK. Mortality rates observed at hospital discharge were 10.7 and 13.0 percent in the SK and control groups, respectively, an 18 percent reduction. At 1 year, the mortality difference persisted with SK and control mortality rates of 17.2 and 19.0 percent, respectively, a 9 percent reduction. Thus for every 1000 patients with acute infarction treated with 1.5 million units of intravenous SK, 23 patients destined to die under conventional management on average survive hospitalization, and at 1 year it falls to 18 additional survivors. An important GISSI finding is the time dependency of the treatment effect; for those treated within 3 hours of onset of chest pain a 23 percent reduction in hospital mortality was observed, and in those treated within 1 hour a 47 percent reduction was noted. These substantial reductions in short-term mortality persisted and are statistically significant at 1 year, 13 percent reduction in those treated within 3 hours (15.1 percent mortality in SK and 17.3 percent in control patients) and

39 percent reduction in those treated within 1 hour (12.9 percent mortality in SK patients and 21.2 percent in controls).

A second large trial, ISIS-II, completed recruitment in December 1987. Although complete details are not available, among approximately 4000 patients randomized to SK or placebo within 4 hours the short-term mortality observed was 8 and 12 percent in SK and placebo groups, respectively, a 33 percent reduction [16]. In addition, trials reported from The Netherlands, West Berlin, and Seattle support the GISSI and ISIS-II results [17–21]. These large mortality trials provided the crucial bit of evidence that closed the causal link between the formation of an occlusive coronary clot and subsequent mortality. Interruption of the infarction process by earlier treatment and the development of more effective thrombolytic regimens promise substantial myocardial salvage and attendant reduction in subsequent mortality and morbidity.

Early rt-PA Trials

There have been a number of trials designed to evaluate the comparative efficacy of rt-PA and SK [7, 22–25]. In addition, several trials designed to assess the effect of rt-PA compared with placebo on subsequent left ventricular function have been reported [26, 27]. Two independent trials—Thrombolysis in Myocardial Infarction (TIMI-I) in the United States and the European Collaborative Study—compared the thrombolytic efficacy of rt-PA and SK in patients with acute infarction [7, 23]. In TIMI-I, 290 patients with acute infarction were randomly assigned to 1.5 million units of intravenous SK (147 patients) given over 1 hour or to 80 mg of rt-PA (143 patients) given intravenously over 3 hours (40, 20, and 20 mg over the first, second, and third hours, respectively). Treatment assignment was masked, with all patients receiving two infusions, either rt-PA and SK placebo or the reverse. All patients underwent pretreatment coronary arteriography. Among 233 patients with closed coronary arteries prior to treatment, 62 percent of those treated with rt-PA and 31 percent

of those treated with SK demonstrated reperfusion at 90 minutes. The proportion of infarct-related arteries open 90 minutes after initiation of rt-PA or SK in all 290 randomized patients, irrespective of pretreatment arteriographic findings, was 70 and 42 percent, respectively. The mean time from onset of chest pain to start of treatment was 285 minutes. The TIMI investigators concluded that rt-PA was about twice as effective as SK for opening closed coronaries [23].

The European Collaborative Group conducted a similar trial comparing rt-PA and SK [7]. Trial design was similar to TIMI-I except that a slightly smaller dose of rt-PA was used (0.75 mg/kg), and there was no pretreatment coronary arteriography permitting initiation of therapy at an average of 2.8 hours after onset of chest pain, in contrast to the TIMI-I study in which mean time to treatment was 4.8 hours. A total of 129 patients were randomized, 64 to rt-PA and 65 to SK. Coronary patency rates at coronary arteriography approximately 90 minutes after the start of intravenous rt-PA and SK were 70 and 55 percent, respectively. Thus the European Collaborative Group reported patency of the infarct-related artery approximately 90 minutes after initiation of rt-PA infusion in exactly the same percentage as was found in TIMI-I (70 percent). The patency rate after the same dose of intravenous SK was higher in the European trial (55 percent) than in TIMI-I (42 percent). This difference may be related to the time from onset of chest pain to initiation of SK infusion. Reperfusion rates after intravenous SK dropped with increasing duration of chest pain prior to initiation of treatment, whereas no such relation is observed with rt-PA [23]. Thus both TIMI-I and the European Collaborative Group found substantial differences in the rates of coronary patency rates between groups assigned to intravenous rt-PA and SK. The dose of SK used in both trials was identical to that used in the GISSI and ISIS-II trials.

In both the European collaborative study and TIMI-I, mean fibrinogen levels fell by two-thirds in patients randomized to SK and by one-third in patients randomized to rt-PA

[7, 23]. Measurement of plasminogen and fibrin(ogen) degradation products provided consistent data. Plasminogen levels fell by approximately one-half in the rt-PA group and by 80 percent in the SK group. Fibrinogen degradation products increased two- to threefold more in the SK than in the rt-PA group. The European study group noted appreciably fewer bleeding complications in the rt-PA patients, whereas bleeding complications were similar in the rt-PA and SK groups in TIMI-I. There were no intracranial hemorrhages reported in TIMI-I; in the European study, one transient ischemic attack occurred in an rt-PA patient and one cerebrovascular accident in an SK-treated patient. Thus the two trials reported similar findings in SK and rt-PA patients with respect to clotting system changes. Transfusions were given in TIMI-I in 29 percent of rt-PA patients and 27 percent of those treated with SK. Transfusions were given to 6 and 8 percent of the rt-PA and SK groups, respectively, in the European study. Approximately 75 percent of transfusions in TIMI-I were related to bleeding at the catheterization site and were therefore an artifact of the experimental protocol. The rather large contrast in transfusion rates between TIMI-I and the European trial is unexplained but may relate to the degree of instrumentation, the intensity of the anticoagulation regimen, and population differences. Whatever the reason, vascular invasion should be kept to an absolute minimum with thrombolytic therapy.

New rt-PA Preparation

The rt-PA preparation (G11021) used in both TIMI-I and the European study was provided by Genentech, which shortly after completion of these trials changed the rt-PA production process, resulting in a preparation with slightly different pharmacokinetic properties (G11044). Given the promise of rt-PA noted in TIMI-I and the European Collaborative Study, the TIMI investigators subsequently conducted a series of investigations with increasing doses of the new rt-PA preparation [6]. During the same series of investigations,

they explored the feasibility of applying percutaneous transluminal coronary angioplasty (PTCA) over the several days following rt-PA treatment in an effort to determine the feasibility of applying PTCA to reduce the occurrence of reocclusion [28].

The proportion with reperfusion at 30, 60, and 90 minutes following doses of 50, 70, and 100 mg of rt-PA over 90 minutes as part of a total dose of 80, 100, and 150 mg, respectively, is displayed in Figure 25-3 and compared with that observed after administration of 50 mg of G11021 over 90 minutes. The reperfusion rate at 90 minutes is similar for the higher two doses. The 150-mg dose results in a higher proportion with reperfusion at 30 minutes. Although the 150 mg given with a 9-mg bolus and a total of 90 mg during the first hour, 20 mg during the second hour, and 10 mg during each of the subsequent 4 hours results in earlier re-

Fig. 25-3
Coronary reperfusion at 30, 60, and 90 minutes after initiation of intravenous rt-PA. Doses at each time point are as follows: (□) 20, 40, and 50 mg of G11021 rt-PA; (△) 20, 40, and 50 mg of G11044 rt-PA; (○) 33, 60, and 70 mg of G11044 rt-PA; (●) 50, 90, and 100 mg of G11044 rt-PA. (From H. Mueller et al. Thrombolysis in myocardial infarction (TIMI): Comparative studies of coronary reperfusion and systemic fibrinogenolysis with two forms of recombinant tissue-type plasminogen activator. *J. Am. Coll. Cardiol.* 10:479, 1987. With permission.)

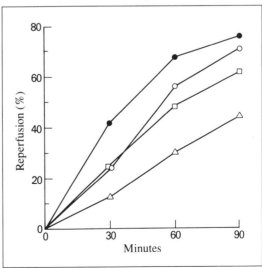

perfusion, it is associated with an observed rate of intracranial hemorrhage of 1.6 percent. The rate with the 100-mg dose is 0.6 percent [29]. Thus it appears that the optimum dose of commercially available rt-PA is 100 mg given over a period of 3 to 6 hours. This dose results in reperfusion rates similar to that observed with intracoronary delivery of thrombolytic drugs. This 80 percent patency rate may represent a structural limit on drug-induced coronary reperfusion.

The risks of the new rt-PA preparation are confined to hemorrhage. The risk of hemorrhage increases with the dose of rt-PA and probably with the intensity of the concomitant heparin administration and the degree of instrumentation of the patient [29]. Approximately three-fourths of hemorrhagic complications are related to femoral arterial puncture carried out prior to or shortly after administration of rt-PA coupled with withdrawal of substantial amounts of blood for diagnostic purposes. In addition, 5 to 10 percent of patients have been noted to have some evidence of gastrointestinal hemorrhage, most without clinical consequence.

These rates of hemorrhagic complications were observed in patients who were selected for treatment after application of the exclusion factors listed in Table 25-1. The occurrence of hemorrhagic complications in patients given thrombolytic therapy can be related to one of two mechanisms or a combination of the two: (1) dissolution of a clot that is maintaining vascular competence, for example, a clot formed at the site of arterial puncture or in the base of a duodenal ulcer; (2) consumption of important components of the clotting system with ultimate compromise of hemostasis.

It is unlikely that new thrombolytic drugs or conceivable combinations of such drugs will dissolve occlusive coronary clots without attacking thrombi serving to maintain vascular integrity. However, as noted above, clinically effective doses of rt-PA result in much less perturbation of the clotting system. It is likely that manipulation of the intensity of heparin administration, further refinement of patient selection, and reduction of vascular invasion to a minimum can further reduce hemorrhagic complications with rt-PA.

Table 25-1
Contraindications to thrombolytic therapy

| Active hemorrhage or hemorrhagic diathesis |
| History of cerebrovascular event |
| Intracranial neoplasm, arteriovenous malformation or aneurysm |
| Uncontrolled hypertension (>180/110 mm Hg) |
| Major surgical procedure or other severe trauma within 10 days |
| Cardiopulmonary resuscitation |

Left Ventricular Function Trials

Two placebo-controlled trials of rt-PA utilizing subsequent left ventricular function as the primary endpoint have demonstrated substantial myocardial salvage. The first, done in Australia, randomized 136 patients who presented with ST segment elevation within 2.5 hours of the onset of chest pain [27]. The mean time from onset of chest pain to initiation of intravenous infusion of rt-PA (100 mg over 3 hours) was 1.9 hours in these patients with first infarction. The left ventricular ejection fraction, as assessed by contrast left ventriculography at 21 days, was 0.62 in patients treated with rt-PA compared with 0.54 in those treated with placebo, a statistically significant and biologically meaningful improvement.

A similar placebo-controlled trial, carried out by investigators at Johns Hopkins University, randomized 138 patients with chest pain and ST elevation to rt-PA or placebo [26]. Left ventricular ejection fraction determined by radionuclear ventriculography at hospital discharge was 0.54 compared with 0.48 in placebo patients. The dose used in this trial was 80 mg over 3 hours of the first rt-PA preparation (G11021) in the initial one-third of patients recruited and 100 mg of the new rt-PA preparation over 3 hours in the last two-thirds of patients. This trial accepted patients with prior infarction and included a second randomization to PTCA in those thought to be candidates.

These two placebo-controlled trials demonstrating important improvements in left ventricular ejection fraction in the wake of acute infarction and were important elements in the November 1987 Federal Drug Administration

(FDA) decision to approve rt-PA for use in patients with myocardial infarction.

Patient Selection

A major advance in clinical cardiology over the past two decades has been the identification of easily measured risk factors for subsequent mortality and morbidity in patients during the early hours of myocardial infarction. Advancing age, female sex, anterior electrocardiographic location of ST segment elevation, presence of rales, presence of hypotension, and history of prior infarction are important indicators of an increased likelihood of subsequent mortality. After exclusion of patients likely to suffer serious bleeding complications, use of rt-PA should be predicated on the intention to interrupt infarction in patients likely to suffer major myocardial loss if rt-PA is not given. A spectrum of patients with varying need of rt-PA can be constructed ranging from the patient with anterior ST segment elevation seen within 30 minutes of onset to the patient with inferior ST elevation arriving 5 hours after onset of symptoms.

In the first instance, in the absence of contraindications, rt-PA should almost invariably be given; in the second, it should be considered only under certain circumstances (e.g., persistance of severe pain). In patients with inferior ST segment elevation who arrive at the hospital within the first 2 to 4 hours and those with anterior ST segment elevation who arrive within 4 hours after onset, rt-PA might be given if the clinician believes that substantial amounts of myocardium are salvageable and if the risk of hemorrhagic complications are low.

It is likely that the risk of hemorrhagic complications with rt-PA is not related to the time elapsed from onset of chest pain to initiation of infusion. However, substantial experimental and clinical data support the notion that, in general, myocardial necrosis after coronary occlusion is rapid, and this hypothesis is supported by data from independent clinical trials.

Thrombolytic therapy for selected patients with acute infarction has been clearly established with the publication of GISSI and ISIS-II, with supportive data from other trials assessing SK and the Australian and Johns Hopkins studies of rt-PA demonstrating drug-induced preservation of left ventricular function. The direct comparison of thrombolytic efficacy of SK and rt-PA carried out in TIMI-I and in the European Collaborative Study. Cost considerations aside, rt-PA is the preferred agent of many cardiologists based on higher reperfusion rates, lack of hemodynamic changes, and far less perturbation of the clotting system. There remain, however, a number of important questions that are the subject of intense investigation at present.

Future Research Directions

Refinement of thrombolytic regimens for acute infarction patients to improve reperfusion rates and, more importantly, reduction of the risk of hemorrhagic complications is a major goal. It is unlikely that foreseeable regimens will result in major improvement in the current patency rate of 75 to 85 percent observed with rt-PA. However, as noted above, intracranial hemorrhage occurs in an estimated 0.6 percent of patients treated with rt-PA with application of current exclusion criteria, and gastrointestinal hemorrhage is noted in an additional 5 to 10 percent [7, 23, 25, 29]. Furthermore, some of the one in eight acute infarction patients with contraindications to thrombolytic therapy might be treated with safer regimens; and patients over age 75 who have heretofore not been intensely studied and who account for 50 percent of in-hospital acute myocardial infarction mortality might be considered as well. Research interest is now focused on combinations of thrombolytic agents in hopes that low doses of each individual agent will deliver high reperfusion rates with less risk of bleeding [30–32].

A second important area of investigation includes the addition of nonthrombolytic drugs to improve reperfusion rates, increase the time from coronary occlusion to irreversible myocardial necrosis, blunt reperfusion injury, and reduce reocclusion rates. The optimal use of heparin, antiplatelet agents, and other anticoagulants in the wake of thrombolytic therapy for acute infarction patients has not been carefully studied. The goal of administration of these agents would be to improve reperfusion rates and reduce the incidence of reocclusion. The need for and optimal mix of these anticoagulants with thrombolytic drugs are unknown.

Prolongation of the interval between coronary occlusion and myocardial necrosis may be possible with the use of agents that reduce myocardial oxygen demands, including such drugs as vasodilators, calcium channel blockers, and beta blockers. The use of intravenous beta blockers appears to have a favorable influence on nonfatal reinfarctions and recurrent ischemic episodes according to the results of the TIMI phase II trial [33].

Determination of the importance of reperfusion injury and estimation of the likelihood of reducing this injury by means of free radical scavengers are areas of active research [34–36]. Whether these agents, which include superoxide dismutase and others, and improve outcome over and above simple reperfusion is at present unknown.

A major unknown is whether the infarct-related lesion can be stabilized by means of drug therapy or all or most patients treated with thrombolytic therapy require cardiac catheterization and either PTCA or coronary artery bypass graft surgery (CABG) to consolidate and perhaps improve gains derived from coronary clot dissolution. The use of PTCA and CABG in GISSI was limited (PTCA, 0.25 percent; CABG, 2.9 percent). Thus the use of SK without further invasive efforts appears to deliver a modest benefit if given within 6 hours of onset and a major mortality reduction if given within 1 hour of onset of pain. Whether general or selective use of PTCA or CABG, or both, during the days and weeks following thrombolytic therapy can improve mortality outcome is at present still debated. It appears that rt-PA followed by immediate PTCA is no more beneficial than rt-PA followed by elective PTCA [37], or PTCA only if there is spontaneous or exercise-induced ischemia following infarction [33].

Preferable Thrombolytic Agent

It is clear that the ideal thrombolytic drug is not yet available. Such an agent would be inexpensive, effective, and safe and its use predicated on large, carefully performed, randomized clinical trials. There are at present two extensively studied candidates, SK and rt-PA. SK reduced mortality in two large intravenous trials, with supporting data from other smaller trials. The drug is relatively inexpensive. However, it is only modestly effective in opening closed coronaries (31 percent reperfusion in TIMI-I) and in observed patency (42 percent in TIMI-I and 55 percent in the European Collaborative Study.) Given in the dose used in these studies (1.5 million units over 1 hour), it results in a profound, prolonged disruption of the clotting system. Streptokinase is often associated with hypotension, occasionally with fever and chills, and rarely with severe allergic reactions. Physicians are reluctant to repeat SK administration, as it is a foreign protein and likely to elicit an immune response.

The newer agent, rt-PA, is expensive, and it has not been shown to reduce mortality in large placebo-controlled trials. Placebo-controlled mortality trials have not been done because of ethical constraints against randomization of early infarction patients to placebo given the clear-cut GISSI and ISIS-II findings. However, rt-PA is a more effective coronary clot thrombolytic and is effective in doses that result in only modest disruption of the clotting system. Moreover, two carefully done placebo-controlled trials have demonstrated substantial myocardial salvage, as demonstrated by improved left ventricular ejection fractions [26, 27]. There are only rare hemodynamic changes associated with administration, virtually no allergic reactions, and no immune response that has been noted. A number of European trials in the planning stages may carry out large direct randomized comparison of rt-PA and SK using a mortality endpoint. Data from these trials will help guide drug choice in the future.

Early Treatment

Whatever thrombolytic agent or agents are ultimately shown to be most effective with the least side effects, and whatever adjuncts are used, the major limiting feature of this form of therapy for patients with acute myocardial infarction is delay to initiation of treatment. Myocardial necrosis occurs with varying rapidity in various animal models. In humans, necrosis is probably complete by 6 hours and is largely completed by 3 hours. However, recent data indicate that mortality may be improved when lytic agents are used up to 24 hours after the clinical onset of myocardial infarction [38].

Delay in initiation of treatment is due to patient delay in seeking medical therapy and then delay in diagnosis, screening, and initiation of treatment when the patient enters the health care system. It is important that potential infarction patients be made aware of the signs and symptoms of acute infarction and the emergency systems be prepared to expeditiously screen patients complaining of these symptoms. Patients with acute myocardial infarction can never be treated too early given accurate diagnosis and careful exclusion of those with contraindications.

Editorial Comments

Passamani has been a principal figure in the development of the NIH-sponsored TIMI trials. These important trials have established the safety and efficacy of rt-PA as lytic therapy for patients with acute myocardial infarction and have refined our knowledge of dosing requirements. Certain important questions remain, however. Are there definite advantages of rt-PA over less expensive lytic agents? Can new generations of rt-PA be made more clot-specific with a reduction in bleeding complications? Can improvement in regional wall motion activity be translated into a clear-cut improvement in survival? Can the rather narrow "therapeutic window" be widened to broaden the application of therapy? Are ancillary measures such as aspirin, heparin, beta blockers, and angioplasty of major importance? Answers to these and other questions must await future controlled trials. G.S.F.

References

1. Rijken, D. C., Wijngaards, G., and Welbergen, J. Relationship between tissue plasminogen activator and the activators in blood and vascular wall. *Thromb. Res.* 18:815, 1982.
2. Hoylaerts, M., Rijken, D. C., Lijnen, H. R., et al. Kinetics of the activation of plasminogen by human tissue plasminogen activator: Role of fibrin. *J. Biol. Chem.* 257:2912, 1982.
3. Pennica, D., Holmes, W. E., Kohr, W. J., et al. Cloning and expression of human tissue-type plasminogen activator cDNA in E. coli. *Nature* 301:214, 1983.
4. Ny, T., Elgh, F., and Lund, B. The structure of the human tissue-type plasminogen activator gene: Correlation of intron and exon structures to functional and structural domains. *Proc. Natl. Acad. Sci. U.S.A.* 81:5355, 1984.
5. Holvoet, P., Lijnen, H. R., and Collen, D. Characterization of functional domains in human tissue-type plasminogen activator with the use of monoclonal antibodies. *Eur. J. Biochem.* 158:173, 1986.
6. Mueller, H. S., Rao, A. K., Forman, S. A., and the TIMI investigators. Thrombolysis in myocardial infarction (TIMI): Comparative studies of coronary reperfusion and systemic fibrinogenolysis with two forms of recombinant tissue-type plasminogen activator. *J. Am. Coll. Cardiol.* 10:479, 1987.
7. Verstraete, M., Bernard, R., Bory, M., et al. Randomised trial of intravenous recombinant tissue-type plasminogen activator versus intravenous streptokinase in acute myocardial infarction. *Lancet* 1:842, 1985.
8. Tiefenbrunn, A. J., Graor, R. A., Robinson, A. K., et al. Pharmacodynamics of tissue-type plasminogen activator characterized by computer-assisted simulation. *Circulation* 73:1291, 1986.
9. Herrick, J. B. Clinical features of sudden obstruction of the coronary arteries. JAMA 59:2015, 1912.
10. Friedberg, C. K., and Horn, H. Acute myocardial infarction not due to coronary artery occlusion. JAMA 112:1675, 1939.

11. Miller, R. D., Burchell, H. B., and Edwards, J. E. Myocardial infarction with and without acute coronary occlusion; a pathologic study. *Arch. Intern. Med.* 88:597, 1951.

12. DeWood, M. A., Spores, J., Notske R., et al. Prevalence of total coronary occlusion during the early hours of transmural myocardial infarction. *N. Engl. J. Med.* 303:897, 1980.

13. Rentrop, P. K. Thrombolytic therapy in patients with acute myocardial infarction. *Circulation* 71:627, 1985.

14. GISSI. Effectiveness of intravenous thrombolytic treatment in acute myocardial infarction. *Lancet* 1:377, 1986.

15. GISSI. Long-term effects of intravenous thrombolysis in acute myocardial infarction: Final report of the GISSI study. *Lancet* 2:871, 1987.

16. ISIS. Intravenous streptokinase given within 0–4 hours of onset of myocardial infarction reduced mortality in ISIS-2. *Lancet* 1:502, 1987.

17. Simoons, M. L., van der Brand, M., De Zwann, C., et al. Improved survival after early thrombolysis in acute myocardial infarction. *Lancet* 2:578, 1985.

18. Simoons, M. L., Serruys, P. W., van der Brand, M., et al. Early thrombolysis in acute myocardial infarction: Limitation of infarct size and improved survival. *J. Am. Coll. Cardiol.* 7:717, 1986.

19. ISAM Study Group. A prospective trial of intravenous streptokinase in acute myocardial infarction (ISAM): Mortality, morbidity, and infarct size at 21 days. *N. Engl. J. Med.* 314:1465, 1986.

20. Schroder, R., Neuhaus, K. L., Leizorovicz, A., et al. A prospective placebo-controlled double-blind multicenter trial of intravenous streptokinase in acute myocardial infarction (ISAM): Long-term mortality and morbidity. *J. Am. Coll. Cardiol.* 9:197, 1987.

21. Martin, G. V., Stadius, M. L., Davis, K. B., et al. The Western Washington intravenous streptokinase trial: Effects of intravenous streptokinase on vessel patency and left ventricular function (Abstract) *Circulation* 74(Suppl II):11, 1986.

22. The TIMI Study Group. The thrombolysis in myocardial infarction (TIMI) trial: Phase I findings. *N. Engl. J. Med.* 312:932, 1985.

23. Chesebro, J. H., Knatterud, G., Roberts, R., et al. Thrombolysis in myocardial infarction (TIMI) trial: Phase I: a comparison between intravenous tissue plasminogen activator and intravenous streptokinase clinical findings through hospital discharge. *Circulation* 76:142, 1987.

24. Sheehan, F. H., Braunwald, E., Canner P., et al. The effect of intravenous thrombolytic therapy on left ventricular function: A report on tissue plasminogen activator and streptokinase from the thrombolysis in myocardial infarction (TIMI phase I) trial. *Circulation* 75:817, 1987.

25. Rao, A. K., Pratt, C., Berke, A., et al. The thrombolysis in myocardial infarction trial: Phase I: hemorrhagic, manifestations, complications, and changes in plasma fibrinogen and fibrinolytic system. *J. Am. Coll. Cardiol.* (in press).

26. Guerci, A., Gerstenblith, G., Brinker, J., et al. A double-blinded, placebo-controlled, randomized trial of rt-PA with subsequent randomization to elective PTCA for acute MI. *N. Engl. J. Med.* (in press).

27. O'Rourke, M., Baron, D., Keogh, A., et al. Randomized, placebo-controlled, double blind trial of intravenous tissue-type plasminogen activator initiated within 2½ hours of symptom onset in acute coronary occlusion. *Circulation* (in press).

28. Williams, D. O., Ruocco, N. A., Forman, S., and the TIMI investigators. Coronary angioplasty following recombinant tissue-type plasminogen activator in acute myocardial infarction: A report from the thrombolysis in myocardial infarction trial. *J. Am. Coll. Cardiol.* 10(Suppl):45B, 1987.

29. Braunwald, E., Knatterud, G., Passamani, E., et al. Update from the thrombolysis in myocardial infarction trial. *J. Am. Coll. Cardiol.* 10:970, 1987.

30. Collen, D., Strassen, J., Stump, D. C., et al. Synergism of thrombolytic agents in vivo. *Circulation* 74:838, 1986.

31. Collen, D., Stump, D. C., and Van de Werf, F. Coronary thrombolysis in patients with acute myocardial infarction by intravenous infusion of synergic thrombolytic agents. *Am. Heart J.* 112:1083, 1986.

32. Gurewich, V., and Pannel, R. A comparative study of the efficacy and specificity of tissue and plasminogen activator and pro-urokinase: Demonstration of synergism and of different thresholds of nonselectivity. *Thromb. Res.* 44:217, 1986.

33. The TIMI Study Group. Comparison of invasive and conservative strategies after treatment with intravenous tissue plasminogen activator in acute myocardial infarction. *N. Engl. J. Med.* 320:618, 1989.

34. Werns, S. W., Shea, M. J., Driscoll, C., et al. The independent effects of oxygen radical scavengers on canine infarct size: Reduction by superoxide dismutase but not catalase. *Circ. Res.* 56:895, 1985.

35. Ambrosio, G., Becker, L. C., Hutchins, G. M., et al. Reduction in experimental infarct size by recombinant human superoxide dismutase: Insights into the pathophysiology of reperfusion injury. *Circulation* 74:1424, 1986.

36. Ambrosio, G., Weisfeldt, M. W., Jacobus, W. E., et al. Evidence for a reversible oxygen radical-mediated component of reperfusion injury: Reduction by recombinant human superoxide dismutase administered at the time of reflow. *Circulation* 75:282, 1987.

37. Topol, E. S., Califf, R. M., George, B. S., et al. A multicenter randomized trial of intravenous tissue plasminogen activator and immediate versus elective angioplasty in acute myocardial infarction. *N. Engl. J. Med.* 317:581, 1987.

38. ISIS-2 (Second International Study of Infarct Survival) Collaborative Group. Randomised trial of intravenous streptokinase, oral aspirin, both, or neither among 17,187 cases of suspected acute myocardial infarction: ISIS-2. *Lancet* 2:349, 1988.

26
Echocardiography in Acute Myocardial Infarction

WILLIAM F. ARMSTRONG

Acute myocardial infarction is a leading cause of morbidity and mortality in the United States and other industrialized nations. Modern therapy includes emergent hospitalization with stabilization of hemodynamics and close observation for arrhythmias and other complications of myocardial infarction. Moreover, today, emergent intervention in an effort to reverse the course of acute myocardial infarction is often undertaken. Because of the immediate and dramatic sequelae of acute coronary occlusion, speed of diagnosis and institution of therapy is of utmost importance, and diagnostic studies that allow rapid assessment of myocardial infarction location and size and the likelihood of complications are of paramount importance in the initial management of these patients. In most institutions this assessment is performed by a combination of studies, including electrocardiography, enzyme determinations, and some form of cardiac imaging.

Because cardiac imaging provides a direct assessment of myocardial infarction size and location, it is playing an increasing role in evaluating patients and decision making regarding emergent therapy. Multiple forms of cardiac imaging can be used to this end. Of all forms of cardiac imaging, two-dimensional echocardiography is probably the one most often associated with cardiology but, paradoxically, in many institutions the one least often used in patients with coronary artery disease. Although the ability of two-dimensional echocardiography to accurately diagnose congenital, pericardial, valvular, and primary myocardial disease is well known, its utility in patients with acute and chronic manifestations

of coronary artery disease is less well appreciated by those not intimately involved in the technique.

In this chapter we first review the principles of registering a two-dimensional echocardiogram for those not acquainted with the technique and then review the practical data that can be gained from the examination in patients with known or suspected myocardial infarction. Finally, we review some investigational techniques that may have future applicability in patients with coronary disease.

Two-Dimensional Echocardiographic Examination

The echocardiographic examination involves the combined utilization of three interdependent modalities. The primary imaging technique is two-dimensional echocardiography, which serves as the routine screening tool for defining chamber size, anatomic abnormalities, and detection and quantification of wall motion abnormalities. M-mode echocardiography, the older imaging technique, provides only a limited "ice pick" view of the heart and plays little or no role at this time in the evaluation of patients with coronary artery disease. Doppler ultrasound techniques allow determination of the direction and velocity of blood flow, from which information concerning intracardiac physiology can be deduced. The newer technique of color Doppler flow imaging allows visualization of intracardiac shunts and can be used to detect ventricular septal defects and regurgitant valvular lesions developing as a consequence of myocardial infarction.

The echocardiographic examination can be performed using equipment of only moderate cost and with relatively small commitments to personnel requirements and laboratory space. Modern echocardiographic equipment is portable, and the examination can be performed in the emergency room, coronary care unit, catheterization laboratory, echocardiography laboratory, or office. The examination is highly versatile, as not only information concerning left ventricular mechanics as they relate to ischemic heart disease can be evaluated, but the diagnosis of virtually any other form of anatomic heart disease can be made as well. Such information concerning coincident valvular, pericardial, myocardial, or congenital heart disease is immediately obtained with a high degree of accuracy. Because the examination affords an excellent view of all areas of the heart, two-dimensional echocardiography combined with Doppler interrogation can be used for detection of any and all mechanical complications of myocardial infarction.

The echocardiographic examination is generally performed by a single sonographer-technician who directs an array of ultrasound beams into the chest. These rays are then reflected from intracardiac structures and converted into a real-time two-dimensional image of the beating heart. This examination is performed in multiple views. Most diagnoses rely on a series of parasternal long- and short-axis views and apical two- and four-chamber views. The orientation of the more common echocardiographic views with respect to external cardiac anatomy is presented in Figures 26-1 and 26-2. An example of a normal two-dimensional echocardiogram is presented in Figures 26-3 and 26-4. It should be noted that the illustrations in this chapter are all taken from the frozen image of a video screen. In reality, interpretation of the echocardiographic examination is done in real time from the videotaped image of the beating heart. The latter real-time image is of higher visual quality than the single frozen frame images presented here and generally contains substantially more diagnostic information.

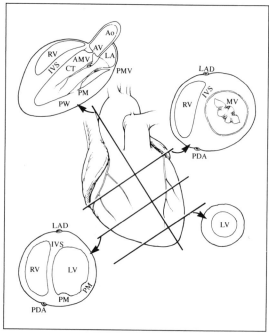

Fig. 26-1
Parasternal echocardiographic imaging planes. The topography of the heart is illustrated along with the plane of imaging for the parasternal long-axis view (*upper left*) and parasternal short-axis views at the mitral level (*upper right*), papillary muscle level (*middle right*) and apical level (*lower right*). Ao = aorta; LA, RA = left and right atria; LV, RV = left and right ventricles; MV = mitral valve; AV = aortic valve; IVS = intraventricular septum; PW = posterior wall; AMV, PMV = anterior and posterior mitral valves; CT = chordae tendineae; LAD = left anterior descending artery; PDA = posterior descending artery.

ADVANTAGES AND LIMITATIONS OF ECHOCARDIOGRAPHY

Echocardiography has several advantages compared to other imaging modalities often used in patients with acute myocardial infarction. Among these advantages are its relatively low cost, the versatility of the examination with respect to being able to assist in the diagnosis of virtually any form of heart disease, the portability of the equipment, the short time required to accomplish an examination, and the totally noninvasive and risk-free nature of the examination, which allows it to be repeated at

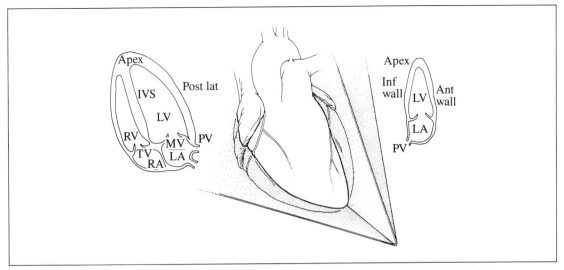

Fig. 26-2
Apical imaging planes. The two traditional apical views are the four-chamber and
two-chamber views and are schematized to the left and right of the heart,
respectively. See Figure 26-1 for abbreviations.

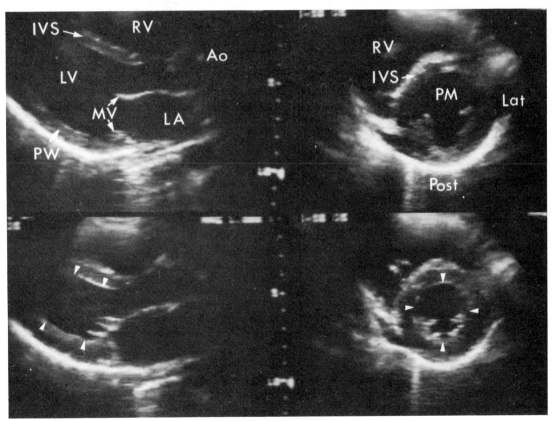

Fig. 26-3
Normal parasternal long- and short-axis views of the left ventricle. Note the
normal thickness of all regions of visualized myocardium and the inward motion
and thickening of the myocardium that has occurred with systole. See Figure 26-1
for abbreviations.

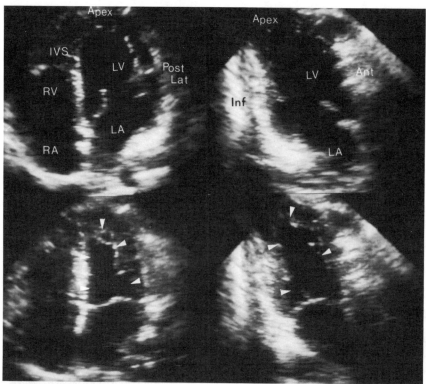

Fig. 26-4
Normal four- and two-chamber apical views. Note the normal "bullet" shape of
the left ventricle and the more triangular geometry of the right ventricle during
both diastole and systole. All regions of myocardium appropriately thicken and
move inward with ventricular systole. See Figure 26-1 for abbreviations.

short intervals if necessary. Disadvantages include the user-interactive nature of the examination, which requires skilled sonographers
to perform the examination and highly trained
personnel for interpretation. The success with
which the complete examination is adequately
accomplished in older patients is less than it is
in pediatric populations; however, in most experienced laboratories diagnostic information
is available in more than 90 percent of patients.

Principles of Echocardiography and Coronary Disease

The premise underlying the utilization of
echocardiography for coronary disease is that
myocardial ischemia or infarctions results in
abnormal left ventricular wall motion that can
then be detected by echocardiography. That
the wall motion becomes abnormal almost immediately after onset of myocardial ischemia
was first described by Tennant and Wiggers in
1935 [1]. Abnormal wall motion with ischemia
or infarction has subsequently been documented by a number of other techniques
including ventriculography, radionuclide angiography, and echocardiography [2–4]. As
is further discussed below, two-dimensional
echocardiography can detect wall motion abnormalities associated with transient myocardial ischemia or acute myocardial infarction,
or that result from established remote myocardial infarction.

The advent of percutaneous balloon angioplasty has afforded the opportunity to evaluate the timing of onset of wall motion abnor-

malities after interruption of coronary flow in patients. These studies have confirmed earlier animal work, which showed almost immediate onset of wall motion abnormalities following coronary occlusion. Following balloon coronary occlusion at the time of angioplasty, wall motion becomes almost immediately abnormal, preceding the onset of electrocardiographic changes or angina [4–7]. In this setting wall motion abnormalities may also occur in the absence of typical symptoms or electrocardiographic changes.

As imaged with two-dimensional echocardiography, normal left ventricular wall motion includes two interrelated phenomena—endocardial thickening and concurrent motion of the endocardial border toward the center of the left ventricle—both of which contribute to shrinking of the ventricular cavity and ejection of blood during systole. Myocardial thickening and endocardial motion can be detected with echocardiography. With mild degrees of ischemia, myocardial thickening is diminished and, coincident with the inward endocardial motion, the affected segment first diminishes (hypokinesis) and then moves paradoxically (dyskinesis) with more advanced stages of ischemia [8–13]. As is discussed subsequently, this two-stage abnormality of wall motion is a simplification; in reality, there is marked heterogeneity over the time course of systole such that the wall may initially move paradoxically but later during systole have more appropriate motion [14].

RELATION TO INFARCT SIZE

The ability of echocardiography to detect wall motion abnormalities of myocardial infarction has been evaluated in numerous studies. When experimentally controlled and evaluated with high-resolution techniques such as sonomicrometry, abnormalities of left ventricular wall motion occur with reductions in resting coronary flow of 20 percent or more [8]. Further reduction in flow results in more marked abnormalities, including systolic thinning of the myocardium and endocardial

dyskinesis [8–11]. It should be noted that the subtle abnormalities present with reductions of only 20 percent or less may not be detectable with two-dimensional echocardiography. Acute flow reductions of 50 percent or more probably result in wall motion abnormalities of sufficient magnitude to be visually detected with two-dimensional scanning [10–15].

Weiss and colleagues directly compared the extent of left ventricular akinesis or dyskinesis in 11 patients whose hearts were subsequently examined pathologically at autopsy [2]. They found a correlation of $r = .9$ for pathologic percent circumference of the left ventricle infarcted versus the percent circumference that was akinetic or dyskinetic on echocardiography (Fig. 26-5). As with experimental animal studies, echocardiography tended to overestimate the anatomic myocardial infarction size.

Both myocardial thickening and endocardial motion have been evaluated with two-dimensional echocardiography and compared to myocardial infarction size experimentally

Fig. 26-5
Comparison of the extent of the left ventricular circumference demonstrating akinesis or dyskinesis on an antemortem echocardiogram and the percent of transmurally infarcted left ventricular circumference by postmortem examination in 11 patients subsequently examined at autopsy. (From J. L. Weiss et al. Two-dimensional echocardiographic recognition of myocardial injury in man: Comparison with postmortem studies. *Circulation* 63:401, 1981. By permission of the American Heart Association Inc.)

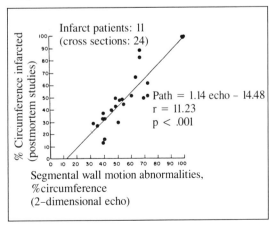

Infarct patients: 11
(cross sections: 24)

Path = 1.14 echo – 14.48
r = 11.23
p < .001

% Circumference infarcted (postmortem studies)

Segmental wall motion abnormalities, %circumference (2–dimensional echo)

[11–13, 16–20]. Virtually all studies are in concurrence that the extent of abnormal wall motion overestimates the anatomic size of myocardial infarction [11–13, 19]. It has been well demonstrated that normally perfused viable myocardium at the border of ischemic or infarcted myocardium may have abnormal systolic function [21–24]. Thus although there is generally good correlation between histologic infarct size and distribution of wall motion abnormalities, the echocardiographic technique detects functionally abnormal border areas resulting in overestimation of the anatomic infarct size. The most likely explanation for this adjacent abnormality is that the adjacent, non-ischemic areas are "tethered" to the ischemic region and passively reflect the abnormal motion of the infarct area [21]. The method of wall motion analysis can also introduce errors that add to this overestimation because of their dependence on a fixed or floating reference point to which the endocardial motion is then referenced. As the infarct or ischemic area expands and moves during systole, the center of the mass shifts; and nonequivalent areas may then be compared, resulting in overestimation of the ischemic zone [25].

Just as the degree of flow reduction required to produce abnormal wall motion is of importance, so is the absolute size of myocardial infarction. Pandian and his colleagues have evaluated this phenomenon in an animal model and demonstrated that small subendocardial myocardial infarctions, involving 1 to 6 percent of the left ventricular mass, were not likely to be associated with wall motion abnormalities of sufficient magnitude to be detected by routine echocardiography [20]. The clinical correlate of this situation is that smaller myocardial infarctions may not be detected by two-dimensional echocardiography in patients.

The role of the extent of transmural involvement has been specifically investigated by several investigators. Lieberman and colleagues demonstrated that regions of myocardium with 1 to 20 percent of transmural involvement had reduced thickening when compared to noninfarcted remote segments.

They furthermore showed a threshold effect, such that segments with in excess of 20 percent myocardial involvement showed frank systolic thinning and that the degree of thinning did not increase with increasing degrees of transmural involvement above 21 percent of wall thickness [12]. It thus appears from an experimental standpoint that myocardial infarction is reflected accurately by the presence of echocardiographic wall motion abnormalities. There are thresholds with respect to the degree of flow reduction required before wall motion abnormalities develop. Furthermore, thresholds exist with respect to the absolute amount of myocardium as well as the transmural degree of involvement required to produce abnormalities detectable with echocardiography.

COMPARISON WITH OTHER TECHNIQUES

Two-dimensional echocardiography has been compared to other imaging techniques for detection of abnormal wall motion. The first large comparative study of echocardiography and biplane angiography was performed in 105 patients by Kisslo et al. [26]. Using early-generation scanning equipment they were able to obtain images adequate for analysis in 430 of 525 (82 percent) cardiac regions in their study patients. Comparing the two techniques, they noted concordance of observations with respect to the presence or absence of wall motion abnormalities in 375 of the 430 analyzable regions. Similar studies have been repeated by other investigators who have also included radionuclide techniques for comparison [3, 27–31]. Nixon and colleagues compared the presence of left ventricular wall motion abnormalities and the distribution of thallium perfusion deficits in 32 consecutive patients admitted with acute myocardial infarction [31]. They found close correlations between two-dimensional echocardiographic wall motion scores and estimates of myocardial infarction by both thallium scintigraphy and technetium pyrophosphate scanning.

METHODS OF WALL MOTION ANALYSIS

The early studies relied on visual assessment of wall motion abnormalities and division by subjective criteria into normal, hypokinetic, akinetic, or dyskinetic wall motion. The exact methodology for analyzing and quantifying wall motion is not uniformly accepted among echocardiographers, and so reports are often generated using different schemes for analysis of wall motion.

Figure 26-6 outlines several such methods. The simplest is obviously visual assessment of normal versus akinetic, dyskinetic, or hypokinetic motion, which can then be semiquantified by dividing the left ventricle into predefined regions and assigning a numerical hierarchy to increasing degrees of wall motion abnormality in each of the regions. These numbers can be summed to form a wall motion score or indexed to the number of segments to form a wall motion score index [32]. Figures 26-7 and 26-8 are examples of the wall motion score index generated for two patients with small inferior and large anteroapical infarctions, respectively. This semiquantitative method for quantifying wall motion abnormalities thus takes into account both the severity of the abnormality and its extent in the left ventricle. It is this technique of determining a wall motion score that has found the most practical use in clinical assessment of patients with acute myocardial infarction. Superimposed on any of these schemes is the understanding that left ventricular regions are perfused by different coronary arteries. The general relation of the perfusion beds of the three major epicardial coronary arteries to the echocardiographic walls is presented in Figure 26-9.

More detailed and quantitative schemes have also been developed, and generally they rely on outlining the endocardial border at end-diastole and end-systole and then creating a series of radians from the center of the mass of the left ventricle. This maneuver then divides the left ventricle into any number of regions (typically 16 to 100), which can then be quantitatively evaluated by shortening the individual radians or shrinking individual subtended areas [33, 34]. Methodologic problems arise when defining the center of the mass of the ventricle during diastole and systole. Additionally, the left ventricle rotates around both its long and short axes during contraction, which may cause nonequivalent regions to be compared during diastole and systole. Several methods have been advanced to correct for this phenomenon, none of which has been uniformly accepted by echocardiographers [35].

The two newest methods for analyzing wall motion include analysis of the entire contrac-

Fig. 26-6
Multiple algorithms by which wall motion can be graded. An example of anterior dyskinesis is presented that can be described in a purely descriptive manner as dyskinetic or quantified by any of the five demonstrated algorithms. See text for full details. (From W. F. Armstrong. *Progress in Cardiovascular Disease*, January/February 1988. With permission.)

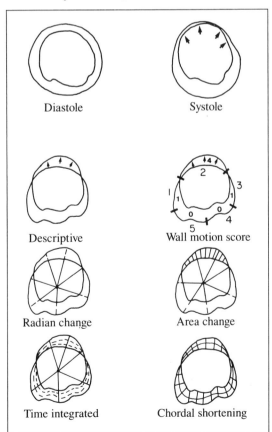

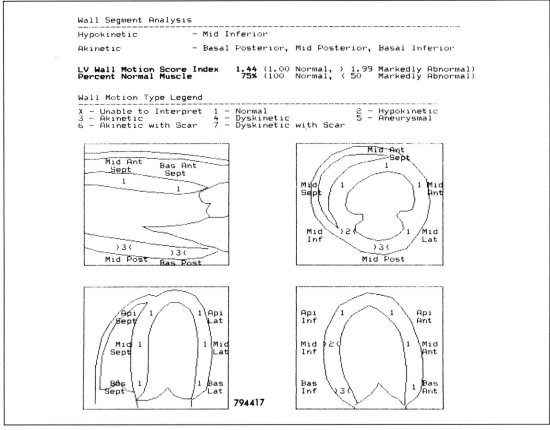

Fig. 26-7
Wall motion score generated by the patient presented in Figure 26-11. Note in the schematic portion that the inferoposterior and inferior walls are either hypokinetic (score 2) or akinetic (score 3) and that the remaining wall motion is normal. This pattern is consistent with a limited-extent electrocardiographic inferior infarction.

tion sequence as suggested by Weyman and his colleagues [14, 36, 37] and the center line chord shortening method originally developed for angiography [38] but subsequently applied to two-dimensional echocardiography [4]. The detailed studies of Weyman and colleagues explain many of the problems previously encountered with wall motion analysis. These workers have demonstrated that there is a temporal heterogeneity to left ventricular wall motion in the presence of myocardial ischemia. When the entire contraction sequence of the left ventricle is analyzed at 17-msec intervals from end-diastole to end-systole, it becomes apparent that dyskinesis occurs at different points during systole depending on the

duration of myocardial ischemia. It results in a phenomenon in which endocardial position may be frankly dyskinetic during early systole but move to appropriate end-systolic points later in the contraction sequence. It has the effect of masking areas of wall motion abnormality present during early systole but not present at end-systole.

Abnormal Wall Motion in Clinical Syndromes

As previously noted, experimentally induced myocardial ischemia results in abnormal left

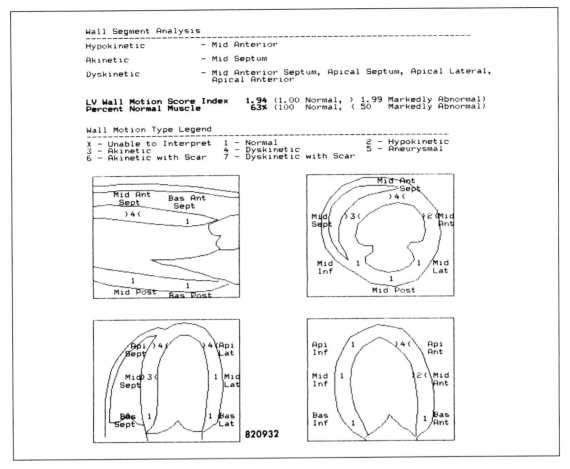

Fig. 26-8
Wall motion score generated in the patient presented in Figures 26-12 and 26-13.
A large anteroapical infarction is present with a wall motion score index of 1.94.

ventricular wall motion. Identical abnormalities occur with spontaneous ischemia in patients with coronary disease. Wall motion abnormalities associated with transient myocardial ischemia and infarction are identical in quality, the only difference being that those associated with myocardial infarction persist, whereas those associated with transient ischemia (as seen with angina pectoris) are transient.

Several centers have evaluated two-dimensional echocardiography at the time of attacks of variant angina, either spontaneous or induced with ergonovine [39–42]. The most extensive experience in this field is that of Distante and his colleagues from Pisa [41]. They

noted that each of 37 spontaneous and 18 ergonovine-induced attacks of angina were associated with abnormalities of left ventricular wall motion, which generally preceded the onset of chest pain. Wall motion abnormalities were occasionally seen in the absence of chest pain or diagnostic electrocardiographic changes. Their data suggested that detection of wall motion abnormalities might be an early indicator of myocardial ischemia in these patients and that echocardiographic monitoring during ergonovine challenge may allow detection of coronary spasm at a point prior to establishment of more advanced stages of ischemia required when traditional endpoints are used.

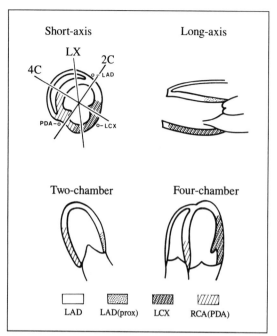

Short-axis   Long-axis

LX   2C
4C

PDA-o   o-LCX

Two-chamber   Four-chamber

LAD   LAD(prox)   LCX   RCA(PDA)

Fig. 26-9
General distribution of the coronary arteries
versus the echocardiographic wall segments.
(From H. Feigenbaum. *Echocardiography* [4th
ed.]. Philadelphia: Lea & Febiger, 1986. With
permission.)

Abnormal wall motion is often seen in patients presenting with unstable angina. Unlike
variant angina, which has a clear onset and
resolution of both the clinical syndrome and
the wall motion abnormalities, unstable angina tends to be associated with more profound and long-lasting ischemia. Nixon and
colleagues have demonstrated that many of
these patients have persistent wall motion abnormalities [43]. Some of these more long-lasting abnormalities may represent subclinical
myocardial infarction rather than active transient ischemia. Unlike the profound ischemia
of unstable or preinfarction angina, milder
attacks of angina may be associated with
shorter-lived periods of abnormal wall motion, which are more difficult to detect because of their transient nature. Figure 26-10
was recorded in a patient with a spontaneous
episode of angina during the echocardiographic examination and demonstrates a reversible wall motion abnormality of the anterior ventricular septum.

DIAGNOSIS OF ACUTE MYOCARDIAL INFARCTION

Given the sensitivity of echocardiographic
scanning to detect ischemia-induced wall motion abnormalities, one obvious utilization of
echocardiography is to assist in the initial diagnosis of acute myocardial infarction in the
patient presenting with chest pain. One of
the earliest demonstrations of this use was
by Heger et al. from our institution who
performed two-dimensional echocardiograms
within 48 hours of admission in 44 patients
with chest pain and acute myocardial infarction [44]. Using early-generation equipment,
wall motion abnormalities were identified in
all 37 patients in whom complete echocardiographic studies could be recorded. There
was generally good agreement between the
electrocardiographic location of the myocardial infarction and echocardiographic wall motion abnormality. Those patients with inferior
myocardial infarctions (manifested by electrocardiographic changes in leads II, III, and
aVF) had wall motion abnormalities bordering
on the posterior interventricular groove in the
basal and mid portions of the left ventricle.
Those patients with either inferoposterior or
inferolateral myocardial infarctions on the
echocardiogram had wall motion abnormalities in the contiguous posterolateral regions of
the left ventricle. Those patients with anteroseptal myocardial infarctions (Q waves in
leads V_1–V_4) had apical, anterior wall, and
septal involvement at the level of the mid ventricle. Those with anterolateral involvement
(Q waves in V_3–V_6) had anterior septal, apical,
and lateral wall involvement. Three patients
with both anterior and inferior electrocardiographic changes had diffuse wall motion abnormalities, including in all cases the apex, inferior wall, septum, lateral and anterior walls
at the mid ventricle, and the more proximal
lateral and inferior walls.

In a similar study, Stamm and his colleagues
evaluated 51 patients with recent myocardial
infarctions and single-vessel coronary disease
at subsequent angiography [45]. Using a more
detailed 11-segment ventricular model, they
demonstrated a similar distribution of wall

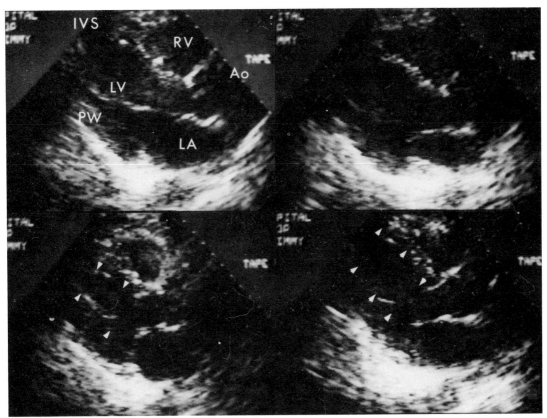

Fig. 26-10
Two-dimensional echocardiogram recorded in a patient with spontaneous angina.
The parasternal long axis views during diastole (*upper panels*) and systole (*lower
panels*) in a pain-free state (*left panels*) and during a spontaneous episode of
angina (*right panels*) are shown. During angina the distal anterior septum is
dyskinetic, whereas wall motion remains normal in the inferoposterior wall.

motion abnormalities. In their study patients
with single-vessel left anterior descending coronary artery disease had anteroseptal and anterolateral wall motion abnormalities as well
as apical abnormalities. Of note in their study,
patients with right and left circumflex coronary artery occlusions occasionally demonstrated apical wall motion abnormalities. The
most common site of abnormality in right coronary occlusions was at the base of the left
ventricular inferior wall, adjacent to the posterior interventricular groove. Circumflex coronary obstructions tended to be less specifically localized and generally involved the
inferior posterior wall in a region overlapping
that of a right coronary obstruction and the
posterolateral wall in an area often overlap-

ping that seen in left anterior descending coronary artery obstruction. Their patients with
single-vessel disease had localized wall motion abnormalities, whereas 17 of 20 patients
with multivessel disease at subsequent cardiac
catheterization had multiple regions of wall
motion abnormality. The regions of remote
wall motion abnormalities often normalized
over the course of myocardial infarction. The
authors termed this phenomenon "remote
asynergy" and demonstrated a link between
this phenomenon and adverse clinical outcome. In a subsequent study from this same
group the presence of remote asynergy statistically correlated with subsequent angina,
reinfarction, congestive failure, arrhythmia,
and death [46].

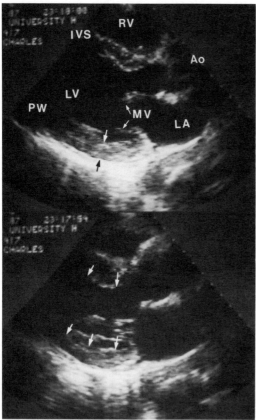

Fig. 26-11
Parasternal long-axis views recorded in a patient
with an acute inferoposterior myocardial
infarction. *Upper panel.* Note the full thickness of
the inferoposterior wall during diastole (*black and
white arrows*). *Lower panel.* With systole the
anterior septum thickens and moves downward
(*white arrows*), but the inferoposterior wall moves
posteriorly and thins (*white arrows*). The wall
motion score for this patient is presented in Figure
26-7.

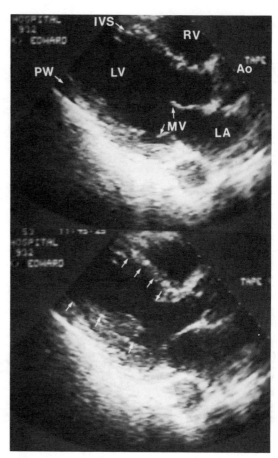

Fig. 26-12
Parasternal long-axis view during diastole (*upper
panel*) and systole (*lower panel*) recorded in a
patient presenting with a large anterior myocardial
infarction. Note the preserved thickness of the
ventricular septum and that the distal 90 percent
of the anterior septum is dyskinetic during systole
(*upward-pointing white arrows*), whereas the
proximal portion of the ventricular septum moves
normally.

Horowitz and colleagues from Philadelphia
have evaluated the ability of two-dimensional
echocardiography to assist in the initial diagnosis of acute myocardial infarction in
patients presenting with chest pain [47].
Their study was performed in 80 consecutive
patients, 65 of whom (81 percent) had adequate two-dimensional echocardiograms recorded within 8 hours of admission. Abnormal regional wall motion was found in 36 of
these patients, 31 of whom developed clinical
myocardial infarction by routine enzymatic

and electrocardiographic criteria. Five patients with wall motion abnormalities failed to
develop clinical myocardial infarction; three
of them subsequently underwent angiography,
and coronary disease was demonstrated in
each. These patients in all likelihood had unstable angina with wall motion abnormalities.
Left ventricular wall motion was normal in 29
patients presenting with chest pain, and in 27
no clinical myocardial infarction developed.
Two patients developed small subendocardial

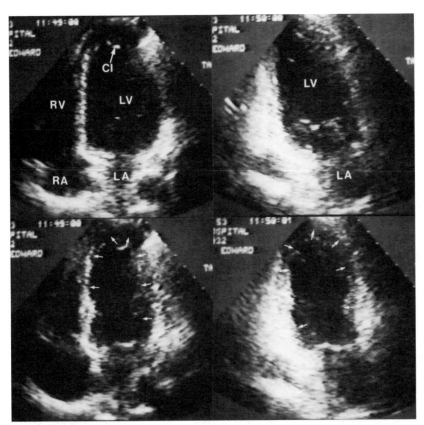

Fig. 26-13
Apical four- and two-chamber views in the patient presented in Figure 26-12, demonstrating dyskinesis of the anterior wall, anterior septum, and apex (*arrows*). The wall motion score for this patient can be found in Figure 26-8.

(non-Q-wave) myocardial infarctions. Cardiac complications occurred in ten patients in this cohort, all of whom had abnormal regional wall motion on echocardiography performed early after admission. Figures 26-11 through 26-15, recorded in patients with either acute or remote myocardial infarction, demonstrate the range of abnormalities seen in myocardial infarction.

Patients presenting with typical chest pain and classic electrocardiographic changes of Q-wave myocardial infarction rarely present a diagnostic dilemma. Those patients with smaller non-Q-wave myocardial infarction remain problematic by all techniques. It is a subset that has been specifically evaluated with echocardiography by several investigators [48–51]. As noted earlier in the section on ex-

perimental background for use of echocardiography in coronary disease, there is a threshold mass of myocardium and degree of transmural infarction that must be exceeded before abnormal wall motion is detected by echocardiography. As such, the frequency of wall motion abnormalities in non-Q-wave infarct is expected to be less than that seen in Q-wave myocardial infarction.

Loh et al. evaluated this problem in 30 patients studied within 12.5 hours following the onset of chest pain [51]. Wall motion abnormalities were seen in 10 of 12 (83 percent) patients subsequently demonstrated to have myocardial necrosis and were absent in all 18 patients who failed to develop clinical myocardial infarction. A similar study was undertaken in 50 patients by Arvan and Varat [50].

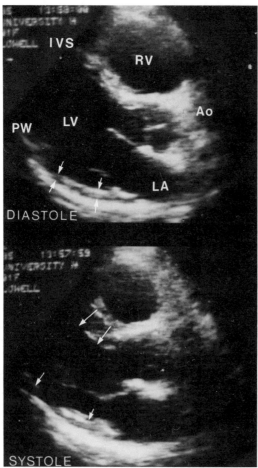

Fig. 26-14
Parasternal long-axis view recorded in a patient with a remote inferior myocardial infarction. During diastole (*upper panel*) note the normal-thickness ventricular septum with a thin, scarred inferoposterior wall (*arrows*). With systole the anterior septum thickens and moves normally, whereas the inferoposterior wall remains pathologically thinned and is dyskinetic.

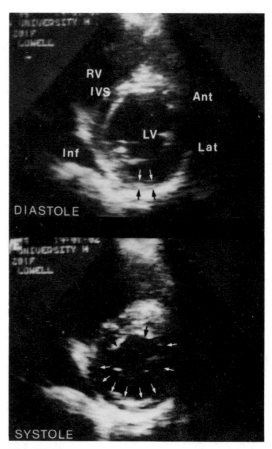

Fig. 26-15
Parasternal short-axis views in a patient with a remote inferior myocardial infarction (same as in Figure 26-14). Note the full thickness of the septum and the anterior and lateral walls and the pathologically thinned and scarred inferoposterior wall (*white and black arrows*). With systole (*lower panel*) the inferoposterior and inferior walls are dyskinetic.

Sensitivity for identifying patients who subsequently developed enzymatic evidence of a non-Q-wave myocardial infarction was 67 percent for echocardiographic imaging versus 52 percent for the electrocardiogram; respective specificities were 91 and 95 percent. By combining the two studies the sensitivity for detecting non-Q-wave myocardial infarction increased to 76 percent.

It thus appears that wall motion abnormalities are often present in non-Q-wave myocar-

dial infarction, but that as with either other imaging techniques or electrocardiography the diagnosis of myocardial infarction is less precise for non-Q-wave infarct than it is for Q-wave infarct. Although wall motion abnormalities, once established, tend to persist in Q-wave infarct [48], there may be spontaneous improvement in patients with non-Q-wave infarctions [49]. This observation has been associated with a higher risk of reinfarction during the ensuing 6 months.

The problem of perioperative myocardial infarction has been addressed by Force and his colleagues [52, 53]. As expected, Q-wave myocardial infarctions following coronary artery bypass surgery are associated with a high likelihood of wall motion abnormalities. These authors noted a similar severity of wall motion abnormality in those patients with perioperative non-Q-wave infarcts as well.

There has been substantial interest in the problem of reciprocal ST segment depression seen in the anterior leads in patients with acute inferior myocardial infarction. The two possible explanations for the reciprocal precordial ST segment depression are that it represents a pure reciprocal phenomenon from the inferior ST segment elevation or that it represents concurrent anterior myocardial ischemia. Analysis of left ventricular wall motion with echocardiography suggests that the ST segment depression seen in the anterior precordium is most often a reflector of larger inferior myocardial infarctions generally with some posterolateral extension and not due to coincident anterior wall ischemia [54, 55].

Persistent ST segment elevation following acute anterior myocardial infarction has also been evaluated with two-dimensional echocardiography. In a limited series of patients this observation appears to correlate with marked dyskinesis of the anterior and apical wall segments rather than frank aneurysm formation [56, 57].

ASSESSMENT OF PROGNOSIS AFTER ACUTE MYOCARDIAL INFARCTION

Although simple detection of wall motion abnormalities in a patient with chest pain implies coronary artery disease, their mere presence does not assist in the assessment of prognosis. For the latter analysis, the distribution of wall motion abnormalities must be quantified. It should be stressed that when it is done with echocardiography (or any other imaging technique which relies on ventricular function) what is assessed is the functional extent of the wall motion abnormality and not necessarily the anatomic extent of infarction, which often tends to be somewhat smaller. As noted previously under the discussion of methods for wall motion analysis, multiple schemes for quantitation of wall motion abnormalities have been proposed by numerous investigators. The scheme that has been utilized most often in studies evaluating prognosis is the generation of a wall motion score or score index, in which the motion of multiple predefined ventricular wall areas is graded along a hierarchical score [32]. These scores are then summed and indexed to the number of segments evaluated. The more diffuse and extensive the wall motion abnormalities, the higher is the wall motion score or score index. Examples of this type of wall motion score were presented in Figures 26-7 and 26-8, which were derived from the patients presented in Figures 26-11, 26-12, and 26-13.

The first attempt at correlating the extent of left ventricular wall motion abnormalities with clinical outcome was reported by Heger et al. in 1980 [32]. This study comprised 44 consecutive patients with acute myocardial infarction evaluated with early-generation two-dimensional scanning equipment. The left ventricle was divided into nine predefined segments and the wall motion characterized as normal (score 0) to dyskinetic (score 3). These individual scores were then summed for all nine segments into a wall motion score. Analysis of the two-dimensional echocardiograms revealed that regional wall motion abnormalities were present in all 44 patients. Uncomplicated clinical courses were seen in 13 patients who had a mean wall motion score of 3.2 ± 2.4. This wall motion score was statistically less ($p < .001$) than that seen in the 12 patients with pulmonary congestion (9.7 ± 3.1), or with hypotension and pulmonary congestion (10.6 ± 4.8).

A similar study was performed in 75 patients by Gibson et al. [46]. Their patients underwent echocardiographic imaging an average of 7.9 hours after admission for acute myocardial infarction, and the results of the echocardiograms were analyzed in a fashion similar to that noted above. The authors used a more complicated 11-segment scheme and indexed the wall motion scores to the number of segments. This initial wall motion score in-

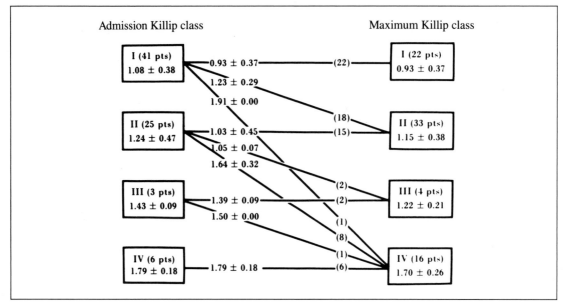

Fig. 26-16
Correlation of the echocardiographically derived wall motion index (mean ±
standard deviation) with admission and maximal Killip classes (I–IV). The
number of patients (pts) in each subgroup appears in parentheses. See text for
further details. (From R. S. Gibson et al. Value of early two dimensional
echocardiography in patients with acute myocardial infarction. *Am. J. Cardiol.*
49:110, 1982. With permission.)

dex was then correlated with the admission
and maximum Killip classification experienced by the patient during hospitalization. In
their study 41 patients were classified on admission as Killip I, and their initial wall motion score index was 1.08 ± 0.38. Twenty-two
patients with a mean wall motion score of 0.93
± 0.37 remained in Killip class I during their
hospitalization. Eighteen patients initially in
Killip class I progressed to Killip class II, and
a single patient progressed from Killip class I
to Killip class IV. The wall motion score indices in these patients were 1.23 ± 0.29 and
1.91, respectively. The data from this study
are presented in Figure 26-16. The higher wall
motion score indices were seen in patients
with large infarctions and in those with remote
areas of wall motion abnormality in addition
to the index infarction. Remote wall motion
abnormalities were seen in 32 patients; and as
previously noted, their presence had a statistical association with a number of complications, including, death, cardiogenic shock,

reinfarction, progression of Killip classification, and postinfarct angina.

The ability of two-dimensional echocardiography to assess prognosis following myocardial infarction has been demonstrated in
numerous other laboratories [58–63]. Table 26-
1 summarizes results of some studies in which
two-dimensional echocardiography was used
to assess patient prognosis following acute
myocardial infarction.

DOPPLER ASSESSMENT OF
SYSTOLIC FUNCTION

The above discussion dealt with direct visualization of wall motion abnormalities and their
implication for detection and quantification of
myocardial infarction. Infarct size was expressed as a function of the amount of muscle
with abnormal motion. Information concerning overall systolic function of the left ventri-

Table 26-1
Echocardiographic assessment of prognosis following myocardial infarction

Study	No. of pts.	Timing[a]	Endpoint[b]	Analysis[c]	N[d]	Adverse outcome	Analysis	N	Adverse outcome
Heger [32]	39	E	C,D HP	WMS ≥ 8	19	18 (95%)	WMS < 8	18	6 (33%)
Horowitz [62]	43	E	C,D,MA HP,	WMS ≥ 8	16	11 (69%)	WMS < 8	27	2 (7%)
Abrams [63]	23	E	C,D,A, MI	WMS ≥ 2 EF < 40%	12 9	7 (58%) 7 (78%)	WMS < 2 EF > 40%	11 14	0 (0%) 0 (0%)
VanReet [30]	93	E	D	WMS < 0.5 EF < 35%	25 27	10 (40%) 10 (37%)	WMS > .5 EF ≥ 95%	68 60	1 (2%) 1 (2%)
Nishumura [59]	61	E	C,D,MA	WMS ≥ 2	27	24 (89%)	WMS < 2	34	6 (18%)
Bhatnagar [61]	47	P	A,MI	WMS ≥ 8	16	14 (89%)	WMS < 8	31	3 (10%)
Nishumura [60]	46	P	D,MI,C,A	WMS ≥ 2	24	15 (63%)	WMS < 2	22	2 (9%)

[a]Timing = time frame for obtaining echocardiographic study. E = early: echocardiogram performed at time of presentation and short follow-up period (generally in hospital); P = predischarge echocardiogram and longer outpatient follow-up.

[b]D = death; MI = recurrent myocardial infarct; A = angina; C = congestive heart failure; HP = hypoperfusion/shock; MA = malignant arrhythmias or heart block.

[c]Analysis = type of echocardiographic analysis and threshold for favorable or adverse outcome. EF = ejection fraction; WMS = wall motion score (scoring systems are different for each study; therefore absolute numbers are *not* interchangeable among studies for WMS).

[d]N = number of patients in each subset.

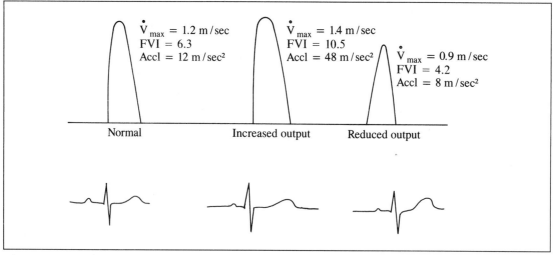

Fig. 26-17
Aortic flow velocity under baseline circumstances (*left*), with increased cardiac output (*middle*) or with diminished output (*right*). Note that peak velocity, acceleration, and area under the curve increase with an increase in stroke volume and diminish with reduced left ventricular systolic function. (From W. F. Armstrong. *Progress in Cardiovascular Disease,* January/February 1988. With permission.)

cle can be obtained from Doppler recordings of the aortic outflow. Stroke volume and cardiac output can be calculated as the product of left ventricular outflow tract (or aortic) cross sectional area and the systolic velocity integral [64, 65]. As such, in any given patient when outflow tract or aortic dimensions are constant, global systolic performance is directly proportional to the Doppler-derived aortic flow velocity integral. In addition to the overall velocity integral, other parameters (e.g., peak acceleration and velocity) reflect systolic performance of the ventricle. The behavior of these parameters is shown in Figure 26-17. The behavior of the aortic flow velocity signals under different conditions of contractility and loading conductions has been experimentally evaluated [65]. Similar observations have been made in the clinical arena in patients with ventricular dysfunction undergoing therapy for congestive failure [66, 67]. This application of Doppler ultrasound has thus far seen only limited clinical utilization in the United States. Because of substantial deviation from cardiac output measured by thermodilution or other standard techniques when

group data are compared, its role for precise prediction of output is limited. Doppler evaluation of the aortic flow velocity may play a valuable role in detecting serial changes in a given patient, however.

Complications of Myocardial Infarction

Modern two-dimensional imaging combined with Doppler techniques allows the rapid noninvasive diagnosis of virtually any complication of myocardial infarction with the exception of an isolated rhythm disturbance. Table 26-2 outlines the common complications of myocardial infarction that can be detected with cardiac ultrasound. The following discussion further outlines many of these applications.

PERICARDIAL EFFUSION

Perhaps the most common complication of myocardial infarction is the development of transient pericarditis with effusion. When

Table 26-2
Complications of myocardial infarction that can be
detected with echocardiography and Doppler

Pericardial effusion (acute or delayed)
Aneurysm formation
Mural thrombus
Pseudoaneurysm
Infarct expansion
Papillary muscle rupture
Functional mitral regurgitation
Tricuspid regurgitation
Right ventricular infarction
Reinfarction

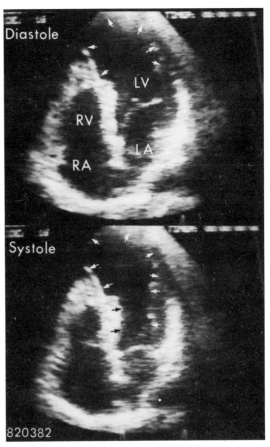

Fig. 26-18
Apical four-chamber view in a patient with
anteroapical aneurysm. Note the full thickness of
the myocardium at the base with a distinct break
from normal geometry (*arrows*) present during
diastole and systole. (From W. F. Armstrong.
Progress in Cardiovascular Disease. January/
February 1988. With permission.)

evaluated with serial echocardiograms, this
complication occurs after 26 to 37 percent of
myocardial infarctions, usually 1 to 3 days after the acute event [68, 69]. The etiology of
this type of pericarditis is an associated epicardial infarction and inflammation, and as
such it is a complication of transmural myocardial infarction. Acute pericarditis following myocardial infarction has been associated
with a worse prognosis and more extensive infarction [69].

ANEURYSM FORMATION

The definition and detection of aneurysms by
two-dimensional echocardiography is based
on the same criteria as for contrast ventriculography. Left ventricular aneurysm refers to
the formation of an area of myocardial scar
with distinctly abnormal geometry during both
diastole and systole compared to the normal
left ventricular configuration [70–72]. This
complication is more common after anterior
and apical myocardial infarctions, occurring in
20 to 40 percent of cases [71, 73]. Figure 26-18
illustrates a large anteroapical aneurysm in a
patient following an anterior myocardial infarction.

The detection of left ventricular aneurysm
by two-dimensional echocardiography was
first demonstrated by Weyman and colleagues
in 1976 [70]. In this small retrospective study
there was excellent agreement between single-
plane angiography and two-dimensional echo-

cardiography for localizing left ventricular
aneurysms. Similar reports have been generated in other laboratories [71–74]. The largest
study comparing catheterization and echocardiography for detection of left ventricular
aneurysm was reported by Visser et al. in 422
consecutive patients with documented myocardial infarction [71]. Using more recent generation equipment these authors obtained adequate two-dimensional echocardiograms in
91 percent of their patients. Left ventricular
aneurysm was present by echocardiography in
111 patients and by cineangiography in 118 patients. Concordance of the two studies was

seen in 103 patients thought to have aneurysm and in 260 thought not to have aneurysm. Compared to cineangiography, echocardiography was 93 percent sensitive and 94 percent specific for detection of left ventricular aneurysm.

It should be noted that many of the discrepancies in studies such as this one probably arise from the different loading conditions under which the examinations are performed rather than true discrepancies of data. The adverse loading conditions present at the time of cardiac catheterization generally tend to exacerbate wall motion abnormalities compared to the noninvasive and the truly resting echocardiographic examinations.

These same authors evaluated the time course of aneurysm formation after myocardial infarction in 158 patients in whom serial studies were available [74]. Aneurysms formed in 35 of 158 (22 percent) patients, and importantly all formed within the first 3 months after myocardial infarction. The patient most likely to form an aneurysm was described as that patient with marked anterior dyskinesis acutely following myocardial infarction. Aneurysms formed in 27 of 84 patients (32.1 percent) with anterior wall motion abnormalities and in only 6 of 68 patients (8.8 percent) with posterior wall motion abnormalities. Marked anterior dyskinesis was present in 25 of the 27 patients who proceeded to form an aneurysm but in only 5 of the 57 with anterior infarcts not forming aneurysms. Of particular note in this study, 15 patients formed aneurysms within the first 5 days after myocardial infarction. This early aneurysm formation probably represents infarct expansion (to be discussed subsequently) rather than formation of a true fibrous aneurysm. Other investigators have previously suggested that this factor carries a poor prognosis for spontaneous myocardial rupture [75]. In the Visser et al. study the 3-month mortality was 66 percent and the 1-year mortality 80 percent in those patients with early aneurysm formation [74].

The size of the left ventricular aneurysm can be quantified by defining the boundary between normal and abnormal wall motion and then measuring the normal and abnormal areas either linearly or as a function of the circumference of the ventricle. With this procedure, an index of the residual myocardium can then be generated. Those patients with greater amounts of residual normal myocardium tend to have a better prognosis [72, 73]. The ability of echocardiography to predict surgical survival and improvement following aneurysmectomy has also been investigated [76, 77]. We have reported 37 patients studied with two-dimensional echocardiography prior to aneurysmectomy and demonstrated that an echocardiographic index of functioning myocardium at the base of the heart accurately separated those patients likely to survive surgery and to be improved by at least one clinical classification from those who either died at surgery or were not improved [77]. In comparison, global ejection fraction from angiography did not distinguish those with favorable outcomes from those with poor clinical outcomes. Virtually identical data were reported by Visser et al. in a cohort of 56 patients [76]. These workers calculated an index of aneurysm size versus normal functioning muscle by quantifying the linear extent of normal muscle along the anterior, posterior, lateral, and septal walls of the ventricle. From this index they calculated a percent of functioning muscle. Their data suggested that those patients with less than 40 percent functioning muscle were at high risk for aneurysm resection.

For those patients who are not undergoing surgical resection, echocardiographic aneurysm size also correlates with the clinical status. This parameter has been retrospectively evaluated by Motsomoto et al. in 68 patients studied with serial echocardiograms following their first myocardial infarction [73]. These investigators noted a significantly higher incidence of heart failure and mortality in those patients with large aneurysms (functioning muscle <40 percent) than in those with small aneurysms.

Infarct Expansion

Formation of a true ventricular aneurysm with a fibrous wall generally occurs over a period of weeks to several months following myocardial infarction. A second, superficially similar phenomenon is that of infarct expansion [75, 78–81]. This term refers to the acute thinning and stretching of infarcted myocardium, which from a cardiac imaging standpoint produces an abnormality suggestive of ventricular aneurysm acutely rather than more slowly after myocardial infarction. Clinically, this phenomenon is suggested when a patient has

Fig. 26-19
Apical four-chamber views in a patient with acute infarct expansion. During diastole the left ventricle is clearly dilated, and there is abnormal geometry of the left ventricle (*arrowheads*) produced by acute dilation and thinning of the distal septum and apex. During systole the abnormal geometry is more marked.

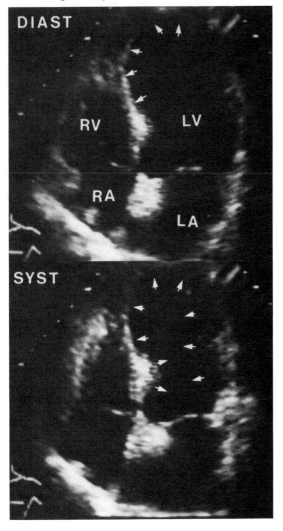

recurrent pain and increasing ST segment elevation without enzymatic evidence of reinfarction [81]. Pathologically, it is associated with an acutely thinned area of necrotic myocardium devoid of a dense fibrous wall, as seen in chronically forming aneurysms. It has been associated with a higher likelihood of rupture in the zone of expansion [80]. Infarct expansion can be recognized by two-dimensional echocardiography when wall dilation occurs within the first several days following myocardial infarction [78, 79]. An example of acute aneurysm formation 1 day after anterior myocardial infarction is shown in Figure 26-19. This patient subsequently experienced rupture near the apex.

Infarct expansion can be quantified in the short axis of the left ventricle using internal landmarks such as the papillary muscles and then quantifying the circumferential distance between them or the arc subtended by their centers. Using this technique, investigators from Johns Hopkins University have demonstrated that acute expansion and dilation of the infarct segment is a not uncommon cause of global cardiac enlargement during the first 3 days after myocardial infarction [79]. Recent data suggest that development of myocardial expansion, independent of electrocardiographic or enzyme estimates of myocardial infarction size, predicts a greater short-term mortality, specifically with the likelihood of frank myocardial rupture being substantially greater in these patients [75, 78–80].

PSEUDOANEURYSM

A pseudoaneurysm is the short-term result of a walled-off or contained myocardial rupture. In contrast with true aneurysm, which has a fibrous wall of high tensile strength and which is unlikely to rupture, a pseudoaneurysm represents a walled-off myocardial rupture that has a low strength wall and a reasonably high likelihood of recurring rupture leading to cardiac tamponade and death. Both true and pseudoaneurysms cause an abnormal bulge of the ventricular contour when imaged by echocardiography and other imaging techniques. Pathologically, a pseudoaneurysm is connected to the left ventricular cavity by a narrow orifice. Because of the high-resolution and tomographic imaging nature of echocardiography, this diagnostic feature of a pseudoaneurysm can be accurately identified [82, 83]. It has been suggested that aneurysms that appear external to the cardiac silhouette and that connect with the left ventricular cavity by a narrow orifice (less than one-third the maximum dimension of the body of the aneurysm) represent a false aneurysm rather than a true aneurysm. These aneurysms are frequently filled with fresh thrombus. Figure 26-20 was recorded in a patient with a posterior wall

Fig. 26-20
Parasternal long-axis and apical two-chamber views in a patient with an inferior myocardial infarction 3 months prior to admission. Rupture of the inferior wall leading to pseudoaneurysm formation is evident. Note the communication between the cavity of the left ventricle and the extra cardiac space (*long white arrow*) and the border of the pseudoaneurysm (*small white arrows*), which is partially filled with thrombus.

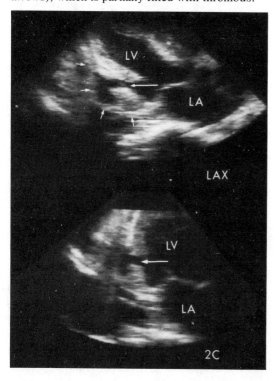

pseudoaneurysm detected 2 months after a clinical inferior infarction.

Mural Thrombus

Two-dimensional echocardiography is an excellent tool for evaluating intracardiac masses. It extends not only to intracardiac tumors but also to mural thrombi following acute myocardial infarction. Its sensitivity, specificity, and overall accuracy compare favorably to postmortem examination [84, 85], direct examination in the operating room [85, 86], contrast ventriculography [85], or indium 113 labeled platelet studies [84, 85]. Because echocardiography allows simultaneous assessment of left ventricular wall motion and the remainder of the cardiac anatomy, it is probably the preferred examination when screening for mural thrombi. Its sensitivity is reported as 97 percent in experimentally induced thrombus [85] and 95 percent in patients [84, 86]. Specificity has ranged from 86 percent [89] to 92 percent [86]. Experimentally, early abnormalities of blood flow suggesting stasis occur within minutes to hours of coronary occlusion [87]. Mural thrombi are most likely to form within the first 72 hours after myocardial infarction [88–89] and may form during administration of therapeutic anticoagulation [90–92]. They are found after approximately 40 percent of anterior myocardial infarctions and are rarely seen after inferior myocardial infarction [88, 89, 93, 94]. Figure 26-21 illustrates the range of thrombus formation seen with myocardial infarction.

The likelihood of clinical embolization is greater in those patients with echocardiographically demonstrated mural thrombi than in those without [84, 93, 95, 96]. Additional characteristics of the thrombus can be defined by echocardiography, including its size, whether it is sessile or protruding, and if it has mobility within the cavity. Subsequent embolization is more likely if the underlying ventricular thrombus is either pedunculated (protruding into the cavity) or mobile [96–98]. Therapeutic anticoagulation, although having

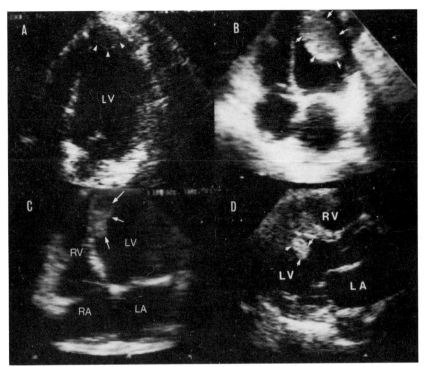

Fig. 26-21
Two-dimensional echocardiograms from four patients with mural thrombi complicating infarction or aneurysm. *A.* There is a small round filling defect in the apex of the left ventricle that is neither pedunculated nor mobile. *B.* There is a larger mass filling approximately one-third of the ventricular cavity. *C.* Pedunculated apical thrombus with free edges. Note that this thrombus is not adherent along its entire length and that it protrudes into the ventricular cavity. *D.* Pedunculated and mobile thrombus. This thrombus has a free edge that during the real-time examination was mobile. (From W. F. Amstrong. *Progress in Cardiovascular Disease.* January/February 1988. With permission.)

only a minimal effect on thrombus formation, may protect from embolic events [95, 99].

RIGHT VENTRICULAR INFARCTION

Right ventricular infarction is a relatively common complication seen almost exclusively in the presence of inferior rather than anterior myocardial infarction. It generally occurs in the presence of proximal right coronary artery lesions, often in patients with transient heart block and large inferior myocardial infarctions [100]. It should be suspected clinically when hypotension out of proportion to the suspected infarct size is seen in a patient with an inferior myocardial infarction. From an echo-

cardiographic standpoint right ventricular infarction is diagnosed when the right ventricle is dilated and wall motion abnormalities are present in both the inferior wall and the right ventricular free wall [101–104]. Figure 26-22 shows a right ventricular infarction diagnosed with two-dimensional echocardiography. Right ventricular infarct consists of a spectrum of abnormalities ranging from subclinical right ventricular dysfunction to marked right ventricular dilation with necrosis of the entire right ventricular wall [100, 104]. Right ventricular infarctions with only subtle degrees of systolic dysfunction may not be detected with echocardiography. In addition to the obvious primary problems with right ventricular systolic function, right ventricular in-

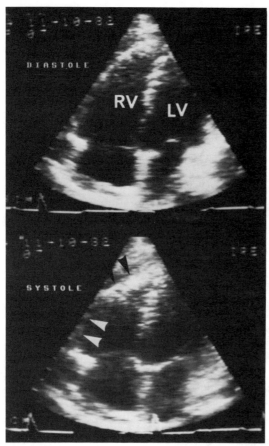

Fig. 26-22
Apical four-chamber view of a patient with a right
ventricular infarction. During systole the more
apical portions of the right ventricle appropriately
move inward (*black arrowheads*) whereas the
more basal portion of the wall is frankly
dyskinetic (*white arrows*). (From W. F.
Armstrong. *Progress in Cardiovascular Disease.*
January/February 1988. With permission.)

farction may be associated with more subtle
abnormalities. Among them is transient right-
to-left intracardiac shunting through a patent
foramen ovale, which manifests only after
right ventricular and right atrial pressures rise.
It results in systemic hypoxia and can be documented using contrast echocardiography
[105, 106].

VENTRICULAR SEPTAL DEFECT

Rupture of infarcted myocardium can occur in
one of three general areas. The first is rupture

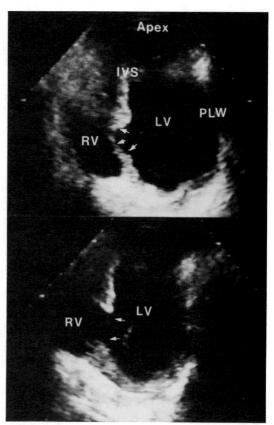

Fig. 26-23
Apical views in a patient with an inferior
myocardial infarction and an acute ventricular
septal defect. In the view at the left there is an
area of distinct thinning and aneurysm formation
in the proximal ventricular septum (*arrows*). With
a slightly different angulation a large ventricular
septal defect is seen (*arrows*).

of the free wall, which usually results in immediate cardiac tamponade and death but in a
minority of patients results in formation of a
pseudoaneurysm. In the usual case, in which
rupture leads to tamponade and death, two-dimensional echocardiography may be used to
visualize the point of rupture [107], but because of the rapid downhill course of these patients it rarely has any practical impact. The
second form of myocardial rupture is that of
the ventricular septum, leading to an acquired
ventricular septal defect; and the third is a
rupture of a papillary muscle (most commonly
of the mitral valve), resulting in severe valvular regurgitation.

Ventricular septal rupture or papillary mus-

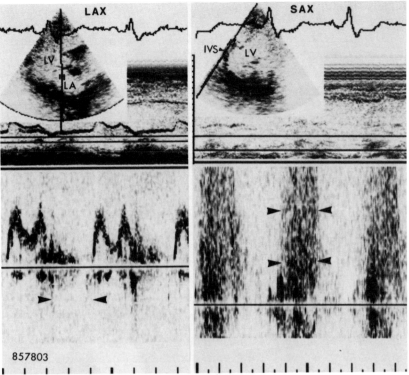

Fig. 26-24
Doppler examination of a patient with acute myocardial infarction and a new holosystolic murmur. (No anatomic defect was visualized with two-dimensional imaging.) On Doppler interrogation of the left atrium, no abnormal flow could be seen during systole (*left panel between the arrows*), excluding a diagnosis of mitral regurgitation. On careful scanning of the ventricular septum in the region of the wall motion abnormality (*right panel*), abnormal high velocity flow directed from left to right was detected. It is noted between the arrows in the right-hand panel and is diagnostic of a ventricular septal defect as the source of the new murmur. (From W. F. Armstrong. *Progress in Cardiovascular Disease*. January/February 1988.)

cle rupture should be suspected in a patient with acute myocardial infarction who develops a new loud holosystolic murmur. Often the two entities can be accurately distinguished by echocardiography when one is directly imaged [108–111]. Figure 26-23 shows a large ventricular septal defect that occurred after an inferior myocardial infarction.

Most ventricular septal defects are associated with aneurysm formation, and early rupture usually occurs at the margin of the aneurysm. As such, the area of rupture is usually immediately adjacent to a major wall motion abnormality [108–111]. Using modern scanning equipment and multiple views, most of the larger (i.e., >1 cm) ventricular septal de-

fects should be directly imaged. These defects occur in locations different from congenital ventricular septal defects, and the scanning planes for their detection are different than those used for the congenital defects. Careful attention is required to scan all areas of the ventricular septum, especially along regions of wall motion abnormality.

If the defect is anatomically small, it may evade detection by routine two-dimensional echocardiography. In these cases contrast echocardiography has diagnosed many of the acquired septal defects by detection of right-to-left shunting, which is often present to a mild degree during diastole [108, 112]. More recently, the Doppler ultrasound examination has been used to accurately identify the source of the new murmur by localizing the abnormal flow pattern [109, 113–118]. In the case of mitral regurgitation, an abnormal systolic flow signal is detected in the left atrium [116, 118]. If a ventricular septal defect is present, an abnormal high-velocity left-to-right flow is detected along the ventricular septum [113–115]. Figure 26-24 shows a patient with a new loud holosystolic murmur following a myocardial infarction. Direct imaging failed to detect any defect in the ventricular septum or abnormality of the mitral valve. Doppler interrogation, however, documented the presence of an abnormally high-velocity jet from the left to the right ventricle consistent with a ventricular septal defect. Even more recently the newly developed color flow imaging systems have been used to detect acquired ventricular septal defects [119]. An example is presented in Figure 26-25. In addition to establishing the diagnosis of ventricular septal defect, echocardiography may play a role in determining prognosis. Those patients with well preserved ventricular function and

normal hyperdynamic wall motion outside the infarct zone have a better prognosis than those with diffuse wall motion abnormalities and depressed systolic function [108].

Complications Involving the Mitral Apparatus

As with the free wall and septum, necrosis of the papillary muscle can lead to rupture of that structure. Frank rupture of a papillary muscle is generally associated with immediate onset of severe mitral regurgitation and pulmonary edema. The papillary muscles are complicated structures with multiple heads, and rupture can produce variable degrees of papillary muscle disruption. It leads to a spectrum of mitral regurgitation dependent on the exact location of rupture. Mitral valve papillary muscle rupture should be clinically suspected in those patients with acute pulmonary edema, hypotension, recurrent chest pain, and a new murmur following myocardial infarction. From an echocardiographic standpoint a spectrum of abnormalities can be visualized including actual rupture of the papillary muscle body (Fig. 26-26) and detection of a flail mitral valve leaflet (Fig. 26-27) [111, 120, 121]. When

Fig. 26-25

Doppler flow imaging in a patient with an inferior septal infarct and a loud holosystolic murmur. The dark area represents a systolic jet of blood moving from the left to the right ventricle through the ventricular septal defect. (From H. Feigenbaum. *Echocardiography* [4th ed.]. Philadelphia: Lea & Febiger, 1986. With permission.)

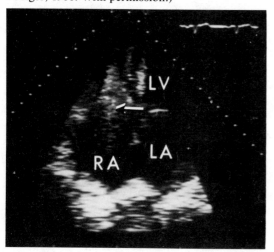

Fig. 26-26

Apical four-chamber view in a patient with flail mitral valve due to acute myocardial infarction. The papillary muscle has ruptured, and the tip of the muscle can be seen as a free-floating structure attached only by its chordae (*arrowhead*) in the cavity of the left ventricle.

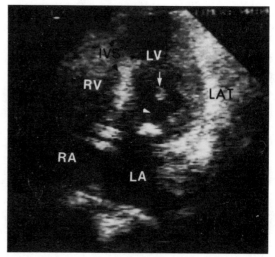

either of these entities is noted in the presence of an acute myocardial infarction and a loud systolic murmur, a diagnosis of rupture of the papillary muscle can be established. When technical considerations preclude adequate imaging or when the rupture involves only one small head of a papillary muscle, two-dimensional imaging may not be diagnostic. In these cases Doppler interrogation along the plane of the mitral valve documents the presence of mitral regurgitation as the cause of newly noted murmur [118].

A chronically infarcted papillary muscle may not demonstrate frank rupture but, rather, only reduction in its length leading to functional papillary muscle dysfunction. Echocardiographically, it causes abnormal closure of the mitral valve such that it tends to bow into the cavity of the left ventricle and become functionally incompetent [122, 123]. This form of papillary muscle dysfunction can be accurately identified with two-dimensional echocardiography; furthermore, the degree of

mitral regurgitation can be assessed using Doppler interrogation. Figure 26-28 shows a patient with a known inferior myocardial infarction and a loud holosystolic murmur. No abnormalities of the ventricular septum were visualized. The mitral valve had abnormal coaptation, and Doppler interrogation revealed abnormal systolic flow in the left atrium consistent with mitral regurgitation.

The above discussion was based on the evaluation of a murmur in a patient with a known myocardial infarction. The role of cardiac ultrasound is actually more extensive than presented above, as many if not all of the

Fig. 26-28
Apical four-chamber view recorded in a patient with a remote myocardial infarction and a holosystolic murmur. Note the abnormal mitral valve closure with bowing of the leaflets toward the ventricular cavity during systole. With the Doppler sample volume immediately behind the mitral valve, an abnormal high velocity regurgitant jet is noted that is diagnostic of mitral regurgitation.

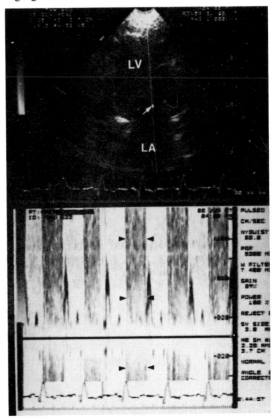

Fig. 26-27
Parasternal long-axis view during systole in a patient with a inferoapical myocardial infarction and papillary muscle rupture. The cross marks note the diastolic position of the ventricular endocardium. Note that during systole the anterior septum has moved appropriately, as has the proximal inferoposterior wall. There is dyskinesis of the inferoapical area (*outward-pointing arrows*). The anterior mitral valve leaflet is flail, and its tip (*small white arrow*) can be seen in the left atrium behind the mitral annulus (*white arrowhead*).

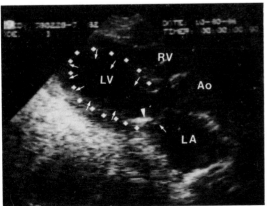

Table 26-3
Clinical syndromes associated with chest
discomfort and a murmur

Associated with myocardial infarction
   Ventricular septal rupture[a]
   Papillary muscle rupture (mitral)[a]
   Papillary muscle dysfunction without rupture[a]
   Acute tricuspid regurgitation[a]
   Free wall rupture[a]
Nonischemic syndromes
   Valvular aortic stenosis[a]
   Bacterial endocarditis[b]
   Hypertrophic myopathy[a]
   Acute myocarditis with mitral regurgitation[b]
   Chordal rupture (spontaneous or traumatic)[a]
   Pulmonary embolus with tricuspid regurgitation[b]
   Mitral valve prolapse[a]

---

[a]Entities for which echocardiography/Doppler provides
definitive data.
[b]Entities for which echocardiography/Doppler provides
supportive data.

clinical events or illnesses for which a patient
may present with the combination of chest
pain and a murmur can be accurately diagnosed with the combination of two-dimensional imaging and Doppler. Table 26-3 outlines many of these entities.

ECHOCARDIOGRAPHY IN
ACUTE INTERVENTIONS

Modern therapy for acute myocardial infarction includes not only observation and maintenance of hemodynamics during the natural
history of the ischemic event but often urgent
efforts at reperfusion. It is currently done via
thrombolysis with either tissue plasminogen
activator/streptokinase or emergent balloon
dilation of a coronary artery (or both). Two-
dimensional echocardiography can be used to
document the return of function following
such an intervention.

The study by Topol and colleagues was one
of the first using echocardiography to document return of function following reperfusion
[124]. These authors demonstrated that left
ventricular wall motion was more likely to improve in those segments distal to coronary arteries that not only had been subject to thrombolysis but also acute dilation with balloon
angioplasty.

Data from our institution are similar with respect to demonstration of myocardial salvage
following emergent balloon angioplasty [125].
We have performed serial two-dimensional
echocardiograms in 19 patients who underwent emergent reperfusion and in eight patients
who received only conventional noninterven-
tional therapy. Examples of echocardiograms
from such patients are presented in Figures 26-
29, 26-30, and 26-31. Figures 26-29 and 26-30
are two-dimensional echocardiograms recorded in patients at the time of presentation
and again several days after reperfusion via
coronary angioplasty. Both studies demonstrate return of left ventricular function
following reperfusion. Figure 26-31 is a
computer-generated outline of the diastolic-
systolic endocardial contours before and after
angioplasty of the case presented in Figure 26-
30. The global ejection fraction has been calculated and is shown to increase following return of ventricular function. Overall results of
this study, presented in Figure 26-32, demonstrate that in those patients who did not receive any form of reperfusion therapy the wall
motion abnormalities, as quantified by a wall
motion score index, remain stable over a minimum 6-day period, whereas there was a statistically significant improvement in wall motion in the patients undergoing reperfusion. In
this study a wall motion score index was generated that confirmed return of regional function; however, a return of global function has
also been demonstrated by other investigators
by calculation of the ejection fraction from
echocardiograms [126, 127]. In addition to its
role in demonstrating return of function following reperfusion, two-dimensional echocardiography may play a role in identifying
patients who are appropriate for aggressive
therapy [128]. As previously discussed, echocardiography can make the initial diagnosis of
infarction and estimate its size. As such, an
earlier diagnosis is feasible, and those patients
with large infarcts who are most likely to benefit from aggressive management can be immediately identified.

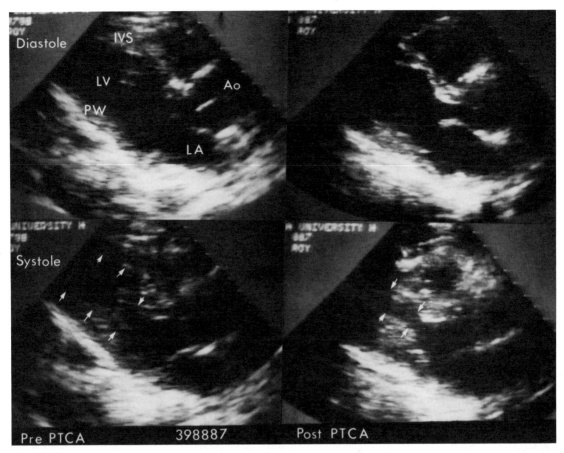

Fig. 26-29
Parasternal long-axis views during diastole and systole recorded in a patient with
impending anterior myocardial infarction. The figures on the left were recorded at
the time of presentation and those on the right 5 days after successful angioplasty
of the left anterior descending coronary artery. Note that at the time of
presentation the distal septum is dyskinetic (*upward-pointing arrows*), and the
inferoposterior wall is relatively hypokinetic. Five days after successful
angioplasty the inferoposterior wall moves normally and there has been
restitution of normal wall motion in the entire ventricular septum. (From W. F.
Armstrong. Echocardiography in acute myocardial infarction. In: *Cardiac
Imaging 1988*. Chicago: Year Book Medical Publishers, 1988. With permission.)

EXERCISE ECHOCARDIOGRAPHY AFTER MYOCARDIAL INFARCTION

The resting echocardiogram provides valuable
prognostic information in patients following
myocardial infarction. It is done on the basis
of the established wall motion abnormalities.
Exercise echocardiography refers to the technique of echocardiographic imaging in conjunction with stress to detect inducible wall
motion abnormalities that imply exercise-
induced ischemia and further myocardium in
jeopardy. This technique has been shown by a
number of investigators to be an accurate
means of detecting patients with coronary artery disease [129, 130]. More recently it has
been performed in conjunction with low level
exercise in patients recovering from myocardial infarction [131–133].

Jaarsma et al. have reported results in 49 patients [131] in which new exercise-induced
wall motion abnormalities during the conva-

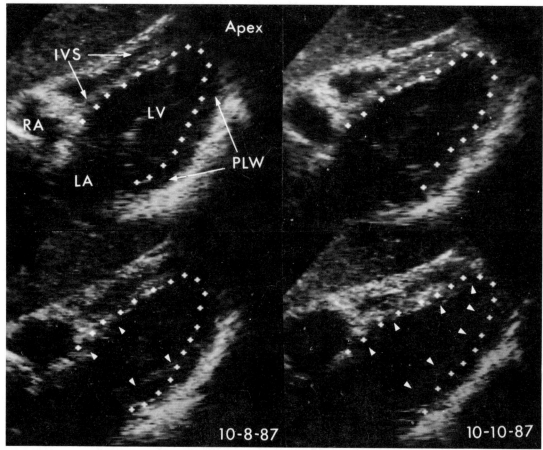

Fig. 26-30
Subcostal two-dimensional echocardiograms in a patient with impending
myocardial infarction. The upper panels are end-diastolic images. The lower
panels are recorded at end-systole. The asterisks outline the endocardial position
at end-diastole. At presentation (*left panels*) only the basal septum and proximal
posterolateral wall (PLW) move inward with systole (*arrows*). Two days after
angioplasty (*right panels*) there has been return of normal systolic function of the
distal septum, apex, and posterolateral wall (*arrows*). See Figure 26-1 for
abbreviations. (From W. F. Armstrong. *Progress in Cardiovascular Disease*.
January/February 1988. With permission.)

lescent period were associated with a higher
likelihood of recurrent angina or infarction.
Results from our institution are virtually identical [133]. In our study 16 of 17 patients with
new or worsening abnormalities postexercise
experienced a complication versus 4 of 23 patients with stable wall motion abnormalities.
Figure 26-33 shows a patient with a non-Q-
wave infarct evaluated during the convalescent period. Wall motion is preserved in the
septum at rest but becomes markedly abnormal after only low intensity exercise.

Future Developments

The current capabilities of two-dimensional
echocardiography and Doppler ultrasound
techniques in patients with chest pain syndromes who develop acute myocardial infarction are outlined above. Other applications
currently under investigation include attempts
at tissue characterization, myocardial perfusion contrast echocardiography, and direct
coronary visualization.

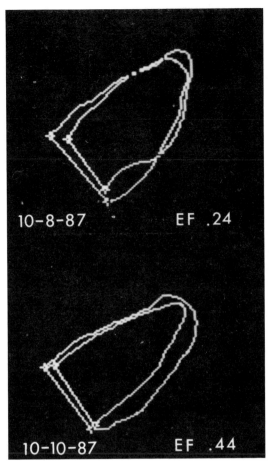

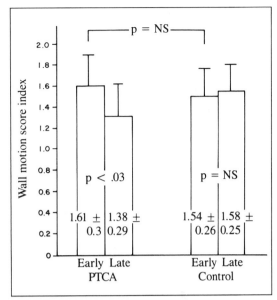

Fig. 26-31
Computer-generated endocardial outlines for the patient in Figure 26-30. The ejection fraction (EF) increased from 0.24 to 0.44 between the two studies. The apex is no longer dyskinetic, and there is normal motion of the lateral wall.

Fig. 26-32
Changes in wall motion score index in patients undergoing emergent percutaneous balloon coronary angioplasty (PTCA) and a control group of patients without intervention. There were 19 patients in the PTCA group and 8 in the control group. (From W. F. Armstrong. Echocardiography and coronary artery disease. *Int. J. Cardiac Imaging* 2:241, 1987. With permission.)

TISSUE CHARACTERIZATION

Tissue characterization relies on a computerized analysis of the gray levels of myocardium in an effort to detect ischemic or necrotic myocardium [134–137]. Multiple algorithms have been used successfully to this end, although they all appear closely linked to wall motion. To provide truly valuable information, tissue characterization parameters must be developed that allow demonstration of functionally abnormal but potentially viable ischemic myocardium, which would then assist in decisions for emergent reperfusion.

DIRECT CORONARY VISUALIZATION

The proximal right and left coronary arteries can be imaged by transthoracic ultrasound, and this imaging plays a role in the pediatric population for diagnosing aberrant coronary arteries and coronary arterial aneurysm [138]. In the adult population the feasibility of detecting atherosclerotic plaque in the proximal coronary arteries has been demonstrated by ourselves and in other laboratories [139–141]; however, its clinical impact is yet to be defined. The technique may eventually play a role in screening patients for high risk lesions such as left main or proximal left anterior descending coronary artery obstructions.

DIASTOLIC PROPERTIES OF THE LEFT VENTRICLE

Although the abnormalities of systolic function are often thought of as the major abnor-

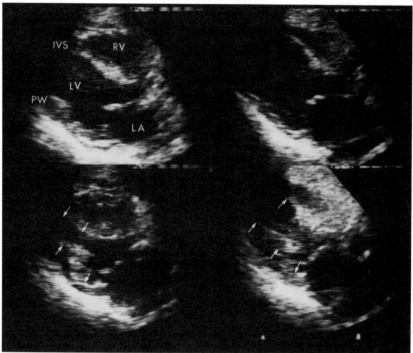

Fig. 26-33
Rest and postexercise echocardiograms recorded in the parasternal long axis view. The study was performed 14 days after an uncomplicated myocardial infarction. At rest the proximal inferoposterior wall is akinetic. With exercise the patient developed no chest pain, and the test was stopped for fatigue and dyspnea. After exercise the entire inferoposterior wall and distal ventricular septum become dyskinetic, implying multivessel coronary disease, which was confirmed at subsequent catheterization.

mality produced by myocardial ischemia, abnormalities of diastolic relaxation occur almost universally with ischemia and may play a role in clinical deterioration [142–146]. These abnormalities are reflected in the pattern of left ventricular inflow through the mitral valve. With normal left ventricular compliance, mitral inflow is biphasic with more rapid early than late inflow velocities. There is an immediate reversal in this ratio with the onset of myocardial ischemia. This picture is seen experimentally in the animal laboratory [142] and at the time of balloon angioplasty in patients [143]. Although these changes are generally thought to reflect altered diastolic compliance of the left ventricle, they do not correlate highly with any of the more well accepted hemodynamic parameters of a diastolic function [142], and their magnitude is highly dependent on ventricular loading conditions. At least one preliminary report has suggested that the magnitude of these changes reflects patient prognosis in the acute setting [146].

MYOCARDIAL PERFUSION/ CONTRAST ECHOCARDIOGRAPHY

Contrast echocardiography was initially developed for assessing chamber boundaries and intracardiac shunts. Development of new myocardial contrast agents now allows assessment of myocardial perfusion with two-dimensional echocardiography [147–150]. This technique, initially developed in the animal laboratory, has been demonstrated to be an accurate means of determining myocardial infarction size [148] and, more recently, an

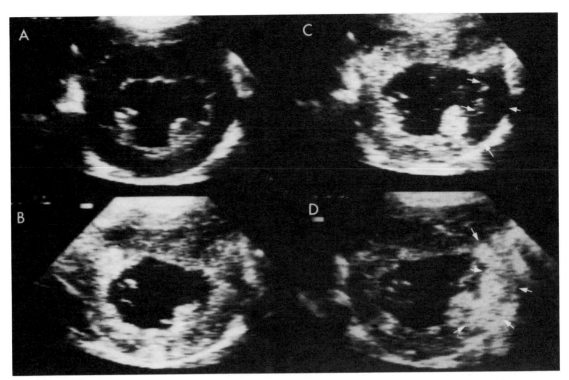

Fig. 26-34
Myocardial contrast echocardiograms recorded at baseline (*B*), during coronary
occlusion (*C*), and immediately after release of the occlusion, demonstrating
reactive hyperemia (*D*). *A*. Recorded at baseline prior to contrast injection or any
coronary manipulation. *C*. There is an area (*arrows*) that has not increased in
image intensity and that corresponds to a nonperfused region of myocardium.
This same area shows preferential uptake of the contrast during the phase of
reactive hyperemia.

accurate means of identifying reperfusion
hyperemia [151]. Figure 26-34 is a composite
showing the range of observations that have
been noted with myocardial contrast echocardiography. The ultimate goal of this technique
would be to develop contrast agents and methodology for determining absolute myocardial
perfusion levels. Although it has been approximated in animal laboratories [149], it is not
yet feasible to precisely determine perfusion
levels with this technique.

Myocardial contrast echocardiography has
been used in patients on an investigational basis and was demonstrated to be safe [152–154].
Newer agents currently under development
will increase the margin of safety for this technique. Preliminary data suggest that the distribution of coronary arteries can be determined

with myocardial perfusion contrast echocardiography [152], that severe coronary artery
narrowings can be documented, and that return of flow following reperfusion can be
demonstrated [153]. This technique shows
tremendous promise for allowing simultaneous assessment of perfusion and ventricular
function using echocardiography.

Summary/Conclusion

Modern ultrasound techniques are highly versatile, relatively inexpensive, and noninvasive, and they allow visualization of all areas
of the human heart. When dealing with patients with coronary artery disease, wall motion abnormalities are the hallmark of myocar-

dial ischemia and can be accurately identified and quantified. Echocardiography may provide the initial diagnosis of acute ischemic syndromes, quantitation of myocardial infarction size, and assessment of short- and long-term prognosis. Additionally, two-dimensional echocardiography combined with Doppler techniques can diagnose most complications arising after myocardial infarction. Future developments may allow assessment of the diastolic properties of the heart and of myocardial perfusion itself.

Editorial Comments

The group from Indiana University, including Dr. Armstrong, has long been at the forefront of echocardiography research. Echocardiographic analysis is of extraordinary value in acute ischemic syndromes, including acute myocardial infarction. It is our practice to perform careful echocardiographic assessment of nearly all patients with acute infarction, particularly those with complicated courses, where its value cannot be overstated. G.S.F.

References

1. Tennant, R., and Wiggers, C. J. The effect of coronary occlusion on myocardial contraction. *A.J.P.* 112:351, 1935.
2. Weiss, J. L., Bulkley, B. H., Hutchins, G. M., and Mason, S. J. Two-dimensional echocardiographic recognition of myocardial injury in man: Comparison with postmortem studies. *Circulation* 63:401, 1981.
3. Hecht, H. S., Taylor, R., Wong, M., and Shah, P. M. Comparative evaluation of segmental asynergy in remote myocardial infarction by radionuclide angiography, two-dimensional echocardiography, and contrast ventriculography. *Am. Heart J.* 101:740, 1981.
4. Wohlgelernter, D., Cleman, M., Highman, H. A., et al. Regional myocardial dysfunction during coronary angioplasty: Evaluation by two-dimensional echocardiography and 12 lead electrocardiography. *J. Am. Coll. Cardiol.* 7:1245, 1986.
5. Labovitz, A. J., Lewen, M. K., Kern, M., et al. Evaluation of left ventricular systolic and diastolic dysfunction during transient myocardial ischemia produced by angioplasty. *J. Am. Coll. Cardiol.* 10:748, 1987.
6. Hauser, A. M., Gangadharan, V., Ramos, R. G., et al. Sequence of mechanical, electrocardiographic and clinical effects of repeated coronary artery occlusion in human beings: Echocardiographic observations during coronary angioplasty. *J. Am. Coll. Cardiol.* 5:193, 1985.
7. Visser, C. A., David, G. K., Kan, G., et al. Two-dimensional echocardiography during percutaneous transluminal coronary angioplasty. *Am. Heart J.* 111:1035, 1986.
8. Vatner, S. F. Correlation between acute reductions in myocardial blood flow and function in conscious dogs. *Circ. Res.* 47:201, 1980.
9. Banka, V. S., Bodenheimer, M. M., and Helfant, R. H. Relation between progressive decreases in regional coronary perfusion and contractile abnormalities. *Am. J. Cardiol.* 40:200, 1977.
10. Wyatt, H. L., Forrester, J. S., and Tyberg, J. V. Effect of graded reductions in regional coronary perfusion on regional and total cardiac function. *Am. J. Cardiol.* 36:185, 1975.
11. Buda, A. J., Zotz, R. J., Pace, D. P., and Krause, L. C. Comparison of two-dimensional echocardiographic wall motion and wall thickening abnormalities in relation to the myocardium at risk. *Am. Heart J.* 111:587, 1986.
12. Lieberman, A. N., Weiss, J. L., and Jugdutt, B. I. Two-dimensional echocardiography and infarct size relationship of regional wall motion and thickening to the extent of myocardial infarction in the dog. *Circulation* 63:739, 1981.
13. Nieminen, M., Parisi, A. F., and O'Boyle, J. E. Serial evaluation of myocardial thickening and thinning in acute experimental infarction: Identification and quantification using two-dimensional echocardiography. *Circulation* 66:174, 1982.
14. Weyman, A. E., Franklin, T. D., and Hogan, R. D. Importance of temporal heterogeneity in assessing the contraction abnormalities associated with acute myocardial ischemia. *Circulation* 70:102, 1984.
15. Kerber, R. E., Marcus, M. L., Ehrhardt, J., et al. Correlation between echocardiographically demonstrated segmental dyskinesis and regional myocardial perfusion. *Circulation* 52:1097, 1975.
16. O'Boyle, J. E., Parisi, A. F., Nieminen, M., et al. Quantitative detection of regional left ventricular contraction abnormalities by 2-dimensional echocardiography. *Am. J. Cardiol.* 51:1732, 1985.
17. Pandian, N. G., Koyanagi, S., Skorton, D. J., et al. Relations between 2-dimensional echocardiographic wall thickening abnormalities,

myocardial infarct size and coronary risk area in normal and hypertrophied myocardium in dogs. *Am. J. Cardiol.* 52:1318, 1983.

18. Ellis, S. G., Henschke, C. I., Sandor, T., et al. Relation between the transmural extent of acute myocardial infarction and associated myocardial contractility two weeks after infarction. *Am. J. Cardiol.* 55:1412, 1985.

19. Wyatt, H. L., Meerbaum, S., Heng, M. K., et al. Experimental evaluation of the extent of myocardial dyssynergy and infarct size by two-dimensional echocardiography. *Circulation* 63:607, 1981.

20. Pandian, N. G., Skorton, D. J., Collins, S. M., et al. Myocardial infarct size threshold for two-dimensional echocardiographic detection: Sensitivity of systolic wall thickening and endocardial motion abnormalities in small versus large infarcts. *Am. J. Cardiol.* 55:551, 1985.

21. Wyatt, H. L., Forrester, J. S., da Luz, P. L., et al. Functional abnormalities in nonoccluded regions of myocardium after experimental coronary occlusion. *Am. J. Cardiol.* 37:366, 1976.

22. Homans, D. C., Asinger, R., Elsperger, K. J., et al. Regional function and perfusion at the lateral border of ischemic myocardium. *Circulation* 71:1038, 1985.

23. Guth, B. D., White, F. C., Gallagher, K. P., and Bloor, C. M. Decreased systolic wall thickening in myocardium adjacent to ischemic zones in conscious swine during brief coronary artery occlusion. *Am. Heart J.* 107:458, 1984.

24. Lima, J. A. C., Becker, L. C., Melin, J. A., et al. Impaired thickening of nonischemic myocardium during acute regional ischemia in the dog. *Circulation* 71:1048, 1985.

25. Force, T., Kemper, A., Perkins, L., et al. Overestimation of infarct size by quantitative two-dimensional echocardiography: The role of tethering and of analytic procedures. *Circulation* 73:1360, 1986.

26. Kisslo, J. A., Robertson, D., Gilbert, B. W., et al. A comparison of real-time, two-dimensional echocardiography and cineangiography in detecting left ventricular asynergy. *Circulation* 55:134, 1977.

27. Linduall, K., Hamsten, A., Landou, C., et al. Comparative study of echo- and angiocardiographically determined regional left ventricular wall motion in recent myocardial infarction. *Eur. Heart J.* 5:533, 1984.

28. Erbel, R., Schweizer, P., Meyer, J., et al. Sensitivity of cross-sectional echocardiography in detection of impaired global and regional left ventricular function: Prospective study. *Int. J. Cardiol.* 7:375, 1985.

29. Freeman, A. P., Giles, R. W., Walsh, W. F., et al. Regional left ventricular wall motion assessment: Comparison of two-dimensional echocardiography and radionuclide angiography with contrast angiography in healed myocardial infarction. *Am. J. Cardiol.* 56:8, 1985.

30. VanReet, R. E., Quinones, M. A., Poliner, L. R., et al. Comparison of two-dimensional echocardiography with gated radionuclide ventriculography in the evaluation of global and regional left ventricular function in acute myocardial infarction. *J. Am. Coll. Cardiol.* 3:243, 1984.

31. Nixon, J. V., Narahara, K. A., and Smitherman, T. C. Estimation of myocardial involvement in patients with acute myocardial infarction by two-dimensional echocardiography. *Circulation* 62:1248, 1980.

32. Heger, J. J., Weyman, A. E., Wann, L. S., et al. Cross-sectional echocardiographic analysis of the extent of left ventricular asynergy in acute myocardial infarction. *Circulation* 61:1113, 1980.

33. Moynihan, P. F., Parisi, A. F., and Feldman, C. L. Quantitative detection of regional left ventricular contraction abnormalities by two-dimensional echocardiography. *Circulation* 63:752, 1981.

34. Parisi, A. F., Moynihan, P. F., Folland, E. D., and Feldman, C. L. Quantitative detection of regional left ventricular contraction abnormalities by two-dimensional echocardiography. *Circulation* 63:761, 1981.

35. Mann, D. L., Gillam, D., and Weyman, A. E. Cross-sectional echocardiographic assessment of regional left ventricular performance and myocardial perfusion. *Prog. Cardiovasc. Dis.* 29:1, 1986.

36. Gillam, L. D., Hogan, R. D., Foale, R. A., et al. A comparison of quantitative echocardiographic methods for delineating infarct-induced abnormal wall motion. *Circulation* 70:113, 1984.

37. Gillam, L. D., Franklin, T. D., Foale, R. A., et al. The natural history of regional wall motion in the acutely infarcted canine ventricle. *J. Am. Coll. Cardiol.* 7:1325, 1986.

38. Bolsono, E. L., Kliman, S., Sheehan, F. H., and Dodge, H. T. Left ventricular segmental wall motion: A new method using local direction information. *IEEE Comput. Cardiol.* 1982.

39. Gerson, M. C., Noble, R. J., Wann, L. S., et al. Noninvasive documentation of Prinzmetal's angina. *Am. J. Cardiol.* 43:329, 1979.

40. Widlansky, S., McHenry, P. L., Corya, B. C., and Phillips, J. F. Coronary angiographic, echocardiographic and electrocardiographic studies on a patient with variant angina due to coronary artery spasm. *Am. Heart J.* 90:631, 1975.

41. Distante, A., Rovai, D., Picano, E., et al. Transient changes in left ventricular mechan-

ics during attacks of Prinzmetal angina: A two-dimensional echocardiographic study. *Am. Heart J.* 108:440, 1984.

42. Distante, A., Picano, E., Moscarelli, E., et al. Echocardiographic versus hemodynamic monitoring during attacks of variant angina pectoris. *Am. J. Cardiol.* 55:1319, 1985.

43. Nixon, J. V., Brown, C. N., and Smitherman, T. C. Identification of transient and persistent segmental wall motion abnormalities in patients with unstable angina by two-dimensional echocardiography. *Circulation* 65:1497, 1982.

44. Heger, J. J., Weyman, A. E., Wann, L. S., et al. Cross-sectional echocardiography in acute myocardial infarction: Detection and localization of regional left ventricular asynergy. *Circulation* 60:531, 1979.

45. Stamm, R. B., Gibson, R. S., Bishop, H. L., et al. Echocardiographic detection of infarct-localized asynergy and remote asynergy during acute myocardial infarction: Correlation with the extent of angiographic coronary disease. *Circulation* 67:233, 1983.

46. Gibson, R. S., Bishop, H. L., Stamm, R. B., et al. Value of early two dimensional echocardiography in patients with acute myocardial infarction. *Am. J. Cardiol.* 49:1110, 1982.

47. Horowitz, B. S., Morganroth, J., Parrotto, C., et al. Immediate diagnosis of acute myocardial infarction by two-dimensional echocardiography. *Circulation* 65:323, 1982.

48. Jaarsma, W., Visser, C. A., Van Eengie, M. J., and Roos, J. P. Left ventricular wall motion with and without Q-wave disappearance after acute myocardial infarction. *Am. J. Cardiol.* 59:516, 1987.

49. Mahias-Navarte, H., Adams, K. F., and Willis, P. W. Evolution of regional left ventricular wall motion abnormalities in acute Q and non-Q wave myocardial infarction. *Am. J. Heart* 113:1369, 1987.

50. Arvan, S., and Varat, M. A. Two-dimensional echocardiography versus surface electrocardiography for the diagnosis of acute non-Q wave myocardial infarction. *Am. J. Heart* 110:44, 1985.

51. Loh, I. K., Charuzi, Y., Beeder, C., et al. Early diagnosis of nontransmural myocardial infarction by two-dimensional echocardiography. *Am. Heart J.* 104:963, 1982.

52. Force, T., Kemper, A. J., Bloomfield, P., et al. Non-Q wave perioperative myocardial infarction: Assessment of the incidence and severity of regional dysfunction with quantitative two-dimensional echocardiography. *Circulation* 72:781, 1985.

53. Force, T., Bloomfield, P., O'Boyle, J. E., et al. Quantitative two-dimensional echocardiographic analysis of regional wall motion in patients with perioperative myocardial infarction. *Circulation* 70:233, 1984.

54. Camara, E. J., Chandra, N., Ouyang, P., et al. Reciprocal ST change in acute myocardial infarction: assessment by electrocardiography and echocardiography. *J. Am. Coll. Cardiol.* 2:251, 1983.

55. Pierard, L. A., Sprynger, M., Gilis, F., and Carlier, J. Significance of precordial ST-segment depression in inferior acute myocardial infarction as determined by echocardiography. *Am. J. Cardiol.* 57:82, 1986.

56. Diamond, T. H., Steingo, L., Davidoff, R., et al. Persistent ST-segment elevation in patients with anterior myocardial infarctions. *S. Afr. Med. J.* 68:94, 1985.

57. Arvan, S., and Varat, M. A. Persistent ST-segment elevation and left ventricular wall abnormalities: A 2-dimensional echocardiographic study. *Am. J. Cardiol.* 53:1542, 1984.

58. Kan, G., Visser, C. A., Lie, K. I., and Durrer, D. Early two-dimensional echocardiographic measurement of left ventricular ejection fraction of acute myocardial infarction. *Eur. Heart J.* 5:210, 1984.

59. Nishimura, R. A., Tajik, A. J., Shub, C., et al. Role of two-dimensional echocardiography in the prediction of in-hospital complications after acute myocardial infarction. *J. Am. Coll. Cardiol.* 4:1080, 1984.

60. Nishimura, R. A., Reeder, G. S., Miller, F. A., et al. Prognostic value of predischarge 2-dimensional echocardiogram after acute myocardial infarction. *Am. J. Cardiol.* 53:429, 1984.

61. Bhatnagar, S. K., Moussa, M. A. A., and Al-Yusuf, A. R. The role of prehospital discharge two-dimensional echocardiography in determining the prognosis of survivors of first myocardial infarction. *Am. Heart J.* 109:472, 1985.

62. Horowitz, R. S., and Morganroth, J. Immediate detection of early high-risk patients with acute myocardial infarction using two-dimensional echocardiographic evaluation of left ventricular regional wall motion abnormalities. *Am. Heart J.* 103:814, 1982.

63. Abrams, D. S., Starling, M. R., Crawford, M. H., and O'Rourke, R. A. Value of noninvasive techniques for predicting early complications in patients with clinical class II acute myocardial infarction. *J. Am. Coll. Cardiol.* 2:818, 1983.

64. Huntsman, L. L., Stewart, D. K., Barnes, S. R., et al. Noninvasive Doppler determination of cardiac output in man. *Circulation* 67:593, 1983.

65. Wallmeyer, K., Wann, L. S., Sagar, K. B., et al. The influence of preload and heart rate on Doppler echocardiographic indexes of left

ventricular performance: Comparison with invasive indexes in an experimental preparation. *Circulation* 74:181, 1986.

66. Buchtal, A., Hanson, G. C., and Pleisach, A. R. Transcutaneous aortovelography—potentially useful technique in management of critically ill patients. *Br. Heart J.* 38:451, 1976.

67. Mehta, N., and Bennett, D. E. Impaired left ventricular function in acute myocardial infarction assessed by Doppler measurement of ascending aortic blood velocity and maximum acceleration. *Am. J. Cardiol.* 57:1052,1986.

68. Kaplan, K., Davison, R., Parker, M., et al. Frequency of pericardial effusion as determined by M-mode echocardiography in acute myocardial infarction. *Am. J. Cardiol.* 55:335, 1985.

69. Pierard, L. A., Albert, A., Henrard, L., et al. Incidence and significance of pericardial effusion in acute myocardial infarction as determined by two-dimensional echocardiography. *J. Am. Coll. Cardiol.* 8:517, 1986.

70. Weyman, A. E., Peskoe, S. M., Williams, E. S., et al. Detection of left ventricular aneurysms by cross-sectional echocardiography. *Circulation* 54:936, 1976.

71. Visser, C. A., Kan, G., David, G. K., et al. Echocardiographic-cineangiographic correlation in detecting left ventricular aneurysm: A prospective study of 422 patients. *Am. J. Cardiol.* 50:337, 1982.

72. Barrett, M. J., Charuzi, Y., and Corday, E. C. Ventricular aneurysm: Cross-sectional echocardiographic approach. *Am. J. Cardiol.* 46:1133, 1980.

73. Matsumoto, M., Watanabe, F., Goto, A., et al. Left ventricular aneurysm and the prediction of left ventricular enlargement studied by two-dimensional echocardiography: quantitative assessment of aneurysm size in relation to clinical course. *Circulation* 72:280, 1985.

74. Visser, C. A., Kan, G., Meltzer, R. S., et al. Incidence, timing and prognostic value of left ventricular aneurysm formation after myocardial infarction: A prospective, serial echocardiographic study of 158 patients. *Am. J. Cardiol.* 57:729, 1986.

75. Eaton, L. W., Weiss, J. L., Bulkley, B., et al. Regional cardiac dilatation after acute myocardial infarction. *N. Engl. J. Med.* 300:57, 1979.

76. Visser, C. A., Kan, G., Meltzer, R. S., et al. Assessment of left ventricular aneurysm resectability by two-dimensional echocardiography. *Am. J. Cardiol.* 56:857, 1985.

77. Ryan, T., Petrovic, O., Armstrong, W. F., et al. Quantitative two-dimensional echocardiographic assessment of patients undergoing left ventricular aneurysmectomy. *Am. Heart J.* 111:714, 1986.

78. Erlebacher, J. A., Weiss, J. L., Eaton, L. W., et al. Late effects of acute infarct dilation on heart size: A two dimensional echocardiographic study. *Am. J. Cardiol.* 49:1120, 1982.

79. Erlebacher, J. A., Weiss, J. L., Weisfeldt, M. L., and Bulkley, B. H. Early dilation of the infarcted segment in acute transmural myocardial infarction: Role of infarct expansion in acute left ventricular enlargement. *J. Am. Coll. Cardiol.* 4:201, 1984.

80. Schuster, E. H., and Bulkley, B. H. Expansion of transmural myocardial infarction: A pathophysiologic factor in cardiac rupture. *Circulation* 60:1532, 1979.

81. Hutchins, G. M., and Bulkley, B. H. Infarct expansion versus extension: Two different complications of acute myocardial infarction. *Am. J. Cardiol.* 41:1127, 1978.

82. Gatewood, R. P., and Nanda, N. C. Differentiation of left ventricular pseudoaneurysm from true aneurysm with two dimensional echocardiography. *Am. J. Cardiol.* 46:869, 1980.

83. Catherwood, E., Mintz, G. S., Kotler, M. N., et al. Two-dimensional echocardiographic recognition of left ventricular pseudoaneurysm. *Circulation* 62:294, 1980.

84. Stratton, J. R., Lighty, G. W., Pearlman, A. S., and Ritchie, J. L. Detection of left ventricular thrombus by two-dimensional echocardiography: Sensitivity, specificity, and causes of uncertainty. *Circulation* 1:156, 1966.

85. Seabold, J. E., Schroder, E., Conrad, G. R., et al. Indium-111 platelet scintigraphy and two-dimensional echocardiography for detection of left ventricular thrombus: Influence of clot size and age. *J. Am. Coll. Cardiol.* 9:1057, 1987.

86. Pechacek, L. W., Lazar, A. V., Sonnemaker, R. E., et al. Comparison of two-dimensional echocardiography, radionuclide ventriculography and cineangiography in detecting surgically documented left ventricular thrombi. *Texas Heart Inst. J.* 11:118, 1984.

87. Mikell, F. L., Asinger, R. W., Elsperger, K. J., et al. Tissue acoustic properties of fresh left ventricular thrombi and visualization by two dimensional echocardiography: Experimental observations. *Am. J. Cardiol.* 49:1157, 1982.

88. Spirito, P., Bellotti, P., Chiarella, F., et al. Prognostic significance and natural history of left ventricular thrombi in patients with acute anterior myocardial infarction: A two-dimensional echocardiographic study. *Circulation* 72:774, 1985.

89. Visser, C. A., Kan, D. G., Meltzer, R. S., et al. Long-term follow-up of left ventricular thrombus after acute myocardial infarction. *Chest* 86:532, 1984.

90. Gueret, P., Dubourg, O., Ferrier, A., et al. Effects of full-dose heparin anticoagulation on

the development of left ventricular thrombosis in acute transmural myocardial infarction. *J. Am. Coll. Cardiol.* 8:419, 1986.

91. Arvan, S., and Boscha, K. Prophylactic anticoagulation for left ventricular thrombi after acute myocardial infarction: A prospective randomized trial. *Am. Heart J.* 113:688, 1987.

92. Sharma, B., Carvalho, A., Wyeth, R., and Franciosa, J. A. Left ventricular thrombi diagnosed by echocardiography in patients with acute myocardial infarction treated with intracoronary streptokinase followed by intravenous heparin. *Am. J. Cardiol.* 56:422, 1985.

93. Weinreich, D. J., Burke, J. F., and Pauletto, F. J. Left ventricular mural thrombi complicating acute myocardial infarction. *Ann. Intern. Med.* 100:789, 1984.

94. Asinger, R. W., Mikell, F. L., Elsperger, J., and Hodges, M. Incidence of left-ventricular thrombosis after acute transmural myocardial infarction. *N. Engl. J. Med.* 305:297, 1981.

95. Keating, E. C., Gross, S. A., Schlamowitz, R. A., et al. Mural thrombi in myocardial infarctions. *Am. J. Med.* 74:989, 1983.

96. Stratton, J. R., and Resnick, A. D. Increased embolic risk in patients with left ventricular thrombi. *Circulation* 75:1004, 1987.

97. Visser, C. A., Kan, G., Meltzer, R. S., et al. Embolic potential of left ventricular thrombus after myocardial infarction: A two-dimensional echocardiographic study of 119 patients. *J. Am. Coll. Cardiol.* 5:1276, 1985.

98. Meltzer, R. S., Visser, C. A., and Fuster, V. Intracardiac thrombi and systemic embolization. *Ann. Intern. Med.* 104:689, 1986.

99. Tramarin, R., Pozzoli, M., Opasich, F. C., et al. Two-dimensional echocardiographic assessment of anticoagulant therapy in left ventricular thrombosis early after acute myocardial infarction. *Eur. Heart J.* 7:482, 1986.

100. Isner, J. M., and Roberts, W. C. Right ventricular infarction complicating left ventricular infarction secondary to coronary heart disease. *Am. J. Cardiol.* 42:885, 1978.

101. Panidis, I. P., Kotler, M. N., Mintz, G. S., et al. Right ventricular function in coronary artery disease as assessed by two-dimensional echocardiography. *Am. Heart J.* 107:1187, 1984.

102. Lopez-Sendon, J., Garcia-Fernandez, A., Coma-Canella, I., et al. Segmental right ventricular function after acute myocardial infarction: Two-dimensional echocardiographic study in 63 patients. *Am. J. Cardiol.* 51:390, 1983.

103. Jugdutt, B. I., Haraphongse, M., Basualdo, C. A., and Rossall, R. E. Evaluation of biventricular involvement in hypotensive patients with transmural inferior infarction by two-dimensional echocardiography. *Am. Heart J.* 108:1417, 1984.

104. Dell'Italia, L. J., Starling, M. R., Crawford, M. H., et al. Right ventricular infarction: Identification by hemodynamic measurements before and after volume loading and correlation with noninvasive technique. *J. Am. Coll. Cardiol.* 4:931, 1984.

105. Rietveld, A. P., Merrman, L., Essed, C. E., et al. Right to left shunt, with severe hypoxemia, at the atrial level in a patient with hemodynamically important right ventricular infarction. *J. Am. Coll. Cardiol.* 4:776, 1983.

106. Bansal, R. C., Marsa, R. J., Holland, D., et al. Severe hypoxemia due to shunting through a patent foramen ovale: A correctable complication of right ventricular infarction. *J. Am. Coll. Cardiol.* 5:188, 1985.

107. Desoutter, P., Halphen, C., and Haiat, R. Two-dimensional echographic visualization of free ventricular wall rupture in acute anterior myocardial infarction. *Am. Heart J.* 108:1360, 1984.

108. Bishop, H. L., Gibson, R. S., Stamm, R. B., et al. Role of two-dimensional echocardiography in the evaluation of patients with ventricular septal rupture postmyocardial infarction. *Am. Heart J.* 102:965, 1981.

109. Smith, G., Endresen, K., Sivertssen, E., and Semb, G. Ventricular septal rupture diagnosed by simultaneous cross-sectional echocardiography and Doppler ultrasound. *Br. Heart J.* 6:631, 1985.

110. Rogers, E. W., Glassman, R. D., Feigenbaum, H., et al. Aneurysms of the posterior interventricular septum with postinfarction ventricular septal defect. *Chest* 78:741, 1980.

111. Mintz, G. S., Victor, M. F., Kotler, M. N., et al. Two-dimensional echocardiographic identification of surgically correctable complications of acute myocardial infarction. *Circulation* 64:91, 1981.

112. Drobac, M., Gilbert, B., Howard, R., et al. Ventricular septal defect after myocardial infarction: Diagnosis by two-dimensional contrast echocardiography. *Circulation* 67:335, 1983.

113. Recusani, F., Raisaro, A., Sgalambro, A., et al. Ventricular septal rupture after myocardial infarction: Diagnosis by two-dimensional and pulsed Doppler echocardiography. *Am. J. Cardiol.* 54:277, 1984.

114. Keren, G., Sherez, J., Roth, A., et al. Diagnosis of ventricular septal rupture from acute myocardial infarction by combined 2-dimensional and pulsed Doppler echocardiography. *Am. J. Cardiol.* 53:1202, 1985.

115. Come, P. A. Doppler detection of acquired ventricular septal defect. *Am. J. Cardiol.* 55:586, 1985.

116. Eisenberg, P. R., Barzilai, B., and Perez, J. E. Noninvasive detection by Doppler echocardiography of combined ventricular septal rup-

ture and mitral regurgitation in acute myocardial infarction. *J. Am. Coll. Cardiol.* 4:617, 1984.

117. Miyatake, K., Okamoto, M., Kinoshita, N., et al. Doppler echocardiographic features of ventricular septal rupture in myocardial infarction. *J. Am. Coll. Cardiol.* 5:182, 1985.

118. Loperfido, F., Biasucci, L. M., Pennestri', F., et al. Pulsed Doppler echocardiographic analysis of mitral regurgitation after myocardial infarction. *Am. J. Cardiol.* 58:692, 1986.

119. Kapur, K. K., Nanda, N. C., Fan, P-H., et al. Color Doppler evaluation of acute ventricular septal rupture (Abstract). *Circulation* 76(Suppl IV):527, 1987.

120. Erbel, R., Schweizer, P., Besdos, P., and Meyer, J. Two-dimensional echocardiographic diagnosis of papillary muscle rupture. *Chest* 79:595, 1981.

121. Come, P. C., Riley, M. F., and Weintraub, R. Echocardiographic detection of complete and partial papillary muscle rupture during acute myocardial infarction. *Am. J. Cardiol.* 56:787, 1985.

122. Godley, R. W., Wann, L. S., Rogers, E. W., et al. Incomplete mitral leaflet closure in patients with papillary muscle dysfunction. *Circulation* 63:565, 1981.

123. Ogawa, S., Hubbard, F. E., Mardelli, T. J., et al. Cross-sectional echocardiographic spectrum of papillary muscle dysfunction. *Am. Heart J.* 97:312, 1979.

124. Topol, E. J., Weiss, J. L., Brinker, J. A., et al. Regional wall motion improvement after coronary thrombolysis with recombinant tissue plasminogen activator: Importance of coronary angioplasty. *J. Am. Coll. Cardiol.* 6:426, 1985.

125. Presti, C. F., Gentile, R., Armstrong, W. F., et al. Demonstration of myocardial salvage by percutaneous transluminal coronary angioplasty using two-dimensional echocardiography (Abstract). *Clin. Res.* 35:315A, 1987.

126. Lambertz, H., Schweizer, P., Krebs, W., et al. Echokardiographische verlaufskontrolle des akuten myokardinfarktes nach intrakoronarer streptolysebehandlung. *Z. Kardiol.* 73:321, 1984.

127. Charuzi, Y., Beeder, C., Marshall, L. A., et al. Improvement in regional and global left ventricular function after intracoronary thrombolysis: Assessment with two-dimensional echocardiography. *Am. J. Cardiol.* 53:622, 1984.

128. Oh, J. K., Miller, F. A., Shub, C., et al. Evaluation of acute chest pain syndromes by two-dimensional echocardiography: Its potential application in the selection of patients for acute reperfusion therapy. *Mayo Clin. Proc.* 62:59, 1987.

129. Limacher, M. C., Quinones, M. A., Poliner,

L. R., et al. Detection of coronary artery disease with exercise two-dimensional echocardiography. *Circulation* 67:1211, 1983.

130. Armstrong, W. F., O'Donnell, J., Ryan, T., and Feigenbaum, H. Effect of prior myocardial infarction and extent and location of coronary disease on accuracy of exercise echocardiography. *J. Am. Coll. Cardiol.* 10:531, 1987.

131. Jaarsma, W., Visser, C. A., Funke Kupper, A. J., et al. Usefulness of two-dimensional exercise echocardiography shortly after myocardial infarction. *Am. J. Cardiol.* 57:86, 1986.

132. Applegate, R. J., Dell'Italia, L. J., and Crawford, M. H. Usefulness of two-dimensional echocardiography during low-level exercise testing early after uncomplicated acute myocardial infarction. *Am. J. Cardiol.* 60:10, 1987.

133. Ryan, T., Armstrong, W. F., O'Donnell, J., and Feigenbaum, H. Risk stratification following myocardial infarction using exercise echocardiograpy. *Am. Heart J.* (in press).

134. Rasmussen, S., Lovelace, D. E., Knoebel, S. B., et al. Echocardiographic detection of ischemic and infarcted myocardium. *J. Am. Coll. Cardiol.* 3:733, 1984.

135. Glueck, R. M., Mottley, J. G., Miller, J. G., et al. Effects of coronary artery occlusion and reperfusion on cardiac cycle-dependent variation of myocardial ultrasonic backscatter. *Circ. Res.* 56:683, 1985.

136. Skorton, D. J., Melton H., Pandian, N. G., et al. Detection of acute myocardial infarction in closed-chest dogs by analysis of regional two-dimensional echocardiographic gray-level distributions. *Circ. Res.* 52:36, 1983.

137. Haendchen, R. V., Ong, K., Fishbein, M. C., et al. Early differentiation of infarcted and noninfarcted reperfused myocardium in dogs by quantitative analysis of regional myocardial echo amplitudes. *Circ. Res.* 57:718, 1985.

138. Caldwell, R. L., Hurwitz, R. A., Girod, D. A., et al. Two-dimensional echocardiographic differentiation of anomalous left coronary artery from congestive cardiomyopathy. *Am. Heart J.* 106:710, 1983.

139. Rogers, E. W., Feigenbaum, H., Weyman, A. E., et al. Evaluation of left coronary artery anatomy in vitro by cross-sectional echocardiography. *Circulation* 62:782, 1980.

140. Ryan, T., Armstrong, W. F., and Feigenbaum, H. Prospective evaluation of the left main coronary artery using digital two-dimensional echocardiography. *J. Am. Coll. Cardiol.* 7:807, 1986.

141. Chen, C. C., Morganroth, J., Ogawa, S., and Mardelli, T. J. Detecting left main coronary artery disease by apical, cross-sectional echocardiography. *Circulation* 62:288, 1980.

142. Armstrong, W. F., Ryan, T., and Feigenbaum,

H. Doppler evaluation of left ventricular inflow during transient myocardial ischemia (Abstract). *J. Am. Coll. Cardiol.* 9:213A, 1987.

143. Klodnicki, W., Sokil, A. B., Paul, J., et al. Doppler evaluation of left ventricular filling dynamics during coronary angioplasty (Abstract). *J. Am. Coll. Cardiol.* 9:213A, 1987.

144. Friedman, B. J., Drinkovic, N., Miles, H., et al. Assessment of left ventricular diastolic function: Comparison of Doppler echocardiography and gated blood pool scintigraphy. *J. Am. Coll. Cardiol.* 8:1348, 1986.

145. Fujii, J., Yaxaki, Y., Sawada, H., et al. Noninvasive assessment of left and right ventricular filling in myocardial infarction with a two-dimensional Doppler echocardiographic method. *J. Am. Coll. Cardiol.* 5:1155, 1985.

146. Visser, C. A., deKoning, H., Delemarre, B., et al. Pulsed Doppler-derived mitral inflow velocity in acute myocardial infarction: An early prognostic indicator (Abstract). *J. Am. Coll. Cardiol.* 7:136A, 1986.

147. Armstrong, W. F., Mueller, T. M., Kinney, E. L., et al. Assessment of myocardial perfusion abnormalities with contrast-enhanced two-dimensional echocardiography. *Circulation* 66:166, 1982.

148. Armstrong, W. F., West, S. R., Dillon, J. C., and Feigenbaum, H. Assessment of location and size of myocardial infarction with contrast-enhanced echocardiography. II. Application of digital imaging techniques. *J. Am. Coll. Cardiol.* 4:141, 1984.

149. Kemper, A. J., Force, T., Kloner, R., et al. Contrast echocardiographic estimation of regional myocardial blood flow after acute coronary occlusion. *Circulation* 72:1115, 1985.

150. Armstrong, W. F. Assessment of myocardial perfusion with contrast enhanced echocardiography. *Echocardiography* 3:355, 1986.

151. Gage, S., Vasey, C. G., Dillon, J. C., et al. Reactive hyperemia evaluation with myocardial contrast echocardiography (Abstract). *J. Am. Coll. Cardiol.* 7:189A, 1986.

152. Moore, C. A., Smucker, M. L., and Kaul, S. Myocardial contrast echocardiography in humans. I. Safety—a comparison with routine coronary arteriography. *J. Am. Coll. Cardiol.* 8:1066, 1986.

153. Lang, R. M., Feinstein, S. B., Feldman, T., et al. Contrast echocardiography for evaluation of myocardial perfusion: Effects of coronary angioplasty. *J. Am. Coll. Cardiol.* 8:232, 1986.

154. Feinstein, S. B., Lang, R. M., Dick, C., et al. Contrast echocardiographic perfusion studies in humans. *Am. J. Cardiac Imaging* 1:29, 1986.

27
Nuclear Medicine Procedures Used in Acute Myocardial Infarction

JAMES T. WILLERSON AND JAMES R. CORBETT

The detection of acute myocardial infarction ordinarily relies on a classic clinical history, a typical evolution of cardiac enzymes, and diagnostic changes in the electrocardiogram. However, some patients delay their hospital admissions or are unable to provide an accurate history, making recognition of myocardial infarction more difficult. In some of these same circumstances, the temporal limitations related to infarct detection by the cardiac enzyme measurements make them unreliable for establishing if an infarct has occurred. Some patients have preexisting electrocardiographic (ECG) alterations that preclude using the ECG to detect acute myocardial infarction, including patients with left bundle branch block and those with several previous infarcts. Moreover, patients with non-Q-wave myocardial infarcts do not demonstrate diagnostic ECG changes; the best one can hope for is ST–T wave changes that are typical of non-Q-wave infarction, but similar ECG alterations sometimes occur in patients with subendocardial ischemia, rapid heart rates, ventricular hypertrophy, electrolyte abnormalities, subarachnoid hemorrhage, and intracardiac conduction abnormalities. Thus it is important to have alternative means for detecting myocardial infarction when it occurs. Moreover, because infarct size is an important determinant of future prognosis, one also wishes to have methods that allow accurate estimates of infarct size to be made independent of its location.

Infarct-Avid Myocardial Scintigraphy

Technetium 99m stannous pyrophosphate (^{99m}Tc-PPi) has been shown to be a sensitive method for detecting acute myocardial infarcts [1–18]. ^{99m}Tc-PPi is incorporated into regions of myocardial necrosis with some residual myocardial blood flow (10–40 percent of control values) and increased calcium concentration in the hours to days following myocardial infarction (Figs. 27-1 and 27-2). With permanent coronary artery occlusion, ^{99m}Tc-PPi deposition increases in the irreversibly injured myocardial cells between 10 to 12 hours and 24 to 72 hours after myocardial infarction. Approximately one-half of the ^{99m}Tc-PPi myocardial scintigrams become negative within 5 days of the event. The sequence of events correlates with calcium deposition and increases in coronary blood flow to the damaged area followed by the resorption of calcium during the reparative phase following the infarct (Fig. 27-1). With temporary coronary artery occlusion and reperfusion, such as occurs with thrombolytic therapy, the ^{99m}Tc-PPi myocardial scintigrams become abnormal within 1 to 2 hours of the event and may return to a normal pattern within 2 to 3 days. The more rapid deposition of ^{99m}Tc-PPi is associated with the increased coronary blood flow to the damaged myocardial region as part of thrombolytic therapy, thus emphasizing that any delay in the development of an abnormal ^{99m}Tc-PPi

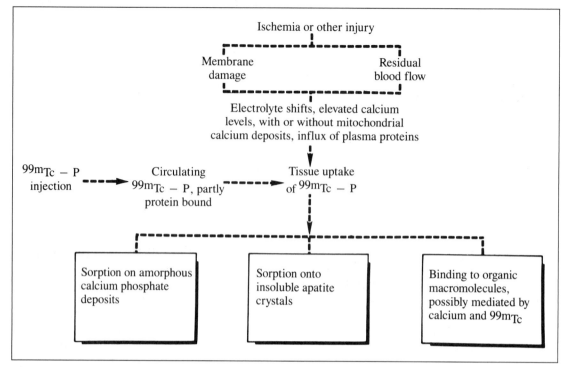

Fig. 27-1
Scheme for explaining abnormal technetium 99m stannous pyrophosphate (^{99m}Tc-P) myocardial scintigrams following the onset of acute myocardial infarction (or other injury). With severe ischemia or other cellular injury, there are alterations in membrane permeability followed by the entry of excess calcium into irreversibly damaged myocardial cells where it is deposited in mitochondria. Subsequently, the intravenous injection of ^{99m}Tc-P is bound to albumin and taken up in the injured myocardial cells where it complexes with calcium phosphate in soluble and insoluble form. (Reproduced from *The Journal of Clinical Investigation*, 1977, 60:724, by copyright permission of The American Society for Clinical Investigation.)

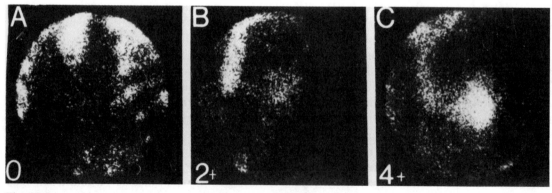

Fig. 27-2
Varying intensity of technetium 99m stannous pyrophosphate from faintly positive (2 +) to intensely positive (4 +). Typically, acute myocardial infarcts associated with adequate flow to the area of necrosis show the intensely positive pattern, but infarcts with very severely reduced residual myocardial flow show the faintly positive patterns. Often the faintly positive pattern of abnormal technetium 99m stannous pyrophosphate uptake is found during the first 10 to 24 hours after a Q-wave infarct followed by a more intense uptake of the radiopharmaceutical at 2–4 days after the event. With non-Q-wave infarcts, perhaps 33 to 40 percent have the faintly positive pattern.

496

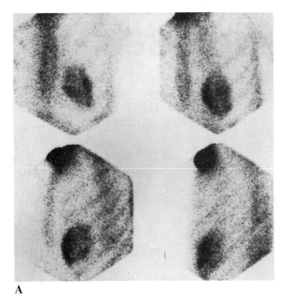
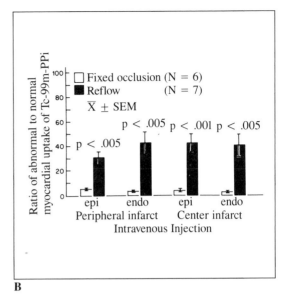

A   B

Fig. 27-3

A. A markedly abnormal technetium 99m stannous pyrophosphate myocardial scintigram may occur with immediate reperfusion of an acute anterolateral infarct in the anterior (*top left*), slight left anterior oblique (*top right*), steep left anterior oblique (*bottom left*), and left lateral (*bottom right*) imaging projection images. *B.* Effect of blood flow on accumulation of technetium 99m stannous pyrophosphate in acutely infarcted canine myocardium after an intravenous injection. Open bars represent pyrophosphate uptake in animals with permanent left anterior descending coronary artery occlusions for 3 hours; filled bars represent pyrophosphate uptake in animals that had reperfusion after 3 hours of temporary coronary artery occlusion. There was a marked increase in pyrophosphate uptake by the injured tissue when reflow was provided, such that mean technetium 99m stannous pyrophosphate uptake in the damaged tissue was 40 times that in normal myocardium in the reflow model. (*B* from R. W. Parkey et al., Effect of coronary blood flow and site of injection on Tc99m-PPi detection of early canine myocardial infarcts. *J. Nucl. Med.* 22:134, 1981. With permission.)

myocardial scintigram relates to the relative inadequacy of coronary blood flow to the damaged region within the first few hours to days after the event. With thrombolytic therapy or spontaneous thrombolysis, improved coronary blood flow to the damaged myocardial region allows early detection of the region of myocardial infarction by ^{99m}Tc-PPi (Fig. 27-3).

Planar (two-dimensional) ^{99m}Tc-PPi myocardial scintigraphy generally detects infarcts 3 gm in size and larger, but it may fail to detect smaller infarcts, especially those that are subendocardial or inferior in location. However, single photon emission computed tomography (SPECT) imaging allows the detection of infarcts as small as 1 gm in size, including most subendocardial and inferior infarcts after permanent or temporary coronary artery occlusion followed by reperfusion. An overlay of the ^{99m}Tc-PPi myocardial scintigram against the blood pool background using SPECT imaging allows one to more precisely identify myocardial infarcts and eliminate blood pool activity as a cause of an apparently abnormal ^{99m}Tc-PPi study. However, acute myocardial necrosis of any etiology that results in confluent necrosis of more than 1 gm of myocardial tissue may be detected by ^{99m}Tc-PPi myocardial scintigraphy with SPECT. Thus trauma, infection, cardioversion-induced myocardial injury, and an invasive tumor may all cause abnormal ^{99m}Tc-PPi myocardial scintigrams.

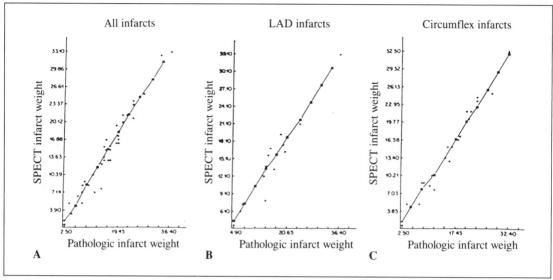

Fig. 27-4
Scatter plots of scintigraphic (SPECT) versus postmortem determined infarct
weight in dogs with the corresponding data fit by linear regression for all infarcts
(A), infarcts caused by left anterior descending coronary artery occlusions (B),
and infarcts caused by circumflex coronary artery occlusions (C). (From S. E.
Lewis et al. Measurement of infarct size in acute canine myocardial infarction by
single photon emission computed tomography with technetium-99m
pyrophosphate. *Am. J. Cardiol.* 54:195, 1984. With permission.)

^{99m}Tc-PPi to Size Myocardial Infarcts

^{99m}Tc-PPi has been used to estimate the extent of myocardial infarction with SPECT. ^{99m}Tc-PPi myocardial scintigraphy with SPECT provides an accurate estimate of the size of myocardial infarcts with permanent coronary artery occlusion (Fig. 27-4) [14, 15, 17] and with temporary coronary artery occlusion followed by reperfusion (Fig. 27-5) [18]. With reperfused infarcts, it is important to inject the ^{99m}Tc-PPi approximately 90 minutes after reperfusion to avoid overestimation of infarct size (Fig. 27-5) [18].

We have demonstrated that it is possible to measure infarct size using ^{99m}Tc-PPi and express the measurement as a percentage of total left ventricular mass or as the "infarction fraction" [15]. Using this approach, one may estimate the extent of normally perfused left ventricular myocardium using a perfusion marker such as thallium 201 and the size of the myocardial infarction using ^{99m}Tc-PPi. SPECT measurements and an overlay of the ^{201}Tl and ^{99m}Tc-PPi myocardial scintigrams allow one to estimate infarct size as a percentage of the left ventricular mass (Fig. 27-6) [15]. This approach allows one to normalize infarct size for the size of the heart.

Radionuclide Ventriculography

Radionuclide ventriculography (RVG) is used to evaluate global and segmental left and right ventricular function (Fig. 27-7) [19–29]. Technical details relative to methodology for performing RVGs are given elsewhere [19–29], but it should be emphasized that an RVG may be obtained after one intravenous injection and that technetium 99m pertechnetate is used to label the patient's red blood cells following administration of stannous pyrophosphate. Technetium-labeled red blood cells allow visualization of the cardiovascular blood pool and the subsequent measurement of right and

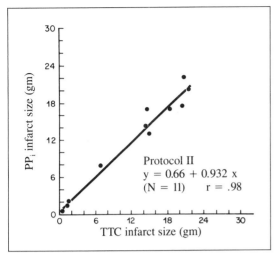

Fig. 27-5
Comparison of infarct size as estimated by the triphenyltetrazolium chloride (TTC) method and by technetium 99m stannous pyrophosphate myocardial scintigraphy with SPECT (PPi infarct size) in anesthetized dogs with a temporary occlusion (3 hours) of the left anterior descending coronary artery followed by 2 hours of reflow. The pyrophosphate was injected in 11 dogs 90 minutes after reflow. Using SPECT imaging, an excellent estimate of infarct size was obtained. (From D. E. Jansen et al., Quantification of myocardial injury produced by temporary coronary artery occlusion and reflow with technetium-99m-pyrophosphate. *Circulation* 75:613, 1987. By permission of the American Heart Association, Inc.)

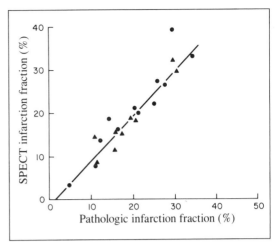

Fig. 27-6
Correlation between postmortem determined "infarction fraction" and SPECT determinations of "infarction fraction" in 21 dogs with circumflex (12 dogs) or left anterior descending (9 dogs) coronary artery occlusions. Myocardial imaging for detection of "infarction fraction" was done with a combination of thallium 201 and technetium 99m stannous pyrophosphate with overlay images. See reference 15 for details. (Reprinted with permission from the American College of Cardiology. *J. Am. Coll. Cardiol.* 6:149, 1985.)

left ventricular ejection fractions and volumes using an interactive computer (Fig. 27-7).

We have used RVG to estimate the functional impact of myocardial infarction on left and right ventricular performance in patients during the first few hours following their infarcts (Fig. 27-8) [26]. Using these methods, we have found that an early RVG (within the first 8 hours from the onset of symptoms suggestive of infarction) adds to the discriminate power of clinical and radiographic characterization of ventricular function in these patients [26]. Moreover, some patients with clinical evidence suggestive of left ventricular failure had well preserved left ventricular function on the RVG, whereas others without clinical evidence of heart failure sometimes had moderate or severe left ventricular dysfunction identified by the RVG (Table 27-1; Fig. 27-8) [26]. Thus objective estimates of the severity of left ventricular dysfunction with myocardial infarction are superior to clinical assessments, especially the chest radiograph, physical examination, and estimation of severity of left ventricular dysfunction by Killip classification [26]. RVG allows relatively rapid evaluation of the extent of left (or right) ventricular dysfunction, and these estimates may be repeated serially over time as one attempts to determine if thrombolytic therapy (or another intervention) improves ventricular function.

ASSESSMENT OF PROGNOSIS AFTER MYOCARDIAL INFARCTION

Nuclear cardiology tests are of value for predicting prognosis in patients after myocardial

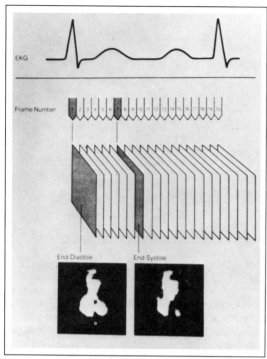

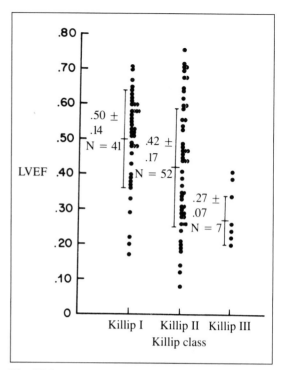

Fig. 27-7
Radionuclide ventriculogram obtained by summing radionuclide counts from various portions of the cardiac cycle from the subsequent display of the radionuclide ventriculogram and end-diastolic (*bottom left*) and end-systolic (*bottom right*) frames. This type of imaging is often referred to as MUGA imaging.

Fig. 27-8
Left ventricular ejection fraction (LVEF) determined by MUGA imaging compared to the clinical Killip classification. Mean values ± standard deviation are presented for each classification. A higher Killip classification is associated with a significantly lower mean ejection fraction ($p < .001$). Please note, however, that some patients with Killip I classification have severe impairment of their LVEFs and a few patients with Killip III classification have relatively well preserved LVEFs. (From C. F. Sanford et al. Value of radionuclide ventriculography in the immediate characterization of patients with acute myocardial infarction. *Am. J. Cardiol.* 49:637, 1982. With permission.)

infarction [23, 26, 27, 30]. The early assessment of the severity of left ventricular dysfunction using RVGs as described above is useful in that regard. However, one may also use selected nuclear cardiology tests close to the time of hospital discharge in association with submaximal exercise testing to predict prognosis [23, 27, 30]. Specifically, we have used RVGs with submaximal exercise testing and shown that patients developing reductions in their left ventricular ejection fractions or increases in their left ventricular end-systolic volumes at low levels of exercise are at risk for future coronary heart disease events, including myocardial infarction, sudden death, refractory heart failure, or new myocardial ischemia requiring some form of surgical intervention (Fig. 27-9; Tables 27-2 and 27-3).

The assessment of global left ventricular function by RVG coupled to submaximal exercise provided better prognostic insight than obtained by evaluating only the electrocardiographic responses to exercise [23, 27]. Thus in the patient without valvular heart disease or underlying cardiomyopathy, assessments of residual myocardium at risk because of additional important coronary heart disease provide a valuable means to estimate prognosis during the 8 months following myocardial infarction [23, 27].

Table 27-1
Radionuclide left ventricular volumes and ejection fraction according to Killip classification

Killip class	LVEF		LVEDVI (ml/m²)	LVESVI (ml/m²)
	All patients	Patients with volume data		
I	0.50 ± 0.14 (N = 41)	0.52 ± 0.14 (N = 27)	75 ± 29 (N = 27)	39 ± 24 (N = 27)
II	0.42 ± 0.17 (N = 52)	0.43 ± 0.17 (N = 43)	82 ± 33 (N = 43)	49 ± 28 (N = 43)
III	0.27 ± 0.07 (N = 7)	0.27 ± 0.07 (N = 6)	110 ± 52 (N = 6)	80 ± 41 (N = 6)

LVEDVI and LVESVI = left ventricular end-diastolic and left ventricular end-systolic volume index, respectively;
LVEF = left ventricular ejection fraction; N = number of patients.
Source: C. F. Sanford et al. Value of radionuclide ventriculography in the immediate characterization of patients
with acute myocardial infarction. *Am. J. Cardiol.* 49:637, 1982. With permission.

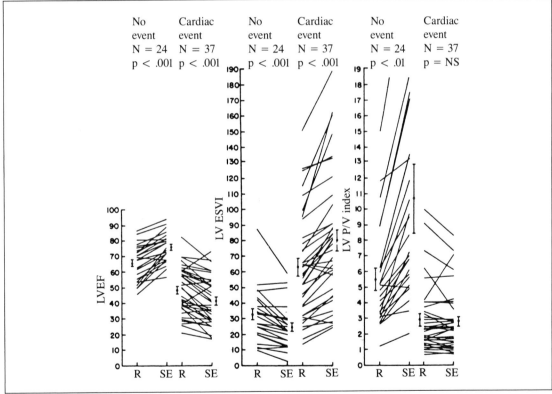

Fig. 27-9
Left ventricular ejection fraction (LVEF), end-systolic volume index (*middle panel*), and pressure voluem (P/V) index (*right panel*) at rest (R) and during peak submaximal exercise (SE) in patients with and without cardiac events during the 8 months after myocardial infarction. Note that patients who did not have future cardiac events usually had normal left ventricular global functional responses to submaximal exercises, whereas patients destined to have future cardiac events usually had abnormal left ventricular functional responses to low-level exercise. (From J. R. Corbett et al. Prognostic value of submaximal exercise radionuclide ventriculography following acute transmural and nontransmural myocardial infarction. *Am. J. Cardiol.* 52:82A, 1983. With permission.)

Table 27-2
Results of multivariate, discriminant-function analysis according to degree of left ventricular dysfunction

	LVEF <40% (N = 29)		LVEF ≥40% (N = 88)	
No event versus any event	1. Peak LVEF	90%	1. ΔLVEF	89%
	2. ΔESVI	97%	2. Peak LVEF	93%
	3. Killip class	100%		

ESVI = left ventricular end-systolic volume index; LVEF = left ventricular ejection fraction; MI = myocardial infarction; SE = submaximal exercise.
Source: J. R. Corbett et al. Prognostic value of submaximal exercise radionuclide ventriculography following acute transmural and nontransmural myocardial infarction. *Am. J. Cardiol.* 52:82A, 1983. With permission.

Thallium 201 Myocardial Scintigraphy

Perfusion imaging using thallium 201 myocardial scintigraphy or, perhaps in the future, the technetium-labeled isonitrile analogs with submaximal exercise testing also provides a means to predict prognosis in patients after myocardial infarction. Gibson et al. have shown that patients developing reversible perfusion defects using thallium imaging and submaximal exercise are at risk for future coronary events, including myocardial infarction, death, and the need for a future surgical intervention (coronary artery bypass surgery or percutaneous transluminal coronary angioplasty) because of recurrent acute coronary heart disease syndromes [30]. Thallium 201 myocardial scintigraphy and submaximal exercise testing might be especially valuable in the patient with underlying cardiomyopathy or valvular heart disease, in whom abnormal global left ventricular functional responses to exercise might be expected to be independent of the presence or absence of additional important coronary heart disease. Thus thallium-201 myocardial scintigraphy and submaximal exercise provide a relatively noninvasive means to assess prognosis in patients after myocardial infarction. Moreover, estimates of the extent of the thallium perfusion defect, especially with SPECT imaging, provide an estimate of prognosis in hospital and following discharge, as old and new myocardial infarcts may be detected by this form of perfusion imaging and the extent of myocardial infarction is an important predictor of the prognosis [31].

Alternatives for Infarct-Avid Myocardial Scintigraphy in the Future

Haber et al. in Boston have developed a specific monoclonal antibody against cardiac myosin and have shown that myocardial scintigraphy using technetium- or indium-labeled monoclonal antibody to myosin allows the noninvasive detection of myocardial infarction and relative estimates of its size [32, 33]. Extensive studies have been performed in experimental animals, and substantial numbers of patients have been studied with this imaging technique. Anti-myosin antibody scintigraphy coupled with SPECT appears to be an alternative to ^{99m}Tc-PPi myocardial scintigraphy for purposes of infarct detection and sizing.

EVALUATION OF THROMBOLYTIC THERAPY

Perfusion imaging should be useful for detecting the success of thrombolytic therapy in regard to improved coronary blood flow to viable myocardium. Thallium 201 myocardial scintigraphy at rest has been used for this purpose, but there is substantial concern that thallium may enter some myocardial regions where necrosis exists but some coronary flow persists after thrombolytic therapy [5]. The technetium-labeled isonitrile analogs may be an alternative to thallium 201 for estimating the extent of reperfused but viable myocardium after thrombolytic therapy, but additional studies are necessary to evaluate this

Table 27-3
Results of multivariate, discriminant-function analysis of all clinical, exercise, and scintigraphic variables at 6-month follow-up

	All patients (N = 117)		Anterior TM (N = 33)		Inferior TM (N = 39)		Limited NT (N = 18)		Extensive NT (N = 24)	
No event versus any event	1. ΔLVEF	89%	1. Peak LVEF	84%	1. ΔLVEF	87%	1. ΔESVI	84%	1. ΔESVI	96%
	2. Peak LVEF	91%	2. Age	90%	2. WMS	90%	2. SE pain	89%	2. ΔWMS	96%
			3. ΔLVEF	94%			3. ST changes	89%	3. SE pain	100%
							4. ST ↓ 0.1 mV	94%		
							5. ΔBP	94%		
							6. ΔWMS	100%		

BP = systolic blood pressure; ESVI = left ventricular end-systolic volume index; LVEF = left ventricular ejection fraction; NT = nontransmural; SE = submaximal exercise; ST = ST segment; TM = transmural; WMS = wall motion score; Δ = change with exercise; ↓ = depression.
Source: J. R. Corbett et al. Prognostic value of submaximal exercise radionuclide ventriculography following acute transmural and nontransmural myocardial infarction. *Am. J. Cardiol.* 52:82A, 1983. With permission.

possibility. Alternatively, some combination of perfusion and metabolic imaging [34, 35] or perfusion and infarct-avid myocardial scintigraphy should provide a good estimate of the extent of myocardial necrosis and of remaining relatively normal myocardial perfusion or metabolic function. As mentioned above, combinations of thallium 201 (or isonitrile analogs) and an infarct-avid imaging technique (either ^{99m}Tc-PPi or perhaps the anti-myosin antibody) with SPECT imaging provide an estimate for the extent of myocardial infarction and of remaining relatively normal myocardial perfusion. The synthetic fatty acid phenylpentadecanoic acid labeled with ^{123}I allows the detection of metabolic abnormalities with coronary artery stenoses and myocardial infarction, and it may be possible to utilize this metabolic probe with either perfusion or infarct-avid imaging for purposes of estimating the extent of myocardial infarction and for identifying regions of relatively normal myocardial perfusion in the future.

Positron-Emitting Radionuclides

Selected positron-emitting radionuclides have been shown to be useful for the evaluation of patients with acute myocardial infarction [36–40]. Sobel et al. have demonstrated the utility of ^{11}C palmitate for the detection and estimation of the extent of myocardial infarction and for the evaluation of thrombolytic therapy [36, 37]. ^{11}C-labeled palmitate uptake occurs in viable myocardium, and it has been a useful probe of relatively normal myocardial metabolism. Ischemic myocardium preferentially utilizes ^{18}F-2-deoxyglucose as a preferred metabolic substrate rather than fatty acids, and infarcted myocardium fails to utilize either glucose or fatty acids as substrates [38]. Thus a combination of ^{11}C-labeled palmitate and ^{18}-F 2-deoxyglucose may be useful for identifying regions of myocardium with normal metabolic capabilities, ischemic myocardium, and areas of infarction, and it should also be useful for following the efficacy of thrombolytic intervention. However, a general utilization of the positron emitters requires a cyclotron on site and expensive equipment, and it usually proves expensive in terms of maintenance requirements as well. Thus only a relatively few medical institutions in the world have the resources to allow these studies to be done.

Summary

Previous studies have suggested that myocardial infarcts may be detected and sized accurately using technetium 99m stannous pyrophosphate (^{99m}Tc-PPi) and single photon emission computed tomography (SPECT). The most accurate measurements of infarct size with SPECT and ^{99m}Tc-PPi following reperfusion are made when the ^{99m}Tc-PPi is injected at approximately 90 minutes following reperfusion. ^{99m}Tc-PPi with SPECT detects infarcts as small as 1 to 3 gm in size and allows an accurate estimate of the size of infarcts occurring with permanent and temporary coronary artery occlusion followed by reperfusion.

Radionuclide ventriculography may be used to provide an accurate estimate of the functional impact of acute myocardial infarction on global ventricular performance during the acute phases of myocardial infarction and to estimate the beneficial effect of any therapeutic interventions, including thrombolytic therapy and percutaneous transluminal coronary angioplasty in the days to weeks following myocardial infarction. Furthermore, submaximal exercise testing coupled with radionuclide ventriculography may be used to identify patients at risk for future myocardial infarction, sudden death, heart failure, and recurrent severe myocardial ischemia. Alternatively, perfusion imaging with thallium 201 may also be used with submaximal exercise testing at hospital discharge to predict prognosis in patients after myocardial infarction. Patients with reversible myocardial ischemia as detected by thallium 201 imaging are those most likely to have a new myocardial infarction or complications of their coronary heart disease over the subsequent few months.

Thus nuclear cardiology tests provide means to detect and size myocardial infarcts, estimate the functional impact of myocardial infarction on ventricular performance, and predict prognosis at hospital discharge.

Acknowledgments

This work was supported in part by NHLBI Ischemic SCOR grant HL-17669 and the Moss Heart Fund, Dallas, Texas.

Editorial Comments

Nuclear medicine techniques are now established as uniquely helpful in the management of patients with acute myocardial infarction. Certain issues remain, however, primarily related to cost-effectiveness and the appropriate timing of the tests in relation to the infarction. For example, a radionuclide left ventriculogram performed within 24 hours of the onset of infarction may not be representative of findings at 2 weeks postinfarction, largely due to temporary "stunning" of the myocardium, which may resolve over time. Likewise, whether to use a standard graded exercise test or a thallium perfusion scanning technique with exercise for patients following a myocardial infarction has not been rigorously tested from a cost-effectiveness standpoint. Despite these uncertainties, the value of nuclear cardiology is unquestioned in the postinfarction patient and will likely continue to expand. G.S.F.

References

1. Bonte, F. J., Parkey, R. W., Graham, K. D., et al. A new method for radionuclide imaging of myocardial infarcts. *Radiology* 110:473, 1974.
2. Willerson, J. T., Parkey, R. W., Bonte, F. J., et al. Technetium stannous pyrophosphate myocardial scintigrams in patients with chest pain of varying etiology. *Circulation* 51:1046, 1975.
3. Willerson, J. T., Parkey, R. W., Bonte, F. J., et al. Acute subendocardial myocardial infarction in patients: Its detection by technetium 99m stannous pyrophosphate myocardial scintigrams. *Circulation* 51:436, 1975.
4. Buja, L. M., Parkey, R. W., Stokely, E. M., et al. Pathophysiology of technetium-99m stannous pyrophosphate and thallium-201 scintigraphy of acute anterior myocardial infarcts in dogs. *J. Clin. Invest.* 57:1508, 1976.
5. Buja, L. M., Tofe, A. J., Kulkarni, P. V., et al. Sites and mechanisms of localization of technetium-99m phosphorus radiopharmaceuticals in acute myocardial infarcts and other tissues. *J. Clin. Invest.* 60:724, 1977.
6. Buja, L. M., Poliner, L. R., Parkey, R. W., et al. Clinicopathologic study of persistently positive technetium-99m stannous pyrophosphate myocardial scintigrams and mycocytolytic degeneration after acute myocardial infarction. *Circulation* 56:1016, 1977.
7. Poliner, L. R., Buja, L. M., Parkey, R. W., et al. Clinicopathologic findings in 52 patients studied by technetium-99m stannous pyrophosphate myocardial scintigrams. *Circulation* 59:257, 1979.
8. Willerson, J. T., Parkey, R. W., Bonte, F. J., et al. Pathophysiologic considerations and clinicopathological correlates of technetium-99m stannous pyrophosphate myocardial scintigraphy. *Semin. Nucl. Med.* 10:54, 1980.
9. Chien, K. R., Reeves, J. P., Buja, L. M., et al. Phospholipid alterations in ischemic myocardium: Temporal and topographical correlations with Tc-99m-PPi accumulation and an in vitro sarcolemmal Ca^{2+} permeability defect. *Circ. Res.* 48:711, 1981.
10. Parkey, R. W., Kulkarni, P., Lewis, S., et al. Effect of coronary blood flow and site of injection on Tc99m-PPi detection of early canine myocardial infarcts. *J. Nucl. Med.* 22(2):133, 1981.
11. Lewis, S. E., Devous, M. D., Sr., Corbett, J. R., et al. Measurement of infarct size in acute canine myocardial infarction by single photon emission computed tomography with technetium-99m pyrophosphate. *Am. J. Cardiol.* 54:193, 1984.
12. Croft, C., Rude, R. E., Lewis, S. E., et al. Comparison of left ventricular function and infarct size in patients with and without persistently positive technetium-99m pyrophosphate myocardial scintigrams after myocardial infarction: Analysis of 357 patients. *Am. J. Cardiol.* 53:421, 1984.
13. Corbett, J. R., Lewis, M., Willerson, J. T., et al. Technetium-99m pyrophosphate imaging in patients with acute myocardial infarction: Comparison of planar images with single-photon tomography with and without blood pool overlay. *Circulation* 69:1120, 1984.
14. Corbett, J. R., Lewis, S. E., Wolfe, C. L., et al. Measurement of myocardial infarct size in patients by technetium pyrophosphate single photon tomography. *Am. J. Cardiol.* 54:1231, 1984.

15. Wolfe, C. L., Lewis, S. E., Corbett, J. R., et al. Measurement of infarction fraction using single photon emission computed tomography. *J. Am. Coll. Cardiol.* 6:145, 1985.

16. Wheelan, K., Wolfe, C., Corbett, J., et al. Early positive technetium-99m stannous pyrophosphate images as a marker of reperfusion in patients receiving thrombolytic therapy for acute myocardial infarction. *Am. J. Cardiol.* 56:252, 1985.

17. Jansen, D. E., Corbett, J. R., Lewis, S. E., et al. Quantification of myocardial infarction: A comparison of single photon emission computed tomography with pyrophosphate to serial plasma MB-CK measurements. *Circulation* 72:327, 1985.

18. Jansen, D. E., Corbett, J. R., Buja, L. M., et al. Quantification of myocardial injury produced by temporary coronary artery occlusion and reflow with technetium-99m-pyrophosphate. *Circulation* 75:611, 1987.

19. Borer, J. S., Bacharach, S. L., Green, M. U., et al. Real-time radionuclide cineangiography in non-invasive evaluation of global and regional left ventricular function at rest and during exercise in patients with coronary artery disease. *N. Engl. J. Med.* 296:839, 1977.

20. Poliner, L. R., Dehmer, G. H., Lewis, S. E., et al. Left ventricular performance in normal subjects: A comparison of the responses to exercise in the upright and supine positions. *Circulation* 65:528, 1980.

21. Dehmer, G. J., Lewis, S. E., Hillis, L. D., et al. Exercise induced alterations in left ventricular volumes in man: Usefulness in predicting the relative extent of coronary artery disease. *Circulation* 63:1008, 1981.

22. Dehmer, G. J., Falkoff, M., Lewis, S. E., et al. Effect of oral propranolol on rest and exercise left ventricular ejection fraction, volumes and segmental wall motion in patients with angina pectoris: Assessment with equilibrium gated blood pool imaging. *Br. Heart J.* 45:656, 1981.

23. Corbett, J., Dehmer, G. J., Lewis, S. E., et al. The prognostic value of submaximal exercise testing with radionuclide ventriculography prior to hospital discharge in patients with recent myocardial infarction. *Circulation* 64:535, 1981.

24. Dehmer, G. J., Firth, B. G., Lewis, S. E., et al. Direct measurement of cardiac output by gated equilibrium blood pool scintigraphy: Validation of scintigraphic volume measurements by a nongeometric technique. *Am. J. Cardiol.* 47:1061, 1981.

25. Dehmer, G. J., Firth, B. G., Hillis, L. D., et al. Alterations in left ventricular volumes and ejection fraction at rest and during exercise in patients with aortic regurgitation. *Am. J. Cardiol.* 48:17, 1981.

26. Sanford, C. F., Corbett, J., Curry, G. L., et al. Value of radionuclide ventriculography in the immediate characterization of patients with acute myocardial infarction. *Am. J. Cardiol.* 49:637, 1982.

27. Corbett, J. R., Nicod, P., Lewis, S. E., et al. Prognostic value of submaximal exercise radionuclide ventriculography following acute transmural and nontransmural myocardial infarction. *Am. J. Cardiol.* 52:82A, 1983.

28. Corbett, J. R., Jansen, D. E., Lewis, S. E., et al. Tomographic gated blood pool radionuclide ventriculography: Analysis of wall motion and left ventricular volumes in patients with coronary artery disease. *J. Am. Coll. Cardiol.* 6:349, 1985.

29. Wolfe, C. L., Jansen, D. E., Corbett, J. R., et al. Determination of left ventricular mass using single photon emission tomography. *Am. J. Cardiol.* 56:761, 1985.

30. Gibson, R. S., Watson, D. D., Craddock, G. B., et al. Prediction of cardiac events after uncomplicated myocardial infarction: A prospective study comparing predischarge exercise thallium-201 exercise testing with thallium-201 myocardial scintigraphy. *Circulation* 61:729, 1981.

31. Silverman, K. J., Becker, L. C., Bulkley, B. H., et al. Value of early thallium-201 scintigraphy for predicting mortality in patients with acute myocardial infarction. *Circulation* 61:996, 1980.

32. Khaw, B. A., Beller, G. A., Haber, E., et al. Localization of cardiac myosin-specific antibody in myocardial infarction. *J. Clin. Invest.* 58:439, 1976.

33. Khaw, B. A., Scott, J., Fallon, J. T., et al. Myocardial injury: Quantitation by cell sorting initiated with antimyosin fluorescent spheres. *Science* 217:1050, 1982.

34. Kennedy, P. L., Corbett, J. R., Kulkarni, P. V., et al. I-123 phenylpentadecanoic acid myocardial scintigraphy: Usefulness in identifying myocardial ischemia. *Circulation* 74:1007, 1986.

35. Hansen, C. L., Corbett, J. R., Pippin, J., et al. I-123 phenylpentadecanoic acid and single photon emission computed tomography in identifying LV regional metabolic abnormalities in patients with coronary heart disease: Comparison with thallium-201 myocardial scintigraphy. *J. Am. Coll. Cardiol.* 12:78, 1988.

36. Sobel, B. E., Geltman, E. M., Tiefenbrunn, A., et al. Improvement of regional myocardial metabolism after coronary thrombolysis induced with tissue-type plasminogen activator or streptokinase. *Circulation* 69:983, 1984.

37. Ter-Pogossian, M. M., Klein, M. S., Markham, et al.: Regional assessment of myocardial metabolic integrity in vivo by positron-emission to-

mography with ^{11}C-labeled palmitate. *Circulation* 61:242, 1980.

38. Phelps, M. E., Hoffman, E. J., Selin, C., et al. Investigation of [^{18}F]2-fluoro-2-deoxyglucose for the measurement of myocardial glucose metabolism. *J. Nucl. Med.* 19:1311, 1978.

39. Marshall, R. C., Tillisch, J. H., Phelps, M. E., et al. Identification and differentiation of resting myocardial ischemia and infarction in man with positron computed tomography, ^{18}F-labeled fluorodeoxyglucose and N-13 ammonia. *Circulation* 67:766, 1983.

40. Schelbert, H. R., Wisenberg, G., Phelps, M. E., et al. Noninvasive assessment of coronary stenoses by myocardial imaging during pharmacologic coronary vasodilation. VI. Detection of coronary artery disease in human beings with N-13 ammonia and positron computed tomography. *Am. J. Cardiol.* 49:1197, 1982.

VII
Therapeutic Interventions During and After Acute Myocardial Infarction

28
Beta Blockers During and After Acute Myocardial Infarction

ROBERT P. BYINGTON AND CURT D. FURBERG

Coronary heart disease continues to occupy a position of prominence as a cause of death in the United States and other Western nations. Although a reduction in coronary heart disease mortality was observed and well documented during the 1970s and 1980s [1], the acute and chronic sequelae of coronary atherosclerosis are still responsible for more than 540,000 deaths annually in the United States [2]. Sudden cardiac death represents a major factor in these statistics. Furthermore, survivors of a documented myocardial infarction are known to have an increased risk of premature death relative to the general population.

In 1986 there were 758,000 patients in the United States alone admitted to a hospital with the primary diagnosis of acute myocardial infarction [3], and 640,000 were discharged alive [4]. Thus 118,000 patients died during hospitalization, which corresponds to an overall in-hospital mortality rate of 15.6 percent. More than 90 percent of the patients with an acute myocardial infarction who survive the hospital phase and who eventually die, die of cardiac causes [5]. Identifying preventive interventions that can reduce this toll represents a major public health challenge.

Morbid Mechanisms Behind Coronary Deaths of Postmyocardial Infarction Patients and Interventions Aimed at These Mechanisms

It is apparent that to effectively improve survival, either during the acute event itself or in the long term following a myocardial infarction, an intervention must favorably influence one or more of the morbid mechanisms behind the coronary deaths. In principle, there are five morbid mechanisms behind these deaths.

1. Progressive coronary atherosclerosis
2. Coronary thrombosis
3. Electrical complications (e.g., ventricular fibrillation)
4. Mechanical complications (e.g., congestive heart failure)
5. Recurrent ischemia (resulting from an imbalance between oxygen supply and demand)

These mechanisms are related and often overlapping. Progression of the underlying coronary atherosclerosis operates only in the long term, whereas the other mechanisms operate both acutely and over the long term.

Interventions with the potential for counteracting these morbid mechanisms have been and continue to be evaluated in a large number of randomized clinical trials. Extensive review articles are available that provide detailed information concerning the interventions and the findings of the trials [6–11]. These interventions may be summarized as follows:

1. The most fundamental cause of myocardial infarction is coronary atherosclerosis. Lipid-lowering regimens of diet, or medication, or both have been tested with the hope of retarding the rate of progression via a reduction in serum cholesterol levels. The benefits of treatment are a function of the

magnitude of the reduction in serum cholesterol and the duration of treatment. The LRC trial of cholestyramine [12] and the Finnish trial of gemfibrozil [13] have demonstrated the primary preventive effects of lipid-lowering, but secondary effects have yet to be demonstrated in postmyocardial infarction patients.

2. Three types of intervention have been explored aimed at preventing extension of an existing thrombus or achieving thrombolysis. These interventions are conventional anticoagulants (e.g., heparin), platelet-active drugs (e.g., aspirin, sulfinpyrazone, dipyridamole), and thrombolytic agents (e.g., TPA and streptokinase). As acute interventions, all three classes have well documented effects on survival [7, 10, 11, 14–16], although there is no clear evidence that thrombolytic therapy benefits the patient during the first day postmyocardial infarction. Furthermore, it appears that their mechanisms are different and that the effects of a platelet-active agent (e.g., aspirin) and a thrombolytic agent (e.g., streptokinase) are additive [16]. Although aspirin appears to have a small beneficial long-term effect on survival in myocardial infarction patients, there is no strong evidence for the long-term beneficial effects of the other agents.

3. With the observation that more than one-half of all deaths among coronary patients are sudden, presumably due to ventricular arrhythmias, various classes of antiarrhythmic agents have been tested. Intravenous and oral agents have been tested with the expectation of reducing the risk of ventricular fibrillation. Unfortunately, antiarrhythmic drugs can paradoxically also be arrhythmogenic, and their use can lead to serious adverse effects. Overall, a reduction in short- or long-term mortality has not been demonstrated for antiarrhythmics [8], possibly because (1) a reduction in ventricular arrhythmias does not translate into a reduction in mortality (an explanation that is contrary to other experimental evidence), (2) a true beneficial effect is hidden by the deficiencies in the methodology of

the conducted studies, or (3) the arrhythmogenic effect outweighs the antiarrhythmic effect.

4. Until recently, limited attention has been paid to patients with the most complicated myocardial infarctions, primarily because it was difficult enough to find appropriate treatment for patients with uncomplicated infarctions. These patient groups include those with congestive heart failure, hypotension, and shock. Of potential interest are the direct-acting vasodilators (e.g., nitrates/nitroglycerin) [11] and the ACE inhibitors (e.g., enalapril and captopril). The roles of alpha blockers, diuretics, and inotropic agents (e.g., digitalis) in secondary prevention following a myocardial infarction are still unclear. It is known, however, that long-term therapy with high-dose thiazide diuretics may lead to K^+ and Mg^+ depletion, which in turn can lead to serious arrhythmias.

5. Because it is known that an improvement in the balance between oxygen supply and demand can reduce the risk of recurrent ischemic events as well as of certain arrhythmias and mechanical failure, interventions that may improve this balance have been sought. Three types of such intervention have been evaluated in patients with acute myocardial infarction: physical exercise, calcium channel blockers, and beta blockers. Favorable evidence exists for the beneficial effects of moderate physical exercise, but the major problems with this intervention is the cooperation of the patient. Calcium channel blockers (e.g., nifedipine, verapamil, diltiazem, and lidoflazine) have the ability to reduce vasospasm, but there is no proved benefit on short- or long-term mortality. In fact, pooled analyses suggest there is a slight increased risk of death with these agents [11]. On the other hand, a great deal of evidence has accrued demonstrating that beta blockers are the most effective prophylactic agents for the short- and long-term treatment of myocardial infarction patients. If given within the first 24 hours of an acute myocardial infarction, first as an intravenous bolus then

orally, beta blockers have been shown to reduce in-hospital mortality [9, 11, 17]. In the long term, these agents have also been shown to be the most effective treatment for patients who have survived the acute phase of the myocardial infarction.

Thus the presumed major mechanisms for increased coronary mortality during the postinfarction period include cardiac arrhythmias, left ventricular dysfunction, and persistent myocardial ischemia. Increased levels of circulating catecholamines or enhanced sympathetic drive can increase both the severity of myocardial ischemia and the frequency of ventricular arrhythmias. After the clinical introduction of the beta blocker propranolol for angina pectoris and arrhythmias in 1963, it was conceived that beta blocker administration might favorably influence the acute and long-term course of myocardial infarction patients by attenuating the undesirable consequences of increased sympathetic nervous system activity. However, because these drugs could also depress left ventricular function, another major factor contributing to mortality after a myocardial infarction, beta blockers were initially avoided in patients with acute myocardial infarction or were used in small doses for fear of causing, or aggravating existing, congestive heart failure.

Treatment During the Early 1970s: Recognized Need for a Prophylactic Agent

Through the middle of the twentieth century and up to and during the early 1970s, the primary treatment for a myocardial infarction patient (who survived long enough to make it to the hospital) was bed rest. Drugs such as nitroglycerin were given symptomatically to alleviate pain, and early antiarrhythmics were given to reduce ventricular arrhythmias. New diagnostic and monitoring procedures were becoming available and more widely used. Innovative monitoring strategies such as the coronary care unit were also becoming more widely available. However, even as late as the early 1970s there still was no proved medical therapy available with a documented effect on the improved survival of myocardial infarction patients.

In 1976 an international panel of experts in the field of coronary heart disease was brought together by the National Heart, Lung, and Blood Institute (NHLBI) to consider primary and secondary prevention strategies aimed at dealing with coronary heart disease mortality [18]. Particular emphasis was placed on the prevention of sudden cardiac death. A number of therapeutic regimens were considered, all of which were directed toward either the treatment and prevention of arrhythmias or the use of agents that might limit the extent of myocardial ischemia.

The panel recommended examining the possible effectiveness of the long-term administration of a beta-blocking agent in survivors of an acute myocardial infarction. The panelists recognized, as noted above, that an agent that could block the sympathetic nervous activity thought to be involved in precipating sudden death and that also had nonneurologic antiarrhythmic properties would be of value to myocardial infarction patients. In fact, beta blockers were already being prescribed for angina and arrhythmias. Moreover, a number of small clinical trials conducted primarily in Europe had already suggested that beta-blocking agents may have a beneficial effect on the mortality rate (particularly the rate of sudden death) in patients who had experienced an acute myocardial infarction. However, clear proof of efficacy was lacking because of the small sample size and some methodologic deficiencies of these first-generation trials.

Based on the recommendation of the panel, the NHLBI initiated the Beta-Blocker Heart Attack Trial (BHAT) in 1977 [18]. This trial was to be a large-scale (about 4000 patients), double-blind, placebo-controlled, multicentered, long-term (up to 4 years) clinical trial of the efficacy of a particular beta blocker, propranolol (the only approved beta blocker in the United States at that time), given to survivors of acute myocardial infarction.

At approximately the same time a number of other second-generation, large-scale, long-term studies of other beta blockers in post-myocardial infarction patients were also beginning or were just under way. For example, Merck Sharp & Dohme was beginning a large trial of timolol in Norway [19]; Julian and co-workers were examining the effects of sotalol [20]; and Taylor and coworkers were studying oxprenolol [21]. (These and other trials are described below.) Also, investigators were examining the short-term effects of beta-blocker therapy and the effects of different modes of administration.

As has been noted above and is described in more detail below, the results of all of these investigations have indicated that beta blockers are effective prophylactic agents in post-myocardial infarction patients in both the short and the long term.

Pharmacology of Beta Blockers

The pharmacodynamic properties and cardiac effects of most of the commonly used and studied beta blockers are listed in Table 28-1 [22]. The differences in the agents may be useful for explaining the observed differences in the short- and long-term effects of the agents. It is clear now that, although there is a general class effect for beta blockers, this effect may be improved or diminished by the properties of a particular beta blocker, as is described below in the section outlining the results of the clinical trials of the drugs.

Beta blockers, also referred to as beta-adrenergic receptor blockers, are competitive inhibitors of the adrenergic receptors in the body. Two properties shared by all the agents are the ability to lower resting blood pressure and the existence of an antiarrhythmic effect. Three other important properties that a beta-blocking agent may or may not have are cardioselectivity, intrinsic sympathomimetic activity, and membrane stabilizing activity.

Cardioselectivity refers to the ability of some beta blockers to preferentially block the adrenergic receptors of the heart (the beta-1 receptors). Other beta blockers block the ad-

renergic receptors of both the heart (beta-1 receptors) and the bronchi and blood vessels (beta-2 receptors). These substances are often referred to as "unselective" agents.

Although at first blush it may appear that a cardioselective beta blocker is preferable (to avoid the known effects of beta-2 blockers, which can depress left ventricular function and can cause or aggravate pulmonary problems), it may still be possible that the generalized effect of the beta-2 blockers is also of benefit to the myocardial infarction patient. For example, it has been speculated that the hypokalemic effect of stress-induced adrenaline release and diuretic use could reduce serum potassium to dangerously low levels, which in turn could elicit potentially life-threatening ventricular arrhythmias [23]. Through beta-2-receptor blockade, a nonselective blocker could theoretically prevent these hypokalemic effects by slowing the cellular uptake of potassium.

The intrinsic sympathomimetic activity (ISA) of beta blockers refers to the ability of some of the agents to partially stimulate the adrenergic receptors. These agents are still referred to as receptor antagonists because while bound to the receptors (and partially stimulating them) they prevent the binding of more powerful stimulators, e.g., epinephrine and norepinephrine.

The theoretical advantages of beta blockers with ISA may be noted in Table 28-1. Note in Table 28-1 that all beta blockers can lower (or at least leave unchanged) the resting heart rate, myocardial contractility (i.e., cardiac output), and resting atrioventricular conduction. However, the agents with at least a moderate ISA effect may or may not lower these parameters. Thus it may be hypothesized that patients on these agents would have a lower incidence of cardiac mechanical problems compared to patients on beta blockers without ISA.

The membrane-stabilizing activity of a beta blocker refers to the ability of the agent to retard the rate of the rise of the intracardiac action potential while leaving the resting potential and the spike duration unchanged. This anesthetic, electrophysiologic effect is not me-

Table 28-1
Pharmacodynamic properties and cardiac effects of beta-blocking drugs

β-blocker	Cardioselectivity[a]	ISA[b]	Membrane stabilizing activity	Resting heart rate	Myocardial contractility	Resting AV conduction	Antiarrhythmic effect	Potency ratio[c]
Acebutolol	Yes	+	+	→	→	→	+	0.3
Alprenolol	No	++	+	↔	↔	↔	+	0.3
Atenolol	Yes	0	0	→	→	→	+	1.0
Metoprolol	Yes	0	±	→	→	→	+	1.0
Oxprenolol	No	++	+	↔	↔	↔	+	0.7
Pindolol	No	+++	+	↔	↔	↔	+	6.0
Practolol	Yes	++	0	↔	↔	↔	+	0.3
Propranolol	No	0	++	→	→	→	+	1.0
Sotalol	No	0	0	→	→	→	+	0.3
Timolol	No	±	0	→	→	→	+	6.0

+ = β-blocker has a positive effect; ± = β-blocker has mixed effects; ↓ = β-blocker decreases the activity; ↔ = β-blocker has no effect on the activity

[a] Cardioselectivity is generally noted only at therapeutic doses.

[b] ISA = intrinsic sympathomimetic activity.

[c] β-blockade potency ratio (propranolol = 1.0).

Source: W. H. Frishman and R. Silverman. Physiologic and metabolic effects. In W. H. Frishman (ed.). *Clinical Pharmacology of the β-Adrenoceptor Blocking Drugs* (2nd ed.). Norwalk, CN: Appleton-Century-Crofts, 1984. With permission.

diated via beta receptors. Although a number of the agents can produce this effect, no beta blocker at therapeutic doses exhibits this activity. It is therefore questionable if it is of any clinical or therapeutic use.

Review of Clinical Trials of Postmyocardial Infarction Patients

METHODS

The major outcome data of beta-blocker trials in acute myocardial infarction and over the long term following hospital discharge are presented below. We chose to consider those trials reported prior to March 1988 in which both intervention and follow-up were carried out during or beyond the time of hospital discharge. Mortality trials were included in this review if they met the following criteria: (1) random assignment of subjects to either a beta blocker or a control group, and (2) a total sample size of at least 100. These criteria were chosen for two important reasons. First, we wanted to restrict this review to trials that incorporated in their design some protection against treatment group allocation bias. Randomization provides this protection. Second, we wanted to focus on trials that could have possibly had sufficient statistical power, as judged by a relatively large sample size, to discern a clinically important effect or trend.

Total mortality has been used whenever possible as the primary response variable in this review, regardless of whether it was the choice in the published report. This point minimizes the potential bias inherent in endpoint determination, as total mortality relies only on a simple count, with no element of judgment.

To reduce the bias that may come about from the differential withdrawal of patients, we have followed the "intention-to-treat principle" for the analyses. That is, all patients who were randomized in a trial were included in the mortality estimates (to the extent the data were available).

Because many of the trials presented only the number of deaths for each treatment group, classic survival curves could not be computed. We chose therefore to compare the proportion of deaths in each treatment group by a χ^2 test so that there might be some consistency in the analyses. We recognize that it is only an approximation to the comparison of survival curves, but it is our experience that the results are usually similar.

Other endpoints presented in this review are serum enzyme levels (as a surrogate for infarct size) and nonfatal reinfarction. Because the trials that examined the effect of a beta blocker on serum enzymes were not always large, we did not restrict the trials we present to only those with more than 100 patients.

When differences for endpoints other than total mortality are said in this review to be statistically significant, it is in most instances the conclusion of the published report and usually denotes a conventional p value of $< .05$.

In this review we also present data examining the short-term versus the long-term effects of beta-blocker administration, as well as data examining the differences between the intravenous and oral administration of the agents.

RESULTS

Short-Term Oral Trials

Eight published trials meeting the review criteria [24–31] evaluated the effect of short-term, oral administration of beta blockers (Table 28-2). In three of the trials, treatment continued beyond the hospital stay or for more than 28 days. The early trials represent the first-generation beta-blocker trials. The beta-blocking doses were generally low compared to those shown to be effective in subsequent trials. In seven of the eight trials the patients were enrolled within 24 hours of the onset of symptoms. The other trial enrolled patients within 72 hours. Propranolol was tested in five trials; alprenolol, practolol, atenolol, and oxprenolol were tested in one trial each. One trial evaluated two beta blockers. All the trials were fairly small, the largest enrolling 454 patients.

In none of the trials was beta-blocker therapy shown to be effective (Table 28-3). Over-

Table 28-2
Eight short-term mortality trials of oral beta blockers

Investigator	Year of report	β-blocker	Dose (mg)	Initiation of treatment	Days of treatment
Balcon [24]	1966	Propranolol	20 qid	Admission	28
Clausen [25]	1966	Propranolol	10 qid	Pain <24 hr	14
Multicentre [26]	1966	Propranolol	20 qid	Pain <24 hr	28
Norris [27]	1968	Propranolol	20 qid	Pain <72 hr	21
Briant [28]	1970	Alprenolol	100 qid	Admission	3 (mean)
Barber [29]	1976	Practolol	300 bid	Admission	90
Wilcox [30]	1980	Propranolol/ Atenolol	40 tid 50 bid	Pain <24 hr	42
Wilcox [31]	1980	Oxprenolol	40 tid	Pain <24 hr	42

Table 28-3
Eight short-term mortality trials of oral beta blockers: Mortality experience

Investigator	β-blocker	Control group		β-blocker group		Absolute efficacy (/100)	Relative efficacy (%)	p
		Deaths/no. of pts.	%	Deaths/no. of pts.	%			
Balcon	Propranolol	15/58	25.9	14/56	25.0	0.9	− 3	NS
Clausen	Propranolol	19/64	29.7	18/66	27.3	2.4	− 8	NS
Multicentre	Propranolol	12/95	12.6	15/100	15.0	−2.4	+19	NS
Norris	Propranolol	24/228	10.5	21/226	9.3	1.2	−12	NS
Briant	Alprenolol	4/57	7.0	5/62	8.1	−1.1	+15	NS
Barber	Practolol	15/228	6.6	14/221	6.3	0.3	− 4	NS
Wilcox	Propranolol/atenolol	7/129	5.4	8/259	3.1	2.3	−43	NS
Wilcox	Oxprenolol	4/158	2.5	6/157	3.8	−1.3	+51	NS
Total		100/1017	9.8	101/1147	8.8	1.0	−10	NS

all, there were 101 deaths among 1147 patients (8.8 percent) allocated to the beta-blocker groups compared to 100 deaths among 1017 control patients (9.8 percent). The overall relative efficacy is thus a 10 percent difference in mortality among the beta-blocker patients (not statistically significant).

Five other published and unpublished trials did not meet review criteria. However, their overall mortality trends were similar to that of the reviewed trials.

Short-Term Intravenous/Oral Trials: Mortality and Serum Enzyme Changes

In 14 trials that met our review criteria for mortality analysis [17, 32–44], an initial loading dose was given intravenously during the acute phase of the myocardial infarction and was followed by oral medication for the remainder of the trial (Table 28-4). The trials, reported between 1979 and 1986, comprise the second-generation beta-blocker trials. In contrast to the previous trials, which initiated treatment with an oral dose generally within 24 hours of symptoms, the patients in these new trials were enrolled as early as possible, usually within 6 to 8 hours. Although treatment varied from 27 hours to 1 year for these

trials, the data presented below reflect 7-day mortality. Seven beta blockers were tested. The differences in drug dosages reflect varying beta-blocking potency.

The results of our review are presented in Table 28-5. Two trials reported a statistically significant benefit of beta-blocker use. In the larger (ISIS), 317 of the 8037 patients allocated to receive atenolol died (3.9 percent) compared to 367 of the 7990 control patients (4.6 percent), a 14 percent relative reduction in mortality. A pooled analysis shows that in the 14 reviewed trials 497 of 13,442 beta-blocker patients died (3.7 percent) compared to 569 of 13,358 control patients (4.3 percent). Thirteen trials that did not meet our review criteria would have added a total of approximately 700 patients to the database. Their overall mortality trends were similar to that of the reviewed trials.

Further analyses of the ISIS data and of pooled trial results indicate that the benefit of intravenous/oral beta-blocker use in acute myocardial infarction patients is seen primarily within the first 24 hours when the mortality rate is the highest.

Low 7-day mortality rates may be noted among the control patients with an acute myo-

Table 28-4
Fourteen short-term mortality trials of IV/oral beta blockers

Investigator	Year of report	β-blocker	Dose (mg)		Initiation of treatment (hr)	Duration of treatment
			IV	PO (daily)		
Andersen [32]	1979	Alprenolol	5	400	6 (median)	1 year
Hjalmarson [33]	1983	Metoprolol	15	200	11.3 (mean)	3 months
Yusuf [34]	1983	Atenolol	5	100	<12	10 days
UKCSG [35]	1984	Timolol	2 + 14[a]	10	<6	In hosp.
ICSG [36]	1984	Timolol	2 + 14[a]	10	<6	In hosp.
Federman [37]	1984	Timolol	5.5	20	<6	28 days
Heber [38]	1984	Labetalol	[b]	[b]	<6	5 days
Norris [39]	1984	Propranolol	0.1/kg	320	<6	27 hours
MILIS [40]	1984	Propranolol	0.1/kg	[c]	8 (mean)	9 days
Owensby [41]	1984	Pindolol	3	15	<12	3 days
MIAMI [42]	1985	Metoprolol	15	200	<24	16 days
Salathia [43]	1985	Metoprolol	15	200	<6	1 year
TIARA [44]	1986	Timolol	5.5	20	<6	1 month
ISIS [17]	1986	Atenolol	5–10	100	<12	7 days

[a]Infused over 24 hours.
[b]Dose-dependent on blood pressure
[c]Dose-dependent on blood pressure and heart rate.

Table 28-5
Fourteen short-term mortality trials of IV/oral beta blockers: Mortality experience

Investigator	β-blocker	Control group		β-blocker group		Absolute efficacy (/100)	Relative efficacy (%)	p
		Deaths/no. of pts.	%	Deaths/no. of pts.	%			
Andersen	Alprenolol	24/242	9.9	28/238	11.8	−1.9	+19	NS
Hjalmarson	Metoprolol	23/697	3.3	18/698	2.6	0.7	−22	NS
Yusuf	Atenolol	16/233	6.9	6/244	2.5	4.4	−64	<.05
UKCSG	Timolol	5/52	9.6	4/56	7.1	2.5	−26	NS
ICSG	Timolol	4/71	5.6	3/73	4.1	1.5	−27	NS
Federman	Timolol	0/51	0.0	1/50	2.0	—	—	—
Heber	Labetalol	0/83	0.0	3/83	3.6	—	—	—
Norris	Propranolol	10/371	2.7	12/364	3.3	−0.6	+22	NS
MILIS	Propranolol	4/135	3.0	4/134	3.0	0.0	0	NS
Owensby	Pindolol	1/50	2.0	1/50	2.0	0.0	0	NS
MIAMI	Metoprolol	93/2901	3.2	79/2877	2.7	0.5	−14	NS
Salathia	Metoprolol	17/384	4.4	18/416	4.3	0.1	−2	NS
TIARA	Timolol	5/98	5.1	3/102	2.9	2.2	−42	NS
ISIS	Atenolol	367/7990	4.6	317/8037	3.9	0.7	−14	<.05
Total		569/13,358	4.3	497/13,422	3.7	0.6	−13	

Table 28-6
Effects of IV beta blockade on serum enzyme levels in short-term trials

Investigator	β-blocker	Entered pts. within 12 hr of pain	No. on β-blocker	Enzyme	Observed reduction (%)	p
Waagstein [45]	Practolol or H87/07 or metoprolol	Yes	39	Max GOT	−5 (increase)	NS
Evemy [46]	Practolol	No	46	AST	0	NS
Peter [47]	Propranolol	Yes	47	CK	10	NS
Norris [48]	Propranolol	Yes	20	CK	52	NS
Norris [49]	Propranolol	Yes	33	CK	25	<.05
Mueller [50]	Propranolol	Yes	44	CK, CK-MB	"No change"	NS
Azancot [51]	Acebutolol	No	14	CK-MB	0	NS
Yusuf [34]	Atenolol	Yes	244	CK-MB	30	<.001
ICSG [36]	Timolol	Yes	73	CK	30	<.05
MILIS [40]	Propranolol	No	134	CK-MB	−2 (increase)	NS
MIAMI [42]	Metoprolol	Yes	2877	ASAT	11	<.05

cardial infarction in these trials (Table 28-5). This finding may be explained by the trial eligibility criteria that were employed. As many as one-half of the patients admitted to a hospital with an acute myocardial infarction had absolute or relative contraindications to beta-blocker therapy. For example, the excluded patients had a higher prevalence of congestive heart failure.

Unfortunately, the data do not allow a comparison of the effects on mortality among the various beta blockers. It may be said, however, that atenolol had a well documented benefit, and that there is no evidence that metoprolol, a beta blocker without ISA, is more effective than other beta blockers without this activity.

A previous review of beta blockers presented data on the effects of intravenous beta blockade on serum enzyme levels (as a surrogate for infarct size) in 28 short-term trials [9]. Eleven of the trials met our review criteria [34, 36, 40, 42, 45–51] and are presented in Table 28-6. Eight of the eleven trials began beta-blocker treatment within 12 hours of the onset of pain. Most of the trials were small, with fewer than 50 patients allocated to the beta-blocker group.

Overall, beta blockers appear to have a moderate effect on enzyme levels. It is especially true for those trials that began beta-blocker therapy within 12 hours. For the three

trials that began therapy after 12 hours, there was no reduction in the level of the serum enzymes. Also, the wide variety of such agents that produce the observed effect suggests that it is a function of beta blockade in general and not a function of cardioselectivity or ISA.

For the 17 trials that did not meet our strict review criteria, the overall trends in enzyme reduction were almost identical to that of the reviewed trials.

Long-Term Oral Trials: Mortality and Reinfarction

Nineteen published and unpublished randomized controlled trials have evaluated the long-term effect of beta blockers on all-cause mortality [19–21, 29, 30, 32, 43, 52–63]. For this review, long-term has arbitrarily been defined as at least 1 year of treatment and follow-up. Again, our review was restricted to trials that had a total sample size of more than 100 patients. Thus four trials were excluded because they were less than a year in duration, and two were excluded because they had fewer than 100 patients.

The 19 trials we selected were reported between the years 1974 and 1987 and are described in Table 28-7. Treatment was usually initiated prior to hospital discharge. Only four trials had a mean duration of treatment of more than 2 years. Nine beta blockers have been tested, although the largest databases ex-

Table 28-7
Nineteen long-term (1 year or longer) mortality trials of oral beta blockers

Investigator	Year of report	β-blocker	Daily dose (mg)	Initiation of treatment post-MI	Duration of treatment
Wilhelmsson [52]	1974	Alprenolol	400	6 weeks	2 years
Ahlmark [53]	1974	Alprenolol	400	2 weeks	2 years
Barber [29]	1976	Practolol	600	3 hr (median)	2 years
Multicentre [54]	1977	Practolol	400	13 days (mean)	15 mo (mean)
Andersen [32]	1979	Alprenolol	400	6 hr (median)	1 year
Wilcox [30]	1980	Propranolol/atenolol	120 100	<24 hr	1 year
Rehnqvist [55]	1980	Metoprolol	200	Discharge	1 year
Norwegian [19]	1981	Timolol	20	7–28 days	17 mo (mean)
Taylor [21]	1982	Oxprenolol	80	13 mo (mean)	4 years (mean)
Hansteen [56]	1982	Propranolol	160	5 days (mean)	1 year
BHAT [57]	1982	Propranolol	180/240	10 days (mean)	25 mo (mean)
Julian [20]	1982	Sotalol	320	5 days	1 year
Australian-Swedish [58]	1983	Pindolol	15	2–21 days	2 years
Manger Cats [59]	1983	Metoprolol	200	4 weeks (mean)	1 year
EIS [60]	1984	Oxprenolol	320	24 days (median)	1 year
Olsson [61]	1985	Metoprolol	200	Before discharge	3 years
Salathia [43]	1985	Metoprolol	200	<6 hr	1 year
Schwartz [62]	1985	Oxprenolol	160	Not available	~ 4 years
LIT [63]	1987	Metoprolol	200	10 days (mean)	1 year

ist for propranolol, metoprolol, oxprenolol, practolol, and timolol.

The mortality results are presented in Table 28-8. Four trials showed a statistically significant reduction in all-cause mortality: the Norwegian Timolol Trial, the Beta-Blocker Heart Attack Trial, or BHAT (propranolol), the trial by Schwartz and coworkers (oxprenolol), and the trial by Salathia and coworkers (metoprolol). In the last trial the statistical significance emerges only if deaths during the first week of therapy are excluded.

Overall, there were 1008 deaths among 10,171 control patients. This figure corresponds to an average mortality of 9.9 percent. The mortality was 21 percent lower among the beta-blocker-treated patients. Among the 10,723 beta-blocker patients there were 841 deaths, corresponding to an average mortality rate of 7.8 percent. The average relative mortality reduction in the trials of beta blockers without ISA was 66 percent higher than that of the trials with ISA (25 percent reduction versus 15 percent reduction). The average

mortality reduction of the unselective beta blockers was only slightly higher than that of the selective beta blockers (23 percent reduction versus 19 percent reduction).

The long-term effect of oral beta blockers on the rates of nonfatal reinfarction have also been examined. Fourteen of the long-term mortality trials that met our review criteria also presented reinfarction data [19–21, 29, 52–56, 58–61, 64]. The results are presented in Table 28-9. (Descriptions of the trials are found in Table 28-7.)

Most trials found a favorable trend with long-term oral beta blocker use. Four trials showed a statistically significant reduction in events among the beta-blocker patients. In pooled analysis, there was an overall 24 percent reduction in the incidence of nonfatal reinfarction.

General Comments
The accumulation of data from all the short- and long-term trials indicates clearly that the beta blockers, whether given acutely or over

Table 28-8
Nineteen long-term (1 year or longer) mortality trials of oral beta blockers: Mortality experience

Investigator	β-blocker	Control group		β-blocker group		Absolute efficacy (/100)	Relative efficacy (%)	p
		Deaths/no. of pts.	%	Deaths/no. of pts.	%			
Wilhelmsson	Alprenolol	14/116	12.1	7/114	6.1	6.0	−49	NS
Ahlmark	Alprenolol	11/93	11.8	5/69	7.2	4.6	−39	NS
Barber	Practolol	38/213	17.8	33/207	15.9	1.9	−11	NS
Multicentre	Practolol	127/1520	8.4	102/1533	6.7	1.7	−20	NS
Andersen	Alprenolol	40/218	18.3	32/209	15.3	3.0	−17	NS
Wilcox	Propranolol/atenolol	12/122	9.8	28/251	11.2	−1.4	+13	NS
Rehnqvist	Metoprolol	6/52	11.5	4/59	6.8	4.7	−41	NS
Norwegian	Timolol	152/939	16.2	98/945	10.4	5.8	−36	<.001
Taylor	Oxprenolol	48/471	10.2	60/632	9.5	0.7	−7	NS
Hansteen	Propranolol	37/282	13.1	25/278	9.0	4.1	−31	NS
BHAT	Propranolol	188/1921	9.8	138/1916	7.2	2.6	−26	<.01
Julian	Sotalol	52/583	8.9	64/873	7.3	1.6	−18	NS
Australian-Swedish	Pindolol	47/266	17.7	45/263	17.1	0.6	−3	NS
Manger Cats	Metoprolol	16/293	5.5	9/291	3.1	2.4	−43	NS
EIS	Oxprenolol	45/883	5.1	57/858	6.6	−1.5	+30	NS
Olsson	Metoprolol	31/147	21.1	25/154	16.2	4.9	−23	NS
Salathia	Metoprolol	43/364	11.8	27/391	6.9	4.9	−42	<.05
Schwartz	Oxprenolol	39/488	8.0	17/485	3.5	4.5	−56	<.01
LIT	Metoprolol	62/1200	5.2	65/1195	5.4	−0.2	+5	NS
Total		1008/10,171	9.9	841/10,723	7.8	2.1	−21	NS

Table 28-9
Nonfatal reinfarction experience in 14 long-term (1 year or longer) trials of oral beta blockers

Investigator	β-blocker	Control group		β-blocker group		Absolute efficacy (/100)	Relative efficacy (%)	p
		Events/no. of pts.	%	Events/no. of pts.	%			
Wilhelmsson [52]	Alprenolol	18/116	15.5	16/114	14.0	1.5	−10	NS
Ahlmark [53]	Alprenolol	14/93	15.1	3/69	4.3	10.8	−71	<.05
Barber [29]	Practolol	21/226	9.3	9/222	4.1	5.2	−56	<.05
Multicentre [54]	Practolol	97/1520	6.4	75/1533	4.9	1.5	−23	NS
Rehnqvist [55]	Metoprolol	5/52	9.6	3/59	5.1	4.5	−47	NS
Norwegian [19]	Timolol	131/939	14.0	90/945	9.5	4.5	−32	<.01
Taylor [21]	Oxprenolol	58/471	12.3	67/632	10.6	1.7	−14	NS
Hansteen [56]	Propranolol	21/282	7.4	16/278	5.8	1.6	−23	NS
BHAT [64]	Propranolol	121/1921	6.3	103/1916	5.4	0.9	−15	NS
Julian [20]	Sotalol	22/583	3.8	24/873	2.7	1.1	−27	NS
Australian-Swedish [58]	Pindolol	28/266	10.5	25/263	9.5	1.0	−10	NS
Manger Cats [59]	Metoprolol	20/293	6.8	16/291	5.5	1.3	−19	NS
EIS [60]	Oxprenolol	38/883	4.3	36/858	4.2	0.1	−3	NS
Olsson [61]	Metoprolol	31/147	21.1	18/154	11.7	9.4	−45	<.05
Total		625/7792	8.0	501/8207	6.1	1.9	−24	

the long term, reduce all-cause mortality and nonfatal reinfarction. Specifically, whereas there is no specific evidence that short-term oral therapy alone is effective, there is strong evidence that a combination of intravenous (especially soon after the onset of symptoms) and oral beta blockers effectively prevents premature mortality. There is also evidence that in the short term beta blockers can reduce serum enzymes, a finding suggestive that beta blockers can reduce infarct size. Finally, there is overwhelming scientific evidence that in the long term these agents reduce both the incidence of nonfatal reinfarction and the occurrence of all-cause mortality.

The trials have also raised several questions, many of which relate directly to clinical care. Data from the trials may be used in an attempt to address the questions.

Beta Blockers During and After Acute Myocardial Infarction: Evidence from Trials

WHAT ARE THE MECHANISMS OF BETA-BLOCKER ACTION?

As might have been expected, the reduction in all-cause mortality is due to a reduction in atherosclerotic cardiovascular deaths. The benefit is explained particularly by prevention of sudden cardiac deaths. For example, the mortality experience of the BHAT is presented in Table 28-10 [57]. These data are typical of the long-term trials and demonstrate that not only do postmyocardial infarction patients die more frequently of cardiovascular problems than of noncardiovascular problems but that propranolol is significantly effective in reducing the absolute and relative risks of atherosclerotic death in general and sudden atherosclerotic death in particular.

These data suggest that beta blockers exert their favorable effect by reducing the frequency and severity of arrhythmias. Such a statement is further supported in Table 28-11 by an examination of the instantanous death rates in the BHAT [65], the Norwegian Timo-

lol Trial [19], and a propranolol study reported by Hansteen et al. in 1982 [56]. In all three trials, there is again a large reduction in both the absolute and relative risks due to beta blocker use.

Furthermore, the prevalence of ventricular arrhythmias at baseline and 6 weeks postrandomization was examined by treatment group in a sample of the BHAT patients [66] (Table 28-12). Although the prevalence of arrhythmia at 6 weeks was higher in both treatment groups among patients with arrhythmias at baseline, there was still an overall 40 percent reduction of arrhythmia among the propranolol patients (19.9 percent prevalence among the propranolol patients versus 33.0 percent prevalence among the placebo patients).

Stratifying the BHAT patients by the presence or absence of complex ventricular premature beats (VPBs) at baseline reveals that there is a greater relative reduction in mortality among patients with VPBs [67]. As may be noted in Figure 28-1, there is a 31 percent propranolol-attributable reduction in total mortality among patients with complex VPBs and a 28 percent reduction in sudden death. For patients without the arrhythmia, the respective figures are lower: 25 and 16 percent.

Finally, experimental studies have shown that beta blockers raise the threshold for ventricular fibrillation in ischemic myocardium. A reduction in the incidence of ventricular fibrillation (cardiac arrest) during beta blockade has also been noted in some trials (Table 28-13), although the effect in two of the trials is small.

There is much evidence that beta blockers exert their effect via an antiarrhythmic mechanism, but it should be noted that there is also evidence that other mechanisms may be operating as well. For example, the observed reductions in nonsudden death (Table 28-10) and nonfatal reinfarctions (Table 10-9) suggest an anti-ischemic effect. This mechanism may be separate from the antianginal effect of the beta blockers, as other compounds with antianginal properties do not influence survival (e.g., calcium channel blockers).

Other mechanisms for the beta blockers have also been hypothesized, although there is

Table 28-10
Cause-specific mortality by treatment group: BHAT[a]

Cause of death	Placebo group (N = 1921)		Propranolol group (N = 1916)		Absolute efficacy (/100)	Relative efficacy (%)	p
	No. of deaths	Rate (%)	No. of deaths	Rate (%)			
Total mortality	188	9.8	138	7.2	2.6	−26	<.01
Noncardiovascular	17	0.9	11	0.6	0.3	−35	NS
Cardiovascular	171	8.9	127	6.6	2.3	−26	<.01
Nonatherosclerotic	7	0.4	8	0.4	0.0	0	NS
Atherosclerotic	164	8.5	119	6.2	2.3	−27	<.01
Nonsudden	75	3.9	55	2.9	1.0	−26	NS
Sudden[b]	89	4.6	64	3.3	1.3	−28	<.05

[a] Average length of follow-up was 25 months.
[b] Atherosclerotic death within 1 hour of symptoms.
Source: Beta-Blocker Heart Attack Trial Research group. A randomized trial of propranolol in patients with acute myocardial infarction. I. Mortality results. *J.A.M.A.* 247:1707, 1982. Copyright 1982, American Medical Association.

Table 28-11
Instantaneous death rates in three long-term beta-blocker trials

| Trial | Year of report | β-blocker | Instantaneous death rate (%) | | Absolute efficacy (/100) | Relative efficacy (%) |
			Control group	β-blocker group		
Norwegian [19]	1981	Timolol	4.7	1.9	2.8	−60
Hansteen [56]	1982	Propranolol	6.0	3.2	2.8	−47
BHAT [65]	1987	Propranolol	3.5	2.2	1.3	−37
Total			4.1	2.2	1.9	−46

Table 28-12
Prevalence of ventricular arrhythmia at 6 weeks postrandomization by presence of ventricular arrhythmia at baseline and by treatment group: BHAT

| VA at baseline | Placebo group | | Propranolol group | | % difference in VA |
	VA at 6 wk/no. of pts.	%	VA at 6 wk/no. of pts.	%	
Yes	44/59	74.6	25/52	48.1	−36
No	92/353	26.1	60/376	16.0	−39
Total	136/412	33.0	85/428	19.9	−40

VA = ventricular arrhythmia (defined as at least 10 VPBs/hr on a 24-hour ambulatory electrocardiogram).
Source: J. Morganroth et al. Beta-Blocker Heart Attack Trial—impact of propranolol therapy on ventricular arrhythmias. *Prev. Med.* 14:346, 1985. With permission.

no experimental evidence for them [9]. They include an infarct reduction mechanism, increased vascularity mechanisms, scar reduction mechanisms, and antiplatelet mechanisms.

Who Should Get a Beta Blocker?

For a myocardial infarction patient who does not have any contraindication to a beta blocker (discussed below), the question naturally arises: Which of these patients would benefit the most from beta-blocker therapy and which would benefit the least? The overall clinical trial experience indicates that these agents have a greater effect in some patients than in others and that it is, to a large extent, a function of how complicated the myocardial infarction is.

For example, post hoc analyses of the BHAT data suggest that the patients with uncomplicated myocardial infarctions (and an al-

ready low annual mortality) benefit to a small degree from propranolol therapy [68]. The BHAT all-cause mortality rates are stratified by treatment group and by the presence or absence of transient electrical or mechanical cardiac complications at baseline in Table 28-14. In the large subgroup of patients with no complications, the observed relative benefit of propranolol was only 6 percent (relative risk 0.94). The most pronounced relative difference in mortality between the two study groups was observed in the subgroup with electrical problems only. Here the mortality in the propranolol group was roughly one-half of that in the placebo group (relative risk 0.48). In the two risk groups with mechanical complications, the relative difference in mortality was 38 and 25 percent, respectively. These relative differences remained basically unchanged after adjustment for possible confounding variables. The highest absolute risk reduction was found in the subgroup with either electrical or mechanical problems: four

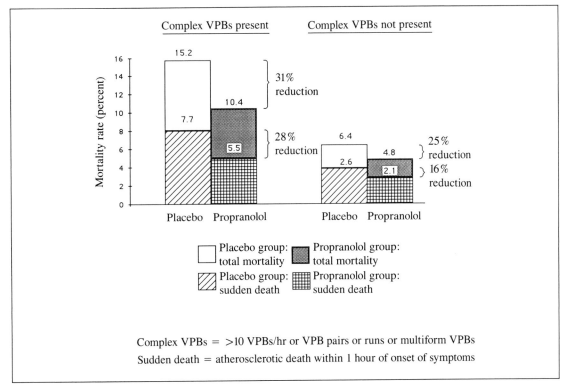

Fig. 28-1
Total mortality and sudden death rates (percent) by the presence of complex
ventricular premature beats (VPBs) at baseline, by treatment group in the Beta-
Blocker Heart Attack Trial. The average length of follow-up was 25 months.
Complex VPBs = >10 VPBs/hr or VPB pairs or runs or multiform VPBs.
Sudden death = atherosclerotic death within 1 hour of onset of symptoms. (From
L. M. Friedman et al. Effect of propranolol in patients with myocardial infarction
and ventricular arrhythmia. *J. Am. Coll. Cardiol.* 7:1, 1986. With permission.)

to six lives were prolonged for every 100 patients treated over an average period of 25
months.

A more detailed analysis of the individual
electrical and mechanical complications in
these patients is shown in Table 28-15. Patients who had suffered an episode of ventricular tachycardia during hospitalization made
up the single largest subgroup. Among these
patients, mortality was 44 percent lower in the
propranolol group than in the control group.
The greatest absolute efficacy and the lowest
relative risk, which suggest that patients received special benefit from propranolol therapy, were observed in the small subgroup of
patients who had experienced ventricular fibrillation (23 lives prolonged for every 200

such patients treated, or a 63 percent reduction in mortality). The smallest absolute efficacy and the highest relative risk, which suggest little benefit from propranolol therapy,
were observed in the small subgroup of patients who had experienced pulmonary edema
(only one life prolonged for every 200 such
patients treated, or a 2 percent reduction in
mortality).

The cumulative life table curves for these
BHAT data stratified by treatment group and
by the presence/absence of any electrical/me-
chanical problem are shown in Figure 28-2.
The difference in the treatment group curves
for the high risk patients is dramatic, whereas
there is little difference in the treatment group
curves for the low risk patients.

Table 28-13
Incidence of ventricular fibrillation in acute beta-blocker trials

Investigator (length of follow-up)	β-blocker	Control group		β-blocker group		Absolute efficacy (/100)	Relative efficacy (%)
		Events/no. of pts.	%	Events/no. of pts.	%		
ISIS [17] (7 days)	Atenolol	198/7990	2.5	189/8037	2.4	0.1	− 5
MIAMI [42] (15 days)	Metoprolol	52/2901	1.8	48/2877	1.7	0.1	− 7
Norris [39] (48 hr)	Propranolol	14/371	3.8	2/364	0.5	3.3	−85

Table 28-14
All-cause mortality by risk and treatment groups: BHAT[a]

Risk group	Placebo group		Propranolol group		Absolute efficacy (/100)	Relative efficacy (%)	Adjusted relative efficacy[b] (%)
	No. of pts.	Mortality rate (%)	No. of pts.	Mortality rate (%)			
No electrical or mechanical complications	1079	6.6	1047	6.2	0.4	− 6	− 4
Electrical complications only	423	10.9	443	5.2	5.7	−52	−57
Mechanical complications only	202	16.8	201	10.4	6.4	−38	−43
Both electrical and mechanical complications	217	17.1	225	12.9	4.2	−25	−30

[a] Average length of follow-up was 25 months.
[b] Adjusted for 13 variables predictive of mortality.
Source: C. D. Furberg et al. Effect of propranolol in post-infarction patients with mechanical or electrical complications. *Circulation* 69:761, 1984.
By permission of the American Heart Association, Inc.

Table 28-15
All-cause mortality by reported complication during hospitalization before enrollment and by treatment group: BHAT*

Complication	Placebo group		Propranolol group		Absolute efficacy (/100)	Relative efficacy (%)
	No. of pts.	Mortality rate (%)	No. of pts.	Mortality rate (%)		
Electrical						
Ventricular fibrillation	99	18.2	104	6.7	11.5	−63
Ventricular tachycardia	446	12.1	441	6.8	5.3	−44
Complete AV block	44	15.9	54	9.3	6.6	−42
Incomplete AV block	153	12.4	158	8.9	3.5	−28
Atrial fibrillation	109	14.7	131	11.5	3.2	−22
Mechanical						
Pulmonary edema	51	19.6	52	19.2	0.4	−2
Cardiogenic shock	21	14.3	29	10.3	4.0	−28
Persistent hypotension	133	12.0	142	9.2	2.8	−23
Basilar rales	57	22.8	58	13.8	9.0	−39
Signs/symptoms of CHF	287	17.4	274	13.5	3.9	−22

*Average length of follow-up was 25 months.
Source: C. D. Furberg et al. Effect of propranolol in post-infarction patients with mechanical or electrical complications. *Circulation* 69:761. 1984. By permission of the American Heart Association, Inc.

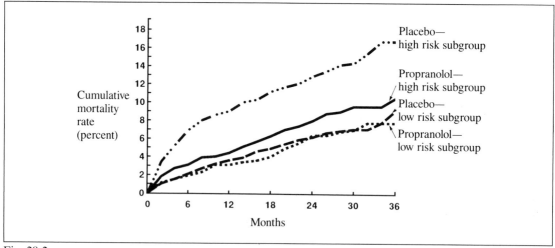

Fig. 28-2
Cumulative life table mortality curves by risk group and by treatment group in the Beta-Blocker Heart Attack Trial. High risk = presence of any of the following at baseline: complete or incomplete AV block, ventricular fibrillation or tachycardia, atrial fibrillation, pulmonary edema, cardiogenic shock, persistent hypotension, congestive heart failure, or basilar rales. (From C. D. Furberg et al. Effect of propranolol in post-infarction patients with mechanical or electrical complications. *Circulation* 69:761, 1984. By permission of the American Heart Association, Inc.)

Similar observations have been noted in other trials, although a common problem in all the trials is inadequate subgroup design and the lack of statistical power to detect real benefit in any subgroup of patients. The Beta-Blocker Pooling Project (BBPP) published its results in 1988 [69]. The overall goals for the BBPP were to overcome the problems inherent in the analysis of one trial and to combine the results of the nine largest long-term secondary-prevention trials of beta blockers to determine if there were subgroups of myocardial infarction patients who benefited the most from beta blocker therapy.

The investigators of the BBPP found, when the results of nine large trials were combined, that patients with a high risk of mortality were those most likely to benefit both absolutely and relatively from beta-blocker therapy. All the trials specifically included patients with nonsevere electrical or mechanical complications at the time of their infarction. Furthermore, the investigators found that lower-risk myocardial infarction patients also benefited from beta-blocker therapy, although the absolute and relative benefits were small.

The clinical trial experience of beta-blocker use in the elderly is limited, but there seems to be good rationale to extrapolate overall results to this population, if only because the proportion of complicated myocardial infarction increases with age. For example, in the BHAT a trend toward an even greater benefit has been observed in patients 60 years of age or older when compared to myocardial infarction patients under 60 [70]. Table 28-16 presents the BHAT mortality statistics for myocardial infarction patients 30 to 59 years of age (N = 2589) and 60 to 69 years of age (N = 1248). For the patients under 60 years of age, approximately 90 percent of all deaths were atherosclerotic in nature, and the observed benefit from propranolol was largely due to a decrease in sudden deaths. For patients 60 years or older, approximately 83 percent of all deaths were atherosclerotic in nature, and the overall reduction in mortality in the propranolol group was due primarily to a large reduction of atherosclerotic sudden and nonsudden deaths.

The BBPP produced similar results [69], with some refinement. For patients under 50

Table 28-16
Cause-specific mortality by age and treatment groups: BHAT[a]

Cause of death	Mortality rate (%)		Absolute efficacy (/100)	Relative efficacy (%)
	Placebo group	Propranolol group		
Age 30–59 years				
Total mortality	7.4	6.0	1.4	−19
Cardiovascular	6.8	5.7	1.1	−16
Atherosclerotic	6.5	5.5	1.0	−15
Nonsudden	2.7	2.5	0.2	−7
Sudden[b]	3.8	3.1	0.7	−18
Age 60–69 years				
Total mortality	14.7	9.8	4.9	−33
Cardiovascular	13.1	8.6	4.5	−34
Atherosclerotic	12.6	7.6	5.0	−40
Nonsudden	6.3	3.7	2.6	−41
Sudden[b]	6.3	3.9	2.4	−38

Propranolol group 30–59 years = 1301 patients; propranolol group 60–69 years = 615 patients; placebo group 30–59 years = 1288 patients; placebo group 60–69 years = 633 patients.
[a]Average length of follow-up was 25 months.
[b]Atherosclerotic death within 1 hour of symptoms.
Source: From C. M. Hawkins et al. Effect of propranolol in reducing mortality in older myocardial infarction patients. *Circulation* 67(Suppl I):94, 1983. By permission of the American Heart Association, Inc.

years of age, the pooled data provided no evidence of beta-blocker benefit (relative risk 0.97, only a 3 percent reduction in mortality). For patients 60 years old or more, there was evidence of a moderate benefit (relative risk 0.83, or a 17 percent reduction in mortality). For patients 50 to 59 years of age, however, there was evidence of relatively large benefit (relative risk 0.63, or a 37 percent reduction in mortality).

Finally, when deciding which patients to treat prophylactically, one should keep in mind that there are other indications for long-term beta-blocker use, e.g., angina pectoris, hypertension, and the presence of ventricular arrhythmias.

WHO SHOULD NOT GET A BETA BLOCKER?

From the early Phase I and II trials of beta blockers, it is known that approximately one-half of all patients admitted early with an acute myocardial infarction and about 20 percent of those surviving 1 to 3 weeks have relative or absolute contraindications to beta-blocker treatment. These contraindications include hypotension, bradycardia, severe congestive heart failure, atrioventricular conduction disorders, and obstructive lung disease.

Although most of the large clinical trials actively avoided recruiting myocardial infarction patients who had any of the above problems to a severe extent, the results from the trials can still be instructive. For example, most of the nine trials comprising the BBPP excluded patients with such problems as severe failure and severe hypotension. With the remaining patient population, the question arises: Is there a subgroup of beta-blocker patients who experience greater mortality than the control patients? The BBPP investigators found that of the 36 patient subgroups examined for beta-blocker benefit only one small subgroup had a relative risk greater than 1, indicating a possible contraindication to the agents [69]. However, even this difference was not statistically significant. The investigators concluded that they could not find, among the patients enrolled into the trials, any subgroup in which beta-blocker therapy was conclusively a problem.

It should also be noted that not all patients with a "contraindication" should be excluded from beta-blocker treatment a priori. It is a

Table 28-17
Cause-specific mortality by history of CHF and by treatment group: BHAT*

Cause of death	Placebo group		Propranolol group		Absolute efficacy (/100)	Relative efficacy (%)
	Deaths/no. of pts.	%	Deaths/no. of pts.	%		
Total mortality						
Hx of CHF	67/365	18.4	46/345	13.3	5.1	−27
No Hx of CHF	121/1556	7.8	92/1571	5.9	1.9	−25
Atherosclerosis						
Hx of CHF	65/365	17.8	40/345	11.6	6.2	−35
No Hx of CHF	99/1556	6.4	79/1571	5.0	1.4	−21
Sudden death (< 1 hr of symptoms)						
Hx of CHF	38/365	10.4	19/345	5.5	4.9	−47
No Hx of CHF	51/1556	3.3	45/1571	2.9	0.4	−13

Hx = history; CHF = congestive heart failure.
*Average length of follow-up was 25 months.
Source: K. Chadda et al. Effect of propranolol after myocardial infarction in patients with congestive heart failure. *Circulation* 73:503, 1986. By permission of the American Heart Association, Inc.

Table 28-18
Incidence of CHF during the follow-up period, by treatment group: BHAT

History of CHF	Placebo group		Propranolol group		Absolute efficacy (/100)	Relative efficacy (%)	p
	Events/no. of pts.	%	Events/no. of pts.	%			
Yes	46/365	12.6	51/345	14.8	−2.2	+17	NS
No	82/1556	5.3	78/1571	5.0	0.3	−6	NS
Total	128/1921	6.7	129/1916	6.7	0.0	0	NS

Source: K. Chadda et al. Effect of propranolol after myocardial infarction in patients with congestive heart failure. *Circulation* 73:503, 1986. By permission of the American Heart Association, Inc.

question of degree. For example, if we again examine the mortality data from the BHAT, we can see that patients with a history of mild or moderate congestive heart failure (CHF) can also benefit from beta-blocker therapy [71]. In Table 28-17 we see that the placebo patients consistently had the higher mortality rate. In fact, the results mirror what was seen in Table 28-14: The patients with CHF actually experienced greater benefit from beta blockade than did patients without failure.

We can also examine the incidence of CHF during the course of a trial. In Table 28-18 we find that overall in the BHAT there was no difference in the incidence of CHF between the propranolol and placebo groups. Both groups had a 25-month incidence of 6.7 percent. If we

stratify by history of CHF, we see that among the patients with a history of CHF the propranolol patients did have a 17 percent higher rate of recurrent CHF (14.8 percent versus 12.6 percent), but this difference is not statistically significant. In fact, a life table analysis of these data indicates that the recurrent failure was more frequent early on and that after 5 months the rates began to approach each other.

WHAT ARE THE ADVERSE EFFECTS OF BETA-BLOCKER THERAPY?

Related to the issue of who not to give a beta blocker is the issue of the possible risks among the patients to whom you do give a beta blocker. When deciding to treat patients with beta blockers after a myocardial infarction, the risks of therapy must be weighed against the potential benefits. In studies of patients with no absolute or relative contraindications to beta-blocker treatment, severe adverse reactions leading to discontinuation of therapy were fairly infrequent. The proportion of patients taken off active treatment for medical reasons ranged from 5 to 20 percent. However, the composition of the patient populations, the drug dosages and duration of treatment, and the methods of ascertaining and reporting adverse effects are factors that need to be considered when comparing these percentages. A notable finding in these reports, however, is the observation that so-called side effects are also common among placebo patients. Often we attribute signs and symptoms to a patient's treatment rather than to the condition being treated.

Beta-blocker adverse effects have been categorized into two types: those pharmacologically related to beta blockade and those not [72]. Reactions of the first type are more common, simply because of the importance of the sympathetic nervous system in controlling our metabolic functions. Related to the pharmacology of the beta blockers, there is still little evidence whether the cardioselective beta blockers or those with partial ISA are associated with a lower incidence of adverse reactions than are the nonselective beta blockers or those without ISA.

Review of the large beta-blocker clinical trials reveals that cardiovascular problems account for the largest number of severe reactions in the beta-blocker groups. These problems include symptomatic CHF, hypotension with and without dizziness, bradycardia, and atrioventricular block. Heart failure, as noted above, is less common than expected, perhaps because most of the trials exclude from participation those patients with moderate to severe heart failure.

The trials also showed a higher frequency among beta-blocker patients of minor side ef-

Fig. 28-3
Incidence of congestive heart failure (leading to temporary or permanent discontinuation of treatment), according to the presence of complications at baseline, by treatment group, in the Beta-Blocker Heart Attack Trial. The average length of follow-up was 25 months. Hatched bars = placebo group; dotted bars = propranolol group. (From C. D. Furberg et al. Effect of propranolol in post-infarction patients with mechanical or electrical complications. *Circulation* 69:761, 1984. By permission of the American Heart Association, Inc.)

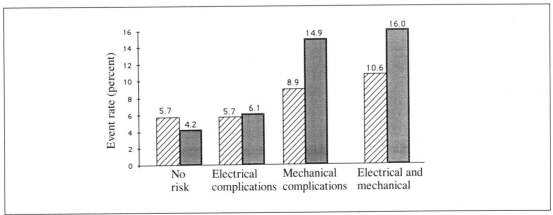

fects that did not lead to discontinuation of the treatment. It included cases of cold extremities, nausea, constipation, asthma, fatigue, mental depression, impotence, and dry eyes.

If we accept that high risk patients are the prime candidates for preventive therapy, we must be prepared to pay a price: a higher incidence of adverse effects. Figure 28-3 presents BHAT data, stratifying the incidence of CHF leading to discontinuation of treatment by treatment group and risk group. We can see that the incidence of CHF in the uncomplicated group and the group with electrical complications was only about 4 to 6 percent over 25 months, regardless of whether they received a beta blocker. Among the patients with a history of mechanical complications and assigned to the placebo group, the risk of CHF was about twice these rates (9–11 percent). If these patients were on propranolol, the rates increased to 15 to 16 percent. However, this figure is outweighed by the 30 to 40 percent reduction in mortality among these patients attributed to beta-blocker therapy (Table 28-14).

CHOOSING A BETA BLOCKER AND ITS DOSAGE

The questions of which beta blocker to use and its dosage are difficult because no large clinical trial has formally compared the preventive and adverse effects of two beta blockers given to postmyocardial infarction patients. Comparing trials can be problematic because several nonpharmacologic factors can explain observed numerical differences in treatment effects across trials. For example, inclusion of a high proportion of low risk, uncomplicated infarctions would tend to dilute the benefit in the high risk groups. True equipotency is also difficult to determine. It is clearly possible that for some beta blockers and some trials (particularly the early ones), a less than optimal dose was tested. Statistically, chance is an important factor to consider when comparing relative and absolute risks and benefits.

However, there may be ancillary pharmacologic properties that could be important. It appears that beta blockers with intrinsic sympathomimetic activity are slightly less effective than those without. For example, of the nine trials in Table 28-8 studying a beta blocker with ISA (e.g., alprenolol and oxprenolol), the pooled relative benefit is a 15 percent reduction in mortality. Of the ten trials studying a beta blocker without ISA (e.g., propranolol, timolol, and metoprolol), the pooled relative benefit is a 25 percent reduction in deaths. Also, there is no scientific evidence that the cardioselective blockers (e.g., atenolol and metoprolol) are more effective than the nonselective blockers (e.g., propranolol and timolol). In fact, the strongest data on the favorable long-term mortality effects come from trials of propranolol and timolol. As noted above, there is some speculation that beta-2 blockade could enhance the antiarrhythmic action of beta-1 blockade.

Reviews of the clinical trial evidence can offer more unbiased insights into drug mechanisms and how the drugs compare than can individual trial reports. Based on the review presented here, the beta blockers recommended for the prophylactic treatment of a myocardial infarction are timolol, propranolol, atenolol, and metoprolol. The side effect profile may be most favorable for atenolol [73]. The recommended daily doses would be those evaluated in the trials: timolol 20 mg/day, propranolol 180 to 240 mg/day, atenolol 100 mg/day, and metoprolol 200 mg/day.

WHEN TO BEGIN AND END BETA-BLOCKER THERAPY

Review of the acute short-term trials (Tables 28-4 and 28-5) clearly indicates that if beta-blocker therapy is contemplated it should be initiated with an intravenous bolus within 6 to 8 hours of the onset of pain. However, the relatively low 7-day mortality among patients without complications to beta blockers (approximately 4 percent, Table 28-5) and the small relative benefit (approximately 13 percent, Table 28-5) raises the issue of cost versus benefit. In light of the larger benefit associated with thrombolytic therapy and aspirin [16], the role of beta blockers in the early phase of a myocardial infarction is debatable. However, because it turns out that there is no clear benefit of thrombolytic therapy during the first day postinfarction and because it is known that a beta blocker such as atenolol has its primary effect during the first day, it makes scientific sense to combine beta-blocker and thrombolytic therapies. In fact, there are trials currently under way to assess this hypothesis.

For the long term, the choices are limited at this time because no intervention other than beta-blocker therapy has a documented effect on survival and risk of reinfarction. In most of the long-term trials, beta-blocker therapy was started 1 to 3 weeks after the infarction, while the patient was still hospitalized (Table 28-7). It was a clear advantage in these trials to initiate treatment by the time the patient had begun to recover, was in a stable condition, and could be observed.

It seems prudent to recommend that oral beta-blocker therapy be initiated 6 to 9 days after the acute event in patients who are hemodynamically stable, have no major contraindications to beta blockers, and are at increased risk of mortality. These patients are prime candidates for beta-blocker therapy. There are no trials that have compared the value of acute versus delayed initiation of beta-blocker therapy.

With respect to the duration of treatment, the long-term trials provide substantial data for the assessment of treatment benefit up to 2 years. Beyond this time, the data are limited, and a recommendation for continued treatment would have to be based on the extrapolation of the 2-year data. Because the cumulative mortality curves for the propranolol and placebo groups continue to diverge even at 36 months for patients with a complicated myocardial infarction in the BHAT (Fig. 28-2), and because most postinfarction patients have angina pectoris and ventricular arrhythmias, it seems prudent, in the absence of any troublesome adverse reaction, to continue treatment indefinitely.

Clinical Impact and Public Health Impact of Beta Blockers

To the clinician and the patient, the absolute benefit of a preventive measure appears to be more important than the relative treatment effect. Table 28-19 demonstrates this principle. In a low-risk population, a reduction of the annual mortality from 2.0 percent to 1.5 percent means that 200 such patients would have to be treated for 1 year to prolong one life. The relative benefit is 25 percent (i.e., the relative risk is 0.75). A similar relative benefit in a high risk population with a 20 percent annual mortality rate would reduce this mortality rate to 15 percent, which corresponds to five lives prolonged for every 100 such patients treated. Thus a 25 percent relative mortality reduction in a high risk group is preferable to a 25 percent reduction in a low-risk group. In fact, among high risk patients a lower relative reduction can actually translate to a greater absolute efficacy. An apparent paradox is that among high risk patients a smaller (10 percent) relative reduction (from 20 to 18 percent) still gives us a better absolute reduction (two lives prolonged for every 100 treated) than a 25 per-

Table 28-19
Efficacy measures and their clinical usefulness (hypothetical data)

Population	Annual mortality rate (%)		Relative efficacy (%)	Absolute efficacy (efficacy by no. of pts. treated)
	Placebo	Intervention		
Low risk	2.0	1.5	−25	0.5/100 = 1/200
High risk	20.0	15.0	−25	5/100
High risk	20.0	18.0	−10	2/100

cent relative reduction in a low risk group (from 2.0 to 1.5 percent mortality, or one life prolonged for every 200 treated.)

We have already seen this principle at work in Table 28-14, where the greatest absolute benefit of propranolol therapy was among those patients with transient mechanical problems. We conclude that, clinically, beta blockers exert their greatest benefit on those patients at high risk of death.

The public health implications are clear. As noted at the beginning of the chapter, there are approximately 120,000 in-hospital heart attack deaths in the United States each year and 640,000 patients who survive hospitalization. Based on the available data from the assembled beta-blocker trials, it is conservatively estimated that among the hospital survivors 16,000 deaths could be postponed during the first year postinfarction and that more than 50,000 deaths could be averted over the first 5 years postinfarction. Furthermore, a cost-effectiveness analysis indicated that there is clear evidence of benefit from beta-blocker treatment of medium to high risk myocardial infarction hospital survivors and suggestive evidence of benefit for the treatment of some low risk patients [74].

For the first time in medical history, a pharmaceutical agent has become available with a demonstrated effect on mortality following a myocardial infarction. Our next goals are now to reduce this toll even more through improved secondary prevention and, more importantly, to engage in research aimed at the primary prevention of coronary disease.

Editorial Comments

The long-term use of beta blockers is securely established in selected patients following acute myocardial infarction. Patients with electrical instability or left ventricular dysfunction (but not overt heart failure) derive the most benefit. Recent data from the TIMI phase II trial indicate that 15 mg of intravenous metoprolol given at the time of lytic therapy followed by oral metoprolol (50 mg twice a day on the first hospital day followed by 100 mg twice a day thereafter), if tolerated, significantly reduced nonfatal reinfarction and recurrent ischemic episodes within 6 days of entry into the trial, but not within 42 days. (The TIMI Study Group. Comparison of invasive and conservative strategies after treatment with intravenous tissue plasminogen activator in acute myocardial infarction. N. Engl. J. Med. 320:618, 1989.) G.S.F.

References

1. Stamler, J. The marked decline in coronary heart disease mortality rates in the United States, 1968-1981: Summary of findings and possible explanations. *Cardiology* 72:11, 1985.
2. American Heart Association: *1988 Heart Facts.* Dallas: AHA, 1988.
3. National Center for Health Statistics: Detailed diagnoses and procedures for patients discharged from short-stay hospitals, United States 1986. *Vital Health Stat.* [13] No. 95, May 1988.
4. National Center for Health Statistics: *Utilization of Short-Stay Hospitals, United States 1986 Summary.* DHHS Publication No. 96, (PHS) 88-1757.
5. Canner, P. L., Berge, K. G., Wenger, N. K., et al. Fifteen year mortality in Coronary Drug Project patients—long-term benefit from niacin. *J. Am. Coll. Cardiol.* 8:1245, 1986.
6. May, G. S., Eberlein, K. A., Furberg, C. D., et al. Secondary prevention after myocardial infarction: A review of long-term trials. *Prog. Cardiovasc. Dis.* 24:331, 1982.
7. May, G. S., Furberg, C. D., Eberlein, K. A., and Geraci, B. Secondary prevention after myocardial infarction: A review of short-term acute phase trials. *Prog. Cardiovasc. Dis.* 25:335, 1983.
8. Furberg, C. D. Effect of antiarrhythmic drugs on mortality after myocardial infarction. *Am. J. Cardiol.* 52:32C, 1983.
9. Yusuf, S., Peto, R., Lewis, J., et al. Beta-blockade during and after myocardial infarction—an overview of the randomized trials. *Prog. Cardiovasc. Dis.* 27:335, 1985.
10. Yusuf, S., Collins, R., Peto, R., et al. Intravenous and intracoronary fibrinolytic therapy in acute myocardial infarction—overview of results on mortality, reinfarction and side-effects from 33 randomized controlled trials. *Eur. Heart J.* 6:556, 1985.
11. Yusuf, S. Interventions that potentially limit myocardial infarct size: Overview of clinical trials. *Am. J. Cardiol.* 60:11A, 1987.

12. Lipid Research Clinics Coronary Primary Prevention Trial Results. I. Reduction in incidence of coronary heart disease. *J.A.M.A.* 251:351, 1984.

13. Frick, M. H., Elo, O., Haapa, K., et al. Helsinki Heart Study—primary prevention trial with gemfibrozil in middle-aged men with dyslipidemia. *N. Engl. J. Med.* 317:1237, 1987.

14. Gruppo Italiano Per Lo Studio Della Streptochinasi Nell' Infarto Miscardico (GISSI): Effectiveness of intravenous thrombolytic treatment in acute myocardial infarction. *Lancet* 1:397, 1986.

15. Antiplatelet trialists' collaboration: Secondary prevention of vascular disease by prolonged antiplatelet treatment. *Br. Med. J.* 296:320, 1988.

16. ISIS Collaborative Group: Results of a large randomized trial of intravenous streptokinase and oral aspirin in acute myocardial infarction (Abstract). *J. Am. Coll. Cardiol.* 11:232A, 1988.

17. ISIS-1 (First International Study of Infarct Survival) Collaborative Group: Randomised trial of intravenous atenolol among 16,027 cases of suspected acute myocardial infarction: ISIS-1. *Lancet* 2:57, 1986.

18. Byington, R. P. for the Beta-Blocker Heart Attack Trial Research Group: Beta-Blocker Heart Attack Trial: Design, methods, and baseline results. *Controlled Clin. Trials* 5:382, 1984.

19. Norwegian Multicenter Study Group: Timolol-induced reduction in mortality and reinfarction in patients surviving acute myocardial infarction. *N. Engl. J. Med.* 304:801, 1981.

20. Julian, D. G., Prescott, R. J., Jackson, F. S., et al. Controlled trial of sotalol for one year after myocardial infarction. *Lancet* 1:1142, 1982.

21. Taylor, S. H., Silke, B., Ebutt, A., et al. A long-term prevention study with oxprenolol in coronary heart disease. *N. Engl. J. Med.* 307:1293, 1982.

22. Frishman, W. H., and Silverman, P. Physiologic and metabolic effects. In W. H. Frishman (ed.), *Clinical Pharmacology of the β-Adrenoceptor Blocking Drugs* (2nd ed.). Norwalk, CN: Appleton-Century-Crofts, 1984.

23. Furberg, C. D., Byington, R. P., Prineas, R. J., et al. Potassium, beta-2 receptor blockade and mortality: The BHAT experience (Abstract). *Circulation* 70(Suppl II):7, 1984.

24. Balcon, R., Jewitt, D. E., Davies, J. P. H., et al. A controlled trial of propranolol in acute myocardial infarction. *Lancet* 2:917, 1966.

25. Clausen, J., Felsby, M., Jorgensen, F. S., et al. Absence of prophylactic effect of propranolol in myocardial infarction. *Lancet* 2:920, 1966.

26. Multicenter Trial: Propranolol in acute myocardial infarction. *Lancet* 2:1435, 1966.

27. Norris, R. M., Caughey, D. E., and Scott, P. J. Trial of propranolol in acute myocardial infarction. *Br. Med. J.* 2:398, 1968.

28. Briant, R. B., and Norris, R. M. Alprenolol in acute myocardial infarction: Double-blind trial. *N.Z. Med. J.* 71:135, 1970.

29. Barber, J. M., Boyle, D. M., Chaturvedi, N. C., et al. Practolol in acute myocardial infarction. *Acta Med. Scand.* [Suppl] 587:213, 1976.

30. Wilcox, R. G., Roland, J. M., Banks, D. C., et al. Randomised trial comparing propranolol with atenolol in immediate treatment of suspected myocardial infarction. *Br. Med. J.* 280:885, 1980.

31. Wilcox, R. G., Rowley, J. M., Hampton, J. R., et al. Randomised placebo-controlled trial comparing oxprenolol with disopyramide phosphate in immediate treatment of suspected myocardial infarction. *Lancet* 2:765, 1980.

32. Andersen, M. P., Bechsgaard, P., et al. Effect of alprenolol on mortality among patients with definite or suspected acute myocardial infarction, preliminary results. *Lancet* 2:865, 1979.

33. Hjalmarson, A., Herlitz, J., Holmberg, S., et al. The Goteborg Metoprolol Trial: Effects on mortality and morbidity in acute myocardial infarction. *Circulation* 67(Suppl I):26, 1983.

34. Yusuf, S., Sleight, P., Rossi, P., et al. Reduction in infarct size, arrhythmias and chest pain by early intravenous beta-blockade in suspected acute myocardial infarction. *Circulation* 67(Suppl I):32, 1983.

35. UK Collaborative Study Group: Mortality results from timolol trials in various British hospitals. Personal communication from W. D. Cooper, MSD Coordinator, and E. J. Flint to the authors of reference 9, 1984.

36. The International Collaborative Study Group: Reduction of infarct size with the early use of timolol in acute myocardial infarction. *N. Engl. J. Med.* 310:9, 1984.

37. Federman, J., Pitt, A., Harris, P., et al. Mortality results from Australian Timolol Trial. Personal communication to authors of reference 9, 1984.

38. Heber, M. E., Rosenthal, E., Thomas, N. B., et al. Effect of labetalol on indices of myocardial necrosis in patients with suspected acute infarction. Unpublished manuscript, results presented in reference 9, 1984.

39. Norris, R. M., Barnaby, P. F., Brown, M. A., et al. Prevention of ventricular fibrillation during acute myocardial infarction by intravenous propranolol. *Lancet* 2:883, 1984.

40. Roberts, R., Croft, C., Gold, H. K., et al. Effect of propranolol on myocardial infarct size in a randomized blinded multicenter trial. *N. Engl. J. Med.* 311:218, 1984.

41. Owensby, D. A., and O'Rourke, M. F. Failure of pindolol to alter determinants of myocardial oxygen requirements, enzyme release or clinical course in acute myocardial infarction (ab-

stract). *Circulation* 70(Suppl II):156, 1984.

42. The MIAMI Trial Research Group: Metoprolol in Acute Myocardial Infarction (MIAMI): A randomised placebo-controlled international trial. *Eur. Heart J.* 6:199, 1985.

43. Salathia, K. S., Barber, J. M., McIlmoyle, E. L., et al. Very early intervention with metoprolol in suspected acute myocardial infarction. *Eur. Heart J.* 6:190, 1985.

44. Roque, F., for the TIARA Group Investigators. Limitation of infarct size and reduction of late ventricular arrhythmias with early administered timolol in acute myocardial infarction: A one-month follow-up study (Abstract). *J. Am. Coll. Cardiol.* 7:67A, 1986.

45. Waagstein, F., and Hjalmarson, A. C. Double-blind study of the effect of cardioselective beta-blockade on chest pain in acute myocardial infarction. *Acta Med. Scand.* [Suppl] 587:201, 1975.

46. Evemy, K. L., and Pentecost, B. L. Intravenous and oral practolol in the acute stages of myocardial infarction. *Eur. J. Cardiol.* 7:391, 1978.

47. Peter, T., Norris, R. M., Clarke, E. D., et al. Reduction of enzyme levels by propranolol after acute myocardial infarction. *Circulation* 57:1091, 1978.

48. Norris, R. M., Clarke, E. D., Sammel, N. J., et al. Protective effect of propranolol in threatened myocardial infarction. *Lancet* 2:907, 1978.

49. Norris, R. M., Sammel, N. L., Clarke, E. D., et al. Treatment of acute myocardial infarction with propranolol: Further studies on enzyme appearance and subsequent left ventricular function in treated and control patients with developing infarcts. *Br. Heart J.* 43:617, 1980.

50. Mueller, H. S., and Ayres, S. M. Propranolol decreases sympathetic nervous activity reflected by plasma catecholamines during evolution of myocardial infarction in man. *J. Clin. Invest.* 65:338, 1980.

51. Azancot, I., Lorente, P., Georgiopoulis, G., et al. Effects of acebutolol on myocardial infarct extension: A randomized electrocardiographic, enzymatic, and angiographic study. *Circulation* 66:986, 1982.

52. Wilhelmsson, C., Vedin, J. A., Wilhelmsen, L., et al. Reduction of sudden deaths after myocardial infarction by treatment with alprenolol. *Lancet* 2:1157, 1974.

53. Ahlmark, G., Saetre, H., and Korsgren, M. Reduction of sudden deaths after myocardial infarction. *Lancet* 2:1563, 1974.

54. Multicentre International Study: Supplementary report: Reduction in mortality after myocardial infarction with long-term beta-adrenoreceptor blockade. *Br. Med. J.* 2:419, 1977.

55. Rehnqvist, N., Ahnve, S., Erhardt, L., et al. Effect of metoprolol after acute myocardial infarction (Abstract). *Proc. Eur. Cong. Cardiol.* 16:16, 1980.

56. Hansteen, V., Moinichen, E., Lorentsen, E., et al. One year's treatment with propranolol after myocardial infarction: Preliminary report of Norwegian Multicentre Trial. *Br. Med. J.* 284:155, 1982.

57. Beta-Blocker Heart Attack Trial Research Group: A randomized trial of propranolol in patients with acute myocardial infarction. I. Mortality results. *J.A.M.A.* 247:1707, 1982.

58. Australian and Swedish Pindolol Study Group: The effect of pindolol on the two years mortality after complicated myocardial infarction. *Eur. Heart J.* 4:367, 1983.

59. Manger Cats, V., van Capelle, F. J. L., Lie, K. I., et al. Effect of treatment with $2 \times$ 100 mg metoprolol on mortality in a single-center study with low placebo—mortality rate after infarction (Abstract). *Circulation* 68(Suppl III):181, 1983. Also personal communication to authors of reference 9.

60. European Infarction Study Group: A secondary prevention study with slow-release oxprenolol after myocardial infarction: Morbidity and mortality. *Eur. Heart J.* 5:189, 1984.

61. Olsson, G., Rehnqvist, N., et al. Long-term treatment with metoprolol after myocardial infarction: Report on 3 year mortality and morbidity. *J. Am. Coll. Cardiol.* 5:1428, 1985.

62. Schwartz, P. J., Motolese, M., Pollavini, G., et al. Surgical and pharmacological antiadrenergic interventions in the prevention of sudden death after a first myocardial infarction (Abstract). *Circulation* 72(Suppl III):358, 1985.

63. The Lopressor Intervention Research Group. The Lopressor Intervention Trial: Multicentre study of metoprolol in survivors of acute myocardial infarction. *Eur. Heart J.* 8:1056, 1987.

64. Beta-Blocker Heart Attack Trial Research Group: A randomized trial of propranolol in patients with acute myocardial infarction. II. Morbidity results. *J.A.M.A.* 250:2814, 1983.

65. Peters, R. W., Byington, R., Arensberg, D., et al. Mortality in the Beta-Blocker Heart Attack Trial: The circumstances surrounding death. *J. Chronic Dis.* 40:75, 1987.

66. Morganroth, J., Lichstein, E., Byington, R., et al. Beta-Blocker Heart Attack Trial: Impact of propranolol therapy on ventricular arrhythmias. *Prev. Med.* 14:346, 1985.

67. Friedman, L. M., Byington, R. P., Capone, R. J., et al. Effect of propranolol in patients with myocardial infarction and ventricular arrhythmia. *J. Am. Coll. Cardiol.* 7:1, 1986.

68. Furberg, C. D., Hawkins, C. M., Lichstein, E., et al. Effect of propranolol in post-infarction patients with mechanical or electrical complications. *Circulation* 69:761, 1984.

69. Beta-Blocker   Pooling   Project   Research

Group: The Beta-Blocker Pooling Project (BBPP): Subgroup findings from randomized trials in post-infarction patients. *Eur. Heart J.* 9:8, 1988.

70. Hawkins, C. M., Richardson, D. W., Vokonas, P. S., et al. Effect of propranolol in reducing mortality in older myocardial infarction patients. *Circulation* 67(Suppl I):94, 1983.

71. Chadda, K., Goldstein, S., Byington, R., and Curb, J. D. Effect of propranolol after myocardial infarction in patients with congestive heart failure. *Circulation* 73:503, 1986.

72. Frishman, W. H. Beta-adrenergic receptor blockers: Adverse effects and drug interactions. *Hypertension* (Suppl II):21, 1988.

73. Kostis, J. B., and Rosen, R. C. Central nervous system effects of β-adrenergic-blocking drugs: The role of ancillary properties. *Circulation* 75:204, 1987.

74. Goldman, L., Benjamin Sia, S. T., Cook, E. F., et al. Costs and effectiveness of routine therapy with long-term beta-adrenergic antagonists after acute myocardial infarction. *N. Engl. J. Med.* 319:152, 1988.

29
Anticoagulant and Platelet Inhibitor Agents for Myocardial Infarction

Valentin Fuster, Marc Cohen, Bernardo Stein, Douglas H. Israel, and James H. Chesebro

The goals of antithrombotic therapy during and after acute myocardial infarction include (1) prevention of deep venous thrombosis and pulmonary embolism, (2) prevention of arterial embolism, (3) reduction of early recurrence or extension of myocardial infarction, (4) reduction of early reocclusion after successful reperfusion with thrombolytic therapy, and (5) secondary prevention of myocardial infarction and cardiovascular mortality.

Prevention of Deep Vein Thrombosis and Pulmonary Embolism

Clinically obvious pulmonary emboli occurred in 5 percent of nonanticoagulated patients (0.6 percent fatal) in the Veterans Administration Cooperative Clinical Trial of anticoagulants for acute myocardial infarction [1]. Similarly, clinical evidence of pulmonary emboli was present in 4 percent of nonanticoagulated patients in a trial of intravenous streptokinase for acute myocardial infarction [2]. These studies were done, however, prior to the current practice of early mobilization after myocardial infarction. Because most pulmonary emboli originate in the veins of the legs, rather than the pelvis [3], and can be prevented with low dose heparin, it is important to review the relation between deep venous thrombosis and pulmonary embolism in acute myocardial infarction and the effect of anticoagulants.

The best noninvasive test for determining the incidence of early, asymptomatic deep vein thrombosis in the popliteal and more dis-

tal veins of the legs is ^{125}I-labeled fibrinogen scanning, as fibrinogen is incorporated into actively growing thrombi [4]. This noninvasive method correlates well with the presence or absence of new venous thrombi by venography [4–6] and thus has been used to relate the presence and incidence of deep venous thrombosis to the risk of pulmonary embolism. The following conclusions were reached after extensive studies by Kakkar and colleagues [4, 7]: (1) Most thrombi in veins of the calf (75 to 80 percent) remain confined to the calf but do extend proximally into veins of the popliteal, femoral, or iliac system in 20 percent of cases. (2) Thrombus extension occurs more than 3 days after initial formation in the calf. (3) Fifty percent of thrombi that extend above the calf embolize to the lungs. (4) Iliofemoral thrombi result almost exclusively from calf vein extension. Thus pulmonary embolism occurs in approximately 10 percent of patients who develop deep venous thrombosis in the calf (unless the patient's condition changes, e.g., early mobilization or institution of anticoagulant therapy), and approximately one-third of them are fatal [7].

The incidence of deep venous thrombosis in the lower extremities of patients with acute myocardial infarction ranges from 17 to 38 percent [8–17] (Table 29-1), which is similar to the incidence in patients after surgery [18]. These observations, coupled with the increased risk of recurrent myocardial infarction within 3 months of an initial infarction in patients undergoing noncardiac surgery [19], suggest the presence of a hypercoagulable state early after acute myocardial infarction similar to that after major surgery [20]. Deep venous thrombi form early after myocardial infarction (one-half or more within 3 days) [9, 10, 13], and the incidence is greater following a large or recurrent infarction with heart failure or cardiogenic shock [10, 14, 21], prolonged immobilization [21], and certain patient characteristics, especially age of more than 70 years [14, 22] (Table 29-1).

Clinical trials have shown that a reduction in the rate of venous thrombosis by anticoagulation also results in a decreased incidence of pulmonary embolism. Acute intravenous heparinization followed by oral anticoagulation

reduced the incidence of venous thrombi to 6 percent or less [9, 11, 13]. It also decreased the incidence of pulmonary embolism from 5 percent to less than 2 percent in clinical studies [1, 23] and from 6 to 32 percent to 0 to 5 percent at autopsy [1, 23, 24].

Low dose heparin (5000 U subcutaneously every 8 or 12 hours) was first introduced in 1962 for the prevention of perioperative venous thromboembolism [25]. Its effectiveness depends on minor alterations in the first steps of the coagulation cascade, which profoundly affect reaction rates of subsequent steps due to the biologic amplification of the system. The main effect of low dose heparin is to increase the rate at which antithrombin III combines with and inactivates activated factor X [25]. It does not increase the risk of bleeding because there is no effect on the clotting time and only a minimal effect on the activated partial thromboplastin time (APTT) [15, 26]. Thus laboratory monitoring is not required. Low dose heparin is effective for prevention of thrombus formation but cannot eliminate the already established thrombotic process [26]. Clinical trials with low dose heparin have shown a reduction in pulmonary embolism and no increased bleeding risk in patients undergoing major surgery [18, 27]. Similarly, low dose heparin started within 12 to 18 hours of the onset of symptoms of acute myocardial infarction and continued for 10 days has successfully reduced the incidence of venous thrombosis in three randomized trials from a mean of 23 percent to 4 percent [15–17] (Table 29-2). This significant benefit is particularly apparent in high risk subgroups. One small trial of low dose heparin following myocardial

Table 29-1
Incidence of deep venous thrombosis in patients admitted for acute myocardial infarction

Conclusion	Proportion with DVT (%)
Chest pain, no myocardial infarction [4, 8, 9]	7–10
Myocardial infarction [8–17]	17–38
Within 72 hours [9, 10, 13]	50–60
Within 5–7 days [9, 10, 13]	75
Mobilization within 1–3 days [21]	
No heart failure	9
With heart failure	22
Restricted to bed rest for 5 days [21]	
No heart failure	63
With heart failure	80
Age < 50 [14, 22]	13
Age > 70 [14, 22]	70

DVT = deep venous thrombosis.

Table 29-2
Low dose heparin for prevention of deep vein thrombosis with acute myocardial infarction

Study	Dose frequency	No. of patients	DVT (%)	
			Control	Heparin
Gallus et al. [15]	q8h	78	23	3
Warlow et al. [16]	q12h	127	17	3
Emerson et al. [17]	q12h	78	34	5
Handley et al. [11]	q12h	50	29	23

DVT = deep venous thrombosis (assessed by fibrinogen 125 scan).

infarction showed no benefit, but the time of initiation of therapy in relation to the onset of symptoms was unclear [11].

CURRENT RECOMMENDATIONS

After acute myocardial infarction early mobilization within 1 to 3 days is important in the prevention of deep venous thrombosis and pulmonary embolism. Immediate subcutaneous heparin (5000 U every 8 to 12 hours) should be given to high risk patients defined as having one or more of the following characteristics: age over 70 years, large acute myocardial infarction, previous myocardial infarction, heart failure or shock, necessity for prolonged immobilization for more than 3 days, prior deep venous thrombosis or pulmonary emboli, obesity, or varicose veins. Some of these patients are good candidates for high dose anticoagulation aimed at preventing systemic embolization from left ventricular thrombus (see below).

Prevention of Arterial Embolism

The primary cause of arterial embolism during acute myocardial infarction is left ventricular mural thrombus [27–32] (Table 29-3). The common predisposing factors of mural thrombus formation include [27–32] the following: (1) location: more than 90 percent of mural

thrombi follow acute transmural anterior myocardial infarction that involves the *apex* with aneurysm formation; (2) infarct size: usually *large* often resulting in peak creatine kinase elevations of more than 1000 IU/L; (3) presence of regional akinesis or dyskinesis, where circulatory stasis and endocardial inflammatory changes occur [33]; and (4) presence of a hypercoagulable state, which perhaps is present in the early days after acute infarction.

Two-dimensional echocardiography is the most accurate method for detecting left ventricular mural thrombus, with a sensitivity of 77 to 92 percent and a specificity of 85 to 94 percent [34–38]. Left ventricular cineangiography may also be used; however, this invasive technique has only 31 percent sensitivity and 75 percent specificity [39–42]. Thrombi, which actively incorporate platelets, may be imaged using indium-111-labeled platelets [37]. Two to four days must elapse to allow sufficient platelets to accumulate on the thrombus for imaging. Despite this limitation, it provides unique information, and false-positive results are unusual; it remains to be seen if actively growing thrombi have an increased tendency to embolize.

Most left ventricular mural thrombi develop within the first 5 to 7 days after acute infarction; 50 to 75 percent may develop within the first 48 hours. In patients anticoagulated for 1 to 3 months, most thrombi resolve, organize, or become undetectable by two-dimensional echocardiography [27, 28, 42]. Furthermore,

Table 29-3
Left ventricular thrombi by two-dimensional echocardiography after acute myocardial infarction: incidence of embolism and effect of anticoagulation

Study	Year	Number of patients with emboli (LV thrombi)	
		Not anticoagulated	Anticoagulated
Asinger et al. [27]	1981	0/2	0/7
Keating et al. [28]	1983	6/7	0/10
Kohari et al. [29]	1984	1/8	1/11
Weinreich et al. [30]	1984	7/18	0/25
Spirito et al. [31]	1985	1/24	—
Funke-Kupper et al. [32]	1985	1/8	0/9
Total		16/67 (24%)	1/62 (2%)

LV = left ventricular.

spontaneous resolution may occur in 20% of untreated patients, particularly when apical dyskinesis resolves, and in the absence of a dilated and diffusely dysfunctional left ventricle [27, 28, 31, 32, 43]. Patients with left ventricular mural thrombus detected during hospitalization for acute myocardial infarction appear to be at particular risk for postinfarction arterial embolism (Table 29-3) [27–32, 34, 43]. Furthermore, echocardiographically diagnosed thrombus protrusion and mobility has been identified as the greatest risk factor for embolism [44–46]. The role of echocardiography in decision-making regarding anticoagulation is discussed below.

The overall incidence of mural thrombus with acute myocardial infarction is about 20%; with anterior myocardial infarction the incidence increases to 40 percent and is as high as 60 percent with large anterior infarctions. Because the incidence of systemic emboli is about 10 percent to that of mural thrombosis, the embolic rates are approximately 2, 4, and 6 percent in each of the three mentioned groups [42] (Table 29-4). The incidence of left ventricular mural thrombus at postmortem examination after acute myocardial infarction was 42 to 58 percent in those not treated with anticoagulants but much lower (22 to 24 percent) in treated patients [1, 2, 24] (Table 29-5). High dose subcutaneous heparin (12,500 U q12h) has been found to be significantly more beneficial than low dose heparin (5000 U q12h) for the prevention of mural thrombus over a 10-day period [47]. With regard to systemic emboli, patients treated with anticoagulant therapy had a reduction in cerebral embolism from 2.3 to 4.0 percent to 0.7 to 1.7 percent compared to controls (Table 29-6) [1, 23, 48, 49]. Such reduction in the incidence of emboli has also been observed in other arterial regions [1, 22, 36–42]. Most systemic emboli occur within the first 3 months after acute myocardial infarction [27–32, 34, 40]. A retrospective study suggests that failure to anticoagulate patients with large anterior infarctions during the first 4 to 6 weeks predisposes them to embolism only within the first 2 months after infarction [40]. These observations are consistent with the low incidence of systemic

Table 29-4
Acute myocardial infarction: mural thrombus and arterial embolism

Condition	Infarct location (%)		
	All	Anterior	Large anterior
Mural thrombus	20	40	60
Emboli	2	4	6

emboli (0.35 percent per year) in patients with chronic left ventricular aneurysm who were not treated with oral anticoagulants [50]. There is, however, a moderate long-term risk of systemic embolism (3.5 percent per year) in nonanticoagulated patients with dilated cardiomyopathy, in whom there is diffuse rather than regional ventricular hypokinesis; this risk is reduced by oral anticoagulation [51]. The results of this study may be extrapolated to patients with coronary disease and poorly contractile left ventricle, who may also benefit from chronic anticoagulation [43].

What is the role of echocardiography in the decision to anticoagulate early after myocardial infarction? Anticoagulation has been effective if given on admission to the hospital. Delay until a mural thrombus is demonstrated echocardiographically may miss the time when therapy can be most valuable. In one study, warfarin was administered only after echocardiographic demonstration of thrombus and was ineffective in preventing embolism [52]. In this context, the use of thrombolytic therapy for lysis of persistent intracardiac thrombus cannot be recommended at present, as the risk-benefit ratio of such strategy has not been determined. Although 16 patients with ventricular thrombi received thrombolytic therapy without complicating embolism [53], lytic therapy in patients with thrombosed left-sided prosthetic valves has been associated with systemic embolism [54]. In a small, nonrandomized study [55], early systemic thrombolytic therapy combined with intravenous heparin therapy within 3 hours of acute anterior myocardial infarction was as-

Table 29-5
Left ventricular mural thrombi at postmortem examination after acute myocardial infarction

| | No. of patients with mural thrombus | |
Study	Nonanticoagulated	Anticoagulated
Aber et al. [2]	10/24 (42%)	—
VACS [1]	15/31 (48%)	5/23 (22%)
Hilden et al. [24]	53/92 (58%)	20/84 (24%)

VACS = Veterans Administration Cooperative Study.

Table 29-6
Cerebral emboli in acute myocardial infarction

| | | Incidence of emboli (%) | |
Study	No. of patients	Control	Anticoagulated
Wright et al. [48]	800	4.0	0.7
BMRC [23]	1,427	2.5	1.1
VACS [1]	999	3.8	0.8
BMH [49]	1457	2.3	1.7

BMRC = British Medical Research Council; VACS = Veterans Administration Cooperative Study; BMH = Bronx Municipal Hospital.

sociated with a low incidence of mural thrombosis compared to an untreated, concurrent, control group.

CURRENT RECOMMENDATIONS

Without waiting for echocardiography, patients with a large anterior transmural myocardial infarction (peak creatine kinase level > 1000 IU/L) or a large transmural infarction in any other location that involves the apex of the heart should receive immediate intravenous heparin (5000 U bolus followed by a continuous infusion of 1000 U/hr, adjusted to prolong the APTT to 1.5 to 2.0 times control) or high dose subcutaneous heparin (12,500 U q12h). Warfarin should subsequently be administered at a dose sufficient to prolong the prothrombin time to 1.5 to 2.0 times control (Standard International Normalized Ratio [INR] = 3.0 to 4.5). It has been suggested that a prothrombin time of 1.3 to 1.5 times control (INR 2.0–3.0) is adequate [56]. In accordance with major prospective studies, the preventive benefit of anticoagulants can be accomplished

at a low risk of minor bleeding and almost absent risk of major hemorrhage [57]. Warfarin can be discontinued after approximately 3 months unless there is evidence of heart failure or a diffusely dilated and poorly contractile left ventricle.

Reduction of Early Recurrence (Extension) of Myocardial Infarction

The quantitative measurement of creatine kinase MB isoenzyme (CK-MB) is the most sensitive and specific method for diagnosing extension or recurrence of myocardial infarction, which occurs in 14 to 30 percent of patients, an incidence comparable to that found at necropsy (17%) [58–66]. The incidence of reinfarction during the hospitalization is much higher in patients with non-Q-wave myocardial infarction (approximately 40%) than in those with Q-wave infarction (approximately 10 percent) [62]; moreover, it is higher in patients with small infarctions than large ones [58]. More than one-half of early recurrences occur within 10 days and the remainder within

14 to 18 days after the initial infarction [62]. Chest pain and ST–T changes in the electrocardiogram are sensitive indicators of recurrence (90 and 80 percent, respectively) but are nonspecific (46 and 36 percent, respectively). Early recurrence can be associated with ST segment elevation in 70% of patients. However, only 20 percent of patients with recurrence after an initial non-Q-wave infarction developed new Q waves [58]. In other studies, one-third to more than one-half of patients with infarct extension or recurrence were not detected clinically [59, 61, 63–65]. In most studies, the electrocardiographic site of early recurrent infarction was the same as the initial site in more than 85 percent of patients. Thus early recurrence and extension of infarction are nearly synonymous.

The clinical impact of early recurrence of myocardial infarction is great because it results in significant reduction in left ventricular function [58] and survival [58, 59, 61–65]. Clinical risk factors associated with reinfarction in patients with non-Q-wave infarction are female sex, obesity (weight over 25 percent of ideal body weight), and recurrent chest pain (at least three episodes during hospitalization) preceding infarct extension, with associated ST–T changes [58, 62, 64]. The reason for instability in patients with non-Q-wave infarction may be partly related to the high incidence of subtotal occlusion of the infarct-related artery, leaving an area of myocardium at ischemic jeopardy [67]. Indeed, the earlier rise in peak creatine kinase and the better preservation of left ventricular function in non-Q-wave infarction compared to Q-wave infarction support the hypothesis that coronary occlusion followed by early reperfusion plays an important pathogenetic role in the former [68]. In addition, high grade residual lesions predispose to reocclusion after successful reperfusion with thrombolytic agents following acute myocardial infarction [69]. The reason for reocclusion may be related to the association of high grade complex lesions with ruptured plaque and thrombus, both serving as a thrombogenic surface [70–73], and the apparent hypercoagulable state that may follow acute infarction [19, 74, 75]. Vasoconstriction may

play an additional role in reocclusion, which may explain the reduction in early reinfarction (from 9.0 percent to 5.2 percent) in patients with non-Q-wave infarctions treated with diltiazem [76]).

The role of platelet inhibitor therapy in patients with acute myocardial infarction was addressed by the second International Study of Infarct Survival (ISIS-2) [77]. In this study, more than 17,000 patients with suspected myocardial infarction were randomized to intravenous streptokinase (1.5 million U), oral aspirin (160 mg daily), both, or neither, within 24 hours of the onset of symptoms. In this remarkably large trial, aspirin alone reduced vascular mortality by 23 percent compared to placebo, as assessed at 5 weeks ($2p < .0001$). The beneficial effect of aspirin was probably related to a reduction in early reinfarction rate once spontaneous or streptokinase-induced vessel recanalization had occurred. Indeed, aspirin reduced the rates of nonfatal reinfarction and stroke by approximately 50 percent. This benefit was maintained after a median 15 months of follow-up [77]. The effects of the combination of aspirin and streptokinase are addressed in the next section.

Can the early recurrence and extension of infarction be prevented by short-term anticoagulant therapy? This question has been reviewed in detail by Harlan and Harker [78]. During the late 1940s and the 1950s, a number of trials were done to evaluate the effect of short-term anticoagulation on mortality and reinfarction in patients with acute myocardial infarction. Many of these studies were not randomized and used historical, alternate, or simultaneously collected controls. Methodologic difficulties of these trials precluded any definite conclusions.

During the 1970s and 1980s there have been several randomized, controlled studies of short-term anticoagulation following acute infarction [79]. Only three of them were of sufficient size to detect a significant effect of therapy: British Medical Research Council (BMRC) [23], Bronx Municipal Hospital [49], and Veterans Administration Hospital (VAH) [1] studies. Mortality and reinfarction rates were not significantly different from controls

Table 29-7
Short-term anticoagulation in acute myocardial infarction

Study	No. of patients	Mortality (%)		Reinfarction (%)	
		Control	Treated	Control	Treated
BMRC [23]	1427	18	16	13	9.7
BMH [49]	1136				
Men	745	16	15	10.3	11.0
Women	391	31	15	18.6	13.4
VACS [1]	999	11	10	6.0	4.0

BMRC = British Medical Research Council; VACS = Veterans Administration Cooperative Study; BMH = Bronx Municipal Hospital.

except for women in the BMH study (Table 29-7). Thus it appeared that high-dose anticoagulation did not significantly reduce in-hospital mortality or reinfarction.

The failure of anticoagulation to reduce mortality is not surprising, as most of the early deaths following myocardial infarction are due to dysrhythmias and pump failure. These events are usually consequences of the initial infarct, rather than of subsequent, recurrent thrombotic events, and would not be affected by anticoagulant therapy [80]. The failure of anticoagulants to reduce early reinfarction, a true thrombotic event, was disappointing. These observations led to the general feeling that short-term, in-hospital anticoagulation after myocardial infarction was not worthwhile.

Three studies during the 1970s attempted to generate new enthusiasm for the short-term use of anticoagulants. In these retrospective epidemiologic studies from Israel and Maryland, it was reported that hospitalized patients treated with anticoagulants had a two- to three-fold lower mortality than those who were untreated [81–83]. A significant criticism of these retrospective studies is related to patient selection bias. In another similar retrospective study, the differences between treatment groups disappeared when groups were controlled for the severity of myocardial infarction [84]. Although admitting that prospective randomization is a more valid study procedure, the authors of these retrospective studies concluded that their data were strong enough to justify a reevaluation of short-term anticoagulation in patients with myocardial in-

farction. Chalmers and coworkers [79] reanalyzed the randomized, controlled trials of anticoagulants for acute infarction and found that, when case fatality ratios were pooled, anticoagulants reduced mortality by a significant 21 percent. They urged that all patients without specific contraindications be given anticoagulants during hospitalization for myocardial infarction. However, the problem of combining data from studies of variable design that span a 10- to 15-year period is obvious. The scientific limitations of pooling data and the fact that percentages rather than exact numbers were pooled have prompted this approach to be described as "pooling, drowning, and floating" [85]. Nevertheless, in our view this pooled approach is helpful for detecting beneficial trends, which, if not convincing, may at least serve as guidelines for future prospective and better designed trials.

CURRENT RECOMMENDATIONS

Based on the data from the ISIS-2 trial [77], patients with acute myocardial infarction should receive aspirin at a dose of 325 mg daily, regardless of whether thrombolytic therapy is planned. There are no convincing data to indicate that short-term anticoagulation following myocardial infarction prevents early recurrence or extension of the infarction or mortality. Nevertheless, because anticoagulation appears to have some beneficial trend, future trials aimed at evaluating the effects of short-term antithrombotic regimens, e.g., anticoagulants plus platelet inhibitors, should be considered.

Reduction in Early Reocclusion After Successful Reperfusion with Thrombolytic Therapy

Following thrombolysis, residual thrombus contributes to residual stenosis visualized at angiography [86]. Based on observations in the porcine model, the high shear rate at the area of stenosis promotes platelet deposition, which is also enhanced by the highly active thrombogenic surface of the residual thrombus [87]. Both these mechanisms may contribute to the relatively high incidence of post-thrombolysis reocclusion seen clinically. Indeed, we postulate that the increase in platelet activation seen after thrombolysis [88] is related to the effects of residual high grade stenosis and thrombogenicity of the residual thrombus, rather than to a direct action of various thrombolytic agents on platelets. Reocclusion following thrombolysis averages 5 to 20 percent during hospitalization, is not significantly different with any particular thrombolytic agent, and appears to be associated with the angiographic severity of the residual lesion in the infarct-related artery (Table 29-8) [69, 89–93]. In the Thrombolysis in Myocardial Infarction (TIMI-I) trial, the incidence of reocclusion after thrombolysis was significantly related to the minimal luminal diameter of the infarct-related artery 90 minutes after lytic therapy [90, 94]. That is, the reocclusion rate

was 28 percent when the minimal stenosis diameter was less than 0.6 mm, but much lower, 3 percent, when the minimal diameter was more than 0.6 mm. Although percutaneous transluminal coronary angioplasty (PTCA) can be accomplished successfully in more than 90 percent of residual lesions with suitable anatomy, immediate catheterization and angioplasty was associated with a higher risk of clinical events, such as emergency coronary artery bypass surgery, reinfarction, and blood transfusion requirements, and was not associated with improvement in left ventricular function or reduction of reocclusion [95–97]. In addition, a certain proportion of patients with severe stenosis on initial angiogram had a nonsignificant stenosis (< 60 percent) on delayed angiography; thus if patients are stable, delaying coronary intervention can avoid the need for angioplasty in some cases [96].

Improved antithrombotic therapy aimed at preventing new thrombus formation has become an important priority in thrombolytic therapy. Thrombolytic agents dissolve fibrin thrombi but do not prevent their formation. Evidence for ongoing thrombosis during administration of thrombolytic therapy has been suggested by the release of platelet-derived prostanoids [88] as well as biochemical markers of thrombin activation, such as fibrinopeptide A [98, 99]. Reduction of this dynamic process, as evidenced by reduction in these biochemical markers, can be achieved by the administration of aspirin [88] and heparin [98, 99]. The effects of combined aspirin and streptokinase in suspected myocardial infarction were analyzed in the ISIS-2

Table 29-8
Relation of reocclusion rate to residual coronary artery stenosis after successful thrombolysis

	Reocclusion rate					
	Low risk			High risk		
Study	No./total	%	Stenosis	No./total	%	Stenosis
Harrison et al. [69]*	0/12	0	> 0.4 mm^2	7/13	54	≤ 0.34 mm^2
Brown et al. [92]*	0/11	0	> 0.25 mm^2	4/7	57	≤ 0.25 mm^2
Cowley [93]	3/22	14	< 90%	10/14	71	> 90%

*By quantitative angiography.

study, mentioned above. Streptokinase alone reduced the 5-week vascular mortality by 25 percent ($2p < .00001$). The combination of aspirin and streptokinase decreased the death rate by an impressive 42 percent, and the beneficial effects of either agent appeared independent of one another. As previously stated, the salutory effects of aspirin were probably due to prevention of coronary reocclusion after vessel patency was achieved through spontaneous or pharmacologic lysis of the occlusive thrombus.

With respect to the use of anticoagulants after thrombolysis, there is experimental evidence suggesting that heparin enhances streptokinase- and urokinase-induced lysis of thrombus [100]. Furthermore, higher doses of heparin (≥ 3.1 U/kg/min) especially when administered as a bolus just before acute and deep experimental arterial injury, reduced quantitative platelet and fibrin deposition and mural thrombus formation [101, 102]. That is, reduction of thrombin generation may be of critical importance in minimizing not only fibrin formation but also acute platelet deposition, as thrombin is the most potent known stimulus for platelet activation. On the other hand, the TIMI-I investigators observed that reocclusion after thrombolysis occurred despite continuous heparin infusion aimed at an APPT of 1.5 to 2.0 times control [90]. Reocclusion was not concentrated to the first few days, but, rather, occurred throughout the study period. In a Johns Hopkins University study, however, no reocclusion occurred during hospitalization, when therapy with heparin (APPT range 2.0 to 3.0 times control) plus aspirin (325 mg/day) and a calcium blocker was used [103]. Therefore it is possible that adequate doses of heparin suppress new thrombus formation during and after thrombolysis and are necessary for prevention of reocclusion. Furthermore, a retrospective study suggested that intravenous heparin is necessary for at least 3 days to minimize the risk of reocclusion after successful thrombolysis [104]. Aspirin at a dose of 1 mg/kg/day greatly enhanced the antithrombotic effect of heparin in an experimental model of acute arterial injury [105]. Thus low dose aspirin combined with

heparin appears to be beneficial and is not associated with a significant risk of gastrointestinal bleeding.

CURRENT RECOMMENDATIONS

Reduction in the incidence of reocclusion after successful thrombolytic therapy is of paramount importance and deserves the following considerations: (1) Rapid and complete clot lysis with an effective thrombolytic agent decreases the residual luminal stenosis and thrombus, which predispose to platelet aggregation and rethrombosis. (2) New thrombus formation should be prevented by adequate anticoagulation with heparin plus a platelet inhibitor, e.g., aspirin (325 mg daily). Heparin should be given after thrombolysis; an intravenous bolus of 5000 U followed immediately by a continuous infusion of 1000 U/h to prolong the APTT to 2.0 to 3.0 times control for 3 to 5 days is recommended. This therapy may be followed by subcutaneous heparin at a dose of 12,500 U every 12 hours; this dosage is safe and was found to reduce left ventricular mural thrombosis in patients with anterior myocardial infarction [47]. No randomized trials to determine the optimal dosage of heparin have been conducted. Platelet-inhibitor therapy with 80 mg of aspirin per day (a dosage effective in reducing ^{111}In-labeled platelet deposition after acute arterial injury [76], without associated gastrointestinal toxicity) should be started upon admission and continued daily for 5 days. Aspirin at a dose of 160 to 325 mg daily is recommended upon discharge [77, 106].

Secondary Prevention of Late Recurrence of Myocardial Infarction and Mortality

We have speculated that there is a greater degree of plaque damage in non-Q-wave infarction than in unstable angina, with persistence of thrombotic occlusion but of insufficient duration to produce Q-wave infarction [73].

Table 29-9
Comparison of platelet inhibitor drugs after myocardial infarction in nine prospective, randomized, double-blind placebo-controlled trials

Study[a]	Interval between MI and entry (months)	Duration of follow-up (months)	Drug[b]	Dosage (mg/day)	No. of pts.	Results of therapy
MRC-I [109]	2⅓	12	ASA	300	1239	Trend toward reduced total death
Coronary Drug Project [110]	3	22	ASA	927	1529	Trend toward reduced total and cardiovascular mortality
GARS [111]	1⅓	24	ASA	1500	946	Trend toward lower MI and cardiac death
MRC-II [112]	¼	12	ASA	900	1682	Trend toward reduced total and coronary mortality
AMIS [113]	25	38	ASA	1000	4524	No benefit
PARIS-I [114]	20	41	ASA	972	2026	Trend toward reduced total and coronary mortality
			ASA + Dip	972 + 225		Same as above
ART [115]	1	16	Sulf	800	1558	Reduction in sudden death only
ARIS [108]	⅔	19	Sulf	800	727	Decreased reinfarction only
PARIS-II [107]	2	23	ASA + Dip	972 + 225	3128	Decreased reinfarction; trend toward lower total and coronary death

[a]MRC = Medical Research Council; GARS = German-Austrian Reinfarction Study; AMIS = Aspirin Myocardial Infarction Study; PARIS = Persantine-Aspirin Reinfarction Study; ART = Anturane Reinfarction Trial; ARIS = Anturane Reinfarction Italian Study.
[b]ASA = aspirin; Dip = dipyridamole; Sulf = sulfinpyrazone.

Given the high incidence of subsequent Q-wave infarction and sudden death in these patients [58, 62, 64, 68], not unlike those with unstable angina, long-term antithrombotic therapy is probably indicated. Indeed, treatment with aspirin and dipyridamole produced a 53 percent reduction in coronary events in patients with non-Q-wave myocardial infarction in one study [107]. With respect to secondary prevention of cardiovascular disease, nine large, randomized, placebo-controlled trials of platelet inhibitor drugs following myocardial infarction have been conducted [107–115] (Table 29-9). In seven of them, aspirin (at a dose of 300–1500 mg daily) was used alone or in combination with dipyridamole. Sulfinpyrazone was used in the other two. Although no significant differences among the various platelet inhibitor regimens used were found [116], available data do not support the additional cost and increased frequency of administration of dipyridamole or sulfinpyrazone. The pooled analysis of these trials concluded that platelet inhibitors significantly reduced vascular mortality by 13 percent, nonfatal reinfarction by 31 percent, nonfatal stroke by 42 percent, and all important vascular events by 25 percent [116, 117].

During the 1950s and 1960s many trials were performed to test the hypothesis that long-term anticoagulation prevents reinfarction and death in patients following a myocardial infarction. Because the incidence of these events decreases after the patient is discharged from the hospital, long-term trials require a large number of patients to detect benefit. Unfortunately, most of the early trials had inadequate numbers of patients.

In 1970 an International Anticoagulant Review Group attempted to overcome the problem of inadequate study size by pooling data from nine controlled, long-term anticoagulant trials involving 2205 men and 282 women [118]. This collective review group concluded that mortality was reduced by 20 percent in men given long-term anticoagulants; however, given the problem of trial heterogeneity and inadequate design, these results must be interpreted with caution.

In 1980 the Sixty-Plus Reinfarction Study from The Netherlands revived the value of long-term anticoagulation after myocardial infarction [119]. Ambulatory patients over the age of 60 years were studied; all patients had been receiving anticoagulants following documented myocardial infarction, which occurred a minimum of 6 months earlier. Eligible patients were randomized to continue anticoagulants or to substitute placebo. The median interval from the time of the initial infarction was 6 years. There was a dramatic 55 percent reduction in the incidence of fatal and nonfatal recurrent myocardial infarction in the anticoagulated group as well as a trend toward lower mortality (Table 29-10). The greater benefit of anticoagulant in this trial was probably related

Table 29-10
Sixty-plus reinfarction study

Parameter	Placebo	Anticoagulant	Significance (p)
No. of patients	439	439	
Mean age (years)	67	67	
Time since first infarction (years)	5	6	
Total recurrent infarction	64	29	.0005
Fatal recurrent infarction	28	11	
Total deaths	69	51	.071
Sudden deaths	20	22	
Total cerebrovascular events	21	13	.16
Intracerebral hemorrhage	1	9	
Nonhemorrhagic event	13	2	
Not identified	6	1	

to the better control of anticoagulant dosage therapy and to the fact that in this relatively stable group of patients studied 6 years postinfarction recurrent thrombotic events were important determinants of survival. Despite the impressive results reported in this study, it is unlikely that clinicians will be enthusiastic about routine use of long-term anticoagulation following myocardial infarction.

CURRENT RECOMMENDATIONS

Aspirin appears to have a protective effect for the prevention of coronary and cerebrovascular events in patients after myocardial infarction. Aspirin, at a dose of 325 mg daily, is devoid of significant side effects and therefore is recommended. Furthermore, the long-term benefit of aspirin in patients in the chronic phase after unstable angina [106, 120] supports this recommendation. Chronic anticoagulant therapy may also reduce the rates of reinfarction and death in patients following a myocardial infarction. This therapy is, however, associated with significant cost, patient discomfort, and potential for hemorrhagic sequelae.

Editorial Comments

Careful consideration should be given to the anticoagulant status of every patient admitted with acute myocardial infarction. Patients undergoing thrombolytic therapy require full-dose heparin plus a platelet inhibitor (low dose aspirin) to prevent new thrombus formation. Patients with large anterior infarctions or large transmural infarctions involving the apex should be fully anticoagulated with heparin and then switched to warfarin. A clear trend seems to be emerging whereby anticoagulation is once again an important part of the therapy of acute myocardial infarction. Selected subsets of patients clearly benefit. An improved understanding of the role of thrombus formation in the pathogenesis of acute myocardial infarction has prompted this renewed interest in anticoagulation. G.S.F.

References

1. Veterans Administration Cooperative Investigators. Anticoagulants in acute myocardial infarction: Results of a cooperative clinical trial. *J.A.M.A.* 225:724, 1973.
2. Aber, C. P., Bass, N. M., Berry, C. L., et al. Streptokinase in acute myocardial infarction: A controlled multicenter study in the United Kingdom. *Br. Med. J.* 2:1100, 1976.
3. Wessler, S., Kleiger, R. E., Cornfield, J. et al. Coumarin therapy in acute myocardial infarction. *Arch. Intern. Med.* 134:774, 1974.
4. Kakkar, V. The diagnosis of deep vein thrombosis using the ^{125}I fibrinogen test. *Arch. Surg.* 104:152, 1972.
5. Negus, D., Pinto, D. J., Le Quesne, L. P., et al. ^{125}I-labeled fibrinogen in the diagnosis of deep vein thrombosis and its correlation with phlebography. *Br. J. Surg.* 55:835, 1968.
6. Lambie, J. M., Mahaffy, R. G., Barber, D. C., et al. Diagnostic accuracy in venous thrombosis. *Br. Med. J.* 2:142, 1979.
7. Kakkar, V. V., Howe, C. T., Flanc, C., et al. Natural history of postoperative deep-vein thrombosis. *Lancet* 2:230, 1969.
8. Murray, T. S., Lorimer, A. R., Cox, F. C., et al. Leg-vein thrombosis following myocardial infarction. *Lancet* 2:792, 1970.
9. Nicolaides, A. N., Kakkar, V. V., Renney, J. T. G., et al. Myocardial infarction and deep-vein thrombosis. *Br. Med. J.* 1:432, 1971.
10. Maurer, B. J., Wray, R., and Shillingford, J. P. Frequency of venous thrombosis after myocardial infarction. *Lancet* 2:1385, 1971.
11. Handley, A. J., Emerson, P. A., and Fleming, P. R. Heparin in the prevention of deep vein thrombosis after myocardial infarction. *Br. Med. J.* 2:436, 1972.
12. Handley, A. J. Low-dose heparin after myocardial infarction. *Lancet* 2:623, 1972.
13. Wray, R., Maurer, B., and Shillingford, J. Prophylactic anticoagulant therapy in the prevention of calf-vein thrombosis after myocardial infarction. *N. Engl. J. Med.* 288:815, 1973.
14. Simmons, A. V., Sheppard, M. A., and Cox, A. F. Deep venous thrombosis after myocardial infarction predisposing factors. *Br. Heart J.* 35:623, 1973.
15. Gallus, A. S., Hirsh, J., Tuttle, R. J., et al. Small subcutaneous doses of heparin in prevention of venous thrombosis. *N. Engl. J. Med.* 288:545, 1973.
16. Warlow, C., Beattie, A. G., Terry, G., et al. A double-blind trial of low doses of subcutaneous heparin in the prevention of deep-vein thrombosis after myocardial infarction. *Lancet* 2:934, 1973.
17. Emerson, P. A., and Marks, P. Preventing

thromboembolism after myocardial infarction: Effect of low-dose heparin or smoking. *Br. Med. J.* 1:18, 1977.

18. International Multicenter Trial. Prevention of fatal postoperative pulmonary embolism by low doses of heparin. *Lancet* 2:45, 1975.

19. Tarhan, S., Moffitt, E. A., Taylor, W. F., et al. Myocardial infarction after general anesthesia. *J. Am. Coll. Cardiol.* 220:1451, 1972.

20. Ygge, J. Changes in blood coagulation and fibrinolysis during the postoperative period. *Am. J. Surg.* 119:225, 1970.

21. Miller, R. R., Lies, J. E., Carretta, R. F., et al. Prevention of lower extremity venous thrombosis by early mobilization: Confirmation in patients with acute myocardial infarction by ^{125}I-fibrinogen uptake and venography. *Ann. Intern. Med.* 84:700, 1976.

22. Emerson, P. A. Teather, D., and Handley, A. J. The application of decision theory to the prevention of deep vein thrombosis following myocardial infarction. *Q. J. Med.* 43:389, 1974.

23. Report on the Working Party on Anticoagulant Therapy in Coronary Thrombosis to the Medical Research Council: Assessment of short-term anticoagulant administration after cardiac infarction. *Br. Med. J.* 1:335, 1969.

24. Hilden, T., Iversen, K., Raaschou, F., et al. Anticoagulants in acute myocardial infarction. *Lancet* 2:327, 1961.

25. Sharnoff, J. G., Kass, H. H., and Mistica, B. A. A plan of heparinization of the surgical patient to prevent postoperative thromboembolism. *Surg. Gynecol. Obstet.* 115:75, 1962.

26. Wessler, S. Prevention of venous thromboembolism by low-dose heparin. *Mod. Concepts Cardiovasc. Dis.* 45:105, 1976.

27. Asinger, R. W., Mikell, F. L., Eisperger, J., et al. Incidence of left ventricular thrombosis after acute transmural myocardial infarction serial evaluation by two-dimensional echocardiography. *N. Engl. J. Med.* 305:297, 1981.

28. Keating, E. C., Gross, S. A., Schiamowitz, R. A., et al. Mural thrombi in myocardial infarctions: Prospective evaluation by two-dimensional echocardiography. *N. Engl. J. Med.* 74:989, 1983.

29. Kohari, A. J., Paczkowski, K., Baker, K. M., et al. Ventricular thrombi in acute myocardial infarction incidence, complications and effects of anticoagulation (Abstract). *J. Am. Coll. Cardiol.* 3:601, 1984.

30. Weinrich, D. J., Burke, J. F., and Pauletto, F. J. Left ventricular mural thrombi complicating acute myocardial infarction: Long-term follow-up with serial echocardiography. *Ann. Interm. Med.* 100:789, 1984.

31. Spirito, P., Bellotu, P., Chiarella, F., et al. Prognostic significance and natural history

of left thrombi or patients with acute anterior myocardial infarction, a two-dimensional echocardiographic study. *Circulation* 72:774, 1985.

32. Funke-Kupper, A. J., Freek, W. A., Verbeugt, F. W. A., et al. Long-term treatment with oral anticoagulants in patients with left ventricular thrombosis after myocardial infarction (Abstract). *Circulation* 72(Suppl III):458, 1985.

33. Hoehman, J. S., Plati, E. B., and Bulkley, B. H. Endocardial abnormalities in left ventricular aneurysms: A clinicopathologic study. *Ann. Intern. Med.* 100:29, 1984.

34. DeMaria, A. N., Bommer, W., Neumann, A., et al. Left ventricular thrombi identified by cross-sectional echocardiography. *Ann. Intern. Med.* 90:14, 1979.

35. Reeder, G. S., Tajik, A. J., and Seward, J. B. Left ventricular mural thrombus: Two-dimensional echocardiographic diagnosis. *Mayo Clin. Proc.* 56:82, 1981.

36. Asinger, R. W., Mikell, F. L., Sharma, B., et al. Observations on detecting left ventricular thrombus with two-dimensional echocardiography: Emphasis on avoidance of false positive diagnoses. *Am. J. Cardiol.* 47:145, 1981.

37. Ezekowitz, M. D., Wilson, D. A., Smith, E. O., et al. Comparison of indium-111 platelet scintigraphy and two-dimensional echocardiography in the diagnosis of left ventricular thrombi. *N. Engl. J. Med.* 306:1509, 1982.

38. Visser, C. A., Kan, G., David, G. K., et al. Two-dimensional echocardiography in the diagnosis of left ventricular thrombus: A prospective study of 67 patients with anatomic validation. *Chest* 83:228, 1983.

39. Swan, J. H. C., Magnusson, P. T., Buchbinder, N. A., et al. Aneurysm of the cardiac ventricle: Its management by medical and surgical intervention. *West. J. Med.* 129:26, 1978.

40. Reeder, G. S., Lengyel, M., Tajik, A. J., et al. Mural thrombus in left ventricular aneurysm: Incidence, role of angiography, and relation between anticoagulation and embolization. *Mayo Clin. Proc.* 56:77, 1981.

41. Simpson, M. T., Oberman, A., Kouchoukos, N. I. T., et al. Effect of anticoagulation on the incidence of mural thrombi and systemic embolization in patients with left ventricular aneurysm (Abstract). *Am. J. Cardiol.* 41:398, 1978.

42. Meltzer, R. S., Visser, C. A., and Fuster, V. Intracardiac thrombi and systemic embolization. *Ann. Intern. Med.* 104:689, 1986.

43. Stratton, J. R., and Resnick, A. D. Increase embolic risk in patients with left ventricular thrombi. *Circulation* 75:1004, 1987.

44. Meltzer, R. S., Visser, C. A., Kan, G., et al. Two-dimensional echocardiographic appearance of left ventricular thrombi with systemic

emboli after myocardial infarction. *Am. J. Cardiol.* 53:1511, 1984.

45. Haugland, J. M., Asinger, R. W., Mikell, F. L., et al. Embolic potential of left ventricular thrombi detected by two-dimensional echocardiography. *Circulation* 70:588, 1984.

46. Visser, C. A., Kan, G., Meltzer, R. S., et al. Embolic potential of left ventricular thrombus after myocardial infarction: A two dimensional echocardiographic study of 119 patients. *J. Am. Coll. Cardiol.* 5:1276, 1985.

47. Turpie, A. G. G., Robinson, J., Mulji, S., et al. Prevention of left ventricular mural thrombosis in acute myocardial infarction with low dose subcutaneous calcium heparin (Abstract). *J. Am. Coll. Cardiol.* 11(Suppl A):26A, 1988.

48. Wright, I. S., Marple, C. D., and Beck, D. F. Report of the committee for the evaluation of anticoagulants in the treatment of coronary thrombosis with myocardial infarction. *Am. Heart J.* 36:801, 1948.

49. Drapkin, A., and Merskey, C. Anticoagulation therapy after acute myocardial infarction: Relation of therapeutic benefit to patient's age, sex, and severity of infarction. *J.A.M.A.* 222:541, 1972.

50. Lapeyre III, A. C., Steele, P. M., Kazmier, F. J., et al. Systemic embolism in chronic left ventricular aneurysm: Incidence and the role of anticoagulation. *J. Am. Coll. Cardiol.* 6:534, 1985.

51. Fuster, V., Gersh, B. J., Giuliani, E. R., et al. The natural history of idiopathic dilated cardiomyopathy. *Am. J. Cardiol.* 47:525, 1981.

52. Johannessen, K. A., Nordrehaug, J. E., and von der Lippe G. Left ventricular thrombus and cerebrovascular accident in acute myocardial infarction. *Br. Heart J.* 51:553, 1984.

53. Kremer, P., Fiebig, R., Tilsner, V., et al. Lysis of left ventricular thrombi with urokinase. *Circulation* 72:112, 1985.

54. Ledian, L. D., Ohayan, J. P., Colle, J. P., et al. Acute thrombotic obstruction with disc valve prostheses: Diagnostic considerations and fibrinolytic treatment. *J. Am. Coll. Cardiol.* 7:743, 1986.

55. Eigle, N., Maurer, G., and Shah, P. K. Effect of early systemic thrombolytic therapy on left ventricular mural thrombus formation in acute anterior myocardial infarction. *Am. J. Cardiol.* 54:261, 1984.

56. Hirsch, J., Deykin, D., and Poller, L. "Therapeutic range" for oral anticoagulant therapy. *Chest* 89(Suppl):11S, 1986.

57. Deykin, D. Anticoagulants in acute myocardial infarction. In S. Wessler, C. G. Becker, and Y. Nemerson (eds.), *The New Dimension of Warfarin Prophylaxis.* New York: Plenum, 1987.

58. Marmor, A., Sobel, B. E., and Roberts, R. Factors presaging early recurrent myocardial infarction ("extension"). *Am. J. Cardiol.* 48:603, 1981.

59. Rothkopf, M., Boerner, J., Stone, M. J., et al. Detection of myocardial infarct extension by CKB radioimmunoassay. *Circulation* 59:268, 1979.

60. Fraker Jr., T. D., Wagner, G. S., and Rosati, R. Extension of myocardial infarction incidence and prognosis. *Circulation* 60:1126, 1979.

61. Nasser, F. N., Chesebro, J. H., Homburger, H. A., et al. Myocardial infarct extension diagnosis by CK-MB radioimmunoassay and clinical significance. *Clin. Res.* 29:226, 1981.

62. Marmor, A., Geltman, E. M., Schechuman, K., et al. Recurrent myocardial infarction: Clinical predictors and prognostic implications. *Circulation* 66:415, 1982.

63. Baker, J. T., Bramlet, D. A., Lester, R. M., et al. Myocardial infarct extension: Incidence and relationship to survival. *Circulation* 65:918, 1982.

64. Strauss, H. D. Myocardial infarction extension: Clinical significance. *Primary Cardiol.* 8:14, 1982.

65. Buda, A. J., MacDonald, I. L., Dubbin, J. D., et al. Myocardial infarct extension: Prevalence, clinical significance, and problems in diagnosis. *Am. Heart J.* 105:744, 1983.

66. Hutchins, G. M., and Bulkley, B. H. Infarct expansion versus extension: Two different complications of acute myocardial infarction. *Am. J. Cardiol.* 41:1127, 1978.

67. DeWood, M., Stifter, W. F., Simpson, C. S., et al. Coronary arteriographic findings soon after non-Q wave myocardial infarction. *N. Engl. J. Med.* 315:417, 1986.

68. Gibson, R. S. Clinical, functional, and angiographic distinctions between Q wave and non-Q wave myocardial infarction: Evidence of spontaneous reperfusion and implications for intervention trials. *Circulation* 75(Suppl V):128, 1987.

69. Harrison, D. G., Ferguson, D. W., Collins, S. M., et al. Rethrombosis after reperfusion with streptokinase: Importance of geometry of residual lesions. *Circulation* 69:991, 1984.

70. Falk, E. Plaque rupture with severe pre-existing stenosis precipitating coronary thrombosis: Characteristics of coronary atherosclerotic plaques underlying fatal occlusive thrombi. *Br. Heart J.* 50:127, 1983.

71. Davies, M. J., and Thomas, A. C.: Plaque fissuring—the cause of acute myocardial infarction, sudden ischemic death, and crescendo angina. *Br. Heart J.* 53:363, 1985.

72. Ambrose, J. A., Monsen, C., Borrico, S., et al. Angiographic demonstration of a common

link between unstable angina pectoris and non-Q wave acute myocardial infarction. *Am. J. Cardiol.* 61:244, 1988.

73. Fuster, V., Badimon, L., Cohen, M., et al. Insights into the pathogenesis of acute ischemic syndromes. *Circulation* 77:1213, 1988.

74. Fuster, V., and Chesebro, J. H. Pharmacologic effects of platelet inhibitor drugs. *Mayo Clin. Proc.* 56:185, 1981.

75. Chesebro, J. H., Fuster, V., Pumphrey, C. W., et al. Improvement of shortened platelet survival half-life from the early to the late phase of myocardial infarction. *Circulation* 64(Suppl IV):197, 1981.

76. Gibson, R. S., Boden, W. E., Theroux, P., et al. Diltiazem and reinfarction in patients with non-Q-wave myocardial infarction: Results of a double-blind, randomized, multicentered trial. *N. Engl. J. Med.* 315:423, 1986.

77. ISIS-2 (Second International Study of Infarct Survival) Collaborative Group. Randomised trial of intravenous streptokinase, oral aspirin, both or neither among 17,187 cases of suspected acute myocardial infarction: ISIS-2. *Lancet* 2:349, 1988.

78. Harlan, J. M., and Harker, L. A. Thrombosis and coronary artery disease. In *Current Concepts.* Kalamazoo, MI: Upjohn Company, 1983.

79. Chalmers, T. C., Matta, R. J., Smith Jr., H. et al. Evidence favoring the use of anticoagulants in the hospital phase of acute myocardial infarction. *N. Engl. J. Med.* 297:1091, 1977.

80. Mitchell, J. R. A. Anticoagulants in coronary heart disease—retrospect and prospect. *Lancet* 1:257, 1981.

81. Modan, B., Shani, M., Schor, S., et al. Reduction of hospital mortality from acute myocardial infarction by anticoagulant therapy. *N. Engl. J. Med.* 292:1359, 1975.

82. Tonascia, J., Gordis, L., and Schmerler, H. Retrospective evidence favoring use of anticoagulants for myocardial infarction. *N. Engl. J. Med.* 292:1362, 1975.

83. Szklo, M., Tonascia, J. A., Goldberg, R., et al. Additional data favoring use of anticoagulant therapy in myocardial infarction: A population-based study. *J.A.M.A.* 242:1261, 1979.

84. Ravid, M., Kleiman, N., Shapira, J., et al. Anticoagulant therapy in acute myocardial infarction: Demonstration of a selection bias in a retrospective study. *Thromb. Res.* 18:753, 1980.

85. Goldman, L., and Feinstein, A. R. Anticoagulants and myocardial infarction: The problems of pooling, drowning, and floating. *Ann. Intern. Med.* 90:92, 1979.

86. Brown, B. G., Gallery, C. A., Badger, R. S., et al. Incomplete lysis of thrombus in the moderate underlying atherosclerotic lesion during intracoronary infusion of streptokinase for acute myocardial infarction: Quantitative angiographic observations. *Circulation* 73:653, 1986.

87. Badimon, L., Badimon, J. J., Turitto, V. T., et al. Mechanism of arterial thrombosis: Platelet thrombus deposition in areas of stenosis (Abstract). *Circulation* 76(Suppl IV):102, 1987.

88. Fitzgerald, D. J., Catella, F., Roy, L., et al. Marked platelet activation in vivo after intravenous streptokinase in patients with acute myocardial infarction. *Circulation* 77:142, 1988.

89. Anderson, J. L., Marshall, H. W., Bray, B. E., et al. A randomized trial of intracoronary streptokinase in the treatment of acute myocardial infarction. *N. Engl. J. Med.* 308:1312, 1983.

90. Chesebro, J. H., Knatterud, G., Roberts, R., et al. Thrombolysis in myocardial infarction (TIMI) trial, Phase I: A comparison between intravenous tissue plasminogen activator and intravenous streptokinase. *Circulation* 76:142, 1987.

91. Leiboff, R. H., Katz, R. J., Wasserman, A. G., et al. A randomized angiographically controlled trial of intracoronary streptokinase in acute myocardial infarction. *Am. J. Cardiol.* 53:404, 1984.

92. Brown, B. G., Mathey, D. G., Sheehan, F. H., et al. Personal communication.

93. Cowley, M. J. Personal communication.

94. Chesebro, J. H. Personal communication.

95. TIMI Research Group. Immediate versus delayed catheterization and angioplasty following thrombolytic therapy for acute myocardial infarction: TIMI II A results. *J.A.M.A.* 260:2849, 1988.

96. Topol, E. J., Califf, R. M., George, B. S., et al. A randomized trial of immediate versus delayed elective angioplasty after intravenous tissue plasminogen activator in acute myocardial infarction. *N. Engl. J. Med.* 317:581, 1987.

97. Simoons, M. L., Betriu, A., Col, J., et al. Thrombolysis with tissue plasminogen activator in acute myocardial infarction: No additional benefit from immediate percutaneous coronary angioplasty. *Lancet* 1:197, 1988.

98. Eisenberg, P. R., Sherman, L., Rich, M., et al. Importance of continued activation of thrombin reflected by fibrinopeptide A to the efficacy of thrombolysis. *J. Am. Coll. Cardiol.* 7:1255, 1986.

99. Eisenberg, P. R., Sherman, L. A., and Jaffe, A. S. Paradoxic elevation of fibrinopeptide A after streptokinase: Evidence for continued thrombosis despite intense fibrinolysis. *J. Am. Coll. Cardiol.* 10:527, 1987.

100. Cercek, B., Lew, A. S., Hod, H., et al. En-

hancement of thrombolysis with tissue-type plasminogen activator by pretreatment with heparin. *Circulation* 74:583, 1986.

101. Heras, M., Chesebro, J. H., Penny, W. J., et al. Importance of adequate heparin dosage in arterial angioplasty in a porcine model. *Circulation* 78:654, 1988.

102. Heras, M., Chesebro, J. H., Penny, W. J., et al. Dose dependent inhibitor by heparin of acute platelet-thrombus deposition during angioplasty (Abstract). *J. Am. Coll. Cardiol.* 11(Suppl A):30A, 1988.

103. Guerci, A. D., Gerstenblith, G., Brinker, J. A., et al. A randomized trial of intravenous tissue plasminogen activator for acute myocardial infarction with subsequent randomization to elective coronary angioplasty. *N. Engl. J. Med.* 317:1613, 1987.

104. Chandler, J. W., Nath, H. P., and Rogers, W. J. Heparin and antiplatelet drugs following streptokinase in acute myocardial infarction: What are their effects on vessel patency? *J. Am. Coll. Cardiol.* 3:600, 1984.

105. Lam, J. Y. T., Chesebro, J. H., Steele, P. M., et al. Is vasospasm related to platelet deposition? Relationship in a porcine preparation of arterial injury in vivo. *Circulation* 75:243, 1987.

106. Lewis Jr., H. D., Davis, J. W., Archibald, D. G., et al. Protective effects of aspirin against acute myocardial infarction and death in men with unstable angina: Results of a Veterans Administration Cooperative Study. *N. Engl. J. Med.* 309:396, 1983.

107. Klimt, C. R., Knatterud, G. L., Stamler, J., et al. Part II. Secondary coronary prevention with persantine and aspirin. *J. Am. Coll. Cardiol.* 7:251, 1986.

108. Report from the Anturane Reinfarction Italian Study: Sulfinpyrazone in post-myocardial infarction. *Lancet* 1:237, 1982.

109. Elwood, P. C., Cochrane, A. L., Burr, M. L., et al. A randomized controlled trial of acetyl salicylic acid in the second prevention of mortality from myocardial infarction. *Br. Med. J.* 1:436, 1974.

110. Coronary Drug Project Group: Aspirin in coronary heart disease. *J. Chronic Dis.* 29:625, 1976.

111. Breddin, K., Loew, D., Lechner, K., et al. Secondary prevention of myocardial infarction: Comparison of acetylsalicylic acid, phenprocoumon and placebo: A multicenter two-year prospective study. *Thromb. Haemost.* 40:225, 1979.

112. Elwood, P. C., and Sweetnam, P. M. Aspirin and secondary mortality after myocardial infarction. *Lancet* 2:1313, 1979.

113. Aspirin Myocardial Infarction Study Research Group. A randomized, controlled trial of aspirin in persons recovered from myocardial infarction. *J.A.M.A.* 243:661, 1980.

114. Persantine-Aspirin Reinfarction Study Research Group: Persantine and aspirin in coronary heart disease. *Circulation* 62:449, 1980.

115. Anturane Reinfarction Trial Research Group. Sulfinpyrazone in the prevention of sudden death after myocardial infarction. *N. Engl. J. Med.* 302:250, 1980.

116. Antiplatelet Trialists' Collaboration. Secondary prevention of vascular disease by prolonged antiplatelet treatment. *Br. Med. J.* 296:320, 1988.

117. Canner, P. L. Aspirin in coronary heart disease: Comparison of six clinical trials. *Isr. J. Med. Sci.* 19:413, 1983.

118. International Anticoagulant Review Group: Collaborative analysis of long-term anticoagulant administration after acute myocardial infarction. *Lancet* 1:203, 1970.

119. Report of the Sixty Plus Reinfarction Study Research Group. A double-blind trial to assess long-term oral anticoagulant therapy in elderly patients after myocardial infarction. *Lancet* 2:989, 1980.

120. Cairns, J. A., Gent, M., Singer, J., et al. Aspirin, sulfinpyrazone, or both in unstable angin. *N. Engl. J. Med.* 313:1369, 1985.

30
Possible Adverse Effect of Digitalis Therapy After Myocardial Infarction

J. Thomas Bigger, Jr., Linda M. Rolnitzky, and Joseph L. Fleiss

Digitalis glycosides have been in common use for more than 200 years, primarily to treat the symptoms of congestive heart failure and to reduce the ventricular rate during atrial fibrillation [1, 2]. Digitalis was used for well over 100 years before myocardial infarction was described. The chronicles of success for treatment of congestive heart failure with digitalis were written at a time when rheumatic heart disease was a common etiologic cause of the heart failure syndrome. The effects of digitalis in patients with myocardial infarction and in animals with experimental models of myocardial infarction were not intensively investigated until the 1960s and 1970s [3–9]. Several concerns have been raised about the risk associated with the use of digitalis during the acute phase of myocardial infarction: (1) the increased contractility produced by digitalis increases myocardial oxygen and may thereby increase infarct size; (2) the ischemic myocardium is more susceptible to the arrhythmogenic effects of digitalis; and (3) intravenous digitalis often causes a substantial increase in systemic arterial resistance and left ventricular afterload. The hemodynamic benefit to be gained from digitalis is not certain because the increased myocardial contractility may be dissipated by systolic bulging in the infarcted region and by increased aortic impedance.

Morrison et al. showed that the usual effect of digitalis in acute myocardial infarction is to increase left ventricular ejection fraction slightly without increasing myocardial infarct size [10]. However, the inotropic effect of digitalis is smaller than that of the catecholamine-like drugs such as dobutamine [11]. There is even a question about the efficacy of digitalis

treatment for acute atrial fibrillation. One study showed no difference between intravenous digoxin and placebo for conversion of atrial fibrillation to sinus rhythm during acute myocardial infarction [12]. The risk-benefit ratio of digitalis treatment of chronic congestive heart failure in patients with sinus rhythm is undergoing reexamination. Lee et al. performed a small study that suggested digitalis treatment was beneficial for patients with dilated left ventricles and S_3 gallop rhythm [13]. Conversely, Gheorghiade and Beller [14] and Fleg et al. [15] showed that patients with coronary heart disease and stable congestive heart failure who were in sinus rhythm could have digitalis discontinued without suffering any long-term adverse effects.

With enhanced awareness of adverse effects and the advent of effective alternative treatments, such as short-acting arterial and venous vasodilators and inotropic agents for intravenous use, the use of digitalis in the coronary care unit (CCU) has declined substantially. However, an interesting new mode of digitalis use developed during that period. Patients who showed evidence of significant left ventricular dysfunction during the CCU phase of myocardial infarction, i.e., those with S_3 gallops, pulmonary rales, or pulmonary vascular congestion on chest radiograph, were treated acutely with vasodilators or catecholamine-like inotropic drugs and were digitalized later during the hospitalization. During the early 1980s, about 25 to 30 percent of patients hospitalized for acute myocardial infarction were discharged from hospital on digitalis. Nearly all were digitalized during that admission.

557

Table 30-1
Comparison of seven nonrandomized studies of the effect of digitalis on survival after acute myocardial infarction

Parameter	U. Rochester Heart Attack Follow-up Program [19] 1981	Coronary Artery Surgery Study [20] 1983	U. California (San Diego) Myocardial Infarction Study [22] 1984
Duration of enrollment	1973–1976	1974–1979	1969–1982
Inclusion criteria	Definite or probable AMI	Definite AMI; chest pain syndrome	Definite AMI
Time of enrollment	Within 3 weeks of AMI	Within 2 months of AMI	Within 3 weeks of AMI
No. of patients analyzed	812	892/1592	1300
Duration of follow-up	4 months	55 months (av.)	12 months
Mortality endpoint	All causes	All causes	All causes
Percent on digitalis	19	21	37
Survival at 1 year (%)	—	90	86
Method for choosing confounding variables	Variables significantly associated with digitalis use	Variables significantly associated with digitalis use	Variables significantly associated with digitalis use
Significant independent predictors of survival	Female sex, cigarette smoking, diabetes, previous infarction, NYHA functional class	Age, rales, edema, left ventricular wall motion score, no. of diseased vessels	Age, previous angina, previous infarction, CHF in hospital, maximal heart rate in hospital
Statistical method used	Modified logistic regression	Cox survival analysis	Cox survival analysis
p value	$<.01$ ($\chi^2 = 9.9$, d.f. $= 1$)	$<.10$ ($\chi^2 = 3.1$, d.f. $= 1$)	$<.10$ ($\chi^2 = 2.8$, d.f. $= 1$)

AMI = acute myocardial infarction; BUN = blood urea nitrogen; CCU = coronary care unit; NYHA = New York Heart Association; VPC = ventricular premature complexes; χ^2 = chi square; CHF = congestive heart failure; LVEF = left ventricular ejection fraction; no. = number.

As the pathophysiology of acute myocardial infarction became better understood, the rationale for this practice was questioned. Almost one-half of the patients who have rales or pulmonary vascular congestion by chest radiograph in the CCU have reasonably good left ventricular ejection fractions 5 to 21 days after myocardial infarction [16, 17]. There is no good rationale for the policy of treating all patients who have evidence of left ventricular dysfunction in the CCU with digitalis because, in many, left ventricular dysfunction is transient and due to myocardial ischemia resulting from multivessel coronary heart disease. During the acute phase of myocardial infarction, the noninfarcted portion of the left ventricle often becomes hypercontractile, and, if served by a critically stenotic vessel, may become ischemic. During the period of ischemia, the functional defect in left ventricular performance worsens and usually becomes symptomatic. In such patients, left ventricular dysfunction may improve substantially after a few days, and diagnostic pursuit of ischemic issues is much more important than digitalis treatment [16–18]. Patients who have clinical evidence of left ventricular dysfunction during their CCU stay (i.e., S_3 gallop, rales, or pul-

Presbyterian Hospital Myocardial Infarction Study [23] 1985	β-Blocker Heart Attack Trial [25] 1985	Multicenter Investigation of the Limitation of Infarct Size [26] 1986	Multicenter Post Infarction Program [30] 1987
1974–1980	1978–1980	1978–1983	1979–1980
Definite AMI	Definite AMI	Definite AMI	Definite AMI
Within 3 weeks of AMI	Within 3 weeks of AMI	Within 18 hr of onset of chest pain	Within 3 weeks of AMI (9±5 days)
504	1921/3837	903	728
23 months (av.)	25 months (av.)	25 months (av.)	22 months (av.)
All causes	All causes	All causes	All causes
45	13	31	31
86	95	91	91
Variables significantly associated with and indications for digitalis use	Variables predictive of mortality	Variables significantly associated with digitalis use	Variables significantly associated with digitalis use
Left ventricular failure in CCU, atrial fibrillation in CCU, enlarged heart on chest radiograph, VPC frequency, repetitive VPC	16 Variables	LVEF, diuretics, age, β-blockers, ST elevation, diabetes, complex VPC	LVEF, NYHA class, VPC frequency, BUN, rales, age, leg edema, diabetes, repetitive VPC
Cox survival analysis	Logistic regression	Cox survival analysis	Cox survival analysis
$<.10$ ($Z = 1.84$)	$>.05$ (value of χ^2 not given)	$>.30$ ($\chi^2 = 0.9$, d.f. $= 1$)	$<.001$ ($Z = 3.4$)

monary vascular congestion in the chest radiograph) and continue to have left ventricular dysfunction later in the hospital course have a rationale for digitalis treatment. However, there is no definitive evidence that treating patients who have persistent signs of left ventricular failure with digitalis improves survival or reduces the incidence of symptomatic heart failure during follow-up.

Beyond the weak rationale for long-term digitalis treatment for most patients after myocardial infarction, the question of harm from such treatment has been raised. We discuss here the studies that have addressed this question (Table 30-1). All of these studies were retrospective, and each used multivariate statistical techniques to adjust for the greater severity of illness in the patients who took digitalis. Obviously, this adjustment can involve only the variables collected in the study, and the best variable(s) for adjustment may not be available. This and other statistical issues are discussed later in the chapter. Although all studies evaluated patients after myocardial infarction, it is likely that some of the differences in results can be attributed to differences in the populations served by the hospitals conducting the studies, differences in the eligibility and exclusion criteria, and differences in the statistical adjustment procedures.

Heart Attack Follow-up Program

A study conducted by Moss et al. [19] was the first large retrospective study to suggest a possible harmful effect of digitalis. These authors examined the effect of digitalis on 4-month mortality in a group of 812 patients who were participating in a longitudinal natural history study. Because no experimental treatments were being used, there was no bias due to treatment-related exclusion criteria. However, the patients were recruited from two community hospitals in Rochester, New York, and the overall mortality was low, indicating a low level of illness in the group recruited to the study. The effect of digitalis on 4-month all-cause mortality was examined. A multivariate analysis suggested that there was an adverse effect of digitalis in one subgroup, consisting of patients with congestive heart failure (defined as rales, leg edema, or both) as well as ventricular arrhythmias found in a 6-hour continuous electrocardiographic (ECG) recording done about 3 weeks after myocardial infarction. In patients with congestive heart failure and ventricular arrhythmias, but not on digitalis, the 4-month mortality rate was 1.8 percent (1 of 56); those in the same category but treated with digitalis had a 38.5 percent (10 of 26) mortality rate (Table 30–2).

It may well be that chance as well as systematic errors in the adjustment procedures worked their mischief in this study. The low mortality rate in this study suggests that the sample may well not have faithfully reflected the population from which it was taken. Ventricular arrhythmias and congestive heart failure were worse in the digitalis-treated group. Also, the unorthodox definition of congestive heart failure and the inclusive definition of "complex" ventricular premature complexes may have selected a peculiar sample of the subgroup of interest. Moreover, given the definitions of congestive heart failure and "complex" ventricular arrhythmias that were used, it is possible that patients in the "high risk" subgroup who were treated with digitalis had lower average left ventricular ejection fractions and a greater prevalence of repetitive ventricular premature complexes than comparably classified patients who were not treated with digitalis.

Coronary Artery Surgery Study

The Coronary Artery Surgery Study (CASS) investigators retrospectively examined the data in their registry of 14,547 patients to determine if any detrimental effects of digitalis could be detected during 5 years of follow-up [20]. The primary objective of the CASS registry was to examine the natural history of patients with angiographically proved coronary heart disease. They evaluated the effects of digitalis on outcome in four groups: (1) the entire sample; (2) 974 patients with congestive heart failure; (3) a subgroup of 1183 patients who had a history of cardiac arrest or were taking antiarrhythmic drugs on entry to the study; and (4) a subgroup of 892 patients who had myocardial infarction within 2 months of enrollment. The last group is most germane to the question being addressed. In their report, the CASS investigators said there were 1592 patients who had myocardial infarction 2 months or less before their entry into the study. For reasons not given, only 892 were used in their analysis. The Cox regression model was used to identify variables that had independent value for predicting survival [21]. Also, a single linear discriminant variable, dubbed P-dig, was constructed from the individual variables that made a significant contribution to predicting digitalis use. P-dig was used as an additional adjustment variable in subsequent analyses.

For the subgroup of CASS patients who had a recent myocardial infarction, the significant independent determinants of mortality were age, presence of pretibial edema, left ventricular wall motion score, number of coronary vessels with significant disease, and presence of rales. After adjusting for all of these variables, adding digitalis use to the Cox regression model did not significantly improve the prediction of mortality over 5 years of follow-up. The χ^2 value was 3.1 ($p < .10$), a borderline result.

Because Moss et al. reported that digitalis

Table 30-2

Association between digitalis treatment after myocardial infarction and 4-month mortality in a high risk subgroup (CHF and ventricular arrhythmias): Comparison of seven retrospective studies

Study	Digitalis		No digitalis		χ^2	p
	No.	Mortality rate (%)	No.	Mortality rate (%)		
University of Rochester Heart Attack Follow-up Study [19]	26	38	56	2	17.5	<.001
Coronary Artery Surgery Study [20]	57	9	22	14	0.4	n.s.
University of California (San Diego) Myocardial Infarction Study [22]	54	15	25	12	0.1	n.s.
Presbyterian Hospital Myocardial Infarction Study [23]	51	24	4	50	0.3	n.s.
Beta-Blocker Heart Attack Trial [25]	63	6	79	6	0	n.s.
Multicenter Investigation of the Limitation of Infarct Size [26]	46	17	33	3	2.6	n.s.
Multicenter Post Infarction Program [30]	84	14	100	5	3.7	<.1

n.s. = not significant.

had an especially adverse effect in patients with congestive heart failure and complex ventricular arrhythmias, the CASS investigators attempted to perform a similar analysis. The label congestive heart failure was assigned if patients complained of dyspnea with mild exercise, orthopnea, or paroxysmal nocturnal dyspnea, or if they had S_3 gallop, pulmonary rales, or pedal edema on physical examination. Because data from Holter recordings were not available to classify the patients as to presence or absence of ventricular arrhythmias, the investigators used a history of cardiac arrest or antiarrhythmic drug use on entry into the study to classify the patients with respect to arrhythmias. The 4-month mortality rate for the 79 postinfarction patients who had congestive heart failure and ventricular arrhythmias was not significantly different between the 57 patients who took digitalis (9 percent) and the 22 who did not (14 percent) (Table 30-2).

The CASS investigators discussed why their results were different from those of Moss et al. Their main hypothesis for the difference was that adjustment for angiographic descriptors of the severity of coronary heart disease and of left ventricular dysfunction permitted improved adjustment for differences in the extent of disease between those treated with digitalis and those not. Thus the CASS investigators concluded that the digitalis effect found by Moss et al. could be attributed to underadjustment for the difference in severity of illness between patients treated with digitalis and those not treated with digitalis. They also noted the peculiarity in the University of Rochester Heart Attack Follow-up Program of having an adverse digitalis effect in patients with two risk factors when there was no significant adverse effect in patients with either one separately. They suggested that the 38.5 percent mortality rate found by Moss et al. in the patients who had congestive heart failure and complex ventricular arrhythmias, and were treated with digitalis, was a spurious finding; and they further suggested that it resulted from a disproportionate distribution of confounding variables between the patients analyzed and those who were excluded from

analysis. Otherwise, they stated, it would be difficult to understand why, among patients not taking digitalis, those who had congestive heart failure and ventricular arrhythmias but were not treated with digitalis had a mortality rate lower than patients who did not have congestive heart failure.

Aside from the explanation given by the CASS investigators, it is possible that their results differed from those of Moss et al. because of the methods and criteria used to select the patients and because of the possibility that the P-dig analytic strategy led to overadjustment. The problem of statistical overadjustment is discussed later.

University of California (San Diego) Study

Madsen et al. from the Special Center for Research in Ischemic Heart Disease, University of California (San Diego) reviewed their postinfarction database derived from three hospitals in San Diego and one in Vancouver [22]. Patients were enrolled over a long period of time, 1969 to 1982, and 1599 were available for a retrospective review. There were marked variations among the four hospitals that contributed patients to the study with respect to the proportion of patients who were treated with digitalis (29 to 50 percent) and to the 1-year mortality rates (11 to 25 percent). A 24-hour continuous ECG recording was available for 432 patients, about one-half of the patients who enrolled after 1978. As with all of the retrospective studies, the digitalis-treated patients were sicker than those not treated, and adjustment for severity of illness decreased the difference between them. There were a number of interesting features of the University of California (San Diego) study that may have importantly influenced its outcome. The overall unadjusted difference in 1-year mortality rate between the digitalis-treated group and the group that was not treated with digitalis was smaller than in most of the other studies. There was no restriction on age for entry into the study so that this group was older than the patients who participated in the other studies. Only clinical variables were available to adjust for differences in the severity of illness: age, congestive heart failure during hospitalization, previous myocardial infarction, maximal heart rate during hospitalization, and history of angina pectoris before the index infarct. No laboratory measures were available to assess the extent of coronary artery disease, left ventricular dysfunction, or ventricular arrhythmias except for 24-hour continuous ECG recordings done in about 25 percent of patients. The overall result, relating digitalis treatment to 4-month and 1-year mortality, was borderline ($\chi^2 = 2.8$; $p < .10$).

The group of about 300 patients who had 24-hour ECG recordings as well as each of the clinical variables selected for adjustment were analyzed. One subgroup, those with congestive heart failure but no complex ventricular arrhythmias, showed a significant association between digitalis treatment and both 4-month and 1-year mortality rates. The subgroup identified by Moss et al. as being at especially high risk of harm from digitalis treatment, those with congestive heart failure and ventricular arrhythmias, were not at increased risk from digitalis in the University of California (San Diego) study. Four-month mortality in the patients with congestive heart failure and ventricular arrhythmias was not influenced by digitalis treatment; it was 12 percent in those not treated with digitalis and 15 percent in those treated with digitalis.

The Presbyterian Hospital Myocardial Infarction Study

Bigger et al. reviewed the postinfarction database of The Presbyterian Hospital in the City of New York over the period of 1974 to 1980 to evaluate the possible adverse effects of digitalis after myocardial infarction [23]. Case finding was done in the CCU, and 504 patients under 70 years of age were hospitalized for myocardial infarction during this period; all had a 24-hour continuous ECG recorded and analyzed by an accurate computer program.

Left ventricular function was assessed clinically; most of the patients did not have left ventricular ejection fraction measured or coronary angiography done. Of the 229 patients (45 percent) who were discharged on digitalis, 91 percent had digitalis treatment initiated during the hospitalization for the index myocardial infarction. There was a strong association between events in the CCU and the initiation of digitalis treatment: If a diagnosis of left ventricular dysfunction was made by the attending cardiologist in the CCU, the odds of digitalis being given increased 8.2-fold; if atrial fibrillation occurred in the CCU, the odds of digitalis being given increased 7.3-fold. There was a significant association between digitalis treatment and older age, previous myocardial infarction, angina pectoris, diabetes mellitus, left ventricular failure, enlarged heart, pulmonary congestion by chest radiograph, frequency and complexity of ventricular arrhythmias, diuretic treatment, and antiarrhythmic drug treatment. The unadjusted association between digitalis treatment and mortality during follow-up was strong; digitalis increased the odds of dying 5.2-fold. After adjustment for atrial fibrillation, left ventricular failure, and ventricular arrhythmias, the association of digitalis with mortality over 3 years of follow-up was borderline ($p < .10$), a result similar to that of Madsen et al.

Several additional analyses were done. First, the relation between serum digoxin concentration and subsequent mortality was examined in the patients who were treated with digitalis. The group was divided into three subgroups based on serum digoxin concentration, and the 3-year survival rates were determined. There was a monotonic increase in mortality rate as a function of increasing serum digoxin concentration. It is not possible to distinguish between an adverse effect of digitalis on mortality rate and the possibility that serum digoxin concentration is higher in sicker patients.

Second, The Presbyterian Hospital investigators considered the possibility of overadjustment in the Cox regression model, i.e., that adjustment for some of the effects of digitalis had weakened the association between digitalis and death [23]. It is known that digitalis can increase ventricular arrhythmias, so a covariate adjustment was carried out that excluded ventricular arrhythmias. When this measure was taken, the association of digitalis treatment and mortality was significant.

Third, these investigators searched for the subset effect reported by Moss et al., i.e., an adverse effect of digitalis in patients with congestive heart failure and ventricular arrhythmias. They did not find it.

Fourth, The Presbyterian Hospital investigators pooled their results with three previous studies using a method proposed by Fisher [24] and found that, taken together, the studies showed that digitalis significantly increased mortality in postinfarction patients even after adjustment for inequalities in the severity of illness between those who were treated with digitalis and those who were not.

Beta Blocker Heart Attack Trial Study

Byington et al. did a retrospective analysis of patients in the Beta Blocker Heart Attack Trial (BHAT) placebo group to evaluate possible adverse effects of digitalis treatment on survival after myocardial infarction [25]. Between 1978 and 1980 a total of 3837 patients were enrolled in 31 centers; they were randomized to propranolol or placebo a median of 9 days (range 5 to 21) after hospitalization, and were followed for an average of 25 months (range 12 tó 40). It is important to recall that severe congestive heart failure was an exclusion criterion for BHAT. The overall mortality rate was low, indicating that the exclusion criteria selected a study group with mild coronary heart disease. Accordingly, only 250 of the 1921 patients in the placebo group (13 percent) were treated with digitalis. The investigators thought that exclusion of the patients who had severe congestive heart failure from the trial might make it easier to evaluate an adverse effect of digitalis.

Overall, the mortality of patients treated with digitalis was 2.5 times as great as the mortality of those who were not (20.4 percent versus 8.2 percent). After adjustment for his-

tory of heart failure and ventricular arrhythmias, the association between digitalis treatment and mortality during follow-up was still statistically significant. After simultaneous adjustment for 17 variables that were associated with mortality, the relation between digitalis treatment dropped to a level that was not statistically significant. Two of the covariates used to adjust for differences between those treated with digitalis and those not treated can be caused by digitalis treatment, ST depression in the resting ECG, and complex ventricular arrhythmias defined as repetitive or multiform ventricular arrhythmias. Using this type of variable may overadjust and spuriously reduce the strength of association between digitalis treatment and mortality. During follow-up, furthermore, about 30 percent of those taking digitalis on the day of randomization stopped digitalis treatment (most by 3 months) and about 10 percent of those who were not initially on digitalis started treatment. The drop-in and drop-out rates and the time of dropping out would tend to weaken the measured association between digitalis treatment with mortality.

As the previous studies did, the BHAT digitalis study examined the group proposed by Moss et al. as being at high risk of adverse effects from digitalis treatment and could not confirm this finding.

Multicenter Investigation of the Limitation of Infarct Size Study

Muller et al. performed a retrospective analysis of 903 patients in the Multicenter Investigation of the Limitation of Infarct Size (MILIS) to evaluate the possible adverse effect of digitalis treatment on survival after myocardial infarction [26]. Between 1978 and 1983 a total of 958 patients, aged less than 76 years, were enrolled in five centers within 18 hours of the onset of symptoms suggesting myocardial infarction; they were randomized to propranolol, hyaluronidase, or placebo and were followed an average of 25 months (6 days to 40 months). Patients who met exclusion criteria for propranolol treatment were randomized to hyaluronidase or placebo. Intervention trials always have the potential for bias owing to treatment-determined exclusion criteria. Given the randomization strategy for MILIS, one would not expect much bias. Also, MILIS had the advantages of enrolling patients early and of having excellent measurement of left ventricular dysfunction. MILIS [27] and MPIP [28, 29], to be described next, were the first studies that recruited patients in the CCU and had both radionuclide ventriculograms to evaluate left ventricular function and 24-hour continuous ECG recordings analyzed by accurate digital computer programs to quantify ventricular arrhythmias. In MILIS, both measures were scheduled for the tenth hospital day. The crude 25-month mortality rate of 16 percent indicates that a relatively sick group of patients were enrolled. Overall, the mortality of the 281 patients treated with digitalis at the time of discharge was 2.5 times as high as the mortality of those who were not (27.7 percent versus 10.8 percent; $p < .001$).

Two strategies were used to select covariates for adjustment using the Cox proportional hazards regression model: (1) a subset of the variables used by the CASS investigators (age, history of previous myocardial infarction, congestive heart failure score, left ventricular ejection fraction, left ventricular regional wall motion score, left ventricular diastolic volume index); and (2) adjustment for all 19 variables for which the digitalis and the no-digitalis groups differed in univariate analyses. For adjustment, the CASS coronary artery score was not available for any patient, and 220 patients were excluded because of missing information about other CASS variables. After adjustment, the association between digitalis treatment and mortality during follow-up was not significant ($p = .14$). For adjustment by the second strategy, 164 patients were excluded because of missing information. After simultaneous adjustment for the 19 variables that were in imbalance between the group treated with digitalis and the group that was not, the relation between digitalis treatment and mortality was even less significant ($p = .34$). The MILIS investigators were

concerned that they had overadjusted in their Cox regression model, but they did not rerun their analyses dropping covariates that may have been caused by treatment with digitalis.

Interestingly, the drop-in/drop-out ratio in MILIS was similar to that found in the BHAT study. During the 25 months average follow-up, 125 of the 622 patients (20 percent) who were discharged without digitalis treatment subsequently were started on digitalis, and 74 of the 281 (26 percent) patients who were discharged on digitalis treatment subsequently had digitalis terminated.

Like the previous studies, the MILIS digitalis study examined the group proposed by Moss et al. as being at high risk of adverse effects from digitalis treatment (congestive heart failure and ventricular arrhythmias) and could not confirm this finding ($\chi^2 = 2.6$; $p > .1$).

Multicenter Post Infarction Program Study

The Digitalis Subcommittee of the Multicenter Post Infarction Program Study (MPIP) did a retrospective analysis to evaluate possible adverse effects of digitalis treatment on survival after myocardial infarction [30]. Between 1979 and 1980 a total of 867 patients were enrolled at nine participating hospitals 9 ± 4 days after hospitalization and were followed for an average of 31 months (range 24 to 48) [28]. The primary objective of MPIP was to determine the natural history of myocardial infarction and to evaluate risk attributable to myocardial ischemia, left ventricular dysfunction, and ventricular arrhythmias [28, 29]. Therefore there was no bias in enrollment attributable to exclusions related to treatment. Patients were recruited on discharge from the CCU or soon thereafter, and three special tests were obtained prior to discharge: (1) radionuclide left ventricular ejection fraction; (2) 24-hour continuous ECG recording; and (3) exercise test. The prevalence of digitalis use varied considerably among the participating hospitals (Fig. 30-1). The crude 31-month mortality rate of 17 percent indicates that a relatively sick group

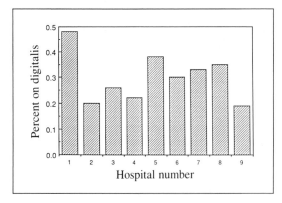

Fig. 30-1
Patients discharged on digitalis from the nine
hospitals that participated in the MPIP.

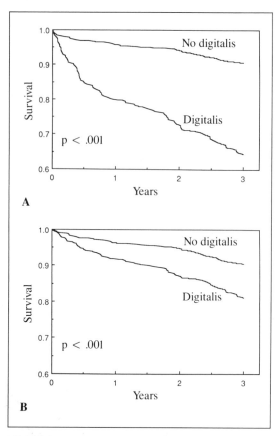

Fig. 30-2
A. Survival of the 599 MPIP patients who were
not given digitalis at the time of hospital discharge
after myocardial infarction compared to the
survival of the 268 patients who were. No
adjustment has been made for covariates. B. Same
survival comparison after adjustment for nine
covariates: age, history of diabetes mellitus,
NYHA functional class before the index
myocardial infarction, rales in the CCU, leg
edema, blood urea nitrogen, left ventricular
ejection fraction, frequency of ventricular
premature complexes, and repetitive ventricular
complexes.

of patients were enrolled; 268 patients (31 percent) were taking digitalis at the time of hospital discharge. At the MPIP 1-year follow-up,
20 percent of those discharged on digitalis had
stopped treatment and 14 percent of those discharged off digitalis had started treatment.

Figure 30-2A compares the time course of
survival for the group treated with digitalis
with the curve of the group that was not.
Overall, the mortality rate of patients treated
with digitalis was nearly four times as great as
the rate of those who were not (34 percent versus 9 percent; $p < .001$). This finding is one of
the strongest unadjusted associations between
digitalis treatment and mortality among all of
the retrospective studies that are available for
review.

The primary adjustment was for the variables that were significantly ($p < .10$) and independently related to mortality as judged by
Cox regression analysis. Two additional strategies were used to adjust for covariates using
the Cox regression method: (1) an adjustment
for any variable that was different ($p <
.05$) between the digitalis and the nondigitalis
groups; and (2) an "efficacy analysis" in
which actual treatment with digitalis during
the course of follow-up was related to mortality rather than the treatment assignment at the
beginning of the study. Differences among the
enrolling centers were adjusted for by using
centers as a stratifying variable in all of the

Cox regression model analyses. Twenty-two
risk predictors were chosen as candidates for
adjustment in the Cox regression analysis on
the basis of: (1) prior publications; (2) a priori
identification of important clinical factors
likely to be associated with advanced cardiovascular disease and mortality; and (3) retrospective identification of univariate factors
significantly ($p < .10$) associated with digitalis

treatment. Nine risk predictors were significantly and independently associated with total mortality before digitalis was added to the Cox regression model: age 60 years or more, history of diabetes mellitus, New York Heart Association (NYHA) functional class III or IV before the index infarct, rales in the CCU, leg edema on the enrollment physical examination, blood urea nitrogen of 35 mg/dl or more, left ventricular ejection fraction, ventricular arrhythmia frequency, and repetitive ventricular arrhythmias. After adjustment for all nine of these covariates simultaneously, digitalis treatment at hospital discharge was still significantly associated with mortality (Z = 3.4; $p < .001$); the relative risk was 2.3 (Fig. 30–2B). Digitalis treatment also was significantly associated with mortality after adjusting for all imbalances. The association between digitalis treatment and mortality was strengthened by the efficacy analysis, which takes account of patients dropping in and dropping out.

For this chapter, we examined the MPIP subgroup that corresponded to the one proposed by Moss et al. as being at high risk of adverse effects from digitalis treatment (congestive heart failure and ventricular arrhythmias). The difference between the two mortality rates (Table 30-2) was borderline significant ($\chi^2 = 3.7$; $p < .1$).

Commentary on the Retrospective Studies

SELECTION OF THE POPULATION

For a study of the relation between digitalis treatment and mortality following myocardial infarction, the patients should be enrolled as early as possible after infarction so that the effect of digitalis on early as well as late mortality can be observed. All of the studies listed in Table 30-1 except the CASS study meet this criterion. For generalizability, the sample studied should reflect the postinfarction population as a whole; i.e., patients should not be selected because they have more or less severe disease or because they are or are not

suitable for some treatment. The University of Rochester Heart Attack Follow-up Study, University of California (San Diego) Myocardial Infarction Study, The Presbyterian Hospital Myocardial Infarction Study, and MPIP meet this criterion.

COVARIATES FOR ADJUSTMENT

When examining retrospectively the relation between digitalis treatment and mortality, it is necessary to adjust for imbalances in factors that are known to influence mortality after myocardial infarction. Quantitative continuous measures permit better adjustment than qualitative measures. For example, two groups might have the same percentage of patients with congestive heart failure but very different average values for left ventricular ejection fraction. The major functional risk factors after myocardial infarction are left ventricular dysfunction, ventricular arrhythmias, and myocardial ischemic jeopardy [17, 18]. Left ventricular dysfunction has the strongest association with mortality. Only CASS, MILIS, and MPIP had quantitative measures of left ventricular ejection fraction and wall motion scores available for adjustment procedures. Quantitatively analyzed 24-hour Holter recordings were available on most subjects in The Presbyterian Hospital, MILIS, and MPIP studies. The only studies with measures of ischemia available for covariate adjustment were the CASS and MPIP studies; CASS had coronary angiograms available (all patients had symptomatic ischemia) [20], and MPIP had exercise test variables available on 667 of its 867 patients [31].

PROBLEMS WITH STATISTICAL ADJUSTMENT FOR COVARIATES

It is striking that the studies that showed the strongest unadjusted association between digitalis treatment and mortality were the most likely to show a significant relation that persisted after adjustment. The University of

Rochester Heart Attack Follow-up Program, The Presbyterian Hospital Myocardial Infarction Study, and the MPIP study all showed a fivefold increase in mortality in the digitalis-treated group and showed significance or borderline significance after adjustment. Adjustment for covariates in retrospective "database" studies is subject to underadjustment or overadjustment and requires superb judgment plus good luck to achieve success. The problem of undercorrection by covariate adjustment was discussed by Yusuf et al. in connection with retrospective studies of digitalis treatment after infarction [32]. They contended that *underadjustment* is likely in database studies because when a confounding variable is measured with random error its statistical control results in removal of only a fraction of its effect on the association between the risk factor under study and the outcome variable [32]. The errors inherent in databases thus make it difficult to assess treatment effects (e.g., digitalis) reliably. Furthermore, important variables bearing on outcome but not available in the database obviously cannot be used for adjustment, which also leads to underadjustment.

Overadjustment consists in controlling for factors whose presence may be caused by the hypothesized risk indicator and that may themselves be associated with the outcome. The consequence of controlling for such factors, whether by matching, stratification, or regression techniques, is to reduce or eliminate a causal effect of the hypothesized risk indicator on the outcome. For example, digitalis excess may cause ventricular arrhythmias, and ventricular arrhythmias are in turn associated with mortality. A regression model that adjusted for ventricular arrhythmias would attenuate the effect of digitalis. This effect was suggested in The Presbyterian Hospital Study [23]. The MILIS investigators were also concerned about the possibility of overadjustment [26]. The difficulty posed by the adjustment for covariates in retrospective database studies makes the results of any one study subject to uncertainty. However, the fact that seven independent studies all trended in the direction of showing harmful effects of digitalis must cause concern [23, 30]. The likelihood that such a trend would occur by chance alone is less than 1 in 50. The data required for a formal meta-analysis [33] of all the results were not available.

SUBSET ANALYSES

Moss et al. found the harmful effects of digitalis to be concentrated in a particular subgroup: patients with congestive heart failure and ventricular arrhythmias [19]. Remarkably, none of the other six retrospective studies reviewed here could confirm this finding with a statistically significant difference, nor did the combination of the results from the six studies after that of Moss et al. by means of a meta-analysis [33] attain statistical significance ($\chi^2 = 1.3$, n.s.) (Table 30-2). Thus the original finding can be considered a quirk of chance. Although the results of subset analyses of the kind reported by the University of Rochester Heart Attack Follow-up Program are intriguing, they often cannot be confirmed and should always be viewed with reservation [34].

WHAT IS THE NEXT STEP?

All seven retrospective studies acknowledged that the only strictly valid way to arrive at a definitive conclusion about whether digitalis has harmful effects in patients who have recently experienced myocardial infarction is to conduct a randomized controlled study [19, 20, 22–26, 30, 35]. The MPIP investigators planned and initiated a randomized study in which patients who had been placed on digitalis by their primary physician were withdrawn from open label digitalis treatment and were placed either on the same dose of digoxin they had taken before or on placebo. After a year, fewer than 30 patients had been enrolled in the seven participating hospitals, and the study was therefore terminated. One of the principal difficulties was the reluctance of the primary physician to discuss the potential harm of a recently prescribed medication with a patient who was recovering from myocardial infarction. Interestingly, the prevalence of digitalis prescription after infarction in the seven hospitals fell during the course of the 1-year study from about 30 percent to about 15 percent. The reason for this large reduction in digitalis use is uncertain. The change could be attributable to the educational aspect of the study: Each primary physician in the participating hospitals had the background and rationale of the study explained to him or her in detail when there was a potentially eligible patient. Another factor that may have contributed to the reduction in digitalis use is the emergence of effective alternate treatments for left ventricular dysfunction, e.g., vasodilators.

The failure of this one attempt to do a controlled study of the effect of digitalis after myocardial infarction does not mean that the question is not subject to study. Designs that randomize patients with congestive heart failure to digitalis treatment or placebo or another active treatment could be used. However, designs of this kind have problems too. First, it is awkward to explain the objective of the trial to a candidate in terms of the evaluation of the harm of a medication rather than the benefit. Second, active control therapy would logically be vasodilators, which have already been shown to improve symptoms and to prolong life in patients with NYHA class II–IV congestive heart failure [36–41]. A difference between treatment arms could result from the harmful effects of digitalis or from the beneficial effects of the vasodilator.

RECOMMENDATIONS FOR MANAGEMENT OF DIGITALIS THERAPY AFTER MYOCARDIAL INFARCTION

Acknowledging the lack of definitive information on the benefit or harm of digitalis treatment after myocardial infarction, Bigger et al. [23] and Muller et al. [26] made similar recommendations. First, when contemplating treatment with digitalis after myocardial infarction, the clinician should consider whether

treatment for left ventricular dysfunction is really necessary. For example, rales and S_3 gallop during the first 36 hours of acute myocardial infarction often resolve satisfactorily without drug treatment. Assessment of symptoms, physical findings, and left ventricular diastolic volume index, ejection fraction, and wall motion scores is indicated before making a decision about treatment. Those who have persistent dyspnea, S_3 gallop, rales, pulmonary vascular congestion, and increased left ventricular diastolic volume index should be treated with digitalis or another drug. Second, the clinician may consider if some alternate therapy might have a better risk-benefit ratio than digitalis. Vasodilators—hydralazine combined with nitrates and enalapril—have been shown to improve symptoms and prolong life in patients with congestive heart failure [36–41]. The use of captopril or enalapril for heart failure or hypertension has been shown to be well tolerated [42–50].

The results of the first randomized comparison of an angiotensin converting enzyme inhibitor and digitalis have been reported [51]. A randomized, double-blind, placebo-controlled trial enrolled 300 patients with class II or III congestive heart failure and randomized them to treatment with captopril, digoxin, or placebo; 62 percent had coronary heart disease. All patients were withdrawn from digitalis and vasodilator treatment and were stabilized on oral diuretics during a prerandomization run-in period; the protocol permitted adjustment of the diuretic dosage during the trial. The increase in exercise duration in a standardized treadmill test and the improvement in NYHA functional class were greater in the captopril group than in the digoxin or placebo groups even though the left ventricular ejection fraction increased most in the digoxin-treated group. Relative to the placebo group, the captopril group showed a substantial decrease in the frequency and complexity of spontaneous ventricular arrhythmias, whereas the group treated with digoxin showed an increase. Diuretic use was greater in the placebo- and digoxin-treated groups. Thus captopril is likely to produce a more favorable neurohumoral profile than digitalis treatment; i.e., it is probably associated with less hypokalemia and lower serum concentrations of renin, angiotensin, and norepinephrine. The Captopril-Digoxin Multicenter Research Group suggested that captopril was an effective alternative to digoxin treatment in patients with mild to moderate congestive heart failure [51].

Acknowledgments

Supported in part by NIH grant HL-70204 from the National Heart, Lung, and Blood Institute; grant RR-00645 from the Research Resources Administration, Bethesda, MD; and funds from the Henry and Shirley Benach Foundation, New York.

References

1. Withering, W., *An Account of the Foxglove and Some of Its Medical Uses: With Practical Remarks on Dropsy and Other Diseases*. London: G.G.J. and J. Robinson, 1785.
2. Fisch, C. William Withering: An account of foxglove and some of its medical uses 1785–1985. *J. Am. Coll. Cardiol.* 5(Suppl A):1A, 1985.
3. Dodek, A. Digitalis use in acute myocardial infarction: Current concepts. *Can. Med. Assoc. J.* 111:561, 1974.
4. Marcus, F. Use of digitalis in acute myocardial infarction (Editorial). *Circulation* 62:17, 1980.
5. Rahimtoola, S. H., and R. M. Gunnar. Digitalis in acute myocardial infarction: Help or hazard? *Ann. Intern. Med.* 82:234, 1982.
6. Mason, D. T., and Braunwald, E. Effects of ouabain on forearm vascular resistance and venous tone in normal subjects and in patients with heart failure. *J. Clin. Invest.* 43:532, 1964.
7. Vatner, S. F., Higgins, C. B., Franklin, D., and Braunwald, E. Effects of digitalis glycoside on coronary and systemic dynamics in conscious dogs. *Circ. Res.* 28:470, 1971.
8. Morris, J. J., Taft, C. V., Whalen, R. E., and McIntosh, H. D. Digitalis and experimental myocardial infarction. *Am. Heart J.* 77:342–55, 1969.
9. Ku, D. D., and Lucchesi, B. R. Ischemic induced alterations in cardiac sensitivity to digitalis. *Eur. J. Pharmacol.* 57:135, 1979.
10. Morrison, J., Coromilas, J., Robbins, M., et al.

11. Digitalis and myocardial infarction in man. *Circulation* 62:8, 1980.
11. Goldstein, R. A., Passamani, E. R., and Roberts, R. A comparison of digoxin and dobutamine in patients with acute infarction and cardiac failure. *N. Engl. J. Med.* 303:846, 1980.
12. Falk, P. H., Knowlton, A. A., Bernard, S. A., et al. Digoxin for converting recent onset atrial fibrillation to sinus rhythm: A randomized, double-blind trial. *Ann. Intern. Med.* 106:503, 1987.
13. Lee, D. C., Johnson, R. A., Bingham, J. B., et al. Heart failure in outpatients: A randomized trial of digoxin versus placebo. *N. Engl. J. Med.* 306:699, 1986.
14. Gheorghiade, M., and Beller, G. A. Effects of discontinuing maintenance digoxin therapy in patients with ischemic heart disease and congestive heart failure in sinus rhythm. *Am. J. Cardiol.* 51:1242, 1983.
15. Fleg, J. L. Gottlieb, S. H., and Lakatta, E. G. Is digoxin really important in the treatment of compensated heart failure? A placebo-controlled crossover study in patients in sinus rhythm. *Am. J. Med.* 73:244, 1982.
16. Greenberg, H. M., McMaster, P., Dwyer, E. M., et al. Left ventricular dysfunction after acute myocardial infarction: Results of a prospective multicenter study. *J. Am. Coll. Cardiol.* 5:867, 1984.
17. Bigger Jr., J. T. Risk stratification after myocardial infarction. *Z. Kardiol.* 74(Suppl 6):147, 1985.
18. Warnowicz, M. A., Parker, H., and Cheitlin, M. D. Prognosis of patients with acute pulmonary edema and normal ejection fraction after acute myocardial infarction. *Circulation* 67:330, 1983.
19. Moss, A. J., Davis, H. T., Conard, D. L., et al. Digitalis associated cardiac mortality after myocardial infarction. *Circulation* 64:1150, 1981.
20. Ryan, T. J., Bailey, K. R., McCabe, B. S. et al. The effect of digitalis on survival in high risk patients after coronary artery disease. *Circulation* 67:735, 1983.
21. Cox, D. R. Regression models and life tables. *J. R. Statist. Soc.* [B] 34:187, 1972.
22. Madsen, E. B., Gilpin, E., Henning, H. et al. Prognostic importance of digitalis after acute myocardial infarction. *J. Am. Coll. Cardiol.* 3:681, 1984.
23. Bigger Jr., J. T., Fleiss, J. L., Rolnitzky, L. M., et al. Effect of digitalis treatment on survival after acute myocardial infarction. *Am. J. Cardiol.* 55:623, 1985.
24. Fisher, R. A. *Statistical Methods for Research Workers* (13th ed.). New York: Hafner, 1958. Pp. 99–101.
25. Byington, R., Goldstein, S., for the BHAT Re-

search Group. Association of digitalis therapy with mortality in survivors of acute myocardial infarction: Observations in the Beta-Blocker Heart Attack Trial. *J. Am. Coll. Cardiol.* 6:976, 1985.

26. Muller, J. E., Turi, Z. G., Stone, P. H., et al. Digoxin therapy and mortality after myocardial infarction: Experience in the MILIS study. *N. Engl. J. Med.* 314:265, 1986.

27. Mukharji, J., Rude, R. E., Poole, W. K., et al. Risk factors for sudden death after acute myocardial infarction: Two-year follow-up. *Am. J. Cardiol.* 54:31, 1984.

28. Multicenter Postinfarction Research Group. Risk stratification and survival after myocardial infarction. *N. Engl. J. Med.* 309:331, 1983.

29. Bigger, J. T., Fleiss, J. L., Kleiger, R., et al. The relationships among ventricular arrhythmias, left ventricular dysfunction, and mortality in the 2 years after myocardial infarction. *Circulation* 69:250, 1984.

30. Digitalis Subcommittee of the Multicenter Post-Infarction Research Group. The mortality risk associated with digitalis treatment after myocardial infarction. *Cardiovasc. Drugs Ther.* 1:125, 1987.

31. Krone, R. J., Gillespie, J. A., Weld, F. M., et al. Low-level exercise testing after myocardial infarction: Usefulness in enhancing clinical risk stratification. *Circulation* 71:80, 1985.

32. Yusuf, S., Wittes, J., Bailey, K., and Furberg, C., Digitalis—a new controversy regarding an old drug: The pitfalls of inappropriate methodology. *Circulation* 73:14, 1986.

33. Light, R. J. Accumulating evidence from independent studies: What we can win and what we can lose. *Statist. Med.* 6:221, 1987.

34. Meier, P. Statistical analysis of clinical trials. In S. H. Shapiro and T. A. Louis (eds.), *Clinical Trials, Issues and Approaches*. New York: Marcel Dekker, 1983. Pp. 155–189.

35. Fleiss, J. L., Bigger Jr., J. T., and Rolnitzky, L. M. Is catch-22 alive and well and living at NHLBI? Reactions to "Digitalis—a new controversy regarding an old drug." *Circulation* 73:19, 1986.

36. Conradson, T. B., Ryden, L., Ahlmark, G., et al. Clinical efficacy of hydralazine in chronic heart failure: One year double blind placebo controlled study. *Am. Heart J.* 108:1001, 1984.

37. Poyhonen, L. Supine and sitting maximal workload difference and response to long term enalapril therapy in congestive heart failure. *Clin. Physiol.* 5:173, 1985.

38. Sharpe, D. N., Murphy, J., Coxon, R., and Hannan, S. F. Enalapril in patients with chronic heart failure: A placebo controlled, randomized, double blind study. *Circulation* 70:271, 1984.

39. Cohn, J. N., Archibald, D. G., Ziesche, S., et al. Effect of vasodilator therapy on mortality in chronic congestive heart failure: Results of a Veterans Administration Cooperative Study. *N. Engl. J. Med.* 314:1547, 1986.

40. Cohn, J. N., Archibald, D. G., Francis, G. S., et al. Veterans Administration cooperative study on vasodilator therapy on heart failure: Influence of prerandomization variables on the reduction of mortality by treatment with hydralazine and isosorbide dinitrate. *Circulation* 75(Suppl IV):49, 1987.

41. CONSENSUS Trial Study Group. Effects of enalapril on mortality in severe congestive heart failure: Results of the Cooperative North Scandinavian Enalapril Survival Study (CONSENSUS). *N. Engl. J. Med.* 316:1429, 1987.

42. Packer, M., Medina, N., and Yushak, M. Comparative hemodynamic and clinical effects of long-term treatment with prazosin and captopril for severe chronic congestive heart failure secondary to coronary artery disease or idiopathic dilated cardiomyopathy. *Am. J. Cardiol.* 57:1323, 1986.

43. Packer, M., Lee, W. H., Yushak, M., and Medina, N. Comparison of captopril and enalapril in patients with severe chronic heart failure. *N. Engl. J. Med.* 315:847, 1986.

44. Hollenberg, N. K. Initial therapy in hypertension: Quality-of-life considerations. *J. Hypertens.* 5(Suppl):3, 1987.

45. Croog, S. H., Levine, S., Testa, M. A., et al. The effects of antihypertensive therapy on the quality of life. *N. Engl. J. Med.* 314:1657, 1986.

46. Yodfat, Y., Fidel, J., and Bloom, D. S. Captopril as a replacement for multiple therapy in hypertension: A controlled study. *J. Hypertens.* 3(Suppl):155, 1985.

47. Bulpitt, C. J., and Fletcher, A. E. Quality of life in hypertensive patients on different antihypertensive treatments: Rationale for methods employed in a multicenter randomized controlled trial. *J. Cardiovasc. Pharmacol.* 7(Suppl 1):137, 1985.

48. Canadian Enalapril Study Group. Comparison of monotherapy with enalapril and atenolol in mild to moderate hypertension. *Can. Med. Assoc. J.* 137:803, 1987.

49. Edmonds, D., Vetter, H., and Vetter, W. Angiotensin converting enzyme inhibitors in the clinic: Quality of life. *J. Hypertens.* 5(Suppl):31, 1987.

50. Chatellier, G., Sassano, P., Amiot, A. M., et al. Efficacy and influence on quality of life of enalapril as a first step treatment of hypertension. *Clin. Exp. Hypertens.* 9:513, 1987.

51. Captopril-Digoxin Multicenter Research Group. Comparative effects of therapy with captopril and digoxin in patients with mild to moderate heart failure. *J.A.M.A.* 259:539, 1988.

31
Management of Persistent Heart Failure After Acute Myocardial Infarction

Milton Packer

Patients who develop congestive heart failure during the acute phase of a myocardial infarction have three possible clinical outcomes. They may die as a result of progressive heart failure or a malignant ventricular tachyarrhythmia. Alternatively, the hemodynamic and clinical manifestations of heart failure may resolve because of the administration of effective therapy or due to spontaneous resolution of the systolic or diastolic abnormalities seen in the acutely ischemic left ventricle. Finally, the heart failure state may persist, even though the patient has received (and may be continuing to receive) appropriate therapy with intravenous diuretics, vasodilators, and positive inotropic agents.

Management of the patient with persistent heart failure following an acute myocardial infarction is more difficult than treatment of the patient with chronic heart failure. The course of patients with persistent postinfarction heart failure is characterized by a striking degree of instability. Their clinical status may deteriorate rapidly and with little warning; hence drugs that require days to weeks to exert their beneficial effects may fail to act with sufficient rapidity to be clinically useful in this setting. The postinfarction patient may also be particularly susceptible to the side effects of pharmacologic interventions; as a result, orally active agents must be used cautiously, as their actions (if unfavorable) cannot be rapidly terminated. Finally, compared to the patient with chronic heart failure, postinfarction patients are more likely to be receiving drugs that may adversely affect left ventricular function. All of these factors make management of the postinfarction patient with persistent heart failure a special therapeutic challenge.

Pathophysiology of Postinfarction Heart Failure

In postinfarction patients the hemodynamic abnormalities that underlie the syndrome of heart failure may result from loss of viable myocardium, mechanical stresses that increase loading conditions in the heart, impaired ventricular relaxation, or a combination of these mechanisms. It is important to elucidate the contribution of each of these factors to the development of heart failure in each patient becuse each mechanism responds differently to therapeutic interventions. Fortunately, the pathophysiology of postinfarction heart failure can be characterized in most patients with the use of noninvasive cardiac imaging techniques.

Two-dimensional echocardiography or radionuclide ventriculography (or both) should be performed in every patient with persistent heart failure after an acute myocardial infarction. These techniques can detect and quantify the loss of functioning myocardium [1, 2]; patients whose heart failure is the result of systolic dysfunction generally have a left ventricular ejection fraction less than 35 percent [3]. These noninvasive techniques can also be used to confirm the presence and estimate the severity of mechanical lesions that may contribute importantly to the development of heart failure, such as the occurrence of mitral regurgitation in patients with papillary muscle rupture or the presence of an intracardiac left-to-right shunt in patients with ventricular septal rupture [4, 5]. Every effort should be made to detect such structural defects, as they are amenable to surgical correction and respond poorly to medical therapy [6–8]. Such defects must be considered in any patient with postinfarction heart failure who develops a new systolic murmur or whose left ventricular ejection fraction is more than 35 percent. Although the heart failure state in patients with preserved systolic function may be related to abnormalities of diastolic function (which may also be qualified by noninvasive techniques), such diastolic abnormalities improve rapidly during the first week of the infarction and require no specific therapy [9–11]. In contrast, mechanical defects produce a precarious hemodynamic state that is likely to deteriorate (rather than resolve) with time [6–8]. Because the presence of a structural defect cannot be ruled out by bedside examination, echocardiography provides essential information in every patient with persistent heart failure and preserved systolic function. If any doubt exists about the diagnosis, right heart catheterization should be performed immediately to look for the presence of regurgitant waves on the pulmonary wedge pressure tracing or to detect a large increase in oxygen saturation in blood collected from the right ventricle and pulmonary artery compared with that obtained from the right atrium.

Factors Contributing to the Development of Postinfarction Heart Failure

Factors that may exacerbate the development of heart failure are more likely to be present in the patient who develops the syndrome immediately after an acute myocardial infarction than in the patient who develops heart failure gradually over long periods of time.

CARDIAC ARRHYTHMIAS

Most of the arrhythmias that can worsen the hemodynamic and clinical status of patients with heart failure are supraventricular in origin and include sinus tachycardia, paroxysmal supraventricular or junctional tachycardia, atrial flutter, and atrial fibrillation. These tachyarrhythmias reduce the time available for ventricular filling, an event that is particularly deleterious in patients with impaired ventricular relaxation. Tachycardias may also increase myocardial oxygen consumption and decrease the time available for myocardial perfusion; these factors may act in concert to exacerbate myocardial ischemia. The most common causes of sinus and supraventricular tachycardias are anxiety, persistent pain, fever, pericarditis, atrial infarction, and pulmonary embolism. Most importantly, the occurrence of supraventricular tachyarrhythmias may be the only clue to the presence of left ventricular failure. Hence attempts to treat supraventricular arrhythmias in the postinfarction patient must address the underlying cause and must assume (unless proved otherwise) that left ventricular function is markedly impaired.

MYOCARDIAL ISCHEMIA

The poor systolic function that is seen in some patients following an acute myocardial infarction may not only be the result of myocardial necrosis but may occur as a consequence of reversible myocardial ischemia. Such ischemia may manifest as episodes of typical angina, or it may occur without symptoms [12, 13]. An aggressive approach to the treatment of recurrent angina in patients with left ventricular dysfunction is warranted [14], but the therapeutic implications of silent ischemia in this patient subset remain unclear. Although some investigators would differ [15], silent ischemia appears to be a rare event in patients with severe left ventricular dysfunction following an acute myocardial infarction. Fewer than 5 percent of such patients have evidence of asymptomatic ST segment changes during ambulatory monitoring (M. Pfeffer, personal communication). Nevertheless, recurrent ischemic events are likely to be an important cause of disease progression in patients with postinfarction heart failure. This point may explain why coronary artery bypass surgery favorably modifies the long-term outcome of patients with multiple-vessel disease and left ventricular dysfunction [14].

PHARMACOLOGIC AGENTS

Several agents that are commonly used in patients with an acute myocardial infarction may exacerbate the symptoms of heart failure.

Anti-inflammatory drugs that are commonly given for the treatment of pericarditis may contribute to the development of heart failure. Corticosteroids as well as nonsteroidal anti-inflammatory drugs may cause sodium retention; the latter may also antagonize the compensatory actions of endogenous vasodilators and reduce the efficacy of diuretic drugs [16, 17]. Both steroids and nonsteroidal agents may increase the severity of infarct expansion, an event that may contribute importantly to the development of heart failure [18, 19]. Low-dose aspirin therapy does not produce such deleterious hemodynamic effects, however, and may be particularly useful in preventing the recurrence of myocardial ischemic events [20].

Antiarrhythmic drugs are commonly given for the treatment of asymptomatic ventricular arrhythmias in patients with left ventricular dysfunction, even though nearly all antiarrhythmic drugs exert important cardiodepressant effects. The negative inotropic actions of agents such as disopyramide and flecainide are well established [21–23], but cardiac performance may also deteriorate following the administration of encainide, mexiletene, tocainide, procainamide, and lidocaine [23–27]. All antiarrhythmic drugs may exacerbate ventricular arrhythmias [28], especially in patients with left ventricular dysfunction. The established risks of antiarrhythmic drug therapy outweigh the unproved benefits of these agents in preventing sudden death in most patients with postinfarction heart failure.

Calcium channel blocking drugs may be used in postinfarction patients for the treatment of myocardial ischemia or supraventricular arrhythmias. All calcium channel blocking drugs (including the dihydropyridines), however, exert important negative inotropic effects and may exacerbate the symptoms of heart failure in patients with advanced left ventricular dysfunction [29]. This observation may explain why the administration of these agents to patients with postinfarction heart failure appears to affect their long-term outcome unfavorably [30].

Beta-adrenergic blocking drugs may be used during the postinfarction period for the treatment of myocardial ischemia and the prevention of future ischemic events. Beta blockers, however, may exacerbate the heart failure state in patients with impaired left ventricular dysfunction after an acute myocardial infarction [31]. If the beta blockers are withdrawn as a consequence of this adverse reaction, attempts should be made to reinstitute therapy with these drugs once the heart failure state is under better control because the long-term prognosis of such patients may be altered favorably by interventions that interfere with the activity of the sympathetic nervous system [31, 32].

Treatment of Postinfarction Heart Failure

The major goals of the treatment of patients with persistent heart failure following an acute myocardial infarction are to improve functional capacity and reduce long-term morbidity and mortality. The treatment of the postinfarction patient with heart failure can be divided into three phases: the first 7 days, 7 to 21 days, and more than 3 weeks after the acute infarction.

FIRST 7 DAYS

Patients with heart failure after an acute myocardial infarction are usually treated acutely with short-acting intravenous drugs in an effort to achieve rapid hemodynamic stability. Should the syndrome of heart failure persist despite intravenous therapy or recur when intravenous drugs are withdrawn, the patient will require long-term treatment with oral agents. The concurrent use of intravenous drugs, however, considerably complicates the initiation of oral therapy, as the actions of and reactions to oral agents may be enhanced or obscured by concurrently administered intravenous drugs. Hence before the initiation of oral therapy, it is advisable to discontinue the use of intravenous agents whenever possible. Fortunately, this can be done in most patients with postinfarction heart failure.

Withdrawal of Intravenous Vasodilators

Nitroglycerin and nitroprusside are used to lower cardiac filling pressures in patients with acute heart failure following a myocardial infarction, but the need for these drugs commonly wanes within 72 hours of the acute event. Cardiac filling pressures may decline because of diuretic therapy or because the diastolic abnormalities seen during the acute phase subside [6, 7]. Hence cardiac filling pressures are frequently low 48 hours after an acute infarction regardless of whether the patient has been treated with nitroprusside [33]. In addition, patients may develop tolerance to intravenous vasodilators, especially nitroglycerin, when they are administered continuously; under such circumstances, these drugs can be tapered without incident [34, 35]. The rapid withdrawal of intravenous vasodilators should always be avoided, however, as the abrupt discontinuation of both nitroprusside and nitrates can produce rebound hemodynamic and clinical events [36, 37]. The increases in cardiac filling pressures that are occasionally seen when these drugs are withdrawn in the postinfarction patient can usually be controlled with intravenous diuretic therapy.

Withdrawal of Intravenous Positive Inotropic Agents

Dobutamine and amrinone can be used to enhance the inotropic state and improve the hemodynamic condition of patients with heart failure after a myocardial infarction [38, 39]. Many patients lose their dependency on these drugs, however, as the function of the acutely ischemic myocardium recovers [40]. Tolerance may also develop to the actions of continuous intravenous dobutamine, probably owing to a progressive decrease in the density of myocardial beta receptors [41]. Consequently, the gradual withdrawal of intravenous positive inotropic agents usually produces few adverse hemodynamic and clinical effects. This is fortunate because no oral substitute for dobutamine or amrinone is presently available. Orally active beta agonists and phosphodiesterase inhibitors have yet to been to be proved clinically useful during long-term treatment [42–44].

Withdrawal of Intravenous Vasoconstrictors

The most difficult challenge in the management of the postinfarction patient with heart failure is the withdrawal of drugs used to support systemic blood pressures, e.g., dopamine and norepinephrine. Orally active substitutes for these agents are not available, and the results of studies with experimental drugs (levodopa and ibopamine) that generate circulating levels of dopamine and its analogs have been disappointing [45, 46]. Occasionally, dopamine therapy can be successfully withdrawn only when the function of the ischemic myocardium can be improved with the use of surgical or nonsurgical revascularization techniques [47].

Days 7 to 21 After Infarction

Once therapy with an intravenous agent is withdrawn, treatment should be immediately initiated with long-term oral agents. The drugs of choice that should be considered in every patient with postinfarction heart failure are (1) digitalis, (2) diuretics, (3) converting-enzyme inhibitors, and (4) isosorbide dinitrate.

Digitalis

Digitalis produces little hemodynamic effect within the first hours of an experimental or clinical myocardial infarction, especially when ventricular function is not impaired [38, 48–50]. As time passes from the onset of the acute event, however, the ability of digitalis to produce favorable hemodynamic effects becomes more apparent [48, 50, 51]. What may account for this observation? Digitalis is most effective in patients with the most marked ventricular dilatation [52, 53], but patients within hours of an acute infarction have insufficient time for ventricular enlargement to occur. As the left ventricle dilates during the first week after the acute event, however, digitalis may begin to produce important hemodynamic benefits [48].

Are these hemodynamic effects translated into clinical improvement? Several controlled trials have now shown that digitalis is an effective agent for the treatment of patients with chronic heart failure in normal sinus rhythm [44, 52, 54]. Digoxin improves exercise tolerance and reduces the need for diuretics, hospitalization, and emergency care for worsening heart failure [54]; when digoxin is withdrawn, the clinical status of the patient deteriorates [44, 55]. These benefits have been observed primarily in patients with systolic dysfunction (as evidenced by a low ejection fraction, left ventricular dilatation, and a third heart sound) [52, 53]. In contrast, digoxin appears to be ineffective in patients with preserved systolic function, regardless of the severity of symptoms [56, 57]. This observation underscores the importance of characterizing the pathophysiology of heart failure before deciding what drugs the patient should receive.

Despite concerns about its toxicity, digoxin appears to be well tolerated by most patients with chronic heart failure. Although there have been concerns about the potential of digoxin to produce arrhythmias in subjects with acute ischemia, this risk appears to subside during the first week after the acute myocardial infarction [48]. In fact, digoxin may be less arrhythmogenic than other positive inotropic agents, particularly those that act by increasing intracellular cyclic AMP [44].

Diuretics

Diuretics produce symptomatic benefits in patients with heart failure following an acute myocardial infarction. Their major advantage is their rapidity of effect. Diuretics can relieve dyspnea and edema within hours or days, whereas the responses to many other therapeutic agents may take weeks or months. Diuretics alone appear to be insufficient to control the symptoms of heart failure in most patients, however. A high proportion of patients whose symptoms are stabilized on diuretics alone deteriorate clinically during long-term follow-up, unless they also receive concurrent therapy with digitalis or converting-enzyme inhibitors [54]. Increments in the dose of diuretics may produce little hemodynamic benefit, perhaps because such high doses activate endogenous neurohormonal vasoconstrictor systems that may limit the benefits of these drugs [58]. Furthermore, the electrolyte depletion that may result from aggressive diuretic therapy may exacerbate the ventricular arrhythmias seen in patients with an acute myocardial infarction [59]. Hence in most patients it seems preferable to add a second drug than to use high doses of diuretics.

Converting-Enzyme Inhibitors

The renin-angiotensin system is activated following an acute myocardial infarction and contributes importantly to the increase in ventricular wall stress that is seen in these patients [60]. Such augmented wall stress may initiate a process of ventricular enlargement that can lead to a progressive deterioration of left ventricular function [61]. This sequence of events, however, can be interrupted by therapy with a converting-enzyme inhibitor [61, 62]. Patients with heart failure following an acute myocardial infarction experience important hemodynamic benefits when treated with converting-enzyme inhibitors; early therapy appers to attenuate the development of ventricular enlargement and, thereby, acts to preserve ventricular function and improve exercise performance [63–65]. Similar benefits may not be achieved, however, if ventricular volumes are reduced by agents that stimulate endogenous neurohormonal systems (e.g., furosemide) [65].

Even if converting-enzyme inhibitors are not initiated early after an acute infarction, they can be beneficial during the chronic phase—after ventricular dilatation has occurred. Converting-enzyme inhibitors reduce the symptoms of heart failure and enhance exercise tolerance; this improvement is seen in patients with mild, moderate, or severe symptoms [54, 66–69]. Converting-enzyme inhibitors, however, cannot control the symptoms of heart failure in the absence of diuretic therapy [70]. Fortunately, captopril and enalapril can antagonize many of the adverse neurohormonal and metabolic effects of diuretics [68, 69]. On the other hand, diuretics appear to potentiate the side effects of the converting-enzyme inhibitors [71, 72]. These observations suggest that although these two classes of drugs should almost always be combined, caution should be exercised (particularly in the postinfarction patient) to titrate the dose of diuretics so as to minimize the occurrence of symptomatic hypotension and functional renal insufficiency.

Nitrates
In patients with postinfarction heart failure, nitroglycerin and isosorbide dinitrate produce hemodynamic effects similar to those seen with the converting-enzyme inhibitors, but it is unknown if long-term nitrate therapy can favorably modify the ventricular remodeling process. When the results of large-scale trials with nitrates are pooled, treatment with nitates appears to reduce mortality in patients with an acute myocardial infarction [72], but this effect may be related to the ability of these drugs to alleviate ischemia rather than improve the hemodynamic status of patients with heart failure.

Once the acute phase of ischemia has passed, the role of nitrates in the management of patients with persistent heart failure remains uncertain. In the placebo-controlled trials carried out to date, long-term treatment with oral isosorbide dinitrate has produced some favorable effects, but nitrates failed to produce an increase in exercise capacity that was consistently better than placebo, and nitrate therapy was not reliably accompanied by the relief of symptoms [37, 73, 74]. Even when combined with hydralazine, isosorbide dini-

trate failed to improve the clinical status or exercise tolerance of patients with chronic heart failure after 2 and 6 months of therapy [75]. It is possible, therefore, that the benefits of nitrates in patients with an acute infarction may be relate to their anti-ischemic effects; indeed such benefits are apparent in patients with and without left ventricular dysfunction [72].

AFTER 3 WEEKS

One of the major goals of long-term therapy in the patient with postinfarction heart failure is to prolong life. Agents that may affect survival (favorably or unfavorably) include digitalis, direct-acting vasodilators, converting-enzyme inhibitors, beta blockers, and calcium channel blockers.

Digitalis
We know little about the effect of digitalis on the survival of patients with heart failure following an acute myocardial infarction, as controlled trials with this agent have not been carried out. Retrospective analyses have identified digitalis therapy as a risk factor for enhanced mortality [76], but it is possible that this adverse association was related to the severity of heart failure in treated patients and not to therapy with the drug. Large-scale trials to evaluate the impact of digitalis on survival are now being planned by the National Heart, Lung and Blood Institute.

Direct-Acting Vasodilators
The Veterans Administration Vasodilator Heart Failure Trial (V-HeFT) reported that a combination of hydralazine and isosorbide dinitrate can reduce mortality in patients with mild to moderate symptoms [77]. The combination of the two vasodilators was poorly tolerated, however. During the period of follow-up, one or both drugs were discontinued in 38 percent of patients because of side effects, and only 55 percent of patients were taking full doses of both drugs at the end of 6 months. These side effects appeared to be more frequent with hydralazine than with isosorbide dinitrate; hydralazine may also exacerbate

ischemia in patients with heart failure and active angina [78]. Consequently, many physicians have prescribed isosorbide dinitrate alone in an effort to gain the prognostic benefits reported in V-HeFT. Isosorbide dinitrate alone may not prolong life in patients with heart failure, however. The reduction in mortality seen in V-HeFT was related to an increase in the left ventricular ejection fraction [79], but such an increase is more likely to be seen with hydralazine than with isosorbide dinitrate [80]. In addition, the regression of cellular hypertrophy seen when the two vasodilators are combined can be achieved with hydralazine alone but not with isosorbide dinitrate alone [81]. Therefore although one retrospective study noted an association between nitrate therapy and prolonged survival of patients after an acute myocardial infarction [82], the role of nitrate monotherapy in preventing future cardiovascular events in these patients remains uncertain.

Converting-Enzyme Inhibitors
Because converting-enzyme inhibitors prolong life in patients with chronic heart failure, they appear to play an important role in the management of all postinfarction patients with heart failure. In the CONSENSUS study [83] long-term treatment with enalapril markedly reduced the mortality of patients with severe (class IV) symptoms; the available data suggest a similar beneficial effect of captopril on the survival of patients with more moderate symptoms [84]. Captopril and enalapril may reduce the incidence of death from progressive heart failure as well as decrease the incidence of sudden arrhythmic deaths.

Beta-Adrenergic Blockers
Beta blockers have particular appeal in the postinfarction patient because they interfere with the potentially deleterious effects of adrenergic stimulation on the failing heart. A variety of beta blockers (primarily those without intrinsic sympathomimetic activity) have been shown to prolong life in patients following an acute myocardial infarction; this reduction in mortality appears to be most marked in patients with a history of heart failure prior to or

during their acute myocardial infarction [31, 32]. Despite these benefits, however, few physicians are using beta blockers in patients with left ventricular dysfunction following an acute infarction because of fears that these drugs may aggravate the symptoms of heart failure. Although this complication could conceivably be avoided by incorporating beta-agonist activity into the pharmacologic profile of the drug, the presence of such activity could potentially abolish the ability of a beta blocker to prolong survival [85].

Calcium Channel Blocking Drugs
Calcium channel blockers at first appear to be advantageous in patients with postinfarction heart failure, as their anti-ischemic effects might prevent the development of ischemic necrosis and their ability to retard entry of calcium into the cell might exert favorable long-term effects on the progression of heart failure [86, 87]. Calcium channel blockers, however, exert important negative inotropic effects in patients with left ventricular dysfunction [29]. Furthermore, their ability to stimulate neurohormonal systems may contribute to disease progression. These factors may explain why the administration of a calcium channel blocker to patients with postinfarction heart failure was associated with an increase (rather than a decrease) in recurrent cardiac events and mortality [30]. These observations indicate that calcium channel blockers should be avoided in patients with postinfarction heart failure.

Conclusion

The patient who develops congestive heart failure after an acute myocardial infarction presents a special challenge to the practicing physician. Every effort should be made to alleviate reversible causes of heart failure in these patients and to minimize the contribution of potentially deleterious factors. A variety of pharmacologic interventions are available that can improve the hemodynamic status and the functional capacity of these patients; in addition, drugs have been developed that can reduce long-term morbidity and mortality in this disease. Above all, we must attempt to reduce the recurrence of future ischemic events in these high-risk patients with aspirin and by the judicious use of coronary artery bypass surgery in patients with multivessel disease [14, 20]. The benefits of surgery appear to be particularly striking in postinfarction patients with left ventricular dysfunction [14].

References

1. Sanford, G. F., Corbett, J., Nicod, P., et al. Value of radionuclide ventriculography in the immediate characterization of patients with an acute myocardial infarction. *Am. J. Cardiol.* 49:637, 1982.
2. Nishimura, R. A., Tajik, A. J., Shub, C., et al. Role of two-dimensional echocardiography in the prediction of in-hospital complications after acute myocardial infarction. *J. Am. Coll. Cardiol.* 4:1080, 1984.
3. Mangschau, A., Rollag, A., Jonsbu, J., and Lund-Karlsen, R. Congestive heart failure and ejection fraction in acute myocardial infarction. *Acta Med. Scand.* 220:101, 1986.
4. Come, P. C., Riley, M. F., Weintraub, R., et al. Echocardiographic detection of complete and partial papillary muscle rupture during acute myocardial infarction. *Am. J. Cardiol.* 56:787, 1985.
5. Barzilai, B., Bessler, C., Jr., Perez, J. E., et al. Significance of Doppler-detected regurgitation in acute myocardial infarction. *Am. J. Cardiol.* 61:220, 1988.
6. Miller, D. C., and Stinson, E. B. Surgical management of acute mechanical defects secondary to myocardial infarction. *Am. J. Surg.* 141:677, 1981.
7. Scanlon, P. J., Montoya, A., Johnson, S. A., et al. Urgent surgery for ventricular septal rupture complicating acute myocardial infarction. *Circulation* 72(Suppl II):185, 1985.
8. Pinwica, A., Menasche, P., Beaufils, P., and Julliard, J. M. Long-term results of emergency surgery for postinfarction ventricular septal defect. *Ann. Thorac. Surg.* 44:274, 1987.
9. Murray, D. P., Corbei, H. M., Dunselman, P. H., et al. Natural evolution of left ventricular haemodynamics following uncomplicated acute myocardial infarction. *Int. J. Cardiol.* 11:175, 1986.
10. Pirzada, F. A., Ekong, E. A., Vokonas, P. S., et al. Experimental myocardial infarction. XIII. Sequential changes in left ventricular pressure-

length relations in the acute phase. *Circulation* 53:970, 1976.
11. Fletcher, P. J., Pfeffer, J. M., Pfeffer, M. A., and Braunwald, E. Left ventricular diastolic pressure-volume relations in rats with healed myocardial infarction: Effects on systolic function. *Circ. Res.* 49:618, 1981.
12. Tavazzi, L., Giannuzzi, P., Giordano, A., et al. Is post-infarction angina related to poor residual left ventricular function? *Eur. Heart J.* 7(Suppl C):25, 1986.
13. Chierchia, S., Lazzari, M., Freedman, B., et al. Impairment of myocardial perfusion and function during painless myocardial ischemia. *J. Am. Coll. Cardiol.* 1:924, 1983.
14. Luchi, R. J., Scott, S. M., and Deupree, R. H. Comparison of medical and surgical treatment for unstable angina pectoris: Results of a Veterans Adminstration Cooperative Study. *N. Engl. J. Med.* 316:977, 1987.
15. Cohn, P. F. Silent myocardial ischemia. *Ann. Intern. Med.* 109:312, 1988.
16. Dzau, V. J., Packer, M., Lilly, L. S., et al. Prostaglandins in severe heart failure: Relation to activation of the renin-angiotensin system and hyponatremia. *N. Engl. J. Med.* 310:347, 1984.
17. Oliw, E., Kover, G., Larsson, C., and Anggard, E. Reduction by indomethacin of furosemide effects in the rabbit. *Eur. J. Pharmacol.* 38:95, 1976.
18. Mannisi, J. A., Weisman, H. F., Bush, D. E., et al. Steroid administration after myocardial infarction promotes early infarct expansion: A study in the rat model. *J. Clin. Invest.* 79:1431, 1987.
19. Hammerman, H., Schoen, F. J., Braunwald, E., et al. Drug-induced expansion of infarct: Morphologic and functional correlations. *Circulation* 69:611, 1984.
20. Lewis, H. D., Davis, J. W., Archibald, D. G., et al. Protective effects of aspirin against acute myocardial infarction and death in men with unstable angina. *N. Engl. J. Med.* 309:396, 1983.
21. Jackson, N., Verma, S. P., Frais, M. A., et al. Hemodynamic dose-response effects of flecainide in acute myocardial infarction with and without left ventricular decompensation. *Clin. Pharmacol. Ther.* 37:619, 1985.
22. Cohen, A. A., Daru, V., Covelli, G., et al. Hemodynamic effects of intravenous flecainide in acute noncomplicated myocardial infarction. *Am. Heart J.* 110:1193, 1985.
23. Silke, B., Frais, M. A., Verna, S. P., et al. Comparative hemodynamic effects of intravenous lignocaine, disopyramide and flecainide in uncomplicated acute myocardial infarction. *Br. J. Clin. Pharmacol.* 22:707, 1986.
24. MacMahon, B., Bakshi, M., Branagan, P., et al. Pharmacokinetics and haemodynamic effects of tocainide in patients with acute myo-

cardial infarction complicated by left ventricular failure. *Br. J. Clin. Pharmacol.* 19:429, 1985.

25. Lotto, A., Finzi, A., Massari, F. M., et al. Hemodynamic effects of antiarrhythmic drugs in acute myocardial infarction. *G. Ital. Cardiol.* 14:762, 1984.

26. Gottlieb, S. S., Kukin, M. L., Yushak, M., et al. Cardiodepressant effects of encainide in patients with severe left ventricular dysfunction. *Ann. Int. Med.* 110:505, 1989.

27. Gottlieb, S. S., Kukin, M. L., Wilson, P. B., et al. Loading doses of oral procainamide exert cardiodepressant effects and activate neurohormones in patients with left ventricular dysfunction (Abstract). *J. Am. Coll. Cardiol.* 11:91A, 1988.

28. Velebit, V., Podrid, P., Lown, B., et al. Aggravation and provocation of ventricular arrhythmias by antiarrhythmic drugs. *Circulation* 65:886, 1982.

29. Packer, M., Kessler, P. D., and Lee, W. H. Calcium channel blockade in the management of severe chronic congestive heart failure: A bridge too far. *Circulation* 75(Suppl V):56, 1987.

30. Multicenter Diltiazem Post-Infarction Research Group. The effect of diltiazem on mortality and reinfarction after myocardial infarction. *N. Engl. J. Med.* 319:385, 1988.

31. Chadda, K., Goldstein, S., Byington, R., and Curb, J. D. Effect of propranolol after acute myocardial infarction in patients with congestive heart failure. *Circulation* 73:503, 1986.

32. Olsson, G., and Rehnqvist, N. Effect of metoprolol in postinfarction patients with increased heart size. *Eur. Heart J.* 7:468, 1986.

33. Cohn, J. N., Franciosa, J. A., Francis, G. S., et al. Effect of short-term infusion of sodium nitroprusside on mortality rate in acute myocardial infarction complicated by left ventricular failure. *N. Engl. J. Med.* 306:1129, 1982.

34. Roth, A., Weber, L., Friedenberger, L., et al. Hemodynamic effects of intravenous isosorbide dinitrate and nitroglycerin in acute myocardial infarction and elevated pulmonary artery wedge pressure. *Chest* 91:190, 1987.

35. Packer, M., Lee, W. H., Kessler, P. D., et al. Prevention and reversal of nitrate tolerance in patients with congestive heart failure. *N. Engl. J. Med.* 317:799, 1987.

36. Packer, M., Meller, J., Medina, N., et al. Rebound hemodynamic events after the abrupt withdrawal of nitroprusside in patients with severe chronic heart failure. *N. Engl. J. Med.* 301:1193, 1979.

37. Franciosa, J. A., Nordstrom, L. A., and Cohn, J. N. Nitrate therapy for congestive heart failure. *J.A.M.A.* 240:443, 1978.

38. Goldstein, R. A., Passamani, E. R., and Roberts, R. A comparison of digoxin and dobutamine in patients with acute infarction and cardiac failure. *N. Engl. J. Med.* 303:846, 1980.

39. Taylor, S. H., Verma, S. P., Hussain, M., et al. Intravenous amrinone in left ventricular failure complicated by acute myocardial infarction. *Am. J. Cardiol.* 56:29B, 1985.

40. Braunwald, E., and Kloner, R. A. The stunned myocardium: Prolonged, postischemic ventricular dysfunction. *Circulation* 66:1150, 1982.

41. Unverferth, D. V., Blanford, M., Kates, R. E., and Leier, C. V. Tolerance to dobutamine after a 72 hour continuous infusion. *Am. J. Med.* 69:262, 1980.

42. Roubin, G. S., Choong, C. Y., Devenish-Meares, S., et al. Beta-adrenergic stimulation of the failing left ventricle: A double-blind, randomized trial of sustained oral therapy with prenalterol. *Circulation* 69:955, 1984.

43. Weber, K. T., Andrews, V., Janicki, J. S., et al. Pirbuterol, an oral beta-adrenergic receptor agonist, in the treatment of chronic cardiac failure. *Circulation* 66:1262, 1982.

44. DiBianco, R., Shabetai, R., Kostuk, W., et al. Oral milrinone and digoxin in heart failure: Results of a placebo-controlled, prospective trial of each agent and the combination (Abstract). *Circulation* 76(Suppl IV):256, 1987.

45. Kasper, W., Meinertz, T., Busch, W., et al. Does long term oral levodopa therapy improve cardiac function in congestive heart failure? (Abstract). *Circulation* 72(Suppl III):302, 1985.

46. Rajfer, S. I., Rossen, J. D., Douglas, F. L., et al. Effects of long-term therapy with oral ibopamine on resting hemodynamics and exercise capacity in patients with heart failure: Relationship to the generation of N-methyldopamine and to plasma norepinephrine levels. *Circulation* 73:740, 1986.

47. Heuser, R. R., Maddoux, G. L., Goss, J. E., et al. Coronary angioplasty for acute mitral regurgitation due to myocardial infarction: A nonsurgical treatment preserving mitral valve integrity. *Ann. Intern. Med.* 107:852, 1987.

48. Kumar, R., Hood Jr., W. B., Joison, J., et al. Experimental myocardial infarction. VI. Efficacy and toxicity of digitalis in acute and healing phase in intact conscious dogs. *J. Clin. Invest.* 49:358, 1970.

49. Balcon, R., Hoy, J., and Sowton, E. Haemodynamic effects of rapid digitalization following acute myocardial infarction. *Br. Heart J.* 30:373, 1968.

50. Marchionni, N., Pini, R., Vannucci, A., et al. Hemodynamic effects of digoxin in acute myocardial infarction in man: A randomized controlled trial. *Am. Heart J.* 109:636, 1985.

51. Kurogane, K., Fujitani, K., and Fukuzaki, H. Hemodynamic effects of digoxin on congestive heart failure in old myocardial infarction, dilated cardiomyopathy, acute myocardial infarc-

tion and mitral stenosis. *Jpn. Heart J.* 26:155, 1985.

52. Guyatt, G. H., Sullivan, M. J. J., Fallen, E. L., et al. A controlled trial of digoxin in congestive heart failure. *Am. J. Cardiol.* 61:371, 1988.

53. Lee, D. C., Johnson, R. A., Bingham, J. B., et al. Heart failure in outpatients: A randomized trial of digoxin versus placebo. *N. Engl. J. Med.* 306:699, 1982.

54. Captopril-Digoxin Multicenter Research Group. Comparative effects of captopril and digoxin in patients with mild to moderate heart failure. *J.A.M.A.* 259:539, 1988.

55. Arnold, S. B., Byrd, R. C., Meister, W., et al. Long-term digitalis therapy improves left ventricular function in heart failure. *N. Engl. J. Med.* 303:1443, 1980.

56. Fleg, J. L., Gottlieb, S. H., and Lakatta, E. G. Is digoxin really important in treatment of compensated heart failure? A placebo-controlled crossover trial in patients with sinus rhythm. *Am. J. Med.* 73:244, 1982.

57. Gheorghiade, M., and Beller, G. A. Effects of discontinuating maintenance digoxin therapy in patients with ischemic heart disease and congestive heart failure in sinus rhythm. *Am. J. Cardiol.* 51:1243, 1983.

58. Larsen, F. F. Haemodynamic effects of high or low doses of furosemide in acute myocardial infarction. *Eur. Heart J.* 9:125, 1988.

59. Nodrehaug, J. E., and von der Lippe, G. Hypokalemia and ventricular fibrillation in acute myocardial infarction. *Br. Heart J.* 50:525, 1983.

60. Dargie, H. J., McAlpine, H. M., and Morton, J. J. Neuroendocrine activation in acute myocardial infarction. *J. Cardiovasc. Pharmacol.* 9(Suppl):S21, 1987.

61. Pfeffer, J. M., Pfeffer, M. A., and Braunwald, E. Influence of chronic captopril therapy on the infarcted left ventricle of the rat. *Circ. Res.* 57:84, 1985.

62. Pfeffer, M. A., Pfeffer, J. M., Steinberg, C., and Finn, P. Survival after an experimental infarction: Beneficial effect of long-term therapy with captopril. *Circulation* 72:406, 1985.

63. McAlpine, H. M., Morton, J. J., Leckie, B., and Drgie, H. J. Haemodynamic effects of captopril in acute left venticular failure complicating myocardial infarction. *J. Cardiovasc. Pharmacol.* 9(Suppl 2):S25, 1987.

64. Pfeffer, M. A., Lamas, G. A., Vaughn, D. E., et al. Effect of captopril on progressive ventricular dilatation after anterior myocardial infarction. *N. Engl. J. Med.* 319:80, 1988.

65. Sharpe, N., Murphy, J., Smith, H., and Hannan, S. Treatment of patients with symptomless left ventricular dysfunction after myocardial infarction. *Lancet* 1:255, 1988.

66. Captopril Multicenter Research Group. A placebo-controlled trial of captopril in refractory chronic congestive heart failure. *J. Am. Coll. Cardiol.* 2:755, 1983.

67. Sharpe, D. N., Murphy J., Coxon, R., and Hannan, S. F. Enalapril in patients with chronic heart failure: A placebo-controlled, randomized, double-blind study. *Circulation* 70:271, 1984.

68. Cleland, J. G. F., Dargie, H. J., Hodsman, G. P., et al. Captopril in heart failure: A double-blind controlled trial. *Br. Heart J.* 52:530, 1984.

69. Cleland, J. G. F., Dargie, H. J., Ball, S. G., et al. Effects of enalapril in heart failure: A double blind study of effects on exercise performance, renal function, hormones, and metabolic state. *Br. Heart J.* 54:305, 1985.

70. Richardson, A., Bayliss, J., Scriven, A., et al. Double-blind comparison of captopril alone against furosemide plus amiloride in mild heart failure. *Lancet* 2:709, 1987.

71. Packer, M., Lee, W. H., Medina, M., et al. Functional renal insufficiency during long-term therapy with captopril or enalapril for severe chronic heart failure. *Ann. Intern. Med.* 106:346, 1987.

72. Yusuf, S., Collins, R., MacMahon, S., and Peto, R. Effect of intravenous nitrates on mortality in acute myocardial infarction: An overview of the randomized trials. *Lancet* 1:1088, 1988.

73. Leier, C. V., Huss, P., Magorien, R. D., and Unverferth, D. V. Improved exercise capacity and differing arterial and venous tolerance during chronic isosorbide dinitrate therapy for congestive heart failure. *Circulation* 67:817, 1983.

74. Franciosa, J. A., Goldsmith, S. R., and Cohn, J. N. Contrasting immediate and long-term effects of isosorbide dinitrate on exercise capacity in congestive heart failure. *Am. J. Med.* 69:559, 1980.

75. Cohn, J. N., Archibald, D. G., and Johnson, G. Effects of vasodilator therapy on peak exercise oxygen consumption in heart failure: V-HeFT (Abstract). *Circulation* 75(Suppl II):443, 1987.

76. Bigger Jr., J. T., Fleiss, J. L., Rolnitzky, L. M., et al. Effect of digitalis treatment on survival after acute myocardial infarction. *Am. J. Cardiol.* 55:623, 1985.

77. Cohn, J. N., Archibald, D. G., Ziesche, S., et al. Effect of vasodilator therapy on mortality in chronic congestive heart failure: Results of a Veterans Administration Cooperative Study. *N. Engl. J. Med.* 314:1547, 1986.

78. Packer, M., Meller, J., Medina, N., et al. Provocation of myocardial ischemic events during initiation of vasodilator therapy for severe chronic heart failure: Clinical and hemodynamic evaluation of 52 consecutive patients with ischemic cardiomyopathy. *Am. J. Cardiol.* 48:939, 1981.

79. Archibald, D. G., and Cohn, J. N. A treatment-

associated increase in ejection fraction predicts long-term survival in congestive heart failure: The V-HeFT study (Abstract). *Circulation* 75(Suppl II):309, 1987.

80. Unverferth, D. V., Mehegan, J. P., Magorien, R. D., et al. Regression of myocardial cellular hypertrophy with vasodilator therapy in chronic congestive heart failure associated with idiopathic cardiomyopathy. *Am. J. Cardiol.* 51:1392, 1983.

81. Magorien, R. D., Unverferth, D. V., and Leier, C. V. Hydralazine therapy in chronic congestive heart failure: Sustained central and regional hemodynamic responses. *Am. J. Med.* 77:267, 1984.

82. Rapaport, E. Influence of long-acting nitrate therapy on the risk of reinfarction, sudden death, and total mortality in survivors of acute myocardial infarction. *Am. Heart. J.* 110:276, 1985.

83. CONSENSUS Trial Study Group. Effect of enalapril on mortality in severe congestive heart failure: Results of the Cooperative North Scandinavian Enalapril Survival Study (CONSENSUS). *N. Engl. J. Med.* 316:1429, 1987.

84. Newman, T. J., Maskin, C. S., Dennick, L. G., et al. Effects of captopril on survival in patients with heart failure. *Am. J. Med.* 84(3A):140, 1988.

85. Yusuf, S., Peto, R., Lewis, J., et al. Beta blockade during and after myocardial infarction: An overview of the randomized trials. *Prog. Cardiovasc. Dis.* 27:335, 1985.

86. Sonnenblick, E. H., Fein, F., Capasso, J. M., and Factor, S. M. Microvascular spasm as a cause of cardiomyopathies and the calcium-blocking agent, verapamil, as potential primary therapy. *Am. J. Cardiol.* 55:179B, 1985.

87. Garrett, J. S., Wikman-Coffelt, J., Sievers, R., et al. Verapamil prevents the development of alcoholic dysfunction in hamster myocardium. *J. Am. Coll. Cardiol.* 9:1326, 1987.

32
Psychosocial and Behavioral Factors During Recovery from Myocardial Infarction

IRA S. OCKENE, LEONARD A. DOERFLER, AND JUDITH K. OCKENE

Improvements in medical therapy have led to increased survival among myocardial infarction (MI) patients, but many patients who survive experience social and psychological problems that can be as severe as or even worse than the physical disease itself [1–4]. Immediately after infarction, fear, anger, depression, and guilt are commonplace. Most patients experience rapid psychological recovery, but as many as one-third continue to suffer negative psychological effects that impair their quality of life [5]. For some patients the emotional distress is so pronounced that psychological intervention in the coronary care unit is necessary [6]. After the initial distress associated with the infarction subsides, most patients function well psychosocially [7, 8]. A significant minority, however, continue to experience marked psychosocial difficulties as much as 2 years later [9–11].

Several reports indicate that patients who experience psychological problems (especially anxiety and depression) during early convalescence continue to demonstrate considerable long-term impairment [11–14]. Moreover, features of "invalidism" such as cessation of sexual activity and failure to return to work for nonphysical reasons generally develop during early convalescence. These psychosocial problems do not appear to be strongly related to the severity of acute MI [15]. Therefore psychological intervention should be initiated early, with specific attention paid to anxiety and depression.

Medical and psychosocial factors interact in a complex manner to influence the recovery process. Symptoms such as angina, dyspnea, and easy fatiguability attendant to an MI can produce deterioration in vocational (e.g., unemployment) or psychological (e.g., anxiety, depression) domains. Such manifestations of coronary heart disease as arrhythmias or tachycardia, particularly when linked by the patient to the possibility of sudden death, can produce hypervigilance to body sensations, hypochondriasis, or a sense of "walking on egg shells." Medications that are commonly used to treat coronary heart disease can also impair psychosocial functioning. For example, antihypertensive and beta-blocking medications have the potential to cause depression or impair sexual performance [16].

Conversely, evidence suggests that psychosocial factors can adversely affect cardiac functioning after an MI. Immediately after an MI, the psychological state of the patient can influence physiologic events. During the hours and days following the infarction there is an increase in plasma levels of catecholamines, free fatty acids, and cortisol [17], which can contribute to potentially lethal complications (e.g., ventricular arrhythmias, cardiogenic shock, left ventricular failure). During this critical period, patients who are less anxious and more effectively cope with the stress of the event have lower elevations of catecholamines and free fatty acids [18]. Later during convalescence, prolonged depression and anxiety can lead to long-term invalidism because of unnecessary restriction of social and physical activity. Such inactivity may contribute to a decline in cardiac functioning due to the physiologic effects of deconditioning [19]. Social isolation, which is often a feature of depression, also appears to be related to increased rates of mortality and sudden death in patients who survive an MI [20]. Another factor that has been reported to affect physical condition after an MI is type A behavior. In a study of men with established coronary disease, those with type A behavior were at a significantly higher risk of subsequent coronary events than men who were type B, although these findings remain controversial (see p. 593) [21].

The occurrence of an MI is a serious life crisis that often dramatically alters the lives of patients and their families. Because many patients have been active and in fairly good health, the diagnosis of a myocardial infarction suddenly arouses concerns about death and long-term disability. In the midst of such a crisis, emotional reactions such as anxiety, helplessness, despondency, and denial are to be expected [22]. As the patient's medical condition stabilizes and the fear of death recedes, other concerns emerge. Prominent among them are the financial drain of hospitalization, the ability to return to work, resumption of physical and sexual activity, and the necessity of making life style changes to reduce the risk of reinfarction [15, 23–26].

Clearly, recovery from MI requires complex social, vocational, and psychological adjustment for patients and their families. Although most MI patients adjust well to their illness after a period of disruption and distress [15, 22, 27, 28], some, perhaps as many as 25 percent, experience long-standing emotional distress, family turmoil, and occupational problems [1, 2, 15, 24, 28, 29]. Failure to recognize and intervene when such problems persist may lead to the development of serious disability and invalidism.

In addition to the direct behavioral effects of an infarct, the recovered patient must deal with the heightened need to address risk factor modification. Clear evidence exists that secondary prevention of coronary heart disease (CHD) is of value, even if the patient has had an infarct or has already undergone coronary artery bypass surgery [30, 31]. The patient is therefore under considerable pressure, both self-generated and from without, to quit smoking, change diet, exercise, and modify a stressful life style. This pressure has its own behavioral consequences, but the alteration of risk factors is in fact desirable, so the health care provider must have the skills needed to help the patient make appropriate changes without causing undue anxiety and stress.

The present chapter, which focuses on psychosocial problems that arise in the course of recovery after a myocardial infarction, is organized into three sections: problems during the acute phase (hospitalization), problems after return to home and during the early convalescent period, and problems during the late convalescent/rehabilitation period. Because of the diversity of factors that have been related to recovery, we limit our discussion to problems that occur relatively frequently or that are particularly deleterious.

Psychological and Behavioral Adjustment During Hospitalization

EMOTIONAL STATUS

The symptoms of myocardial infarction, especially chest pain and shortness of breath, usually arouse intense anxiety. The patient fears disability and death. Upon arrival at the hospital, the often previously well patient is suddenly immersed in the disorienting activity of the hospital. Coming to the coronary care unit (CCU) via the emergency room, the patient is rapidly interviewed, examined, and monitored while an intravenous line is placed, oxygen is administered, and blood samples are drawn, often from an artery as well as a vein. People and machinery swirl about the patient, and the disorientation is accentuated by the drugs used to treat anxiety and pain—sedatives such as diazepam (Valium) and potent narcotics such as morphine.

After initial evaluation in the emergency room, the patient is transferred to the CCU. In the past, therapy of myocardial infarction was largely expectant, with the patient who was doing well being placed in bed and observed, but during the last few years interventional therapies to minimize infarct size (e.g., thrombolytic therapy and coronary angioplasty) have increasingly filled the patient's early hours in the hospital with procedures and discomfort. In the CCU itself the patient finds an unfamiliar environment filled with an array of distracting sounds, alarms, and lights.

For most patients, the procedures involved in the initial evaluation and admission to the CCU temporarily intensify emotional distress [32]. However, after becoming familiar with their surroundings, most patients are reassured by their treatment in the unit [2, 12].

Prior to arrival in the CCU, there is little opportunity to address the patient's emotional distress. In the emergency room the first priority is to manage the medical situation and stabilize the patient's medical condition. Treatment of fear and anxiety is usually limited to explaining the problem, administering medication to control ischemia and pain, and reassuring the patient [15]. Additional simple interventions that do not interfere with emergency room activities are possible.

If possible, the patient should not be left unattended. When left alone, the patient may imagine the worst, creating in his or her mind a situation far gloomier than reality. Anxiolytic medication should be provided to those patients who are unduly distressed, rather than waiting until they arrive in the CCU.

Anxiety
Once the patient arrives in the CCU, emotional distress can be more thoroughly assessed. The characteristics of anxiety (Fig. 32–1) that are frequently observed in MI patients include fear of death and disability, a sense of dread and foreboding, tremulousness, restlessness, and insomnia. Increased sympathetic nervous system activity is also observed, which can produce increased levels of catecholamines, resulting in tachycardia, tachypnea, diaphoresis, hypertension, or ventricular ectopy. Increases in cardiac output, peripheral resistance, and myocardial oxygen consumption may also result [33].

It is important to familiarize the patient with the CCU. This measure involves explaining equipment that is used, restrictions that are imposed (e.g., bed rest), and the unit's routine (e.g., regular monitoring of vital signs during

Fig. 32-1
Typical time course of emotional reaction to a myocardial infarction. (From N. H. Cassem and T. P. Hackett. Psychiatric consultation in a coronary care unit. *Ann. Intern. Med.* 75:9, 1971. With permission.)

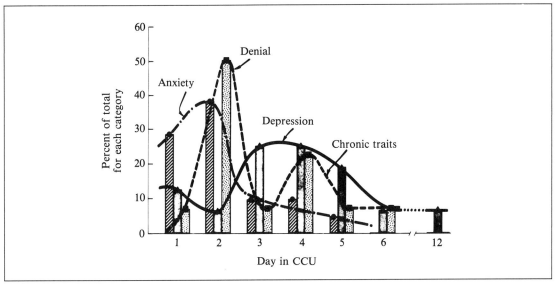

the night). The patient is likely to be easily distracted and may have a short attention span. Therefore short, simple explanations are preferred. Even simple explanations may have to be repeated several times before they are comprehended.

Listening to the patient and providing appropriate reassurance is also important. Patients often harbor unrealistic fears that can be debilitating. Sometimes these fears are expressed directly, but more commonly they are expressed indirectly in comments about the need for others to care for the children or discussion of a will. The patient may not be immediately receptive to support and reassurance and may require encouragement to express his or her concerns.

Pharmacologic treatment of anxiety should also be considered, especially for patients who exhibit heightened autonomic responses to stressful stimuli [15, 32]. Benzodiazepines are the drugs of choice for the treatment of anxiety. Diazepam 5 to 10 mg orally every 8 hours is recommended for MI patients [32]. When benzodiazepines are used, they should be ordered on a fixed-dose schedule rather than on an as-needed schedule because many patients who need medication fail to request it.

Overall, most patients cope with the emotional ordeal of the MI well. Elevated anxiety typically continues for the first day or two and then diminishes as the patient's medical condition stabilizes [6, 12, 18, 34]. As chest pain and shortness of breath decrease, fear of death abates and concern about the future begins to emerge. With the realization that he or she is physically limited and that life style changes are necessary, the patient may experience sadness and a sense of loss [6, 12, 34].

Depression

Depression is a common reaction to severe illness and is probably seen in about 50 percent of MI patients [35], but the depression observed at this early point in recovery is usually transient (Fig. 32-1). Sometimes, however, the patient becomes despondent, pessimistic about the future, hopeless, or withdrawn. Often it is difficult to recognize that the patient is depressed because he or she does not complain about the symptoms or even denies the depression. If the patient is pessimistic about recovery or is withdrawn and inactive, rehabilitation may be compromised.

Patients' perceptions of their health status strongly influence depression. If they believe they will be severely restricted in their activities, they are more likely to become depressed. This situation is especially likely to occur if fatigue and weakness are interpreted as evidence of cardiac decline. For most patients, depression can be alleviated by education, early ambulation, involvement in rehabilitation activities, and reassurance from the medical staff [15]. Aside from preventing deconditioning and other complications of prolonged bed rest, early ambulation provides a clear message that patients are expected to regain their health and to become active again. With early ambulation, the patients' emotional status and self-image generally improve [4, 36, 37]. Early involvement in rehabilitative activities emphasizes that the patient is expected to recover and return to a normal or near-normal life style. Education should be initiated early, with the goal of helping the patient understand the infarction and its management. Information about the anatomy and function of the heart should be provided so that patients can understand why the infarct occurred and how healing takes place. Coronary risk factors must be discussed, with an emphasis on modifiable risk factors. The activities involved in rehabilitation should also be explained (exercise, smoking cessation, diet and weight control, medication).

Patients also should be given the opportunity to discuss their fears and concerns. During this early stage of recovery, worry about ability to support a family, resumption of sexual activity, loss of autonomy, and restriction of leisure activities are common. Patients often have misconceptions about the MI that contribute to depression [38]. Chief among them is the belief that the heart is fragile after infarction and that it will "give out" if subjected to stress [15]. Patients who harbor this belief are reluctant to exert themselves and consequently severely restrict their activities.

DENIAL

Denial of illness has been reported to be a common response to an acute MI (Fig. 32-1) [2, 3, 6, 27, 28]. According to Cassem and Hackett [6], denial is mobilized as a reaction to heightened anxiety and fear of death and plays an important role in keeping the patient's emotional distress in check. An implication of this argument is that patients who use denial experience less anxiety and depression than those who do not. Moreover, Hackett and Cassem [39] argued that deniers have better survival records in the CCU than non-deniers, although the studies done to date have insufficient statistical power to establish this point with certainty. Consistent with this position, research indicates that patients who use denial during hospitalization tend to be less anxious and have less morbidity and mortality in the CCU [34, 40, 41]. However, excessive use of denial is probably maladaptive for long-term recovery [42]. Interestingly, Hackett and Weisman [43] found no differences in the use of denial between patients with heart disease and those with cancer.

Tesar and Hackett [32] have distinguished between two types of denial. Denial of illness occurs when patients contend that they have not sustained an MI or that their illness is not serious. This type of denial is maladaptive and sets the stage for noncompliance and inappropriate behavior. With the second type of denial, the patient accepts that he or she has sustained an MI but denies fear of its consequences. Patients who use denial in this manner cope by minimizing their fear.

Some of the maladaptive behaviors that have been linked to denial of illness are insistence on return to normal activities, inappropriate behavior (e.g., smoking, sexually provoking the nurses), and hostility [6]. When such problems arise, a concerted effort must be made to elicit the patient's cooperation [32]. Sometimes reassurance and clarification of misconceptions is sufficient to solve the problem. Repeated efforts to convince the patient of the gravity of the situation are rarely effective, however, and can exacerbate the problem. When such efforts fail, tactful confrontation may be necessary to change the inappropriate behavior. Caution must be exercised, however, so that staff do not express anger and frustration when confronting a problematic patient. Working with the staff to help them develop a constructive approach to this type of patient is productive.

INFREQUENT PSYCHOSIS-LIKE FEATURES

Some seriously ill patients become agitated or delirious while in the CCU (Fig. 32-1) [15, 32]. For some patients, delirium or agitation is a manifestation of extreme anxiety. Other determinants of these problems include metabolic disturbances, insufficient cerebral blood flow secondary to dropping cardiac output, hypoxia, adverse medication effects (including lidocaine toxicity, and the "paradoxical" agitation sometimes seen with sedatives and opiates), sleep deprivation, or environmental factors such as noise or monotony [3, 15, 32].

Appropriate intervention for these conditions depends on identification of the underlying cause. Depending on the etiology, treatment usually involves one or more of the following: discontinuing toxic drugs, correcting metabolic abnormalities, using neuroleptic medication, or ameliorating environmental factors.

INITIAL RISK FACTOR MANAGEMENT

Studies have demonstrated that interventions for risk factor change (e.g., smoking cessation), which are initiated while the patient is in the hospital, and in many cases have already made a change (either because of hospital policy or because of the impact of the recent event), produce higher continued cessation or maintenance rates than when counseling is delayed until after discharge [44–46]. As change has already often been initiated, the interventions used must include those oriented toward helping the patient to develop the skills needed to resist returning to old behaviors, i.e., "relapse prevention" skills [47, 48]. Perhaps most importantly for the health care provider, it is essential that he or she deliver a strong message advising change. Without it the patient is likely to think that a risk factor change such as smoking cessation is not especially important, as the physician did not give the issue any weight. The physician and other health care providers can also spend a few minutes assisting the patient to decide on an appropriate approach to making or maintaining the change and to develop a plan. The more input and assistance provided by the physician and the health care team, the greater is the likelihood of change [49]. Perhaps the most important factor in change of behavior is the patient's commitment to change, and the health care team can provide support to facilitate this commitment. The topic of risk factor modification is more extensively discussed in the next section.

Psychological Adjustment During Early Convalescence

EMOTIONAL STATUS

Depression is one of the most significant problems confronted by MI patients during the weeks following discharge from the hospital [2, 15, 28, 38, 50]. Cessation of sexual activity, unwarranted restriction of activity, social withdrawal, insomnia, and failure to return to work are some of the problems that are related to depression [38]. The physical inactivity that often accompanies depression also may contribute to deterioration in medical status because of physical deconditioning [4, 37]. Early rehabilitation efforts instill optimism about a quick recovery, but this optimism may quickly dissipate when patients begin to confront the realities of their disability and struggle to implement life style changes. Patients test their physical capacities and reassess their health status [51]. During these early weeks following discharge, complaints about anxiety and nervousness, weakness, tearfulness, diminished appetite, fear of sexual arousal, social withdrawal, disturbed sleep, pessimism about the future, and a sense of uselessness are common [2, 15, 29, 38].

The patient may experience weakness and fatigue with increased activity [4, 37]. When patients return home, they are usually deconditioned because of extended bed rest. As a result, they may fatigue with ordinary activities, such as walking around the yard. Unaware that weakness is due to muscle atrophy and other effects of immobilization, MI patients attribute these symptoms to a damaged heart.

Unless patients are forewarned to expect this weakness and fatigue, they are likely to worry that their disease is more severe than they believed. When even minimal activity produces noticeable fatigue and weakness, it is difficult for the uninformed patient to imagine a return to normal activities. Coupled with the often severe restrictions on smoking, diet, and alcohol, patients may perceive a future marked by limitations.

DENIAL

As already discussed, denial can be a useful protective mechanism whereby the individual minimizes the importance of the cardiac event and can thereby more easily get on with life. Once the patient is beyond the acute event, however, he or she must deal with the need to go through an appropriate rehabilitation process and alter risk factors to diminish the likelihood of a recurrence. At this point denial beyond a level needed to minimize anxiety becomes counterproductive, with the individual resisting making necessary changes (continuing to smoke, permitting excessive physical stress) because "it isn't that serious," and avoiding problem-solving behavior [52, 53].

Levine et al. [42] developed a new scale for assessing denial that built on the Hackett–Cassem denial scale [54]. Using this instrument they demonstrated that increased denial led to more rapid recovery early on, but that these patients had more difficulty during the following year, being less compliant with rehabilitation regimens and requiring more days of hospitalization. Levine et al. concluded:

Denial of illness is adaptive as a coping response in emergency situations when the cardiovascular system is dysfunctional or excessively stressed and no immediate action is necessary or possible. Under these conditions denial of illness blocks added stressor input. However, when the patient's medical condition has become stabilized, denial of illness is maladaptive because continued blocking or distortion of cognitive and affective processes prevents realistic appraisal and motivation for necessary action.

SOCIAL SUPPORT AND FAMILY DISTRESS

Social support has in recent years taken on increasing significance as a major determinant of psychological outcome of disease [55–58]. A complex interaction occurs between patient, family, and professional staff. The family's ability to provide support to the patient is to a large extent dependent on family members' own psychological strength, the distress they are experiencing, and their assessment of the gravity of the patient's illness. The skill of the professional staff in providing support and information to the family members may significantly affect the latter's ability to provide the patient with much-needed support [59]. Family members also benefit from the opportunity to discuss their fears and concerns about caring for the MI patient.

Studies of social support in myocardial infarction are relatively limited. Speedling [57] found that spouses were often more distressed than patients during the acute hospitalization and suggested that the medical structure may have a negative effect on families, restricting access to the patient by limiting visiting hours and surrounding the patient with layers of formidable technology and busy caregivers. Lack of control and unavailability of adequate information, fear of the hospital environment, and concern over changing family roles and altered finances also play important roles as family stressors [60, 61].

Sociocultural factors are also important. Ell and Haywood [62] looked at socioeconomic status and other variables among Blacks, Hispanics, and Anglos as they related to coping mechanisms following an MI. In general, family support was associated with improved

function, but among the Hispanic patients a supportive family and close attachments were most positively correlated with self-esteem and positive well-being but negatively associated with personal functioning, suggesting that perhaps the cared-for individual was being *overly* cared for. Although social networking was in general salutary, other cultural differences were seen. The authors emphasized the need to take cultural considerations into account when planning rehabilitative programs and pointed out the need for further research in this area.

It seems clear that family members should be incorporated into the therapeutic environment of the patient and given the information necessary so that they can play an informed, nonconflicting role. This point is true while the patient is in the hospital [58] and is even more evident once the patient returns home. Spouses and other family members can offer important support and understanding at a crucial time and be effective advocates for life style change to alter risk factor levels [62]. Often, however, the convalescent period is marked by conflict between the patient and spouse, with differing opinions on the timing of the patient's resumption of activity being the most common area of friction [63]. Again, providing adequate and clear information and guidance to both patient and family during the days prior to discharge is valuable and important. The entire team—physician, nurses, rehabilitation personnel—should be involved, with appropriate coordination so that different caregivers deliver the same message. Nothing causes more confusion and family friction than a conservative rehabilitation team saying "no driving for a month" whereas the patient's physician, unaware, says "you can drive in a week." Patients and families often have a sense of having been cast adrift during the first few weeks after discharge as they make the adjustment from intense contact and supervision in the hospital to the far more infrequent caregiver contact once the patient is home. The specific importance of the nurse in assisting the spouse and the specific opportunity provided by the peridischarge period were emphasized by Bramwell [61], who noted that the receptiveness of patient and spouse during this critical time should be effectively utilized.

In an interesting 3-year follow-up study of 2330 post-MI patients, Ruberman et al. [20] found that two major psychosocial factors affected subsequent mortality: stress level related to such traumatic events as marital separation, forced retirement, or financial difficulty; and social isolation, with a lack of contact with family, friends, or social organizations. Individuals with high levels of either stress or social isolation suffered an approximately twofold increase in mortality, especially that due to sudden death, and the two factors demonstrated an additive effect. Marital status alone also is associated with post-MI survival, with married patients having significantly better survival rates than nonmarried individuals [64].

The beneficial effect of social support may manifest through such "physical" forms as providing transportation, cooking heart-healthy meals, doing household work, providing financial support; through "moral support" mechanisms such as encouraging and supporting risk-factor alteration, stress reduction, and healthier work patterns; through the direct psychological effects of companionship; or through a combination of these mechanisms. More research is needed in this area.

Interventions directed at the family must be done with care and sensitivity lest they cause more harm than good. It is considered important to train family members of patients with CHD in resuscitative techniques [65]. However, in an interesting study Dracup et al. [66] demonstrated that patients whose family members had been taught cardiopulmonary resuscitation (CPR) were more anxious at 3 month's follow-up than were those whose family members had not been given such training, and the family members themselves derived no psychological benefit from the training. Thus breaking through a denial mechanism or increasing dependency/responsibility feelings of patients and family members may be counterproductive and must be done carefully.

On a more promising note, Taylor et al. [67] carried out an interesting intervention study

directed at reducing spouse anxiety. During the patient's week 3 exercise test, spouses were randomized either to wait in the waiting room or to attend the exercise test and then go on the treadmill themselves for 3 minutes at their husband's maximum workload. The wives who experienced their husband's workload capabilities increased their ratings of their husbands' ability to handle exercise and stress. This type of intervention should narrow the gap between husband's and wife's perceptions of what the post-MI patient can and cannot do.

RISK FACTOR MODIFICATION

Although the best prevention is primary prevention, the increasing success of our treatment of acute MI is resulting in a large pool of individuals who have had an infarct and in whom prevention of another clinical event is a primary goal. Within 5 years of an infarction, 13 percent of men and almost 40 percent of women suffer a second infarction [68]. The evidence in favor of the important role of risk factor modification in primary prevention of CHD is overwhelming [69]. Although the evidence in favor of secondary prevention is not as strong, numerous studies suggest that post-MI patients benefit from risk factor intervention. Cessation of cigarette smoking results in a 50 percent reduction of mortality in post-MI patients compared to those who continue to smoke [70–72]. Progression of coronary artery disease (CAD) as measured by quantitative angiography is significantly reduced by cholesterol reduction in patients with clinical CAD [31]. Although trials demonstrating a clear benefit of antihypertensive therapy in post-MI patients do not yet exist, such therapy appears logical in view of the known potency of hypertension as a risk factor for CHD and the increased risk of post-MI patients for congestive heart failure and stroke.

Smoking Cessation
Cigarette smoking is one of the most important modifiable risk factors for CAD in the United States today [73]. Certainly it is in the

best interest of the post-MI patient to stop smoking, and fortunately as many as 50 percent do stop immediately after an infarction. However, many eventually resume smoking [74]. An important role of a cardiac rehabilitation program is to help those who have already quit to stay quit and to assist those who have not yet stopped in their efforts at cessation. A variety of smoking cessation techniques, ranging from individual and group sessions to aversive therapy, are available, with all having some short-term success [75–79]. The most effective methods are the multicomponent or "broad spectrum" approaches, which incorporate interventions to deal with the psychological, physiologic, and social aspects of smoking. Although there are many approaches available, most smokers do not go to formal smoking cessation programs, with fewer than 10 percent of smokers who quit having "attended" a special program. Thus the health care team and the setting to which the patient is exposed become important channels for intervention. Patients who are committed to change generally adhere to prescribed regimens and are more often successful. The health care provider may find a number of excellent self-help booklets available from the American Heart Association, the American Lung Association, and the American Cancer Society, all of which are of use to the patient and discuss available alternative options, such as formal smoking cessation programs. Other risk factors, such as nutrition, exercise, and stress, are also behaviorally related, and similar techniques should be of value for all [80].

"Type A" Personality

No discussion of psychological factors and myocardial infarction would be complete without mention of the "type A" controversy. Since the 1950s Rosenman and Friedman and others [21, 81, 82] have put forward the thesis that individuals who are "type A"—defined as hard-driving, competitive, time-oriented, and aggressive—are at increased risk for the development of CAD. An independent panel in 1981 recognized type A behavior as a risk factor for CHD [83]. Nonetheless, other studies have failed to replicate these findings, including the Multiple Risk Factor Intervention Trial, the Aspirin Myocardial Infarction Study, and the Beta Blocker Heart Attack Trial [20, 84, 85]. The proponents of the type A hypothesis have claimed methodologic error in these negative studies. In an especially interesting study, Friedman et al. [86] reported on the results of a controlled study of a program (the Recurrent Coronary Prevention Program) designed to modify the type A characteristics of individuals post-MI. They found that type A behavior could be modified, and that individuals exhibiting such behavior modification had significantly fewer recurrences of nonfatal infarction than the control subjects given only cardiac counseling. At 4.5-years of follow-up, a significant difference in cardiac deaths was also noted. In a later report [87] it was noted that the individuals who had been in the type A counseling group maintained their lowered intensity of type A behavior and their lowered cardiac recurrence rates for the 1-year follow-up period after the end of the counseling program.

To date, the results of the Recurrent Coronary Prevention Program have not been reproduced, although there have been no attempts to do so. The study is of considerable importance, and an effort to confirm its findings is needed.

More recently, Ragland and Brand [88] returned to the original Western Collaborative Group Study [82] and looked at the survival patterns of 257 men from the original group. The average follow-up was 12.7 years among the 160 type A patients and 11.5 years among the 71 type B patients. Unexpectedly, the subsequent mortality in patients surviving more than 24 hours following the myocardial infarction was significantly lower in the type A patients. An editorial accompanying that article [89] summarized the available literature, and concluded, "It is important to acknowledge that *something* is going on in terms of the relation between personality and heart disease. However, the nature of that influence is far more complex than is conveyed by the simple assertion that type A behavior is a risk factor for coronary heart disease."

Psychological and Behavioral Adjustment During Late Convalescence Rehabilitation

MAINTENANCE OF RISK FACTOR MODIFICATION

Relapse or return to old behaviors is common among individuals who have made changes, even among those who had had an MI. Thus continued support and interventions aimed at maintenance of risk factor change continue to be important even after a year of maintained change. Several patterns of relapse occur. Typical patterns include the presence of extended withdrawal effects leading to a conscious decision to return to smoking; a slip under unusual circumstances (e.g., a family crisis) followed by a quick relapse; a gradual return to regular smoking following rationalized use ("one won't hurt"). Smokers are often consistent in their relapse patterns; thus these patterns can be identified, and counseling can be directed toward their prevention.

Steps can be taken to ensure a greater likelihood of maintained cessation. First, the former smoker can identify previous "high-risk" situations that triggered smoking and prepare for them. Next, the former smoker can practice ways of dealing with these situations without cigarettes. Helping patients to develop healthy behaviors (e.g., exercise) in place of unhealthy behaviors such as smoking facilitates maintenance of risk factor change.

SEXUAL ADJUSTMENT

Sexual dysfunction following myocardial infarction is common, occurring to some degree in as many as 50 percent of patients [2, 90]. Reasons for sexual dysfunction include fear of inducing another infarction during intercourse, fear that sexual activity may be excessively stressful, and a general spousal oversolicitousness that may contribute to the patient's lowered self-esteem [91]. Although physical causes for sexual dysfunction are also possible (decreased cardiac output, progressive atherosclerosis, drug effects such as beta-blocker-induced impotence), they are considerably less common than psychogenic causes [92]. Also mentioned as a possible etiology for post-MI sexual dysfunction is the desire by one or both partners to use the infarction for discontinuing what was already an unsatisfactory relationship [93].

Providing adequate information and giving patients and their spouses permission to resume sexual activity is important. Excellent discussions of sex and the cardiac patient can be found in books written for the lay public by Alpert [93] and Cambre [94]. Patients and their partners need to understand that:

1. The risk of death during sexual activity is low. In a study of 5559 cases of sudden death, only 0.6 percent were related to sexual activity, and most of these deaths involved extramarital partners averaging 20 years younger than the victim and occurring in unfamiliar surroundings [95].
2. Sexual activity is normally "moderate" in intensity, comparable to climbing stairs, as an exercise [96]. Peak heart rates rarely exceed 120 beats per minute and maintain this level for only 10 to 15 seconds. Therefore sexual activity can be resumed at about the same time stairclimbing can be resumed, generally 2 to 4 weeks after the infarction.
3. Although it is common for cardiac patients to be advised to assume the bottom position during sexual activity, there is little evidence that body position affects heart rate or blood pressure [97]. Therefore there is no reason to advise the patient and spouse to add the stress of unfamiliar positions.
4. Many of the normal physiologic consequences of sexual activity produce sensations that the patient is apt to interpret as related to heart disease. Heavy breathing, a rapid heart rate, a sense of congestion in the chest, and sweating are normal accompaniments of lovemaking, but the sensitized patient is liable to be frightened by them [50].

Other reasonable recommendations include avoiding sexual activity immediately after food or alcohol consumption, as both increase heart rate; avoiding temperature extremes; and avoiding sex when fatigued or upset [92].

Intervention Programs

Psychosocial intervention programs are an accepted part of present-day cardiac rehabilitation services, yet there are few well controlled studies to support their use. Several studies have suggested reduced morbidity and mortality from psychological intervention [98, 99]. In Rahe et al.'s study [99] patients in the intervention group attended six biweekly sessions beginning 1 month after hospital discharge. Spouses attended only one session. Patients who received group therapy were described as having significantly lower morbidity and mortality, although there was no difference in risk factor alteration. Educational information given to the intervention group was forgotten at follow-up. Of interest, and common to many studies of this type, was the small sample size: 22 patients in each group. In addition, the authors chose to define significance at the .15 level (the mortality difference was $p = .12$). Mumford et al. [100] reviewed 34 controlled studies of intervention in surgical and myocardial infarction patients and concluded that the provision of information and emotional support during a medical crisis resulted in a shorter hospital stay than did routine medical care alone. In recent years, with increasing emphasis being placed on the cost-effectiveness of interventions, there has been an increasing tendency to shift from time- and personnel-intensive psychotherapy toward more broadly diffusible behavioral and educational interventions. Education alone can be effective in allaying patients' anxieties and fear: Mazzuca [101] concluded that patient education alone can be as therapeutic as more expensive psychological interventions.

Oldenburg et al. [102] carried out a controlled study in post-MI patients that compared two in-hospital interventions, education and counseling, with routine medical and nursing care. The educational intervention consisted of relaxation procedures and the provision of information about heart disease and its treatment. The counseling intervention

included the educational interventions as well as six to ten counseling sessions. All of these interventions took place while the patient was in the hospital; no further intervention was provided once the patient was discharged. At 3, 6, and 12 months of follow-up, both intervention groups did significantly better than the control group on tests of psychological and life style functioning, and they were also less symptomatic and less dependent on medical treatment. The authors suggested that these results compare favorably with those seen in outpatient cardiac rehabilitation programs.

In a particularly interesting study, Stern et al. [103] randomized 106 post-MI patients to one of three groups: exercise therapy, group counseling, or control. Subjects who failed to reach a workload of 7 METs (multiples of resting oxygen consumption) on exercise testing were rated as anxious, depressed, or both. Each intervention lasted 12 weeks, with follow-up for 1 year. Exercise increased mean work capacity, decreased fatigue, lessened anxiety and depression, and promoted independence and sociability. Counseling substantially reduced depression, decreased interpersonal friction, and led to greater independence and sociability. The control group showed no significant changes. No mortality differences were seen. With time, however, these differences narrowed, and by the end of the follow-up period there was little difference between the three groups. The authors note that an optimum rehabilitation program would probably include both exercise and counseling interventions.

The best cardiac rehabilitation programs do not separate behavioral interventions but integrate them into an interdisciplinary program that combines physical activity, risk factor intervention, education, nutrition, networking, and emotional support [104].

RETURN TO WORK

Within the first 6 months after an acute MI approximately 75 percent of previously employed individuals return to work [2, 105]. A number of factors, including medical complications during hospitalization, higher age, lower education, higher perceived pre-MI job stress, and rural residence were found to correlate with a lesser likelihood of returning to work [107]. In a later study Mæland and Havik [106] evaluated the relation between likelihood of return to work (RTW) 6 months after an MI and a series of psychological and other factors in 249 patients under 67 years of age, with a number of interesting findings.

Patients characterized by marked hopelessness were less likely to return to work than those less pessimistic. Interestingly, there was a significant negative correlation between years of education and levels of hopelessness; both were independently related to RTW. Denial showed a bipolar response; patients in the lowest and the highest quartiles were less likely to return to work than were patients with moderate denial scores. The RTW rate was strongly related to levels of anxiety and depression as reported by the patients during hospitalization and at 6 weeks' follow-up, and it was independent of age, educational level, or severity of infarction.

The patients' basic knowledge about heart disease was unrelated to RTW, but levels of cardiac life style knowledge (risk factors, behavioral factors) were strongly related to RTW. However, the significance of this relationship disappeared when educational levels were taken into account; education and cardiac life style knowledge were closely related.

Expectation of future work capacity was strongly and linearly related to RTW; patients who anticipated few problems had a nearly threefold higher RTW rate than those who expected the greatest reduction in work capacity. This relationship was also independent of the patient's age or the severity of the infarction. Although expectation of future work capacity was correlated with educational level and level of perceived job stress, the association between expectation of future work capacity and RTW remained highly significant even after controlling for these potential confounders. This central role of patient expectation in predicting RTW has been noted by others for both myocardial infarction and coronary artery bypass surgery [35, 107, 108].

The lack of relation of expectation of return to work to severity of MI and to work-related factors makes it unlikely that the patients' expectations simply reflect the underlying reality of their situation; negative expectations may act as self-fulfilling prophecies by leading to passivity and feelings of helplessness.

In summary, discriminant function analysis reduced the number of variables independently predictive of failure to return to work to three: negative expectations, the experience of negative moods, and insufficient knowledge of the effect of life style on heart disease. Each represents a different set of the patient's psychological make-up: attitude, emotion, and knowledge. The best clinical predictor of return to work is the simple maneuver of asking the patient his or her own opinion of the likelihood of such an event occurring; such a finding is also seen in other areas of patient behavior, such as smoking cessation, where a potent predictor of success is a similar "do you believe you will be smoking one year from now" type of question [109]. In these areas, the patient knows him- or herself best.

Mæland and Havik concluded that the patient's perceived illness plays a central role in the coping and readaptation process that occurs after the acute event. They suggested that early rehabilitative intervention may successfully alter the patient's initial expectations and facilitate recovery.

Summary

In the process of caring for a patient with a serious organic illness such as a myocardial infarction, the attention given to psychosocial and behavioral factors is often inadequate. Yet such critical factors as the patient's quality of life, return to work, and even the likelihood of recurrent infarction depend to a large extent to the attention given these issues immediately after the infarction and during the entire rehabilitative process. The physician and health care team not only must deliver adequate care in these areas but must also learn to work together in a coordinated manner, so that the whole patient, mind and body, derives maximum benefit.

References

1. Croog, S. H. Recovery and rehabilitation of heart patients: Psychosocial aspects. In D. S. Krantz, A. Baum, and J. E. Singer (eds.), *Handbook of Psychology and Health* (Vol. 3). Hillsdale, N.J.: Erlbaum, 1983. Pp. 295–334.
2. Doehrman, S. R. Psycho-social aspects of recovery from coronary heart disease: A review. *Soc. Sci. Med.* 2:199, 1977.
3. Razin, A. M. Psychosocial intervention in coronary artery disease: A review. *Psychosom. Med.* 44:363, 1982.
4. Wenger, N. K., and Hellerstein, H. K. (eds.). *Rehabilitation of the Coronary Patient* (2nd ed.). New York: Wiley, 1984.
5. Mayou, R., Williamson, B., and Foster, A. Outcome two months after myocardial infarction. *J. Psychosom. Res.* 22:439, 1978.
6. Cassem, N. H., and Hackett, T. P. Psychiatric consultation in a coronary care unit. *Ann. Intern. Med.* 75:9, 1971.
7. Ott, C., Sivarajan, E. S., Newton, K. M., et al. A controlled randomized study of early cardiac rehabilitation: The sickness impact profile as an assessment tool. *Heart Lung* 12:162, 1983.
8. Stern, M., Pascale, L., and Ackerman, A. Life adjustment post-myocardial infarction: Determining predictive variables. *Arch. Intern. Med.* 137:1680, 1977.
9. Byrne, D. G. Psychological responses to illness and outcome after survived myocardial infarction: A long term follow-up. *J. Psychosom. Res.* 26:105, 1982.
10. Mayou, R., Foster, A., and Williamson, B. Medial care after myocardial infarction. *J. Psychosom. Res.* 23:23, 1979.
11. Wiklund, I., Sanne, H., Vedin, A., and Wilhelmsson, C. Psychosocial outcome one year after a first myocardial infarction. *J. Psychosom. Res.* 28:309, 1984.
12. Cay, E. L., Vetter, N., Philip, A. E., and Dugard, P. Psychological status during recovery from acute heart attack. *J. Psychosom. Res.* 16:425, 1972.
13. Mayou, R. Prediction of emotional and social outcome after a heart attack. *J. Psychosom. Res.* 28:17, 1984.
14. Stern, M. J., Pascale, L., and McLoone, J. B. Psychosocial adaptation following an acute myocardial infarction. *J. Chronic Dis.* 29:513, 1976.
15. Stern, M. J. Psychosocial rehabilitation following myocardial infarction and coronary artery bypass surgery. In N. K. Wenger and H. K. Hellerstein (eds.), *Rehabilitation of the Coronary Patient* (2nd ed.). New York: Wiley, 1984. Pp. 453–471.
16. Zelnik, T. Depressive effects of drugs. In N. Cameron (ed.), *Presentations of Depression*. New York: Wiley, 1987. Pp. 355–400.
17. Vetter, N. J., Strange, R. C., Adams, W., and Oliver, M. F. Initial metabolic and hormonal response to acute myocardial infarction. *Lancet* 1:284, 1974.
18. Klein, R. F., Garrity, T. F., and Gelein, J. Emotional adjustment and catecholamine excretion during early recovery from myocardial infarction. *J. Psychosom. Res.* 18:425, 1974.
19. Wenger, N. K. Early ambulation after myocardial infarction: Rationale, program components, and results. In N. K. Wenger and H. K. Hellerstein (eds.), *Rehabilitation of the Coronary Patient* (2nd ed.). New York: Wiley, 1984. Pp. 97–113.
20. Ruberman, W., Weinblatt, E., Goldberg, J. D., and Chaudhary, B. S. Psychosocial influences on mortality after myocardial infarction. *N. Engl. J. Med.* 311:552, 1984.
21. Jenkins, C. D., Zyzanski, S. J., and Rosenman, R. H. Risk of new myocardial infarction in middle aged men with manifest coronary heart disease. *Circulation* 53:342, 1976.
22. Moos, R. H. Coping with acute health crisis. In T. Millon, C. Green, and R. Meagher (eds.), *Handbook of Clinical Health Psychology*. New York: Plenum, 1982. Pp. 129–151.
23. Argondizzo, N. T. Education of the patient and family. In N. K. Wenger and H. K. Hellerstein (eds.), *Rehabilitation of the Coronary Patient* (2nd ed.). New York: Wiley, 1984. Pp. 161–178.
24. Bilodeau, C. B., and Hackett, T. P. Issues raised in a group setting by patients recovering from myocardial infarction. *Am. J. Psychiatry* 128:73, 1971.
25. Skelton, M., and Dominian, J. Psychological stress in wives of patients with myocardial infarction. *Br. Med. J.* 2:101, 1983.
26. Stern, M. J. and Pascale, L. Psychosocial adaptation post-myocardial infarction: The spouse's dilemma. *J. Psychosom. Res.* 23:83, 1979.
27. Krantz, D. S., and Deckel, W. Coping with coronary heart disease and stroke. In T. G. Burish and L. A. Bradley (eds.), *Coping with Chronic Disease*. New York: Academic Press, 1983. Pp. 85–112.
28. Razin, A. M. Coronary artery disease: Reducing risk and aiding recovery. In A. M. Razin (ed.), *Helping Cardiac Patients*. San Francisco: Jossey-Bass, 1985. Pp. 157–193.
29. Gulledge, A. D. The psychological aftermath of a myocardial infarction. In W. D. Gentry

and R. B. Williams (eds.), *Psychological Aspects of Myocardial Infarction and Coronary Care*. St. Louis: Mosby, 1975. Pp. 107–123.

30. Weinblatt, E., Shapiro, S., Frank, C. W., and Sagar, R. V. Prognosis of men after myocardial infarction: Mortality and first recurrence in relation to selected parameters. *Am. J. Public Health* 58:1329, 1968.

31. Blankenhorn, D. H., Nessim, S. A., Johnson, R. L., et al. Beneficial effects of combined colestipol-niacin therapy on coronary atherosclerosis and coronary venous bypass grafts. *J.A.M.A.* 257:3233, 1987.

32. Tesar, G. E., and hackett, T. Psychiatric management of the hospitalized cardiac patient. In D. S. Krantz and J. A. Blumenthal (eds.), *Behavioral Assessment and Management of Cardiovascular Disorders*. Sarasota, FL: Professional Resource Exchange, 1987. Pp. 67–80.

33. Tolson, W. W., Mason, J. W., Sachar, E. J., et al. Urinary catecholamine responses associated with hospital admission in normal human subjects. *J. Psychosom. Res.* 8:365, 1965.

34. Hackett, T. P., Cassem, N. H., and Wishnie, H. A. The coronary-care unit: An appraisal of its psychologic hazards. *N. Engl. J. Med.* 279:1365, 1968.

35. Croog, S. H., and Levine, S. *The Heart Patient Recovers*. New York: Human Sciences Press, 1977. Pp. 102–106.

36. Sivarajan, E. S., Bruce, R. A., Almes, M. J., et al. In-hospital exercise after myocardial infarction does not improve treadmill performance. *N. Engl. J. Med.* 305:357, 1981.

37. Wenger, N. K. Rehabilitation of the patient with acute myocardial infarction during hospitalization: Early ambulation and patient education. In M. L. Pollock and D. H. Schmidt (eds.), *Heart Disease and Rehabilitation* (2nd ed.). New York: Wiley, 1986. Pp. 405–421.

38. Hackett, T. P. Depression following myocardial infarction. *Psychosomatics* 26 (Suppl): 23, 1985.

39. Hackett, T. P., and Cassem, N. H. Psychological adaptation to convalescence in myocardial infarction patients. In J. P. Naughton, H. K. Hellerstein, and I. C. Mohler (eds.), *Exercise Testing and Experience Training in Coronary Heart Disease*. New York: Academic Press, 1973.

40. Froese, A., Hackett, T. P., Cassem, N. H., and Silverberg, E. L. Trajectories of anxiety and depression in denying and nondenying acute myocardial infarction patients during hospitalization. *J. Psychosom. Res.* 18:413, 1974.

41. Gentry, W. D., Foster, S., and Haney, T. Denial as a determinant of anxiety and perceived health status in the coronary care unit. *Psychosom. Med.* 34:39, 1972.

42. Levine, J., Warrenburg, S., Kerns, R., et al. The role of denial in recovery from coronary heart disease. *Psychosom. Med.* 49:109. 1987.

43. Hackett, T. P., and Weisman, A. D. Denial as a factor in patients with heart disease and cancer. *Ann. N.Y. Acad. Sci.* 164:802, 1969.

44. Burt, A., Thornley, P., Illingworth, D., et al. Stopping smoking after myocardial infarction. *Lancet* 1:304, 1974.

45. Pozen, M. W., Steckmiller, J. A., Harris, W., et al. A nurse rehabilitator's impact on patients with myocardial infarction. *Med. Care* 15:830, 1977.

46. Johnson, B. L., Cantwell, J. D., and Fletcher, G. F. Eight steps to inpatient cardiac rehabilitation: The team effort—methodology and preliminary results. *Heart Lung* 5:97, 1976.

47. Marlatt, G., and Gordon, J. Determinants of relapse: Implications for the maintenance of behavior change. In W. Davidson (ed.), *Behavioral Medicine: Changing Health Lifestyles*. New York: Brunner/Mazel, 1979.

48. Shiffman, S. Relapse following smoking cessation: A situational analysis. *J. Consult. Clin. Psychol.* 500:71, 1982.

49. Ockene, J. K. Physician-delivered interventions for smoking cessation: Strategies for increasing effectiveness. *Prev. Med.* 16:723, 1987.

50. Hackett, T. P., and Cassem, N. H. Psychologic aspects of rehabilitation after myocardial infarction and coronary artery bypass surgery. In N. K. Wenger and H. K. Hellerstein (eds.), *Rehabilitation of the Coronary Patient* (2nd ed.). New York: Wiley, 1984. Pp. 437–471.

51. Garrity, T. F. Behavior adjustment after myocardial infarction: A selective review of recent descriptive, correlational, and intervention research. In S. M. Weiss, J. A. Herd, and B. H. Fox (eds.), *Perspectives on Behavioral Medicine*. New York: Academic Press, 1981. Pp. 67–87.

52. Lazarus, R. S. The costs and benefits of denial. In S. Breznitz (ed.), *The Denial of Stress*. New York: International Universities Press, 1983.

53. Janis, I. L. Preventing pathogenic denial by means of stress inoculation. In S. Breznitz (ed.), *The Denial of Stress*. New York: International Universities Press, 1983.

54. Hackett, T. P., and Cassem, N. H. Development of a quantitative rating scale to assess denial. *J. Psychosom. Res.* 18:93, 1974.

55. Bruhn, J. G. Effects of chronic illness on the family. *J. Fam. Pract.* 4:1057, 1977.

56. Davidson, D. M. The family and cardiac rehabilitation. *J. Fam. Pract.* 8:253, 1979.

57. Speedling, E. F. *Heart Attack: The Family Response at Home and in the Hospital*. New York: Tavistock, 1982.

58. Waltz, M. Type A, social context, and adaptation to serious illness: A longitudinal investigation of the role of the family in recovery from myocardial infarction. In T. H. Schmidt, T. M. Dembroski, and G. Blumchen (eds.), *Biological and Psychological Factors in Cardiovascular Disease*. Berlin: Springer-Verlag, 1986.

59. Unger, D. G., and Powell, D. R. Supporting families under stress: The role of social networks. *Fam. Relat.* 29:566, 1980.

60. Bedsworth, J. A., and Molen, M. T. Psychological stress in spouses of patients with myocardial infarction. *Heart Lung* 11:450, 1982.

61. Bramwell, L. Wives' experiences in the support role after husbands' first myocardial infarction. *Heart Lung* 15:578, 1986.

62. Ell, K. O., and Haywood, L. J. Social support and recovery from myocardial infarction: A panel study. *J. Soc. Service Res.* 4:1, 1984.

63. Wishnie, H. A., Hackett, T. P., and Cassem, N. H. Psychological hazards of convalescence following myocardial infarction. In R. H. Moos (ed.), *Coping with Physical Illness*. New York: Plenum Press, 1977.

64. Chandra, V., Szklo, M., Goldberg, R., and Tonascia, J. The impact of marital status on survival after an acute myocardial infarction: A population-based study. *Am. J. Epidemiol.* 117:320, 1983.

65. Goldberg, R. J. Physicians and CPR training in high-risk family members. *Am. J. Public Health* 77:671, 1987.

66. Dracup, K., Guzy, P. M., Taylor, S. E., and Barry, J. Cardiopulmonary resuscitation (CPR) training: Consequences for family members of high-risk cardiac patients. *Arch. Intern. Med.* 146:1757, 1986.

67. Taylor, C. B., Bandura, A., Ewart, C. K., et al. Exercise testing to enhance wives' confidence in their husbands cardiac capability soon after clinically uncomplicated acute myocardial infarction. *Am. J. Cardiol.* 55:635, 1985.

68. Kannel, W. B., Thom, T. J., and Hurst, J. W. Incidence, prevalence, and mortality of cardiovascular diseases. In J. W. Willis (ed.), *The Heart* (6th ed.). New York: McGraw-Hill, 1986. P. 560.

69. Goldman, L., and Cook, E. F. The decline in ischemic heart disease mortality rates. *Ann. Intern. Med.* 101:825, 1984.

70. Mulcahy, R., Hickey, N., Graham, I., et al. Factors influencing long-term prognosis in male patients surviving a first coronary heart attack. *Br. Heart J.* 37:158, 1975.

71. Wilhelmsson, C., Vedin, J. A., Elmfeldt, D., et al. Smoking and myocardial infarction. *Lancet* 1:415, 1975.

72. Sparrow, D., Dawber, T., and Colson, T. Influence of cigarette smoking on prognosis after first myocardial infarction. *J. Chronic. Dis.* 31:425, 1978.

73. *The Health Consequences of Smoking: Cardiovascular Disease. A Report of the Surgeon General*. U.S. Department of Health, Education and Welfare, Public Health Service, 1983.

74. Burt, A., Thornley, P., Illingworth, D., et al. Stopping smoking after myocardial infarction. *Lancet* 1:304, 1974.

75. Pechacek, T. F., and McAlister, A. Strategies for the modification of smoking behavior: Treatment and prevention. In J. Ferguson and B. Taylor (eds.), *A Comprehensive Handbook of Behavior Medicine*. New York: Spectrum, 1979.

76. Lichtenstein, E., and Danaher, B. G. Modification of smoking behavior: A critical analysis of theory, research and practice. In M. Hersen, R. M. Eisler, and P. M. Miller (eds.), *Advances in Behavior Modification*. New York: Academic Press, 1976. Pp. 79–132.

77. Bernstein, D. A., and Glasgow, R. E. The modification of smoking behavior. In O. F. Pomerleau and J. P. Brady (eds.), *Behavioral Medicine: Theory and Practice*. Baltimore: Williams & Wilkins, 1979.

78. Syme, S., and Alcahay, R. Control of cigarette smoking from a social perspective. *Annu. Rev. Public Health*. 3:101, 1982.

79. Ockene, J. K., and Ockene, I. S. Nine ways to help your patient stop smoking. *Your Patient and Cancer* 2:47, 1982.

80. Suinn, R. M. Behavior therapy for cardiac patients. *Behav. Res. Ther.* 5:569, 1974.

81. Friedman, M., and Rosenman, R. H. *Type A Behavior and Your Heart*. New York: Alfred A. Knopf, 1974.

82. Rosenman, R. H., Brand, R. J., Jenkins, C. D., et al. Coronary heart disease in the Western Collaborative Group Study: Final follow-up experience of 8.5 years. *J.A.M.A.* 233:872, 1975.

83. Review Panel on Coronary-Prone Behavior and Coronary Heart Disease. Coronary-prone behavior and coronary heart disease: A critical review. *Circulation* 63:1199, 1981.

84. Shekelle, R. B., Hulley, S. B., Neaton, J. D., et al. The MRFIT behavior pattern study. II. Type A behavior and incidence of coronary heart disease. *Am. J. Epidemiol.* 122:559, 1985.

85. Shekelle, R. B., Gale, M., and Norusis, M. Type A score (Jenkins Activity Survey) and risk of recurrent coronary heart disease in the Aspirin Myocardial Infarction Study. *Am. J. Cardiol.* 56:221, 1985.

86. Friedman, M., Thoresen, C. E., Gill, J. J., et al. Alteration of type A behavior and its effect upon cardiac recurrences in post myocardial

infarction subjects: Summary results of the Recurrent Coronary Prevention Project. *Am. Heart J.* 112:653, 1986.

87. Friedman, M., Powell, L. H., and Thoresen, C. E. Effect of discontinuance of type A behavioral counseling on type A behavior and cardiac recurrence rate of post myocardial infarction patients. *Am. Heart J.* 114:483, 1987.

88. Ragland, D. R., and Brand, R. J. Type A behavior and mortality from coronary heart disease. *N. Engl. J. Med.* 318:65, 1988.

89. Dimsdale, J. E. A perspective on type A behavior and coronary disease. *N. Engl. J. Med.* 318:110, 1988.

90. Hellerstein, H. K., and Friedman, E. H. Sexual activity and the post-coronary patient. *Arch. Intern. Med.* 125:987, 1970.

91. Sanders, J. D., and Sprenkle, D. H. Sexual therapy for the post coronary patient. *J. Sex Marital Ther.* 6:174, 1980.

92. Bloch, A., Maeder, J., and Haissly, J. Sexual problems after myocardial infarction. *Am. Heart J.* 90:536, 1975.

93. Alpert, J. S. *The Heart Attack Handbook* (2nd ed.). Boston: Little, Brown, 1985.

94. Cambre, S. *The Sensuous Heart*. Atlanta: Pritchett & Hull, 1978.

95. Ueno, M. The so-called coition death. *Jpn. J. Legal Med.* 17:535, 1963.

96. Hellerstein, H. K., and Friedman, E. H. Sexual activity and the post-coronary patient. *Med. Aspects Hum. Sexuality* 3:70, 1969.

97. Kavanaugh, T., and Shephard, R. J. Sexual activity after myocardial infarction. *Can. Med. J.* 116:1250, 1977.

98. Ibrahim, M. A., Feldman, J. G., Sultz, H. A., et al. Management after myocardial infarction: A controlled trial of the effect of group psychotherapy. *Int. J. Psychiatry Med.* 5:253, 1974.

99. Rahe, R. H., Ward, H. W., and Hayes, V. Brief group therapy in myocardial infarction rehabilitation: Three to four-year follow-up of a controlled trial. *Psychosom. Med.* 41:229, 1979.

100. Mumford, E., Schlesinger, H. J., and Glass, G. The effect of psychological intervention on recovery from surgery and heart attacks: An analysis of the literature. *Am. J. Public Health* 72:141, 1982.

101. Mazzuca, SA. Does patient education in chronic disease have therapeutic value? *J. Chronic Dis.* 35:521, 1982.

102. Oldenburg, B., Perkins, R. J., and Andrews, G. Controlled trial of psychological intervention in myocardial infarction. *J. Consult. Clin. Psychol.* 53:852, 1985.

103. Stern, M. J., Gorman, P. A., and Kaslow, L. The group counseling v exercise therapy study. *Arch. Intern. Med.* 143:1719, 1983.

104. Davidson, D. M., and Maloney, C. A. Recovery after cardiac events. *Phys. Ther.* 65:1820, 1985.

105. Mæland, J. G., and Havik, O. E. Return to work after a myocardial infarction: The influence of background factors, work characteristics and illness severity. *Scand. J. Soc. Med.* 14:183, 1986.

106. Mæland, J. G., and Havik, O. E. Psychological predictors for return to work after a myocardial infarction. *J. Psychosom. Res.* 31:471, 1987.

107. Mayou, R. The course and determinants of reactions to myocardial infarction. *Br. J. Psychiatry* 134:588, 1979.

108. Stanton, B. A., Jenkins, C. D., Denlinger, P., et al. Predictors of employment status after cardiac surgery. *J.A.M.A.* 249:907, 1983.

109. Ockene, J. K., Benfari, R C., Hurwitz, I., et al. Relationship of psychosocial factors to smoking behavior change in an intervention program. *Prev. Med.* 11:13, 1982.

VIII
Postmyocardial Infarction Considerations

33
Exercise Testing After Acute Myocardial Infarction

PIERRE THÉROUX

Exercise testing is now widely used in the investigation of the postmyocardial infarction patient. A Task Force of the American College of Cardiology and of the American Heart Association recently concluded that the test was indicated to evaluate prognosis and functional capacity soon after an uncomplicated myocardial infarction [1]. Ten years ago exercise testing was considered contraindicated in that clinical setting [2].

Pioneer work originating from the Scandinavian countries documented the applicability and the safety of the exercise test performed during the early rehabilitation period [3–6]. Subsequent studies have confirmed the absence of complications and have further described a prognostic implication of the various findings of the test, setting the stage for programs of active management of patients [7–20]. More recent studies have refined the analyses of the various information provided by exercise testing, integrating them with results of other available investigational procedures [21–36]. Concomitant with these developments, therapeutic strategies have been tested to improve prognosis, and emphasis has been put on the positive aspects of early rehabilitation. In recent yers, the management of myocardial infarction has become aggressive, with widespread use of acute interventional procedures. The impact of these procedures on prognosis and risk stratification is now being studied.

Ten years later, exercise testing during the early postinfarction period is not only a method for risk stratification but, more importantly, a tool for direct care of patients.

Factors Influencing Prognosis After Myocardial Infarction

Table 33-1 summarizes the cardiovascular variables associated with a poor prognosis after myocardial infarction and how they can be evaluated.

Myocardial dysfunction, the direct consequence of cell loss, is the main determinant of prognosis [26, 37–39]. The presence of electrical instability not only worsens prognosis [40, 41] it provides independent information [42]. Mechanical dysfunction is conveniently quantified by the ejection fraction and electrical instability via the mean hourly ventricular premature complex (VPC) count on a 24-hour Holter recording.

The third determinant of prognosis is residual ischemia. One manifestation, early spontaneous ischemia during hospitalization for an acute myocardial infarction, occurs in 18 percent of patients and is associated with a high rate of subsequent cardiac complications [43, 44]. The ischemia may be located in the infarct zone or at a distance. In one-third of the patients it is located at a distance from the infarct zone and is associated with multivessel disease. Most often, however, early ischemia is manifested in the infarct zone. It is then more frequent in anterior and non-Q-wave myocardial infarction; multivessel disease is not a prerequisite in this situation, but the artery responsible for the infarct is often patent, suggesting early reperfusion and salvage of myocardium, which remains at risk [45, 46]. Indeed, non-Q-wave myocardial infarction may be considered an unstable state be-

Table 33-1
Predictors of prognosis after myocardial infarction
and their investigation

Left ventricular dysfunction
  Indices of infarct size
  Physical examination
  Radionuclide ventriculography
  Contrast ventriculography
  Echocardiographic studies
Residual ischemia
  Early spontaneous ischemia
  Treadmill exercise test
  Thallium scintigraphy during exercise
  Dipyridamole test
  Exercise radionuclide ventriculography
  Coronary angiography
Ventricular arrhythmias
  Holter monitoring
  Electrophysiologic testing

Table 33-2
Prognostic information derived
from exercise testing

Left ventricular dysfunction
  Tolerance to exercise
  Blood pressure response
  Heart rate response
  ST segment elevation
Residual ischemia
  ST segment depression
  Anginal pain
Ventricular arrhythmias
  Exercise-induced VPCs

cause of the high risk of recurrent infarction
during follow-up [47].

Information Derived from
Exercise Testing

Exercise testing yields information on parameters of cardiac function related to prognosis
(Table 33-2). Thus chest pain and ST segment
depression are usually associated with residual ischemia and more extensive coronary disease [15, 18]. ST segment elevation may occur
in regions of akinetic and dyskinetic wall motion and is often associated with a high QRS
score [48]. Poor left ventricular function also
influences exercise heart rate and blood pressure responses and reduces exercise tolerance. Exercise-induced ventricular premature
beats are associated with more severe regional
wall motion abnormalities in the infarcted area
[49].

None of the above findings, including ST
segment changes, is highly specific because
each can be influenced by a variety of other
factors. The physician should thus consider not a single parameter but the whole patient and all of the data related to him or
her.

HEART RATE

The heart rate and blood pressure responses
during exercise are complex; they are influenced by the level of physical fitness before
the infarction, the deconditioning effect of bed
rest, and the intensity of the early program or
rehabilitation. The physiologic responses may
also be influenced by the altered autonomic
responsiveness often found during the early
postinfarction period and by the various medications. One important determinant, however, is cardiac reserve; the heart with
compromised function reacts excessively, increasing its rate in order to maintain cardiac
output. Various definitions of an inappropriate
increase in heart rate have been used. Among
the studies showing prognostic value, some
have used a heart rate response of more than
125 or 130 beats per minute (bpm) at predefined workloads [6, 16]; others have used the
increase in heart rate from the preexercise
value [17]. In a predischarge, symptom-limited test, the mean heart rate achieved was
greater in nonsurvivors than in survivors [31].
Most of the studies, however, have not found
prognostic value in the increase in heart rate.
Obviously, the heart rate response to exercise
is not be the best indicator of compromised
left ventricular function, and use of this parameter for prognostic value would require
strict, standardized protocols, which is not
now the case. Medications would have to be
avoided, particularly beta blockers [11, 29].
The timing of the test would also have to be

defined, as peak heart rate increases significantly between weeks 3 and 7 after the infarction but not thereafter [50].

BLOOD PRESSURE

Exertional hypotension is an indicator of physiologically severe myocardial ischemia in patients with chronic ischemic disease. The specificity of this finding has been questioned early after myocardial infarction because the 15 percent incidence of hypotension during early testing decreases markedly over the following 4 to 11 weeks [51]. It was suggested that the attenuated heart rate and blood pressure response in patients with well preserved left ventricular function could be caused by stimulation of left ventricular baroreceptors [1].

Many studies, however, have described a worse prognosis when the blood pressure rise was inadequate [12, 17, 20]. In some of these studies, particularly those done more recently, the abnormal response was an independent predictor of prognosis when analyzed jointly with other parameters [29, 31–36]. This prognostic sign did not appear to be significantly influenced by the administration of beta blockers [31, 33–36]. Again a lack of standardization is present because different criteria were used to define the inadequate rise in blood pressure: an increase of less than 5 mm Hg [7], 10 mm Hg [33–35], or 30 mm Hg [31]. In other studies it was defined as a blood pressure below 110 mm Hg [29].

FUNCTIONAL CAPACITY

Reduced exercise capacity is defined as failure to reach a predetermined target workload or heart rate, or in a symptom-limited test a certain level or duration of exercise. The reasons for this failure are usually cardiac and consist of any symptom the patient describes as uncomfortable (e.g., chest pain, dyspnea, fatigue) or an abnormal sign (e.g., marked ST segment depression, a fall in blood pressure, or significant arrhythmias). Reduced exercise capacity is nonspecific and can be related to any of the determinants of prognosis. However, it is sensitive to all the determinants; and, not surprisingly, it is a predictor of prognosis in many studies [11, 14, 21–23, 28, 29, 31–34]. The timing of the test may be important when assessing this parameter, as functional capacity increases markedly during the weeks following an acute myocardial infarction [52] even though left ventricular ejection fraction changes little [53].

ANGINA PECTORIS

The prognostic value of angina pectoris was emphasized mainly in early studies [6, 12, 13, 16–18]. More recent studies have not confirmed these observations [31–36]. Angina pectoris is the classic manifestation of coronary artery disease, and its occurrence during the exercise test is likely to be associated with its occurrence during follow-up [18], particularly when it is present before the infarction [54]. In the presence of both preinfarction angina and a positive test, angina during follow-up was diagnosed in 96 percent of patients; in the absence of these two predictors, it occurred in only 26 percent of patients. Thus the main predictive value of angina relates to the need of subsequent treatment, particularly coronary artery bypass surgery [11, 18, 28, 29]. In one study, surgery was performed in 20 percent of patients with angina during the exercise test compared to 9 percent of the patients without ($p < .001$) [29]. Angina during the test correlates with multivessel disease [18, 55].

The frequency of angina pectoris can vary depending on the protocol used and the timing of the exercise test after myocardial infarction [12, 17]. Angina pectoris occurred in 15 (21 percent) of 70 patients submitted to a symptom-limited protocol before hospital discharge; only nine of these patients had recurrent angina at a test repeated after 6 weeks, whereas 12 others developed new angina [12]. Angina appears to be reproducible at tests performed 3, 7, and 11 weeks after myocardial infarction [50].

Table 33-3
Prognostic value of parameters of exercise tests in various series (1972–1986)

First author	No. of pts.	% With CABG	Heart rate	Blood pressure	Tolerance	Angina	ST segment shift	VPCs	Events Death	Events MI	Events Angina
Granath [6]	205	0	*	—	—	*	—	*	X		
Markiewicz [7]	46	8.7	NS	NS	NS	—	*	*	X		
Théroux [8]	210	5.7	—	—	—	NS	*	*	X	X	
Smith [9]	62	?	—	—	—	—	*	NS	X	X	
Sami [10]	200	9.5	NS	NS	NS	NS	*	*	X	X	
Davidson [11]	195	9.7	—	*	*	*	*	NS	X	X	X
Starling [12]	89	0	—	—	—	*	*	*	X		X
Koppes [13]	90	?	—	—	—	—	*	—	X	X	X
Madsen [14]	205	0	NS	NS	*	*	NS	NS	X		
Schwartz [15]	48	?	NS	NS	NS	—	NS	NS	X		
Lindvall [16]	76	0	*	—	—	*	*	*	X	X	X
Velasco [17]	200	0	*	*	—	*	*	NS	X		
Fuller [18]	40	7.5	—	—	—	*	*	NS	X	X	X
Scrinivasan [19]	154	0	—	—	—	—	*	—	X		
Saunamäki [20]	317	0	*	*	—	—	NS	*	X		
Weld [21]	236	0	—	—	*	—	NS	*	X	X	
Corbett [22]	60	?	NS	NS	*	*	*	NS	X	X	X
De Feyter [23]	179	13.4	—	—	*	NS	NS	NS	X	X	
Gibson [24]	165	15.2	NS	—	NS	*	*	NS	X	X	X
Rapaport [25]	75	?	—	—	—	—	NS	—	X	X	
Norris [26]	325	23.7	—	—	NS	NS	NS	—	X	X	
Dwyer [27]	658	12.8	—	—	NS	NS	NS	—	X	X	
Hung [28]	117	7.7	—	—	*	*	*	*	X	X	
Krone [29]	667	12	*	*	*	*	NS	—	X	X	X
Jespersen [30]	126	1	—	*	—	NS	NS	NS	X	X	
Fioretti [31]	300	15	*	*	*	NS	NS	NS	X		
Madsen [32]	466	0	—	NS	*	NS	NS	*	X	X	
Waters [33]	225	16	NS	*	*	NS	*	*	X		
Handler [34]	222	9	—	*	*	NS	NS	NS	X		
Starling [35]	72	15	—	*	NS	NS	*	NS	X	X	
Fioretti [36]	351	21.7	NS	*	*	NS	NS	NS	X		

NS = nonsignificant; * = denotes statistical significance; X = event considered; — = not analyzed; ? = not reported; CABG = coronary artery bypass grafting; VPCs = ventricular premature complexes; MI = myocardial infarction.

ST Segment Depression

ST segment depression during exercise is observed in 30 to 40 percent of patients. It is associated with extensive coronary artery disease [15, 18, 56–59] and is the single most useful prognostic parameter (Table 33-3). The prognostic value can be influenced by the clinical characteristics of the patient population, the protocol used, the time the test is performed after infarction, and the endpoints analyzed. ST segment depression can predict mortality [8, 20, 30], recurrent myocardial infarction [27, 35], and bypass surgery [29, 34–36]. Its occurrence at low level exercise is associated with a worse prognosis [11]. The magnitude of ST segment depression can also be important [7], and repeated tests may yield more prognostic data than a single test [10]. A symptom-limited exercise test more commonly results in ST segment depression [17], and results are generally reproducible [10, 12, 50].

ST segment depression is often not a specific finding. The use of radionuclide techniques during the treadmill test can distinguish ischemic from nonischemic ST depression, as discussed below.

ST Segment Elevation

ST segment elevation during the exercise testing occurs mainly in electrocardiogram leads overlying the infarct area; its magnitude tends to decrease with time [3]. It is associated with pathologic Q waves, lower ejection fractions, and a greater number of akinetic or dyskinetic segments [15, 60]. It is not an indicator of residual ischemia [60]. The prognostic value associated with ST segment elevation may thus be related more to left ventricular dysfunction than to residual ischemia [15, 33, 60, 61]. As a consequence, it is a weak predictor with no independent value if more accurate parameters of left ventricular function are available.

Ventricular Arrhythmias

Many studies have documented a prognostic value of exercise-induced ventricular arrhyth-mias for predicting mortality during follow-up [6, 7, 21, 29, 33]—more specifically, sudden death [8]. The independent prognostic value of exercise-induced ventricular arrhythmias has been confirmed in multivariate analysis that included clinical and other exercise test data [21, 29, 33]. The frequency of ventricular premature beats increases between tests performed at 3 and 11 weeks after infarction [62] and are stable thereafter [50] in concordance with Holter recording results. The principal pathophysiologic determinant of the ventricular premature beat could be more severe regional wall motion abnormalities in the infarct zone rather than either the number of diseased vessels or global left ventricular dysfunction [49].

Prognostic Value of Exercise Testing

The Confusion

Some of the published results of the prognostic value of exercise testing after myocardial infarction are shown in Table 33-3. At first glance, these results appear confusing. For example, heart rate is predictive of future events in six studies and not predictive in eight; ten studies reported a predictive value for blood pressure response and six no value; exercise tolerance had prognostic value in 12 studies and no value in seven; angina is predictive in one-half the studies; the respective figures for ST segment shifts are 17 and 12 and for VPCs 9 and 14.

Thus the results of exercise testing are clearly influenced by a variety of confounding factors and should be interpreted with caution. On the other hand, exercise testing provides information on the various pathophysiologic factors influencing prognosis, and integration of these data can be useful for the overall assessment of patients. The data content varies, depending on the characteristics of the populations studied, the protocol used, the parameters most clearly scrutinized, the endpoints used, and the concomitant medication being administered. Other factors such as the influence of test results on patient management, the cardiac events considered during follow-up, and the duration of the follow-up also influence the conclusions.

Toward Cohesion

Despite the apparent confusion, many conclusions can be drawn from the available data. First, among the nine studies showing prognostic value for ventricular premature beats, six had as an endpoint mortality alone, whereas eight of the 14 negative studies had multiple endpoints including myocardial infarction and angina. Moreover, some of the positive studies included a multivariate analysis that documented the independent prognostic value of VPCs. The presence of VPCs increased the mortality risk two- to threefold. As indicated in Table 33-3, the prognostic value of VPCs has not changed through the years, probably because no well defined therapeutic strategies exist for management of ventricular beats after myocardial infarction. Studies are now being conducted to determine if control of arrhythmias reduces mortality [63].

Such a time-independent distribution is not found when the prognostic value of ST segment depression is examined. Eighteen of the 26 studies show prognostic value: 75 percent of the 13 published before 1982 and 43 percent of those published since 1982. This apparently decreasing value of ST segment depression can easily be correlated with an increasing use of bypass surgery during follow-up. In the studies performed before 1982, coronary artery surgery, when reported, had been performed in 0 to 9.7 percent of patients, with a mean of 3 percent; the studies performed after 1982 reported an incidence of bypass surgery up to 24 percent with an average of 12.6 percent. In the study by Fuller et al., 8 of the 15 (53 percent) patients with a positive test had bypass surgery compared to 2 of the 25 (8 percent) patients with a negative test [18]; in Norris et al.'s study the respective figures were 40 and 11 percent [26]. Medical treatment, which has changed enormously during these years—with control of risk factors, rehabilitation programs, more liberal use of medication (particularly beta blockers) and the advent of cor-

onary angioplasty—could have had even more impact on prognosis than surgical treatment.

Over this interval, the prognostic value of parameters related to ventricular function has increased; thus an inadequate blood pressure response was reported predictive of cardiac events in 60 percent of the studies performed before 1982 and in 86 percent of the studies performed since.

Additional Information Provided by Radionuclide Studies

Radionuclide techniques can be used in conjunction with exercise testing to provide additional data. Thallium scintigraphy permits detection of transient regional perfusion defects, and radionuclide ventriculography yields information on global and regional wall motion.

Gibson et al. have demonstrated that the presence of multiple thallium defects involving different vascular regions, thallium 201 redistribution, or increased lung uptake secondary to left ventricular dysfunction identified the high risk patient. The sensitivity and specificity of these findings were superior to those provided by exercise testing and coronary angiography [24]. Other investigations have documented a high sensitivity of thallium exercise testing for detecting more extensive coronary artery disease [64, 65].

The exercise ventriculogram can also help identify the patient at high risk. In one study comparing the prognostic value of reversible perfusion defect, time on the treadmill, and a decrease in ejection fraction, the only two independent predictors of prognosis were peak treadmill work load of 4 METs or less and a decrease of 5 percent or more in the ejection fraction [28]. In another study, the change in ejection fraction, end-systolic volume, and ratio of systolic blood pressure to end-systolic volume were predictive of subsequent cardiac events [22]. Resting ejection fraction may be more predictive of mortality and the changes during exercise more predictive of subsequent ischemic events [66]. The sensitivity and specificity of the exercise ventriculogram to detect multivessel disease seem as high as with thallium perfusion scintigraphy [67]. The specificity of both tests for detecting multivessel disease is reduced in the presence of anterior myocardial infarction [64, 67].

Studies published to date with radionuclide techniques have been limited to small numbers of patients and have included multiple cardiac events as endpoints to evaluate prognosis. The yield of the routine use of these tests for evaluation of the postmyocardial infarction patient has not yet been determined. However, their advantage in many clinical circumstances is obvious. Thallium scans and exercise ventriculograms can be used when the ST segments changes are nonspecific, as with bundle branch block, left ventricular hypertrophy, Wolf-Parkinson-White syndrome, digitalis effect, and abnormal resting ST segment abnormalities caused by the myocardial infarction. They can also be useful in the presence of chest pain without ST segment changes or when the ST changes are borderline.

The additional information provided by radionuclide studies may not justify their routine use when the exercise test is completely negative at a high workload or when obvious ischemic ST segment shifts occur at a low workload. In the latter circumstance, however, thallium scintigraphy may be helpful for localizing the site of ischemia and thus influence the selection of therapy.

Exercise Test Protocols

Standard exercise protocols are used. The Naughton protocol is generally selected for the exercise test performed before hospital discharge and the Bruce protocol for tests performed at 2 to 3 weeks. The workload equivalent calculated in multiples of resting oxygen consumption (MET) is the most useful criterion for comparing results of various tests in the same patient and results from various studies. When the test is performed early, the endpoint is generally preset at 5 MET; otherwise symptom-limited tests are performed.

The advantages of an in-hospital test are pa-

tient convenience, early detection of high risk, promotion of self-confidence for the patient and reassurance for the family, and the potential to institute earlier, more definitive medical or surgical treatment and a rehabilitation program. The late test, however, may provide more data on overall cardiovascular status and serve as a guideline for more intensive rehabilitation and return to work. Timing of the test is not a critical issue, as both the early and late tests can be used to provide complementary information.

No serious complications have been reported from the early exercise test. However, selection of patients is important, and close observation during the test to stop it if abnormalities are detected.

Selection of Patients

Patients can be selected on the basis of a careful history and physical examination. The two cardiac contraindications to exercise testing are chest pain occurring at rest or during mild exercise and clinical signs of congestive failure, such as pulmonary rales, presence of a third heart sound, and sinus tachycardia. Some patients are excluded because of other medical conditions, such as chronic obstructive lung disease, peripheral vascular disease, orthopedic conditions, or other severe medical illness. Age per se is not a contraindication. In patients unable to exercise because of a physical condition, an alternative method to unmask ischemia, such as the dipyridamole test [68] or atrial pacing [69], can be used.

EXERCISE TEST AND THE PATIENT: GLOBAL APPROACH

All patients recovering from myocardial infarction should be considered for exercise testing. Indeed the test provides information on prognosis not otherwise available [13, 14, 20, 35, 36, 70]. The presence of a cardiac contraindication to the test is already predictive of a poor prognosis [14, 29, 36]. The associated risk varies depending on the severity of the exclusion criteria used but can be as high as 56 percent.

Good tolerance to exercise without ischemia and with a normal hemodynamic response is associated with a mortality risk less than 2 percent a year [1, 8, 11, 14, 16, 23, 29, 31]. This point could be the most positive aspect of exercise testing. Indeed the asymptomatic patient with a low risk would likely not benefit from additional investigation or treatment. On the contrary, this patient is a candidate for a positive rehabilitation program and early return to work [71]. A positive exercise test is an indication for further investigation to establish the most appropriate treatment.

Because myocardial ischemia is associated with a high risk of recurrent angina, myocardial infarction, and death, a clear ischemic response is an indication for coronary angiography often followed by more intensive medical therapy or a revascularization procedure. If myocardial ischemia is suspected but not documented, further investigation should be carried out with radionuclide techniques. This aggressive attitude for the control of ischemia will hopefully reduce as much as possible the devastating prognostic impact of this parameter.

Poor tolerance to exercise and an abnormal hemodynamic response should also be more fully investigated to determine the cause, whether it is ischemia-related or due to permanent left ventricular dysfunction. Echocardiographic and radionuclide studies are then indicated. Depressed left ventricular function should be managed in light of the recent reports of improved prognosis in patients with congestive heart failure treated with afterload reducing agents [72, 73]. The pressure of ventricular premature beats during exercise is also an indication for investigating left ventricular function; beta blockers should then be considered if they are not contraindicated.

EXERCISE TESTING AFTER MYOCARDIAL INFARCTION: CHANGING ROLE

Fibrinolysis and angioplasty are now widely used for the acute management of myocardial infarction. This form of treatment is associated with improved survival, particularly when applied early after the onset of pain [74]. Changes in our scheme of risk stratification and in the relative frequency of the various determinants of prognosis have already been observed [75]. Successful thrombolysis improves left ventricular function; ventricular arrhythmias are less frequent [75] and less severe [76]. Residual ischemia, however, is a more frequent finding, particularly when a residual stenosis is present [77]. This ischemia may have an impact on prognosis by increasing the incidence of subsequent angina and recurrent myocardial infarction in patients treated with fibrinolysis compared to nontreated patients [78].

Exercise testing for the specified goal of detecting ischemia thus assumes more importance in an era of aggressive management of myocardial infarction. The test can be used to select low risk patients for early discharge and high risk patients for more aggressive interventional procedures [79].

Acknowledgment

The superb secretarial work of Luce Bégin is gratefully acknowledged.

Editorial Comments

Nearly every patient should have a symptom-limited exercise test after a myocardial infarction, unless there is recurrent chest pain, an unstable electrical or hemodynamic state, or an orthopedic problem that precludes walking on a treadmill. The test is most useful when it is normal, as it then largely predicts an uncomplicated course for the patient. When the exercise test is abnormal, management strategy, including further testing, is still largely judgmental and depends on many factors, particularly the individual circumstances of the patient. G.S.F.

When it is not possible for the patient to exercise (e.g., because of amputation or arthri-

tis) the dipyridamole thallium test can be used to aid in planning further therapeutic intervention. When the scan shows a reversible perfusion deficit (i.e., myocardial ischemia) the patient should be considered for coronary angiography with an eye to angioplasty or coronary bypass surgery. J.S.A.

References

1. Report of the American College of Cardiology/American Heart Association: Guidelines for exercise testing. *J. Am. Coll. Cardiol.* 8:725, 1986.
2. Fortuin, N. J., and Weiss, J. L. Exercise stress testing. *Circulation* 56:699, 1977.
3. Atterhög, J. H., Ekelund, L. G., and Kaijser, L. Electrocardiographic abnormalities during exercise 3 weeks to 18 months after anterior myocardial infarction. *Br. Heart J.* 33:871, 1971.
4. Ericsson, M., Granath, A., Ohlsen, P., et al. Arrhythmias and symptoms during treadmill testing three weeks after myocardial infarction in 100 patients. *Br. Heart J.* 35:787, 1973.
5. Ibsen, H., Kjoller, E., Styperek, J., and Pedersen, A. Routine exercise ECG three weeks after acute myocardial infarction. *Acta Med. Scand.* 198:463, 1975.
6. Granath, A., Södermark, T., Winge, T., et al. Early workload tests for evaluation of long-term prognosis of acute myocardial infarction. *Br. Heart J.* 39:758, 1977.
7. Markiewicz, W., Houston, N., and DeBusk, R. Exercise testing soon after myocardial infarction. *Circulation* 56:26, 1977.
8. Théroux, P., Waters, D. D., Halphen, C., et al. Prognostic value of exercise testing soon after myocardial infarction. *N. Engl. J. Med.* 301:341, 1979.
9. Smith, J., Dennic, C., Gassman, A., et al. Exercise testing three weeks after myocardial infarction. *Chest* 75:12, 1979.
10. Sami, M., Kraemer, H., and DeBusk, R. F. The prognostic significance of serial exercise testing after myocardial infarction. *Circulation* 60:1238, 1979.
11. Davidson, D. M., and DeBusk, R. F. Prognostic value of a single exercise test 3 weeks after uncomplicated myocardial infarction. *Circulation* 61:236, 1980.
12. Starling, M. R., Crawford, M. H., Kennedy, G. T., and O'Rourke, R. A. Treadmill exercise tests predischarge and six weeks post-myocardial infarction to detect abnormalities of known prognostic value. *Ann. Intern. Med.* 94:721, 1981.
13. Koppes, G. M., Kruyer, W., Beckmann, C. H., and Jones, F. G. Response to exercise early after uncomplicated acute myocardial infarction in patients receiving no medication: Long-term follow-up. *Am. J. Cardiol.* 46:764, 1980.
14. Madsen, E. B., Rasmussen, S., and Svendsen, T. L. Multivariate long-term prognosis index from exercise ECG after acute myocardial infarction. *Eur. J. Cardiol.* 11:435, 1980.
15. Schwartz, K. M., Turner, J. D., Sheffield, L. T., et al. Limited exercise testing soon after myocardial infarction. *Ann. Intern. Med.* 94:727, 1981.
16. Lindvall, K., and Kaijser, L. Early exercise tests after uncomplicated acute myocardial infarction before early discharge from hospital. *Acta Med. Scand.* 210:257, 1981.
17. Velasco, J. A., Tormo, V., Ridocci, F., and Blanch, S. Early load-limited versus symptom-limited exercise testing: Prognostic value in 200 myocardial infarction patients. *Cardiology* 68(Suppl 2):44, 1981.
18. Fuller, C. M., Raizner, A. E., Verani, M. S., et al. Early post-myocardial infarction treadmill stress testing. An accurate predictor of multivessel coronary artery disease and subsequent cardiac events. *Ann. Intern. Med.* 94:734, 1981.
19. Srinivasan, M., Young, A., Baker, G., et al. The value of postcardiac infarction exercise stress testing: Identification of a group at high risk. *Med. J. Aust.* 2:466, 1981.
20. Saunamäki, K. I., and Andersen, J. D. Early exercise test in the assessment of long-term prognosis after myocardial infarction. *Acta Med. Scand.* 209:185, 1981.
21. Weld, F. M., Chu, K. L., Bigger, J. T., and Rolnitzky, L. M. Risk stratification with low level exercise testing 2 weeks after acute myocardial infarction. *Circulation* 64:306, 1981.
22. Corbett, J. R., Dehmer, G. J., Lewis, S. E., et al. The prognostic value of submaximal exercise testing with radionuclide ventriculography before hospital discharge in patients with recent myocardial infarction. *Circulation* 64:535, 1981.
23. De Feyter, P. J., van Eenige, M. J., Dighton, D. H., et al. Prognostic value of exercise testing, coronary angiography and left ventriculography 6–8 weeks after myocardial infarction. *Circulation* 66:527, 1982.
24. Gibson, R. S., Watson, D. D., Craddock, G. B., et al. Reduction of cardiac events after uncomplicated myocardial infarction: A prospective study comparing predischarge exercise thallium-201 scintigraphy and coronary angiography. *Circulation* 68:321, 1983.
25. Rapaport, E., and Remedios, P. The high risk patient after recovery from myocardial infarction: Recognition and management. *J. Am. Coll. Cardiol.* 1:391, 1983.
26. Norris, R. M., Barnaby, P. F., Brandt, P. W. T., et al. Prognosis after recovery from first acute

myocardial infarction: Determinants of rein-farction and sudden death. *Am. J. Cardiol.* 54:408, 1984.

27. Dwyer Jr., E. M., McMaster, P., Greenberg, H., et al. Non-fatal cardiac events and recurrent infarction in the year after acute myocardial infarction. *J. Am. Coll. Cardiol.* 4:695, 1984.

28. Hung, J., Goris, M. L., Nash, E., et al. Comparative value of maximal treadmill testing, exercise thallium myocardial perfusion scintigraphy and exercise radionuclide ventriculography for distinguishing high- and low-risk patients soon after myocardial infarction. *Am. J. Cardiol.* 53:1221, 1984.

29. Krone, R. J., Gillespie, J. A., Weld, F. M., et al. Low-level exercise testing after myocardial infarction: Usefulness in enhancing clinical risk stratification. *Circulation* 71:80, 1985.

30. Jespersen, C. M., Kassis, E., Edeling, C. J., and Madsen, J. K. The prognostic value of maximal exercise testing soon after first myocardial infarction. *Eur. Heart J.* 6:769, 1985.

31. Fioretti, P., Brower, R. W., Simoons, M. L., et al. Prediction of mortality during the first year after acute myocardial infarction from clinical variables and stress test at hospital discharge. *Am. J. Cardiol.* 55:1313, 1985.

32. Madsen, E. B., Gilpin, E., Ahnvee, S., et al. Prediction of functional capacity and use of exercise testing for predicting risk after acute myocardial infarction. *Am. J. Cardiol.* 56:839, 1985.

33. Waters, D. D., Bosch, X., Bouchard, A., et al. Comparison of clinical variables and variables derived from a limited predischarge exercise test as predictors of early and late mortality after myocardial infarction. *J. Am. Coll. Cardiol.* 5:1, 1985.

34. Handler, C. E. Submaximal predischarge exercise testing after myocardial infarction: Prognostic value and limitations. *Eur. Heart J.* 6:510, 1985.

35. Starling, M. R., Crawford, M. H., Henry, R. L., et al. Prognostic value of electrocardiographic exercise testing and noninvasive assessment of left ventricular ejection fraction soon after acute myocardial infarction. *Am. J. Cardiol.* 57:532, 1986.

36. Fioretti, P., Brower, R. W., Simoons, M. L., et al. Relative value of clinical variables, bicycle ergometry, rest radionuclide ventriculography and 24-hour ambulatory electrocardiographic monitoring at discharge to predict 1 year survival after myocardial infarction. *J. Am. Coll. Cardiol.* 8:40, 1986.

37. Sanz, G., Castaner, A., Betriu, A., et al. Determinants of prognosis in survivors of myocardial infarction: A prospective clinical angiographic study. *N. Engl. J. Med.* 306:1065, 1982.

38. Multicenter Postinfarction Research Group.

Risk stratification and survival after myocardial infarction. *N. Engl. J. Med.* 309:331, 1983.

39. Taylor, G. J., Humphries, J. D., Mellits, E. D., et al. Predictors of clinical course, coronary anatomy and left ventricular function after recovery from acute myocardial infarction. *Circulation* 62:960, 1980.

40. Schulze, R., Strauss, H., and Pitt, B. Sudden death in the year following myocardial infarction. *Am. J. Med.* 62:192, 1977.

41. Mukharji, J., Rude, R. E., Poole, K., et al. Risk factors for sudden death after acute myocardial infarction: Two-year follow-up. *Am. J. Cardiol.* 54:31, 1984.

42. Bigger, J. T., Fleiss, J. L., Kleiger, R., et al. The relationships among ventricular arrhythmias, left ventricular dysfunction, and mortality in the 2 years after myocardial infarction. *Circulation* 69:250, 1984.

43. Schuster, E. H., and Bulkley, B. H. Early postinfarction angina: Ischemia at a distance and ischemia in the infarct zone. *N. Engl. J. Med.* 305:1101, 1981.

44. Bosch, X., Théroux, P., Waters, D. D., et al. Early postinfarction ischemia: Clinical, angiographic and prognostic significance. *Circulation* 75:988, 1987.

45. Gibson, R. S., Beller, G. A., Gheorghiade, M., et al. The prevalence and clinical significance of residual myocardial ischemia two weeks after uncomplicated non-Q wave infarction: A prospective natural history study. *Circulation* 73:1186, 1986.

46. Théroux, P., Kouz, S., Bosch, X., et al. Clinical and angiographic features of non-Q wave myocardial infarction. *Circulation* 74(Suppl II):303, 1986.

47. Théroux, P. A pathophysiologic basis for the clinical classification and management of unstable angina. *Circulation* 75(Suppl V):103, 1987.

48. Palmieri, S. T., Harrison, D. G., Cobb, F. R., et al. QRS scoring system for assessing left ventricular function after myocardial infarction. *N. Engl. J. Med.* 306:4, 1982.

49. Bosch, X., Moise, A., Roy, D., et al. Clinical and angiographic correlates of ventricular premature beats occurring during an exercise test early after myocardial infarction. *Circulation* 70(Suppl II):422, 1984.

50. Haskell, W. L., and DeBusk, R. Cardiovascular responses to repeated treadmill exercise testing soon after myocardial infarction. *Circulation* 60:1247, 1979.

51. DeBusk, R. F., and Haskell, W. Symptom-limited vs heart-rate-limited exercise testing soon after myocardial infarction. *Circulation* 61:738, 1980.

52. DeBusk, R. F., Houston, M., Haskell, W., et al. Exercise training soon after myocardial infarction. *Am. J. Cardiol.* 44:1223, 1979.

53. Wohl, A. J., Lewis, H. R., Campbell, W., et al. Cardiovascular function during early recovery from acute myocardial infarction. *Circulation* 56:931, 1977.

54. Waters, D. D., Théroux, P., Halphen, C., and Mizgala, H. F. Clinical predictors of angina following myocardial infarction. *Am. J. Med.* 66:991, 1979.

55. Midwall, J., Ambrose, J., Pichard, A., et al. Angina pectoris before and after myocardial infarction: Angiographic correlations. *Chest* 81:681, 1982.

56. Dillahunt II, P. H., and Miller, A. B. Early treadmill testing after myocardial infarction: Angiographic and hemodynamic correlations. *Chest* 76:150, 1979.

57. Patterson, R. E., Horowitz, S. F., Eng, C., et al. Can noninvasive exercise test criteria identify patients with left main or 3-vessel coronary disease after a first myocardial infarction? *Am. J. Cardiol.* 51:361, 1983.

58. Benjamin, S. T., MacDonald, P. S., Horowitz, J. D., et al. Usefulness of early exercise testing after non-Q wave myocardial infarction in predicting prognosis. *Am. J. Cardiol.* 57:738, 1986.

59. Benjamin, S. T., MacDonald, P. S., Horowitz, J. D., et al. Usefulness of early exercise testing after non-Q wave myocardial infarction in predicting prognosis. *Am. J. Cardiol.* 57:738, 1986.

60. Haines, D. E., Beller, G. A., Watson, D. D., et al. Exercise-induced ST segment elevation 2 weeks after uncomplicated myocardial infarction: Contributing factors and prognostic significance. *J. Am. Coll. Cardiol.* 9:996, 1987.

61. Stone, P. H., Turi, Z. G., Muller, J. E., et al. Prognostic significance to the treadmill exercise test performance 6 months after myocardial infarction. *J. Am. Coll. Cardiol.* 8:1107, 1986.

62. Sami, M., Kraemer, H., and DeBusk, R. The reproducibility of exercise-induced ventricular arrhythmias following myocardial infarction. *Am. J. Cardiol.* 43:724, 1979.

63. CAPS Investigators. The Cardiac Arrythmia Pilot Study. *Am. J. Cardiol.* 57:91, 1986.

64. Turner, J. D., Schwartz, K. M., Logic, J. R., et al. Detection of residual jeopardized myocardium 3 weeks after myocardial infarction, by exercise testing with thallium-201 myocardial scintigraphy. *Circulation* 61:729, 1980.

65. Rigo, P., Bailey, I. K., Griffith, L. S. C., et al. Stress thallium-201 myocardial scintigraphy for the detection of individual coronary arterial lesions in patients with and without previous myocardial infarctions. *Am. J. Cardiol.* 48:209, 1981.

66. Morris, K. G., Palmeri, S. T., Califf, R. M., et al. Value of radionuclide angiography for predicting specific cardiac events after acute myocardial infarction. *Am. J. Cardiol.* 55:318, 1985.

67. Wasserman, A. G., Katz, R. J., Cleary, P., et al. Non-invasive detection of multivessel disease after myocardial infarction by exercise radionuclide ventriculography. *Am. J. Cardiol.* 50:1242, 1982.

68. Leppo, J. A., O'Brien, J., Rothendler, J. A., et al. Dipyridamole–thallium-201 scintigraphy in the prediction of future cardiac events after acute myocardial infarction. *N. Engl. J. Med.* 310:1014, 1984.

69. Tzivoni, D., Gottlieb, S., Keren, A., et al. Early right atrial pacing after myocardial infarction. I. Comparison with early treadmill testing. *Am. J. Cardiol.* 53:414, 1984.

70. Hugenholtz, P. G., Fioretti, P., Simoons, M. L., et al. Improved prognosis during and after myocardial infarction: A plea for an integrated and stratified approach. *Can. J. Cardiol.* 6:345, 1986.

71. De Busk, R. F., Blomqvist, C. G., Kouchoukos, N. T., et al. Identification and treatment of low risk patients after acute myocardial infarction and coronary artery bypass graft surgery. *N. Engl. J. Med.* 314:161, 1986.

72. Cohn, J. M., Archibald, D. G., Ziesche, S., et al. Effect of vasodilator therapy on mortality in chronic congestive heart failure. *N. Engl. J. Med.* 314:1547, 1986.

73. CONSENSUS Trial Study Group. Effects of enalapril on mortality in severe congestive heart failure: Results of the Cooperative North Scandinavian Enalapril Survival Study. *N. Engl. J. Med.* 316:1429, 1987.

74. GISSI—Gruppo Italiano per lo Studio della Streptochinasi nell'Infarto Miocardico. Effectiveness of intravenous thrombolytic treatment in acute myocardial infarction. *Lancet* 1:397, 1986.

75. Théroux, P., Morissette, D., de Guise, P., et al. Aggressive management of myocardial infarction modifies predischarge risk evaluation. *Circulation* 76(Suppl II):502, 1987.

76. Sager, P., Perlmutter R., Rosenfeld, L., et al. Thrombolysis decreases sudden death and arrhythmogenic potential after anterior myocardial infarction with aneurysm formation. *Circulation* 76(Suppl II):261, 1987.

77. Melin, J. A., De Coster, P. M., Renkin, J., et al. Effect of intracoronary thrombolytic therapy on exercise-induced ischemia after acute myocardial infarction. *Am. J. Cardiol.* 56:705, 1985.

78. Schaer, D. H., Ross, A. M., and Wasserman, A. L. Reinfarction, recurrent angina, and reocclusion after thrombolytic therapy. *Circulation* 76(Suppl II):56, 1987.

79. Topol, E. J., Juni, J. E., O'Neill, W. W., et al. Exercise testing three days after onset of acute myocardial infarction. *Am. J. Cardiol.* 60:958, 1987.

34
Rehabilitation After Acute Myocardial Infarction

CHARLES A. DENNIS

Although physicians are more sophisticated than ever in terms of the management of acute myocardial infarction and its complications, individual patients remain ill-equipped to manage the medical and functional aspects of recovery that significantly disrupt their lives for the weeks to months after hospital discharge. Even the uncomplicated patient faces medical restrictions on the most routine of activities, such as driving, climbing stairs, lifting, and sexual activity. These restrictions are reinforced by family, friends, and coworkers who generally perceive a poor prognosis and are concerned that physical activity can harm the heart. Because patients have an incomplete understanding of their illness, they fear recurrent cardiac problems. This fear can engender a sense of isolation and loss of control as well as a lack of confidence to resume customary activities.

Rehabilitation after myocardial infarction must address medical, physical, emotional, educational, and perceptual problems. Although rehabilitation means literally to restore a former capacity, cardiac rehabilitation should seek larger goals. The short-term goal is to return patients to their normal physical, emotional, functional, and occupational state as soon as possible. The long-term goals are to optimize physical conditioning, educate the patient and the family about coronary heart disease, and slow or reverse the pathophysiologic processes that led to the myocardial infarction.

This chapter reviews the pathophysiology of acute myocardial infarction and aspects of treatment that affect physical capacity. The role of risk factors in the progression of coronary disease and its late complications are described, and the resumption of customary activities is discussed. Finally, the risks and benefits of rehabilitation after myocardial infarction are presented with recommendations for rehabilitation services.

Structure of Cardiac Rehabilitation Programs

Cardiac rehabilitation programs are widely available across the United States, but their services are underutilized. It is estimated that only 15 percent of patients recovering from myocardial infarction participate in formal rehabilitation programs [1]. Individual physicians can provide rehabilitation services to patients effectively but generally do not have the expertise or time to provide the broad-based treatment that is given over a short period by cardiac rehabilitation programs.

PHASED REHABILITATION

Cardiac rehabilitation programs are usually centered on physical conditioning with related efforts directed toward risk factor modification, patient education and counseling, and disability assessment. Although there is variability among programs, most endorse the concept of phased rehabilitation. Phase I programs are hospital-based, treating patients soon after myocardial infarction or coronary surgery. Inpatient programs focus primarily on education and counseling with limited efforts in physical reconditioning. The patient and family receive fundamental information regarding cardiac disease, symptoms, and risk factors. Counseling concerning the psychological impact of myocardial infarction is often provided. Structured programs of increasing physical activity prepare patients for hospital discharge. A low level treadmill test before discharge may be provided.

Phases II to IV are outpatient programs distinguished by the time since the acute cardiac event and the type of exercise training provided. Although this chapter deals primarily with rehabilitation after myocardial infarction, most outpatient programs enroll patients with all types of cardiac conditions. Phase II rehabilitation is the first outpatient level; it generally begins soon after hospital discharge and lasts 8 to 12 weeks. A symptom-limited treadmill test should be performed at entry to assess physical capacity and screen for high risk patients requiring further treatment. Supervised exercise, often employing electrocardiographic monitoring, is begun at a low level based on the treadmill test. Exercise duration and intensity are gradually increased over the 3-month program. Individual and group education regarding risk factor modification is provided. Counseling to assist in social and emotional adjustment to myocardial infarction may be performed individually or in groups.

Phase III rehabilitation follows the early reconditioning and allows patients to exercise in a supervised setting with less intensive monitoring. Patients learn how to self-monitor higher intensity exercise. In addition, skills involved in smoking abstinence, dietary modification, and stress management are reinforced. Phase III programs usually last 6 to 12 months but may continue indefinitely. Phase IV rehabilitation refers to unsupervised physical activity. The skills involved in self-monitoring of exercise and in risk factor modification may be reinforced by periodic visits to the rehabilitation center.

ORGANIZATION OF PROGRAMS

Most cardiac rehabilitation programs use a team approach. Whether the program is inpatient, outpatient, or combined, key personnel with specific roles are identified. The two central figures in any program are the medical director and the program director. The medical director is a primary link to the medical community. The medical director is crucial in the intake evaluation of the clinical status of patients, communication with referring physicians, development of the complete rehabilitation program, and maintenance of the quality of the medical aspects of the program. As is true for any form of consultative service, the medical director must ensure that high quality services are provided to patients without jeopardizing the autonomy of the primary physicians' clinical prerogatives.

The program director is responsible for the organizational, administrative, and operational aspects of the rehabilitation program and is an additional link to the medical and lay community. The program director must be well grounded in all aspects of the rehabilitation process in addition to being skilled in administration and management. The program director must recruit and coordinate the efforts of a highly skilled team. Other members of the multidisciplinary team include nurses, physical therapists, exercise physiologists, exercise leaders, dietitians, vocational counselors, psychologists, a business manager, and clerical help. The size and complexity of the rehabilitation program dictate the number of employees and their time commitments.

The facilities and equipment of a particular program vary depending on the size of the program and the range of services provided. Inpatient programs have limited equipment for exercise training because of the low volume of patients hospitalized at any particular time and the limited exercise training provided. Outpatient programs necessarily have more elaborate exercise equipment. All programs that provide exercise training have emergency resuscitation equipment. Small and large conference rooms meet the needs of group and individual programs for education and counseling.

No two cardiac rehabilitation programs are identical in structure or services provided. Subsequent sections provide guidelines for rehabilitation of patients recovering from myocardial infarction that may be incorporated into individual programs. Five major areas of rehabilitative efforts are discussed: physical conditioning, clinical evaluation, secondary prevention, psychological evaluation, and resumption of customary activities, including return to work.

Physical Conditioning

Physical capacity is reduced in virtually all patients after acute myocardial infarction. The degree of physical incapacity is related to several factors: the physical condition of the patient prior to infarction; the influence of some standard treatments for myocardial infarction, such as bed rest; the extent of myocardial necrosis and residual myocardial ischemia after infarction; medications; age; other noncardiac medical conditions; and the symptoms experienced by the patient while performing physical activity. Distinguishing these effects can be difficult in the individual patient. However, an understanding of each of these effects is paramount to minimizing the iatrogenic causes of physical impairment and to developing a conditioning program.

EXERCISE CAPACITY IN NORMAL INDIVIDUALS

To understand the mechanisms that influence physical capacity after myocardial infarction, one must understand the determinants of physical capacity in normal individuals. In healthy individuals the *peak exercise capacity* is a measure of the ability of the cardiovascular system to deliver oxygen to exercising skeletal muscle and the ability of the exercising muscle to extract oxygen from blood. The ability of the cardiovascular system to deliver oxygen is most simply defined as the *cardiac output*. The ability of skeletal muscle to extract oxygen is most simply defined as *arteriovenous oxygen difference* (a-vO_2 difference). No matter what the physical condition of a healthy individual, these two factors deter-

mine peak exercise capacity. Peak exercise capacity can be increased with exercise training by adaptations in cardiac performance and skeletal muscle oxygen extraction.

Normal Responses to Exercise
Exercise capacity is commonly measured for research purposes using the *maximal oxygen uptake* ($\dot{V}O_2$max). $\dot{V}O_2$max represents the liters of oxygen transported from the lungs and used by skeletal muscle at peak exercise. $\dot{V}O_2$max may be increased by exercise training and decreased by many factors, such as physical deconditioning or cardiac illness. Because measurement of $\dot{V}O_2$max is cumbersome, other estimates of exercise capacity are used clinically. The most common clinical measurement of exercise capacity is multiples of resting oxygen consumption (MET); 1 MET equals 3.5 ml oxygen uptake/kg body weight/min and represents the approximate metabolic cost to stand quietly. Treadmill tests have been calibrated to give approximate MET requirements for each stage, although there is some variability for each patient. MET capacity on treadmill testing generally overestimates the $\dot{V}O_2$max for cardiac patients [2, 3].

The measurement of exercise capacity is complex and includes several factors that are defined in Table 34-1. $\dot{V}O_2$max is the product of maximal cardiac output and a-vO_2 difference. Cardiac output is the product of heart rate and stroke volume. *Stroke volume* is the product of end-diastolic volume and ejection fraction. a-vO_2 difference is the difference in the concentration of oxygen per liter of blood between arterial and mixed venous (i.e., pulmonary arterial) blood.

In healthy individuals, the heart rate may increase 100 to 200 percent with exercise, making it quantitatively the most important influence on cardiac output. End-diastolic volume increases from 0 to 15 percent and ejection fraction from 10 to 20 percent with exercise. During exercise, skeletal muscle can increase oxygen extraction 50 to 150 percent, reflected in a widened a-vO_2 difference. The maximal a-vO_2 difference attainable is related to the capillary density and mitochondrial concentration in skeletal muscle [4].

Table 34-1
Formulas and terms used for calculation of maximal oxygen uptake

Formulas	Terms
$\dot{V}O_2max = CO \times$ a-vO$_2$D	$\dot{V}O_2max$ = maximal oxygen uptake (L/min)
CO = HR $\times$ SV	CO = cardiac output (L/min)
	HR = heart rate (beats/minute; bpm)
SV = EDV $\times$ EF	SV = stroke volume (L/beat)
	EDV = end-diastolic volume (L)
a-vO$_2$D = a-O$_2$conc − VO$_2$conc	EF = ejection fraction (%)
	a-vO$_2$D = arteriovenous oxygen difference (L O$_2$/L blood)
	aO$_2$conc = arterial oxygen concentration (L O$_2$/L blood)
	vO$_2$conc = venous oxygen concentration (L O$_2$/L blood)

Adaptations to Exercise Training

Exercise training of healthy individuals causes both cardiac and skeletal muscle adaptations that increase $\dot{V}O_2max$. The maximal heart rate response to exercise in healthy individuals is roughly related to age and does not change with exercise training. Therefore other cardiac adaptations must occur to increase cardiac output with exercise above that in the untrained state. Maximal stroke volume increases with exercise training. The change in maximal stroke volume reflects an increase in both end-diastolic volume and ejection fraction. Exercise training also increases capillary density and mitochondrial density in skeletal muscle, causing an increased a-vO$_2$ difference at maximal exercise [5].

The influence of cardiac and peripheral factors on the exercise capacity of a 50-year-old healthy man in the untrained state and after 4 months of exercise training is shown in Table 34-2. Peak heart rate is unchanged, but increases in end-diastolic volume and ejection fraction lead to a 24 percent increase in cardiac output. Skeletal muscle oxygen extraction is increased, reflected in a widened a-vO$_2$ difference at peak exercise after training. The combination of cardiac and skeletal muscle adaptations to exercise training result in a 42 percent increase in $\dot{V}O_2max$.

Other cardiac effects of exercise training contribute to the increase in $\dot{V}O_2max$ that are not obvious from examining peak exercise data alone. Resting heart rate decreases, and a lower heart rate at any given exercise workload is common. This chronotropic adaptation allows increased diastolic filling time and therefore improved ventricular filling and emptying. Blood pressure is usually lowered by chronic exercise training, especially in hypertensive patients. A lower blood pressure at any given workload results in a lower afterload and increased ejection fraction. All of these effects result in an improved cardiac output at higher levels of work and therefore an improved exercise capacity.

EXERCISE CAPACITY AFTER MYOCARDIAL INFARCTION

The exercise capacity of individuals recovering from myocardial infarction is influenced by both the pathophysiologic effects of the illness and certain effects of treatment. Although the same mechanisms of cardiac output and a-vO$_2$ difference determine $\dot{V}O_2max$, temporally related changes in chronotropic response, intravascular volume, myocardial perfusion and contractility, and skeletal muscle conditioning interact to determine peak exercise capacity at any given time. Normal processes of recovery, even in the absence of exercise training, are important contributors to the increases in exercise capacity during the early postinfarction period.

Effects of Bed Rest

Although current coronary care emphasizes early mobilization of patients after myocardial infarction, patients still spend significant periods at supine bed rest during hospitalization.

Table 34-2
Adaptations in cardiac and peripheral responses to maximum exercise after 4 months of training of a healthy 50-year-old man

Condition	Peak exercise values						
	HR (bpm)	EDV (ml)	EF (%)	SV (ml/beat)	CO (L/min)	a-vO$_2$D (L/L)	V̇O$_2$max (L/min)
Untrained	170	170	60	100	17	0.14	2.4
Trained	170	190	65	124	21	0.16	3.4
% Change	0	+12	+9	+24	+24	+15	+42

Even in healthy individuals, bed rest has a detrimental effect on physical capacity. Several studies have demonstrated that 10 to 30 days of bed rest is associated with decrements in V̇O$_2$max of 9 to 30 percent [6–8], with the largest proportion of loss during the first 10 days.

The etiology of the decrement in V̇O$_2$max is multifactorial. A prolonged absence of orthostatic stress results in a decreased stroke volume due to hypovolemia [9] and diminished control of venous capacitance vessels resulting in a decreased venous return [8]. Blunting of normal postural vasomotor reflexes results in postural tachycardia and hypotension. Losses in skeletal muscle mass of 10 to 15 percent [10] and a shift from aerobic to anaerobic metabolism at moderate levels of exercise [5] also contribute to a diminution of physical capacity. Diminished lung volume, vital capacity, and increased respiratory exchange ratio occur with bed rest, implicating pulmonary mechanisms as well [10].

Vigorous training in the supine position during bed rest fails to prevent the deterioration of upright exercise capacity [11], although as little as 3 hours of daily simulated gravitational stress significantly decreases the deconditioning effect of bed rest [12]. These effects of bed rest resolve spontaneously after hospitalization. This resolution is related primarily to the resumption of upright posture for prolonged periods. The return to normal dietary habits and the conditioning effects of usual activities such as walking also play a role.

Chronotropic Incompetence

Most patients manifest chronotropic incompetence after myocardial infarction. *Chrono-* *tropic incompetence* is the inability to achieve the maximal heart rate response to exercise predicted by age. Maximal heart rate can be decreased by as much as 25 percent during the first weeks after myocardial infarction. Although the etiology of chronotropic incompetence is unknown, one proposed mechanism relates to a loss of normal vagal reflexes during exercise, which has been demonstrated in an animal model [13].

Because the heart rate response to exercise is quantitatively the most important mechanism for increasing cardiac output, chronotropic incompetence can have a significant effect on V̇O$_2$max. Chronotropic incompetence improves spontaneously over the first 3 to 8 weeks after myocardial infarction, as shown in serial exercise testing studies [14]. Therefore even in the absence of formal exercise training, V̇O$_2$max increases during this period.

Left Ventricular Dysfunction

All patients develop some degree of left ventricular dysfunction after myocardial infarction. Although the clinical effects of myocardial necrosis may be obvious by physical examination or noninvasive evaluation of left ventricular function, the effects on exercise performance are variable. A diminished ejection fraction at rest or one that fails to rise normally with exercise might be expected to predict a limited exercise capacity. However, most measures of ventricular performance at rest and with exercise correlate poorly with exercise performance, including left ventricular end-diastolic dimension, velocity of circumferential fiber shortening, systolic time intervals, and ejection fraction [15].

To determine the major factors influencing exercise capacity in patients with left ventricular dysfunction, Higgenbotham compared patients to age-matched sedentary controls. Both patients and controls had a wide range of exercise capacities with significant overlap. Ejection fractions were significantly lower in patients than in controls, and no overlap was present. In both groups, the major determinants of exercise capacity were the same: the heart rate response to exercise and the a-vO$_2$ difference at maximum exercise. Chronotropic incompetence was more common in patients than controls. In the absence of chronotropic incompetence, the onset of anaerobic metabolism was the major limiting effect [16].

Central and peripheral compensatory mechanisms can improve exercise performance even when severe left ventricular dysfunction is present. They include a preserved chronotropic response to exercise, increasing stroke volume with exercise, decreasing peripheral vascular resistance with exercise, ventricular dilation, increased levels of circulating catecholamines at rest and with exercise, and the ability to tolerate markedly elevated pulmonary artery wedge pressures [16–18]. Some of these mechanisms can be stimulated by exercise training, whereas the etiology of others is unclear. The implication of these findings is that the common clinical measures used to evaluate left ventricular function are inadequate to predict exercise capacity, and formal exercise testing should be used.

Myocardial Ischemia

After myocardial infarction, patients may have exercise-induced myocardial ischemia if segments of viable myocardium are served by diseased coronary arteries. Myocardial ischemia can limit exercise tolerance. The first physiologic abnormality caused by myocardial ischemia is a contraction abnormality in the affected segment. If a large segment of myocardium becomes ischemic, filling pressures increase and the ejection fraction and cardiac output decrease. These abnormalities may occur in the absence of angina, and patients may be limited by symptoms of dyspnea and fatigue.

Symptoms of angina may also limit exercise performance even in the absence of evidence of exercise-induced left ventricular dysfunction. Because patients perceive angina differently, the same degree of myocardial ischemia is tolerated by some patients and limits exertion in others. Amelioration of symptoms by medical therapy may improve exercise tolerance even in the absence of formal exercise training.

The effect of the normal recovery process on the coronary circulation is unknown. Spontaneous improvement in myocardial perfusion measured by radionuclide techniques has been demonstrated by several investigators [19–22]. However, these improvements are not reflected in changes in electrocardiographic or symptomatic evidence of myocardial ischemia on serial exercise testing in the absence of treatment [14, 22]. The double product (peak heart rate × peak systolic blood pressure) is a reasonable measure of myocardial oxygen demand. Although exercise capacity may increase spontaneously by the mechanisms described previously, the double product at which ischemia occurs remains relatively constant and reproducible in the absence of medical therapy.

Spontaneous Improvement in Exercise Capacity

The factors discussed previously contribute to spontaneous improvements in exercise capacity in most patients recovering from myocardial infarction. Table 34-3 shows the spontaneous improvement of exercise capacity in a 50-year-old man between 2 and 8 weeks after myocardial infarction in the absence of formal exercise training. Quantitatively, the resolution of chronotropic incompetence is the most important factor. Restoration of intravascular volume and recovery of normal cardiovascular reflexes play a major role during the first several days after hospital discharge. Skeletal muscle reconditioning from the resumption of customary activities contributes to improved physical activity by improving skeletal muscle oxygen extraction, resulting in a widened a-vO$_2$ difference.

These factors should influence evaluation and treatment after myocardial infarction. Early mobilization and prolonged periods of

Table 34-3
Spontaneous improvement in exercise capacity in a 50-year-old man between 2 and 8 weeks after myocardial infarction in the absence of formal exercise training

Time since MI	Peak exercise values						
	HR (bpm)	EDV (ml)	EF (%)	SV (ml/beat)	CO (L/min)	a-vO$_2$D (L/L)	V̇O$_2$max (L/min)
2 Weeks	140	190	45	86	12	0.14	1.7
8 Weeks	170	200	45	90	15	0.16	2.4
% Change	+21	+5	0	0	+25	+14	+41

upright posture should be emphasized during hospitalization, especially in uncomplicated patients. Progressive ambulation in the hospital should precede hospital discharge. The combination of chronotropic incompetence and volume depletion may precipitate a hypotensive response at higher levels of exercise; this physiologic response may be incorrectly interpreted as indicating a poor prognosis, leading to further diagnostic testing and limitation of activity. Physicians performing early exercise testing should plan tests with these considerations in mind.

EXERCISE TRAINING AFTER MYOCARDIAL INFARCTION

The factors influencing physical capacity after myocardial infarction have been presented. Although spontaneous improvement in exercise capacity occurs as a part of the normal recovery process after myocardial infarction, exercise training plays an important role in hastening the return to a normal exercise capacity in uncomplicated patients and improving the exercise capacity and symptomatic state of complicated patients. Exercise testing is the basis for recommendations regarding exercise training.

Exercise Testing
Over the past decade, exercise testing has become a valuable tool for the assessment of prognosis and the determination of functional capacity in patients recovering from myocardial infarction. Any patient being considered for an exercise training program after myocar-

dial infarction should undergo symptom-limited exercise testing. The indications for and the prognostic value of treadmill testing after myocardial infarction are presented in Chapter 33. This section reviews considerations related to using the exercise test for prescription of physical activity.

The timing of exercise testing relates primarily to the condition of patients and their suitability for exercise training. Uncomplicated patients without evidence of significant left ventricular dysfunction, myocardial ischemia, or arrhythmias may be tested soon after myocardial infarction. There is controversy regarding the best timing and type of exercise test to use for prognostication. Exercise testing before hospital discharge is usually performed to a submaximal limit, that is, a target heart rate of 60 percent of predicted maximum or 5 MET. Postdischarge treadmill testing may also use heart rate or workload targets.

The limitations of the predischarge submaximal test for exercise prescription are several. Bed-rest-induced volume depletion, chronotropic incompetence, and loss of physical conditioning may transiently limit exercise capacity. Exercising to a predicted heart rate or workload with submaximal testing underestimates physical capacity and results in an inappropriately low exercise prescription. Delaying treadmill testing until 7 to 14 days after hospital discharge can obviate some of these problems. A symptom-limited test can be performed and a more realistic exercise prescription given.

The Stanford Cardiac Rehabilitation Program has consistently used symptom-limited treadmill testing for exercise prescription after myocardial infarction. Patients exercise to an endpoint of fatigue, dyspnea, moderate angina, leg cramps, abnormal blood pressure response, or ventricular ectopy (triplets or runs). Symptom-limited treadmill testing should be performed when factors such as volume depletion and chronotropic incompetence do not blunt the exercise capacity or limit the test because of exertional hypotension. Symptom-limited testing may be performed soon after hospital discharge in uncomplicated patients [23, 24] but should be delayed in complicated patients.

Complicated postinfarction patients are not candidates for early symptom-limited exercise testing and therefore are not candidates for early exercise training. Patients with evidence of uncompensated left ventricular dysfunction (e.g., rales, jugular venous distention, a third heart sound, and peripheral edema) are at high risk for cardiac death during the 6 months after myocardial infarction [25]. After such patients are stabilized on appropriate medical therapy, exercise testing can be performed safely and can be used as the basis for an exercise training program [26]. Patients with angina at rest or with minimal activity are at high risk for recurrent infarction and death; these patients require more aggressive evaluation, and many will undergo coronary bypass surgery or angioplasty. Exercise testing can be used after a revascularization procedure as the basis for an exercise training program.

Other, less common complications of myocardial infarction decrease the utility of exercise testing after myocardial infarction. Abnormalities of conduction such as complete heart block or pacemaker-dependent rhythms and high grade or symptomatic ventricular arrhythmias limit the performance and value of exercise testing. Hemodynamic abnormalities other than left ventricular dysfunction, such as ischemic mitral regurgitation, can limit exercise performance. Atrial arrhythmias such as atrial fibrillation and flutter can affect both the chronotropic and ventricular loading responses to exercise. Extensive discussion of each of these problems is beyond the scope of this chapter; management of these problems requires careful coordination between the rehabilitation specialist and the primary cardiologist.

In uncomplicated patients, symptom-limited exercise testing has been demonstrated to be safe when performed 10 to 21 days from the date of infarction [27–29]. This timing for testing is optimal because higher risk patients with asymptomatic myocardial ischemia are identified soon after myocardial infarction, and the problems of chronotropic incompetence and volume depletion are sufficiently resolved to obtain a true measure of physical performance. The exercise test should be performed after cardiac medications have been tapered and withdrawn if possible. Medications can mask significant ischemic and arrhythmic abnormalities during exercise that might require further evaluation and more specific therapy [10, 30]. In addition, some patients treated with prophylactic antianginal and antiarrhythmic medications may show no significant abnormalities if tested off medications, and medications may then be discontinued.

Delaying exercise testing for complicated patients for 6 to 8 weeks after myocardial infarction is appropriate. Complicated patients with left ventricular dysfunction or symptomatic myocardial ischemia do not need early exercise testing for prognostication. These clinical syndromes are sufficient to prompt further diagnostic evaluation and therapy with medications or revascularization procedures. Once stabilized, these patients are candidates for exercise testing to establish an exercise prescription.

In all patients recovering from myocardial infarction, a modified Naughton treadmill protocol is a reasonable choice for exercise testing [31]. A comparison of the Bruce and modified Naughton protocols is shown in Table 34-4. The modified Naughton protocol begins at a lower MET level than the Bruce protocol and progresses at 1-MET increments every 3 minutes. The transition between stages is therefore less dramatic, and patients can progress comfortably. Patients ultimately achieve the same peak workload on either protocol, but the longer time of exercise on the modified Naughton protocol can reassure the patients

Table 34-4
Comparison of modified Naughton and Bruce protocols for treadmill exercise testing

Modified Naughton protocol					Bruce protocol				
Stage	Minutes	MET	Speed (mph)	Grade (%)	Stage	Minutes	MET	Speed (mph)	Grade (%)
I	3	3	2.0	3.5					
II	3	4	2.0	7.0					
III	3	5	2.0	10.5	I	3	5	1.7	10
IV	3	6	2.0	14.0					
V	3	7	2.0	17.5	II	3	7	2.5	12
VI	3	8	3.0	12.5					
VII	3	9	3.0	15.0					
VIII	3	10	3.0	17.5	III	3	10	3.4	14

that they are capable of beginning formal exercise training. In addition, patients with significant physical deconditioning or symptoms are not overly stressed during the initial stages of exercise.

Eligibility for Exercise Training

Most patients recovering from myocardial infarction are eligible to undergo exercise training within 3 months after myocardial infarction. Uncomplicated patients eligible for treadmill testing soon after myocardial infarction can begin exercise training as early as 10 days after hospital discharge. Patients with significant myocardial ischemia, presenting as angina or significant ST segment depression at low levels of exercise, are not candidates for exercise training until myocardial ischemia is ameliorated by medical or revascularization therapy. Patients with significant left ventricular dysfunction, manifested by symptoms of exertional dyspnea, physical signs of congestive heart failure, or ejection fractions of less than 30 percent are not candidates for exercise training until their symptoms and signs have been adequately treated.

Other patients are eligible for exercise training with some caveats. Patients with high grade or symptomatic ventricular arrhythmias should undergo evaluation and treatment as outlined in Chapters 10, 35, and 36. Once high grade ventricular arrhythmias have been suppressed, developing an exercise prescription using treadmill testing is appropriate. Patients

with atrial arrhythmias, especially atrial fibrillation, should receive appropriate therapy to suppress an excessive chronotropic response to exercise before beginning exercise training. Exercise testing is a useful tool for assessing such therapy. Patients with electrocardiographic abnormalities that might obscure evidence of myocardial ischemia on exercise testing, such as left bundle branch block, should undergo exercise testing with radionuclides to be certain that significant ischemic abnormalities are not present.

Exercise Prescription

The basic principles that apply to exercise training of healthy adults are applicable in a modified form to patients recovering from myocardial infarction. The modifications include changes in type, frequency, intensity, and duration of training sessions; the rate of progression to higher intensity training; and the level of surveillance of patients. Special considerations are necessary for patients with left ventricular dysfunction, myocardial ischemia, and arrhythmias, both atrial and ventricular.

BASIC PRINCIPLES OF EXERCISE TRAINING
In the healthy adult the recommendations for achieving and maintaining optimal cardiovascular conditioning include training 3 to 5 days per week, a minimum intensity of 60 percent of maximal heart rate, and a duration of 15 to 60 minutes per training session. The inten-

sity and duration of exercise are adjusted to achieve an overall energy expenditure of 300 kilocalories per session. Kilocalorie expenditure is directly related to duration and intensity; the more intense the exercise, the shorter the duration required to expend 300 kilocalories [32–36].

Training sessions are commonly divided into four components: warm-up, muscular conditioning, aerobic exercise, and cooldown. The warm-up and cool-down sessions are important aspects of the conditioning program. An adequate warm-up can decrease the incidence of injury, especially muscle and ligament strains. It may also decrease the incidence of exercise-induced angina. The cooldown is equally important in patients with coronary disease. The immediate cessation of aerobic exercise is commonly associated with precipitation of ventricular arrhythmias and with sensations of lightheadedness. Ventricular arrhythmias are precipitated by the unopposed catecholamine stimulation of abnormal myocardium. Lightheadedness results from a mismatch between the rapid fall in heart rate and cardiac output with cessation of exercise and the slow return of peripheral vasomotor tone from the intense vasodilation induced by exercise.

The muscular conditioning and aerobic components of exercise have the dual goals of optimizing muscular strength for customary activities and developing cardiac and peripheral training effects. Strength training should emphasize large muscle groups in dynamic exercise with as little an isometric component as possible. Isometric exercise, such as weight lifting, and exercise that requires a strong hand grip component are associated with significant increases in blood pressure [37]. The size of the muscle group used during strength training is directly related to the increases in blood pressure. Adequate muscular training can be achieved with a well balanced calisthenic program and the use of light hand weights (3–7 lb) either prior to or during aerobic exercise. Dynamic upper extremity exercise, such as arm ergometry or rowing, can provide a conditioning effect and is not associated with the hypertensive response of static exercise [38].

Aerobic conditioning programs commonly use walking, jogging, bicycling, or swimming as the predominant exercise. For the patient recovering from myocardial infarction, swimming is not recommended during the first 3 to 6 months because of potential difficulties in monitoring heart rate and treatment in the event of a cardiac complication. The intensity and duration of the aerobic portion of exercise training is generally thought of as the *exercise prescription*. Individual prescriptions are developed depending on the timing after myocardial infarction, the presence or absence of symptoms, the degree of left ventricular dysfunction and myocardial ischemia, the level of conditioning, and the presence of other complications such as arrhythmias, conduction abnormalities, and other diseases (e.g., obstructive lung disease, orthopedic abnormalities, and peripheral vascular disease).

The intensity of exercise is most commonly regulated by heart rate. Heart rate can be monitored using pulse counting at either the radial or the carotid artery. Inexpensive heart rate monitors are also available that allow one to set upper and lower heart rate limits; and they give an audible signal to patients when they are out of range. Another method for monitoring exercise intensity is to use the rate of perceived exertion (RPE) scale developed by Borg and Linderholm [39]. The scale originally used numbers between 60 and 200 matched with descriptions such as "very light," "somewhat hard," and so on. The numbers were estimates of heart rate and correlated well with perceived exertion in healthy men undergoing exercise training. The scale has been simplified (Table 34-5) and now ranges from 6 to 20 with the same descriptions. Using the RPE scale during exercise testing allows the prescription of a heart rate range based on the patient's perception of exertion. Matching the prescribed heart rate to the RPE rating and using the RPE for monitoring exercise has been shown to be as reliable as assigning heart rate limits [40].

INPATIENT (PHASE I) EXERCISE TRAINING
Inpatient exercise training should prepare patients for customary activities they will undertake at home. Programs for progressive am-

Table 34-5
Borg RPE scale

Description of exertion	Score
	6
Very, very light	7
	8
Very light	9
	10
Light	11
	12
Somewhat hard	13
	14
Hard	15
	16
Very hard	17
	18
Very, very hard	19
	20

bulation have been published [35, 36] and should serve as general guidelines for gradually increasing patient activity. Complete physical reconditioning before hospital discharge is an unrealistic goal for several reasons. The period for reconditioning is short, generally only 3 to 5 days. Other physiologic abnormalities such as volume depletion and chronotropic incompetence are significant impediments to formal exercise training. Exercise testing is not usually performed before progressive ambulation.

Realistic goals for inpatient exercise training include preparation to perform customary activities during the first days to weeks after hospital discharge, evaluation of symptomatic responses to physical activity, instruction in low level exercise including pulse and symptom monitoring, and determination of the optimal timing of entry into a formal conditioning program. For inpatient and early postdischarge exercise, a heart rate limit of 20 beats per minute (bpm) above the standing resting heart rate is reasonable. This heart rate limit is recommended because most patients do not perform maximal exercise testing before hospital discharge, and the calculation of heart rate targets from predicted maximal heart rates (220 minus the patient's age) may overestimate peak heart rate responses because of the problem of chronotropic incompetence.

OUTPATIENT (PHASE II) EXERCISE TRAINING

Following the performance of a symptom-limited treadmill test, patients may begin formal exercise training. The time of testing and the exercise prescription depend on the condition of individual patients, as discussed below. In general, patients with complications of myocardial ischemia, left ventricular dysfunction, or arrhythmias are tested later and exercise at lower levels. (The issues of safety and supervision are discussed in later sections.)

The exercise prescription is based on the peak heart rate attained on the treadmill test and the symptomatic response. Exercise training is initiated at 60 to 70 percent of the peak treadmill heart rate. Patients should be able to monitor their pulse and understand the concept of a target heart range. Target heart ranges should be given for 10-second counts. For example, if the desired heart rate is 120 bpm, dividing by 6 gives a target of 20 for 10 seconds. The usual target rate is then 20 ± 1, giving an actual minute heart rate range of 114 to 126. Although the 10-second count range of ± 1 seems narrow, it is easily attained after some practice by patients.

The simplest aerobic exercise to perform and monitor is walking. During the initial exercise session, the pulse should be monitored frequently to allow patients to determine the exercise level needed to attain the target heart rate. Some exercise programs begin with a "30–30" program [41]: Patients walk for 30 seconds at a speed sufficient to meet their target and then slow down for 30 seconds to heart rates below target. This technique is valuable for demonstrating how heart rate is a good measure of physical activity. As patients progress, the 30–30 is shifted to a "45–15" programs (45 seconds at target, 15 seconds below target) and then to full aerobic periods at the target heart rate. Uncomplicated patients may make this progression within one or two exercise sessions, whereas complicated patients may require several sessions.

Significant emphasis on pulse and symptom monitoring should be provided during exercise training because most cardiac complications of exercise occur when patients exceed their target heart rates. Patients should be aware that other factors can influence heart rate. Elevated body temperature increases heart rate at any given workload. Factors such as ambient temperature, heavy clothing, and intercurrent febrile illnesses must be considered. Changes in medical condition can influence heart rate response. Worsening left ventricular function, development of atrial or ventricular arrhythmias, and changes in drug therapy can potentially influence heart rate response to exercise. As chronotropic incompetence resolves, the heart rate response changes. Finally, as physical conditioning occurs, the heart rate is lower for any given workload.

UNCOMPLICATED PATIENTS

In the uncomplicated patient without significant abnormalities on the treadmill test, target heart rates during early exercise training should be 70 to 85 percent of the peak heart rate achieved on treadmill testing. During the first 7 weeks after myocardial infarction, the target heart rates should be gradually increased from 70 percent to 85 percent. At the same time the training effect is occurring, chronotropic incompetence is spontaneously resolving. By the eighth week most patients can achieve significantly higher peak heart rates on treadmill testing [14]. The target heart rates can then be increased to 85 to 100 percent of the peak heart rate attained on early testing. This target corresponds to 70 to 85 percent of the peak heart rate, which would be attained by repeated treadmill testing at 8 weeks after myocardial infarction [14]. Uncomplicated patients performing post-infarction treadmill testing and beginning exercise training later (e.g., 6 to 8 weeks after infarction) do not require this adjustment because chronotropic incompetence has resolved. Further adjustments in exercise prescription should be based on repeated treadmill testing. Using the guidelines outlined previously, uncomplicated patients should exercise for 30 to 60 minutes three to five times weekly. Pulse counting and symptom monitoring is a sufficient method to monitor intensity of exercise.

PATIENTS WITH MYOCARDIAL ISCHEMIA

The extent and severity of myocardial ischemia on exercise testing soon after myocardial

infarction should guide therapy and modify the exercise prescription. Several studies have demonstrated that patients with exercise-induced ischemia after myocardial infarction have higher rates of cardiac death, recurrent infarction, and coronary revascularization during the first 6 to 12 months [28, 42–46]. Patients with more than 0.2 mV of ST depression, especially at a low heart rate or workload, have significantly higher event rates [42]. Abnormal blood pressure response [28, 46] or a low exercise tolerance, even in the absence of significant ischemic changes on the electrocardiogram [28, 46], also predict cardiac events.

The best diagnostic and therapeutic approach to patients with exercise-induced myocardial ischemia is unknown. The guidelines for exercise training should be modified depending on the therapy used to treat ischemia. Patients undergoing coronary bypass graft surgery are usually eligible for treadmill testing 4 to 6 weeks after surgery. Treadmill testing should be performed postoperatively even if a preoperative treadmill was performed. Exercise capacity, ischemic threshold, symptoms, heart rate response, medications, and other parameters affecting exercise training can be modified by surgery; and repeat testing is necessary to provide an accurate exercise prescription. The type of exercise postoperative patients perform should be modified initially to avoid stress to the pectoral girdle as the sternum heals. Patients undergoing coronary angioplasty can undergo treadmill testing within 1 week of the procedure and are given an exercise prescription based on the results.

Patients with mild ischemia may receive medical therapy with beta blockers, nitrates, calcium channel blockers, or a combination. Each of these agents has been shown to increase the exercise capacity primarily by decreasing the double-product for any given workload [47–51]. Ideally, exercise prescriptions should be based on treadmill testing performed on treatment. However, patients often receive medical therapy because of an ischemic abnormality on a routine, postinfarction treadmill test, and repeat treadmill testing is not performed. For patients taking antianginal medications other than beta blockers, it is usually reasonable to provide an exercise prescription without repeating the treadmill test. In such patients, and those with treadmill ischemia in whom medical therapy is not prescribed, the target heart rate should be set at 5 to 10 bpm below the heart rate at which ischemia occurs or to 70 to 85 percent of peak heart rate, whichever is lower. For patients who do not undergo repeat testing, this prescription may be conservative in comparison to the target that might be prescribed if the treadmill were repeated.

Because beta blockers can have a profound effect on peak heart rate response to exercise, treadmill testing on medication is ideal for prescribing exercise training [47]. When repeat testing is not feasible, an exercise prescription at 55 to 70 percent of the peak heart rate attained on treadmill testing off medication or 5 to 10 bpm below the heart rate at which ischemia is present may be used. This modification of the prescription was developed empirically in our program and is useful clinically. Exercise testing should be repeated at 4 to 6 weeks after exercise training on beta blockers to ensure that patients are experiencing a training effect and to determine if the target heart rates can be increased safely.

The effect on conditioning of patients receiving anti-ischemic therapy is not clear. Some authors have suggested that beta blockade attenuates training in angina patients [49], whereas others have demonstrated exercise training effects in the presence of beta-blockade therapy [52, 53]. Calcium channel blockers do not appear to attenuate training effects in patients with coronary disease [48, 54]. Most studies of the effects of medications on training are in mixed populations of patients with coronary disease, rather than only patients recovering from recent myocardial infarction.

PATIENTS WITH LEFT VENTRICULAR DYSFUNCTION
Persistent left ventricular dysfunction in the absence of myocardial ischemia occurs in 10 to 15 percent of postinfarction patients. The severity of left ventricular dysfunction and patient symptoms are variable. Although left ventricular dysfunction is the most powerful predictor of a poor prognosis [25], many patients have few symptoms and a preserved functional capacity. Symptoms and signs of congestive heart failure and measurements of ventricular performance are useful for prognostication, but they do not necessarily correlate with exercise capacity, as discussed previously.

Unlike uncomplicated patients and those with mild postinfarction ischemia, patients with left ventricular dysfunction should undergo symptom-limited treadmill testing on maximal medical therapy. When revascularization therapy is not an option, exercise testing should be performed when hemodynamics are optimal. Although significantly more physiologic data can be obtained by combined respiratory and cardiac monitoring during an exercise test [26], a standard treadmill test is usually sufficient to develop an exercise prescription.

In addition to determining if ischemia is present, other specific abnormalities should be looked for during exercise testing in patients with left ventricular dysfunction. The development of mitral regurgitation during exercise testing may reflect either myocardial ischemia and papillary muscle dysfunction or impaired ventricular dynamics. A fall in systolic blood pressure may reflect myocardial ischemia or an inadequate cardiac output response to exercise-induced peripheral vasodilation. Exercise-induced pulmonary congestion may occur because of these and other mechanisms. Exercise prescriptions must be modified in the presence of any of these abnormalities.

Although patients with significant left ventricular dysfunction are frequently excluded from exercise training because of their high risk status, there is clear evidence that exercise training can provide beneficial physiologic effects without increased risk [55–57]. Physiologic changes induced by exercise training include decreased peripheral vascular resistance and improved skeletal muscle oxygen extraction. Even in the absence of major central changes, these peripheral influences can improve ventricular function by reducing afterload and increasing efficiency of skeletal muscle oxygen extraction [58].

The exercise prescription in patients with left ventricular dysfunction uses the same intensity (i.e., 60 to 85 percent of peak heart rate on the treadmill), but shorter duration initially. The "30–30" program can limit the degree of fatigue experienced by the patient. Patients tolerating interval training can gradually increase the duration of higher intensity exercise and decrease the duration of lower intensity exercise. The exercise intensity should be decreased in patients developing any of the hemodynamic abnormalities described previously. Clinically, lowering the prescription by 10 bpm below the heart rate at which the abnormality occurs has been suggested [47].

There is evidence that chronic nitrate therapy improves exercise capacity long term in patients with left ventricular dysfunction, primarily by its effects on the venous circulation [50]. Similarly, long-term improvements in exercise capacity have been demonstrated in patients receiving vasodilator therapy alone and in association with exercise training programs [59, 60]. Significant changes in medical therapy should prompt repeated exercise testing and prescription.

PATIENTS WITH ARRHYTHMIAS

High grade ventricular arrhythmias are common when myocardial infarction is complicated by left ventricular dysfunction. Management of left ventricular dysfunction and ventricular arrhythmias is presented in Chapters 30, 35, and 36. Once arrhythmias are successfully treated, patients should undergo symptom-limited treadmill testing to develop an exercise prescription.

The postinfarction exercise test may reveal previously unsuspected high grade ventricular arrhythmias. Ectopy is common during the early recovery phase after exercise because of high levels of unopposed circulating catecholamines. These arrhythmias should not necessarily prompt more aggressive therapy unless they are high grade, such as Lown class III or IV, or sustained. If exercise-induced arrhythmias are high grade, further evaluation and treatment is needed. Exercise testing should be repeated after therapy is instituted.

Even in patients managed with antiarrhythmic drugs, arrhythmias may occur on treadmill testing. Patients with high grade ventricular arrhythmias, such as triplets or runs, during exercise while on medical therapy should be evaluated further. If antiarrhythmic therapy is deemed adequate, the target heart rates for exercise training should be at least 10 bpm below the heart rate at which arrhythmias occur.

In some patients, complete suppression of all high grade ventricular arrhythmias is not possible. In those patients, the benefit of exercise training should be carefully weighed against the risk. If patients are allowed to exercise, electrocardiographic monitoring should be performed during training to assess the reproducibility and prognostic significance of the arrhythmias. The results of monitoring may be used to guide the clinician in further evaluation and therapy as well as the desirability of continued exercise training.

Atrial arrhythmias may be present after myocardial infarction and should be evaluated and treated as outlined in Chapter 12. The most common atrial arrhythmia that influences the exercise prescription is atrial fibrillation. Even when heart rates are well controlled at rest, patients with atrial fibrillation often have an exaggerated chronotropic response to exercise. This response can impair exercise capacity because of the rate-related loss of diastolic filling time and the absence of the atrial component of ventricular filling. If this exaggerated chronotropic response is present on treadmill testing, consideration should be given to beta blockers or verapamil for rate control and the exercise test repeated.

The development of complete heart block after myocardial infarction usually reflects a large amount of myocardial necrosis, especially if the infarction is anterior. Exercise capacity is more often limited by the concomitant left ventricular dysfunction than the heart block. If left ventricular dysfunction is not severe, consideration of placement of a rate-responsive pacemaker should be considered. The exercise prescription should then be based on exercise testing with the pacemaker in place.

OUTPATIENT (PHASES III AND IV)
EXERCISE TRAINING

After completion of the standard 12-week phase II exercise training program, some patients want or need further exercise training. Uncomplicated patients desiring prolonged exercise training who have progressed well through phase II training should undergo repeated treadmill testing. If the treadmill test is normal, the patient can be given the option of continued supervised group exercise (phase III) or self-monitored home exercise (phase IV). The prescription is similar to that of phase II, but patients should exercise at an intensity closer to 85 percent of peak treadmill heart rate. The four components of exercise (warm-up, muscular conditioning, aerobic exercise, and cool-down) should be emphasized, as should self-monitoring techniques for heart rate response and symptoms.

Complicated patients or those who were severely deconditioned at the beginning of phase II programs may benefit from more prolonged phase III exercise training. These patients should also undergo repeat treadmill testing, and a new exercise prescription should be given based on that test. The same caveats described for phase II training of complicated patients are true for phase III training. Complicated patients with stable symptoms may eventually become candidates for unsupervised, self-monitored exercise training. The decision to advance such patients should be made only after careful medical evaluation by the primary physician and the medical director of the rehabilitation program.

Effects of Exercise Training

The physiologic benefits of exercise training after myocardial infarction are well demonstrated. Training studies consistently demonstrate increased peak heart rates, increased functional capacity, decreased heart rates at rest and submaximal exercise, and decreased systolic blood pressure at submaximal exercise [4, 61]. The immediate response to training is a reduced heart rate and systolic blood pressure for a given workload. These changes lower myocardial oxygen demand at any given level of work.

Whether exercise training causes significant improvement in cardiac function after myocardial infarction is controversial. High intensity exercise and prolonged endurance training have been associated with increases in stroke volume, left ventricular ejection fraction, and myocardial perfusion in some studies [20, 62–64]. However, other investigators have not demonstrated significant changes in cardiac performance despite improvements in exercise capacity [22, 55, 57]. Although exercise-induced angina and ST depression appear at higher workloads after exercise training, they generally occur at a constant double product.

Controversy exists concerning cardiac adaptations to exercise training after myocardial infarction, but peripheral adaptations appear in virtually all patients. The primary peripheral adaptations are in the circulation and in skeletal muscle metabolism, and they include increases in capillary density, skeletal muscle mitochondria, myoglobin content, and oxidative enzymes [58, 65]. These peripheral adaptations lower the double product for a given workload. The workload at which ischemia occurs is therefore increased. Favorable hemodynamic responses, such as lower systolic blood pressure, can decrease myocardial work in patients with left ventricular dysfunction.

These physiologic changes are usually associated with improvements in symptoms. Patients with angina often have their anginal threshold increased, so they can perform more physical activity without ischemia. The lower mean blood pressure with exercise results in a greater exercise capacity for patients with left ventricular dysfunction. The latter patients often have the greatest symptomatic benefit because their exercise capacity is so low initially.

Whether exercise training decreases cardiac mortality after myocardial infarction is controversial. Postinfarction training studies have demonstrated trends toward improved survival in most instances [66–69]. However, design flaws such as an inadequate number of patients or short follow-up limited results in some studies. In other studies, compliance to exercise training was low, and crossovers from the nonexercise to the exercise groups occurred. Despite these flaws, the improvements in physical capacity and hemodynamic response to exercise are significant benefits of exercise training that occurred in most studies [70].

Other benefits of exercise training are related to secondary prevention and psychosocial outcomes, discussed in more detail later in this chapter. Increased caloric expenditure can, with dietary modification, help the patient to achieve ideal body weight. Because energy costs of physical work are proportional to body mass, a loss of fat can reduce the energy requirement of any given activity [36]. Improvements in lipid profiles are associated with exercise training [66, 71]. Reductions in blood pressure occur, especially in hypertensive patients [72]. Psychological benefits include diminished anxiety and depression [73] and improved confidence to undertake physical activity and resume customary activities [74].

SAFETY OF EXERCISE TRAINING

Ensuring that physical training does not harm the patient is a paramount concern during rehabilitation. The most important factors that ensure safety are patient selection, careful intake evaluation, appropriate prescription, and adequate supervision. The risk of exercise for the individual patient is related primarily to the extent and severity of left ventricular dysfunction, myocardial ischemia, and ventricular arrhythmias. In postinfarction patients without significant abnormalities, the risk of exercise is minimal, and rapid progression from supervised to unsupervised exercise is possible. Conversely, in patients with severe manifestations of one or more of these abnormalities, exercise training may be contraindicated or high level surveillance may be appropriate.

Several clinical and exercise test abnormalities are associated with a higher risk for cardiac events during exercise training. Significant left ventricular dysfunction increases the risk of exercise. It may be manifested by multiple prior infarctions; low ejection fraction seen by radionuclide, echocardiographic, or angiographic techniques; symptoms of dyspnea at rest or low levels of exercise; low treadmill exercise tolerance; chronotropic incompetence; and abnormal blood pressure response to exercise. Significant myocardial ischemia may be manifested by frequent angina poorly controlled by medical therapy, significant exercise-induced ST segment depression with or without angina, low exercise tolerance, a declining ejection fraction with exercise, and severe anatomic coronary disease at angiography. Significant electrical instability may be manifested as complex atrial and ventricular arrhythmias at rest, high degree atrioventricular block, and complex ventricular arrhythmias induced by exercise.

If any of these clinical or exercise test abnormalities are present, exercise training should be undertaken with caution after appropriate therapy is begun. The exercise prescription should account for the exercise level at which abnormalities appear. Higher levels of supervision and surveillance should be used in higher risk patients. Complications of exercise training are directly related to the intensity of exercise. To achieve the desired training effect in higher risk patients, the intensity can be lowered and the frequency or duration (or both) of training sessions increased.

In higher risk patients, compliance to the exercise prescription is crucial. Exercising above the prescribed intensity may be due to inaccurate monitoring techniques by the patient, a lack of understanding of techniques for monitoring, inadequate frequency of monitoring, or a disregard for the need for monitoring. In these circumstances, increased surveillance by the exercise leaders may be required. This surveillance might include electrocardiographic monitoring, either continuous or intermittent, increased frequency of pulse monitoring, the use of electronic heart rate monitors, and increased educational efforts [75].

There is considerable debate among rehabilitation specialists regarding the degree and duration of medical supervision needed for patients undergoing exercise training. Individual programs vary from requiring continuous electrocardiographic monitoring of all patients during early exercise training, to frequent pulse and symptom monitoring by patients and supervising personnel, to home exercise training with patient pulse and symptom monitoring. No single set of guidelines has been established unequivocally as appropriate for all programs. Guidelines suggested by individual investigators [35, 36, 75] and professional organizations [32–34] are consistent in matching the intensity of monitoring with the severity of pathophysiologic manifestations of the individual patient.

On-site supervision with continuous electrocardiographic monitoring is recommended for patients at high risk for cardiac arrest or ventricular fibrillation, such as those with prior cardiac arrest, severe congestive heart failure, exercise-induced ventricular tachycardia, or complex ventricular arrhythmias associated with left ventricular dysfunction. At the other end of the spectrum, very low risk patients without left ventricular dysfunction and a peak treadmill capacity of 6 MET or higher without evidence of myocardial ischemia or arrhythmias are recommended for home exercise training with pulse monitoring using an individualized exercise prescription. In the absence of firm guidelines, decisions regarding the degree of medical supervision for exercise must be made by the responsible physician.

Although concerns regarding risks of exercise training are appropriate, supervised exercise training of cardiac patients is associated with a low risk of precipitating cardiac events. A recent survey of 167 cardiac rehabilitation programs evaluated the incidence of major cardiovascular complications over a 4-year period. The level of medical supervision ranged from continuous to limited electrocardiographic monitoring of new patients. The incidence rate per million patient hours of exercise for fatalities was 1.3, for myocardial infarctions 3.4, and for resuscitated cardiac arrests 8.9. There were no significant differences in these event rates for small compared to large programs or for continuously monitored compared to intermittently monitored programs [76].

These rates of major cardiovascular complications are significantly lower than the rates found in a similar study of programs surveyed between 1960 and 1977 [77]. The reasons for the improvement in complication rates are speculative. Improved risk stratification, improved medical and revascularization therapies, more rigorous standards for cardiac rehabilitation programs, and increased awareness of the necessity for monitoring high risk patients may have contributed to this improved safety record.

Secondary Prevention After Myocardial Infarction

Although exercise training is the focus of most rehabilitation programs after myocardial infarction, secondary prevention is at least as important for the long-term health of patients. Secondary prevention measures after myocardial infarction commonly include drug therapy for symptoms and prophylaxis of left ventricular dysfunction and myocardial ischemia, as discussed in Part VII of this book. Other measures include treatment of conventional risk factors, including smoking, lipid abnormalities, hypertension, and type A personality. Smoking cessation has clearly been demonstrated to decrease mortality after myocardial infarction. Treatment of elevated plasma lipid levels has not been shown unequivocally to alter outcome, but elevated lipid levels have been implicated in adverse outcomes. There is no convincing evidence that treating hypertension alters outcome after myocardial infarction, although such treatment is customary. Finally, there is controversy regarding the effect of type A personality on prognosis.

SMOKING

Risk of Smoking

Cigarette smoking is an established risk factor for the development of angina and myocardial infarction and for the recurrence of myocardial infarction [78, 79]. Survivors of myocardial infarction who continue to smoke have approximately twice the rate of recurrent infarction and cardiac death compared to nonsmokers and patients who quit smoking after myocardial infarction [79–82]. Smoking cessation was associated with a 61 percent reduction in mortality rate over 6 years in the Framingham Study [82] and a 55 percent reduction in mortality over 13 years in survivors of unstable angina or myocardial infarction [83]. The Norwegian Multicenter Group Study demonstrated a 45 percent reduction in the reinfarction rate over 17 months after myocardial infarction in patients who quit smoking compared to those who continued to smoke [80]. The risk for cardiac death and reinfarction appears to decline rapidly in smokers who quit after suffering a myocardial infarction compared to those who continue to smoke. Within 3 years of myocardial infarction, ex-smokers have approximately the same risk for reinfarction as survivors of myocardial infarction who never smoked [81].

Pathophysiology of Smoking

The pathophysiology underlying the risk for death and reinfarction in smokers is uncertain. Coronary spasm, platelet aggregation, thrombosis [84], and diminished coronary and collateral reserve [85] have been implicated as possible etiologies. Coronary vascular reserve, the capacity of coronary arteries to dilate and increase blood flow on increased demand, is significantly reduced in smokers compared to that in nonsmokers. Heavy smokers have significantly lower coronary vascular reserve than light smokers [85]. Fibrinogen levels are significantly higher in smokers than nonsmokers and appear to increase the primary risk for myocardial infarction [86]. Although the degree of coronary atherosclerosis does not appear to be strongly correlated to smoking habits [87], the risk for myocardial infarction in smokers appears to be strongly correlated with the degree of underlying coronary disease and the plasma cholesterol level [84]. Although some of these data are derived primarily from patients who have not suffered a previous myocardial infarction, they shed some light on pathophysiologic mechanisms that may be relevant in postinfarction patients.

Factors Influencing Smoking After Myocardial Infarction

The association between smoking and cardiac disease is well known in both medical and lay communities. Myocardial infarction is a sufficient impetus to stop smoking in 20 to 60 percent of patients [88]. Several demographic and psychological factors are associated with continued smoking after myocardial infarction. Lower occupational and educational levels, smoking a higher number of cigarettes per day before myocardial infarction, increasing age [88], and high rates of alcohol consumption [89] are demographic factors associated with continued smoking. Psychological factors such as less negative attitudes regarding smoking, high anxiety levels, and a low sense of personal control of life events identify smokers who are less likely to quit after myocardial infarction [88].

Etiology of Tobacco Dependence

There are several theories that attempt to explain tobacco dependence. No single theory is adequate to explain all aspects of smoking behavior. Smoking is a complex behavior with physiologic, psychological, and sociologic causes. Continued smoking reflects the psychologic dependence on nicotine; abrupt smoking cessation can cause acute craving for cigarettes related to nicotine deprivation [90]. Smoking is also a habit that appears to minimize negative emotions, such as distress, anger and fear. Smoking may be a coping behavior to transform such negative emotions into a socially acceptable habit [91]. Finally, smoking behavior has sociologic origins related to modeling behavior after others, such as parents or peer groups.

Smoking Abstinence

The significantly higher morbidity and mortality rates of postinfarction patients who continue to smoke is the rationale for including smoking abstinence as a part of comprehensive cardiac rehabilitation. Abstinence from cigarette smoking has two components: smoking cessation and relapse prevention. Smoking abstinence is best achieved through structured programs. However, physicians should not discount their influence on patients who smoke. Patients receiving specific advice to stop smoking from health professionals are more likely to quit and remain abstinent than those who do not receive advice [92]. This point is particularly true for individuals who believe that they are at personal risk if they continue smoking [93]. Providing low cost educational materials available from the American Heart Association, American Lung Association, and the American Cancer Society can reinforce the strong medical advice provided during hospitalization for myocardial infarction.

SMOKING CESSATION

Most smokers quit smoking at the time of hospitalization for myocardial infarction. For patients unable to quit on their own, a variety of methods for smoking cessation are available. Although no one method appears significantly more effective than another, the most effective programs focus on the physiologic dependence on nicotine, the psychological need for a coping mechanism, and aspects of the learned behavior of smoking. Nicotine dependence may be approached using tapering techniques by changing cigarette brands, controlling smoking habits, and substituting nicotine gum. Aversive techniques, such as rapid puffing or smoke holding, may also be effective.

The availability of nicotine gum has improved the cessation and abstinence rates of smoking cessation programs [94, 95]. Simple prescription of nicotine gum to smokers without a concomitant program to change behavior has not been effective in maintaining long-term smoking abstinence. Nicotine gum appears to blunt craving for cigarettes by exposing patients to low levels of nicotine. A 2-mg nicotine gum dose gives an average blood nicotine level of 12 ng/ml compared to levels of 35 to 54 ng/ml obtained from cigarette smoking [96]. Nicotine gum is available as 2-mg doses prescribed on an as-needed basis up to 30 pieces per day. Most patients use ten pieces per day. The frequency of use should gradually decrease over a 1- to 3-month period. If smoking cessation has not occurred by 6 months, nicotine gum is most likely being used as a cigarette substitute rather than a cessation aid.

Techniques to eliminate the physiologic dependence on nicotine are most effective when coupled with behavioral counseling such as identifying and avoiding situations in which smoking is likely and substituting behaviors such as exercise. The same behavioral techniques are effective for both smoking cessation and relapse prevention.

RELAPSE PREVENTION

Once patients stop smoking, relapse prevention becomes the goal of smoking abstinence programs. Education of the patient regarding the effects of continued smoking is the first step in relapse prevention. Informing them about symptoms associated with smoking abstinence prepares them for behavior change and allows them to correctly attribute sensations to smoking withdrawal. Intense craving for cigarettes is common and is often behavior-specific (e.g., while drinking coffee or alcohol, while talking on the telephone) and situation-specific (e.g., at parties, in stressful environments). Irritability, emotionality, anxiety, and inability to concentrate are all symptoms of smoking cessation [91]. Physical symptoms such as nausea, headache, increased appetite, and sleep disturbance are common [97, 98].

Teaching patients new ways to deal with situations or behaviors that encourage smoking is the next step in relapse prevention. Having patients identify, list, and carry the list of circumstances in which they are at high risk of relapse is useful. Applying self-control strategies to high risk situations is also useful. For example, if smoking is associated with the morning coffee break, the patient should switch the time or the activity of the break. If smoking is likely in social situations, role-playing cigarette denial or refusal may be helpful. Substituting healthful behaviors, such as a short walk or a short period of reminding themselves that they and not the cigarettes are in control, are effective strategies to prevent relapse [99]. Enlisting social support from spouses, friends, coworkers, or other participants in a cardiac rehabilitation program may help to reinforce nonsmoking behavior.

HYPERCHOLESTEROLEMIA

A large body of basic, clinical, and epidemiologic research support the link between hypercholesterolemia and the development of coronary artery disease. The association between elevated cholesterol levels and the progression of coronary artery disease on coronary arteriography has been established. Most studies investigating the effects of treatment of hypercholesterolemia on coronary disease have used patients who have not suffered myocardial infarction. The results of these primary prevention trials have been consistent: reductions in cholesterol by dietary or drug therapy have reduced cardiovascular morbidity and mortality [100, 101] and have slowed the progression of coronary atherosclerosis [102, 103].

The effect of hypercholesterolemia on morbidity, mortality, and progression of coronary disease in survivors of myocardial infarction is less clear. Several intervention trials have demonstrated a trend toward lower coronary mortality through treatment of hyperlipidemia in postinfarction patients [104, 105], but there is no unequivocal evidence linking treatment to survival. Until such evidence is available, the indirect evidence supports the treatment of elevated plasma cholesterol levels, as suggested at one consensus conference [106].

Metabolism of Plasma Lipids

The absorption, transport, metabolism, and excretion of the plasma lipids—cholesterol, cholesterol esters, triglycerides, phospholipids—is complex and well described in review articles [107]. A comprehensive review of lipid metabolism is beyond the scope of this chapter, but certain concepts are important to the treatment of lipid disorders after myocardial infarction.

Four major families of lipoproteins are defined by density on ultracentrifugation of plasma: chylomicrons, very low-density lipoproteins (VLDL), low-density lipoproteins (LDL), and high-density lipoproteins (HDL). The lipoproteins consist of a hydrophilic coat of associated apoproteins and a neutral lipid core. The apoproteins are functionally important as catalysts for some enzymatic reactions and as recognition sites for binding to specific cellular receptors. At a bonding position between the protein surface and neutral core are the polar head groups of unesterified cholesterol and the fatty acyl chains of phospholipids. The density of the lipoproteins is determined by the relative concentrations of the esterified cholesterol and triglycerides in the core. The structure and functions of the major lipoproteins are outlined in Table 34-6.

Chylomicrons are the largest of the lipoproteins and are responsible for transfer of ingested fats from the intestine into the circulation and to the liver. Lipoprotein lipase, an enzyme in vascular endothelial cells, degrades triglycerides from chylomicrons, leaving remnants that are cleared rapidly by the liver. These cholesterol-rich remnants suppress the de novo synthesis of cholesterol by the liver.

In the liver, VLDL particles are synthesized and released. VLDL particles, which are rich in triglycerides, undergo lipolysis in the circulation by lipoprotein lipase, leaving intermediate lipoproteins, which are converted to LDL in the liver and the peripheral circulation. LDL is the major transport particle for cholesterol, delivering it to both the liver and peripheral cells, including vascular endothelium. LDL uptake occurs through cell-specific receptors; cholesterol absorption suppresses de novo synthesis of cholesterol within cells. Elevated LDL cholesterol is the most important lipid abnormality related to risk for the development of coronary disease.

High-density lipoprotein is synthesized by the liver and is partially responsible for catabolism of VLDL through reactions involving lipoprotein lipase, lecithin-cholesterol acyl transferase (LCAT), and other enzymes that may inhibit hepatic uptake of cholesterol. HDL is postulated to facilitate cholesterol transport from peripheral tissues to the liver. This process may increase cholesterol excretion in the form of bile acids and down-regulate hepatic synthesis of cholesterol by suppressing the rate-limiting step catalyzed by 3-hydroxy-3-methyl-glutamyl coenzyme A (HMG-CoA) reductase.

Table 34-6
Structure and function of major classes of lipoproteins

Lipoprotein	Density	Major lipid constituents	Function	Comment
Chylomicron	0.95	Triglyceride	Transport ingested fat to circulation and liver	Degraded by lipoprotein lipase
VLDL	0.95–1.006	Triglyceride Phospholipid	Transport of endogenous triglyceride and cholesterol	Degraded to LDL by lipoprotein lipase
LDL	1.019–1.063	Esterified cholesterol Triglyceride	Transport of cholesterol to tissues	Uptake by cell-specific receptors
HDL	1.063–1.21	Phospholipid cholesterol	Catabolism of VLDL and transport of cholesterol to liver	Suppresses cholesterol synthesis at HMG-CoA reductase step

The incorporation of cholesterol into bile acids is an important step in cholesterol metabolism. An enterohepatic recirculation mechanism reclaims cholesterol incorporated into bile acids, thereby conserving a portion of biliary cholesterol. This recirculation phenomenon inhibits excretion of cholesterol into bile acids, helping to maintain plasma cholesterol levels. Each of the metabolic pathways discussed is of clinical importance because it can be affected by various therapies.

Definition of Hypercholesterolemia
The definition of hypercholesterolemia has been difficult to establish. The mean plasma total cholesterol level for white men over the age of 30 in the Lipid Research Clinic prevalence study ranged from 192 to 214 mg/dl and approximated the 50th percentile. The 90th percentile ranged from 239 mg/dl at age 30 to 34 to 262 mg/dl at age 55 to 59 [108]. Compared to epidemiologic data from other cultures with substantially lower mortality rates from coronary heart disease, cholesterol levels above the 50th to 75th percentile in American men are associated with an increased risk from coronary heart disease. Using these data, the Consensus Conference of the National Institutes of Health defined a moderate risk and a high risk category of hypercholesterolemia and recommended therapy for each [106].

The moderate risk category is defined as

Table 34-7
Age-adjusted risk categories for total plasma cholesterol suggested by the Consensus Conference [106]

Age (years)	Moderate risk (mg/dl)	High risk (mg/dl)
20–29	>200	>220
30–39	>220	>240
>40	>240	>260

age-adjusted values of total plasma cholesterol in the 75th to 90th percentiles (Table 34-7). The high risk category was defined as age-adjusted values above the 90th percentile. The moderate risk category includes large numbers of individuals with elevated cholesterol levels due at least in part to elevated dietary saturated fats and cholesterol. The high risk category includes most individuals with hereditary forms of hypercholesterolemia [106].

The plasma cholesterol level should be determined with a fasting sample and abnormal values confirmed with repeated samples. Secondary causes of hypercholesterolemia should be sought, such as diabetes, liver disease, nephrotic syndrome, hypothyroidism, and medications such as beta blockers and thiazide diuretics. Fractionation of cholesterol to determine LDL and HDL levels may be helpful for determining therapy. HDL levels below 30 mg/dl appear to be an independent risk factor and might prompt more aggressive therapy for even moderately elevated total or LDL cholesterol. Screening family members for hereditary forms of hypercholesterolemia is indicated in patients with elevated plasma cholesterol.

Goals of Therapy for Hypercholesterolemia

The goals of therapy for hypercholesterolemia have not been explicitly defined. Recognizing the epidemiologic links between cholesterol levels and coronary heart disease in Western cultures, lowering plasma cholesterol levels to at least the 50th percentile for age is a conservative goal. For most patients recovering from myocardial infarction, a total cholesterol level of 200 mg/dl or lower is an appropriate goal. Specific guidelines for LDL and HDL cholesterol levels are not available. However, lowering LDL levels below the 50th percentile (130 mg/dl for men aged 35 to 39) and raising HDL levels above the 50th percentile (43 mg/dl for men aged 35 to 39) are reasonable goals. Some patients, especially those with hereditary forms of hypercholesterolemia, may be unable to reach these goals even with the most aggressive dietary and medical therapy. Clinicians should recognize this limitation, but it should not impede them from attempting to lower total and LDL cholesterol levels as much as possible.

Dietary Treatment of Hypercholesterolemia

In both moderate and high risk patients, dietary therapy is the initial step in management. The goals of dietary therapy are to lower total fat, saturated fat, and cholesterol intake and to achieve ideal body weight in patients who are overweight. The dietary modifications suggested by various groups to achieve these goals differ in regard to the manner in which the diet is undertaken. However, most guidelines recommend an initial approach restricting 30 percent of total caloric intake to fats and no more than 300 mg of cholesterol per day (Table 34-8). The total saturated fat intake should be less than 10 percent of total calories. This limitation on total saturated fats has the most effect on LDL levels.

Table 34-8
Recommended daily restrictions on fat as a percentage of total calories and cholesterol in moderate and high risk hypercholesterolemic patients

Patient risk	Total fat (%)	Saturated fat (%)	Cholesterol (mg)
Moderate	30	10	300
High	20	5–10	100–150

In high risk groups, progressive restrictions to 20 percent of calories as fats and 100 to 150 mg of cholesterol per day are recommended. Total caloric restriction combined with exercise is important in overweight patients.

Life style changes are among the most difficult for patients to make. However, most patients recovering from myocardial infarction are highly motivated to adopt habits that will reduce their risk of subsequent complications of coronary disease. A major effort by the patient, physician, dietitian, and cardiac rehabilitation specialist is necessary to provide the education, motivation, and encouragement needed for dietary modification. The person primarily responsible for food buying and preparation must be actively included in the dietary management.

Drug Therapy for Hypercholesterolemia

For patients failing to achieve the goals for reductions in total and LDL cholesterol with dietary measures within 3 months, several drugs are available that have been demonstrated to lower cholesterol levels (Table 34-9).

BILE ACID SEQUESTRANTS

The bile acid sequestrants, cholestyramine and colestipol, are nonabsorbable resins that have quarternary amine groups that interact with the acidic moiety of bile acids. Taken orally, they interrupt the normal enterohepatic recirculation of bile acids by binding them so they are excreted in the stool. Enhanced bile acid excretion interrupts the feedback inhibition on bile acid synthesis and increases conversion of cholesterol to bile acids. Lower

Table 34-9
Major lipid-lowering drugs: mechanisms of action and effects on lipid levels

Type	Examples	Mechanism	Effect
Bile acid sequestrants	Cholestyramine Colestipol	Bind bile acids in bowel, preventing enterohepatic recirculation of cholesterol	Decreases total cholesterol 8–25%, LDL 12–35%
Nicotinic acid		Inhibit secretion of VLDL and LDL from liver	Decreases total cholesterol 15–25%
Fibric acid derivatives	Clofibrate Gemfibrozil	Promote lipolysis of VLDL by activating lipoprotein lipase	Decreases total cholesterol 7–15%; may increase cholesterol in patients with hypertriglyceridemia
Probucol		Unknown but appears to promote clearance of LDL	Decreases total cholesterol 15–20%; also lowers HDL
HMG-CoA reductase inhibitors	Lovastatin	Inhibits HMG-CoA reductase reaction	Decreases total cholesterol 18–39%; increases HDL

hepatic cellular cholesterol levels result in increased LDL receptor density on hepatocytes and increased LDL extraction from the bloodstream, causing plasma concentrations of LDL cholesterol to fall. Small changes in VLDL and triglyceride levels are sometimes noted.

The usual dose for cholestyramine is 16 to 24 gm daily and for colestipol 20 to 25 gm daily in divided doses, mixed with liquid. Treatment is best initiated at one-half the full dosage and increased gradually over a 1- to 3-week period. The most commonly reported side effects of the resins are gastrointestinal, primarily constipation and heartburn. Other symptoms related to therapy include abdominal pain, diarrhea, bloating, gas, and nausea. Symptoms tend to diminish with prolonged use of the medications and may be ameliorated with antacids and antiflatulents.

In the Coronary Primary Prevention Trial [100, 101], cholestyramine therapy resulted in a mean reduction in total cholesterol of 8.2 percent and in LDL cholesterol of 12 percent. Patients who adhered completely with higher doses of cholestyramine had sustained reductions of 25 and 35 percent, respectively, whereas poor adherers had little or no change in total and LDL-cholesterol levels. Maximum reductions tend to occur early in treatment, and cholesterol levels tend to rise with time. This gradual increase in cholesterol probably reflects lower adherence to diet and drug therapy and the effect of aging.

NICOTINIC ACID
Nicotinic acid lowers plasma cholesterol by inhibiting the secretion of both VLDL and LDL from the liver. It also suppresses free fatty acid mobilization from adipose tissue, which suppresses VLDL synthesis. Nicotinic acid also increases HDL levels, probably secondary to decreased VLDL production. Nicotinic acid use was associated with a decrease in the rate of recurrent myocardial infarction in the Coronary Drug Trial [104].

The usual dosage for nicotinic acid is 2 to 6 gm per day in three divided doses. Side effects of cutaneous flushing due to capillary dilation and pruritus are common and may result in noncompliance if patients are not counseled to expect them. Flushing generally begins 20 minutes after the dose and lasts 30 to 60 minutes. Gastric irritation is common and can be mitigated by taking the medication with meals. Hepatic transaminases may become elevated with the initiation of therapy, but the rise is usually transient. Some impairment of carbohydrate tolerance may occur, which is of clinical significance primarily in insulin-dependent diabetics. Uric acid levels may increase with nicotinic acid ingestion, precipitating gout in some patients. Transient declines in blood pressure may occur, and antihypertensive medications may need to be adjusted as doses of nicotine acid are increased.

Intolerance to side effects is a common reason many patients do not continue nicotinic acid in high doses or for long periods. Side effects can be minimized by several measures. Hot drinks can exacerbate the flushing, and patients should be told to avoid them around the time of dosing. Because capillary dilation appears to be prostaglandin-mediated, pretreatment with aspirin before dosing is helpful. Tachyphylaxis to flushing and pruritus at any given dose level is common; patients can be counseled to expect the side effects to improve. Beginning at extremely low doses, such as 100 to 250 mg three times daily and increasing the dose by 250 mg each week minimizes side effects. Sustained-release preparations are available that may decrease the flushing sensation.

Most patients normalize LDL cholesterol levels with nicotinic acid alone. In patients with extremely high plasma cholesterol levels, the combination of diet, a bile acid sequestrant, and nicotinic acid can reduce LDL cholesterol levels by as much as 50 percent [107]. Patients receiving nicotinic acid should have pretreatment measurements of plasma glucose, hepatic transaminases, and uric acid in addition to lipid screening. Studies should be repeated after titration to moderate doses and then monitored at 3- to 6-month intervals.

FIBRIC ACID DERIVATIVES

Two fibric acid derivatives, clofibrate and gemfibrozil, lower cholesterol by lowering VLDL levels. Clofibrate promotes lipolysis of VLDL triglycerides by activating lipoprotein lipase and reducing hepatic VLDL synthesis. Gemfibrozil appears to reduce hepatic VLDL synthesis as well as to inhibit its secretion. Both drugs reduce triglyceride levels, which is associated with increases in LDL levels in some patients with hypertriglyceridemia.

The usual dose of clofibrate is 1 gm orally twice daily and that of gemfibrozil 600 mg orally twice daily. The most common side effects of clofibrate are nausea, diarrhea, and weight gain. Other important side effects include a rare myositis syndrome, transient hepatic transaminase elevation, and potentiation of the action of warfarin by displacing it from protein-binding sites. A small increase in biliary and gastrointestinal cancers and a failure to decrease cardiac mortality were noted in one primary prevention trial [109]. Gemfibrozil is well tolerated, with the most common side effects being nausea and diarrhea.

The fibric acid derivatives can be expected to lower total cholesterol by 7 to 15 percent and triglycerides by 30 to 50 percent [107]. Both clofibrate and gemfibrozil raise HDL levels. Because these drugs are less effective than either the bile acid sequestrants or nicotinic acid, they should be considered second-line agents. They are the drugs of choice in only a small group of patients with primary elevations of VLDL.

PROBUCOL

Probucol is a relatively new hypolipidemic drug that is structurally dissimilar to the previously described agents. The mechanism of action is not clear, but it appears to promote the clearance of LDL. There is no consistent effect on triglycerides, but the HDL level usually falls. The usual dose of probucol is 500 mg orally twice daily. Side effects are mild, generally consisting of diarrhea, flatulence, and nausea. Total cholesterol lowering of 15 to 20 percent is reported. The lower efficacy compared to the resins and nicotinic acid and the HDL-lowering effect make probucol a second-line agent, to be used in conjunction with the resins or when first-line agents fail.

LOVASTATIN

Lovastatin, a recently released drug, is an inactive lactone that is hydrolyzed to a beta-hydroxy acid form after ingestion. This form is a principal metabolite of HMG-CoA reductase, which is a key enzyme in the biosynthetic pathway of cholesterol. In pharmacologic doses, lovastatin lowers both total and LDL cholesterol by 18 to 39 percent and increases HDL cholesterol by 3 to 13 percent by partially blocking the HMG-CoA reductase reaction. The usual dose of lovastatin is 20 to 80 mg orally in single or divided doses daily. Side effects, which are uncommon, are predominantly gastrointestinal, including constipation, diarrhea, and gas. Persistently elevated hepatic transaminases have been noted in some patients. Others have developed lenticular opacities seen by slit-lamp examination, but no changes in visual acuity have been noted. Baseline and periodic hepatic transaminase measurements and slit-lamp examinations are recommended.

OTHER MEDICATIONS

Other medications that are known to lower plasma cholesterol levels include dextrothyroxine, neomycin, and beta-sitosterol. These drugs have a limited role in most patients recovering from myocardial infarction. Drugs currently under investigation include other inhibitors of HMG-CoA reductase (e.g., compactin and mevinolin) and fibric acid derivatives (e.g., fenofibrate).

HDL CHOLESTEROL

Although low HDL cholesterol levels have been associated with high rates of coronary events in the general population, the influence of HDL cholesterol on the outcome of patients recovering from myocardial infarction is unknown. Several factors may cause HDL levels to be low, including sedentary life style, cigarette smoking, obesity, hypertriglyceridemia, some cholesterol-lowering drugs, and other medications including some beta blockers and thiazide diuretics. Exercise training has been shown to increase HDL levels, but the effects of other interventions are not known. In patients with low HDL cholesterol levels, attention should be directed to factors that lower HDL, and exercise should be prescribed as a means of increasing HDL.

Nonpharmacologic Therapy for Hypercholesterolemia

EXERCISE

The effects of exercise training on plasma lipids is not completely understood. Conflicting reports on the effect of exercise on total cholesterol are probably related to the failure of studies to control for the effects of changes in body weight, diet, and intensity of exercise. In general, low-to-moderate intensity exercise has little influence on total cholesterol [4]. More consistent data are available that demonstrate a beneficial effect of exercise training on HDL levels. Longitudinal training studies have consistently demonstrated increases in HDL cholesterol levels at low, moderate, and high durations and intensities of exercise [71, 110]. Coronary patients with low initial HDL levels show the largest increases with training. These changes appear in the HDL_2 subfraction, which has been epidemiologically associated with lower rates of coronary heart disease.

ALCOHOL

The effect of alcohol consumption on plasma cholesterol levels is not completely understood. Moderate alcohol consumption has been associated with a decreased prevalence of coronary artery disease [111, 112]. This association was initially postulated to be a protective effect of increased HDL concentrations. However, more recent evidence demonstrates that moderate alcohol consumption is associated primarily with increases in the HDL_3 subfraction of cholesterol, which does not appear to have an epidemiologic association with coronary disease [113]. Further study is required to elucidate the effect of alcohol on cholesterol and coronary heart disease.

FISH OILS

The effect of diets rich in fish oils, especially omega-3 fatty acids, on plasma lipid profiles has also been controversial. Evidence suggests that fish oils probably reduce VLDL synthesis in the liver or increase catabolism of VLDL. Through this effect on VLDL metabolism, plasma LDL levels may be decreased [114]. Fish oils may have a role in treating hypercholesterolemic states in which VLDL levels are increased. The influence of dietary fish oils on the development and manifestations of coronary heart disease is unknown.

Resumption of Customary Activities

Whereas health professionals focus on the medical consequences of myocardial infarction, patients are often concerned with the social consequences. Even the uncomplicated patient faces restrictions on activities that days before were performed as a customary part of daily life. In addition to those restrictions, the patient is surrounded by family, friends, and coworkers who have limited information about the effects of heart disease. Americans harbor many misconceptions about myocardial infarction that are translated into attitudes and actions toward patients recovering from heart attack. The most prevalent misconceptions are the beliefs in a dire prognosis for cardiac patients and that physical and mental stress are harmful.

Because of their limited knowledge and misconceptions about myocardial infarction, patients should receive specific advice and education during the early phases of recovery. Even seemingly common sense knowledge should not be presumed by the health professionals caring for the patient. The spouse or primary caretaker should receive the advice along with the patient for two reasons. First, the retention of information by patients is limited, especially during the hospitalization for myocardial infarction. Second, most disagreements between patient and spouse during the early recovery period are related to perceptions of the medical advice given.

HOUSEHOLD ACTIVITIES

In addition to the advice regarding physical activity presented previously, patients should be specifically counseled regarding performance of customary household activities soon after discharge. These activities include climbing stairs, lifting, driving, socializing with visitors, shopping, and walking outdoors. Individual patients may have more specific questions.

A simple approach to providing guidelines for these activities is to treat them as forms of exercise. In the absence of a formal exercise test, limiting patients to a heart rate 20 beats above the standing heart rate is a concrete guideline the patient can grasp and practice before hospital discharge. After teaching patients how to count their pulse, walking different speeds and climbing stairs can be performed with supervision. The patient learns quickly the heart rate response to each activity and so can be confident when undertaking such activities at home.

Other activities that may involve more mental than physical stress, such as driving, socializing, and shopping, are best limited until a more formal exercise evaluation is performed. In studies of patients recovering from myocardial infarction who underwent psychological stress testing using standard techniques, the mean resting heart rate rose less than 10 bpm and the mean systolic blood pressure rose less than 15 mm Hg with the most stressful intervention. In every case, the hemodynamic response to psychological stress was substantially lower than to treadmill exercise. Among a subset of patients with exercise-induced ST segment depression, none developed ischemic responses to psychological stress testing [115]. These data suggest that the psychological stress of usual social activities is unlikely to precipitate significant cardiovascular abnormalities.

Lifting is often proscribed for 6 to 8 weeks after myocardial infarction. The rationale for this restriction is concern that the marked blood pressure response to static, upper extremity exercise might precipitate cardiac rupture during the 6-week healing phase of myocardial infarction. In an evaluation of 40 men after myocardial infarction, static lifting of an average of 36 pounds using one arm was associated with a double product of less than 50 percent of that attained by bicycle ergometry [38, 116]. Combined static lifting and dynamic treadmill walking was not associated with significantly higher double products than walking alone. In both studies, no patient had electrocardiographic evidence of ischemia with static lifting, although 25 percent had ischemic ST segment depression during treadmill testing [116]. These data suggest that lifting 25 to 50 pounds is safe for patients without evidence of severe myocardial ischemia or left ventricular dysfunction. These data also suggest that activities such as carrying moderate loads, such as groceries, should not necessarily be prohibited.

RETURN TO WORK

Most previously employed patients under the age of 60 return to work after myocardial infarction [117]. However, decisions regarding reemployment are complex. Older patients, especially those with accessible retirement benefits are less likely to return to work [118]. Patients with lower educational achievement or blue collar jobs and those unemployed for more than 3 months before myocardial infarction are significantly less likely to be employed after infarction [117, 119, 120]. Patients with severe symptoms of angina or congestive heart failure are less likely to return to work. Rehabilitation efforts alone are unlikely to affect these medical, demographic, and social impediments to reemployment after myocardial infarction.

For younger, employed patients the most important consideration is not if but when the patient should return to work. Concerns by patients, employers, and physicians that occupational work will precipitate a recurrent cardiac event underlie the current recommendations for a convalescent period of 2 to 4 months before return to work. This prolonged convalescence places a significant economic burden on both the patient and the employer. The patient generally lives on more limited disability income, especially during the late convalescence period, and the employer must function without the patient or with less efficient temporary help.

The two primary issues that must be addressed if earlier reemployment is allowed are prognosis and physical capacity. Uncomplicated patients generally have an excellent prognosis and a well preserved physical capacity. Early, symptom-limited treadmill testing in such patients can confirm these findings [42].

In a study to determine if the interval between myocardial infarction and return to work could be shortened, Dennis and coworkers [121] used a predischarge risk stratification model to identify uncomplicated patients [42]. In four community hospitals patients without angina at rest or clinical evidence of congestive heart failure were designated as uncomplicated and comprised 57 percent of all patients and 77 percent of employed patients. Patients who were uncomplicated and under age 60—and therefore most likely to return to work within 6 months—included 64 percent of all employed patients.

Patients with these criteria were randomized to receive either usual care from their primary physicians or to undergo an occupational work evaluation. This evaluation consisted of a symptom-limited treadmill test at 3 weeks after myocardial infarction and specific advice to the patient and primary physician regarding reemployment. The 6 percent of patients demonstrating severe ischemia (e.g., 0.2 mV of ST segment depression at a heart rate less than 135) on their treadmill test were advised to undergo further evaluation with coronary arteriography. The 70 percent of patients without treadmill abnormalities were advised to return to work at 35 days; the 24 percent of patients with mild treadmill abnormalities, most commonly 0.1 to 0.2 mV of ST depression or angina at a heart rate greater than 135, were advised to return to work at 42 days, after beginning antianginal medication.

At a 6-month follow-up, cardiac events were rare. The mortality rate was 1.5 percent and the reinfarction rate 2 percent in the randomized patients without differences between the two groups. Events were more common in patients with severe treadmill ischemia. All but one event occurred before the patient returned to work, and no cardiac events occurred on the job.

At 6 months, 90 percent of patients in both groups were working either full-time or part-time. However, patients who underwent the occupational work evaluation returned to work at a median of 51 days compared to 75 days in patients receiving usual care. This 33 percent reduction of the convalescence period resulted in an average of $2102 per patient more earned income over the 6 months after myocardial infarction by patients who underwent the occupational work evaluation than those who received usual care.

This type of intervention can be employed in outpatient cardiac rehabilitation programs. It may not be sufficient for the evaluation of patients performing heavy manual labor, however. In the cited study, the average peak treadmill capacity at 3 weeks was 7 MET. This capacity is sufficient for most jobs that are sedentary or involve light physical labor, but it may be insufficient for patients performing heavy manual labor. However, only 16 percent of Americans perform manual labor, and that percentage declines with age. Patients performing manual labor or those involved with public safety, e.g., police officers, fire fighters, and pilots, may require more extensive evaluation or prolonged exercise training before return to work.

Conclusions

Rehabilitation after myocardial infarction should be comprehensive and begin during the hospitalization. Medical and surgical therapy may be the first step in rehabilitation of more complicated patients. For uncomplicated patients and after appropriate therapy of complicated patients, a complete evaluation of physical capacity and cardiac risk factors should be the basis for a comprehensive rehabilitation program.

A symptom-limited treadmill test is the basis for recommendations regarding both physical reconditioning and resumption of customary activities. Risk factor evaluation is the basis for recommendations regarding diet, smoking cessation, and medical therapy for hyperlipidemia, hypertension, and diabetes. The medical, physical, and psychological status of the patient can guide the physician who is giving recommendations regarding return to work.

A comprehensive rehabilitation program after myocardial infarction has the potential to improve survival as well as the quality of life. Prompt rehabilitative efforts that include the

features described previously as well as education and counseling can hasten the return to a full and active life style of patients recovering from myocardial infarction.

References

1. DeBusk, R. F. Cardiac rehabilitation: A strategy for the 1990's and beyond. In Tsung Cheng (ed.), *International Practice of Cardiology.* New York: Pergamon Press, 1985.
2. Haskell, W. L., Savin, M., Oldridge, N., and DeBusk, R. Factors influencing estimated oxygen uptake during exercise testing soon after myocardial infarction. *Am. J. Cardiol.* 50:299, 1982.
3. Roberts, J. M., Sullivan, V. F., Froelicher, V. F., et al. Predicting oxygen uptake from treadmill testing in normal subjects and coronary artery disease patients. *Am. Heart J.* 108:1454, 1984.
4. Franklin, B. A., Wrisley, D., Johnson, S., et al. Chronic adaptations to physical conditioning in cardiac patients. *Clin. Sports Med.* 3:471, 1984.
5. Dehn, M. M., Blomquist, C. G., and Mitchell, J. H. Clinical exercise program. *Clin. Sports Med.* 3:319, 1984.
6. Convertino, V., Hung, J., Goldwater, D., and DeBusk, R. F. Cardiovascular responses to exercise in middle-aged men after 10 days of bedrest. *Circulation* 65:134, 1982.
7. Convertino, V. A., Bisson, R., Bates, R., et al. Effects of anti-orthostatic bedrest on the cardiorespiratory responses to exercise. *Aviat. Space Environ. Med.* 251, 1981.
8. Saltin, B., Blomquist, G., Mitchell, J. H., et al. Response to exercise after bedrest and after training. *Circulation* 38(Suppl VII):1, 1968.
9. Fareeduddin, K., and Abelmann, W. H. Impaired orthostatic tolerance after bedrest in patients with acute myocardial infarction. *N. Engl. J. Med.* 280:345, 1969.
10. Wenger, N. K. Cardiovascular drugs: Effects on exercise testing and exercise training of the coronary patient: Exercise and the heart. *Cardiovasc. Clin.* 15:133, 1985.
11. Birkhead, N. C., Blizzard, J. J., Daly, J. W., et al. Cardiodynamic and metabolic effects of prolonged bedrest with daily recumbent or sitting exercise and with sitting inactivity. In *Technical Report No. AMRL-TDR-64-61.* Wright-Patterson Air Force Base, Ohio, 1964.
12. Convertino, V. A., Sandler, H., and Webb, P. The effect of an elastic reverse gradient garment on the cardiorespiratory decondition-

ing following fifteen days bedrest. *Aerospace Med. Assoc. Preprints* 1978, p 148.

13. Thoren, P. N. Activation of left ventricular receptors with nonmedullated vagal afferente fibers during occlusion of a coronary artery in the cat. *Am. J. Cardiol.* 37:146, 1976.

14. Haskell, W. L., and DeBusk, R. Cardiovascular responses to repeated treadmill exercise testing soon after myocardial infarction. *Circulation* 60:1247, 1979.

15. Franciosa, J. A. Lack of correlation between exercise capacity and indexes of resting left ventricular performance in heart failure. *Am. J. Cardiol.* 47:33, 1981.

16. Higginbotham, M. B., Morris, K. G., Conn, E. H., et al. Determinants of variable exercise performance among patients with severe left ventricular dysfunction. *Am. J. Cardiol.* 51:52, 1983.

17. Litchfield, R. L., Kerber, R. E., Benge, W., et al. Normal exercise capacity in patients with severe left ventricular dysfunction: Compensatory mechanisms. *Circulation* 66:129, 1982.

18. Wilson, J. R., and Ferraro, N. Exercise tolerance in patients with chronic left heart failure: Relation to oxygen transport and ventilatory abnormalities. *Am. J. Cardiol.* 51:1358, 1983.

19. Buda, A. J., Dubbin, J. D., McDonald, I. L., et al. Spontaneous changes in thallium-201 myocardial perfusion imaging after myocardial infarction. *Am. J. Cardiol.* 50:1272, 1978.

20. Froelicher, V. F., Jensen, D., Atwood, E., et al. Cardiac rehabilitation: Evidence for improvement in myocardial perfusion and function. *Arch. Phys. Med. Rehabil.* 61:517, 1980.

21. DeBusk, R. F., and Hung, J. Exercise conditioning soon after myocardial infarction: Effects on myocardial perfusion and ventricular function. *Ann. N.Y. Acad. Sci.* 343, 1982.

22. Hung, J., Gordon, E. P., Houston, N., et al. Changes in rest and exercise myocardial perfusion and left ventricular function 3 to 26 weeks after clinically uncomplicated acute myocardial infarction: Effects of exercise training. *Am. J. Cardiol.* 54:943, 1984.

23. DeBusk, R. F. Physical conditioning following myocardial infarction. *Adv. Cardiol.* 31:156, 1982.

24. DeBusk, R. F., Houston, N., Haskell, W., et al. Exercise training soon after myocardial infarction. *Am. J. Cardiol.* 44:1223, 1979.

25. Multicenter Postinfarction Research Group. Risk stratification and survival after myocardial infarction. *N. Engl. J. Med.* 309:331, 1983.

26. Weber, K. T., and Janicki, J. S. Cardiopulmonary exercise testing for evaluation of chronic cardiac failure. *Am. J. Cardiol.* 55:22A, 1985.

27. DeBusk, R. F., and Haskell, W. L. Symptom-limited vs heart-rate-limited exercise testing

soon after myocardial infarction. *Circulation* 61:738, 1980.

28. Madsen, E. B., Gilpin, E., Ahnve, S., et al. Prediction of functional capacity and use of exercise testing for predicting risk after acute myocardial infarction. *Am. J. Cardiol.* 45:839, 1985.

29. Fioretti, P., Brower, R. W., Simoons, M. L., et al. Prediction of mortality during the first year after acute myocardial infarction from clinical variables and stress test at hospital discharge. *Am. J. Cardiol.* 55:1313, 1985.

30. Ho, S.W-C., McComish, M. J., and Taylor, R. R. Effect of beta-adrenergic blockade on the results of exercise testing related to the extent of coronary artery disease. *Am. J. Cardiol.* 55:258, 1985.

31. Naughton, J., Sevelios, G., and Balke, B. Physiological responses of normal and pathological subjects to a modified work capacity test. *J. Sports Med.* 3:201, 1973.

32. American College of Sports Medicine. Position statement on the recommended quantity and quality of exercise for developing and maintaining fits in healthy adults. *Med. Sci. Sports* 10:vii, 1978.

33. Erb, B., Fletcher, J. F., and Sheffield, T. L. Standards for cardiovascular exercise treatment programs. *Circulation* 59:1084A, 1979.

34. Council on Scientific Affairs. Physician supervised exercise programs in rehabilitation of patients with coronary heart disease. *J.A.M.A.* 245:1463, 1981.

35. Pollock, M. L., and Pells III, A. E. Exercise prescription for the cardiac patient: An update. *Clin. Sports Med.* 3:425, 1984.

36. Shephard, R. J. Exercise regimens after myocardial infarction: Rationale and results: Exercise and the heart. *Cardiovasc. Clin.* 15:145, 1985.

37. Bezucha, G. R., Lenser, M. L., Hanson, P. G., et al. Comparison of hemodynamic responses to static and dynamic exercise. *J. Appl. Physiol.* 53:1589, 1982.

38. DeBusk, R., Pitts, W., Haskell, W., and Houston, N. Comparison of cardiovascular responses to static-dynamic effort and dynamic effort alone in patients with chronic ischemic heart disease. *Circulation* 59:977, 1979.

39. Borg, G., and Linderholm, H. Exercise performance and perceived exertion in patients with coronary insufficiency, arterial hypertension and vasoregulatory asthenia. *Acta Med. Scand.* 187:17, 1970.

40. Juneau, M., Rogers, F., deSantos, V., et al. Comparison of the effectiveness of self-monitored home-based moderate-intensity exercise training in middle-aged men and women. *Am. J. Cardiol.* 60:66, 1987.

41. Fry, G., and Berra, K. *YMCArdiac Therapy.*

Chicago: National Council of the Young Men's Christian Associations, 1981.

42. DeBusk, R. F., Kraemer, H. C., Nash, E., et al. Stepwise risk stratification soon after myocardial infarction. *Am. J. Cardiol.* 52:1161, 1983.

43. Koppes, G. M., Kruyer, W., Beckman, C. H., and Jones, F. G. Response to exercise early after uncomplicated acute myocardial infarction in patients receiving no medication: Long-term follow-up. *Am. J. Cardiol.* 46:764, 1980.

44. Miller, D. H., and Borer, J. S. Exercise testing early after myocardial infarction: Risks and benefits. *Am. J. Med.* 72:427, 1982.

45. Weiner, D. A. Predischarge exercise testing after myocardial infarction: Prognostic and therapeutic features: Exercise and the heart. *Cardiovasc. Clin.* 15:95, 1985.

46. Waters, D. D., Bosch, X., Bouchard, A., et al. Comparison of clinical variables and variables derived from a limited predischarge exercise test as predictors of early and late mortality after myocardial infarction. *J. Am. Coll. Cardiol.* 5:1, 1985.

47. Williams, R. S., Miller, H., and Koisch, F. P. Guidelines for unsupervised exercise in patients with ischemic heart disease. *J. Cardiac. Rehabil.* 1:213, 1981.

48. Hossack, K. F., and Bruce, R. A. Improved exercise performance of persons with stable angina pectoris receiving diltiazem. *Am. J. Cardiol.* 47:95, 1981.

49. Hossack, K. F., Bruce, R. A., and Clark, L. J. Influence of propranolol on exercise prescription of training heart rates. *Cardiology* 65:47, 1980.

50. Leier, C. V., Huss, P., Magonen, B. D., et al. Improved exercise capacity and differing arterial and venous tolerance during chronic isosorbide dinitrate therapy for congestive heart failure. *Circulation* 67:817, 1983.

51. Malborg, R., Isaacson, S., and Kallivroussis, G. The effects of beta blockade and/or physical training in patients with angina pectoris. *Curr. Ther. Res.* 16:171, 1974.

52. Gordon, N. F., Kruger, P. E., Hons, B. A., et al. Improved exercise ventilatory responses after training in coronary heart disease during long-term beta-adrenergic blockade. *Am. J. Cardiol.* 51:755, 1983.

53. Pratt, C. M., Welton, D. E., Squires, W. G., et al. Demonstration of training effect during chronic beta-adrenergic blockade in patients with coronary artery disease. *Circulation* 64:1125, 1981.

54. Koiwaya, Y., Nakamura, M., Mitsutake, A., et al. Increased exercise tolerance after oral diltiazem, a calcium antagonist, in angina pectoris. *Am. Heart J.* 101:143, 1981.

55. Cobb, F. R., Williams, P. S., McEwan, P., et al. Effects of exercise training on ventricular function in patients with recent myocardial infarction. *Circulation* 66:100, 1982.

56. Conn, E., Williams, R. S., and Wallace, A. G. Exercise responses before and after conditioning in patients with severely depressed left ventricular function. *Am. J. Cardiol.* 49:296, 1982.

57. Verani, M. S., Hartung, G. H., Hoepfel-Harris, J., et al. Effects of exercise training on left ventricular performance and myocardial perfusion in patients with coronary artery disease. *Am. J. Cardiol.* 47:797, 1981.

58. Ogawa, T., Vyden, J., Rose, H. B., et al. Peripheral circulatory changes after physical conditioning in coronary artery disease patients. *J. Cardiac. Rehabil.* 1:269, 1981.

59. Awan, N. A., Miller, R. R., DeMaria, A. N., et al. Efficacy of ambulatory systemic vasodilator therapy with oral prazosin in chronic refractory heart failure. *Circulation* 56:346, 1977.

60. Goldsmith, S. R., Franciosa, J. A., and Cohn, J. N. Contrasting acute and chronic effects of nitrates on exercise capacity in heart failure. *Am. J. Cardiol.* 43:404, 1979.

61. DeBusk, R. F. Physical conditioning following myocardial infarction. *Adv. Cardiol.* 31:156, 1982.

62. Jensen, D., Atwood, J. E., Froelicher, V., et al. Improvement in ventricular function during exercise studied with radionuclide ventriculography after cardiac rehabilitation. *Am. J. Cardiol.* 46:770, 1980.

63. Williams, R. S., McGinnis, R. D., Cobb, F. C., and Califf, R. C. Enhanced left ventricular ejection fraction during exercise in subjects with coronary artery disease following physical conditioning (Abstract). *Circulation* 68(Suppl III):377, 1983.

64. Paterson, D. H., Shepard, R. J., Cunningham, D., et al. Effects of physical training upon cardiovascular function following myocardial infarction. *J. Appl. Physiol.* 47:487, 1979.

65. Buchwalsky, R. Hemodynamics before and after physical endurance training in patients with myocardial infarction under various physical and psychomotor stress tests. *Clin. Cardiol.* 5:332, 1982.

66. Shaw, L. W. Effects of a prescribed supervised exercise program on mortality and cardiovascular morbidity in patients after a myocardial infarction. *Am. J. Cardiol.* 48:39, 1981.

67. Naughton, J. Contributions of exercise clinical trials to cardiac rehabilitation. *Clin. Sports Med.* 3:545, 1984.

68. Rechnitzer, P. A., Cunningham, D. A., Andrew, G. M., et al. Relation of exercise to the recurrence rate of myocardial infarction in men: Ontario Exercise-Heart Collaborative

Study. *Am. J. Cardiol.* 51:65, 1983.

69. Shaw, L. W. Effects of a prescribed supervised exercise program on mortality and cardiovascular morbidity in patients after a myocardial infarction: The National Exercise and Heart Disease Project. *Am. J. Cardiol.* 48:39, 1981.

70. Prosser, G., Carson, P., and Phillips, R. Exercise after myocardial infarction: Long-term rehabilitation effects. *J. Psychosom. Res.* 29:535, 1985.

71. Heath, G. W., Ehsani, A. A., Hagberg, J. M., et al. Exercise training improves lipoprotein lipid profiles in patients with coronary artery disease. *Am. Heart J.* 105:889, 1983.

72. Boyer, J. L., and Cash, F. W. Exercise therapy in hypertensive men. *J.A.M.A.* 211:1668, 1970.

73. Gentry, W. D., and Stewart, M. A. Psychologic effects of exercise training in coronary-prone individuals and in patients with symptomatic coronary heart disease: Exercise and the heart. *Cardiovasc. Clin.* 15:255, 1985.

74. Ewart, C. K., Stewart, K. J., Gillilan, R. E., et al. Usefulness of self-efficacy in predicting overexertion during programmed exercise in coronary artery disease. *Am. J. Cardiol.* 57:557, 1986.

75. Haskell, W. L. Safety of outpatient cardiac exercise programs. *Clin. Sports Med.* 3:455, 1984.

76. Van Camp, S. P., and Peterson, R. A. Cardiovascular complications of outpatient cardiac rehabilitation programs. *J.A.M.A.* 256:1160, 1986.

77. Haskell, W. L. Cardiovascular complications during exercise training of cardiac patients. *Circulation* 57:920, 1978.

78. Pooling Project Research Group. Relationship of blood pressure, serum cholesterol, smoking habit, relative weight and ECG abnormalities to incidence of major coronary events: Final report of the Pooling Project. *J. Chronic Dis.* 31:201, 1978.

79. Gordon, T., Kannel, W. B., and McGee, D. Death and coronary attacks in men giving up cigarette smoking: A report from the Framingham Study. *Lancet* 2:1345, 1974.

80. Ronnevik, P. K., Gundersen, T., and Abrahamsen, A. M. Effect of smoking habits and timolol treatment on mortality and reinfarction in patients surviving acute myocardial infarction. *Br. Heart J.* 54:134, 1985.

81. Rosenberg, L., Kaufman, D. W., Helmrich, S. P., and Shapiro, S. The risk of myocardial infarction after quitting smoking in men under 55 years of age. *N. Engl. J. Med.* 313:1511, 1985.

82. Sparrow, D., Dawber, T. R., and Colton, T. The influence of cigarette smoking on prognosis after a first myocardial infarction: A report from the Framingham Study. *J. Chronic Dis.* 31:425, 1978.

83. Daly, L. E., Mulcahy, R., Graham, I. M., and Hickey, N. Long-term effect on mortality of stopping smoking after unstable angina and myocardial infarction. *Br. Med. J.* 287:324, 1983.

84. Hartz, A. J., Barboriak, P. N., Anderson, A. J., et al. Smoking, coronary artery occlusion and non-fatal myocardial infarction. *J.A.M.A.* 246:851, 1981.

85. Klein, L. W., Pichard, A. D., Holt, J., et al. Effects of tobacco smoking on the coronary circulation. *J. Am. Coll. Cardiol.* 1:421, 1983.

86. Wilhelmsen, L., Svardsudd, K., Korsan-Bengfsen, K., et al. Fibrinogen as a risk factor for stroke and myocardial infarction. *N. Engl. J. Med.* 311:501, 1984.

87. Vliestra, R. E., Kronmal, R. A., Frye, R. L., et al. Factors affecting the extent and severity of coronary artery disease in patients enrolled in the CASS. *Arteriosclerosis* 2:208, 1982.

88. Ockene, J. K., Hosmer, D., Rippe, J., et al. Factors affecting cigarette smoking status in patients with ischemic heart disease. *J. Chronic Dis.* 38:985, 1985.

89. Taylor, C. B. Alcohol use and smoking relapse in patients recovering from myocardial infarction. In preparation.

90. Sachs, D. P. L. Cigarette smoking: Health effects and cessation strategies. *Clin. Geriatr. Med.* 2:337, 1986.

91. Benfari, R. C., Ockene, J. K., and McIntyre, K. M. Control of cigarette smoking from a psychological perspective. *Annu. Rev. Public Health 1982* (Vol. 3). Washington, DC: Government Printing Office, 1982. Pp. 101–128.

92. Mulcahy, R. Influence of cigarette smoking on morbidity and mortality of stopping smoking after myocardial infarction. *Br. Heart J.* 49:410, 1983.

93. Weinblatt, E., Shapiro, S., and Frank, C. W. Changes in personal characteristics of men over five years following first diagnosis of coronary heart disease. *Am. J. Public Health* 61:831, 1971.

94. Fee, W. H., and Stewart, M. J. A control trial of nicotine chewing gum in a smoking withdrawal clinic. *Practitioner* 226:148, 1982.

95. Hjalmarson, A. I. Effect of nicotine chewing gum in smoking cessation: A randomized, placebo-control double-blind study. *J.A.M.A.* 252:2835, 1984.

96. McNabb, M. E., Ebert, R. V., and McCusker, K. Plasma nicotine levels produced by chewing tobacco gum. *J.A.M.A.* 248:865, 1982.

97. Carney, R. M., and Goldberg, A. P. Weight gain after cessation of cigarette smoking. *N. Engl. J. Med.* 310:614, 1984.

98. Soldatos, C. R., Kales, J. D., Sharf, M. B., et al. Cigarette smoking associated with sleep difficulty. *Science* 207:551, 1980.

99. Marlatt, G. A., and Parks, G. A. Self-management of addictive behaviors. In P. Karoly and F. H. Kanfer (eds.), *Self-Management and Behavior Change.* New York: Pergamon, 1982.

100. Lipid Research Clinics Program. The lipid research clinics coronary primary prevention trial results. I. Reduction in incidence of coronary heart disease. *J.A.M.A.* 251:351, 1984.

101. Lipid Research Clinics Program. The lipid research clinics coronary primary prevention trial results. II. The relationship of reduction in incidence of coronary heart disease to cholesterol lowering. *J.A.M.A.* 251:365, 1984.

102. Brensike, J. F., Levy, R. I., Kelsey, S. F., et al. Effects of therapy with cholestyramine on progression of coronary atherosclerosis: Results of the NHLBI type II coronary intervention study. *Circulation* 69:313, 1984.

103. Artzenius, A. C., Krombout, D., Barth, J. D., et al. Diet, lipoproteins and progression of coronary atherosclerosis: The Leiden intervention trial. *N. Engl. J. Med.* 312:805, 1985.

104. Coronary Drug Project Research Group. Natural history of myocardial infarction in a coronary drug project: Long-term prognostic importance of serum lipid levels. *Am. J. Cardiol.* 41:489, 1978.

105. Leren, P. The effect of plasma cholesterol lowering diet in male survivors of myocardial infarction. *Acta Med. Scand. [Suppl.]* 466:142, 1966.

106. Consensus Development Conference on Lowering Blood Cholesterol to Prevent Heart Disease. *J.A.M.A.* 253:2080, 1985.

107. Gotto Jr., A. M., Jones, P. H., and Scott, L. W. The diagnosis and management of hyperlipidemia. *DM* 32:247, 1986.

108. Lipid Research Clinics Program Epidemiology Committee. Plasma lipid distributions in selected North American populations. The lipid research clinics program prevalence study. *Circulation* 60:427, 1979.

109. Committee of Principal Investigators. WHO Cooperative Trial on primary prevention of ischemic heart disease using clofibrate to lower serum cholesterol: Mortality follow-up. *Lancet* 23:379, 1980.

110. Hartung, G. H., Squires, W. G., and Gotto, A. M. Effect of exercise training on plasma high density, lipoprotein cholesterol and coronary disease patients. *Am. Heart J.* 101:181, 1981.

111. Klatsky, A. L., Friedman, G. D., and Seiglaub, A. B. Alcohol consumption before myocardial infarction: Results from the Kaiser Permanente epidemiologic study of myocardial infarction. *Ann. Intern. Med.* 81:294, 1974.

112. Dyer, A. R., Stamler, J., Paul, O., et al. Alcohol consumption and seventeen year mortality in the Chicago Western Electric Company Study. *Prev. Med.* 9:78, 1980.

113. Haskell, W. L., Camargo Jr., C., Williams, P. T., et al. The effect of cessation and resumption of moderate alcohol intake on serum high-density-lipoprotein subfractions: A controlled study. *N. Engl. Med.* 310:805, 1984.

114. Phillipson, B. E., Rothrock, D. W., Connor, W. E., et al. Reduction of plasma lipids, lipoproteins and apoproteins by dietary fish oils in patients with hypertriglyceridemia. *N. Engl. J. Med.* 312:1210, 1985.

115. DeBusk, R. F., Taylor, C. B., and Agras, W. S. Comparison of treadmill exercise testing and psychologic stress testing soon after myocardial infarction. *Am. J. Cardiol.* 43:907, 1979.

116. DeBusk, R. F., Valdez, R., Houston, N., and Haskell, W. Cardiovascular responses to dynamic and static effort soon after myocardial infarction: Application to occupational work assessment. *Circulation* 58:368, 1978.

117. Wenger, N. K., Hellerstein, H. K., Blackburn, H., and Castranova, S. J. Physician management and the practice of patients with uncomplicated myocardial infarction: Changes in the past decade. *Circulation* 65:421, 1982.

118. Shapiro, S., Weinblatt, E., and Frank, C. W. Return to work after first myocardial infarction. *Arch. Environ. Health* 24:17, 1972.

119. Kjoller, E. Resumption of work after acute myocardial infarction. *Acta Med. Scand.* 199:379, 1976.

120. Weinblatt, E., Shapiro, S., Frank, C. W., and Sager, R. V. Return to work and work status following first myocardial infarction. *Am. J. Public Health* 56:169, 1966.

121. Dennis, C. A., Houston-Miller, N., Schwartz, R. G., et al. Early return to work after uncomplicated myocardial infarction. Results of a randomized trial. *J.A.M.A.* 260:214, 1988.

35
Coronary Artery Surgery in Patients with Recent Myocardial Infarction

BRUCE C. WILSON AND STUART W. JAMIESON

The role of surgical revascularization for a myocardial infarction in progress or for continuing pain after a recent myocardial infarction has been controversial. However, improvements in operative technique over the past years have brought an awareness that revascularization can be performed safely in such patients. The evolution of thought regarding coronary artery surgery in these patients is discussed here. A number of problems can occur after myocardial infarction that require surgical intervention (papillary muscle dysfunction or rupture, septal rupture, free wall rupture), and discussions regarding these complications may be found in other chapters of this text.

Acute Myocardial Infarction

Emergency revascularization for acute myocardial infarction was first achieved during the early 1970s. Originally, the operative mortality and morbidity were believed to be too high for the procedure to be performed except in the most extreme circumstances. It was therefore suggested that a 2- to 4-week waiting period was advisable between infarction and revascularization in order to reduce the operative complications to an acceptable level [1].

By the late 1970s and early 1980s, reports were published in which successful revascularization was performed during the early hours of acute infarction. Berg et al. reported on an aggressive surgical approach to acute infarction within 6 hours after onset of chest pain [2]. In a large series of 260 patients undergoing bypass, their in-hospital mortality was only 1.5 percent. In 1983 DeWood et al. examined their surgical experience with acute myocardial infarction in 701 patients who underwent bypass grafting as treatment for myocardial infarction within 24 hours of peak symptoms [3]. They demonstrated that surgical reperfusion within 6 hours from the onset of symptoms was associated with significantly lower short-term and long-term mortality than reperfusion following this time frame. Although the study was criticized, they emphasized the need for early reperfusion [4]. These observations are in concordance with more recent data accumulated from trials involved in lytic therapy for myocardial infarction.

Flameng et al. published an encouraging report in which emergency bypass grafting was performed during the first 2 to 4 hours of myocardial infarction in 48 patients [5]. Quantitative assessment of myocardium salvaged as evaluated by thallium 201 myocardial scans revealed that the residual infarction was less than 50 percent of that in a matched, medically treated control group. Enhanced recovery of regional and global ejection fraction after operation was demonstrated with technetium 99m blood pool studies when compared to medical treatment for similar infarctions. Patients were divided into low risk and high risk groups according to their preoperative status, those who were in cardiogenic shock comprising the high risk group. Operative mortality was 0 percent in the low risk patients and 18 percent in the high risk patients. This finding is encouraging because 18 percent operative mortality in patients with cardiogenic shock is low. They were also able to save three of four patients with total electrical and mechanical cardiac dysfunction. They correctly observed that the chance of survival in these patients is essentially absent with medical treatment alone.

The above study not only demonstrates that early reperfusion brings about a partial restoration of myocardial function, it also provides evidence for the phenomenon now widely referred to as "stunned myocardium." Patients revascularized *early* demonstrated a delayed recovery of myocardial function that was observed 2 months after operation.

These reports effectively lay to rest the notion that coronary artery bypass surgery in patients experiencing acute myocardial infarction is prohibitively dangerous. In properly selected patients this procedure has become a welcome alternative and one that continues to be used with both safety and efficacy.

Postinfarction Angina

In 1974 an early report by Dawson et al. described the experience from the Texas Heart Institute with 1700 patients who underwent coronary artery bypass surgery [6]. They observed that the early mortality following operation was closely related to the time interval between infarction and surgery. Their operative mortality was twice as high in patients undergoing revascularization within 30 days of infarction as in patients who had suffered an infarction in the remote past (14.5 percent versus 6.9 percent), and three to four times higher than that observed in patients having no previous infarction. Furthermore, patients who underwent operation within the first 7 days after acute infarction had a sixfold risk of early death when compared to patients undergoing bypass operations between days 31 and 60. They recommended that although coronary artery bypass after myocardial infarction could be life-saving it should be reserved until at least 30 days after infarction unless the condition that prompted surgical consideration had not responded to aggressive medical therapy.

A report from the Massachusetts General Hospital reestablished some confidence in performing bypass operations during the postinfarction period by describing 80 patients with unstable angina following infarction that was refractory to maximal medical therapy [7]. Sixty-nine percent of these patients underwent operation during the first 10 days after infarction, and the remaining 31 percent were operated on between days 10 and 30. Seventy-two percent of the overall group required intervention with the intra-aortic balloon pump; 2.5 percent of the patients had a perioperative myocardial infarction, and the mortality rate was approximately 9 percent overall. In a 33-month follow-up period, there was only one late death and one recurrent infarction, and 96 percent of the patients were angina-free. Their conclusion was that patients with continuing ischemia after infarction could undergo myocardial revascularization safely and without further injury to the myocardium. Their long-term results were considered excellent, and new interest was generated in operating on patients with postinfarction angina or hemodynamic instability.

Other groups were quick to reiterate the Boston experience. In 1981 Jones et al. from Emory University reviewed their experience from 1976 until 1980, when 116 patients had undergone urgent coronary artery bypass surgery within 30 days following a myocardial infarction [8]. Although no patient died while in hospital, there was an increased incidence of the need for either intra-aortic balloon pumping or inotropic drugs in the patients operated on before 7 days following infarction. The actuarial survival was 97 percent at 18 months. Seventy-one percent of their patients remained pain-free, and there was a high graft patency rate in patients undergoing repeat catheterization. They observed that both the morbidity and the mortality was essentially the same for patients undergoing bypass surgery within 1 month after myocardial infarction as for those patients undergoing elective revascularization at any time. Similar conclusions were reached by Fudge et al. the following year [9]. This similarity was remarkable because their patient population included not only patients with low ejection fractions but also those who underwent concomitant ventricular aneurysm repair.

Other groups turned their attention to specific timing of surgery after myocardial infarction. Breyer et al. observed that 21 percent of their operations for postinfarction angina during 1982 were performed less than 7 days after the infarction [10]. In a similar period from mid-1983 until mid-1984, the incidence of postinfarction angina as an indication for surgery rose from 8 percent to 18 percent, and 37 percent of these operations were performed during the first week after infarction. These authors found that the only variable correlating with an increased risk of mortality was a decreased ejection fraction.

With a further refinement in time frame, Williams et al. published their experience at the University of Washington with 103 patients who were operated on because they were refractory to medical management [11]. Eleven of these patients were operated on less than 24 hours after their symptoms began, 21 patients underwent bypass surgery between days 1 and 7, and 71 patients between days 7 and 30. Although only 18 percent of the myocardial infarctions in this group overall had transmural damage, more of the patients in the very early group demonstrated this pathologic finding. Most of the patients requiring the intra-aortic balloon or experiencing major arrhythmias were also in the group operated on within 24 hours. It is interesting to note that they have late follow-up in 97 percent of their patients, and there have been no late infarctions. The only two deaths observed were in the group operated on between 7 and 30 days.

Finally, Hochberg et al. observed that in a group of patients undergoing revascularization within 7 weeks after infarction there was a high mortality (46 percent) if the operation was performed within 1 week [12]. It should be noted that 23 percent of these patients were in cardiogenic shock and 62 percent required the intra-aortic balloon pump. Between 4 and 7 weeks after myocardial infarction, the mortality was low compared to their overall group, but it was still 6 percent. Their findings were that if the ejection fraction was greater than 50 percent *no* patient died in the hospital, whereas 22 percent of 124 patients with an ejection fraction below 50 percent died in the hospital. They summarized their experience with the recommendation that patients with ejection fractions more than 50 percent are safe to operate on at *any* time, whereas a delay of at least 4 weeks is preferable in patients with ejection fractions below this level.

We have taken an aggressive position with regard to postinfarction angina. Angina or anginal equivalents that occur following infarction are treated aggressively with medications in order to stabilize the patient. It usually involves therapy with intravenous nitroglycerin. Oral calcium channel blocking agents and oral or intravenous beta blockers may be employed in addition. A vigorous attempt is made to optimize the patient's hemodynamic status, which may require the use of a Swan-Ganz catheter, the assistance of an intra-aortic balloon pump, or both.

Regardless of whether the patient stabilizes, the patient is then brought to the Cardiac Catheterization Laboratory where angiography is performed. Percutaneous transluminal coronary angioplasty (PTCA) is performed when it is deemed to be a feasible solution to the current problem. When angioplasty seems to be neither a thorough enough nor safe enough procedure, the patient is taken to coronary artery bypass surgery. The key to successful management is first to remove the patient from an unstable condition. If it cannot be accomplished with medical therapy or interventions such as intra-aortic balloon pumping or urgent angioplasty, the patient should be surgically revascularized. Only if the patient can be adequately stabilized do we believe that the ideal outcome may be realized after a waiting period of approximately 7 days.

As discussed in other chapters of this text, patients who suffer an uncomplicated infarction and have no chest pain can be safely exercised according to the usual protocols after their infarction. By this method, patients with additional myocardium at risk may be discovered. Patients who have recurrent angina pectoris weeks, months, or years after infarction should also be investigated aggressively in this regard. These patients pose essentially no additional surgical risk above and beyond undergoing elective revascularization.

Cardiogenic Shock

Coronary artery surgery after myocardial infarction is most often due to recurrent angina pectoris. Unfortunately, hemodynamic instability that is characterized by or progresses to cardiogenic shock represents another category of patients in whom revascularization may not only be attempted but be crucial.

Cardiogenic shock is the final stage in 10 to 20 percent of all patients with a myocardial infarction. Despite advances in the medical therapy of this condition, the mortality rate has been described as 86 percent [13]. Thus if a patient is able to undergo angiography (most likely with the support of an intra-aortic balloon pump and inotropic agents), it may be entertained with the idea that a surgical intervention may provide the only chance for survival. Buckley emphasized that patient selection for revascularization is crucial if shock is present [14]. Patients who have collateral flow to native coronary circulation in the area of the recent infarction may be logically considered for surgery. At Buckley's institution, patients without such collateral support to an infarct artery did not survive surgery unless they had an additional surgically correctable defect such as a ventricular aneurysm or septal rupture. Therefore patients without collateral support are considered poor operative candidates.

Finally, Nunley et al. observed that the mortality after bypass surgery (for the indication of cardiogenic shock in 17 percent of patients undergoing this surgery) was only 14 percent [15]. Considering the alternatives, this figure is remarkably low and emphasizes the need to consider revascularization under these conditions.

Transplantation

This discussion of surgical options after recent myocardial infarction would be incomplete were not the therapeutic possibilities for cardiac transplantation mentioned. Obviously, this operation is reserved for patients with no chance of survival without such an intervention, but we have successfully performed transplantations in a small number of patients following myocardial infarction at the Minnesota Heart and Lung Institute. These patients required intervention with left ventricular assist devices after pharmacologic inotropic support and intra-aortic balloon pumping were unsuccessful, and the anatomy was not suitable for bypass surgery. We favor the left ventricular assist device over the total artificial heart because of the many complications associated with the latter device. Urgent transplantation has been successfully accomplished at our institution but of course can be considered only in centers that have a vast experience with the procedure. It is obviously a therapy of last resort and is severely limited by the availability of donor organs.

Conclusion

In otherwise viable patients, further myocardium at risk must be aggressively evaluated following myocardial infarction. Noninvasive evaluation with graded exercise testing is and should be routinely employed in such patients if chest pain does not occur spontaneously. If chest pain does occur soon after myocardial infarction, we believe such patients should undergo angiography and ultimately surgery to revascularize the myocardium if other therapies such as angioplasty would be incomplete. It has become a safe procedure, and coronary artery bypass grafting can be carried out with optimum safety if the patient can be stabilized for approximately 7 days. Even if such a waiting period cannot be accomplished, the morbidity and mortality for such an operation has been drastically reduced and therefore should be considered promptly.

The role for revascularization has also evolved for acute myocardial infarction and cardiogenic shock. In the case of acute infarction, the crucial determinant is time; revascularization is best accomplished within the first few hours of infarction and has been demonstrated to restore both regional and global myocardial function. In the case of cardiogenic shock, there may be no other alternative; and if the patient has amenable coronary artery anatomy, it should be strongly considered.

Cardiac transplantation has been employed successfully at a few centers with a great deal of experience in this procedure. Whether it develops into a more widely used therapy remains to be seen.

Editorial Comments

The group from the University of Minnesota has taken an aggressive posture with regard to coronary artery surgery in patients who develop angina pectoris soon after myocardial infarction. The results at Minnesota and at other major institutions have been reasonably favorable, but these results cannot be necessarily translated to the community at large. The decision to perform surgery obviously depends on multiple factors including local surgical skills and experience, the urgency of operative intervention, whether the patient is truly refractory to medical treatment, and the extent of left ventricular dysfunction. In the final analysis, the decision for operative intervention always rests with the judgment of the attending physician, who is usually in the best position to carefully consider all of these variables. G.S.F.

References

1. Jones, E. L. Surgical revascularization during acute evolving myocardial infarction. *Circulation* 76(Suppl III):146, 1987.
2. Berg Jr., R., et al. Immediate coronary artery bypass for acute evolving myocardial infarction. Presented at Symposium on Coronary Artery Disease Today: Diagnosis, Surgery, and Prognosis. Sponsored by The Netherlands Heart Foundation and American Heart Association, Utrecht, The Netherlands, 27 May 1981.
3. DeWood, M. A., Spores, J., Berg Jr., R., et al. Acute myocardial infarction: A decade of experience with surgical reperfusion in 701 patients. *Circulation* 68(Suppl II):8, 1983.
4. Spencer, F. C. Emergency coronary bypass for acute infarction: An unproved clinical experiment. *Circulation* 68(Suppl II):17, 1983.
5. Flameng, W., Sergeant, P., Vanhacke, J., and Suy, R. Emergency coronary bypass grafting for evolving myocardial infarction: Effects on infarct size and left ventricular function. *J. Thorac. Cardiovasc. Surg.* 94:124, 1987.
6. Dawson, J. T., Hell, R. J., Hallmann, G. L., and Cooley, D. A. Mortality in patients undergoing coronary artery bypass surgery after myocardial infarction. *Am. J. Cardiol.* 33:483, 1974.
7. Levine, F. H., et al. Safe early revascularization for continuing ischemia after acute myocardial infarction. *Circulation* 60(Suppl I):5, 1979.
8. Jones, E. L., et al. Coronary bypass for relief of persistent pain following acute myocardial infarction. *Ann. Thorac. Surg.* 32:33, 1981.
9. Fudge, T. L., et al. Coronary artery bypass after recent myocardial infarction. *Arch. Surg.* 117:1418, 1982.
10. Breyer, R. H., Sagelman, R. M., Rousou, J. A., and Lemeshow, S. Postinfarction angina: An expanding subset of patients undergoing coronary artery bypass. *J. Thorac. Cardiovasc. Surg.* 90:532, 1985.
11. Williams, D. B., et al. Postinfarction angina: Results of early revascularization. *J. Am. Coll. Cardiol.* 2:859, 1983.
12. Hochberg, M. S., et al. Timing of coronary revascularization after acute myocardial infarction. *J. Thorac. Cardiovasc. Surg.* 88:914, 1984.
13. Scheidt, S., Aschein, R., and Killip, T. Shock after acute myocardial infarction: A clinical and hemodynamic profile. *Am. J. Cardiol.* 26:556, 1970.
14. Buckley, M. J. In J. M. Moran and L. L. Michaelis (eds.), *Surgery for Acute Myocardial Infarction: Evolution and Current Status.* Orlando: Grune & Stratton, 1980. P. 247.
15. Nunley, D. L., et al. Coronary bypass operation following acute myocardial infarction. *J. Thorac. Cardiovasc. Surg.* 85:485, 1983.

36
Ambulatory Monitoring After Acute Myocardial Infarction

PASQUALE F. NESTICO AND JOEL MORGANROTH

Myocardial infarction (MI) remains an important cause of death and morbidity in the United States [1] with an average in-hospital mortality of about 12 to 15 percent [2]. Most deaths attributable to MI occur within the first few hours after the onset of symptoms [3–5]. Thereafter, mortality declines steadily [6, 7]. Those fortunate to survive the in-hospital period have a relatively good prognosis. However, after discharge from the hospital, the occurrence of clinically significant nonfatal and fatal cardiac events is greatest during the first few months [8].

During the 1970s and 1980s, mortality rates associated with coronary disease have declined by almost 40 percent in the United States. Reports suggest that this decline results from a combination of improvement in the cardiovascular risk factors in the population, a falling incidence of coronary heart disease (particularly of sudden death), and improved survival [9]. Evidence exists that the presence of ventricular arrhythmias independently influences survival in patients after myocardial infarction; and because the mechanism responsible for sudden death is, in more than 80 percent of patients, a ventricular tachyarrhythmia [10], it is not surprising that the use and complexity of ambulatory (Holter) electrocardiography (ECG) have grown rapidly.

The scope of this report is to: (1) review the basis of Holter monitoring, (2) describe the indications for Holter monitoring in the various stages of MI (early and late in-hospital phase and posthospital phase), and (3) discuss the limitations of Holter monitoring.

History

The first Holter monitoring device was an 85-pound backpack radio transmitter with limited range, and it was followed by a portable magnetic tape "electrocardiorecorder" developed during the mid-1950s that weighed only 4 pounds and could record the ECG for up to 10 hours [11]. Further technologic developments during the 1960s provided a system that allowed for the direct recording of the ECG from electrodes attached to a patient's chest over several hours during the day. Subsequently, the widespread use of Holter monitoring followed the early clinical reports that identified a relation between ventricular arrhythmias and mortality from heart disease [12]. Technologic advancements have increased the accuracy and reliability of the analytic and recording methods [13, 14]. Commercial development has now provided recorders capable of obtaining continuous data, and technologic advancement has consisted of printed circuit boards and small transistors that allow recorders to be of smaller size and capable of longer recording periods (24–48 hours). Advances in playback systems have allowed for a variety of sophisticated and complex data analysis processes. The introduction of solid-state microprocessors, microcomputers, and integrated circuits have further fostered a more flexible and versatile handling of data. Prospective comparative studies are now necessary to evaluate the various Holter systems and to define quantitatively and qualitatively the relative cost–benefit ratio of the various types of equipment.

Indications for Holter Monitoring

The clinical indications for Holter monitoring after an acute MI are to: (1) attempt to define an arrhythmia as the cause of specific patient complaints; (2) detect the presence of ventricular arrhythmias to define those patients at high risk for sudden death; (3) assess the efficacy, inefficacy, or proarrhythmic effect of antiarrhythmic therapy; and (4) evaluate ST segment morphology to define subgroups with ischemia (e.g., silent ischemia, coronary spasm).

Ventricular arrhythmias that occur following an acute MI can be divided into two categories: (1) early-onset arrhythmias that occur within the first 3 days after MI, and (2) late-onset arrhythmias that occur about 6 to 14 days after the MI.

EARLY-ONSET ARRHYTHMIAS

Holter monitoring has a limited role for the detection of arrhythmias during the first 3 days after an acute MI. The reasons are twofold; first, patients admitted to the hospital with an acute MI are usually ECG monitored constantly in the coronary care unit. Second, early-onset ventricular arrhythmias, even ventricular tachycardia or fibrillation, do not influence the postdischarge sudden death prognosis [15].

The principal use of Holter monitoring has been to detect the cardiac rhythm disturbances that mark a patient at increased risk of sudden death. Patients who had cardiac arrest unexpectedly while undergoing ambulatory ECG monitoring have displayed the ECG mechanism of cardiac collapse [10]. In one study [10] of 15 such patients the terminal event at the time of cardiac arrest was a bradyarrhythmia associated with ischemia in about 20 percent with no survivals. A ventricular tachyarrhythmia was the precursor of sudden cardiac death in the remaining 80 percent of patients, with 42 percent of them surviving. Others [16] have reported that sudden cardiac arrest recorded on ambulatory ECG monitoring was associated with bradyarrhythmias in

26 percent and with tachyarrhythmias in 74 percent of patients.

LATE-ONSET ARRHYTHMIAS

After MI, the presence of late ventricular premature complexes (VPCs) on 24-hour Holter monitoring, a mean of more than 6 VPCs/hour or repetitive forms (ventricular couplets or ventricular tachycardia, defined as more than 3 VPCs in a row) increase the risk of sudden cardiac death (Table 36-1). Therefore Holter monitoring has become the main noninvasive modality to detect late-onset ventricular arrhythmias after acute MI and thus define the patient's risk of sudden cardiac death [17, 18].

Analysis of 24-hour Holter recordings in several large studies, performed about 10 days after acute MI, revealed that the frequency of ventricular arrhythmias has a strong association with subsequent cardiac death [19–22]. An S-shaped curve relates VPC frequency rate to risk of mortality. The curve rises steeply between 1 to 10 VPCs/hour. Mortality rates are 2.5 to 4.0 times as high for patients with 10 or more VPCs/hour than for patients with lower VPC frequency.

Several studies have suggested that the occurrence of repetitive VPCs had a more important effect on mortality during follow-up. Early studies proposing this concept used short-duration Holter recordings and variable definitions of complex ventricular arrhythmias [23]. Studies [20, 21, 24] using 24-hour Holter recordings have defined the relation between repetitive VPCs and mortality in large populations of post-MI patients. They concluded that repetitive VPCs have more impact on subsequent mortality then frequent VPCs. In a predischarge 24-hour Holter monitoring study, nonsustained ventricular tachycardia had the strongest relation with subsequent mortality (odds ratio = 4.2) but this arrhythmia occurred in only 12 percent of MI patients [20, 21, 25].

Holter monitoring has also been an important tool for studying the independent relation between ventricular arrhythmias, left ventricular dysfunction, and sudden death after MI.

Interest in this relation stems from a small but provocative study by Schulze and coworkers in which they concluded that ventricular arrhythmias and ventricular dysfunction were not independent risk factors [26, 27]. In their study of 81 patients, left ventricular ejection fractions were measured by radionuclide ventriculography, and ventricular arrhythmia frequency was measured by 24-hour Holter recording. There were only eight deaths, each of which occurred in the subgroup with a left ventricular ejection fraction of less than 0.40 *and* "high grade" arrhythmias. Thus one cannot determine from such data the potential independence of these two variables.

Multicenter studies, using Holter monitoring, have demonstrated that VPCs and ventricular dysfunction are indeed independent predictors of mortality [20, 22, 28]. The Multicenter Post Infarction Program (MPIP) was a nine-hospital natural history study of patients under age 70 who had proved MI. The Multicenter Investigation of the Limitation of Infant Size (MILIS) study was a five-hospital intervention study of the effect of hyaluronidase, propranolol, or both in patients under age 76 with acute MI. Both studies obtained a radionuclide ventriculogram and a 24-hour ECG recording about 10 days after MI. Both used standardized procedures to analyze the radionuclide left ventricular function studies and comparable high quality computer programs to analyze the 24-hour Holter monitoring data [29–31]. In both MPIP and MILIS, repetitive VPCs in patients with left ventricular ejection fractions of less than 40 percent were strongly and independently related to mortality compared to left ventricular dysfunction. In MILIS, the risk of dying was increased about 16-fold when both repetitive VPCs and low left ventricular dysfunction were present. In MPIP, the risk of dying in patients with low left ventricular ejection fractions and high frequency VPCs with repetitive forms was about 12-fold higher.

The Beta Blocker Heart Attack Trial (BHAT) [32] presented the largest body of data yet reported to confirm that in acute MI survivors VPCs predicted mortality independently of other factors. As part of BHAT, 3290 patients had 24-hour Holter monitoring performed before randomization at baseline. As expected, VPCs were significantly related to total mortality in the 1640 BHAT patients randomized to the placebo group over an average follow-up period of 25 months

Studies have been reported with differing viewpoints. Holter monitoring data assessing certain subsets of MI patients with complex ventricular arrhythmias have shown interesting findings. Maisel et al. [33] reported that in a study of 777 patients the presence of complex VPCs at the time of hospital discharge was an important predictor of 1-year mortality in the presence of non-Q-wave MI, but not Q-wave infarctions. Patients with a non-Q-wave MI with complex VPCs on a predischarge Holter recording were at high risk for cardiac death during the subsequent year, irrespective of left ventricular ejection fraction (LVEF). These data require further evaluation and confirmation.

Bigger et al. [34] reported that nonsustained ventricular tachycardia had a strong and statistically significant association ($p < .05$) with all-cause and arrhythmic mortality independent of other risk variables that were associated with ventricular tachycardia. However, the 3-year survival for the group that had neither ventricular tachycardia nor LVEF of less than 30 percent was 0.88 compared with 0.43 for patients who had both of these risk factors, emphasizing the interdependence of these two variables on survival. In contrast, Ahnve et al. [35] noted that VPCs did not yield prognostic information in addition to that supplied by LVEF for sudden death, although it did carry importance for predicting total cardiac mortality. Furthermore, the relative prognostic value of thallium 201 imaging, radionuclide ventriculography, and 24-hour Holter monitoring was compared prospectively in 93 patients after acute MI [36]. Although all three tests were important predictors of survival by univariate Cox survival analysis, only the thallium score was the important predictor of survival by multivariate analysis.

Holter monitoring has been used in several studies comparing beta-adrenergic blocking drugs to placebo in post-MI patients. In the

Table 36-1
Effect of LV dysfunction and VPCs on cardiac mortality and sudden death late after acute MI

First author	Type of population	Size	LVEF (%)	VPC/hr	Holter (hours)
Kotler [17]	Patients	160	—	≥ 1	12
Vismara [18]	Patients	64	—	≥ 1	10
MPIRG [19]	Patients	766	<40	≥ 10	24
Bigger [21]	Patients	55	<30	≥ 3	24
	Controls	476	≥ 30	<3	24
Mukharji [22]	Patients	40	≤ 40	≥ 10	24
	Controls	314	>40	<10	24
Moss [23]	Patients	470	—	≥ 1	6
	Controls	470	—	0	6
Bigger [25]	Patients	50	—	VT	24
	Controls	380	—	No VT	24
Schulze [26]	Patients	14	<40	Lown class II–IV	24
	Controls	22	<40	Lown class 0–I	24
Schulze [27]	Patients	45	<40	Lown class III–V	24
	Controls	36	≥ 40	Lown class 0–II	24
Mukharji [28]	Patients	47	≤ 40	Lown class 4A–4B	24
	Controls	199	>40	Lown class <4A	24

FU (mo)	Time of data (days)	Patients			Comments
		Total[a]	CM[b]	SD (%)	
(30–54)	>90	128	20	14	Complex form of VPCs were associated with an excess risk of SD.
26(13–38)	11(5–14)	49	16	12	In this relatively small number of patients, VPCs late in the hospital course predispose to subsequent SD.
22	—	—	(11)	(4)	Patients with a low LVEF and frequent VPCs had a 3.8-fold increased risk of CM when compared with patients without these risks.
24	—	55	21(38)	—	VPCs and LVEF are independently related to mortality rate. However, the relative risk estimated by multivariate analysis of CM for patients with an LVEF of <30%, at least 3 VPCs/hour, and runs of VPCs was 13 times that of patients without these findings.
24	—	476	31(7)	—	
18 (up to 24)	—	40	16	7(18)	The presence of frequent VPCs (≥10/hour) is an important and independent risk factor for subsequent SD. However, the relative risk of SD for up to 2 years in patients with an LVEF of 40% or less and at least 10 VPCs/hour was reported to be nine times that of patients without these conditions.
18 (up to 24)	—	314	16	5(2)	
36(1–60)	Last 3 days	470	67	37(68)	Complex VPCs made an independent contribution to the risk of CM.
36(1–60)	Last 3 days	470	31	18(32)	
36	10–20	50	27(54)	—	The probability of surviving 36 months in the group with VT was 46% compared with 81% in the group without VT.
36	10–20	380	72(19)	—	
—	14–28	13(93)	—	—	VPCs may not be an independent risk factor for SD in the convalescent phase of MI. Of 14 class II–IV patients, 13 had EF <40% compared with only 8 of 22 class 0–I patients.
—	14–28	8(36)	—	—	
7(2–16)	14	26(58)	—	8(18)	Although a low LVEF may suggest a poor prognosis following MI, the presence of VPCs significantly increases the risk of SD.
7(2–16)	14	3(8)	—	0	
14 (up to 10)	10–12	47	—	12(26)	The combined presence of repetitive VPCs and reduced LVEF define a subgroup of post-MI patients at high risk for SD.
14 (up to 18)	10–12	199	—	3(2)	

Table 36-1
Continued

First author	Type of population	Size	LVEF (%)	VPC/hr	Holter (hours)
Bigger [34]	Patients	26	<30	VT	24
	Controls	588	≥30	No VT	24
Ahnve [35]	Patients	97	<45	Lown class ≥II	24
	Controls	204	≥45	None	24
Maisel [33]	Non-Q-wave MI	191	50 ± 15 (mean)	Complex VPCs	24
Kostis [32]	Q-wave MI	586	43 ± 14 (mean)	Complex VPCs	24

CM = cardiac mortality; FU = follow-up; LVEF = left ventricular ejection fraction; SD = sudden death; VPCs = ventricular premature complexes; VT = ventricular tachycardia.
[a]Patients meeting the criteria of LVEF breakpoint and/or VPCs or VT.
[b]Witnessed deaths.

group randomized to beta blockers, total and sudden death mortality rates were reduced in those treated for 2 years or more after MI [37–39]. It has been shown that the reduction in mortality on beta-blocker treatment is greater in those patients who have substantial reduction in the ventricular arrhythmia frequency on treatment [40].

In summary, Holter monitoring is a valuable tool for detecting frequent and complex ventricular arrhythmias after MI. This noninvasive modality has also enabled investigators to assess the prognostic significance of the presence of these arrhythmias in predicting cardiac death. Holter monitoring is the primary tool used to test the hypothesis that effective reduction in ventricular arrhythmia density may reduce subsequent mortality in post-MI patients. Figure 36-1 details the therapeutic approach we currently recommend for the management of VPCs and ventricular tachycardia after MI. For early-onset ventricular arrhythmias empiric intravenous drug therapy is indicated to stabilize the ventricular arrhythmia. Therapy should be discontinued after transfer from critical care to allow evaluation of late-onset of arrhythmias.

For late-onset ventricular arrhythmias post-MI, ambulatory ECG recordings have shown that simple and complex VPCs are independent predictors of sudden death. In these patients initiation of therapy depends on the frequency and complexity of VPCs, hemodynamic instability, and LVEF. In patients with potentially lethal ventricular arrhythmias and well preserved ventricular function, prophy-

FU (mo)	Time of data (days)	Patients			Comments
		Total[a]	CM[b]	SD (%)	
36	11 ± 3	26	19(73)	—	VT nearly doubled the risk of
36	11 ± 3	588	365(62)	—	dying during the follow-up period. VT had a strong and statistically significant association with CM independent of LV dysfunction. The cumulative 3-year survival for the group that had neither VT nor LVEF less than 30% was 0.88, compared with 0.43 for patients who had both risks.
12	—	97	23(24)	11(11)	VPCs did not yield prognostic
12	—	204	8(4)	1(0.5)	information in addition to that supplied by LVEF for SD, but it did carry importance for total CM.
12			(24) $p<.001$		The presence of complex VPCs at the time of hospital
12			(8)		discharge is an important predictor of 1 year mortality in the presence of non-Q-wave, but not Q-wave, infarction.

lactic use of antiarrhythmic drugs is not indicated, and with left ventricular dysfunction the indication for treatment is not established. Except for beta-adrenergic blockers, no studies have shown that treatment of potentially lethal ventricular arrhythmias with drugs reduces the incidence of sudden cardiac death. Lethal ventricular arrhythmias require aggressive treatment, and we believe that therapy should be guided by electrophysiologic testing.

SYMPTOM EVALUATIONS

After an MI many patients complain of symptoms of altered consciousness (dizziness, lightheadedness, syncope) or palpitations. These symptoms may be due to a variety of mechanisms (i.e., sinus tachycardia, forceful normal heart beats, or dangerous ventricular tachyarrhythmias). Holter monitoring can help ascertain the precise diagnosis, particularly if the standard 12-lead ECG is not diagnostic. Often the ambulatory ECG recording defines no ECG correlates to patient symptoms. Conversely, no symptoms are common in patients with potentially lethal ventricular arrhythmias.

ST SEGMENT ANALYSIS

Holter monitoring is used as the principal technique for identifying silent myocardial ischemia. The poor frequency response of the early Holter recorders led to many false-positive ST segment changes. Because the validity of ST segment changes to define silent myocardial ischemia has now been shown [41, 42], many manufacturers have developed sophisticated computer techniques for recogni-

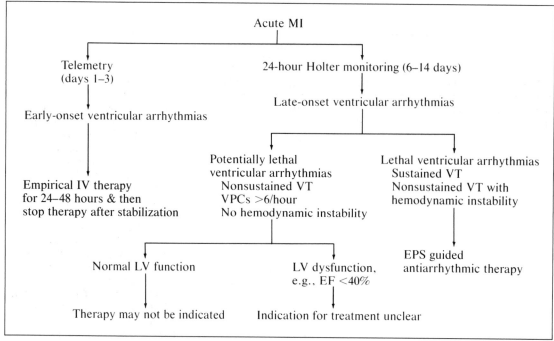

Fig. 36-1
Ventricular arrhythmia onset and its management after acute myocardial
infarction. EPS = electrophysiologic study; IV = intravenous;
LV = left ventricular; MI = myocardial infarction; VPCs = ventricular
premature complexes; VT = ventricular tachycardia; EF = ejection fraction.

tion and quantitation of these changes [13, 14]. Instrumentation capable of simultaneously examining two or more channels of ECG data for ST segment changes with automatic measurement and quantitation of ST segment magnitude, integral area, and slope is now available [43].

Ambulatory ECG recording studies have shown that silent episodes of ST segment depression may greatly outnumber those accompanied by angina pectoris and occur in previously unsuspected circumstances [41, 44]. That these episodes are ischemic and frequently spontaneously reversible may be demonstrated by concomitant radionuclide and metabolic abnormalities [41, 45, 46]. Furthermore, exercise performance and angiographic characteristics of patients with silent myocardial ischemia are similar to those patients with symptomatic ischemia [47]. One study reported that ischemic ST segment changes shown by ambulatory Holter monitoring predicted an increase in 1-year mortality in post-MI patients [48]. In fact, multiple logistic

regression analysis on 17 variables has shown that ST segment change as detected by Holter monitoring was the most predictive variable for 1-year mortality ($p<.03$). Most ST segment changes were silent.

Ambulatory ECG monitoring has also been used to guide drug therapy in patients with "mixed" angina [49, 50]. In one such study, ten patients underwent 48-hour Holter monitoring that recorded 204 ischemic episodes on placebo, of which 79 percent were silent [50]. On atenolol therapy, 98 ischemic events were recorded during ambulatory ECG monitoring, a 63 percent decrease relative to placebo ($p< .01$).

The comparative validity of ambulatory ECG recording and exercise electrocardiography for the detection of ST segment changes reflecting myocardial ischemia has been addressed [51, 52] (Table 36-2). Effort angina pectoris and myocardial ischemia are more reliably detected by exercise electrocardiography, whereas silent myocardial ischemia may be more predictably identified by ambulatory

Table 36-2
Sensitivity and specificity of Holter monitoring and exercise ECG in detecting VPCs

Study	No. of pts.	Holter		Exercise ECG	
		Sensitivity (%)	Specificity (%)	Sensitivity (%)	Specificity (%)
Stern & Tzivoni [51]	48	88	82		
Crawford et al. [52]	70	62	61	67	75

recording. Stern and Tzivoni [51] reported a sensitivity of 88 percent and a specificity of 82 percent for ambulatory ECG recordings in patients with both normal and abnormal exercise tests. Crawford et al. [52] compared exercise electrocardiography with ambulatory ECG recording in 70 patients who subsequently underwent coronary angiography and found the sensitivity of exercise testing to be 67 percent and that of ambulatory ECG recordings 62 percent; the specificity of the two tests was 75 percent and 61 percent respectively. Despite the lower sensitivity and specificity of the ambulatory ECG, it often affords complementary information. For instance, patients with nocturnal angina or variant angina occurring frequently in the early morning hours may demonstrate ST–T abnormalities only on Holter monitoring.

Thus much of the interest in the subject of silent ischemia has resulted from the use of Holter monitoring to detect ST segment changes occurring out of hospital. This technique provides a unique, objective means of evaluating both symptomatic and silent episodes of ischemia during ordinary daily life. However, the value of Holter monitoring in patients with coronary artery disease clearly depends on the reliability of transient ST segment depression as a clinical marker of a myocardial ischemic event. This point assumes use of appropriate equipment (e.g., proper frequency response), optimal lead placement, awareness of changes with posture, effect of hyperventilation, and other physiologic variables [53]. Because of the potential for a high frequency of false-positive ST segment responses in subjects, prospective clinical trials are necessary to define the clinical relevance of silent myocardial ischemia in this setting and the proper approach to therapy.

LIMITATIONS AND COMPARISON

Holter recording is a safe, inexpensive, noninvasive technique. Minor adverse effects consist in skin irritation or hypersensitivity from the electrode gel, which if necessary can be successfully treated with hydrocortisone cream. Holter recorders have standard electrical safety requirements, which should eliminate the possibility of electrical leak.

Problems of analysis of Holter recordings are avoided by sampling the ECG output to ascertain that the lead system provides adequate voltage to "trigger" the system. Extraneous magnetic induction or demagnetization of the recording tape may occur and must be avoided. Errors may result in heart rate and ST segment trends if changes in motor speed or timing are not detected. Equipment malfunction (electrical and mechanical), technician errors, or movement by the patient can produce pseudoectopic beats and pauses. Such artifacts may be identified by the simultaneous use of two ECG channels, knowledge of their previous occurrence, and changes in the ECG complexes, which become either too narrow or wide.

The limitation of Holter monitoring for assessing ventricular ectopy frequency because of a high rate of spontaneous variability is well known [54–58]. Because of this problem, a high rate of suppression (>75 percent) of VPC frequency is necessary to define therapeutic efficacy when comparing one 24-hour ambulatory Holter recording on placebo compared to a second 24-hour recording on therapy.

The duration of the Holter recording and the probability of detecting arrhythmias have been examined [59–61] (Table 36-3). The percent of patients detected with VPCs relate to the duration of the recording: the longer the

Table 36-3
Relation between length of ambulatory recording and ventricular arrhythmias detected

Study	No. of pts.	VPCs detected (%)							VT detected (%)	
		1 min	1 hr	6 hr	12 hr	24 hr	36 hr	48 hr	1 hr	24 hr
Lopes et al. [59]	54				84	100				
Kennedy et al. [60]	35			29	57	83	100	100		
Bigger et al. [61]		11	47	66		84			10	67

recording, the more the likelihood of detecting patients with repetitive arrhythmias. In particular, Bigger et al. [61] examined the relation between the probability of detecting VPCs and the duration of the Holter recording in 200 (24-hour) monitoring sessions in patients 2 weeks after acute MI. The percent of patients detected with VPCs related to the duration of the recording: 11 percent for 1 minute, 47 percent for 1 hour, 66 percent for 6 hours, 84 percent for 24 hours. Detection of repetitive forms of VPCs was also related to the duration of the recording. Furthermore, the incidence of ventricular tachycardia accumulated linearly over the 24-hour period, and only 10 percent of these patients with ventricular tachycardia would have been detected with only a 1-hour ECG recording.

Treadmill exercise test has been compared with Holter monitoring for the detection of ventricular arrhythmias [62, 63]. VPCs are more frequently detected on Holter recordings than on treadmill exercise testing. However, there is a subset of patients who have ventricular arrhythmias only on treadmill exercise testing. Furthermore, in some post-MI patients exercise-induced ventricular ectopic activity is a better predictor of cardiac death than that detected by Holter monitoring [64].

Summary

Holter recording provides an excellent, sensitive, specific noninvasive tool for detecting arrhythmias in post-MI patients. Attention must be given to proper technique and assurance that quantitation is provided to ensure accurate differentiation of efficacy from proar-rhythmic effects of therapy. The role of ambulatory ECG monitoring in post-MI patients to detect silent myocardial ischemia is of great interest but needs further clarification.

Editorial Comments

One of the issues not directly addressed by the authors is the decision as to which patient should have a Holter monitor following a myocardial infarction. At the present time there are cardiologists who would argue that all patients should have Holter monitoring performed prior to discharge, but it is not a common practice. Clearly, there are some patients who benefit more than others from having Holter monitoring. Probably all patients with persistent, frequent, and/or complex ventricular arrhythmias 3 days beyond the acute event should be considered for Holter monitoring. Until more data are available regarding this issue, physicians must rely on their judgment when making decisions about performing this test on patients with acute myocardial infarction. G.S.F.

Ventricular fibrillation and/or ventricular tachycardia requiring cardioversion during the first 3 days after the onset of acute myocardial infarction has traditionally been thought to be without influence of the long-term prognosis of these patients. However, collected data now strongly suggests that survival is better for patients without cardiac arrest within the first 2 days after myocardial infarction than it is for patients who suffer this early complication. Improved survival for patients without cardiac arrest seems to last approximately 4 years after hospital discharge.

Thereafter, no difference is seen with respect to survival in these two groups of patients. J.S.A.

References

1. Pell, S., and Fayerweather, W. E. Trends in the incidence of myocardial infarction and in associated mortality and morbidity in a large employed population, 1957–1983. *N. Engl. J. Med.* 312:1005, 1985.
2. Sobel, B. E., and Braunwald, E. The management of acute myocardial infarction. In E. Braunwald (ed.), *Heart Disease: A Textbook of Cardiovascular Medicine.* Philadelphia: Saunders, 1984. Pp. 1353–1386.
3. Weinblatt, E., Shapiro, S., Frank, C. W., et al. Prognosis of man after first myocardial infarction: Mortality and first recurrence in relation to selected parameters. *Am. J. Public Health* 58:1329, 1968.
4. Crampton, R. S., Aldrich, R. F., Gascho, J. A., et al. Reduction of prehospital, ambulance and community coronary death rates by the community wide emergency cardiac care system. *Am. J. Med.* 58:151, 1975.
5. Colling, A., Dellipiani, A. W., Donaldson, R. J., et al. Teesside coronary survey: An epidemiological study of acute attacks of myocardial infarction. *Br. Med. J.* 2:1169, 1976.
6. Mulcahy, R., Hickey, N., Graham, I., et al. Factors influencing long-term prognosis in male patients surviving a first coronary attack. *Br. Heart J.* 37:158, 1975.
7. Geltman, E. M., Ehsani, A. A., Campbell, M. K., et al. The influence of location and extent of myocardial infarction on long-term ventricular dysrhythmia and mortality. *Circulation* 60:805, 1979.
8. Dwyer, E. M., McMaster, P., Greenberg, H., et al. Non-fatal cardiac events and recurrent infarction in the year after acute myocardial infarction. *J. Am. Coll. Cardiol.* 4:695, 1984.
9. Gomez-Marin, O., Folsom, A. R., Kottke, T. E., et al. Improvement in long-term survival among patients hospitalized with acute myocardial infarction, 1970 to 1980. *N. Engl. J. Med.* 316:1353, 1987.
10. Panidis, I., and Morganroth, J. Sudden death in hospitalized patients: Cardiac rhythm disturbances detected by ambulatory electrocardiographic monitoring. *J. Am. Coll. Cardiol.* 2:798, 1983.

11. Holter, N. J. New methods for heart studies: Continuous electrocardiography of active subjects over long periods is now practical. *Science* 134:1214, 1961.
12. Hinkle Jr., L. E., Carver, S. T., and Stevens, M. The frequency of asymptomatic disturbances of cardiac rhythm and conduction in middle-aged men. *Am. J. Cardiol.* 24:629, 1969.
13. Morganroth, J. Ambulatory Holter electrocardiography: Choice of technologies and clinical uses. *Ann. Intern. Med.* 102:73, 1985.
14. Morganroth, J., and Nestico, P. F. Ambulatory Holter electrocardiography: Technology, clinical applications, and limitations. *Cardiology.* Chicago: Year Book, 1987. Chapter 66.
15. Campbell, R. W. F. Prognostic significance of cardiac arrhythmias recorded during the acute phase of myocardial infarction. In H. E. Kulbeztus and H. J. J. Wellens (eds.), *The First Year After Myocardial Infarction.* Mount Kisco, NY: Futura, 1983. Pp. 43–49.
16. Kempf, F. C., and Josephson, M. E. Cardiac arrest recorded on ambulatory electrocardiograms. *Am. J. Cardiol.* 53:1577, 1984.
17. Kotler, M. N., Tabatznik, B., Mower, M. M., et al. Prognostic significance of ventricular ectopic beats with respect to sudden death in the late postinfarction period. *Circulation* 47:959, 1973.
18. Vismara, L. A., Amsterdam, E. A., and Mason, D. T. Relation of ventricular arrhythmias in the late hospital phase of acute myocardial infarction to sudden death after hospital discharge. *Am. J. Med.* 59:6, 1975.
19. Multicenter Post-Infarction Research Group. Risk stratification and survival after myocardial infarction. *N. Engl. J. Med.* 309:331, 1983.
20. Bigger Jr., T. J., Fleiss, J. L., Kleiger, R., et al. The relationships among ventricular arrhythmias, left ventricular dysfunction, and mortality in the 2 years after myocardial infarction. *Circulation* 69:250, 1984.
21. Bigger Jr., T. J., Weld, F. M., Coromilas, J., et al. Prevalence and significance of arrhythmias in 24-hour ECG recordings made within one month of acute myocardial infarction. In H. Kulbertus and H. J. J. Wellens (eds.), *The First Year After a Myocardial Infarction.* Boston: Martinus Nijhoff, 1983. Pp. 161–175.
22. Mukharji, J., Rude, R. E., Poole, W. K., et al. Risk factors for sudden death after acute myocardial infarction: Two-year follow-up. *Am. J. Cardiol.* 54:31, 1984.
23. Moss, A. J., Davis, H. T., DeCamilla, J., et al. Ventricular ectopic beats and their relation to sudden and nonsudden cardiac death after myocardial infarction. *Circulation* 60:998, 1979.
24. Bigger Jr., T. J., and Weld, F. M. Analysis of prognostic significance of ventricular arrhythmias after myocardial infarction: Shortcomings

*Goldberg, F. J., Gore, J. M., Haffajee, C. I., et al. Outcome after cardiac arrest during acute myocardial infarction. *Am. J. Cardiol.* 59:251, 1987.

of Lown grading system. *Br. Heart J.* 45:717, 1981.

25. Bigger Jr., T. J., Weld, F. M., and Rolnitzky, L. M. Prevalence and significance of ventricular tachycardia (three or more complexes) detected by ambulatory electrocardiographic recording in the late hospital phase of acute myocardial infarction. *Am. J. Cardiol.* 48:815, 1981.

26. Schulze Jr., R. A., Rouleau, J., Rigo, P., et al. Ventricular arrhythmias in the late hospital phase of acute myocardial infarction: Relation to left ventricular function detected by gated cardiac blood pool scanning. *Circulation* 52:1006, 1975.

27. Schulze Jr., R. A., Strauss, H. W., and Pitt, B. Sudden death in the year following myocardial infarction: Relation to ventricular premature contractions in the late hospital phase and left ventricular ejection fraction. *Am. J. Med.* 62:192, 1977.

28. Mukharji, J., Rude, R. E., Poole, K., et al. Late sudden death following acute myocardial infarction: Importance of combined presence of repetitive ventricular ectopy and left ventricular dysfunction (Abstract). *Clin. Res.* 30:208A, 1982.

29. Clark, K. W., Hitchens, R. E., Ritter, J. A., et al. Argus/2H: A dual-channel Holter-tape analysis system. In *Computers in Cardiology.* Long Branch, CA: IEEE Computer Society, 1977. Pp. 191–196.

30. Birman, K. P., Rolnitzky, L. M., and Bigger Jr., J. T. A shape oriented system for automated Holter ECG analysis. In *Computers in Cardiology.* Long Beach, CA: IEEE Computer Society, 1974. Pp. 217–220.

31. Clark, K. W., Rolnitzky, L. M., Miller, J. P., et al. Ambulatory ECG analysis shared by two independent computer labs in a multicenter postinfarction program (MPIP). In *Computers in Cardiology.* Long Beach, CA: IEEE Computer Society, 1981. Pp. 271–275.

32. Kostis, J. B., Byington, R., Friedman, L. M., et al. Prognostic significance of ventricular ectopic activity in survivors of acute myocardial infarction. *J. Am. Coll. Cardiol.* 10:231, 1987.

33. Maisel, A. S., Scott, N., Gilpin, E., et al. Complex ventricular arrhythmias in patients with Q wave versus non-Q wave myocardial infarction. *Circulation* 72:963, 1985.

34. Bigger Jr., J. T., Fleiss, J. L., Rolnitzky, L. M., et al. Prevalence, characteristics and significance of ventricular tachycardia detected by 24-hour continuous electrocardiographic recordings in the late hospital phase of acute myocardial infarction. *Am. J. Cardiol.* 58:1151, 1986.

35. Ahnve, S., Gilpin, E., Henning, H., et al. Limitations and advantages of the ejection fraction for defining high risk after acute myocardial infarction. *Am. J. Cardiol.* 58:872, 1986.

36. Hakki, A. H., Nestico, P. F., Heo, J., et al. Relative prognostic value of rest thallium-201 imaging, radionuclide ventriculography, and 24-hour ambulatory electrocardiographic monitoring after acute myocardial infarction. *J. Am. Coll. Cardiol.* 10:25, 1987.

37. Norwegian Multicenter Study Group: Timolol-induced reduction in mortality and reinfarction in patients surviving acute myocardial infarction. *N. Engl. J. Med.* 304:801, 1981.

38. Beta-Blocker Heart Attack Trial Research Group: A randomized trial of propranolol in patients with acute myocardial infarction. I. Mortality results. *J. Am. Coll. Cardiol.* 247:1707, 1982.

39. May, G. S., Eberlein, K. A., Furberg, C. D., et al. Secondary prevention after myocardial infarction: A review of long-term trials. *Prog. Cardiovasc. Dis.* 24:331, 1982.

40. Lichstein, E., Morganroth, J., Harrist, R., et al. Effect of propranolol on ventricular arrhythmias: The Beta-Blocker Heart Attack Trial Experience. *Circulation* 67(Suppl 1, Part 2):1, 1983.

41. Deanfield, J. E., Maseri, A., Selwyn, A. P., et al. Myocardial ischaemia during daily life in patients with stable angina: Its relation to symptoms and heart rate changes. *Lancet* 2:753, 1983.

42. Biagini, A., Mazzei, M. G., Carpeggionic, C., et al. Vasospastic ischemic mechanism of frequent asymptomatic transient ST-T changes during continuous electrocardiographic monitoring in selected unstable angina pectoris. *Am. Heart J.* 103:13, 1982.

43. Gallino, A., Chierchia, S., Smith, G., et al. Computer system for analysis of ST segment changes on 24-hour Holter monitor types: Comparison with other available systems. *J. Am. Coll. Cardiol.* 4:245, 1984.

44. Stern, S., and Tzivoni, D. Early detection of silent ischemic heart disease by 24-hour electrocardiographic monitoring of active subjects. *Br. Heart J.* 36:481, 1974.

45. Cohn, P. F., Brown, E. J., Wynne, J., et al. Global and regional left ventricular ejection fraction abnormalities during exercise in patients with silent myocardial ischemia. *J. Am. Coll. Cardiol.* 1:931, 1983.

46. Shea, M. J., Deanfield, J. E., Wilson, R., et al. Transient ischemia in angina pectoris: Frequent silent events with everyday activities. *Am. J. Cardiol.* 56:3.4E, 1985.

47. Ouyang, P., Shapiro, E. P., Chandra, N. C., et al. An angiographic and functional comparison of patients with silent and symptomatic treadmill ischemia early after myocardial infarction. *Am. J. Cardiol.* 59:730, 1987.

48. Gottlieb, S. H., Gerstenblith, G., Achuff, S. C., et al. Ischemic ST segment changes by ambulatory Holter predict one year mortality in high

risk post-infarct patients (Abstract). *Circulation* 74(Suppl II):58, 1986.

49. Maseri, A., Chierchia, S., and Kaski, J. C. Mixed angina pectoris. *Am. J. Cardiol.* 56:30E, 1985.

50. Chierchia, S., Glazier, J. J., and Gerosa, S. A single-blind, placebo-controlled study of effects of atenolol on transient ischemia in "mixed angina." *Am. J. Cardiol.* 60:36A, 1987.

51. Stern, S., and Tzivoni, D. Evaluation for ischemic ST-T changes. In N. K. Wenger, M. B. Mock, and I. Ringvist (eds.), *Ambulatory Electrocardiographic Recordings.* Chicago: Year Book Medical Publishers, 1981.

52. Crawford, M. H., Mendoza, C. A., O'Rourke, R. A., et al. Limitations of continuous ambulatory electrocardiogram monitoring for detecting coronary artery disease. *Ann. Intern. Med.* 89:1, 1978.

53. Bragg-Remschel, D. A. Problems with ST-segment analysis in ambulatory ECG monitoring systems. In W. Rutishauser and H. Roskamm (eds.), *Silent Myocardial Ischemia.* Berlin: Springer-Verlag, 1984. Pp. 90–98.

54. Misner, J. E., Imrey, P. B., Smith, L., et al. Secular variations in frequency of premature ventricular contractions in untreated individuals. *J. Clin. Lab. Med.* 92:117, 1978.

55. Winkle, R. A. Antiarrhythmic drug effect mimicked by spontaneous variability of ventricular ectopy. *Circulation* 57:1116, 1978.

56. Morganroth, J., Michelson, E. L., Horowitz, L. N., et al. Limitations of routine long-term electrocardiographic monitoring to assess ventricular ectopic frequency. *Circulation* 58:408, 1978.

57. Michelson, E. L., and Morganroth, J. Spontaneous variability of complex ventricular arrhythmias detected by long-term electrocardiographic recording. *Circulation* 61:690, 1980.

58. Pratt, C. M., Slymen, D. J., Wierman, A.M., et al. Analysis of the spontaneous variability of ventricular arrhythmias: Consecutive ambulatory electrocardiographic recordings of ventricular tachycardia. *Am. J. Cardiol.* 56:67, 1985.

59. Lopes, M. G., Runge, P., Harrison, D. C., et al. Comparison of 24 versus 12 hours of ambulatory ECG monitorings. *Chest* 67:269, 1975.

60. Kennedy, H. L., Chandra, V., Sayther, K. L., et al. Effectiveness in increasing hours of continuous ambulatory electrocardiography in detecting maximal ventricular ectopy: Continuous 48 hour study of patients with coronary heart disease and normal subjects. *Am. J. Cardiol.* 42:925, 1978.

61. Bigger Jr., J. T., Rolnitzky, L. M., Leahey, E. B., et al. Ambulatory ECG recording: Duration of recording and activity protocol. In N. K. Wenger, M. B. Mock, and I. Ringvist (eds.), *Ambulatory Electrocardiographic Recordings.* Chicago: Year Book Medical Publishers, 1981.

62. DeSoyza, N., Murphy, M. L., Bissett, J. K., et al. Detecting ventricular arrhythmia after myocardial infarction: Comparison of Holter monitoring and treadmill exercise. *South Med. J.* 70:403, 1977.

63. Pratt, C. M., Fong, A., DeMazia, A. N., et al. Recent advances in the understanding of ambulatory electrocardiography. *Clin. Cardiol.* 2:56, 1979.

64. Henry, R. L., Kennedy, G. T., and Crawford, M. H. Prognostic value of exercise-induced ventricular ectopic activity for mortality after acute myocardial infarction. *Am. J. Cardiol.* 59:1251, 1987.

37
Programmed Electrical Stimulation After Acute Myocardial Infarction

David A. Rawling and Jay W. Mason

The role of electrophysiologic studies in determining prognosis and guiding therapy in patients who have had a myocardial infarction is undergoing evaluation and evolution. At the present time electrophysiologic studies are used in four situations: (1) to evaluate the need for temporary prophylactic pacing in patients with acute bifascicular block; (2) to evaluate the need for a permanent pacemaker in patients who develop or have progression of conduction disturbances during their myocardial infarction; (3) to evaluate and guide therapy in patients developing sustained ventricular tachycardia or having a cardiac arrest during the postinfarct period (i.e., not occurring during the initial period of the myocardial infarction); and (4) to assess the patient's risk of sudden death after infarction so that those at highest risk can be selected for intervention to reduce their high sudden death risk.

Assessing the Need for Temporary Prophylactic Pacing for Acute Bundle Branch Block

Limited data are available regarding temporary prophylactic pacing for acute bundle branch block. Lie et al. [1] studied 50 consecutive patients with a new right bundle branch block, with or without hemiblock, complicating an acute anteroseptal myocardial infarction. His bundle recordings were made in 35 of these patients at the time of appearance of bundle branch block. Ten patients had only right bundle branch block. Only one had a prolonged H–V interval (defined as an H–V ≥60

msec), and none went on to develop complete heart block. Ten of 25 patients with bifascicular block had a normal H–V interval; only one of these developed complete heart block. Eleven of 15 patients with bifascicular block and prolonged H–V interval developed complete heart block. Thus 11 of 12 patients who developed complete heart block had a prolonged H–V interval. Lie et al. concluded that His bundle recording was useful in patients with a *new* right bundle branch block and hemiblock that occurs during the first 24 hours of acute anteroseptal myocardial infarction as patients in this group with prolonged H–V intervals are at high risk for development of complete heart block and should have a temporary pacemaker placed.

Two important limitations of the above study must be noted: First, Lie et al. specifically excluded patients without anteroseptal infarction; and, second, they excluded patients with left bundle branch block. Thus their results are based on a highly selected group of patients. Also, although the authors thought that 10 of 14 patients who developed complete heart block benefited from temporary pacing (by prevention of Stokes-Adams attacks), all 14 died in hospital. Thus an overall benefit of H–V interval measurement on in-hospital mortality has not been demonstrated.

Lichstein et al. reported two studies [2, 3] in which the H–V interval was measured in patients who developed new bifascicular block as a result of an acute myocardial infarction. Measurements were made at the time of temporary pacemaker insertion, which was placed as soon as an electrocardiographic (ECG) pattern of bifascicular block developed. In the initial report of 15 patients [2], 4 had normal and 11 had prolonged H–V intervals (defined as an H–V interval of $\geq$ 55 msec). None of four patients with normal H–V intervals developed complete heart block, and only 1 of 11 patients with prolonged H–V intervals developed complete heart block. This patient died suddenly 6 weeks later (2 weeks after permanent pacemaker implant).

Lichstein et al. later extended the series to 28 patients [3]. None of the five patients with normal H–V intervals developed complete heart block, and just 4 (17 percent) of 23 patients with prolonged H–V intervals developed complete heart block. Thus in this less selected patient population, Lichstein et al. found a prolonged H–V interval to be less useful. Also, all patients in their study who developed complete heart block died, with an average postinfarct survival of 3 weeks.

In summary, although electrophysiologic studies appear to be useful for identifying those within specific subsets of patients with acute infarction who will develop complete heart block, the overall mortality rate in this group is sufficiently high that the therapeutic value of H–V interval measurement is reduced.

Assessing the Need for Permanent Pacemaker After Myocardial Infarction

Although several groups of investigators have suggested that patients who develop conduction disturbances or advanced degrees of AV block during an acute myocardial infarction require permanent pacing [4–8], the Birmingham pacer trial [9] suggested it was not the case. Given these conflicting opinions, it would be useful to have an objective means to determine which patients need permanent pacemaker placement. In 1973 Lichstein et al. [2] used electrophysiologic studies to assess long-term prognosis in patients who developed conduction abnormalities in association with acute infarction. Patients who developed a new bifascicular block had an H–V interval

measured at the time of temporary pacemaker insertion. In an initial study of 15 patients, Lichstein et al. [2] found that three of four patients with normal H–V intervals (H–V < 55 msec) who survived their infarction remained alive at follow-up, whereas three of six patients with prolonged H–V intervals who survived the acute infarct died early during follow-up. Later the study was extended to 28 patients [3]. Now four of five patients with normal H–V intervals survived the acute infarct and remained alive (3 weeks to 22 months' follow-up), whereas only 8 of 23 patients with prolonged H–V intervals remained alive at an average of 9.2 months' follow-up. Thus all patients who survived an acute infarct and had a normal H–V interval were alive at follow-up, whereas only 53 percent of those with a prolonged H–V interval survived. However, of seven "late" deaths in those with prolonged H–V intervals, only two were sudden, and one of these patients had a permanent pacemaker.

Harper et al. [10] studied 72 patients with atrioventricular (AV) or bundle branch block associated with acute infarction. They divided the patients into three groups: Group 1 consisted of 32 patients with AV block of more than first degree but with no intraventricular conduction defect (i.e., the QRS duration was normal). Group 2 consisted of 18 patients with either complete right or left bundle branch block, with or without hemiblock. Patients with both acute and chronic bundle branch block were included. Group 3 consisted of 22 patients with complete bundle branch block (right or left) *plus* an acute episode of any degree of AV block.

Harper et al. found that 30 of 32 patients in group 1 had normal H–V intervals, including seven of nine in complete heart block at the time of study. Only 5 of these 32 patients died, four in hospital. One-half of the group 2 patients had prolonged H–V intervals; none died in hospital, and there were two late deaths. Seventeen group 3 patients had distal His block; three also had a prolonged A–H interval. Of 14 with distal His block alone, 10 died in hospital. Also 12 of the group 3 patients progressed to second- or third-degree AV block;

nine of them died in hospital despite having a temporary pacemaker in place. Harper et al. concluded that His bundle recording added little in determining the site of the AV block.

The authors repeated His bundle recordings in 19 patients 10 to 14 days after infarction. They found that only two group 3 patients showed a more than 10 msec change in H–V interval over the intervening period.

Pagnoni et al. [11] studied 59 patients at the time they developed a new conduction disturbance (except Mobitz II or third-degree AV block) during an acute infarction. Fourteen patients (24 percent) had a prolonged H–V interval (> 55 msec). Although mortality rate was higher in these patients than in those with a normal H–V interval (50 percent versus 13 percent), those with a prolonged H–V interval had greater cardiac dysfunction. Only one patient (with an H–V interval of 90 msec) progressed to complete heart block. During follow-up there were only three sudden deaths, one in a patient with a normal H–V interval. Thus in this study and that of Lichstein et al. [3] there were only 4 of 78 patients in whom a permanent pacemaker might have influenced outcome.

The Birmingham Trial [9] approached the issue differently. Fifty patients with a new, but persistent, conduction defect after an acute myocardial infarction were randomized either to receive a permanent pacemaker (23 patients) or to a control group. Patients with left bundle branch block were excluded. H–V intervals were measured at the time of randomization. Throughout the follow-up period, up to 5 years, there was no difference in survival between the paced and unpaced groups. Furthermore, no conduction disorder progression was observed, and no significant differences were found in the average H–V interval in the two groups. Thus the H–V interval did not appear predictive of outcome, but few patients in the study had H–V intervals of more than 70 msec, which has been found to identify patients at higher risk by some authors [12, 13].

How does the H–V interval change over time after an acute myocardial infarction? Lichstein et al. [3] repeated H–V measurements in ten patients an average of 18 days af-ter the first measurement. The H–V interval decreased an average of 2 msec between the two recordings. Only one patient had a "significant" (10 msec) increase in H–V interval. Harper et al. [10] found only 2 of 19 patients to have a more than 10 msec H–V interval increase at 10 to 14 days. Pagnoni et al. [11] remeasured the H–V interval in 48 surviving patients an average of 7.2 months after infarction and found no significant change. Overall, the available data, though somewhat limited, suggest that the H–V interval remains relatively constant during the first few weeks to months after myocardial infarction.

In summary, although a prolonged H–V interval in association with a new conduction disturbance occurring during an acute myocardial infarction is associated with a poor prognosis, at present there is insufficient information to determine that H–V interval measurement can be used to decide the need for permanent pacemaker placement. Only a large, prospective study can resolve this issue. Such a study should be patterned after the Birmingham trial [9] and should include both early and late measurement of H–V interval. Also, those patients receiving pacemakers should receive units with rate hysteresis in which the lower rate is set low (e.g., 40 beats per minute); the units should provide a count of pacing events. In contrast to the Birmingham trial, however, patients with new left bundle branch block should be included.

Studies in Patients with Ventricular Tachycardia or Ventricular Fibrillation After Myocardial Infarction

Although most ventricular tachyarrhythmia episodes occur within the first 48 hours of acute myocardial infarction, some patients, usually those with extensive, complicated infarction [14–16], develop recurrent, sustained ventricular tachyarrhythmias after the first 2 days of infarction. The prognosis of these patients is grim. They have a 1-year mortality rate of 50 to 80 percent [14–20]. Because these patients are at high risk, several approaches have been tried to reduce the risk. In a retrospective study, Wald et al. [15] performed coronary artery bypass grafting or aneurysmectomy (or both) in 16 of 25 patients who developed medically intractable ventricular tachyarrhythmias an average of 5 weeks after a large anterior infarction. Survival in the surgically treated group was 62 percent, whereas all nine medically treated patients died either in hospital or within 2 months of hospital discharge. Although Wald et al. concluded that surgery improved survival, their results appear seriously flawed, as surgery was actually offered to *all* patients. Therefore the medically treated group was *not* randomly selected, but was selected by either patient or physician choice, often because of a projected high operative mortality rate.

In another retrospective study Marchlinski et al. [20] used electrophysiologic studies to guide therapy in 40 patients with sustained ventricular tachyarrhythmias early after infarction. Thirty-three patients with inducible ventricular tachyarrhythmias were tried on several "standard" antiarrhythmic agents; if they failed, mexiletine or amiodarone (occasionally with another drug) was tried. If all drugs failed, the patient was referred for surgical management. Patients ultimately received a variety of therapies, including electrophysiologically guided antiarrhythmic therapy (seven patients), amiodarone (eight patients), clinically guided antiarrhythmic therapy (three patients), and guided endocardial resection (11 patients). Also, one patient had a "nondirected" aneurysmectomy, and three patients were discharged without testing of their discharge drug. Finally, two of seven patients not inducible at baseline electrophysiology study received no therapy, three received procainamide, and two had surgery (aneurysmectomy and "guided" endocardial resection).

During 20 months' mean follow-up, one-half of these patients died, 11 suddenly. As subgroup analyses failed to show superior results for any treatment, Marchlinski et al. [20] concluded that prognosis was poor in these patients regardless of therapy. A problem with this interpretation, however, is that patient number in each subgroup was small.

In a subsequent abstract [21] these investigators divided 85 patients into two treatment groups: electrophysiologically guided medical therapy or surgical management. Patients with one or two clinical episodes of ventricular tachycardia prior to their baseline electrophysiology study (group A) were compared with those who had three or more episodes (group B). No difference in survival (78 percent medical, 67 percent surgical) or ventricular tachycardia recurrence/sudden death (22 percent medical, 0 percent surgical) was found between the two treatment modalities in group A patients, but an improvement in ventricular tachycardia recurrence/sudden death rate was seen in surgically treated group B patients (59 percent medical, 22 percent surgical). Thus medical or surgical therapy appeared to work well for patients with less ventricular tachycardia, but surgery was better for those with frequent arrhythmias. However, with the variety of medical therapy probably used, the significance of these findings is questionable.

Finally, DiMarco et al. [16] reported 53 patients who developed sustained ventricular tachyarrhythmias within 2 months of myocardial infarction. Thirty-four patients were considered clinically stable after their initial event and underwent electrophysiology study. Twenty of 29 patients who had ventricular tachyarrhythmias inducible were discharged on antiarrhythmic therapy (14 on amiodarone). Nine underwent elective cardiac surgery because of limiting angina or heart failure and had intraoperative mapping and arrhythmia focus ablation also attempted. Four patients were not inducible and did not receive any antiarrhythmic therapy.

Nineteen patients were considered clinically unstable after their initial event. Three of them died from cardiac arrest; the other 16 underwent emergency cardiac surgery, which included aneurysmectomy, attempted arrhythmia focus ablation, and bypass surgery in 12. There were four operative deaths. Only 13 patients (52 percent) were considered successfully mapped, and five of them required long-term antiarrhythmic therapy. Nevertheless, 19 of the 21 surviving surgically treated patients were alive at 17.9 months' average follow-up. In the medically treated group, 21 of the 24 patients were alive at 15 months' average follow-up. DiMarco et al. concluded that an aggressive medical and surgical approach offered the best chance of survival for these patients.

In summary, electrophysiologic studies have been used in patients with sustained ventricular tachyarrhythmias "early" after myocardial infarction to guide antiarrhythmic or surgical therapy. However, as all reported series are retrospective and have used a variety of therapies, it is difficult to determine how much the electrophysiology studies contributed to improving patient survival. Regardless of the mode of therapy, however, long-term prognosis for these patients appears poor.

Assessing the Risk of Sudden Death After Myocardial Infarction

Sustained ventricular tachyarrhythmias are a major cause of mortality in patients who survive an acute myocardial infarction [22, 23]. As a result, numerous investigators have tried to identify specific risk factors for sudden death [24–41]. Two factors that have been found to provide the greatest prognostic information are (1) left ventricular function and (2) the presence of frequent or complex ventricular arrhythmias, or both [23,25–27, 29–37, 39–43].

Once these prognostic factors were identified, investigators began to look for ways to improve patient survival. In patients with poor left ventricular function inotropes, vasodilators, calcium channel blockers, and even beta blockers [44] have been tried. In patients with frequent or complex ventricular ectopy, or both, several trials of prophylactic antiarrhythmic therapy have been carried out. To date, however, the overall results of these antiarrhythmic trials have been disappointing [45–47].

Several reasons have been proposed to explain the failure of these trials to show benefit: (1) The choice of antiarrhythmic drugs was suboptimal. Two studies used phenytoin and two trials used aprindine. (2) The trials were too small. Only two trials included more than 350 patients. (3) In most studies a fixed drug dose was used. Drug levels therefore varied from subtherapeutic to toxic. (4) In most trials no effort was made to document arrhythmia suppression with the drug. (5) Adverse effects were common and led to withdrawal of a significant portion of patients on active drug. (6) Finally, patient selection was poor as "high risk" patients were not selectively enrolled.

Because of the problems with these studies investigators have been trying to improve antiarrhythmic trial design [48] and find other ways to better identify high risk patients so that future antiarrhythmic drug trials can be better focused. One method currently being explored is electrophysiologic study. The hypothesis is that patients with inducible ventricular arrhythmias are more prone to clinical ventricular tachyarrhythmias and that antiarrhythmic drug therapy will improve survival.

Tables 37-1 and 37-2 highlight the studies published to date. Studies have appeared as full manuscripts (Table 37-1) or as abstracts (Table 37-2). Seven of 14 full manuscript studies have been said to show that electrophysiology studies provide useful prognostic information; two of five studies reported in abstract form reach similar conclusions. Thus one-half of the published studies support electrophysiologic testing, and one-half do not. How can we explain this difference?

We have found six study features that strongly influence the study's results: (1) the time after the acute infarct the patients were studied; (2) the stimulation protocol used; (3) the endpoint for a positive study; (4) the length of follow-up; (5) the number of "events" that occurred; and (6) any treatment modalities patients received that could alter their inherent risk of developing an "event." When we compare the studies in Tables 37-1 and 37-2 the most striking finding is the *lack* of uniformity in study design or method, with the three most consistent studies [49–51] from the same group of investigators.

How might the above features influence the results of the studies? First, let us consider the time after infarct patients were studied. As

Table 37-1
Electrophysiologic studies (published as articles)

Parameter	Greene et al. [73]	Hamer et al. [74]	Richards et al.[a] [49 (100,101)]	Marchlinski et al. [75,102]	Kowey et al. [103]	Somberg et al. [61,63]
No. of pts. studied	48[b]	70[c]	165	46	57[d]	29[e]
No. eligible	?	?	304	?	?	47[e]
Av. time post-MI pts. studied	24 days	11 days (median)	10 days	22 days	12 mo	10–20 days
Age (av.)	51	59	54	57	56	?
S_1–S_1	AP (700)	SR, AP (600,500) VP (500,400)	VP (600)	SR, VP (600,400)	VP (< sinus, 500)	VP (500)
No. of extrastimuli	1	1–2	1–2	1–2	1–3	1–4
Sites stimulated	RVA, RVOT	RVA, RVOT	RVA, RVOT	RVA	RVA	RVA, RVOT
Current strength	2 × DT	2 V, 4–10 V	2 × DT, 20 mA	2 × DT	2 × DT	2 × DT
P.W. (msec)	0.9	2	2	1	2	2
Reproducible?	NS	Yes	NS	NS	Yes	NS
Endpoint for positive study	≥2 RVRs	≥2 RVRs; > 5 RVRs gave better discrimination	>10 sec VT/VF	≥ 2 RVRs	≥ 5 RVRs	≥ 10 beats VT
RVRs	19			13		
NSVT		12	—	5	13	10
Sust VT		8	—	5	5	18
VF		0	—	0	0	0
Pos. study	19	20	38	23	18	28
LVEF (av.)	48%	—	55%	44%	49%	37%
Follow-up (mo)	12 (av.)	12 (av.)	8 (av.)	18 (av.)	None	12.5 (av.)
a.a.	?	26 pts. (37%)	8%	15%	?	96%[f]
β-Block	?	"Some"	20%	39%	51%	17%
CABG or PTCA	?	5 pts. (7%)	13%	9%	?	?
+ pts. - SD	8	4	9	4		0
+ pts. - VT	7	0	4	0		1
− pts. - SD	4	1/17 full study, 4/33 limited studies	1	2		0
− pts. - VT	0		2	0		0
EPS worthwhile	Yes	Yes	Yes	No	?	Yes

AP = atrial paced rhythm; SR = sinus rhythm; VP = ventricular paced rhythm; RVA = right ventricular apex; RVOT = right ventricular outflow tract; LV = left ventricle; P.W. = pulse width; DT = diastolic threshold; NS = not studied; RVRs = repetitive ventricular responses; VT = ventricular tachycardia; VF = ventricular fibrillation; NSVT = nonsustained ventricular tachycardia; LVEF = left ventricular ejection fraction; a.a. = antiarrhythmic therapy; CABG = coronary artery bypass graft; PTCA = percutaneous transluminal coronary angioplasty; + pts. = positive study; − pts. = negative study; SD = sudden death; EPS = electrophysiologic study, VB = ventricular burst pacing.

[a]Large patient overlap between this study and that of Denniss et al. [50].

[b]Patients had ventricular arrhythmias after first 24 hours in CCU.

[c]Patients had mechanical or electrical complications of their AMI.

[d]17 Patients had VF with AMI.

[e]On preentry Holter, 15% had cardiac arrest, 62% had symptomatic ventricular arrhythmias, 15% had asymptomatic ventricular arrhythmias.

[f]Lorcainide in 67%; all but two had EP-guided therapy.

Santarelli et al. [104 (105)]	Waspe et al. [95]	Denniss et al. [50]	Roy et al. [94 (106,107)]	Bhandari et al. [64 (108)]	Breithardt et al. [96,97 (109–111)]	Denniss et al. [51 (112,113)]	McComb et al. [87]
50	50[g]	175	150	45	132	403	92[l]
119	~250[g]	339	320	84	379	495	92
25 days	16 days	1–4 weeks	12 days	14 days	22 days	12 days	12 days
53	65	55	52	52	56	52	52
VP (600,460)	SR, VP (600,425)	VP (600)	VP (600,400)	VP (500,400)	SR, VP (500,430,370,330)	VP (600)	SR, VP (600,500,400)
1–2	1–3[h]	1–2	1–2	1–3, VB	1–2	1–2	SR 1–3; VP 1–2
RVA, RVOT	RVA, RVOT	RVA, RVOT	RVA, RVOT	RVA, RVOT, LV apex	RVA	RVA, RVOT	RVA
2 mA, 10 mA	4 × DT	2 × DT, 20 mA	2 × DT	2 × DT	2 × DT	2 × DT, 20 mA	2.5 mA
2	1	2	1.5	2	1.8	2	2
NS	NS	NS	No	No	NS	No	NSVT only
≥ 10 RVRs	≥ 8 RVRs	> 10 sec VT/VF	≥ 6 RVRs	Sust. VT/VF	≥ 4 RVRs	> 10 sec VT/VF	≥ 5 RVRs
			85	5	27	—	—
13	6	—	17	1	6	—	12
10	11	—	16	13	28	80	20
0	0	—	2	7		56	—
23	17	38	35	20	61	136	32
45%	44%	52%	46%	48%	—	35% (meas. in those with + EPS)	50%
11.2 (av.)	22.8 (av.)	12 (minimum)	10 (av.)	10 (av.)	15 (av.)	12	30
24%	14 (28%)[j]	8 (5%)	5 (3%)	10 (22%)[j]	26 (20%)	63 (16%)[m]	32 (35%)[n]
16%	13 (26%)	48 (27%)	66 (44%)	0	44 (33%)[k]	126 (31%)	35 (38%)
14%	9 (18%)	27 (15%)	21 (14%)	4 (9%)	22 (17%)	66 (16%)	?
0	6	10	1	1	1	0.90 (1 yr actuarial survival)	0
3	1	—	1	1	9		1
0	0	8	1	1	3	0.96 (1 yr actuarial survival)	1
0	0	—	1	0	0		0
Not sure	Yes	Yes	No	No	Probably	Yes	Cannot say

[g] All had complicated MI (new conduction disturbance and/or ventricular tachyarrhythmias and/or CHF).
[h] Varied during study (10-1, 10-2, 30-3).
[i] Some EP-guided therapy; more positive patients got treated.
[j] Given to patients with positive EPS.
[k] Most with positive EPS.
[l] All received thrombolytic therapy for their AMI.
[m] Mostly given to patients with positive EPS.
[n] Given to patients with positive EPS.

Table 37-2
Electrophysiologic studies (published as abstracts)

Parameter	Gonzales et al. [114]	Pumphrey et al. [86]	Korn et al. [62]	Bhandari et al. [83]	Iesaka et al. [115]
No. pts. studied	84	70	38	75	133
No. eligible	?	?	?	?	?
Time post-MI studied	6–8 weeks	≤ 4 weeks	7–10 days	14 days av.	1.8 mo. av.
Age	32–70				
S_1–S_2		SR, VP (600,500)	2 C.L.		
No. extrastimuli	1–2	1–2	1–4, VB	1–3	1–3
Sites stim.	RVA		RVA, RVOT	RVA, RVOT, LV	RVA, RVOT
Current strength	2 × DT		5 mA		
Pulse width			2		
Reproducibility	N.S.	N.S.	N.S.	N.S.	N.S.
Endpoint for positive study	≥ 6 RVRs	≥ 4 RVRs	NSVT or sust. VT	Sust. VT/VF	N.S.
RVRs	29				
NSVT	} 19		} 33		21
Sust. VT	19			19	36
VF				14	57
+ Study	19	16		33	
LVEF (av.)		48%			
Follow-up (mo.)	20	3 mo. (minimum)	12.3	16	20
Other therapy					
a.a.		9 pts.[a]	about 75%		
β-Blocker		2[b]			
CABG					
+ Patients - S.D.	0		} 4 S.D.	} 5	8
+ Patients - V.T.	0				1
− Patients - S.D.	4			} 2	
− Patients - V.T.	0				
EPS of value	No	?	No	Yes	Yes

[a] Given to patients with positive EPS.
[b] Both on sotalol.
See Table 37-1 for key to abbreviations.

summarized in Table 37-3, the time after infarction the patients were studied ranged from 5 days to more than a year, although most were studied during the first 4 weeks. This factor is important, as several studies [52–58] have shown that there is variable concordance between electrophysiologic findings "early" and "late" after myocardial infarction. Kuck et al. [56] studied 18 patients 5 and 24 days after an infarct and found two patients with inducible sustained ventricular tachycardia at day 5, but nine patients inducible at day 24. Also, Aonuma et al. [55] studied 19 patients at three time periods after infarction. A positive study was defined as one in which six or more repetitive ventricular responses (RVRs) were induced. Fifty-three percent of the patients had a positive study 2 to 3 weeks after infarct, 37 percent were positive at 4 to 6 weeks, and 21 percent were positive at 12 to 14 weeks. Furthermore, 80, 85, and 100 percent of patients had sustained ventricular tachycardia induced at the respective intervals. Aonuma et al. [55] concluded that electrophysiologic study results were time-dependent. Roy et al. [57], however, found a 76 percent concordance in 21 patients studied an average of 12 days and 8 months after their infarctions. A group of 150 patients were initially studied; 21 were inducible (2 had ventricular fibrillation, 8 had sustained ventricular tachycardia, and 11 had nonsustained ventricular tachycardia). During the repeat study, six of the ten patients with sustained tachyarrhythmias initially still had a sustained tachycardia, two had nonsustained ventricular tachycardia, and two were not inducible. Eleven patients had nonsustained arrhythmias at the first study; one now had ventricular fibrillation, seven had nonsustained ventricular tachycardia, and three were not inducible. Because 16 patients with inducible tachyarrhythmias at the first study had tachyarrhythmias induced at the second study, Roy et al. calculated the concordance to be 76 percent, although only 60 percent of patients with sustained ventricular arrhythmias and 64 percent of patients with nonsustained ventricular arrhythmias had the same type of arrhythmia induced at the second study. Finally, Bhandari et al. [58] studied 17 patients with inducible sustained ventricular tachyarrhythmias an average of 15 days and 150 days after infarction. Eight patients (47 percent) had a sustained ventricular tachyarrhythmia induced at follow-up study.

These studies show that induction of ventricular tachyarrhythmias changes over time after infarction. This finding should not be surprising as other investigators have reported day-to-day changes in ventricular tachyarrhythmia induction [59, 60]. However, for postinfarction studies, the time after an infarction at which ventricular tachyarrhythmia inducibility stabilizes or the time at which specificity peaks remains unknown. Until this point is known, we must rely on the present method of empiric selection of study time.

The second feature to examine is the stimulation protocol used. Except for studies done by the same investigators, none of the protocols are the same. The basic drive varied from sinus rhythm to an atrial paced rhythm to ventricular paced rhythms; pacing cycle lengths also varied. One to two extrasystoles were used in most studies, but two groups used up to four extrastimuli [61–63] and two groups used ventricular burst pacing [62, 64]. In studies in which four extrastimuli were used, the percentage of positive studies was high (97 and 87 percent, respectively), raising the question of the specificity of the induction protocol, as several groups of investigators have shown that specificity decreases as the number of extrastimuli is increased, especially above two extrastimuli [65–69].

Other stimulation protocol variations included the number of pacing sites used; most groups used two, but a few used only one, and Bhandari et al. [64] performed left ventricular stimulation. Stimulation current strength also varied. Most groups used current strengths of twice diastolic threshold, but some used current strengths of 10 to 20 milliamperes. This point is a concern, as several studies have questioned the sensitivity and specificity of using higher stimulus current strengths [69–72]. Finally, even pulse width varied among studies.

The third feature to examine is the endpoint for a positive study, as it can profoundly influ-

Table 37-3
Time after infarct: Influence on studies

Ref.	No. of pts.	Time after MI studied	Endpoint	No. of pts. with pos. study	% Pos. studies	Av. follow-up (mo)	Pts. with VT/SD No.	%
73	48	24 days	≥ 2 RVRs	19	40	12	19	40
74	70	11 days	≥ 2 RVRs	20	29*	12	9	13
49	165	10 days	≥10 sec VT/VF	38	23	8	16	10
75	46	22 days	≤ 2 RVRs	23	50	18	6	13
103	57	12 months	≥ 5 RVRs	18	32*	—	—	—
61, 63	29	10–20 days	≥10 beats VT	28	97*	12.5	1	3
104	50	25 days	≥10 RVRs	23	46	11.2	3	6
95	50	16 days	≥ 8 RVRs	17	34*	22.8	7	14
50	175	1–4 weeks	>10 sec VT/VF	38	22	min 12	10	6
94	150	12 days	≥ 6 RVRs	35	23	10	4	3
64	45	14 days	Sust. VT/VF	20	44	10	3	7
96, 97	132	22 days	≥ 4 RVRs	61	46	15	13	10
51	403	12 days	>10 sec VT/VF	136	34	12	34	9
87	92	12 days	≥ 5 RVRs	32	35*	30	4	2
114	84	6–8 weeks	≥ 6 RVRs	19	23	20	4	5
86	70	≤4 weeks	≥ 4 RVRs	16	23	min 3	2	3
62	38	7–10 days	?	33	87	12.3	4	11
83	75	14 days	Sust. VT/VF	33	44	16	7	9
115	133	1.8 months	?	57	43	20	9	7
81	72	3–4 weeks	≥ 6 RVRs	53	74	—	—	—
54	70	3–4 weeks	≥ 6 RVRs	33	47	10.3	3	4
56	18	5 days	Sust. VT/VF	2	11	24	0	0
55	19	2–3 weeks	≥ 6 RVRs	10	53	—	—	—
84	84	5–10 days	Sust. VT/VF	18	21*	—	—	—
82	36	26 days	Sust. VT/VF	25	69*	14	1	3
58	62	15 days	Sust. VT/VF	26	42	19	5	8
116	84	4 weeks	≥ 6 RVRs	25	30	—	—	—
117	33	<6 weeks	?	9	27	12	2	6
85	111	2–52 weeks	Sust. VT/VF	92	83	12	2	2
Total (or mean)	2501	34.4		959	38	14.3	166	7.6

*Selected patients studied.
See Table 37-1 for key to abbreviations.

ence the sensitivity and specificity of results. Again, significant variability was present (Table 37-3). In three studies [73–75] induction of two repetitive ventricular responses was classified as a positive result. Although it may have increased study sensitivity, several other reports have raised serious questions about the specificity of using so few repetitive ventricular responses [76–80]. In most studies a minimum of five repetitive ventricular responses had to be induced for a positive result. Several studies, however, required that a sustained ventricular tachyarrhythmia be induced for a positive result [53, 56, 58, 64, 81–85]. Thus it is not surprising that reported ventricular tachyarrhythmia induction varied from 11 percent to 97 percent.

Only three groups reported testing arrhythmia induction reproducibility. Reproducibility was not tested in three studies, and in the rest it could not be determined.

The fourth feature to examine is the length of follow-up. Related to this point is the fifth feature, the number of events that occurred during follow-up. As the cumulative probability of a patient having an event increases with time, the longer the follow-up, the greater the number of events that should occur. This point is important because should no events occur (as in ref. 56) the study does not provide meaningful information. Table 37-3 shows that follow-up varied from a "minimum of 3 months" [86] to a 30-month average follow-up [87]. Because patients are at greatest risk of sudden death during the first 6 to 12 months after infarction [23, 88, 89], a well-designed study should have a minimum of 12 months' follow-up. As can be seen from Table 37-3, however, only 13 of the 29 studies had follow-up times of more than 12 months.

Given the variable follow-up periods, and the recruitment of specific patient groups in some studies, it is not surprising that the incidence of ventricular tachycardia or sudden death was variable (from 0 percent in ref. 56 to 40 percent in ref. 73). This point is a concern because if the event rate is "too low" the power of the study to show that electrophysiologic testing has predictive value is low (a type II error).

The final factor is other therapies that might have altered the subject's risk of having an event and thus biased the outcome of the study. Three such therapeutic interventions and the percentage of patients receiving them are listed in Tables 37-1 and 37-2. The interventions are (1) use of antiarrhythmics, (2) use of beta blockers, and (3) coronary artery bypass surgery or angioplasty. The last is probably least important. Although there are data suggesting bypass surgery can decrease recurrence in patients who have had ventricular tachycardia or a cardiac arrest [90, 91], this effect appears to be uncertain and poorly defined [90–93]; for angioplasty no data are available. Nevertheless, these interventions could alter mortality and, depending on study endpoint, alter the study's conclusions. In the studies cited 7 to 18 percent of patients underwent bypass surgery or angioplasty during follow-up.

In contrast to the above, antiarrhythmic therapy certainly could alter patient outcome, particularly if the results of the electrophysiology study were used to select those who would receive antiarrhythmic therapy. In the listed studies 3 percent [94] to 96 percent [61, 63] of the patients were given antiarrhythmic agents. Although most patients received antiarrhythmics without the results of the electrophysiology study influencing their use, in six studies [51, 61, 63, 64, 86, 87, 95] antiarrhythmics were preferentially given to patients with positive results. For example, Somberg et al. [61, 63] treated all (except one) patients with positive electrophysiology studies. Most were given lorcainide, with therapy guided by electrophysiology testing. McComb et al. [87] placed all 32 patients with positive electrophysiology studies on antiarrhythmic therapy using electrophysiologic testing to determine drug efficacy. Finally, Denniss et al. [51] entered 96 of 136 patients with a positive electrophysiology study into a randomized trial; 49 of the 96 patients received quinidine, disopyramide, or mexiletine at dosages that achieved "therapeutic" serum levels. Denniss et al. [68] found that antiarrhythmic therapy did *not* reduce subsequent events, perhaps because the antiarrhythmics suppressed inducible ventricular arrhythmias in only 31 percent of treated patients. Thus several studies were possibly influenced by patients receiving antiarrhythmic agents, and six studies were definitely tainted as antiarrhythmic agents were selectively given to those with positive electrophysiology studies.

Arguments similar to those above can be made regarding the use of beta blockers. Beta blocker use varied from 0 percent to almost 80 percent, with an average of about one-third of patients in most studies receiving a beta blocker. Also, in one study [96, 97] beta blockers were preferentially given to patients with a positive electrophysiology result. Again, as with antiarrhythmic drugs, the substantial use of beta blockers may have had an important impact on the results of these studies.

Table 37-3 reviews selected aspects of the studies. The percentage of positive electrophysiology studies varied from 11 percent [53, 56] to 97 percent [61, 63], with an average of 38 percent of patients having a positive study. None to 40 percent of patients had a major arrhythmic event during follow-up; the overall average was 7.6 percent during a 14.3-month average follow-up period. The wide percentage range of positive studies suggests that selection of certain patients for study inclusion and the variability in stimulation protocols, as well as the variable definitions of a positive result, significantly influenced the incidence of study positivity. On the other hand, the widely variable incidence of follow-up events suggests that administration of antiarrhythmics and beta blockers may have influenced this figure.

The above considerations suggest that the prognostic usefulness of electrophysiologic testing soon after infarction remains to be established, especially when electrophysiologic testing, an invasive procedure, is compared with other noninvasive risk-assessment techniques.

Table 37-4 provides an overview of several studies that have used other techniques to determine risk after infarction. What is clear in the table is that we are much better at predicting that an event *will not occur* (negative predictive value) than we are at predicting its occurrence (positive predictive value). It pro-

duces a problem in antiarrhythmic therapy, as several patients must be treated to prevent an event in one.

Holter monitoring seems to be the least useful of the other techniques that have been used. Otherwise, there seems to be little difference in the overall usefulness of ejection fraction, presence of late potentials as measured by the signal-averaged ECG, and ventricular tachyarrhythmia induction by electrophysiology testing. For example, in the study by Kuchar et al. [98] information derived from the signal-averaged ECG and measurement of ejection fraction gave similar results, whereas Holter monitoring did less well. In contrast, in the study of Gomes et al. [99] information derived from the signal-averaged ECG did best, whereas measurement of ejection fraction and Holter monitoring indices gave less predictive information.

Studies involving electrophysiologic testing do not show clear superiority for the technique. In the study of Marchlinski et al. [75] the presence of a left ventricular aneurysm gave the best predictive information, followed by ejection fraction. Holter monitoring did less well, and electrophysiologic testing was only marginally useful. In the study of Waspe et al. [95] both electrophysiologic testing and ejection fraction provided highly sensitive results, and Holter monitoring did poorly. Two studies compared electrophysiologic testing with the signal-averaged ECG. Breithardt et al. [96, 97] found that electrophysiologic testing and the signal-averaged ECG provided almost identical prognostic information. In the large study of Denniss et al. [51] the signal-averaged ECG again closely matched electrophysiologic testing for predictive ability. However, if the electrophysiologic results were based on using a stimulus strength of two times diastolic threshold, rather than the results with 20 mA stimulation, electrophysiologic testing did much worse.

In summary, the case for using electrophysiologic testing to help determine prognosis after infarction is weak. The reasons are as follows: First, studies to date give conflicting information about the usefulness of the technique, although part of it may be due to methodologic differences. Second, prognostic

Table 37-4
Several studies using alternate techniques to determine risk after infarction

Ref.	No. of pts.	Test and criteria	Percent				Notes
			Sens.	Spec.	PPV	NPV	
31	430	HM; VT	30	92	38	88	
118	430	HM; ≥ 1 PVC/hr	75	56	23	93	
		HM; ≥ 10 PVC/hr	48	78	27	90	
		HM; ≥ 100 PVC/hr	13	94	26	86	
35	766	HM; ≥ 30 PVC/hr	18	90	19	92	a
		HM; VT	24	90	23	91	
		RNV; EF < 30%	42	88	30	92	
36	533	HM + RNV					b
		EF >40%, <10 PVCs/hr	17	39	2	89	
		EF <40%, ≥10 PVCs/hr	24	93	18	96	
41	1640	HM: >0 PVCs/24 hr	92	16			c
		≥10 PVCs/hr	25	88			
		Pairs or VT	34	81			
		Multiform PVCs	62	69			
		≥10 PVCs/hr or pairs or VT or multiform	67	61			
33	1739	HM; R-on-T or pairs or VT or multiform or bigeminy	56	74	5	99	d
34	139	HM + RNV; complex PVCs, age, EF <50%, anterior MI	85	79			
28	55	QTc > 440 msec on 12-lead	57	81	76	65	e
39	750	RNV or cath					
		EF < 30%	20				
		EF < 40%	57				
		EF < 45%	77				
		RNV or cath + HM: EF <45% + PVCs ≥ Lown grade 2	41				
98	165	SAECG; late potential and/or long QRS	92	62			
		RNV or cath; EF < 40%	92	75			
		HM; Lown grade 3–5 PVCs	73	67			

Table 37-4 (continued)

Ref.	No. of pts.	Test and criteria	Percent				Notes
			Sens.	Spec.	PPV	NPV	
43	200	SAECG; late potential only	93	65			
		SAECG; late potential and/or long QRS	50	90	28		
		SAECG + HM: abn. SAECG and complex PVCs	65	89			
		SAECG + RNV or cath; abn. SAECG and EF < 40%	80	89			
119	138	SAECG; late potentials occurring 350–500 msec after QRS	79	80			
99	102	SAECG; late potentials and/or long-duration low-amp. signals and/or long QRS	87	63	29	96	
		RNV; EF < 40%	80	54	24	94	
		HM; ≥ 10 PVCs/hr and/or couplets and/or NSVT	80	42	23	91	
		SAECG + RNV; abn. SAECG + EF < 40%	100	59	36	100	
		SAECG + HM; abn. SAECG + high grade ectopy (as above)	100	45	35	100	
		HM + RNV; high grade ectopy + EF < 40%	92	44	37	94	
		Abn. SAECG + high grade ectopy + EF < 40%	100	53	50	100	
62	58	EPS; VT	80	28			
73	48	EPS; ≥ 2 RVRs	79	86	79	86	
		HM; Lown grade 4B–5	54	88			
74	70	EPS; ≥ 2 RVRs	44	74	20	90	
49	165	EPS; > 10 sec VT/VF	81	83	65	91	
75	46	EPS; ≥ 4 RVRs	17	82	13	86	b
		EPS; ≥ 2 RVRs	67	55	19	91	
		HM; Lown grade 3–4	50	58	16	88	
		RNV or cath or 2-D echo; EF < 40%	83	70	31	96	
		RNV or cath or 2-D echo; presence of LV aneurysm	83	78	38	97	
		EPS + HM; ≥ 4 RVRs and Lown grade 3–4	17	83	13	87	
		EPS + EF deter.; ≥ 4 RVRs + EF < 40%	17	98	50	89	
		HM + EF deter.; Lown grade 3–4 + EF < 40%	33	87	29	89	

Ref	n	Criteria				
104	50	EPS; ≥ 10 RVRs	100	57	13	100
95	50	EPS; > 7 RVRs	100	57		
		RNV or cath; EF < 40%	100	52		
		RNV or cath; LV aneurysm	50	68		
		HM; Lown grade 4B	33	79		
		Patients receiving antiarrhythmic drug	50	75		
		Patients receiving CABG	17	82		
		Patients not treated	17	70		
50	228	EPS; > 10 sec VT/VF	56	82	26	94
		ETT; ≥ 2 mm ST segment depression or elevation	58	70	11	96
		EPS + ETT; both positive	88	65	13	99
94	150	EPS; ≥ 6 RVRs	50	77	6	98
64	45	EPS; sust. VT/VF	67	57	10	96
96,97	132	EPS; ≥ 4 RVRs	77	57	16	96
		SAECG; presence of late potential	77	59	17	96
		EPS + SAECG; ≥ 4 RVRs + late potential	62	77	23	95
51	403	EPS; > 10 sec VT/VF	57	83		
		SAECG; presence of delayed potentials	65	77		
		EPS + SAECG; > 10 sec VT/VF *and* late potentials	39	92		
		EPS + SAECG; > 10 sec VT/VF *or* late potentials	83	68		
87	92	EPS; > 10 sec VT/VF, 2 × DT current *only*	30	91		98[f]
		EPS; ≥ 5 RVRs	50	66		
Range			13–100	16–98	2–79	65–100

[a]Figured for 2-year follow-up.
[b]Figured for 13-month follow-up.
[c]For sudden death only.
[d]One hour of monitoring; figured for 5-year follow-up.
[e]Figured for 10-year follow-up.
[f]Patients had received thrombolytic therapy.

HM = Holter monitoring; VT = ventricular tachycardia; PVC = premature ventricular contractions; RNV = radionuclide ventriculography; EF = ejection fraction; SAECG = signal-averaged electrocardiography; VF = ventricular fibrillation; RVRs = repetitive ventricular responses; EPS = electrophysiologic study; NSVT = nonsustained ventricular tachycardiac; CABG = coronary artery bypass graft; ETT = exercise treadmill test.

information similar to that obtained from electrophysiologic testing is available from other less invasive and less expensive techniques. Finally, when the results of electrophysiologic testing were used to identify patients needing antiarrhythmic therapy, treatment did not substantially improve survival. To determine the prognostic usefulness of electrophysiologic testing after myocardial infarction, a large, prospective study is required in which other tests thought to provide prognostic information are performed on each patient: Holter monitoring, signal-averaged ECG, radionuclide measurement of ejection fraction, and an exercise test. These tests should all be done 2 to 4 weeks after infarction. Test results should *not* alter therapy. The electrophysiologic testing protocol *must* be standardized; whether to use a high stimulus current could be a major issue. Finally, at least a 12-month follow-up is needed. Such a study should allow determination of the most cost-effective and accurate way to determine prognosis in patients after a myocardial infarction.

Summary

Although electrophysiologic testing has been used for several purposes in patients after infarction, its value in this patient population remains unclear. Part of the reason for uncertainty is the lack of well-designed studies, and part is due to the large methodologic differences that exist among investigators. Until the results of more well-designed studies are available, the use of electrophysiologic testing in this patient population should remain investigational.

Editorial Comments

It seems clear from this careful and thorough review that the routine use of electrophysiologic testing to determine prognosis following myocardial infarction is not yet established. Measurement of left ventricular function and the use of the noninvasive signal-averaged ECG may provide similar prognostic information regarding the chance of death from ventricular arrhythmia in patients after myocardial infarction. Moreover, effective therapy is not defined. This area of cardiology is clearly in search of some answers. It is likely that only a large, randomized, prospective study can supply these answers. G.S.F.

References

1. Lie, K. I., Wellens, H. J., Schuilenburg, R. M., et al. Factors influencing prognosis of bundle branch block complicating acute antero-septal infarction: The value of His bundle recordings. *Circulation* 50:935, 1974.
2. Lichstein, E., Gupta, P. K., Chadda, K. D., et al. Findings of prognostic value in patients with incomplete bilateral bundle branch block complicating acute myocardial infarction. *Am. J. Cardiol.* 32:913, 1973.
3. Lichstein, E., Gupta, P. K., and Chadda, K. D. Long-term survival of patients with incomplete bundle-branch block complicating acute myocardial infarction. *Br. Heart J.* 83:924, 1975.
4. Atkins, J. M., Leshin, S. J., Blomqvist, G., and Mullins, C. B. Ventricular conduction blocks and sudden death in acute myocardial infarction: Potential indications for pacing. *N. Engl. J. Med.* 288:281, 1973.
5. Waugh, R. A., Wagner, G. S., Haney, T. L., et al. Immediate and remote prognostic significance of fascicular block during acute myocardial infarction. *Circulation* 47:765, 1973.
6. Ritter, W. S., Atkins, J. M., Blomqvist, C. G., and Mullins, C. B. Permanent pacing in patients with transient trifascicular block during acute myocardial infarction. *Am. J. Cardiol.* 38:205, 1976.
7. Hindman, M. C., Wagner, G. S., Jaro, M., et al. The clinical significance of bundle branch block complicating acute myocardial infarction. 1. Clinical characteristics, hospital mortality, and one-year follow-up. *Circulation* 58:679, 1978.
8. Hindman, M. C., Wagner, G. S., Jaro, M., et al. The clinical significance of bundle branch block complicating acute myocardial infarction. 2. *Circulation* 58:689, 1978.
9. Watson, R. D. S., Glover, D. R., Page, A. J. F., et al. The Birmingham trial of permanent pacing in patients with intraventricular conduction disorders after acute myocardial infarction. *Am. Heart J.* 108:496, 1984.
10. Harper, R., Hunt, D., Vohra, J., et al. His bundle electrogram in patients with acute

myocardial infarction complicated by atrioventricular or intraventricular conduction disturbances. *Br. Heart J.* 37:705, 1975.

11. Pagnoni, F., Finzi, A., Valentini, R., et al. Long-term prognostic significance and electrophysiological evolution of intraventricular conduction disturbances complicating acute myocardial infarction. *PACE* 9:91, 1986.

12. Scheinman, M. M., Peters, R. W., Sauve, M. J., et al. Value of the H-Q interval in patients with bundle branch block and the role of prophylactic permanent pacing. *Am. J. Cardiol.* 50:1316, 1982.

13. Scheinman, M. M., Peters, R. W., Morady, F., et al. Electrophysiologic studies in patients with bundle branch block. *PACE* 6:1157, 1983.

14. Lie, K. I., Liem, K. L., Schuilenburg, R. M., et al. Early identification of patients developing late in-hospital ventricular fibrillation after discharge from the Coronary Care Unit: A 5 1/2 year retrospective and prospective study of 1,897 patients. *Am. J. Cardiol.* 41:674, 1978.

15. Wald, R. W., Waxman, M. B., Corey, P. N., et al. Management of intractable ventricular tachyarrhythmias after myocardial infarction. *Am. J. Cardiol.* 44:329, 1979.

16. DiMarco, J. P., Lerman, B. B., Kron, K. L., and Sellers, T. D. Sustained ventricular tachyarrhythmias within 2 months of acute myocardial infarction: Results of medical and surgical therapy in patients resuscitated from the initial episode. *J. Am. Coll. Cardiol.* 6:759, 1985.

17. Wilson, C., and Adgey, A. A. J. Survival of patients with late ventricular fibrillation after acute myocardial infarction. *Lancet* 2:124, 1974.

18. Goldberg, R., Szklo, M., Tonascia, J., and Kennedy, H. L. Length of time between hospital admission and ventricular fibrillation or cardiac arrest: complicating acute myocardial infarction: Effect on prognosis. *Johns Hopkins Med. J.* 145:187, 1979.

19. Wellens, H. J. J., Bar, F. W., Vanagt, E. J., and Brugada, P. Medical treatment of ventricular tachycardia: Considerations in the selection of patients for surgical treatment. *Am. J. Cardiol.* 49:186, 1982.

20. Marchlinski, F. E., Waxman, H. L., Buxton, A. D., and Josephson, M. E. Sustained ventricular tachyarrhythmias during the early postinfarction period: Electrophysiologic findings and prognosis for survival. *J. Am. Coll. Cardiol.* 2:240, 1983.

21. Kleiman, R. G., Marchlinski, F. E., Buxton, A. E., and Josephson, M. E. Ventricular tachycardia early after infarct (Abstract). *Circulation* 74(Suppl II):11, 1986.

22. Horowitz, L. N., and Morganroth, J. Can we prevent sudden cardiac death? *Am. J. Cardiol.* 50:535, 1982.

23. Rosenthal, M. E., Oseran, D. S., Gang, E., and Peter, T. Sudden cardiac death following acute myocardial infarction. *Am. Heart J.* 109:865, 1985.

24. Kotler, M. N., Tabatznik, B., Mower, M. M., and Tominaga, S. Prognostic significance of ventricular ectopic beats with respect to sudden death in the late postinfarction period. *Circulation* 47:959, 1973.

25. Ruberman, W., Weinblatt, E., Goldberg, J. D., et al. Ventricular premature beats and mortality after myocardial infarction. *N. Engl. J. Med.* 297:750, 1977.

26. Schulze, R. A., Strauss, H. W., and Pitt, B. Sudden death in the year following myocardial infarction: Relation to ventricular premature contractions in the late hospital phase and left ventricular ejection fraction. *Am. J. Med.* 62:192, 1977.

27. Anderson, K. P., DeCamilla, J., and Moss, A. J. Clinical significance of ventricular tachycardia (3 beats or longer) detected during ambulatory monitoring after myocardial infarction. *Circulation* 57:890, 1978.

28. Schwartz, P. J., and Wolf, S. QT interval prolongation as predictor of sudden death in patients with myocardial infarction. *Circulation* 57:1074, 1978.

29. Hammermeister, K. E., DeRouen, T. A., and Dodge, H. T. Variables predictive of survival in patients with coronary artery disease. *Circulation* 59:421, 1979.

30. Moss, A. J., Davis, H. T., DeCamilla, J., and Bayer, L. W. Ventricular ectopic beats and their relation to sudden and nonsudden cardiac death after myocardial infarction. *Circulation* 60:998, 1979.

31. Bigger, J. T., Weld, F. M., and Rolnitzky, L. M. Prevalence, characteristics and significance of ventricular tachycardia (three or more complexes) detected with ambulatory electrocardiographic recording in the late hospital phase of acute myocardial infarction. *Am. J. Cardiol.* 48:815, 1981.

32. Ruberman, W., Weinblatt, E., Frank, C. W., et al. Repeated 1 hour electrocardiographic monitoring of survivors of myocardial infarction at 6 month intervals: Arrhythmia detection and relation to prognosis. *Am. J. Cardiol.* 47:1197, 1981.

33. Ruberman, W., Weinblatt, E., Goldberg, J. D., et al. Ventricular premature complexes and sudden death after myocardial infarction. *Circulation* 64:297, 1981.

34. Rapaport, E., and Remedios, P. The high risk patient and recovery from myocardial infarction: Recognition and management. *J. Am. Coll. Cardiol.* 1:391, 1983.

35. Bigger, J. T., Fleiss, J. L., Kleiger, R., et al. The relationships among ventricular arrhyth-

mias, left ventricular dysfunction, and mortality in the 2 years after myocardial infarction. *Circulation* 69:250, 1984.

36. Mukharji, J., Rude, R. E., Poole, W. K., et al. Risk factors for sudden death after acute myocardial infarction: Two-year follow-up. *Am. J. Cardiol.* 54:31, 1984.

37. Olson, H. G., Lyons, K. P., Troop, P., et al. Prognostic implications of complicated ventricular arrhythmias early after hospital discharge in acute myocardial infarction: A serial ambulatory electrocardiography study. *Am. Heart J.* 108:1221, 1984.

38. Luria, M. H., Debanne, S. M., and Osman, M. I. Long-term follow-up after recovery from acute myocardial infarction: Observations on survival, ventricular arrhythmias, and sudden death. *Arch. Intern. Med.* 145:1592, 1985.

39. Ahnve, S., Gilpin, E., Henning, H., et al. Limitations and advantages of the ejection fraction for defining high risk after acute myocardial infarction. *Am. J. Cardiol.* 58:872, 1986.

40. Bigger, J. T., Fleiss, J. L., Rolnitzky, L. M., et al. Prevalence, characteristics and significance of ventricular tachycardia detected by 24-hour continuous electrocardiographic recordings in the late hospital phase of acute myocardial infarction. *Am. J. Cardiol.* 58:1151, 1986.

41. Kostis, J. B., Byington, R., Friedman, L. M., et al. Prognostic significance of ventricular ectopic activity in survivors of acute myocardial infarction. *J. Am. Coll. Cardiol.* 10:231, 1987.

42. Moss, A. J., DeCamilla, J., Mietlowski, W., et al. Prognostic grading and significance of ventricular premature beats after recovery from myocardial infarction. *Circulation* 51/52(Suppl III):204, 1975.

43. Kuchar, D. L., Thorburn, C. W., and Sammel, N. L. Prediction of serious arrhythmic events after myocardial infarction: Signal-averaged ECG, Holter monitoring and radionuclide ventriculography. *J. Am. Coll. Cardiol.* 10:531, 1987.

44. Furberg, C. D., and Yusuf, S. Effect of drug therapy on survival in chronic congestive heart failure. *Am. J. Cardiol.* 62:41A, 1988.

45. Furberg, C. D. Effect of antiarrhythmic drugs on mortality after myocardial infarction. *Am. J. Cardiol.* 52:32C, 1983.

46. IMPACT Research Group. International mexilitine and placebo antiarrhythmic coronary trial. I. Report on arrhythmia and other findings. *J. Am. Coll. Cardiol.* 4:1148, 1984.

47. Gottlieb, S. H., Achuff, S. C., Mellits, E. D., et al. Prophylactic antiarrhythmic therapy of high-risk survivors of myocardial infarction: Lower mortality at 1 month but not at 1 year. *Circulation* 75:792, 1987.

48. Cardiac Arrhythmia Pilot Study Investigators. Effects of encainide, flecainide, imipramine, and moricizine on ventricular arrhythmias during the year after acute myocardial infarction: The CAPS. *Am. J. Cardiol.* 61:501, 1988.

49. Richards, D. A., Cody, D. V., Denniss, A. R., et al. Ventricular electrical instability: A predictor of death after myocardial infarction. *Am. J. Cardiol.* 51:75, 1983.

50. Denniss, A. R., Baaijens, H., Cody, D. V., et al. Value of programmed stimulation and exercise testing in predicting one-year mortality after acute myocardial infarction. *Am. J. Cardiol.* 56:213, 1985.

51. Denniss, A. R., Richards, D. A., Cody, D. V., et al. Prognostic significance of ventricular tachycardia and fibrillation induced at programmed stimulation and delayed potentials detected on the signal-averaged electrocardiograms of survivors of acute myocardial infarction. *Circulation* 74:731, 1986.

52. Bhandari, A., Rose, J., Au, P., and Rahimtoola, S. H. Long-term reproducibility of the stimulus induced ventricular arrhythmia during pre-hospital discharge phase of acute myocardial infarction (Abstract). *Circulation* 72(Suppl III):360, 1985.

53. Costard, A., Schluter, M., and Geiger, M. Inducibility of ventricular arrhythmias after acute myocardial infarction: Influence of time on stimulation results and prognostic significance (Abstract). *Circulation* 72(Suppl III):477, 1985.

54. Klein, H., Trappe, H. J., Hartwig, C. A., et al. Repeated programmed stimulation within the first year after myocardial infarction (Abstract). *Circulation* 72(Suppl III):359, 1985.

55. Aonuma, K., Iesaka, Y., Ri, K., et al. Time dependent response to ventricular programmed stimulation in post acute myocardial infarction patients (Abstract). *Circulation* 74(Suppl II):189, 1986.

56. Kuck, K. H., Costard, A., Schluter, M., and Kunze, K. P. Significance of timing programmed electrical stimulation after acute myocardial infarction. *J. Am. Coll. Cardiol.* 8:1279, 1986.

57. Roy, D., Marchand, E., Theroux, P., et al. Long-term reproducibility and significance of provokable ventricular arrhythmias after myocardial infarction. *J. Am. Coll. Cardiol.* 8:32, 1986.

58. Bhandari, A. K., Au, P. K., Rose, J. S., et al. Decline in inducibility of sustained ventricular tachycardia from two to twenty weeks after acute myocardial infarction. *Am. J. Cardiol.* 59:284, 1987.

59. McPherson, C. A., Rosenfeld, L. E., and Batsford, W. P. Day-to-day reproducibility of responses to right ventricular programmed

electrical stimulation: Implications for serial drug testing. *Am. J. Cardiol.* 55:689, 1985.

60. Lombardi, F., Stein, J., Podrid, P. J., et al. Daily reproducibility of electrophysiologic test results in malignant ventricular arrhythmias. *Am. J. Cardiol.* 57:96, 1986.

61. Somberg, J. C., Butler, B., Torres, V., et al. Lorcainide therapy for the high-risk patient post myocardial infarction. *Am. J. Cardiol.* 54:34B, 1984.

62. Kron, J., Li, C., Broudy, D., et al. Lack of prognostic value of programmed electrical stimulation in patients with recent myocardial infarction or unstable angina (Abstract). *J. Am. Coll. Cardiol.* 5:471, 1985.

63. Somberg, J. C., Butler, B., Torres, V., et al. Therapy for late post infarction ventricular tachycardia. *Angiology* 36:181, 1985.

64. Bhandari, A. K., Rose, J. S., Kotlewski, A., et al. Frequency and significance of induced sustained ventricular tachycardia or fibrillation two weeks after acute myocardial infarction. *Am. J. Cardiol.* 56:737, 1985.

65. Mann, D. E., Luck, J. C., Griffin, J. C., et al. Induction of clinical ventricular tachycardia using programmed stimulation: Value of third and fourth extrastimuli. *Am. J. Cardiol.* 52:501, 1983.

66. Brugada, P., Green, M., Abdollah, H., and Wellens, H. J. J. Significance of ventricular arrhythmias initiated by programmed stimulation: The importance of the type of ventricular arrhythmia induced and the number of premature stimuli required. *Circulation* 69:87, 1984.

67. Buxton, A. E., Waxman, H. L., Marchlinski, F. E., et al. Role of triple extrastimuli during electrophysiologic study of patients with documented sustained ventricular tachyarrhythmias. *Circulation* 69:532, 1984.

68. Denniss, A. R., Ross, D. L., Cody, D. V., et al. Randomized trial of antiarrhythmic drugs in patients with inducible ventricular tachyarrhythmias after recent myocardial infarction (Abstract). *Circulation* 74(Suppl II):213, 1986.

69. Herre, J. M., Mann, D. E., Luck, J. C., et al. Effect of increased current, multiple pacing sites and number of extrastimuli on induction of ventricular tachycardia. *Am. J. Cardiol.* 57:102, 1986.

70. Morady, F., DiCarlo, L. A., Liem, L. B., et al. Effects of high stimulation current on the induction of ventricular tachycardia. *Am. J. Cardiol.* 56:73, 1985.

71. Kennedy, E. E., Rosenfeld, L. E., McPherson, C. A., et al. Mechanisms and relevance of arrhythmias induced by high-current programmed ventricular stimulation. *Am. J. Cardiol.* 57:598, 1986.

72. Weissberg, P. L., Broughton, A., Harper, R. W., et al. Induction of ventricular arrhythmias by programmed ventricular stimulation: A prospective study on the effects of stimulation current on arrhythmia induction. *Br. Heart J.* 58:489, 1987.

73. Greene, H. L., Reid, P. R., and Schaeffer, A. H. The repetitive ventricular response in man: A predictor of sudden death. *N. Engl. J. Med.* 299:729, 1978.

74. Hamer, A., Vohra, J., Hunt, D., and Sloman, G. Prediction of sudden death by electrophysiologic studies in high risk patients surviving acute myocardial infarction. *Am. J. Cardiol.* 50:223, 1982.

75. Marchlinski, F. E., Buxton, A. D., Waxman, H. L., and Josephson, M. E. Identifying patients at risk of sudden death after myocardial infarction: Value of the response to programmed stimulation, degree of ventricular ectopic activity and severity of left ventricular dysfunction. *Am. J. Cardiol.* 52:1190, 1983.

76. Mason, J. W. Repetitive beating after single ventricular extrastimuli: Incidence and prognostic significance in patients with recurrent ventricular tachycardia. *Am. J. Cardiol.* 45:1126, 1980.

77. Akhtar, M. The clinical significance of the repetitive ventricular response (Editorial). *Circulation* 63:773, 1981.

78. Ruskin, J. N., DiMarco, J. P., and Garan, H. Repetitive responses to single ventricular extrastimuli in patients with serious ventricular arrhythmias: Incidence and clinical significance. *Circulation* 63:767, 1981.

79. Horowitz, L. N., and Morganroth, J. Can we prevent sudden cardiac death? *Am. J. Cardiol.* 50:535, 1982.

80. Roy, D., Brugada, P., Bar, F. W. H. M., and Wellens, H. J. J. Repetitive responses to ventricular extrastimuli: Incidence and significance in patients without organic heart disease. *Eur. Heart J.* 4:79, 1983.

81. Brugada, P., Waldecker, B., Kersschot, Y., et al. Ventricular arrhythmias initiated by programmed stimulation in four groups of patients with healed myocardial infarction. *J. Am. Coll. Cardiol.* 8:1035, 1986.

82. Kersschot, I. E., Brugada, P., Ramentol, M., et al. Effects of early reperfusion in acute myocardial infarction on arrhythmias induced by programmed stimulation: A prospective, randomized study. *J. Am. Coll. Cardiol.* 7:1234, 1986.

83. Bhandari, A., Hong, R., Au, P., et al. Prognostic significance of programmed ventricular stimulation in patients at "low-risk" two weeks after acute myocardial infarction (Abstract). *J. Am. Coll. Cardiol.* 9:107A, 1987.

84. Grigg, L. E., Chan, W., Hamer, A., et al. Cor-

relation between electrophysiological studies. Holter recordings, and signal-averaged ECGs in the postinfarction period (Abstract). *Circulation* 76(Suppl IV):32, 1987.

85. Zehender, M., Brugada, P., Geibel, A., et al. Programmed electrical stimulation in healed myocardial infarction using a standardized ventricular stimulation protocol. *Am. J. Cardiol.* 59:578, 1987.

86. Pumphrey, C. W., Skehan, J. D., and Rothman, M. T. Responses to ventricular extrastimuli following myocardial infarction are independent of ventricular function and can be modified by therapy (Abstract). *Circulation* 70(Suppl II):401, 1984.

87. McComb, J. M., Gold, H. K., Leinbach, R. C., et al. Electrically induced ventricular arrhythmias in acute myocardial infarction treated with thrombolytic agents. *Am. J. Cardiol.* 62:186, 1988.

88. Moss, A. J., DeCamilla, J., Chilton, J., and Davis, H. T. The chronology and suddenness of cardiac death after myocardial infarction. *Ann. N.Y. Acad. Sci.* 382:465, 1982.

89. Moss, A. J., DeCamilla, J., and Davis, H. Cardiac death in the first 6 months after myocardial infarction: Potential for mortality reduction in the early posthospital period. *Am. J. Cardiol.* 39:816, 1977.

90. Anderson, K. P., and Mason, J. W. Surgical management of ventricular tachyarrhythmias. *Clin. Cardiol.* 6:415, 1983.

91. Garan, H., Ruskin, J. N., DiMarco, J. P., et al. Electrophysiologic studies before and after myocardial revascularization in patients with life-threatening ventricular arrhythmias. *Am. J. Cardiol.* 51:519, 1983.

92. Horowitz, L. N., Harken, A. H., Josephson, M. E., and Kastor, J. A. Surgical treatment of ventricular arrhythmias in coronary artery disease. *Ann. Intern. Med.* 95:88, 1981.

93. Boineau, J. P., and Cox, J. L. Rationale for a direct surgical approach to control ventricular arrhythmias. *Am. J. Cardiol.* 49:381, 1982.

94. Roy, D., Marchand, E., Theroux, P., et al. Programmed ventricular stimulation in survivors of an acute myocardial infarction. *Circulation* 72:487, 1985.

95. Waspe, L. E., Seinfeld, D., Ferrick, A., et al. Prediction of sudden death and spontaneous ventricular tachycardia in survivors of complicated myocardial infarction: Value of the response to programmed stimulation using a maximum of three ventricular extrastimuli. *J. Am. Coll. Cardiol.* 5:1292, 1985.

96. Breithardt, G., Borggrefe, M., and Haerten, K. Role of programmed ventricular stimulation and noninvasive recording of ventricular late potentials for identification of patients at risk of ventricular tachyarrhythmias after acute myocardial infarction. In *Cardiac Electrophysiology and Arrhythmias*. Orlando: Grune & Stratton, 1985. Pp. 553–561.

97. Breithardt, G., Borggrefe, M., and Haerten, K. Ventricular late potentials and inducible ventricular tachyarrhythmias as a marker for ventricular tachycardia and myocardial infarction. *Eur. Heart J.* 7(Suppl A):127, 1986.

98. Kuchar, D. L., Thorburn, C. W., and Sammel, N. L. Late potentials detected after myocardial infarction: Natural history and prognostic significance. *Circulation* 74:1280, 1986.

99. Gomes, J. A., Winters, S. L., Stewart, D., et al. A new noninvasive index to predict sustained ventricular tachycardia and sudden death in the first year after myocardial infarction: Based on signal-averaged electrocardiogram, radionuclide ejection fraction and Holter monitoring. *J. Am. Coll. Cardiol.* 10:349, 1987.

100. Richards, D. A., Cody, D. V., Denniss, A. R., et al. Ventricular electrical instability during the first year following myocardial infarction (Abstract). *Am. J. Cardiol.* 49:929, 1982.

101. Holley, L. K., Denniss, A. R., Cody, D. V., et al. Comparison of clinical significance of programmed stimulation induced ventricular tachycardia and fibrillation in survivors of acute myocardial infarction (Abstract). *PACE* 6:73, 1983.

102. Marchlinski, F. E., Waxman, H. L., Buxton, A. D., and Josephson, M. E. Predictive value of programmed stimulation in determining electrical instability after myocardial infarction (Abstract). *PACE* 6:73, 1983.

103. Kowey, P. R., Friehling, T., Meister, S. G., and Engel, T. R. Late induction of tachycardia in patients with ventricular fibrillation associated with acute myocardial infarction. *J. Am. Coll. Cardiol.* 3:690, 1984.

104. Santarelli, P., Bellocci, F., Loperfido, F., et al. Ventricular arrhythmia induced by programmed ventricular stimulation after acute myocardial infarction. *Am. J. Cardiol.* 55:391, 1985.

105. Santarelli, P., Bellocci, F., Loperfido, F., et al. Ventricular electrical instability in acute myocardial infarction: Clinical, angiographic and electrophysiologic correlations (Abstract). *Circulation* 68(Suppl III):108, 1983.

106. Marchand, E., Roy, D., Theroux, P., et al. Induction of ventricular arrhythmias after myocardial infarction: Relation to other determinants of prognosis (Abstract). *Circulation* 70(Suppl II):19, 1984.

107. Roy, D., Marchand, E., Theroux, P., et al. Reproducibility and significance of ventricular arrhythmias induced after an acute myocardial infarction (Abstract). *Circulation* 70(Suppl II):18, 1984.

108. Bhandari, A., Rose, F., Kotlewski, A., et al. Programmed ventricular stimulation two

weeks after acute myocardial infarction (Abstract). *J. Am. Coll. Cardiol.* 5:471, 1985.

109. Haerten, K., Borggrefe, M., and Breithardt, G. Repetitive ventricular response and late potentials in patients early after myocardial infarction (Abstract). *Circulation* 68(Suppl III):174, 1983.

110. Breithardt, G., Borggrefe, M., and Haerten, K. Programmed ventricular stimulation and recording of late potentials for risk stratification after myocardial infarction (Abstract). *Circulation* 70(Suppl II):19, 1984.

111. Borggrefe, M., Haerten, K., and Breithardt, G. Electrophysiological characteristics of stimulus-induced ventricular tachycardia after myocardial infarction (Abstract). *J. Am. Coll. Cardiol.* 5:471, 1985.

112. Denniss, A. R., Richards, D. A., Cody, D. V., et al. Comparable prognostic significance of delayed potentials and inducible ventricular tachycardia after myocardial infarction (Abstract). *Circulation* 72(Suppl III):359, 1985.

113. Denniss, A. R., Ross, D. L., Cody, D. V., et al. Randomized trial of antiarrhythmic drugs in patients with inducible ventricular tachyarrhythmias after recent myocardial infarction (Abstract). *Circulation* 74(Suppl II):213, 1986.

114. Gonzalez, R., Arriagada, D., Corbalan, R., et al. Programmed electrical stimulation of the heart does not help to identify patients at high risk post myocardial infarction (Abstract). *Circulation* 70(Suppl II):19, 1984.

115. Iesaka, Y., Anuma, K., Nogami, A., et al. Prognostic significance of induced ventricular tachycardia, Holter monitor grade and ejection fraction in recent myocardial infarction patients (Abstract). *Circulation* 76(Suppl IV):33, 1987.

116. Treese, N., Pop, T., Erbel, R., et al. Outcome of primary coronary recanalization and arrhythmia profile in survivors of acute myocardial infarction. *Int. J. Cardiol.* 15:19, 1987.

117. Moses, J. W., Tamari, I., Friedman, C., et al. Arrhythmogenic effects of procainamide in high risk patients after myocardial infarction (Abstract). *Clin. Res.* 32:678A, 1984.

118. Bigger, J. T., Weld, F. M., and Rolnitzky, L. M. Which postinfarction ventricular arrhythmias should be treated? *Am. Heart J.* 103:660, 1982.

119. Potratz, J., Mentzel, H., Djonlagic, H., and Diederich, K. The significance of late potentials in the acute and chronic infarction period (Abstract). *Circulation* 74(Suppl II):470, 1986.

38
Prognosis of Acute Myocardial Infarction

Hartmut Henning

Since 1968 there has been a decline in the mortality from cardiovascular disease and especially coronary artery disease. These declining mortality trends have been confirmed over the subsequent two decades and have been observed in all age groups, in both sexes, and in the major race groups [1, 2]. Data indicate that there has been a more than 25 percent decrease in the overall age-adjusted death rate from coronary heart disease. The causes for this impressive decline in the death rates from coronary artery disease are not unique to the North American continent but are seen as well in other countries including Australia, South America, Europe, and Japan. It remains uncertain whether the decline in coronary artery disease death rates is the result of a decreased incidence of acute myocardial infarction and sudden death or the result of changes in survival in patients with coronary heart disease [3]. Other causes for the decline in coronary heart disease mortality include the development of acute coronary care, noninvasive diagnostic methods for early detection of myocardial infarction, new treatment modalities with drugs as well as coronary artery bypass graft surgery, and lastly the identification and modification of specific cardiovascular risk factors.

The decrease in the incidence rates of coronary artery disease and the associated decrease in mortality could be attributed to changes in prevalence and severity of the major coronary risk factors. However, with an unchanged incidence in coronary heart disease and an associated decline in coronary heart disease death, the progressive decrease in mortality could be related to effects from secondary preventive efforts. It appears that both primary prevention through life style changes and improved treatment regimens have played a role in the decline in mortality in patients with acute myocardial infarction.

With the introduction of prehospital care and greater access and use of emergency medical services, the out-of-hospital death rate in patients with acute myocardial infarction has been reduced. Prior to the development of the coronary care unit (CCU), early mortality after acute myocardial infarction had been approximated at 30 percent. Treatment in the CCU has reduced in-hospital mortality to 10 to 18 percent [4–18]. A further reduction in early mortality to approximately 12 percent has been accomplished with the use of anti-ischemic therapy early in the course of acute myocardial infarction. An approximately 8 percent further reduction has been observed in early and late mortality in acute infarct patients who undergo thrombolysis and invasive reperfusion therapy [19, 20]. However, mortality following discharge from hospital after recovery from acute myocardial infarction remains high, with an approximately 10 percent mortality within the first year after myocardial infarction. Most of these deaths occur within the first 6 months after discharge owing to sudden death, recurrent myocardial infarction, and congestive heart failure [4–6]. A large proportion of cardiac deaths within the first 6 months is due to sudden arrhythmic death. The death rates decline during the second half of the first year after myocardial infarction, further decline to 5 percent during

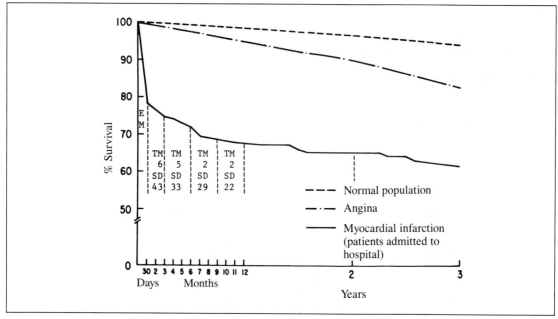

Fig. 38-1
Actuarial survival curve for patients with myocardial infarction (*solid line*). The survival rates of an age- and sex-matched normal population (*dashed line*) and patients with angina pectoris (*dashed/dotted line*) are shown for comparison. The survival rates in the normal population and angina population were significantly higher at 1, 2, and 3 years [7]. EM = early (30-day) mortality; TM = total mortality (%) for time interval; SD = sudden death (% of total mortality) for time intervals during the first year after acute myocardial infarction.

the second year, and subsequently approach 3 to 4 percent annual mortality in the years thereafter [4, 7] (Fig. 38-1).

Prognosis of Myocardial Infarction

The short-term and long-term survival after acute myocardial infarction depends on certain patient characteristics that signify independent risk for morbidity and mortality early and late after acute myocardial infarction. The reported variables that predict high risk after acute myocardial infarction have varied largely because of differences in study design that examined historical and objective information [4–13].

Studies on prognostication and stratification of postinfarction patients have used different patient selection criteria, commonly introducing an age limit to 60 or 65 years or restriction to a specific population criterion that may in-

clude the capability of early postinfarction exercise testing [21] or the availability of rest and exercise perfusion imaging [22]. The eligibility for predischarge exercise stress testing has been shown to define an already lower risk group, as these patients are free of complications that may indicate poor prognosis, such as postinfarction angina, congestive heart failure, or complex ventricular arrhythmias during the postinfarction period. Thus in one study the 1-year mortality in patients who did not undergo exercise testing was 14 percent compared to only a 5 percent mortality in patients who were able to undergo exercise testing [21].

Another factor that may influence the variables and the importance of these variables for prediction of mortality and survival is the era in which the study has been carried out. During the 1950s characteristics from the history and the electrocardiographic, radiographic, and laboratory examinations were available;

during the 1970s more objective parameters were included to define high risk and low risk after myocardial infarction with hemodynamic measurements, accurate assessment of the extent of ischemia by myocardial perfusion imaging, and estimation of left ventricular function by radionuclide angiography or contrast ventriculography. The development of quantitative techniques to accurately determine the extent of continuing myocardial ischemia, the severity of ventricular arrhythmias, and impairment of left ventricular function has provided a better definition of high risk patients and established risk stratification schemes for patients after myocardial infarction. Similarly, early and late mortality after acute myocardial infarction may have been altered by the changing treatment modalities that have become available through the past decades. They have included prophylactic aspirin [23] and beta blockers [24–26], early coronary artery bypass graft surgery [27, 28], and more recently thrombolytic therapy [19, 20]. Such treatment during the acute phase, convalescent phase, and postdischarge period has been shown to improve subsequent morbidity and mortality and is to be taken into account when natural history and outcome are examined in postinfarction patients.

Prognostic variables may vary in terms of their significance of predicting death and survival depending on the timing of the start of the follow-up period after acute infarction. Variables examined at the time of admission with acute myocardial infarction may be a significant predictor for in-hospital mortality but may not predict 1-year or long-term mortality [7]. The mortality rates are highest during the first two 3-month intervals after hospital discharge, and therefore studies showing lower mortality rates may be the result of late enrollment rather than specific therapy. Studies following patients 2 to 10 years after acute myocardial infarction have shown that most deaths occur within the first several months and differing mechanisms of mortality have been implied [4, 7–13]. Beyond the first year after acute infarction, the mortality rate stays relatively constant at about 3 to 5 percent a year, and from there on it may not differ from

mortality rates reported for chronic stable angina pectoris [7]. Certain variables obtained at the time of admission or hospital discharge may be predictive of short-term mortality within 1 month after acute myocardial infarction (AMI) but not beyond this time. Objective patient characteristics obtained at the time of discharge similarly may predict outcome during the first year after AMI but not during the subsequent long-term follow-up period. Complications of recurrent angina pectoris, recurrent myocardial infarction, or need for coronary artery bypass graft surgery are predictive from data obtained at the time of hospital discharge but not from data obtained at the time of admission with acute myocardial infarction [18, 29–38].

The difference in the identification of risk variables after myocardial infarction has also been attributed to the method of statistical analysis applied to the data obtained during the early and late phases after myocardial infarction. More sophisticated statistical techniques have been utilized for risk factor assessment following AMI. Multivariate analytic techniques can define the significant factors that identify death and survivors with high accuracy and correctly classify death in a studied infarct population [7, 39–45]. These methods determine the importance and independence of predictor variables and have been validated in subsequent test populations. The recognition of the similarity of basic characteristics in infarct populations in different institutions and different countries and mortality trends during the time periods after infarction as well as validation of prognostication schemes have provided a means of reliably identifying high risk and low risk patients for decision-making on treatment.

Early Mortality After Acute Myocardial Infarction

Early mortality rates after acute myocardial infarction have shown a wide variability for the early prognosis following acute myocardial infarction. Table 38-1 shows the in-hospi-

Table 38-1
Studies on early mortality after acute myocardial infarction

First author	Study period	Population size	Early mortality rate (%)
Juergens [8]	1935–1951	279	15.8
Honey [9]	1940–1954	543	32.2
Zukel [46]	1943–1944	1090	17.0
Hughes [47]	1953–1960	445	32.8
Pell [10]	1956–1961	1331	30.0
Day [14]	1962–1964	126	15.9
Mosbech [48]	1963	1094	41.0
Norris [11]	1966–1967	757	26.0
Peterson [16]	1966–1969	6955	29.5
Henning [7]	1969–1973	221	21.0
	1973–1976	150	18.0
Gillum [18]	1970	3842	16.7
	1980	3736	11.9
Wolffenbuttel [49]	1977	132	12.1

tal mortality rates from selected studies showing a range from 12 to 41 percent. Studies on mortality and risk stratification have often included different periods after the onset of acute symptoms, including the first day after admission [43] and the hospital period [39], intervals ranging from 2 to 20 days; in other studies early mortality is defined as a death within 30 days after AMI [7]. These defined intervals are the result of an observed mortality pattern in the study population. Early mortality rates and in-hospital mortality during the 1950s and 1960s were high (approximately 28 percent). An improving short-term prognosis has been observed in study populations of different intervals in the same institution showing an early mortality rate of 29 percent in 1967 compared with mortality of 22.4 percent in patients hospitalized in 1971 [50]. In later studies during the 1970s and 1980s, the in-hospital mortality ranged from 9 to 21 percent [7, 17, 18, 49].

Goldberg et al. found a decreasing in-hospital and long-term mortality over consecutive study periods in the Worcester Heart Attack Study [51]. The age-adjusted in-hospital mortality declined by 32 percent over the 10-year period between 1975 (22.2 percent) and 1984 (15.1 percent). A decline of 37 percent was seen in the patients with first myocardial infarction, and a decline of 26 percent was reported for patients with recurrent AMI between 1975 and 1984. Similarly, declining

mortality rates may be related to changes in the extent and severity of AMI. In some studies, an increase in non-Q-wave myocardial infarction has been observed which has a low early mortality as compared with Q-wave infarction [52, 53]. A decrease in the extent of myocardial damage in the acute infarction phase as determined by peak creatinine phosphokinase levels has also been observed when study periods of 1975, 1978, and 1981 were compared. It appears that in-hospital mortality from AMI has declined over time from 24 percent in 1970 to 18 percent in 1977 and 14 percent in 1984.

Long-Term Survival After AMI

The long-term survival rates in patients with AMI discharged from hospital are shown in Table 38-2, demonstrating the highest risk for death within the first year. The 1-year mortality for discharged patients varies between 10 and 15 percent with subsequent annual mortality rates between 4 and 6 percent. Longitudinal studies of cardiac mortality after myocardial infarction have found an exponential fall in mortality for the 6- and 8-month periods after myocardial infarction [4, 57]. In our study of a population of 2290 patients from three geographically different populations, it was observed that 50 percent of all deaths dur-

Table 38-2
Long-term survival rates after acute myocardial infarction

First author	Study period	Population size	Survival rates at follow-up points				
			1 yr	2 yr	3 yr	5 yr	10 yr
Juergens [8]	1935–1951	224	—	—	68.8	55.4	29.2
		1030	—	—	—	59.0	39.0
Beard [55]	1950–1952	427	—	—	—	69.0	44.0
Pell [10]	1956–1961	932	90.5	86.8	81.8	74.0	—
Kjoller [37]	1966–1969	644	84.9	—	67.0	—	—
Goldberg [50]	1966–1967	334	85.0	79.0	—	64.0	—
Martin [56]	1970–1971	666	87.7	80.0	73.6	60.8	—
Luria [34]	1970–1973	143	—	76.9	—	60.1	—
Henning [7]	1969–1973	224	68.5	—	61.0	—	—

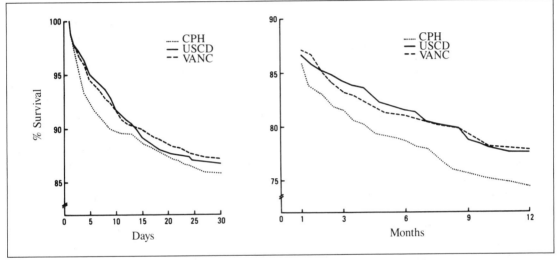

Fig. 38-2
Survival curves for patients with acute myocardial infarction from three
institutions. *Left.* Percent of patients alive at the end of day 1 after admission
with acute myocardial infarction through day 30. *Right.* Percent survival from the
end of 1 month through 12 months. The curves are extensions of those in the left
panel on a different time scale. CPH = Cophenhagen, Denmark; UCSD =
University of California (San Diego); VANC = Vancouver, British Columbia,
Canada.

ing the first year had occurred by day 19 and
70 percent of all deaths by day 100 [4] (Fig. 38-
2). The cardiac mortality between day 2 and 3
weeks was 11.4 percent and for the remainder
of the year 10.5 percent. We found that separate exponential curves best delineate the survival distributions up to 3 weeks and for the
remainder of the first year after myocardial infarction.

Several studies have examined the changes
of long-term mortality in hospital survivors of

AMI to assess improvement over time in the
long-term prognosis of AMI [17, 50, 58]. Studies on hospital survivors of AMI have failed to
observe an improvement in the long-term survival over time, with no differences between
first or recurrent MI [17, 50]. However, after introduction of thrombolytic agents, both
short-term and long-term survival appear to
be improved [19, 20], but these therapeutic
advances require further documentation of
changes in the long-term survival patterns.

Risk factor assessment and prognostication begins at the time of admission with AMI. Data from the patient's history, physical examination, electrocardiogram, chest radiograph, and laboratory examinations, including serum enzyme determinations, are available. During the patient's stay in the CCU, further clinical information becomes available. Clinical data obtained during the patient's stay in the CCU and from the hospital predischarge evaluation by special studies such as exercise testing, radionuclide left ventriculography, 24-hour ambulatory electrocardiographic recording, and coronary angiography are available to derive prognostic information.

Prognostic Indicators for Mortality and Survival

Certain patient characteristics indicate an increased risk for cardiac death and sudden cardiac death during the in-hospital phase and postdischarge phase after AMI. The major risk indicators are related to the reduction in left ventricular performance, ongoing myocardial ischemia, and ventricular arrhythmias after AMI. Many investigations during the past decades have identified many simple independent risk factors for mortality and morbidity. There have been multiple studies on the relation of prognosis to historical and clinical factors prior to the availability of invasive hemodynamic monitoring and techniques of left ventricular function measurement. The historical factors such as age, sex, previous myocardial infarction, previous congestive heart failure, previous angina, and chronic obstructive pulmonary disease have carried a twofold or more mortality compared with infarct patients without the abnormal variable [4, 7–9, 11, 59–61]. The clinical factors and the standard laboratory examinations are often an indirect indication of the extent of myocardial damage and the resulting impairment of myocardial function. Data from the physical examination include heart rate, systolic blood pressure, respiratory rate, temperature, ventricular third heart sound gallop rhythm, bilat-

eral pulmonary rales, and peripheral edema; and these abnormalities contribute to early and late outcome after AMI [4, 7, 9–11, 29, 42, 62, 63]. The initial chest radiograph provides information on cardiac enlargement and the presence and severity of congestive heart failure [64]. Composites of clinical findings relate to left ventricular function and severity of congestive heart failure as devised by Killip and Kimball [65]. Twenty to thirty percent of patients present on admission to the CCU without signs of left ventricular congestive heart failure and have a low 1-month mortality; 40 to 60 percent of patients on admission exhibit mild to moderate left ventricular failure, which carries a twofold mortality (approximately 15 percent) compared with patients who do not show signs of left ventricular failure [7, 65]. A fivefold early mortality is associated with the presence of pulmonary edema and a tenfold early mortality with the presence of cardiogenic shock at the time of admission [7]. Congestive heart failure in AMI has been identified in most prognostication studies as the most important clinical variable [7, 8, 11, 43, 66, 67] even in the presence of quantitative indicators of mechanical or ischemic dysfunction. Clinical and radiologic abnormalities of congestive heart failure have been heavily weighed in composite prognostic schemes [11, 60]. Thus the clinical prognostic indices of Norris and Peel selected congestive heart failure as the most important variable. The Multicenter Postinfarction Research Group reported four independent risk predictors of mortality that ranked the presence of bilateral pulmonary rales above left ventricular ejection fraction, ventricular ectopic depolarization activity, and advanced New York Heart Association (NYHA) functional class before infarction [67].

Other historical and demographic factors are associated with a poor prognosis and have included the female gender [68], a history of diabetes mellitus [69], and prior angina pectoris [70]. Diabetes mellitus affects the risk after an AMI for both early and late mortality [69]. The in-hospital mortality among diabetic patients has been reported to be 30 percent compared with less than 20 percent for non-diabetic patients. Similarly, 1-year mortality after hospital discharge is increased at 20 to 30 percent compared with 8 to 15 percent in non-diabetic patients. The exact mechanism contributing to increased early and late mortality in diabetic patients remains unclear but may possibly be related to more extensive myocardial infarctions, more previous infarctions, and the greater prevalence of heart failure in diabetic infarct patients. Isolated elevation of systolic blood pressure and combined systolic and diastolic hypertension appear to have prognostic indication [71]. Studies on the influence of obesity on early and late prognosis after AMI show that obese patients with a body mass index over 30 have a similar mortality rate of 13 percent when compared with a 14 percent hospital mortality in normal-weight patients [72]. Obese patients over age 65 showed a mortality of 30 percent compared with a 17 percent mortality in patients over 65 years with normal weight. Excessive early mortality was strongly influenced by obesity in older patients, but the obesity appears to have no significant influence on 1-year outcome or on early prognosis in patients younger than age 65.

Laboratory data such as white blood cell count, blood urea nitrogen, serum creatinine, uric acid, and serum enzymes (CK, AST, LDH) have been reported as independent risk predictors for early and late mortality. The electrocardiogram demonstrates multiple indicators of poor prognosis [74, 75]. There is a greater mortality after anterior wall infarction than after inferior infarction even when corrected for infarct size [76, 77]. Further prognostic information can be derived from the QRS duration, the QT interval, the QRS score of electrocardiographic infarct size, ST segment changes, conduction defects, atrial and ventricular arrhythmias, and sinus tachycardia. Early and late prognosis is worsened by the persistence of advanced heart block, new bifascicular or trifascicular block, and preexisting left bundle branch block. The persistence of ischemic ST segment depression on serial electrocardiograms and ischemic ST segment abnormalities found on ECG leads other than leads with new Q waves have a higher subsequent mortality and reinfarction rate compared with patients without persisting ischemic ST abnormality [75]. Similarly, ischemic ST abnormalities developing with recurrent angina early after myocardial infarction distant from the acute infarct have a worse prognosis than angina associated with ischemia in the infarct zone.

The electrocardiogram may be diagnostic of a prior myocardial infarction in the absence of a diagnostic history of infarction. Although the incidence of an unrecognized myocardial infarction is not known, the long-term prognosis after a "silent" infarction is similar to the hospitalized diagnosed infarction [78]. There appears to be a lesser incidence of angina pectoris after silent myocardial infarction. Prognostic importance has been attributed to silent ischemia after previously unrecognized myocardial infarction, which also has a high incidence of congestive heart failure. Estimation of the extent of myocardial damage by serial CK values relates to anatomic infarct size and to the impairment of left ventricular function. In previous studies, CK areas of over 40 IU/L/hr and elevated plasma CK levels over 2000 have been associated with poor prognosis and high incidence of left ventricular failure [7]. Large defects on thallium 201 perfusion scintigrams [79] and large infarcts on technetium 99m scintigrams [80] are associated with increased mortality and recurrent cardiac events. The extent of transmural infarct involvement is characterized by electrocardiographic Q-wave development in contrast to the subendocardial, nontransmural or non-Q-wave infarction. Despite the poor correlation between the electrocardiographic definitions of transmural or subendocardial infarction and the pathologic myocardial findings, marked similarities between the two types of infarction have been found [53, 81]. Many investigations have shown that acute mortality in patients with non-Q-wave infarcts is significantly lower than that in patients with Q-wave infarcts [82–84]. The prevalence of non-Q-wave myocardial infarction has shown a variable incidence of 16 to 36 percent in large infarct populations. Non-Q wave infarction is more common in patients with previous coronary artery bypass graft surgery with an incidence as high as 60 percent in postsurgery patients [85]. Patients with non-Q-wave infarction tend to have smaller infarctions [86]. It is supported by lower CK levels, a lower incidence of heart failure, and a lower average Killip class as well as a mean higher ejection fraction compared with Q-wave infarct patients [85]. Non-Q-wave infarct patients have less commonly total occlusions of the infarct-related coronary artery but may have more than 60 percent critical stenotic lesions in two or three coronary arteries and a higher incidence of left main coronary artery disease [87]. Non-Q-wave infarctions tend to have subtotal but severe stenosis of the infarct-related artery and a high incidence of recurrent angina early after infarction or after hospital discharge; 20 percent of patients develop acute Q-wave infarction within 3 months after the onset of a non-Q-wave infarct [81]. Hutter et al. reported a high recurrence rate of 21 percent at 9 months after initial infarction and 57 percent when patients were followed up to 54 months [84]. Increased complications are found in non-Q-wave infarcts that show large perfusion abnormalities within the infarct zone on thallium 201 perfusion scintigrams [88]. Patients studied in a 30-month follow-up period had a reinfarction rate of 18 percent in non-Q-wave and 6 percent in Q-wave infarction. Eighty-eight percent of recurrent infarctions in non-Q-wave patients related to the previous area of infarct compared with only 20 percent in the Q-wave infarctions.

Comparable late mortalities have been found in patients with both types of infarction [83, 84, 88]. In a collaborative study we studied early and late mortality in 277 patients with non-Q-wave infarction and compared these with 959 patients with Q-wave infarction [53]. One-year cumulative survival rates for patients with Q-wave and non-Q-wave infarcts were nearly identical when patients with infarct extensions were excluded. The hospital mortality in patients with infarct extension was 15 percent in those with Q-wave infarcts, whereas 43 percent in those with non-Q-wave infarcts died. During the follow-up period, there was a significantly higher incidence of infarct extension in the nonsurvivors than the

6 percent incidence in the survivors. For patients with infarct extension, the 1-year survival rate of 66 percent in patients with Q-wave infarction was higher than 35 percent in patients with non-Q-wave infarction. Extension of infarction was a strong predictor of a 1-year mortality in patients with non-Q-wave infarctions. Thus non-Q-wave infarctions are considered relatively unstable situations with a low early mortality rate but a higher risk of infarct extension and later infarction with a high late mortality rate. The recognition of this entity and the associated coronary artery findings provide the basis for early coronary arteriography in this patient group.

Hemodynamic measurements obtained by bedside pulmonary artery catheter monitoring during the acute phase and complications of myocardial infarction have provided quantitative parameters to further define early and late prognosis after AMI. Hemodynamic indices reflect the severity of congestive heart failure and inotropic dysfunction of the left and right ventricles and correlate to early and late mortality after AMI. An elevated left ventricular filling pressure, decreased cardiac output, cardiac index, increased arteriovenous oxygen difference, decreased stroke volume index, and left ventricular stroke work index signify poor early prognosis after AMI [7, 49, 89, 90]. Hemodynamic measurements can be abnormal in the absence of clinical manifestations of pump failure [91]. The presence of acute pulmonary edema that may be associated with normal ejection fraction can further identify patients at high risk of early death after AMI [7, 92]. We found that abnormal invasive measurements yielded a fivefold mortality when left ventricular filling pressure was over 20 mm Hg, cardiac index less than 2 L/min/m², stroke volume index less than 25 ml/beat/m², and arteriovenous oxygen difference over 5.6 ml/dl [7]. Hemodynamic measurements improve the predictive accuracy of early death and survival compared to historical and clinical data. Using discriminant function analysis for the development of a prognostication scheme, the factors from the history, physical examination, and noninvasive assessment correctly classified 73 percent of the deaths. The inclusion of hemodynamic data improved the correct classification of early death to 97 percent. Also, in this study, during a follow-up period of 26 months late mortality was increased twofold in patients with a left ventricular filling pressure over 20 mm Hg. Only the two other indicators of cardiac enlargement and previous myocardial infarction signified a twofold higher late mortality after 30 days and after hospital discharge [7]. The accurate identification of high risk patients by hemodynamic data has been demonstrated in patients with cardiogenic shock [89]. Accurate prediction of in-hospital mortality is improved by admission hemodynamic measurements with the added information on left ventricular failure from the initial chest radiograph and the Peel index [93].

Late Postinfarct Evaluation of Prognosis

During the late postinfarct period, the risk of subsequent cardiac death is the result of recurrent myocardial ischemia, complex or frequent ventricular ectopic activity, and left ventricular dysfunction [42, 67, 94]. It is suggested that the impairment of left ventricular function is the most important indicator for 1-year and 2-year cardiac mortality after myocardial infarction [67, 95]. Depressed left ventricular ejection fraction is often associated with persistent sinus tachycardia, a third heart sound, palpable left ventricular dyssynergy, bibasilar rales, and a murmur of papillary muscle dysfunction after acute myocardial infarction [96]. Significant correlations between both Killip and NYHA classes for congestive heart failure with ejection fraction have been reported [67]. An abnormal chest radiograph after myocardial infarction may predict the presence of depressed left ventricular ejection fraction in more than 50 percent of patients [97]. Dewhurst and Muir reported the relation between rest ejection fraction and infarct location on the discharge electrocardiogram. Patients exhibiting Q waves in the anterior or lateral leads or in both the anterior and inferior leads had the most severely depressed ejection fractions [98]. The same authors reported a significant association between depressed ejection fraction and peak creatinine kinase af-

ter both anterior and inferior infarction. A study on survivors of AMI indicated that abnormal rest or exercise ejection fraction was related to a history of previous infarction, cardiomegaly, functional class for congestive heart failure at the time of discharge, infarct location, and Killip class, whereas depressed ejection fraction did not correlate to significant exercise-induced ST segment depression [99].

It has been suggested that impaired left ventricular performance is related to complex ventricular arrhythmias with ejection fractions of less than 40 percent [95]. Similarly, patients identified with high grade ventricular arrhythmias after acute infarction have lower rest and exercise ejection fractions [93, 100]. The left ventricular ejection fraction (LVEF) within the first 24 hours after admission relates to short-term mortality [91]. Ejection fraction stabilizes within the subsequent 24 to 48 hours [101], and ejection fraction measured during the later hospital stay relates to postdischarge mortality over the subsequent 2 years [67, 94]. Various separation points in the measurement of rest ejection fraction have been reported to best predict in-hospital and postdischarge mortality [102, 103]. Patients with acute infarction and resting ejection fraction of less than 30 percent showed an early mortality of 55 percent [103]; and an ejection fraction of less than 40 percent at the time of discharge has been associated with a 30 percent 1-year mortality [67, 95]. We found that a separation point of 45 percent can provide optimal sensitivity and specificity for cardiac death up to 1 year [92]. Significant differences in mortality are found in patients with abnormal ejection fractions of less than 52 percent (24 percent 1-year mortality) compared with patients with normal values (10 percent 1-year mortality). In our study, an LVEF of less than 45 percent classified 62 percent of deaths correctly and 64 percent of the survivors that had an ejection fraction over 45 percent. Only 19 percent of deaths within the first year had an LVEF of less than 30 percent, but 90 percent of survivors had an LVEF over 30 percent.

The one-year cardiac mortality progressively increases as the ejection fraction decreases below 40 percent, and an LVEF of less than 30 percent carries a fivefold increase in the risk of dying during the first year after infarction [67] (Fig. 38-3). Studies on the role of ejection fraction combined with other prognostic parameters suggest that rest ejection fraction is the most important predictor of mortality after hospital discharge [93, 102].

The Multicenter Postinfarction Research Group reported progressive increases in 1-year mortality in patients with ejection fractions less than 40 percent [67]. Four risk factors were independent predictors of mortality including an ejection fraction below 40 percent, evidence of congestive heart failure with bilateral extensive pulmonary rales in the CCU, ventricular ectopy of 10 beats or more per hour, and advanced NYHA functional class before infarction. These factors were analyzed in a logistic regression analysis for mortality, and the most important independent prognostic factors were pulmonary rales and LVEF. The increasing number of these risk factors have an increasing mortality, the lowest risk group without any prognostic factors having less than 3 percent 2-year mortality, and the highest risk group with all four factors having a 60 percent 2-year mortality (Fig. 38-4). The combination of pulmonary rales and ejection fraction of less than 40 percent identified patients with a 2-year mortality of 38.1 percent, whereas mortality in the remaining patient group was only 8.9 percent, and the combination of pulmonary rales and a history of previous infarction had a high mortality of 39.4 percent within 2 years.

In the Multicenter Investigation of the Limitation of Infarct Size (MILIS), ejection fraction was examined with 15 other variables for prognostic importance in a Cox regression analysis [94]. LVEF of less than 40 percent ranked as the second most important indicator after ventricular premature beats of more than 10 per hour, followed by the use of digitalis at discharge and a history of previous infarction.

The presence or absence of clinical or radiographic heart failure gives further prognostic information in patients with normal or depressed left ventricular ejection fraction [92]. In our multicenter study of 972 patients with AMI, the effect of the presence or absence of in-hospital heart failure on late mortality was

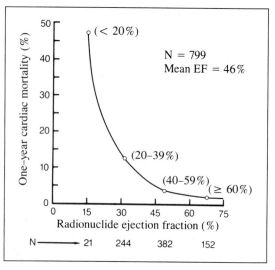

Fig. 38-3
One-year cardiac mortality as a function of left ventricular ejection fraction (EF) during the first year following hospital discharge after acute myocardial infarction. Mortality increases greatly as the ejection fraction before hospital discharge falls below 40 percent. (From The Multicenter Postinfarction Research Group: Risk stratification and survival after myocardial infarction. *N. Engl. J. Med.* 309:331, 1983. With permission.)

studied in three groups divided according to LVEF; group I had an LVEF of 40 percent or less, group II 41 to 50 percent, and group III 51 percent or more. In group I patients with clinical signs of left ventricular failure, 1-year mortality rate after hospital discharge was 26 percent, significantly higher than the 19 percent mortality in group II and the 8 percent mortality in group III. In the absence of left ventricular failure, mortality rates were significantly lower at 12, 6, and 3 percent, respectively. The 1-year mortality was markedly increased for patients who had radiographic signs of congestive heart failure during the CCU period at 36, 24, and 14 percent in groups I, II, and III, respectively, and markedly lower at 13, 9, and 3 percent when no radiographic heart failure was seen. Moderate or severe depression of LVEF in the absence of clinical or radiographic heart failure predicted an increased 1-year mortality compared with patients with a normal LVEF but at much lower mortality levels than when heart failure was present. Patients with a normal ejection frac-

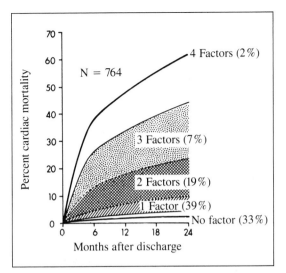

Fig. 38-4
Mortality curves and zones of risk according to the increasing number of risk factors. The risk factors included NYHA functional classes II to IV before hospital admission, pulmonary rales, occurrence of ten or more PVCs per hour, and a left ventricular ejection fraction below 40 percent. The risk zones indicate the spectrum of relative risk for single factors and the range of multiple risks for combinations of two, three, and four factors. The numbers in parentheses indicate the proportions of the population with the specified number of risk factors. (From The Multicenter Postinfarction Research Group: Risk stratification and survival after myocardial infarction. *N. Engl. J. Med.* 309:331, 1983. With permission.)

tion without heart failure had a 1-year mortality of 3 percent, which increased to 8 or 14 percent when clinical or radiologic signs of left ventricular failure were present.

Comparative Prognostic Value of Ejection Fraction with Other Clinical and Laboratory Parameters

Other studies have compared the prognostic value of radionuclide ejection fraction with other clinical and laboratory parameters [98, 104, 105] and suggested that LVEF is a more potent predictor of subsequent mortality and events than those available from history, physical examination, electrocardiogram, and other noninvasive examinations. Similarly, the LVEF was also ranked higher than other clinical variables or the prognostic indices of Peel and Norris [106].

Exercise-induced ST segment abnormalities have been shown not to be as potent predictors of subsequent cardiac events as the radionuclide angiographic variables. Submaximal exercise testing variables such as maximal heart rate, blood pressure, workload, angina, ST segment changes, and arrhythmias were found to be less significantly related to subsequent events than the radionuclide angiographic variables [104, 105].

Thallium 201 myocardial imaging has been used prognostically in survivors of AMI [22]. Prognostic information from the rest and exercise radionuclide ventriculogram has been compared to thallium 201 myocardial perfusion scintigraphy [107]. The results of thallium imaging were significantly related to subsequent combined events, but radionuclide angiographic variables were superior to thallium scintigraphy for predicting cardiac events in post-MI patients.

The prognostic value of exercise radionuclide angiography parameters has been examined [106]. Exercise ejection fraction and the change in ejection fraction was predictive of major cardiac events, which included cardiac death and recurrent myocardial infarction. Rest ejection fraction, left ventricular wall motion score, and left ventricular end-systolic volume index also had significant association with subsequent events. The peak LVEF during exercise was the most important variable in determining the highest risk groups if ventricular ejection fraction at rest was less than 40 percent. The change in the LVEF with exercise distinguished best the patients with minor cardiac events of angina pectoris and congestive heart failure rather than identifying patients with subsequent major events and cardiac death.

Cardiac Arrhythmias

Certain cardiac arrhythmias during the acute phase of myocardial infarction and the late postinfarct phase have been associated with an increased in-hospital and short-term mortality [108–113]. Supraventricular tachyar-rhythmias including atrial fibrillation and si-nus tachycardia, ventricular fibrillation, and complete atrioventricular block have been as-sociated with a more than twofold early mor-tality, and multivariate analyses have identi-fied sinus tachycardia, ventricular fibrillation, and complete atrioventricular block as inde-pendent predictors for poor early prognosis [7, 114]. Other studies have reported that early prognosis with increased in-hospital mortality or 40-day mortality after acute infarction is af-fected by the occurrence of supraventricular tachycardia, atrial fibrillation, sinus bradycar-dia, atrioventricular block, ventricular pre-mature beats, ventricular tachycardia, and ventricular fibrillation [114]. Also, the new occurrence of left bundle branch block, bifas-cicular block, and trifascicular conduction block has been associated with increased early mortality.

Ventricular arrhythmias occurring during the acute phase of myocardial infarction have been established as important predictors of subsequent mortality. Investigations have documented the prognostic value of ventricu-lar arrhythmias that occur before discharge and are associated with an increased risk of cardiac and sudden death after hospital dis-charge [108, 109, 111, 112, 115]. Sudden car-diac death after hospital discharge is attrib-uted to ventricular fibrillation and accounts for a large proportion of cardiac deaths within the first year after myocardial infarction. We have observed an incidence of 45 percent sudden arrhythmic death among all cardiac deaths during the first 2 months after hospital discharge after myocardial infarction with a subsequent decreasing incidence of 33, 29, and 22 percent sudden death for the following 3-month intervals during the first year after myocardial infarction. Frequent and complex ventricular premature beats documented by ambulatory electrocardiographic recordings or telemetry and exercise testing with electrocar-diographic monitoring have been related to prognosis with improved prediction of subse-quent mortality in association with either im-paired left ventricular function or myocardial ischemia [67, 110, 113].

Thus 1-hour electrocardiographic record-ings in postinfarction patients showed that ventricular premature beats in combination with congestive heart failure carried a seven-fold risk of sudden death compared to patients without both findings [115]. Residual ventric-ular ectopic activity after acute myocardial infarction has a more adverse impact on prognosis in the presence of myocardial dys-function [110]. All the patients who died sud-denly in a follow-up study of 81 patients had complex ventricular arrhythmias and a LVEF of less than 40 percent by radionuclide ven-triculography. Taylor et al. documented that complex ventricular arrhythmias during the late hospital phase and after discharge are as-sociated with multivessel coronary artery dis-ease, left ventricular dysfunction, and sudden death [103]. This study defined complex ven-tricular arrhythmias as multiform ventricular premature beats, bigeminy, or runs of ventric-ular beats recorded with a 24-hour Holter monitor 10 to 24 days after AMI. In this study, 60 percent of patients had complex ventricular arrhythmias at some time during the 1-year follow-up period, and their common presence resulted in a low predictive value for morbid-ity and mortality.

Controversy exists concerning whether complex ventricular arrhythmias have prog-nostic value independent of other major risk indicators. Similarly, a uniform definition of "complex" ventricular arrhythmias and the frequency indicative of poor prognosis re-mains undefined. The Multicenter Postinfarc-tion Research Group has established that ten ventricular premature beats per hour indicate an increased risk for subsequent mortality [67]. In this study, 866 patients underwent 24-hour Holter monitoring and determination of the resting radionuclide ventricular ejection fraction; 1-year and 2-year mortality were in-dependently related to ventricular ectopy of ten or more depolarizations per hour but, more importantly, to the ejection fraction of less than 40 percent and the occurrence of ad-vanced left ventricular failure with the pres-ence of extensive pulmonary rales and a his-tory of previous congestive heart failure. A progressive increase in 1-year cardiac mortality was observed as the frequency of ventricular ectopic depolarizations rose above one per hour and the ejection fraction fell below 40 percent. However, ejection fraction had a considerably stronger effect on mortality than did ectopic depolarizations. The same group reported from another study that an ejection fraction of less than 30 percent was significantly more important for the prediction of total cardiac mortality than ventricular ectopic beats of more than three per hour, with a 50 percent mortality in patients with both risks compared to 6 percent of patients without these findings [95]. Similarly, patients with low ejection fractions (< 40 percent) and frequent depolarizations (> 10/hour) had a 3.8-fold increased risk of cardiac death compared with the patient without these risk indicators.

The MILIS identified in 533 patients ventricular ectopic activity of more than ten per hour as the most important type of ventricular arrhythmia and strongest predictor for subsequent sudden death [94]. LVEF of less than 40 percent was identified as the next important predictor among many historical and clinical variables. The occurrence of both ventricular premature beats more than ten per hour and a reduced LVEF of less than 40 percent identified a group of postinfarction patients with a sudden death rate of 18 percent during an 18-month follow-up period compared to only 2 percent for the patients without these findings. Thus the additive risk for sudden death among the group of patients with ventricular premature beats of more than ten per hour was five times that of the group with neither frequent ventricular beats nor left ventricular dysfunction. The additive risk for sudden death was 11 times greater in the group with both left ventricular dysfunction and frequent premature ventricular beats. Patients with good left ventricular function have a relatively low mortality, even in the presence of a high frequency of ventricular ectopic beats. The MILIS study identified ventricular premature beats frequency of more than ten per hour as the most important ventricular arrhythmia, to a lesser degree complex features of premature ventricular contractions (PVCs) including couplets, R on T phenomenon, runs, and mul-

tiform ventricular premature beats, which were also predictive of sudden death.

An association between silent myocardial ischemia after myocardial infarction and arrhythmias has been suggested [116, 117]. Patients with myocardial infarction and ventricular fibrillation had exercise-induced painless myocardial ischemia. Malignant ventricular arrhythmias in patients with prior myocardial infarction were inducible by programmed ventricular stimulation in the presence of ischemia and were not inducible in the absence of ischemia.

Early ventricular fibrillation after AMI has an increased in-hospital mortality rate [118]. In one study we observed a 7 percent incidence of ventricular fibrillation within 48 hours of hospital admission, which carried a 25 percent hospital mortality compared with 13 percent in patients without early ventricular fibrillation. The common causes of death in these patients were congestive heart failure and cardiogenic shock. Multivariate analysis identified ventricular fibrillation as an independent prognostic factor for the in-hospital mortality. The 1-year mortality rate after hospital discharge was not significantly greater in patients with than in those without early ventricular fibrillation (15 percent and 11 percent, respectively), even in the subgroup of patients with anterior myocardial infarction.

In another study, we investigated the relation of complex ventricular arrhythmias including multiform PCVs, couplets, and ventricular tachycardia to infarct location [119]. Sixty-two percent of patients with non-Q-wave infarcts who did not survive 1 year had complex PVCs compared with 32 percent of survivors. No differences were seen in the Q-wave group. In patients with complex PVCs, survival was higher (92 percent) in patients with Q-wave infarction compared to 76 percent in non-Q-wave infarction. For the Q-wave infarcts, survival was similar in patients with and without complex ectopic activity, and the incidence of complex ectopic activity was similar in patients with LVEF above and below 45 percent. Complex PVCs were independent of ejection fraction in patients with non-Q-wave infarction but closely associated with ejection fraction in patients with Q-wave infarction. The presence of complex PVCs at the time of hospital discharge appears to be an important predictor of 1-year mortality in the presence of non-Q-wave infarction.

Exercise Testing

Exercise stress testing soon after recovery from an uncomplicated myocardial infarction has been shown to be a safe and useful technique that aids in patient management and prognostic assessment. The predischarge submaximal or symptom-limited exercise test is useful for the detection of myocardial ischemia and arrhythmias in patients without clinical features apparent during the early hospital stay after acute infarction [120–122]. Furthermore, maximal stress test performed 4 to 6 weeks after the hospital stay may identify a large number of patients with residual myocardial ischemia [123].

Studies have shown that 30 to 40 percent of postinfarction patients demonstrate ischemic electrocardiographic abnormalities during early treadmill exercise testing that relate to the extent of coronary artery disease in the risk area of recent infarction and other sites adjacent or remote from the recent infarct [124, 125]. Even in uncomplicated patients after myocardial infarction who do not exhibit symptoms of residual or recurrent ischemia, exercise testing has identified patients with multiple vessel coronary artery disease. Further methods used to identify residual myocardial ischemia include exercise myocardial imaging with thallium 201, exercise radionuclide angiography, and exercise two-dimensional echocardiography.

Most clinical studies indicate that the ST segment depression or the development of angina during electrocardiographic exercise testing prior to hospital discharge relates to mortality and subsequent reinfarction or unstable angina [120–122, 126]. Other exercise test variables that predict subsequent cardiac events after infarction are the development of angina pectoris [120–122], complex ventricular arrhythmias [120, 127], heart rate response

[128], the blood pressure response [121–129], and the rate pressure product at the time of chest pain or ST depression [129]. In patients unable to increase their systolic blood pressure by at least 10 mm Hg or in whom the systolic blood pressure decreases by 20 mm Hg during continued exercise, a high incidence of severe three-vessel or left main coronary artery disease with a high associated cardiac mortality is found [120, 123]. In such patients, a symptom-limited treadmill exercise test has been shown to demonstrate myocardial ischemia better than a heart-rate-limited exercise test [123]. Most studies have identified the exercise functional capacity to be of predictive value for subsequent mortality as determined by the duration of exercise [129, 130], the early termination of exercise, the maximum accomplished workload in watts [131], and the total cardiac capacity expressed in multiples of resting oxygen consumption (MET) [121, 127]. The more important prognostic indicators from exercise testing largely reflect impaired left ventricular function. Cardiac mortality is high in patients who achieve 4 MET or less of exercise [132]. Patients achieving 4 MET or less had a cardiac event rate of 18 percent with cardiac death or new myocardial infarction within 1 year compared with a 2 percent cardiac event rate in patients with a more than 4 MET exercise capacity. A good functional capacity over 4 MET was predicted from age and ST segment abnormalities at rest. Among the 60 percent of patients who were predicted to have good functional capacity of more than 4 MET, only 15 percent had poor functional capacity at the time of exercise testing. Multivariate analysis identified only functional capacity but not ST depression as a predictor of subsequent death. An important indicator of poor prognosis is the inability to perform an exercise test [132, 133]. Similarly, patients selected for exercise testing have a more favorable prognosis than those who are not tested. Reasons for the inability to perform an exercise test include age, poor general medical condition, severe peripheral vascular disease, congestive heart failure, and markedly impaired left ventricular function. The inability to perform an exercise test has

been identified as the strongest predictor of outcome in a study that examined variables with clinical factors and LVEF [131].

ST segment depression of 1 mm or more during exercise testing has been related to subsequent mortality [120–122, 127]. Studies have reported a significantly higher mortality (4–25 percent) in patients with ST depression in contrast to a low mortality (0–7 percent) in patients without exercise-induced ST depression. Waters et al. investigated 225 patients with a predischarge exercise test to 5 MET or 70 percent of maximum predicted heart rate, and only exercise-induced ST segment abnormality and the failure to increase the systolic blood pressure by 10 mm Hg predicted mortality during the first year after myocardial infarction [134]. Cardiac mortality during the follow-up period after the first year could no longer be predicted by ST segment abnormalities, but exercise-induced ventricular arrhythmias and a history of previous myocardial infarction predicted mortality beyond the first year. Other studies ascribed a high risk to the development of angina during exercise testing in association with ST segment depression [123]. Patients who manifest angina with exercise-induced ST depression have been shown to have an 88 percent prevalence of multivessel coronary artery disease with increased subsequent mortality. In the presence of more marked ST depression of 2 mm or more at peak heart rates of less than 135 per minute a high risk group is identified with a 10 percent mortality, compared to 1.3 percent mortality in patients without these exercise test abnormalities.

Exercise-induced asymptomatic myocardial ischemia has been identified as an important predictor of poor prognosis [135]. In one study, 63 percent of patients who underwent low level exercise treadmill testing early after myocardial infarction had a positive exercise test without angina. The group with anginal chest pain and the group without exercise angina had similar extents of coronary artery disease and left ventricular ejection fraction. Silent myocardial ischemia recorded as intermittent ST depression on ambulatory electrocardiographic recording has been associated with an increased risk of cardiac events during the postinfarction period [136].

Exercise Test Variables and Other Prognostic Variables

The importance of variables from exercise testing has been investigated for the prediction of mortality and other cardiac events [137, 138]. Different multivariate methods ranked exercise duration highest for prediction of death with lesser importance for the heart rate pressure product, exercise-induced ventricular arrhythmias, heart rate, and female gender; but ST segment depression was not selected as a significant predictor of subsequent death [127].

Madsen et al. examined prognosis from both clinical and exercise test variables and ranked heart failure over exercise-induced ventricular ectopic activity and exercise duration [114]. For the endpoints of death and nonfatal new myocardial infarction, exercise duration was most important compared with exercise-induced arrhythmias, female gender, age, and atrioventricular block. In this study, clinical variables alone provided the highest correct prediction of death.

Patients who are able to exercise after myocardial infarction are at a lower risk for subsequent death. The Multicenter Postinfarction Research Group study found a 7.5 percent 1-year mortality in the total study population, but mortality was low, at 5 percent, in patients who were able to perform a low level exercise tolerance test, compared to 17 percent in patients who were unable to exercise [67]. The same study group identified a subgroup of exercised postinfarction patients who had no evidence of congestive heart failure on chest radiograph with an only 1 percent 1-year cardiac mortality.

DeBusk et al. studied postinfarction patients to develop a risk stratification scheme. A high risk group was identified with an 80 percent mortality or recurrent infarction during the subsequent 6 months by the presence of a history of previous infarction or angina and recurrent angina in the CCU [126]. Of the remaining patients, the ineligibility for exercise testing further identified a risk group with a 6.4 percent event rate. Of the patients who performed an exercise test, a positive test of 2 mm or more ST segment depression had a high event rate compared with those with a negative exercise test, indicating the value of exercise testing for defining high and low risk subgroups after myocardial infarction.

Thallium Scintigraphy

Myocardial thallium 201 imaging in conjunction with exercise testing enhances sensitivity and specificity for detection of ischemia in patients with functionally important multivessel coronary artery disease [139]. In patients with negative exercise tests, scintigraphic evidence of residual myocardial ischemia, either within the infarct zone or in myocardial regions remote from infarction, is common. Patients with demonstrated ischemia on thallium 201 testing were found to have a significantly greater mortality, a higher incidence of reinfarction during long-term follow-up, and higher risk of experiencing subsequent cardiac events compared with patients without scintigraphic evidence of residual ischemia [22, 140]. The prognostic value of thallium perfusion imaging has been similarly demonstrated in postinfarction patients with painless ST segment depression during predischarge exercise testing and in patients who exhibit false-positive electrocardiographic responses after recent myocardial infarction [141].

Exercise scintigraphy detects significant disease in the anterior descending coronary artery, right coronary artery, the circumflex coronary artery with a sensitivity of 91, 87, and 63 percent, respectively [139]. The presence of thallium 201 perfusion abnormalities in multiple different vascular distributions allows identification of multivessel and left main coronary artery disease after myocardial infarction.

Gibson et al. compared the results of submaximal exercise testing, thallium 201 scintigraphy, and coronary angiography prior to hospital discharge after myocardial infarction for identification of patients at high risk defined by defects in more than one vascular region, redistribution within or remote from the infarct zone, or abnormal lung uptake [22]. Thallium scintigraphy was more sensitive (95 percent) than either treadmill exercise testing or coronary angiography for identifying nonfatal recurrent myocardial infarction and rehospitalization with class 3 and class 4 angina during a follow-up period of 15 months. Exercise electrocardiographic studies identified only 50 percent of patients with either cardiac death or recurrent infarction. In contrast, total cardiac event rate was 6 percent and cardiac mortality rate 2 percent in patients with normal perfusion or single persistent defects in the infarct zone. All cardiac deaths during the follow-up period had underlying multiple vessel disease, and 90 percent of them had one or more high-risk scintigraphic findings. In patients with single-vessel disease and subsequent cardiac events, 92 percent demonstrated redistribution within the infarct region. However, for the prediction of death, multivessel disease by coronary angiography was a stronger predictor than exercise thallium scintigraphy. Hung et al. reported that the magnitude of exercise-induced thallium-201 defects and the extent of redistribution during symptom-limited exercise testing 3 weeks after infarction were strongly predictive of subsequent events [140]. In a study of 117 men followed over 12 months, variables from exercise thallium scintigraphy, maximal exercise electrocardiographic testing, and radionuclide angiography were examined by regression analysis together with the clinical data. A decreased exercise capacity and an inability to raise ejection fraction by 5 percent with exercise predicted cardiac death, nonfatal recurrent infarction, and ventricular fibrillation better than thallium scintigraphic abnormalities.

Thallium 201 exercise scintigraphy following myocardial infarction may identify 50 percent of postinfarction patients with multivessel disease. In these patients with multiple perfusion defects on exercise scintigrams 3 months after myocardial infarction, 28 percent of patients had a subsequent cardiac event, compared to 6 percent of patients with a monovessel disease pattern on scintigrams [142].

The relative prognostic value of rest thallium 201 imaging, radionuclide ventriculography, and 24-hour ambulatory electrocardiographic monitoring has been studied for the prediction of 1-year mortality after acute myocardial infarction [143]. High risk patients were identified by an abnormal thallium perfusion score, LVEF less than 40 percent, and complex ventricular arrhythmias (three or more consecutive PCVs, paired PCVs, or more than ten PVCs in 1 hour) and were important predictors of survival by univariate Cox survival analysis. The thallium perfusion score, however, was the only important predictor by multivariate analysis, and the predictive power of the thallium perfusion score was comparable to that of combined ejection fraction and ambulatory electrocardiographic monitoring. Conversely, patients with a small, persistent thallium 201 defect in a single region and without increased lung uptake appear at very low risk for a future cardiac event and mortality and are candidates for early hospital discharge and rehabilitation.

Two-Dimensional Echocardiography

Two-dimensional echocardiography at rest and during exercise is useful in the diagnosis of coronary artery disease, left ventricular function, and wall motion abnormalities [144–148]. Two-dimensional echocardiography has been shown to be comparable to radionuclide ventriculography for the quantitation of LVEF and left ventricular wall motion abnormalities in anterior infarction with superior detection of wall motion abnormalities of the inferoposterior wall [149, 150]. Among 93 patients studied with two-dimensional echocardiography and radionuclide ventriculography, high and low risk patients were identified by left ventricular ejection fraction and left ventricular wall motion indices by both techniques. In repeated studies, 10 days after myocardial infarction in 81 survivors, risk groups with similar 1-year mortality rates by either technique were defined.

Two-dimensional echocardiography within 12 hours after admission with acute myocardial infarction has been performed to assess the location and extent of contraction abnormalities [151]. Patients with a high abnormal wall motion score were at high risk of subsequent cardiac death, left ventricular failure, and malignant ventricular arrhythmias during the hospital stay. Of the 27 patients with a high risk echocardiographic wall motion score at 12 hours after infarction, 24 (89 percent) had one or more cardiac events compared to an 18 percent event rate in the low risk group with a low abnormal wall motion score. Patients with a high abnormal wall motion score had a 37 percent in-hospital mortality, and patients with a lesser extent of wall motion abnormalities only a 6 percent mortality.

Ryan et al. examined the value of prognostic information from exercise two-dimensional echocardiography compared to treadmill exercise testing in patients recovering from AMI [152]. During a 10-month follow-up period, 80 percent of patients who had exercise-induced echocardiographic wall motion abnormalities had subsequent cardiac events with cardiac death, readmission with unstable angina, recurrent myocardial infarction, or coronary artery bypass graft surgery. Treadmill exercise tests were positive in only 55 percent of patients with subsequent events. No cardiac deaths occurred in patients with negative exercise echocardiograms, and there was a significant decrease in the event-free survival in those patients without exercise-induced wall motion abnormalities compared to those with new abnormalities. Exercise echocardiography was more sensitive and specific than treadmill exercise testing for the prediction of subsequent cardiac events after AMI.

Cardiac Catheterization, Coronary Angiography

Cardiac catheterization can be safely performed early after an AMI to identify subgroups of patients with variable extent and severity of coronary artery disease and the related prognosis [153–156]. Coronary artery bypass surgery improves survival in certain subgroups with narrowing of the left main coronary artery and in patients with three-vessel coronary artery disease and left ventricular dysfunction. In patients recovering from an AMI, approximately 10 percent of patients have critical stenosis of the left main coronary artery, and 30 to 40 percent have three-vessel disease. Thus a substantial proportion of patients who survive an acute myocardial infarction may be recommended for coronary artery bypass surgery based on the coronary arteriographic findings after infarction.

Clinical features of patients with multivessel disease include advanced age [155], postinfarction angina [155, 157], complex arrhythmias during 24-hour electrocardiographic monitoring [156], ventricular tachycardia and ventricular fibrillation in the CCU [158], congestive heart failure, pulmonary edema, or shock [158]. In other studies, weight, systolic blood pressure, serum cholesterol, and infarct location have been identified as common features in patients with three-vessel disease [157]. Other historical information of previous myocardial infarction [158, 159], history of angina [157, 158] or changing angina prior to infarction [153], family history of coronary artery disease [157], and history of hypertension [103] have been related to the extent of coronary artery disease. Left ventricular function was inversely related to the number of involved arteries [158]. More extensive coronary disease is commonly found in the presence of increased left ventricular end-diastolic pressure, increased end-diastolic volume, and reduced stroke work index [160]. Multivariate statistical techniques have been applied to identify patients with multivessel disease. These variables include the occurrence of postinfarction angina, a family history of coronary disease and a high serum cholesterol level [157], anterior ST and T wave abnormalities, and a positive treadmill exercise test after myocardial infarction [161].

The results from coronary angiography have been examined using multivariate analysis to determine subsequent cardiac events and mortality. In a study of 179 survivors of AMI who underwent coronary angiography and left ventriculography within 8 weeks after infarction, the prevalence of multivessel disease was high (79 percent) in the symptomatic patients [130]. Three-vessel disease or an ejection fraction less than 30 percent identified a subgroup of patients with a high mortality rate (22 percent) during an average 20-month follow-up period, but recurrent myocardial infarction was best predicted from exercise test variables. Another study examined prognosis in relation to the location and severity of coronary artery stenosis defined by a coronary artery jeopardy score [162]. The highest jeopardy score had a 56 percent 5-year survival rate and the low jeopardy scores a 95 percent survival rate. However, the LVEF was more closely related to prognosis than the coronary artery jeopardy score, and only the maximal percent stenosis in the left anterior descending artery added prognostic information to the jeopardy score.

Sanz et al. investigated predictors for late mortality in 259 consecutive patients who underwent coronary arteriography after myocardial infarction [45]. An ejection fraction of 0.50 or less, the number of diseased vessels, and the occurrence of congestive heart failure in the CCU were the only independent predictors of survival. Survival was lowest in patients with ejection fractions between 0.21 and 0.49, and the proportion with three-vessel disease was high in this group, who stand to benefit the most from coronary artery bypass surgery.

The severity of coronary artery disease and the degree of impairment of left ventricular dysfunction have been useful for prognostication and risk stratification up to 5 years after AMI [163]. In this study one-half of the patients had three-vessel disease, and only 7 percent had an LVEF of less than 0.30. Of multiple clinical and angiographic variables, combined right and left anterior descending coronary artery stenosis, ejection fraction, and the presence of myocardial risk segments were significant predictors of subsequent cardiac death, nonfatal reinfarction, or coronary artery bypass surgery over the 5-year follow-up period. These angiographic variables added significant information for prognosis and prediction of cardiac events to the clinical variables over the entire 5-year period after myocardial infarction.

One study identified left ventricular end-systolic volume as a stronger indicator of survival than either ejection fraction or the number of coronary occlusions after myocardial infarction [164]. Left ventricular ejection fraction, however, can be assessed by noninvasive techniques, which may further reduce the indications for cardiac catheterization as a means for risk stratification.

Programmed Electrical Stimulation

Although the prognostic importance of complex ventricular arrhythmias during the in-hospital and postdischarge phase after AMI has been documented, the role of programmed electrical stimulation is uncertain. Provoked ventricular tachyarrhythmias may identify patients with late sudden death and poor prognosis after AMI [165–169]. Patients who develop sustained ventricular tachycardia or ventricular fibrillation spontaneously during the early recovery period after infarction have an increased in-hospital mortality. Electrical instability produced by programmed electrical stimulation (PES) has been related to subsequent sudden death after myocardial infarction, and it is suggested that associated myocardial ischemia may be a requirement for the induction of ventricular tachycardia in patients with coronary artery disease who have survived a "sudden death" event [170]. Patients with AMI who have sustained ventricular tachycardia in hospital or have been resuscitated from ventricular fibrillation have more frequently inducible ventricular tachycardia with a lesser number of premature stimuli required. Forty percent of patients with PES-inducible ventricular tachycardia had also documented spontaneous early ventricular tachycardia or fibrillation after infarction. In contrast, nonsustained ventricular tachyarrhythmia was more frequently induced in patients without earlier ventricular arrhyth-

mias or with nonsustained ventricular tachycardia. The temporal evolution of inducible sustained ventricular arrhythmias after myocardial infarction has been studied in clinically stable patients early and late after myocardial infarction [171]. During the initial programmed ventricular stimulation at an average of 2 weeks after myocardial infarction, sustained ventricular tachycardia or ventricular fibrillation was inducible in most of the patients but was reproduced at an average of 5 months later in only 47 percent of patients. A decrease in late inducibility of the sustained ventricular arrhythmias was greater for those induced during initial programmed ventricular stimulation by triple extra stimuli and burst pacing than for those induced by double extra stimuli; but it appeared to be unrelated to other clinical, hemodynamic, or angiographic variables. Only 7 percent of patients with initially inducible ventricular arrhythmias died during a 1-year follow-up period, and all patients were surviving in the noninducible group. Higher mortality rates have been reported with 32 percent incidence of sudden death in patients with inducible ventricular tachycardia or fibrillation [167], but sudden death rates of 14 percent have been reported for nonresponders during 1-year follow-up periods. Other studies have suggested that ventricular arrhythmias induced early after myocardial infarction can be reproduced late in these survivors of acute infarction, but the persistent electrical instability is not a predictor of the risk of sudden death during the first year after myocardial infarction [172]. Denniss et al. compared the relative prognostic significance of ventricular tachycardia and fibrillation inducible by PES within 1 month after AMI in a prospective study of 403 survivors of transmural myocardial infarction and found that 20 percent of the patients had inducible ventricular tachycardia and 14 percent had inducible ventricular fibrillation [173]. For the patients with inducible ventricular tachycardia, the 1-year probability of survival was significantly lower than the respective probability for patients without inducible arrhythmias, and the probability of remaining incident-free of cardiac death or nonfatal arrhythmia was significantly lower than in the group with no inducible arrhythmias.

The prognostic significance of programmed ventricular stimulation and its usefulness in relation to other forms of invasive and noninvasive testing has been investigated in 150 survivors of myocardial infarction with inducibility of ventricular arrhythmias in 23 percent of these patients [174]. No significant differences existed between patients with or without inducible ventricular tachyarrhythmias in relation to spontaneous ventricular arrhythmias during the acute and recovery phases after infarction, inducible ischemia or arrhythmias on predischarge treadmill exercise testing, severity of coronary artery disease on angiography, or degree of left ventricular dysfunction. A higher incidence of inferior infarction was observed in patients with inducible ventricular tachycardia. Patients with and without inducible ventricular arrhythmias had a similar occurrence of sudden death, cardiac death, and ventricular tachyarrhythmias during the subsequent year. In this population, a low left ventricular ejection fraction, presence of a left ventricular aneurysm, and exercise-induced PVCs were predictors of subsequent death and spontaneous ventricular tachycardia, whereas PES-induced ventricular tachycardia in the patients recovering from infarction could not identify a high risk group for subsequent sudden cardiac death.

The combined use of PES and the exercise test allows definition of high and low risk groups after infarction [169]. In one study, patients with inducible ventricular arrhythmias had a higher mortality than those without inducible arrhythmias (26 percent versus 6 percent). Exercise-induced ST segment change of 2 mm or more had a higher (11 percent) mortality rate than the 4 percent rate in ST changes of less than 2 mm. Of patients who had both tests, 62 percent had no inducible arrhythmia and an ST change of less than 2 mm; only 1 percent died during the first year. Of the patients with inducible ventricular arrhythmias and/or ST segment depression of 2 mm or more, 13 percent died within 1 year. Programmed stimulation and exercise testing together predicted death within the first year

and identified a large group of patients with a low mortality rate.

The contribution of PES to risk assessment in patients after myocardial infarction has been compared to clinical variables, information from exercise testing, and 24-hour ambulatory electrocardiographic recording and radionuclide ejection fraction [175]. In 19 of the 84 patients (23 percent), ventricular tachycardia of more than six repetitive beats was produced, but none of these patients died during an average 20 months of follow-up, whereas 9 percent died in the group without inducible arrhythmias. In the patients with inducible ventricular tachycardia, complex ventricular ectopy and ventricular tachycardia were commonly detected on ambulatory electrocardiographic recording. No relation was found between the response to PES and the abnormalities of exercise testing and radionuclide ejection fraction. All but one of the patients who died had an LVEF under 40 percent, and four of the six patients had ventricular tachycardia on ambulatory electrocardiographic recording. PES at 6 weeks after myocardial infarction appears not to contribute to identification of high risk patients after myocardial infarction; high risk patients were more accurately characterized by ventricular function, exercise testing, and complex ventricular arrhythmias on ambulatory electrocardiographic recording.

The identification of high risk patients with inducible ventricular arrhythmias during the postinfarction period may, however, define a group at high risk for arrhythmic death in whom control of ventricular arrhythmias by medical and surgical therapy may improve long-term mortality and form the basis for a population for controlled randomized antiarrhythmic therapy trials.

Prognostic Indices

Multiple risk factors have been investigated by univariate analyses and found to be important prognostic indicators of mortality and survival after AMI [7, 9, 39, 43, 57, 59, 60, 61, 63,

176]. These univariately significant indicators for prognosis may be selected at different times during and after hospitalization and may differ in their significance, although the importance and independence of such variables cannot be assessed by simple statistical methods [4, 7, 73, 177]. In simple prognostication and stratification schemes, principles of prognostic risk factor selection are used to classify a patient into a high risk or a low risk group. Such prognostic schemes utilize the frequency of risk factors from historical, standard laboratory, and clinical data, which may provide an indirect measure of the extent of myocardial damage and the resulting impairment of cardiac performance [114, 178]. Prognostic information from the physical examination have included heart rate, systolic blood pressure, respiration rate, temperature, shock, S_3 gallop rhythm, pulmonary rales, and peripheral edema [179]. Cardiomegaly and severity of pulmonary congestion on the chest radiograph and laboratory data (including leukocyte count, blood urea nitrogen, serum creatinine, cholesterol, and serum enzymes) have been related to outcome. Prognostic information from the electrocardiogram includes the site of infarction, QRS duration, QT interval, ST segment abnormalities, conduction blocks, atrial and ventricular arrhythmias, and sinus tachycardia [179]. The hemodynamic measurements of compromised left ventricular function during AMI more accurately distinguish death and survivors by such indices as left ventricular filling pressure, stroke volume index, left ventricular stroke work index, cardiac output, cardiac index, arteriovenous oxygen difference, and left ventricular ejection fraction [7, 89, 90].

First prognostic indices were devised by assigning weights to the various factors observed during the first 24 hours after admission [59]. Schnur's pathologic index rating system used 19 historical and clinical variables, some of which were graded according to the severity of the finding. This prognostic scoring system was applied to 230 patients surviving the first 24 hours after hospitalization and allowed distinction of five patient groups. The long-term mortality in the lowest

group was 8 percent and for the highest patient group 95 percent.

Peel et al. developed a prognostic index in 1962 based on assigned weights from the clinical impressions of their relative prognostic importance [60]. Their index assigned numerical values to six factors—age, sex, previous history, shock, heart failure, the electrocardiogram and rhythm disturbances during the first 24 hours after admission—to obtain a patient's prognostic score. The index was applied to 628 patients with five score ranges that produced patient groups with 30-day mortality rates from 2.5 to 88.5 percent. An accurate prediction of early death was obtained only in patients with very high scores, but precise prediction of death and survival was not possible in patients with lower scores. The Peel index has been tested by other investigators and used as a single variable within other multivariate prognostic schemes [39, 93].

The construction of more precise prognostic indices was facilitated by the development of multivariate statistical methodologies and the use of computers, including multiple objective and quantitative indicators, and considering the relative importance and interdependency of risk variables to a final prognostic function. Hughes et al. attempted to predict hospital mortality in a retrospective study of 445 patients from three hospitals using 20 historical, admission, and early postadmission variables in a linear discriminant function analysis [47]. From the variables of age, white blood cell count, temperature, systolic blood pressure, presence of conduction defects, pulmonary infarction, congestive heart failure, and shock, 97 percent of the survivors and 80 percent of the deaths were correctly classified. Lemlish et al. applied multiple linear regression to 368 patients to develop a ranking system of several important factors for 30-day mortality or survival [180]. The relative importance of prognostic indicators was identified by the ranking order of blood pressure, history of a previous myocardial infarction, age, temperature, and duration of elevated temperature. McHugh et al. used multiple linear regression in 42 patients predicting in-hospital mortality by a weighted combination of mixed venous oxygen saturation, chest radiographic determination of left ventricular failure, and the Peel index as an individual variable [93]. Shubin et al. predicted outcome for 20 shock patients by discriminant analysis from stroke volume index and diastolic arterial pressure measured serially over the first 80 hours after admission with a 94 percent predictive accuracy [89].

Norris and associates presented in 1970 a method using discriminant function analysis that had selected indicators from historical and admission data for the prediction of in-hospital and 3-year mortality [11]. Univariately significant factors were further quantitated and discriminant weights computed for index scores that divided patients into six groups, each with increasing mortality. Prognostic indicators for in-hospital outcome included age, location of infarct, admission systolic blood pressure, heart size, and the presence of congestive heart failure from the chest radiograph and the history of infarction or angina. Prognostic indicators for late outcome were only age, heart size and congestive failure on the chest radiograph, and previous infarction or angina. The Norris and Peel indices have been tested by other investigators on various infarct populations [181, 182].

Studies of late outcome after myocardial infarction have utilized historical and clinical variables from the time of admission, from the early hospital course and prior to the time of discharge from the CCU [43, 57, 61], or the entire hospital course [13, 36, 41, 57, 178]. The only prognostic variables consistently identified during the later in-hospital period are pulmonary congestion on the chest radiograph [43, 178, 183] and certain ventricular arrhythmias [13, 36, 39, 41, 43, 57, 61, 112]. However, data from the first 24 to 48 hours after onset of myocardial infarction may allow risk prediction from 6 to 36 months after acute infarction [43, 57, 61]. In one study, linear regression selected from 42 factors from the history and the first 48 hours after admission the ten variables of age, female gender, diabetes, previous angina, blood pressure, clinical and radiographic left ventricular failure, high LDH level, high blood urea nitrogen, and high leukocyte count [43]. The prognostic score from these variables correctly classified 90 percent of the patients at 1 month and 86 percent at 6 months, allowing early in-hospital identification of patients with risk of late death.

In a study from our group, data from the history and the first 24 hours of hospitalization predicted 1-year death and survival; it predicted equally well as the data from the entire hospital course [57]. Discriminant function analysis identified in 818 patients discharged from hospital five important factors from the 24-hour data: maximal level of blood urea nitrogen, previous myocardial infarction, age, displaced left ventricular apex on physical examination, and sinus bradycardia. When data from the entire hospital stay were included, extension of infarction and maximal heart rate in the CCU were also selected. Examining variables including discharge parameters, the presence of S_3 gallop, and abnormal apex were important for prediction of 1-year mortality. Left ventricular ejection fraction and the presence of complex ventricular arrhythmias during a 24-hour ambulatory electrocardiographic recording were independent predictors of 6-month and 1-year mortality, but correct classification of 58 percent of the deaths and 79 percent of the survivors from clinical data alone was not further improved by more than 2 percent with the inclusion of ejection fraction and ambulatory electrocardiographic ECG monitoring.

Studies on risk factor identification, high risk prediction, and stratification have used different infarct populations and different analytic methodologies. The commonly employed multivariate schemes provide similar precise prognostic evaluation with applicability to test populations in the same or a different institution [7, 13, 36, 37, 184]. A reliable risk identification scheme requires validation before its generalization to other populations. These problems have been investigated in one of our studies that used four separate multivariate methodologies for predicting death and survival at 30 days after myocardial infarction [185]. Predictive schemes were constructed using stepwise discriminant analysis, logistic regression, recursive partitioning, and a nearest neighbor procedure. The four methods were then used on a second population, and the reliability of a risk identification scheme within each population was assessed by a cross-validation procedure. Subsequently, each scheme constructed from the data of one population was tested on the data from the other. One study population had 295 patients who were admitted to the University of California (San Diego) Medical Center (UCSD) and the other 407 patients admitted to the Vancouver General Hospital (VGH) in British Columbia [185]. Similar predictors showed the same trends and patterns of significance for both populations. Population differences indicated that the VGH population was older but had a lower incidence of predictive factors of previous myocardial infarction, history of chronic obstructive lung disease, S_3 gallop on admission, rales above the scapula on admission, third-degree atrioventricular block, and anterior infarct location. Maximum heart rate within the first 24 hours and admission heart rate were higher for the UCSD population, whereas respiration rate was higher for the VGH population.

Using stepwise discriminant analysis, logistic regression, and recursive partitioning, the relative importance of each of the candidate predictor variables included in the analyses was identified for both populations. Only one predictor (maximum heart rate during the first 24 hours after admission) played a role in all six analyses. Four other variables were identified in five of the six analyses and included age, third-degree atrioventricular block, pulmonary congestion on chest radiograph, and minimum systolic blood pressure during the first 24 hours after admission. Age and pulmonary congestion on chest radiograph had a high rank in each of the analyses, whereas the importance of the other two factors varied. Variables that were highly significant for one population but not for the other, such as history of congestive heart failure, tended to enter the analysis for that population only and not the other.

CROSS-VALIDATION WITHIN POPULATIONS

The three methodologies cross-validated performed better on the complete UCSD data (a reduction in error risk of close to 50 percent) than on the complete data from VGH (a reduction in error risk of about 30 percent). For both populations, recursive partitioning produced the lowest error risk and correctly classified 72 percent of early deaths and 85 percent of survivors within the UCSD population and 85 percent of early deaths but only 65 percent of survivors within the VGH population [185]. When patients with some missing data for UCSD were included, the error risk increased. However, for the VGH population only a minor increase in the error risk was observed, indicating that some missing data are tolerable but that too much decreases the performance for the method of recursive partitioning.

BETWEEN-POPULATION CLASSIFICATION

When the risk prediction schemes for VGH were used to predict for UCSD, the error risks for the three methods were lower than those when UCSD data were used to predict for VGH. This finding represented a reduction in error risk by 40, 44, 11, and 11 percent for UCSD and by 20, 30, 11, and 3 percent for VGH, similar to the reduction in error risk achieved by cross-validation within each population.

Another study from our institution examined four methodologies for predicting short-term outcome after acute infarction using risk factor selection, discriminant function analysis, recursive partitioning, and Cox multivariate analysis [186]. Similar correct classification rates were obtained in the four multivariate schemes providing equally precise prognostic evaluation. Thus the choice of methodology for prognostication is often based on other considerations, such as ease of use as in the method of recursive partitioning, or the ability to accurately assess individual risk as provided in the Cox models.

Madsen et al. compared linear discriminant analysis, Cox regression, and recursive partitioning for prediction of short-term (36 day) and long-term (1 year) mortality using two independent populations [73]. Each scheme performed similarly for prediction of short-term mortality, with a 90 percent correct classification rate of deaths in the base sample and an 87 percent correct classification rate in a test population by discriminant analysis, and 89 percent for the other two methods. For 1-year mortality, recursive partitioning performed better than the two other methods on the test population using congestive heart failure in the CCU as the first discriminant variable.

VALIDATION STUDIES OF RISK PREDICATION SCHEMES

Previously developed risk prediction schemes have shown good performance in risk identification in the population used to develop such schemes rather than in an independent test population. The need for validation was first developed by Peel et al., who used a cohort of patients admitted to their center from 1958 to 1961 to assess and amend the weightings for each risk factor in their original prognostic index [60]. The factors and their weights were introduced into that prognostic index based on general clinical impressions of their importance for prognosis at 4 weeks. The scheme was then applied to additional earlier cohorts comprised of patients who were admitted from 1946 to 1950 and those admitted from 1951 to 1957. Both the percentages of patients falling in the four prognostic categories established from the index and the mortality for each prognostic group varied, however, by as much as 100 percent among the three cohorts. Other studies have applied the Peel index to their own population groups [93, 181]. The validation studies used small patient samples. The high Peel scores predictive of death were associated with error rates of up to 37 percent for survivors and 21 percent for deaths; similar error rates were seen for the base population used to construct the index, with 31 percent error rate for survivors and 18 percent for deaths.

The Norris index for in-hospital mortality, developed by discriminant function analysis, has been tested in other institutions [181, 184]. In the original population of 757 patients high index scores predictive of death had a 30 percent error rate for deaths and 40 percent for survivors [11, 187]. Error rates in subsequent test populations were lower than those in the original population, ranging from 12 to 22 percent for survivors and 4 to 19 percent for deaths.

Previous studies have attempted to validate the prognostic indices in groups of patients from another institution or new populations from the same institution [8, 13, 36, 75, 178, 184]. Some studies carry low prediction error rates for survivors and others low prediction rates for deaths at the relative cost for misclassification of either deaths or survivors (Table 38-3). The prediction schemes developed by linear discriminant function analysis were associated with overall error rates within 6 percent of that derived from their base population. Habib et al. [182] compared the Norris index developed by discriminant function analysis with the Chapman index [188] developed by multiple regression in a small independent population. They found 88.3 percent total correct classification for the Chapman index and 77.7 percent for the Norris index. However, Rotmensch et al. found a lesser performance for the Norris index, with only 38.6 percent correct classification [181]. This study also tested the Peel index with higher total correct classification but with very low correct classification of the deaths (15 percent).

Moss et al. applied their two prognostic stratification schemes for a 4-month mortality that was developed on a 1973 cohort to patients studied during 1974 [178]. Only one of the schemes performed satisfactorily on the 1974 population, as the mortalities for the low and high risk groups were not statistically different using the other scheme.

The application of prognostic stratification techniques developed by Moss et al. showed high error rates when applied to populations of other institutions [11, 183]. The identified prognostic predictors (20 or more PVCs per hour, history of angina with moderate activity or at rest, and hypotension or heart failure in the CCU) were applied by Bigger et al. [183] without differences in mortality rates when compared to patients in their population with-

Table 38-3
Validation results for risk stratification schemes

First author	Period	Method[a]	No. of pts.[b]	No. of survivors	No. of deaths
Chapelle [184]	14 days	LDF	B 159 (.18)[c]	142 (.18)[c]	17 (.18)[c]
			T 201 (.16)	176 (.15)	25 (.24)
Henning [7]	30 days	LDF	B 177 (.07)	143 (.03)	33 (.27)
			T 150 (.12)	123 (.04)	27 (.48)
Evans [66]	3 months	LDF	B 298 (.29)	249 (.33)	49 (.04)
			T 437 (.35)	362 (.44)	95 (.04)
Moss [178]	4 months	PS	B 269 (.13)	258 (.12)	11 (.36)
			T 234 (.16)	223 (.14)	11 (.55)
Helmers [13]	1 year	AID	B 308 (.24)	255 (.21)	53 (.38)
			T 163 (.21)	141 (.20)	22 (.32)
Luria [36]	2 years	LDF	B 137 (.17)	110 (.06)	27 (.59)
			T 105 (.14)	91 (.08)	22 (.57)

[a]LDF = linear discriminant function analysis; PS = prognostic stratification; AID = automatic interaction detection.
[b]B = base sample; T = test sample.
[c]Numbers in parentheses are the percent error (percent of the group incorrectly classified).

out these predictors. The lack of cross-validation of a prediction scheme in this study was attributed to the discrepancy of the two patient populations with respect to age, mortality at 4 months, cardiac status, and urban versus suburban locale.

In a much larger study involving the placebo group of 2789 patients in the Coronary Drug Project, it was observed that even though very different variables proved important within each of two geographically separated subpopulations, acceptable performance for 3-year mortality was achieved when this scheme was applied to the other population and subsequently to a third group of patients from clinics not part of the Coronary Drug Project [41]. Our studies have indicated that cross-population testing of various prediction schemes produces acceptable classification results for deaths and survivors when applied to new populations, with total correct classification ranging from 50 to 68 percent [185, 186].

Low Risk Identification

The goal of risk stratification and prognostication after AMI is to include a scheme that allows stratification of the individual patient into high risk or low risk status. A low risk status implies a less than 2 percent risk of cardiac death during the first year after myocardial infarction and a reduced probability of recurrent infarction and rehospitalization for new-onset angina [66, 189–191]. Patients after myocardial infarction identified as having low risk status would be candidates for early discharge and early resumption of normal physical activities and reemployment.

There has been a decreasing trend in median hospitalization time for patients with uncomplicated myocardial infarction, from a 21-day average hospital stay in 1970 to 14 days in 1979 [192]. A number of studies have shown that discharge even earlier than days 5 to 9 after acute infarction is feasible for selected patients, with apparently small increase in risk [66, 189, 193, 194]. In a controlled study of 268 patients, which comprised 70 percent of the total studied population randomized to discharge on day 9 or day 16 after admission with acute infarction, no significant differences during a 6 weeks' follow-up were reported for death, chest pain, congestive heart failure, arrhythmias, or readmission [66]. The same authors developed a prognostic index by discriminant function analysis in 298 patients that allocated 56 percent of the total infarct population to a risk group that carried a 3-month mortality of 1.2 percent, in contrast to a high risk group that had a 36 percent mortality and represented 43.6 percent of their study population [189]. The low risk identification required the absence of certain risk variables: electrocardiographic ST segment elevation of more than 2 mm, more than 40 ventricular ectopic beats per hour, the presence of R on T ventricular ectopic beats, persistent sinus tachycardia, blood urea nitrogen over 12 mmol/L, signs of congestive heart failure on chest radiograph, and age. In a smaller study, 67 patients (42 percent of the study population) without serious complications from day 1 to day 4 were randomized to discharge 1 week after admission in the absence of ventricular tachycardia or fibrillation, advanced-degree heart block, pulmonary edema, cardiogenic shock, sinus tachycardia, hypotension, rapid atrial arrhythmias, or extension of infarction [195]. No complications or death occurred in either of these small groups of patients during a 6-month follow-up period. These studies have used insufficient sample sizes to detect an event rate that is significantly greater than the 4 to 6 percent event rate during the first year after myocardial infarction expected in the low risk patients.

Other uncontrolled studies have defined low risk criteria for the selection of patients for early discharge resulting in low event rates of 0 to 2.7 percent during the early postdischarge period of 2 to 6 months [190, 191]. Madsen et al. in a retrospective study of 1140 patients with AMI used a daily risk assessment scheme on a Cox regression analysis that assigned the patient to a low risk of events of death, cardiac arrest, or cardiogenic shock with a projected incidence of less than 2 percent [189]. Of the study population, 47 percent of patients fulfilled early discharge criteria but were kept in hospital until day 18 after admission. Only one death and a 2 percent event rate occurred in this group during a 30-day observation period. The same institution has prospectively discharged 67 percent of 169 consecutive patients that survived day 5, and only 1.7 percent unexpected deaths occurred between 12 and 24 days after discharge. For low risk identification most investigators used a set of exclusion criteria that have included infarct extension, persistent chest pain, signs of congestive heart failure, hypotension or cardiogenic shock, or severe arrhythmias (ventricular tachycardia, ventricular fibrillation, supraventricular tachycardia, atrial fibrillation, atrioventricular block, nodal rhythm, or frequent or complex ventricular ectopic beats). Other studies have also identified elderly patients and those with a history of previous myocardial infarction not suitable for early discharge [66, 196].

Our previous studies identified a group of patients at low risk of cardiac endpoints between days 9 and 90 after acute infarction. Patients with complications from days 1 to 8 that would preclude early discharge were excluded when death, persistent pain beyond the first day after admission, extension of infarct, ventricular tachycardia or fibrillation, cardiac arrest, second- or third-degree heart block or congestive heart failure occurred. Linear discriminant analysis identified a group comprising 25 percent of the total population with a 2.3 percent mortality between days 9 and 90, as well as a 4.6 percent combined death and complication rate during this period. The events in the low risk group included one patient with extension of infarction on day 9, recurrent infarction on days 42 and 45, and one sudden death 23 days after discharge. In this identified low risk group, younger age was observed, a lower incidence of previous congestive heart failure, hypertension, family history, complex Holter arrhythmias, and higher ejection fractions.

Exercise testing [120–123] and exercise thallium 201 scintigraphy testing [139, 141, 142] have been shown to identify low risk patients after myocardial infarction with annual mortality rates of less than 2 percent. Similarly, we identified a low risk group among patients with a first myocardial infarction [197]. Patients with a first myocardial infarction at age less than 50 years with a left ventricular ejection fraction over 40 percent and those patients between 51 and 70 years with a left ventricular ejection fraction over 50 percent had only a 1.2 percent cardiac mortality within the first year. In this study, ejection fraction as the only predischarge test identified a sizable low risk group of patients with a first myocardial infarction that comprised 47 percent of individuals with a first myocardial infarction. Studies on low risk identification in patients undergoing coronary reperfusion therapy by thrombolysis, angioplasty, or both defined low risk in the absence of angina, congestive heart failure, ventricular arrhythmias, and provocable ischemia on exercise testing; and they discharged these patients 3 days after admission without fatal events during the 6-month follow-up period, with a substantial reduction in hospital costs [198].

Further studies on low risk identification and its applicability for early discharge are required to provide general implications for low risk stratification after myocardial infarction and to provide a safe selection procedure for the early discharge of patients after AMI.

References

1. Stern, M. P. The recent decline in ischemic heart disease mortality. *Ann. Intern. Med.* 91:630, 1979.
2. Thom, T. J., and Kannel, W. B. Downward trend in cardiovascular mortality. *Annu. Rev. Med.* 32:427, 1981.
3. Havlik, R. K., and Feinleib, M. *Proceedings of the Conferences on the Decline in Coronary Heart Disease Mortality.* NIH Publication 79:1610. U.S. Department of Health, Education and Welfare, 1979.
4. Gilpin, E. A., Koziol, J. A., Madsen, E. B., et al. Periods of differing mortality distribution during the first year after acute myocardial infarction. *Am. J. Cardiol.* 52:240, 1983.
5. Helmers, C., Lundman, R., Maasing, R., and Wester, P. O. Mortality pattern among initial survivors of acute myocardial infarction using a life table technique. *Acta Med. Scand.* 200:469, 1976.
6. Carlisle, R., and Lewis, A. F. Survival curves applied to acute myocardial infarction. *Am. Heart J.* 94:807, 1977.
7. Henning, H., Gilpin, E., Covell, J. W., et al. Prognosis after acute myocardial infarction: A multivariate analysis of mortality and survival. *Circulation* 59:1124, 1979.
8. Juergens, J. L., Edwards, J. E., and Achor, R. W. Prognosis of patients surviving first clinically diagnosed myocardial infarction. *Arch. Intern. Med.* 105:444, 1960.
9. Honey, G. E., and Truelove, S. C. Prognostic factors in myocardial infarction. *Lancet* 1:1155, 1957.
10. Pell, S., and D'Alonzo, C. A. Immediate mortality and five year survival of employed men with a first myocardial infarction. *N. Engl. J. Med.* 270:915, 1964.
11. Norris, R. M., Caughey, D. E., Deeming, L. W., et al. Coronary prognostic index for predicting survival after recovery from acute myocardial infarction. *Lancet* 2:485, 1970.
12. Norris, R. M., Caughey, D. E., and Deeming, L. W. Prognosis following acute myocardial infarction. *N. Z. Med. J.* 77:12, 1973.
13. Helmers, C. Short and long-term prognostic indices in acute myocardial infarction: A study of 606 patients initially treated in a CCU. *Acta Med. Scand.* [Suppl.] 555:1973.
14. Day, H. W. Effectiveness of an intensive coronary care area. *Am. J. Cardiol.* 15:51, 1965.
15. Goble, A. J., Sloman, G., and Robinson, J. S. Mortality reduction in a coronary care unit. *Br. Med. J.* 1:1005, 1966.
16. Peterson, D. R., Thompson, D. J., and Chinn, N. Ischemic heart disease prognosis: A community-wide assessment (1966–1969). *J.A.M.A.* 219:1423, 1972.
17. Elveback, L. K., Connolly, D. C., and Kurland, L. T. Coronary heart disease in residents of Rochester, Minnesota. II. Mortality, incidence and survivorship 1950–1975. *Mayo Clin. Proc.* 56:665, 1981.
18. Gillum, R. F., Folsom, A., and Luepker, R. V. Sudden death and acute myocardial infarction in a metropolitan area, 1970–1980: The Minnesota Heart Survey. *N. Engl. J. Med.* 309:1353, 1983.
19. Gruppo Italiano per lo Studio delta Streptochinasi nell'Infarto Miocardico (GISS). Effectiveness of intravenous thrombolytic treatment in acute myocardial infarction. *Lancet* 1:397, 1986.
20. ISIS Steering Committee. Intravenous streptokinase given within 0–4 hours of onset of myocardial infarction reduced mortality in ISIS-2. *Lancet* 1:502, 1987.
21. Krone, R. J., Gillespie, J. A., Weld, F. M., et al. Low-level exercise testing after myocardial infarction: Usefulness in enhancing clinical risk stratification. *Circulation* 71:80, 1985.
22. Gibson, R. S., Watson, D. D., Craddock, G. B., et al. Prediction of cardiac events after uncomplicated myocardial infarction: A prospective study comparing predischarge exercise thallium-201 scintigraphy and coronary angiography. *Circulation* 68:321, 1983.
23. Elwood, P. C. Aspirin in the prevention of myocardial infarction: Current status. *Drugs* 28:1, 1984.
24. Norwegian Multicenter Study Group: Timolol-induced reduction in mortality and reinfarction in patients surviving acute myocardial infarction. *N. Engl. J. Med.* 304:801, 1981.
25. Herlitz, J., Elmfeldt, D., Holmberg, S., et

al. Goteborg metoprolol trial: Mortality and causes of death. *Am. J. Cardiol.* 53:9D, 1984.

26. Beta-Blocker Heart Attack Study Group: The Beta-Blocker Heart Attack Trial. *J.A.M.A.* 246:2073, 1981.

27. CASS Principal Investigators and Their Associates. Coronary Artery Surgery Study (CASS): A randomized trial of coronary artery bypass surgery: Survival data. *Circulation* 68:939, 1983.

28. CASS Principal Investigators and Their Associates. Myocardial infarction and mortality in the Coronary Artery Surgery Study (CASS) randomized trial. *N. Engl. J. Med.* 310:750, 1984.

29. Moss, A. J., DeCamilia, J., Davis, H., and Bayer, L. The early posthospital phase of myocardial infarction. *Circulation* 54:58, 1976.

30. Kannel, W. B., Sortic, P., and McNamara, P. M. Prognosis after initial myocardial infarction: The Framingham Study. *Am. J. Cardiol.* 44:53, 1979.

31. Vedin, J. A., Wilhelmsson, C., Elmfeldt, D., et al. Sudden death: Identification of high risk groups. *Am. Heart J.* 86:124, 1973.

32. Jelinek, V. M., McDonald, I. G., Ryan, W. F., et al. Assessment of cardiac risk 10 days after uncomplicated myocardial infarction. *Br. Med. J.* 284:227, 1982.

33. Kjoller, E., Mortensen, L. S., Larsen, S., et al. Long term prognosis after acute myocardial infarction. *Dan. Med. Bull.* 26:199, 1979.

34. Lofmark, R. Clinical features in patients with recurrent myocardial infarction. *Acta Med. Scand.* 206:367, 1979.

35. Kentala, E., Pyorala, K., Heikkila, J., et al. Factors related to long-term prognosis following acute myocardial infarction: Importance of left ventricular function. *Scand. J. Rehabil. Med.* 7:118, 1975.

36. Luria, M. H., Knoke, J. D., Margolis, R. M., et al. Acute myocardial infarction prognosis after recovery. *Ann. Intern. Med.* 85:561, 1976.

37. Vedin, A., Wilhelmsen, L., Wedel, H., et al. Prediction of cardiovascular deaths and nonfatal reinfarctions after myocardial infarction. *Acta Med. Scand.* 201:309, 1977.

38. Davis, H. T., De Camilla, J., Bayer, L. W., and Moss, A. J. Survivorship patterns in the posthospital phase of myocardial infarction. *Circulation* 60:1252, 1979.

39. Moss, A. J., DeCamilla, J., Engstrom, F., et al. The posthospital phase of myocardial infarction: Identification of patients with increased mortality risk. *Circulation* 49:460, 1974.

40. Bay, K. S., Lee, S. J. K., Flathman, D. P., and Roll, J. W. Application of step-wise discriminant analysis and Bayesian classification procedure in determining prognosis of acute myocardial infarction. *Can. Med. Assoc. J.* 115:887, 1976.

41. Coronary Drug Project Research Group. Factors influencing long-term prognosis after recovery from myocardial infarction—three year findings of the coronary drug project. *J. Chronic Dis.* 27:267, 1974.

42. Helmers, C. Assessment of 3-year prognosis in survivors of acute myocardial infarction. *Br. Heart J.* 37:593, 1975.

43. Beaune, J., Touboul, P., Boissel, J. P., and Belhaye, J. P. Quantitative assessment of myocardial infarction prognosis to 1 and 6 months from clinical data. *Eur. J. Cardiol.* 8:629, 1978.

44. Ruberman, W., Weinblatt, E., Goldberg, J. D., et al. Ventricular premature beats and mortality after myocardial infarction. *N. Engl. J. Med.* 297:750, 1977.

45. Sanz, G., Castaner, A., Betriu, A., et al. Determinants of prognosis in survivors of myocardial infarction. *N. Engl. J. Med.* 306:106, 1982.

46. Zukel, W. J., Cohen, B. M., and Mattingly, T. W. Survival following first diagnosis of coronary heart disease. *Am. Heart J.* 78:159, 1969.

47. Hughes, W. I., Kalbfleisch, J. M., Brandt, E. N., and Costiloe, J. P. Myocardial infarction prognosis by discriminant analysis. *Arch. Intern. Med.* 3:120, 1963.

48. Mosbech, J., and Dreyer, K. Coronary occlusion in Denmark: Morbidity and mortality. *Acta Med. Scand.* 180:429, 1966.

49. Wolffenbuttel, B. H. R., Verdouw, P. D., and Hugenholtz, P. G. Immediate and two year prognosis after acute myocardial infarction: Prediction from noninvasive as well as invasive parameters in the same individuals. *Eur. Heart J.* 2:375, 1981.

50. Goldberg, R., Szklo, M., and Tonascia, J. Time trends in prognosis of patients with myocardial infarction: A population-based study. *Johns Hopkins Med. J.* 144:73, 1979.

51. Goldberg, R. J., Gore, J. M., and Alpert, J. S. Recent changes in attack and survival rates of acute myocardial infarction (1975 through 1981): The Worcester Heart Attack Study. *J.A.M.A.* 255:2774, 1986.

52. Goldberg, R. J., Gore, J. M., and Alpert, J. S. Non-Q wave myocardial infarction: Recent changes in occurrence and prognosis—a community-wide perspective. *Am. Heart J.* 113:273, 1987.

53. Maisel, A. S., Ahnve, S., Gilpin, E., et al. Prognosis after extension of myocardial infarct: The role of Q-wave or non-Q-wave infarction. *Circulation* 71:211, 1985.

54. Kjoller, E. The long-term prognosis after

acute myocardial infarction. *Dan. Med. Bull.* 22:202, 1971.

55. Beard, O. W., Hipp, H. R., Robins, M., et al. Initial myocardial infarction among veterans: Ten-year survival. *Am. Heart J.* 73:317, 1967.

56. Martin, C. A., Thompson, P. L., Armstrong, B. K., et al. Long-term prognosis after recovery from myocardial infarction: A nine year follow-up of the Perth Coronary Register. *Circulation* 68:961, 1983.

57. Madsen, E. B., Gilpin, E., Henning, H., et al. Prediction of late mortality after myocardial infarction from variables measured at different times during hospitalization. *Am. J. Cardiol.* 53:47, 1984.

58. Weinblatt, E., Goldberg, J. D., Ruberman, W., et al. Mortality after first myocardial infarction: Search for a secular trend. *J.A.M.A.* 247:1576, 1982.

59. Schnur, S. Mortality rates in acute myocardial infarction. II. A proposed method for measuring quantitatively severity of illness on admission to the hospital. *Ann. Intern. Med.* 39:1018, 1953.

60. Peel, A. A. F., Semple, T., Wang, I., et al. A coronary prognostic index for grading the severity of infarction. *Br. Heart J.* 24:745, 1962.

61. Norris, R. M., Caughey, D. E., Mercer, C. J., et al. Coronary prognostic index for predicting survival after recovery from acute myocardial infarction. *Lancet* 2:485, 1970.

62. Rosenbaum, F. F., and Levine, F. A. Prognostic value of various clinical and electrocardiographic features of acute myocardial infarction. *Arch. Intern. Med.* 68:913, 1941.

63. Cole, D. R., Singian, E. B., and Katz, L. N. The long-term prognosis following myocardial infarction and some factors which affect it. *Circulation* 9:321, 1954.

64. Battler, A., Karliner, J. S., Higgins, C. B., et al. The initial chest x-ray in acute myocardial infarction: Prediction of early and late mortality and survival. *Circulation* 61:1004, 1980.

65. Killip, T., and Kimball, J. I. Treatment of myocardial infarction in a coronary care unit: A two-year experience with 250 patients. *Am. J. Cardiol.* 20:457, 1967.

66. Evans, A. E., Boyle, D. Mc. C., Barber, J. M., et al. Safe selection of coronary patients for early discharge. *Eur. Heart J.* 2:395, 1981.

67. Multicenter Postinfarction Research Group: Risk stratification and survival after myocardial infarction. *N. Engl. J. Med.* 309:331, 1983.

68. Toller, G. H., Stone, P. H., Muller, J. E., et al. Effects of gender and race on prognosis after myocardial infarction: Adverse prognosis for women, particularly black women. *J. Am. Coll. Cardiol.* 9:473, 1987.

69. Smith, J. W., Marcus, F. I., and Serokman, H., et al. Prognosis of patients with diabetes mellitus after acute myocardial infarction. *Am. J. Cardiol.* 54:718, 1984.

70. Merrilees, M. A., Scott, P. J., and Norris, H. M. Prognosis after myocardial infarction: Results of 15-year follow-up. *Br. Med. J.* 288:356, 1984.

71. Coronary Drug Project Research Group: Blood pressure in survivors of myocardial infarction. *J. Am. Coll. Cardiol.* 4:134, 1984.

72. Hoit, B. D., Gilpin, E. A., Maisel, A. S., et al. Influence of obesity on morbidity and mortality after acute myocardial infarction. *Am. Heart J.* 114:1334, 1987.

73. Madsen, E. B., Gilpin, E., and Henning, H. Short-term prognosis in acute myocardial infarction: Evaluation of different prediction methods. *Am. Heart J.* 107:1241, 1984.

74. Coronary Drug Project Research Group: The prognostic importance of the electrocardiogram after myocardial infarction: Experience in the coronary drug project. *Ann. Intern. Med.* 77:677, 1972.

75. Schuster, E. H., and Bulkley, B. H. Early post-infarction angina: Ischemia at a distance and ischemia in the infarct zone. *N. Engl. J. Med.* 35:1101, 1981.

76. Maisel, A. S., Gilpin, E., Hoit, B., et al. Survival after hospital discharge in matched populations with inferior or anterior myocardial infarction. *J. Am. Coll. Cardiol.* 6:731, 1985.

77. Hands, M. E., Lloyd, B. L., Robinson, J. S., et al. Prognostic significance of electrocardiographic site of infarction after correction for enzymatic size of infarction. *Circulation* 73:885, 1986.

78. Kannel, W. B., and Abbott, R. D. Incidence and prognosis of unrecognized myocardial infarction. *N. Engl. J. Med.* 311:1144, 1984.

79. Becker, L. C., Silverman, K. J., Bulkley, B. H., et al. Comparison of early thallium-201 scintigraphy and gated blood pool imaging for predicting mortality in patients with acute myocardial infarction. *Circulation* 67:1272, 1983.

80. Holman, B. L., Chisholm, B. J., and Braunwald, E. The prognostic implications of acute myocardial infarct scintigraphy with 99m Tc-pyrophosphate. *Circulation* 57:320, 1978.

81. Madias, J. E., Chahine, R. A., Gorlin, R., and Blacklow, D. J. A comparison of transmural and nontransmural myocardial infarction. *Circulation* 49:498, 1974.

82. Rigo, P., Murray, M., Taylor, D. R., et al. Hemodynamic and prognostic findings in patient with transmural and nontransmural infarction. *Circulation* 51:1064, 1975.

83. Szklo, M., Goldberg, R., and Kennedy, H. L. Survival of patients with transmural infarction: A population-based study. *Am. J. Cardiol.* 42:648, 1978.

84. Hutter, A. M., DeSanctis, R. W., Flynn, T., and Yeatman, L. A. Nontransmural myocardial infarction: A comparison of hospital and late clinical course of patients with that of matched patients with transmural anterior and transmural inferior myocardial infarction. *Am. J. Cardiol.* 48:595, 1981.

85. Waters, D. D., Pelletier, G. B., and Hache, M. Myocardial infarction in patients with previous coronary artery bypass surgery. *J. Am. Coll. Cardiol.* 3:909, 1984.

86. Nicholson, M. R., Boubin, G. S., Bernstein, L., et al. Prognosis after an initial non-Q-wave myocardial infarction related to coronary arterial anatomy. *Am. J. Cardiol.* 52:462, 1983.

87. Theroux, P., Kouz, S., and Bosch, X. Clinical and angiographic features of non-Q and Q wave myocardial infarction. *Circulation* 74(Suppl II):303, 1986.

88. Gibson, R. S., Beller, G. A., Gheoghiade, M., et al. The prevalence and clinical significance of residual myocardial ischemia 2 weeks after uncomplicated non-Q wave infarction: A prospective natural history study. *Circulation* 73:1186, 1986.

89. Shubin, H., Afifi, A. A., Rand, W. M., and Weil, M. H. Objective index of hemodynamic status for quantification of severity and prognosis of shock complicating myocardial infarction. *Cardiovasc. Res.* 4:329, 1968.

90. Verdouw, P. D., Hagemeijer, F., van Dorp, W. G., et al. Short-term survival after acute myocardial infarction predicted by hemodynamic parameters. *Circulation* 52:413, 1975.

91. Battler, A., Slutsky, R., Karliner, J., et al. Left ventricular ejection fraction and first-third ejection fraction early after acute myocardial infarction: Predictive value for mortality and survival. *Am. J. Cardiol.* 45:797, 1980.

92. Nicod, P., Gilpin, E., Dittrich, H., et al. Influence on prognosis and morbidity of left ventricular ejection fraction with and without signs of left ventricular failure after acute myocardial infarction. *Am. J. Cardiol.* 61:1165, 1988.

93. McHugh, T. J., and Swan, H. J. C. Prognostic indicators in acute myocardial infarction. *Geriatrics* 26:72, 1971.

94. Mukharji, J., Rude, R. E., Poole, W. K., et al. Risk factors for sudden death after acute myocardial infarction: Two-year follow-up. *Am. J. Cardiol.* 54:31, 1984.

95. Bigger, J. T., Fleiss, J. L., Kleiger, R., et al. The relationships among ventricular dysfunction, and mortality in the 2 years after myocardial infarction. *Circulation* 69:250, 1984.

96. Ahnve, S., Gilpin, E., Henning, H., et al. Limitations and advantages of the ejection fraction for defining high risk after acute myocardial infarction. *Am. J. Cardiol.* 58:872, 1986.

97. Madsen, E. B., Gilpin, E., Slutsky, R. A., et al. Usefulness of the chest x-ray for predicting abnormal left ventricular function after acute myocardial infarction. *Am. Heart J.* 108:1431, 1984.

98. Dewhurst, N. G., and Muir, A. L. Comparative prognostic value of radionuclide ventriculography at rest and during exercise in 100 patients after first myocardial infarction. *Br. Heart J.* 49:111, 1983.

99. Morris, K. G., Palmeri, S. T., Califf, R. M., et al. Value of radionuclide angiography for predicting specific cardiac events after acute myocardial infarction. *Am. J. Cardiol.* 55:318, 1985.

100. Kuchar, D. L., Throburn, C. W., and Neville, L. S. Prediction of serious arrhythmic events after myocardial infarction: Signal averaged electrocardiogram, Holter monitoring and radionuclide ventriculography. *J. Am. Coll. Cardiol.* 9:531, 1987.

101. Schelbert, H. R., Henning, H., Ashburn, W. L., et al. Serial measurements of left ventricular ejection fraction by radionuclide angiography early and late after myocardial infarction. *Am. J. Cardiol.* 38:407, 1976.

102. Greenberg, H., McMaster, P., Dwyer, E. M., et al. Left ventricular dysfunction after acute myocardial infarction: Results of a prospective multicenter study. *J. Am. Coll. Cardiol.* 4:867, 1984.

103. Taylor, G. J., Humphries, J. O., Mellits, E. D., et al. Predictors of clinical course, coronary anatomy and left ventricular function after recovery from acute myocardial infarction. *Circulation* 62:960, 1980.

104. Corbett, J. K., Dehmer, G. J., Lewis, S. E., et al. The prognostic value of submaximal exercise testing with radionuclide ventriculography before hospital discharge in patients with recent myocardial infarction. *Circulation* 64:535, 1981.

105. Corbett, J. R., Nicod, P., and Lewis, S. E. Prognostic value of submaximal exercise radionuclide ventriculography after myocardial infarction. *Am. J. Cardiol.* 52:82A, 1983.

106. Morris, K. G., Califf, R. M., and Palmeri, S. T. Independent prognostic value to rest and exercise radionuclide angiography 3 and 8 weeks after infarction. *Circulation* 68:111, 1983.

107. Hung, J., Goris, M. L., Nash, E., et al. Comparative value of maximal treadmill testing, exercise thallium myocardial perfusion scintigraphy and exercise radionuclide ventriculography for distinguishing high- and low-risk patients soon after myocardial infarction. *Am. J. Cardiol.* 53:1221, 1984.

108. Moss, A. J., David, H. T., DeCamilla, J., and Bayer, L. W. Ventricular ectopic beats and

their relation to sudden and nonsudden cardiac death after myocardial infarction. *Circulation* 60:998, 1979.

109. Ruberman, W., Weinblatt, E., Goldberg, J. D., et al. Ventricular premature beats and mortality after myocardial infarction. *N. Engl. J. Med.* 297:750, 1977.

110. Schultze, R. A., Strauss, H. W., and Pitt, B. Sudden death in the year following myocardial infarction: Relation to ventricular premature contractions in the late hospital phase and left ventricular ejection fraction. *Am. J. Med.* 62:192, 1977.

111. Lown, B., and Wolf, M. Approaches to sudden death from coronary heart disease. *Circulation* 44:130, 1971.

112. Vismara, L. A., Amsterdam, E. A., and Mason, D. T. Relationship of ventricular arrhythmias in the late hospital phase of acute myocardial infarction to sudden death after hospital discharge. *Am. J. Med.* 59:6, 1975.

113. Lesch, M., and Kehoe, R. F. Predictability of sudden cardiac death: A partially fulfilled promise. *N. Engl. J. Med.* 310:255, 1984.

114. Madsen, B., Svendsen, L. T., and Rasmussen, S. Multivariate long-term prognostic index from exercise ECG after acute myocardial infarction. *Eur. J. Cardiol.* 11:435, 1980.

115. Coronary Drug Project Research Group: Factors influencing long-term prognosis after recovery from myocardial infarction: Three-year findings of the Coronary Drug Project. *J. Chronic Dis.* 27:267, 1974.

116. Sharma, B., Asinger, R., Francis, G. S., et al. Demonstrations of exercise-induced painless myocardial ischemia in survivors of out-of-hospital ventricular fibrillation. *Am. J. Cardiol.* 59:740, 1987.

117. Morady, F., DiCarlo, L. A., Krol, R. B., et al. Role of myocardial ischemia during programmed stimulation in survivors of cardiac arrest with coronary artery disease. *J. Am. Coll. Cardiol.* 9:1004, 1987.

118. Nicod, P., Gilpin, E., Dittrich, H., et al. Late clinical outcome in patients with early ventricular fibrillation after myocardial infarction. *J. Am. Coll. Cardiol.* 11:464, 1988.

119. Maisel, A. S., Scott, N., Gilpin, E., et al. Complex ventricular arrhythmias in patients with Q wave versus non-Q wave myocardial infarction. *Circulation* 72:963, 1985.

120. Theroux, P., Water, D. D., Halphen, C., et al. Prognostic value of exercise testing soon after myocardial infarction. *N. Engl. J. Med.* 301:341, 1979.

121. Davidson, D. M., and DeBusk, R. F. Prognostic value of a single exercise test 3 weeks after uncomplicated myocardial infarction. *Circulation* 61:236, 1980.

122. Starling, M. R., Crawford, M. H., Kennedy, G. T., and O'Rourke, R. A. Exercise testing early after MI: Predictive value for subsequent unstable angina and death. *Am. J. Cardiol.* 46:909, 1980.

123. Starling, M. R., Crawford, M. H., Kennedy, D. T., and O'Rourke, R. A. Treadmill exercise tests predischarge and six weeks post-myocardial infarction to detect abnormalities of known prognostic value. *Ann. Intern. Med.* 94:721, 1981.

124. Akhras, F., Upward, J., Keates, J., and Jackson, G. Early exercise testing and elective coronary artery bypass surgery after uncomplicated myocardial infarction: Effect on morbidity and mortality. *Br. Heart J.* 52:413, 1984.

125. Akhras, F., Upward, J., Stott, R., and Jackson, G. Early exercise testing and coronary angiography and uncomplicated myocardial infarction. *Br. Med. J.* 284:1293, 1982.

126. DeBusk, R. F., Kraemer, H. C., and Nash, E. Stepwise risk stratification soon after acute myocardial infarction. *Am. J. Cardiol.* 52:1161, 1983.

127. Weld, F. M., Chu, K. L., Bigger, J. T., and Rolnitzky, L. M. Risk stratification with low-level exercise testing 2 weeks after acute myocardial infarction. *Circulation* 64:306, 1981.

128. Jennings, K., Reid, D. S., Hawkins, T., and Julian, D. J. Role of exercise testing early after myocardial infarction in identifying candidates for coronary surgery. *Br. Med. J.* 288:185, 1984.

129. Birk Madsen, E., and Gilpin, E. Prognostic value of exercise test variables after myocardial infarction. *J. Cardiac Rehabil.* 3:481, 1983.

130. DeFeyter, P. J., van Eenige, M. J., Dighton, D. H., et al. Prognostic value of exercise testing, coronary angiography and left ventriculography 6-8 weeks after myocardial infarction. *Circulation* 66:527, 1982.

131. Fioretti, P., Brower, R. W., Simoons, M. L., et al. Prediction of mortality in hospital survivors of myocardial infarction: Comparison of predischarge exercise testing and radionuclide ventriculography at rest. *Br. Heart J.* 52:292, 1984.

132. Birk Madsen, E., Gilpin, E., Ahnve, S., et al. Prediction of functional capacity and use of exercise testing for predicting risk after acute myocardial infarction. *Am. J. Cardiol.* 56:839, 1985.

133. Deckers, W., Fioretti, P., Brower, R. W., et al. Ineligibility for predischarge exercise testing after myocardial infarction in the elderly: Implications for prognosis. *Eur. Heart J.* 5(Suppl E):97, 1984.

134. Waters, D. D., Bosch, X., Bourchard, A., et al. Comparison of clinical variables and variables derived from a limited predischarge ex-

ercise test as predictors of early and late mortality after myocardial infarction. *J. Am. Coll. Cardiol.* 5:1, 1985.

135. Ouyang, P., Shapiro, E. P., Chandra, N. C., et al. An angiographic and functional comparison of patients with silent and symptomatic treadmill ischemia early after myocardial infarction. *Am. J. Cardiol.* 59:730, 1987.

136. Gottlieb, S. H., Gerstenblith, G., Achuff, S. C., et al. Ischemic ST segment changes by ambulatory Holter predict one year mortality in high risk post-infarct patients (Abstract). *Circulation* 74(Suppl II):58, 1986.

137. Jelinek, V. M., McDonald, I. G., Ryan, W. F., et al. Assessment of cardiac risk 10 days after uncomplicated myocardial infarction. *Br. Med. J.* 284:227, 1982.

138. Sami, M., Kraemer, H., and DeBusk, R. F. The prognostic significance of serial exercise testing after myocardial infarction. *Circulation* 60:1238, 1979.

139. Gibson, R. S., Taylor, G. J., and Watson, D. D. Predicting the extent and location of coronary disease during the early post-infarction period by quantitative thallium-201 scintigraphy. *Am. J. Cardiol.* 47:1010, 1981.

140. Hung, J., Goris, M. L., Nash, E., et al. Comparative value of maximal treadmill testing, exercise thallium myocardial perfusion scintigraphy and exercise radionuclide ventriculography for distinguishing high- and low-risk patients soon after acute myocardial infarction. *Am. J. Cardiol.* 53:1221, 1984.

141. Gibson, R. S., Beller, G. A., and Kaiser, D. L. Prevalence and clinical significance of painless ST segment depression during early postinfarction exercise testing. *Circulation* 75(Suppl 2):36, 1987.

142. Smeets, J. P., Rigo, P., and Legrand, V. Prognostic value of thallium-201 stress myocardial scintigraphy with exercise ECG after myocardial infarction. *Cardiology* 68:67, 1981.

143. Hakki, A. H., Nestico, P. F., Heo, J., et al. Relative prognostic value of rest thallium-201 imaging, radionuclide ventriculography and 24 hour ambulatory electrocardiographic monitoring after acute myocardial infarction. *J. Am. Coll. Cardiol.* 10(1):25, 1987.

144. Heger, J. J., Weyman, A. E., Wann, L. S., et al. Cross-sectional echocardiographic analysis of the extent of left ventricular asynergy in acute myocardial infarction. *Circulation* 60:531, 1987.

145. Gibson, R. S., Bishop, H. L., Stamm, R. B., et al. Value of early two dimensional echocardiography in patients with acute myocardial infarction. *Am. J. Cardiol.* 49:1110, 1982.

146. Horowitz, R. S., and Morganroth, J. Immediate detection of early high-risk patients with acute myocardial infarction using two-dimensional echocardiographic evaluation of left ventricular regional wall motion abnormalities. *Am. Heart J.* 103:814, 1982.

147. Horowitz, R. S., Morganroth, J., Parrotto, C., et al. Immediate diagnosis of acute myocardial infarction by two-dimensional echocardiography. *Circulation* 65:323, 1982.

148. Morganroth, J., Chin, C. C., David, D., et al. Exercise cross-sectional echocardiographic diagnosis of coronary artery disease. *Am. J. Cardiol.* 47:20, 1981.

149. Crawford, M. H., Amon, K. W., and Vance, W. S. Exercise 2-dimensional echocardiography: Quantitation of left ventricular performance in patients with severe angina pectoris. *Am. J. Cardiol.* 51:1, 1983.

150. Van Reet, R. E., Quinones, M. A., Poliner, L. R., et al. Comparison of two-dimensional echocardiography with gated radionuclide ventriculography in the evaluation of global and regional left ventricular function in acute myocardial infarction. *J. Am. Coll. Cardiol.* 3:243, 1984.

151. Nishimura, R. A., Tajik, A. J., Shub, C., et al. Role of two-dimensional echocardiography in the predication of in-hospital complications after acute myocardial infarction. *J. Am. Coll. Cardiol.* 4:1080, 1984.

152. Ryan, T., Armstrong, W. F., O'Donnell, J. A., and Feigenbaum, H. Risk stratification after acute myocardial infarction by means of exercise two-dimensional echocardiography. *Am. Heart J.* 114:1305, 1987.

153. Madigan, N. P., Rutherford, B. D., and Frye, R. L. The clinical course, early prognosis and coronary anatomy of subendocardial infarction. *Am. J. Med.* 60:634, 1976.

154. Califf, R. A., Burks, J. M., Behar, V. S., et al. Relationships among ventricular arrhythmias, coronary artery disease and angiographic and electrocardiographic indicators of myocardial fibrosis. *Circulation* 57:725, 1978.

155. Chaitman, B. R., Waters, D. D., Corbara, F., and Bourassa, M. G. Prediction of multivessel disease after inferior myocardial infarction. *Circulation* 57:1085, 1978.

156. Bertrand, M. E., Lefebvre, J. M., Laisne, C. L., et al. Coronary arteriography in acute transmural myocardial infarction. *Am. Heart J.* 97:61, 1979.

157. Vanhaecke, J., Piessens, J., Willems, J. L., and DeGeest, H. Coronary arterial lesions in young men who survived a first myocardial infarction: Clinical and electrocardiographic predictors of multivessel disease. *Am. J. Cardiol.* 47:810, 1981.

158. Roubin, G. S., Harris, P. J., Bernstein, L., and Kelly, D. T. Coronary anatomy and prognosis after myocardial infarction in patients 60 years of age and younger. *Circulation* 67:743, 1983.

159. Turner, J. D., Rogers, W. J., Mantle, J. A., et

al. Coronary angiography soon after myocardial infarction. *Chest* 77:58, 1980.

160. Betriu, A., Castaner, A., Sanz, G. A., et al. Angiographic findings 1 month after myocardial infarction: A prospective study of 259 survivors. *Circulation* 65:1099, 1982.

161. Veenbrink, T. W. G., van der Werf, T., Westerhof, P. W., et al. Is there an indication for coronary angiography in patients under 60 years of age with no or minimal angina pectoris after a first myocardial infarction? *Br. Heart J.* 53:30, 1985.

162. Califf, R. M., Phillips, H. R., Hindman, M. C., et al. Prognostic value of a coronary artery jeopardy score. *J. Am. Coll. Cardiol.* 5:1055, 1985.

163. Schulman, S. P., Achuff, S. C., Griffith, L. S., et al. Prognostic cardiac catheterization variables in survivors of acute myocardial infarction: A five year prospective study. *J. Am. Coll. Cardiol.* 11:1164, 1988.

164. White, H. D., Norris, R. M., Brown, M. A., et al. Left ventricular end-systolic volume as the major determinant of survival after recovery from myocardial infarction. *Circulation* 76:44, 1987.

165. Waspe, L. E., Seinfeld, D., Ferrick, A., et al. Prediction of sudden death and spontaneous ventricular tachycardia in survivors of complicated myocardial infarction: Value of response to programmed stimulation using a maximum of three ventricular extrastimuli. *J. Am. Coll. Cardiol.* 5:1292, 1985.

166. Hammer, A., Vohra, J., Hunt, D., and Sloman, G. Prediction of sudden death by electrophysiologic studies in high risk patients surviving acute myocardial infarction. *Am. J. Cardiol.* 50:223, 1982.

167. Richards, D. A., Cody, D. V., Denniss, A. R., et al. Ventricular electrical instability: A predictor of death after myocardial infarction. *Am. J. Cardiol.* 51:75, 1983.

168. Marchlinski, F. E., Buxton, A. E., Waxman, H. L., and Josephson, M. E. Identifying patients at risk of sudden death after myocardial infarction: Value of the response to programmed stimulation, degree of ventricular ectopic activity and severity of left ventricular dysfunction. *Am. J. Cardiol.* 52:1190, 1983.

169. Denniss, A. R., Baaijens, H., Cody, D. V., et al. Value of programmed stimulation and exercise testing in predicting one-year mortality after acute myocardial infarction. *Am. J. Cardiol.* 56:213, 1985.

170. Morady, F., DiCarlo, L. A., Krol, R. B., et al. Role of myocardial ischemia during programmed stimulation in survivors of cardiac arrest with coronary artery disease. *J. Am. Coll. Cardiol.* 9:1004, 1987.

171. Bhandari, A. K., Au, P. K., Rose, J. S., et al. Decline in inducibility of sustained ventricular tachycardia from two to twenty weeks after acute myocardial infarction. *Am. J. Cardiol.* 59:284, 1987.

172. Roy, D., Marchand, L., Theroux, P., et al. Long-term reproduction and significance of provokable ventricular arrhythmias after myocardial infarction. *J. Am. Coll. Cardiol.* 8:32, 1986.

173. Denniss, A. R., Richards, D. A., Cody, D. V., et al. Prognostic significance of ventricular tachycardia and fibrillation induced at programmed stimulation and delayed potentials detected on the signal-averaged electrocardiograms of survivors of acute myocardial infarction. *Circulation* 74:731, 1986.

174. Roy, D., Marchand, E., Theroux, P., et al. Programmed ventricular stimulation in survivors of an acute myocardial infarction. *Circulation* 72:487, 1985.

175. Gonzalez, R., Arriagada, D., Corbalan, R., et al. Role of programmed electrical stimulation of the heart in risk stratification post-myocardial infarction. *PACE* 11:283, 1988.

176. Rapaport, E., and Remedios, P. The high risk patient after recovery from myocardial infarction: Recognition and management. *J. Am. Coll. Cardiol.* 1:391, 1983.

177. Madsen, E. B., Gilpin, E., and Henning, H. Evaluation of prognosis one year after myocardial infarction. *J. Am. Coll. Cardiol.* 1:985, 1983.

178. Moss, A. J., Decamilla, J., Davis, H., and Bayer, L. The early posthospital phase of myocardial infarction. *Circulation* 54:58, 1976.

179. Gilpin, E. A., Karliner, J. S., and Ross Jr., J. Risk assessment after acute myocardial infarction. In J. S. Karliner and G. Gregoratos (eds.), *Coronary Care.* New York: Churchill Livingstone, 1980. P. 1040.

180. Lemlish, A., Covo, G., and Ziffer, J. Multivariate analysis of prognostic factors in myocardial infarction. In K. Enslein (ed.), *Data Acquisition and Processing in Biology and Medicine. Proceedings* (Vol. 3): Rochester Conference on Data Acquisition and Processing in Biology and Medicine. New York: Macmillan, 1963. P. 65.

181. Rotmensch, H. H., Terdiman, R., Cheffer, M., et al. Dynamic prognostic profile for acute myocardial infarction. *Chest* 76:663, 1979.

182. Habib, T., Taylor, D. J. E., and Dalton, R. Comparison of two coronary prognostic indices. *Postgrad. Med. J.* 55:255, 1979.

183. Bigger, J. T., Heller, C. A., Wengler, T. L., and Weld, F. M. Risk stratification after acute myocardial infarction. *Am. J. Cardiol.* 42:202, 1978.

184. Chapelle, J. P., Albert, A., Smeets, J. P., et al. Early assessment of risk in patient with acute myocardial infarction. *Eur. Heart J.* 2:187, 1981.

185. Gilpin, E., Olshen, R., Henning, H., and Ross Jr., J. Risk prediction after acute myocardial infarction: Comparison of three multivariate methodologies. *Cardiology* 70:73, 1983.

186. Olshen, R. A., Gilpin, E. A., Henning, H., et al. Twelve month prognosis following myocardial infarction: Classification trees, logistic regression, and stepwise linear discrimination. In L. M. LeCam and R. A. Olshen (eds.), *The Proceedings of the Berkeley Conference in Honor of Jerzy Neyman and Jack Kiefer* (Vol. 1). Monterey, CA: Wadsworth Advanced Books and Software, 1985. P. 245.

187. Norris, R. M., Brandt, P. W. T., Caughey, D. E., et al. A new coronary prognostic index. *Lancet* 1:224, 1969.

188. Chapman, B. L., and Gray, C. H. Prognostic index for myocardial infarction treated in a coronary care unit. *Br. Heart J.* 35:135, 1973.

189. Madsen, E. B., Hougaard, P., Gilpin, E., and Pedersen, A. The length of hospitalization after acute myocardial infarction determined by risk calculation. *Circulation* 68:9, 1983.

190. Chaturvedi, N. C., Walsh, M. J., Evans, A., et al. Selection of patients for early discharge after acute myocardial infarction. *Br. Heart J.* 36:533, 1974.

191. Lindvall, K., Erhardt, L. R., Lundman, T., et al. Early mobilization and discharge of patients with acute myocardial infarction. *Acta Med. Scand.* 206:169, 1979.

192. Wenger, N. K., Hellerstein, H. K., Blackburn, H., and Castranova, S. J. Physician practice in the management of patients with uncomplicated myocardial infarction: Changes in the past decade. *Circulation* 65:421, 1982.

193. Hutter Jr., A. M., Sidel, V. W., Shine, K. L., and DeSanctis, R. W. Early hospital discharge after myocardial infarction. *N. Engl. J. Med.* 288:1141, 1973.

194. Hayes, M. J., Morris, G. K., and Hampton, J. R. Comparison of mobilization after two and nine days in uncomplicated myocardial infarction. *Br. Med. J.* 3:10, 1974.

195. McNeer, J. F., Wagner, G. S., Ginsburg, P. B., et al. Hospital discharge one week after acute myocardial infarction. *N. Engl. J. Med.* 298:229, 1978.

196. Birk Madsen, E. Time of discharge for patients with acute myocardial infarction. *Cardiovasc. Rev. Rep.* 4:1301, 1983.

197. Ahnve, S., Gilpin, E., Dittrich, H., et al. First myocardial infarction: Age and ejection fraction identify a low risk group. *Am. Heart J.* 116:925, 1988.

198. Topol, E. J., Burek, K., O'Neill, W. W., et al. A randomized controlled trial of hospital discharge three days after myocardial infarction in the era of reperfusion. *N. Engl. J. Med.* 318:1083, 1988.

39
Overall Risk Stratification and Management Strategies for Patients with Acute Myocardial Infarction

ANDREW A. WOLFF AND JOEL S. KARLINER

Myocardial oxygen demand in excess of supply is the basic pathophysiologic derangement underlying myocardial ischemia, which, when unrelieved, progresses to myocardial infarction. The latter implies myocardial cell death and subsequent necrosis and is, as such, irreversible. It is the goal of the clinician to interrupt ischemia in progress (thus limiting infarction) and to prevent its recurrence. A logical therapeutic strategy is to increase oxygen supply while decreasing demand.

Initial Management

Acutely, the first step in this effort is to provide supplemental inspired oxygen to the patient. Three factors can act, singly or in combination, to reduce the supply of oxygen-rich coronary arterial blood to an area of myocardium: (1) fixed obstruction of the vascular lumen due to atheroma; (2) dynamic reduction of the vessel diameter due to increases in coronary vascular smooth muscle tone (i.e., "coronary spasm"); and (3) intracoronary thrombus formation, usually in an area of fixed obstruction and often with accompanying coronary spasm. Thus subsequent acute and chronic interventions are directed toward reducing the influence of these three factors in decreasing coronary blood flow while striving whenever possible to diminish the myocardial demand for oxygen.

In the most acute setting, little can be done to effect a reduction in the degree of fixed stenosis underlying an episode of myocardial ischemia. Coronary artery bypass surgery and percutaneous transluminal coronary angioplasty are the only proved therapies directed toward rectifying the problems caused by fixed atherosclerotic lesions; and although they may benefit selected patients when they can be expeditiously initiated and undertaken by experienced personnel, the expense of maintaining such sophisticated teams at the ready on a 24-hour basis is far too great to consider these procedures routinely in the first-line management of acute myocardial ischemia and infarction. On the other hand, the definitive nature of coronary artery bypass surgery has rendered the best results in the long-term management of coronary artery disease in certain subsets of patients [1–3]. Similarly, because angioplasty is clearly effective in directly reducing the stenosis underlying ischemia or infarction, the improvement in the systolic motion of jeopardized myocardium offered by this technique may eventually be translated into gains in long-term survival [4].

Several drugs act to reduce coronary arterial tone, thereby increasing coronary flow. Nitrates, administered sublingually or intravenously, represent the mainstay of therapy for acute myocardial ischemia; in their topical and orally active preparations, nitrates are similarly the cornerstone of prophylaxis against recurrent attacks of ischemia. Nitrates cause vascular smooth muscle relaxation by activating the cytosolic enzyme guanylate cyclase, thereby increasing intracellular levels of 5′-cyclic guanosine monophosphate (cGMP). In turn, increased levels of this cyclic nucleotide activate the enzyme protein kinase G, which promotes smooth muscle relaxation both directly, via effects on the contractile apparatus, and indirectly, by reducing the intracellular free calcium ion concentration [5]. In addition to directly relaxing the vascular smooth muscle of the coronary conductance vessel, nitrates exert a similar effect on the systemic capacitance venules and resistance arterioles. This action on the capacitance venules allows some degree of systemic venous pooling, which reduces venous return to the heart, effecting decreases in ventricular end-diastolic volume and pressure, reflected as a reduction in myocardial preload. Similarly, the arteriolar effects of nitrates are translated into a decline in myocardial afterload. Because myocardial preload and afterload are major determinants of myocardial stroke work, which is in turn a major determinant of myocardial oxygen consumption, nitrates act not only to increase myocardial oxygen supply but to decrease myocardial oxygen demands as well.

Calcium channel blockers, such as nifedipine, diltiazem, and verapamil, offer all the beneficial vascular actions of nitrates but act via a separate mechanism; thus their effect, when used in combination with nitrates, is additive. Whereas the effects of nitrates on guanylate cyclase in smooth muscle are limited to this tissue, calcium channel blockers act to reduce the influx of calcium ion across the cell membranes of both smooth muscle cells and cardiac myocytes. The subsequent reduction of intracellular free calcium ion causes a parallel decrease in the resting tension of vascular smooth muscle cells. Secondarily, these agents also decrease intracellular calcium stores available for efflux from the sarcoplasmic reticulum during depolarization of cardiac myocytes; thus cardiac contractility is reduced. This direct negative inotropic effect of calcium channel blockers, which can be titrated to therapeutic benefit, decreases myocardial oxygen consumption, thereby favorably altering the myocardial oxygen supply-demand ratio; however, calcium channel blockers have the potential for precipitating congestive heart failure (CHF). These drugs also exhibit significantly longer half-lives (3–6 hours) than sublingual, intravenous, or topical preparations of nitrates (about 5 minutes). This longer half-life represents a disadvantage in the management of an acutely ill patient, where rapid fluctuations in the clinical situation may necessitate equally rapid adjustments in therapy. Alternatively, the longer half-life constitutes an advantage in prophylaxis against recurrent ischemia in the stable patient [6].

Morphine sulfate, injected intravenously, is used primarily for the relief of anginal pain due to myocardial ischemia. Although this pain relief is largely the result of the central nervous effects of the drug on pain perception, morphine also reduces systemic venous tone, with the attendant beneficial effect on preload described above for nitrates and calcium channel blockers. There is also a modest dilatory effect on the coronary vessels. Perhaps most importantly, the direct pain relief and sedation offered by morphine are themselves often advantageous; pain and anxiety, nearly universal in conscious patients during the acute stages of a myocardial infarction, contribute to elevations in heart rate and blood pressure, which in turn increase myocardial oxygen demands [7].

Beta blockers competitively antagonize the coupling of beta-adrenergic agonists, such as epinephrine and norepinephrine, with their specific cell-surface receptors. Consequently, the ability of beta agonists to activate cellular adenylate cyclase via their receptors is reduced by beta blockade, resulting in a decrease in intracellular levels of the "second messenger" compound, 5′-cyclic adenosine monophosphate (cAMP). In cardiac myocytes, decreased intracellular levels of cAMP in turn decrease the number of calcium channels available for calcium influx, thereby lowering intracellular calcium ion concentrations, with attendant decreases in heart rate and myocardial contractility; thus myocardial oxygen demand is reduced. In contrast, this effect of cAMP on calcium influx does not occur in vascular smooth muscle; in fact, much like cGMP, cAMP acts to decrease vascular smooth muscle tone by activating protein kinase A, which has effects similar to those of protein kinase G [5]. As a result, beta-blocking agents, by reducing intracellular levels of cAMP in coronary vascular smooth muscle, actually function to increase coronary tone and thus decrease myocardial oxygen supply. Fortunately, the beneficial effects of beta blockers on myocardial oxygen demand outweigh their deleterious effects on oxygen supply, and their net effect on the balance between the two is favorable.

Beta blockers are used primarily to prevent recurrent ischemia in patients with coronary artery disease; however, there are two additional uses specific to the treatment of myocardial infarction. Acutely, the intravenous administration of metoprolol or atenolol has been associated with a modest reduction (about 13 percent) in in-hospital mortality [8, 9]. This reduction in mortality appears to be greater (30–50 percent) in older patients with a history of prior myocardial infarction, angina, CHF, hypertension, or diabetes [10]; nonetheless, early intravenous beta blockade as an approach to the management of acute myocardial infarction has not gained widespread acceptance among clinicians. In contrast, therapy with a variety of beta-blocking drugs, begun prior to discharge and continued for at least 1 year thereafter, is frequently prescribed. This treatment has been associated with mean 21 and 24 percent reductions in subsequent mortality and nonfatal reinfarction, respectively, during the first postinfarction year. The effect on mortality is due largely to the prevention of sudden cardiac death [11].

Elimination of intracoronary thrombus represents the newest approach to the early treatment of acute myocardial infarction; prevention of thrombus reformation actually represents the renaissance of an old concept. Studies have shown that the earlier coronary angiography is performed during acute myocardial infarction, the higher is the prevalence of intracoronary thrombus [12]. Thus the involvement of thrombus in most acute infarctions has been widely acknowledged. Accordingly, the development of thrombolytic agents represents a milestone in the treatment of

acute myocardial infarction. The first of these agents to be approved was the bacterial enzyme streptokinase, which binds with circulating plasminogen to form a complex that accelerates the cleavage of unbound plasminogen to its active form, plasmin. Plasmin, in turn, degrades both fibrin and fibrinogen; thus it dissolves formed thrombus but also precipitates a systemic fibrinolytic state predisposing to hemorrhage. The more recently approved recombinant tissue plasminogen activator (rt-PA) is more specific for fibrin, because it cleaves only plasminogen in proximity to fibrin. When administered within 3 hours of the onset of ischemic symptoms, both agents can effect reperfusion of an infarct-related coronary artery with essentially equal efficiency: approximately 80 percent with intracoronary administration, about 65 to 70 percent when given intravenously [13]. By either route, the incidence of successful thrombolysis decreases with time from the onset of symptoms, as do the beneficial effects of thrombolysis on left ventricular ejection fraction and mortality. In this regard, because intravenous administration of these agents can be instituted immediately upon confirming the diagnosis of acute myocardial infarction, and because this route is associated with a somewhat lower rate of complications, the overall benefit from these agents is maximized by giving them intravenously. In general, the greatest salvage of life and ventricular function occurs when these agents can be given within 4 to 6 hours of the onset of symptoms to patients sustaining an anterior myocardial infarction or to those sustaining their first infarction [14, 15].

Although its more specific mechanism suggests that rt-PA should be associated with fewer bleeding complications than streptokinase, to date this suggestion has not been verified in clinical trials [16]. It is probably because once successful reperfusion has been accomplished with either agent systemic anticoagulation must be instituted to prevent early reocclusion of the infarct-related artery [17]. Unfortunately, heparin also increases the rate of hemorrhagic complications associated with thrombolytic therapy [13]; therefore it is usually discontinued within the first several days of reperfusion, once treatment with antiplatelet agents and calcium channel blockers has been instituted to prevent reocclusion.

With these therapeutic principles in mind, strategies for the initial management of patients with acute myocardial infarction can be outlined. When an acute anterior myocardial infarction (or any first myocardial infarction) can be confidently diagnosed in any patient without contraindications to the use of a thrombolytic agent, one should be given intravenously without delay. How this principle can be best implemented is currently a matter of some clinical controversy. For example, if emergency medical personnel begin intravenous thrombolysis in the field, improvement in survival and myocardial salvage might be expected because of shorter elapsed time from the onset of symptoms to the initiation of therapy. It is possible, however, that this benefit would be offset by an increase in serious hemorrhagic complications due to inappropriate administration of these drugs.

While ongoing trials attempt to resolve such issues, there is no doubt that intravenous thrombolysis should be instituted in the emergency department after an initial evaluation by a physician has determined such therapy to be appropriate for the patient. In general, thrombolysis is indicated for a patient under the age of 75 years who is seen within 6 hours of the onset of ischemic symptoms, whose electrocardiogram displays ST segment elevation, who has no history of stroke or recent trauma (including external chest compression during cardiopulmonary resuscitation that has resulted in significant sternocostal damage), and who is not actively bleeding. Successful reperfusion is recognized clinically by relief of chest pain with resolution of ST segment elevation; "reperfusion arrhythmias," typically accelerated idioventricular complexes, may occur at this time [18]. These arrhythmias are rarely associated with hemodynamic compromise but should be monitored because of their occasional degeneration to ventricular tachycardia and fibrillation.

As the decision whether to administer thrombolysis is made, other therapeutic interventions against ischemia can begin. All of the drugs described above can be given concurrently with thrombolytic agents, although extra caution should be exercised when using those that predispose to hypotension, as thrombolytic agents, particularly streptokinase, are also known to lower the blood pressure in some patients. Sublingual nitrates are usually the agents of first choice: They can be administered even before intravenous access is available, act rapidly, and have beneficial effects on both myocardial oxygen supply and demand, without the price of negative inotropy. When anginal pain persists, morphine may be added, and nitrate therapy can be augmented intravenously while the blood pressure is monitored. When a hyperdynamic state is believed to contribute to ongoing ischemia, the negative inotropic effects of calcium channel blockers may be preferable to the use of beta blockers because the favorable effects of the former drugs on coronary tone also act against any component of coronary spasm that may persist in the face of nitrates. Supplemental oxygen should be given to all patients, as should a prophylactic bolus and infusion of lidocaine. Noncardiac factors that may complicate treatment of ischemia by increasing myocardial oxygen demands (e.g., fever causing tachycardia) should receive prompt attention. The goal is a hemodynamically stable patient without ischemic symptoms.

Risk Stratification and Management Strategies for Surviving Patients

Events during the initial hospitalization most accurately predict the subsequent course of patients with acute myocardial infarction. Patients who survive their first myocardial infarction without recurrent chest pain, congestive heart failure, or significant late arrhythmias enjoy a good prognosis, suffering less than 3 percent mortality during the first 2 years after infarction. Unfortunately, each of these complications increases the likelihood of future cardiovascular morbidity and mortality [19, 20]. Data from noninvasive and, where warranted, invasive testing help to further refine the prognosis and aid in the management of each of these groups.

Electrocardiographic infarct localization at admission is of great value in initial risk stratification. When compared to patients with inferior infarctions, patients with anterior infarction experience increases in both in-hospital (12 percent versus 3 percent) and long-term mortality (27 percent versus 11 percent at 2.5 years). This poorer outcome with anterior infarction persists, even when adjustments are made for infarct size [21]. The prognostic value of the electrocardiographic type of infarction (i.e., Q wave versus non-Q wave) continues to be debated. Some studies have found patients with non-Q-wave infarctions to sustain a more benign in-hospital course but to suffer a higher rate of recurrent infarction and mortality after discharge. Such data are consistent with the hypothesis that non-Q-wave infarctions represent "incomplete" infarctions, with substantial viable myocardium remaining at risk in the distribution of the infarcted vessel [22, 23], and they have been used to support an aggressive management strategy for patients with non-Q-wave infarction, including routine predischarge coronary angiography with, when appropriate, subsequent revascularization. Although the non-Q-wave pattern clearly reflects a smaller infarction (assessed by changes in plasma MB-CK activity) attended by fewer in-hospital complications, other studies have found no differences in survival or reinfarction rates after discharge between patients with Q-wave and those with non-Q-wave infarctions [21]. In the midst of this controversy, two definite statements can be made regarding these two electrocardiographic patterns of infarction. First, they are not useful for determining whether an infarction is "transmural" or "nontransmural"; the use of these terms to denote, respectively, Q-wave and non-Q-wave infarctions is inaccurate and should be abandoned [24]. Second, diltiazem treatment of patients surviving non-Q-wave infarctions is associated with a reduction in the rate of reinfarction [6]; this benefit has not been shown to extend to survivors of Q-wave infarctions.

Management of any patient surviving myocardial infarction, whether complicated or not, must include an aggressive program of overall cardiovascular risk reduction. Smokers must be encouraged to quit and obese patients advised to lose weight. When present, hypertension and diabetes should be controlled. Serum cholesterol should be measured and, if elevated, treated with dietary restrictions and, when necessary, drug therapy. In this regard, it is important to remember that any acute intercurrent illness, including myocardial infarction, can abruptly lower serum cholesterol; therefore a normal serum cholesterol level during the initial hospitalization does not rule out clinically significant hypercholesterolemia. Such patients should have their cholesterol levels rechecked at a follow-up visit, 4 to 6 weeks after discharge.

In addition to these major cardiovascular risk factors, nearly any acute medical illness harbors the potential for aggravating the consequences of coronary artery disease by increasing metabolic rates and subsequently the demand on the heart. Obviously, the clinician optimizes the general medical condition of any patient, but particular care must be taken to ensure that the sinus tachycardia, low grade fever, and mild leukocytosis observed frequently during the first days after myocardial infarction do not serve to mask, for instance, an underlying infection or concomitant hyperthyroidism.

The administration of low doses of aspirin has been shown in controlled studies to reduce the reinfarction and cardiovascular death rates in patients after myocardial infarction [25–27]. Its use is associated with few complications, probably because the effective dose appears to be low and administration need not be frequent (as little as 300 mg every day has been beneficial in some studies). Furthermore, enteric-coated preparations can be used with similar benefit. Theoretical concerns that higher doses might prove to be less beneficial (or even deleterious) due to inhibition of synthesis of the vasodilator prostacyclin, in addition to inhibition of synthesis of the potent vasoconstrictor thromboxane A_2, have not been borne out by clinical investigation [28]. In view of this safety and efficacy, all patients who survive myocardial infarction should be discharged on a dose of at least 300 mg of aspirin per day, excluding only those patients with active peptic ulcer disease, a documented history of true aspirin hypersensitivity, or demonstrated gastrointestinal intolerance of 300 mg per day.

The reductions in mortality and reinfarction attendant to beta-antagonist treatment of survivors of acute myocardial infarction have been noted above. Propranolol or timolol probably should be given to most survivors of acute myocardial infarction who can tolerate this therapy without symptomatic bradycardia or CHF. A reduced left ventricular ejection fraction is not itself a contraindication to beta-blocker therapy if symptomatic CHF is absent; indeed, these patients may benefit most from the protective effects of beta blockade. Treatment should be continued for at least 1 year; however, benefit has not been shown to extend beyond 2 years after infarction. In fact, the adverse effects of most beta-adrenergic antagonists on serum lipid profiles argue against indefinite therapy with these agents.

The management strategies outlined below refer only to patients who have not undergone reperfusion with a thrombolytic agent, either because such an agent was not administered, or because thrombolytic therapy was unsuccessful in restoring flow through the involved coronary artery. Strategies for management of the successfully reperfused patient continue to evolve. Early coronary angiography in these individuals has demonstrated a substantial incidence of high grade residual stenosis of successfully reperfused infarct vessels [4] with an appreciable rate of reocclusion/reinfarction in the absence of anticoagulation [17]. These observations support the emerging consensus that patients successfully reperfused with thrombolytic agents should remain anticoagulated until they undergo coronary angiography, anticipating the performance of percutaneous coronary angioplasty on the infarct-related vessel, if the anatomy of the culprit lesion is amenable to this procedure. Although this intervention should occur prior to hospital discharge, there appears to be no ad-

vantage to urgent angiography/angioplasty, as results are equally good when these procedures are delayed until several days after the acute infarction, so long as the patient remains adequately anticoagulated during this interval [29]. At the time of catheterization, angioplasty may be found to be an unfeasable management strategy. The anatomy of the infarct-related stenosis may be unfavorable or the coexistence of multiple critical stenoses may mandate coronary artery bypass grafting. If surgical revascularization is elected, full anticoagulation with heparin should be continued until 4 hours prior to the time of surgery in order to prevent rethrombosis. Patients should be discharged on aspirin and a calcium channel blocker following angioplasty in order to prevent rethrombosis and postangioplasty coronary spasm.

UNCOMPLICATED MYOCARDIAL INFARCTION

Patients with an uncomplicated myocardial infarction include those without recurrent angina or malignant ventricular arrhythmias detected beyond 48 hours after admission to the coronary care unit (CCU) and without clinical evidence of CHF at any time during their hospital course. Clinical experience indicates that mild to moderate chest discomfort frequently persists for some hours after relief of the acute pain that prompted the patient to seek medical attention. This symptom usually does not evoke complaints from the patient but, rather, is elicited by questioning a patient who appears to be resting comfortably. Such discomfort may originate from the irreversibly damaged myocardium as it undergoes necrosis; it generally does not last beyond the first hospital day, is not associated with new electrocardiographic changes, and is not of particular significance. Such discomfort must be distinguished from a recurrence of angina after initial stabilization of the patient, which indicates that further viable myocardium is at risk of infarction and constitutes a complication of the original myocardial infarction. Obviously, when doubt exists regarding the etiology of a patient's chest discomfort after myocardial infarction, recurrent angina must be presumed until proved otherwise. Finally, hemodynamically significant ventricular tachycardia or ventricular fibrillation during the first 48 hours after acute myocardial infarction does not constitute a complication of the myocardial infarction for purposes of risk stratification. Although the occurrence of this dysrhythmia is associated with a doubling of in-hospital mortality (largely due to severe pump failure), it does not affect the long-term prognosis of patients who survive to hospital discharge [30, 31].

Because of their favorable prognosis (approximately 1–2 percent mortality per year [19]), patients surviving an uncomplicated first myocardial infarction require little in the way of "routine testing" before discharge from the hospital; however, because the single objectively quantifiable variable that best predicts reduced survival after acute myocardial infarction is depressed left ventricular (LV) function [19, 32] and because LV function can be accurately measured noninvasively at a relatively low cost, some quantification of this parameter is recommended for all patients surviving acute myocardial infarction prior to hospital discharge. In patients with an LV ejection fraction greater than 0.40, 1-year mortality is 5 percent or less; however, mortality increases sharply as the LV ejection fraction falls below 0.40 [19] (Fig. 39-1). In addition to aiding in prognosis, this measurement provides baseline data for comparison during follow-up evaluation.

The most common methods employed in the noninvasive quantitation of LV function are echocardiography and radionuclide ventriculography; the choice of techniques may be reasonably based on their relative availability or cost at a given institution. Radionuclide ventriculography offers greater accuracy and reproducibility than echocardiography in measuring the ejection fraction but is perhaps less sensitive in identifying regional wall motion abnormalities (especially smaller ones) and cannot assess the structure or function of the cardiac valves, as can echocardiography, par-

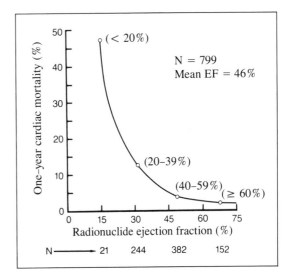

Fig. 39-1
Relation between the predischarge radionuclide ejection fraction and 1-year cardiac mortality after myocardial infarction. (From A. J. Moss for The Multicenter Postinfarction Research Group and the New England Journal of Medicine 309: 331-6, 1983.)

ticularly when Doppler techniques are used. Thus if the clinician expects the predischarge evaluation to disclose some impairment of LV function and anticipates future serial evaluations to discover whether improvement occurs with time or adjustments in therapy, radionuclide ventriculography may be the better choice. If, on the other hand, normal LV function is likely, echocardiography offers a wider "screen" for the unanticipated structural abnormality (e.g., significant LV hypertrophy) and is clearly preferable if any valvular pathology is suspected.

Once adequate global LV function (ejection fraction ≥ 0.40) has been documented in the patient with an uncomplicated myocardial infarction, predischarge submaximal exercise testing is of limited use. Only a few such patients would be found to have severe myocardial ischemia induced by a low level of exercise and would indeed be at high risk for subsequent cardiovascular morbidity and mortality; however, these patients would also be identified by a symptom-limited exercise test at 4 to 6 weeks postinfarction. The risk to this subgroup of interval cardiovascular death or reinfarction associated with delaying the exercise test is well under 1 percent [33]. Later symptom-limited exercise testing identifies those additional patients at risk for recurrent cardiovascular events that the predischarge test would have missed and provides useful information about the functional status of the patient that the submaximal test cannot. It then allows the clinician to prescribe exercise for patients without an early positive result. Therefore a single symptom-limited exercise test, performed 4 to 6 weeks after discharge, constitutes the most effective management of patients with an uncomplicated myocardial infarction and adequate global LV function who have remained angina-free to that time, as well as those who have developed class I or class II angina since discharge that has responded well to medical therapy. This strategy is also rational for patients surviving an uncomplicated myocardial infarction who unexpectedly are found to have an ejection fraction below 0.40 despite the absence of clinically apparent CHF at any time during their hospitalization; however, such patients are clearly at increased risk for subsequent cardiovascular morbidity and mortality, and a substantially larger percentage of them could be expected to have a positive result during a predischarge exercise test compared to patients with a similar hospital course but with adequate LV function. Therefore predischarge exercise testing of patients surviving a clinically uncomplicated myocardial infarction, but with a reduced ejection fraction, should provide early identification of those among this group most likely to benefit from coronary artery bypass grafting (those with three-vessel disease and, by definition of this group, depressed LV function, in addition to those with left main coronary artery disease [1, 2]). Patients with reduced LV function and a positive submaximal exercise test before discharge should undergo early coronary angiography.

Exercise testing should be performed while the patient is on optimal medical therapy, as the issue is not if the patient has coronary disease but, rather, whether medical therapy (if any) allows the patient to tolerate successfully the burden of coronary disease. There is little useful information to be gained from exercise testing a patient on a medical regimen he or she cannot maintain because of unacceptable side effects. If at any time the patient's angina cannot be adequately controlled on well tolerated medicines, referral for coronary angiography is indicated.

Many postmyocardial infarction patients have abnormal resting electrocardiograms; the addition of stress and rest thallium 201 imaging to the exercise test helps to determine how much, if any, myocardium remains jeopardized in these patients, as the exercise electrocardiograms of these patients may be of little use in this regard. In fact, because the severity and extent of reversible perfusion defects detected by exercise thallium 201 scintigraphy is itself of prognostic value [34, 35], it is rational to routinely perform the 6-week postdischarge exercise test with thallium 201 imaging in all patients.

In general, interpretation of the exercise data must be individualized. The patient's desired life style must be considered in concert with such predictors of future cardiovascular morbidity and mortality as objectively measured exercise tolerance and the size and number of myocardial areas made ischemic during exercise. Clearly, large widespread areas of myocardial ischemia warrant referral for coronary angiography; however, one or two ischemic areas of small or moderate size might reasonably prompt continued medical therapy in an elderly patient who achieves a workload significantly in excess of the demands placed on the individual's heart during usual daily activities. Alternatively, if a single, small area of ischemia, associated with limiting angina at a relatively low workload, persists during repeated tests despite an escalation to maximal medical therapy in an otherwise healthy patient wishing to return to a program of regular strenuous physical activity, invasive evaluation with an eye toward revascularization becomes indicated.

With these considerations in mind, one of the three management options presents itself to the clinician after the 6-week postdischarge symptom-limited exercise test in the uncomplicated myocardial infarction patient with adequate global LV function. If the patient performs well, with good exercise tolerance for age, and exhibits little or no evidence of exercise-induced myocardial ischemia, the risk of subsequent cardiovascular morbidity and mortality is low [36], and the patient may be simply followed on the current regimen. Repeat exercise testing every 6 months for 1 year and yearly thereafter is adequate follow-up for patients who remain asymptomatic. In contrast, patients with markedly poor exercise tolerance, with electrocardiographic or scintigraphic evidence suggesting proximal stenosis of the left anterior descending coronary artery, or with large or numerous exercise-induced ischemic defects by thallium 201 scintigraphy should be referred for coronary angiography and, if possible, subsequent revascularization (angioplasty or coronary artery bypass grafting).

The third option, increasing medical therapy followed by repeat exercise testing, should be used sparingly, reserved for three types of patients in this group: (1) those on a minimal to moderate medical regimen who experience early limiting angina from a demonstrably small area of ischemia (particularly inferior ischemia) without evidence of LV dysfunction during the exercise test (i.e., normal blood pressure response to exercise); (2) patients who develop a small to moderate-sized ischemic area in a single coronary distribution but only at a workload clearly in excess of the usual daily activity and again without evidence of LV dysfunction during the test; (3) patients who are poor surgical candidates for a noncardiac reason. Particularly in the group with adequate global LV function, it is prudent to "err" on the side of catheterization. First, the risk of the procedure itself is low. Second, documentation of "surgical disease," where mortality is clearly reduced by surgical revascularization—generally accepted to include significant left main coronary artery disease and severe proximal triple-vessel disease with left ventricular ejection fraction less than 0.50—could be life-saving. Third, coronary artery bypass surgery, if indicated, is of comparatively low risk in patients with preserved LV function.

There is little rationale for routine ambulatory electrocardiographic monitoring of pa-

tients surviving an uncomplicated acute myocardial infarction with adequate global LV function. Only about 10 percent of these patients are found to have frequent ventricular ectopy, defined as a mean of ten or more ventricular premature contractions (VPCs) per hour during 24 hours of ambulatory monitoring [32]. The prognostic value of this finding in the setting of adequate ventricular function is uncertain. In the MILIS study [32], this small subgroup sustained a disturbingly high 18 percent mortality by 1.5 years postinfarction. Other data, however, indicate only 10 percent mortality at 22 months for all patients with ten or more VPCs per hour [19], suggesting that the subgroup with adequate LV function would enjoy an even better prognosis. In a more recent study, no patient with an ejection fraction of more than 0.40 and ten or more VPCs per hour died during a year of follow-up, despite a median frequency of more than 100 VPCs per hour in that group [37]. Beyond this information, there is no evidence that attempts to suppress these ventricular arrhythmias with drug therapy alter subsequent mortality. Thus routine ambulatory electrocardiographic monitoring of patients surviving an uncomplicated acute myocardial infarction with adequate LV function appears to be a low-yield procedure, identifying few patients at an uncertain (but likely low) degree of risk, for whom no proved therapy exists.

MYOCARDIAL INFARCTION COMPLICATED BY CONGESTIVE HEART FAILURE

As demonstrated by Killip and Kimball in 1967 [38], the occurrence of increasingly severe CHF early after myocardial infarction is associated with a parallel increase in hospital mortality. Similarly, late mortality is increased in survivors of myocardial infarction complicated by CHF [19]. These clinical observations reflect the direct relation between the extent of ischemic myocardial dysfunction causing the pump failure and the extent and severity of the underlying coronary disease. Although the occurrence of severe CHF or cardiogenic shock at any point during the course of acute myocardial infarction indicates the presence of widespread coronary disease, all the ischemically dysfunctional myocardium does not necessarily progress irreversibly to infarction and permanent damage [39]. Observations of spontaneous improvement in left ventricular function after CHF due to acute myocardial infarction gave rise to the concept of *stunned myocardium*. This term refers to myocardium depleted of its stores of high-energy phosphates, accumulating excesses of toxic metabolites, and subjected to an acidic pH by a transient ischemic insult; it is thus unable to support normal electromechanical cardiac events but capable of an eventual full recovery given restitution and maintenance of an adequate blood supply [40]. Advances in thrombolytic therapy have improved the salvage of such ischemic myocardium jeopardized during the initial clinical presentation, as reflected by improvement in regional left ventricular function [41] and in both early and late mortality in patients treated with these agents [14, 15, 42].

Thus the first question to be answered in the management of the patient whose myocardial infarction is complicated by CHF is whether the pump failure is a consequence of active, ongoing ischemia or, rather, is it a sequel to some other irreversible cause such as a previous, completed ischemic event. Accordingly, the clinical strategy is, first, to relieve any ischemia contributing to the pump failure; second, to prevent recurrent ischemia; and finally, to provide inotropic support, where necessary, without reaggravating the imbalance between oxygen supply and demand that always underlies myocardial ischemia. In any of these situations, supplemental oxygen should be administered. If the presence of suggestive chest pain, electrocardiographic changes, or other clinical data indicate an acute myocardial infarction, thrombolytic therapy, if not contraindicated, must be instituted as early as possible to maximize its beneficial effects on impaired LV function. If the clinical situation is more compatible with active ischemia than with infarction, or when thrombolytic therapy is not an option, aggressive therapy with nitrates is indicated. By dilating coronary conductance vessels, as well as peripheral arterioles and venules, nitrates favorably alter the myocardial oxygen supply-demand ratio by decreasing preload and afterload while increasing coronary blood flow. In addition to improving ventricular dysfunction by relieving ischemia, the preload reduction itself reduces pulmonary congestion. Beta-adrenergic antagonists and calcium channel blocking agents, though not absolutely contraindicated in this setting, must be used cautiously in order to avoid exacerbating the CHF by their negative inotropic effects. The former class of drugs is useful when inappropriate tachycardia is thought to underlie the ischemia and CHF; the latter can be added to nitrates when hypertension or coronary spasm believed to be aggravating the clinical syndrome does not respond satisfactorily to aggressive nitrate treatment.

As treatment of active ischemia progresses, specific therapy for CHF can be instituted. Gentle diuresis is appropriate. If an inotropic agent is required, intravenous dobutamine or amrinone offer better inotropic support for the same degree of tachycardia compared with dopamine or epinephrine; therefore the former drugs increase myocardial oxygen demands less than the latter. Dobutamine or amrinone are thus the agents of choice when the possibility of inducing recurrent myocardial ischemia with an inotropic drug is a concern. The therapeutic response to these drugs is best evaluated, and they are thus most easily titrated when serial measurements of cardiac output and pulmonary artery pressures are readily available. In view of this point and because patients in CHF due to acute myocardial infarction can deteriorate abruptly, the clinician should have a low threshold for placing a pulmonary artery catheter into these patients. Afterload reduction with nitroprusside is of benefit when the calculated systemic vascular resistance is elevated.

Noninvasive assessment of left ventricular function should be performed as early as is practical to provide a baseline for serial evaluations. Spontaneous improvement in the function of stunned myocardium is most rapid within the first days after the ischemic event and is usually complete within 1 week [40]. As improvement occurs, the patient can be weaned from intravenous inotropic agents and vasodilators and switched to oral digoxin, diuretics, and, when necesssary, vasodilators. The combination of preload reduction with nitrates and afterload reduction with hydralazine improves mortality in patients with congestive heart failure due to a variety of causes, including coronary artery disease and previous myocardial infarction [43]. Treatment with the angiotensin-converting enzyme inhibitor enalapril confers a similar benefit on these patients [44]. Salt restriction should always accompany drug treatment of CHF.

Because serious CHF in the setting of acute myocardial infarction usually indicates the presence of widespread, hemodynamically significant coronary artery stenoses, its occurrence represents a probable indication for coronary angiography. The exceptions to this recommendation include those patients with an LV ejection fraction remaining below 0.30, despite optimal medical therapy, by 6 weeks postinfarction; by this time, further recovery of stunned myocardium is no longer likely [40]. In this subgroup, the risk of coronary artery bypass surgery is greatest and usually outweighs the potential benefits [20]. Continued medical therapy, directed to prevention of ischemia and optimal management of CHF, is appropriate.

In other patients, who survive a myocardial infarction complicated by Killip class III or IV CHF with subsequent improvement in the signs and symptoms of CHF, the incidence of left main or proximal three-vessel coronary artery disease with significant viable but jeopardized myocardium is high [39]. Coronary artery bypass surgery has been shown to decrease mortality in patients with these coronary lesions [1, 2]. In the absence of other contraindications to major thoracic surgery, these patients enjoy an acceptable surgical risk and often display an increase in LV ejection fraction following coronary revascularization. They should therefore undergo coronary angiography followed by coronary artery bypass surgery (when the latter is appropriate).

In order to minimize risk to patients with CHF during an acute myocardial infarction, it is preferable, whenever possible, to delay surgery until at least 2 weeks after the acute event in order to stabilize the patient medically and await maximal spontaneous recovery of ventricular function; indeed, surgical mortality is probably further decreased when more than 6 weeks have elapsed since an acute myocardial infarction. In some patients, however, pump failure is clearly due to recurrent ischemia that cannot be successfully managed by aggressive medical therapy. Definition of the coronary anatomy in anticipation of revascularization offers the only hope for myocardial salvage and must proceed, in the absence of other contraindications, to surgery. In such cases, placement of an intra-aortic balloon pump often can enhance the treatment of both CHF and underlying ischemia by reducing the impedance to ejection during systole and increasing the coronary perfusion pressure during diastole. The balloon pump frequently stabilizes the condition of a critically ill patient, allowing cardiac catheterization to be performed safely and maintaining adequate perfusion of the heart and other vital organs until a definitive myocardial revascularization procedure can be performed. When even intra-aortic balloon pumping leaves a patient in a tenuous hemodynamic state and thus a poor surgical candidate, judicious angioplasty of the most easily approached lesion, although not providing complete revascularization, may allow sufficient improvement to enable the patient to tolerate surgery. Such a strategy should be reserved for patients who would die, despite balloon pumping, without an emergency revascularization procedure.

Finally, many patients whose infarction is complicated only by mild CHF leave the hospital with no congestive signs or symptoms on their medical regimen at that time. Management options at that point are similar to those described earlier for patients who have sustained an uncomplicated myocardial infarction based on the predischarge resting ejection fraction.

The prevalence of malignant ventricular arrhythmias detected by ambulatory electrocardiographic monitoring is known to be significantly increased among patients left with symptomatic CHF after an acute myocardial infarction. Because frequent VPCs ($\geq$10 per hour) documented beyond 48 hours after an acute myocardial infarction pose an independent risk for cardiovascular death [19, 32], routine ambulatory electrocardiographic monitoring of postinfarction patients with CHF should be considered. By 6 weeks after discharge, according to the management strategies discussed above, these patients have undergone either treadmill exercise testing or cardiac catheterization, depending on the severity of the CHF that had complicated their myocardial infarction. If the results of either of these investigations have not suggested the need for further studies or revascularization, it is reasonable to perform ambulatory electrocardiographic monitoring at that time. Otherwise, it is preferable to wait until after revascularization has been completed or the need for it has been excluded.

Once malignant ventricular arrhythmias have been identified in patients with reduced LV function, and treatment of CHF or recurrent ischemia has been optimized with all appropriate pharmacologic and invasive measures, their management should probably involve electrophysiologic testing with programmed electrical stimulation. This study determines the need for, and nature of, further therapy directed against these arrhythmias. The problem of postinfarction ventricular arrhythmias is addressed in a separate section of this chapter.

MYOCARDIAL INFARCTION COMPLICATED BY RECURRENT ISCHEMIA

In general, the problem of recurrent myocardial ischemia can be equated with recurrent angina pectoris; of course, the possibility of "anginal equivalents" as clinical signs of recurrent ischemia must be borne in mind. For example, dyspnea or lightheadedness may be due to left ventricular dysfunction as a result of recurrent ischemia, even in the absence of typical angina pectoris. The clinician must also remember that the character of a patient's angina sometimes changes after an acute myocardial infarction, as myocardium that had previously contributed to symptoms has died and is therefore no longer a source of ischemia. The pharmacologic management of an individual attack of postinfarction angina is no different from that already outlined for the initial ischemic event or for ischemia underlying CHF. As always, the general strategy is to improve myocardial oxygen supply while decreasing the demand.

Patients experiencing ischemic symptoms early after an acute infarction clearly have additional myocardium at risk for reinfarction. Because the 6-month postinfarction mortality exceeds 50 percent in such patients [45], they should undergo coronary angiography prior to discharge from the hospital. Knowledge of the coronary anatomy allows rational management of these patients. Patients with single-vessel coronary artery disease have a good prognosis following an acute myocardial infarction [46]. In one study, none of 97 such patients died during a mean follow-up period of more than 3 years, and only six sustained a recurrent nonfatal infarction. Those patients who displayed thallium redistribution during exercise scintigraphy had a higher incidence of nonfatal infarction and readmission with unstable angina [45]; this subgroup may benefit from prophylactic percutaneous transluminal coronary angioplasty, whereas medical management is sufficient for the others. At the other end of the spectrum, patients with postinfarction angina found at coronary angiography to have significant left main or three-vessel coronary artery disease clearly require coronary artery bypass grafting. When two-vessel coronary disease is found in patients with early postinfarction angina, management may be aided by the location of electrocardiographic changes associated with the postinfarction ischemic events. The 6-month mortality of patients with ischemic changes observed in a distribution different from the electrocardiographic location of the index infarction ("ischemia at a distance") is three times greater than that of patients whose early postinfarction angina is associated with electrocardiographic changes limited to the leads involved by the original infarction [45]; a revascularization procedure (surgery or angioplasty), chosen on the basis of the individual's specific coronary anatomy, is a reasonable strategy. Prognostic information from exercise thallium scintigraphy can also be useful when deciding between medical therapy and a revascularization procedure in patients with two-vessel disease, as the number and severity of reversible defects predict subsequent cardiac events and survival [34, 35]. Finally, guidance comes from the VA Cooperative Study Group; in addition to the well known angiographic criteria for the identification of patients benefiting from bypass surgery with prolonged survival, this study also clinically defined a group that enjoyed an enhanced survival after coronary artery bypass grafting without regard to the angiographically defined coronary anatomy. The latter group included patients with at least two of the following: (1) resting ST depression, (2) a history of myocardial infarction, or (3) a history of hypertension [1].

MYOCARDIAL INFARCTION COMPLICATED BY COMPLEX VENTRICULAR ARRHYTHMIAS

The results of several large studies of postinfarction patients leave little doubt that an average of ten or more VPCs per hour (documented over 24 hours of ambulatory electrocardiographic monitoring performed more than 48 hours after the infarction) is associated with an increased risk of overall cardiac mortality [19] and sudden death [32]. Unfortunately, what impact these associations should have on the care of postinfarction patients is far less clear.

First, frequent and complex ventricular ectopy is so common after myocardial infarction that its predictive value for morbidity is relatively low [47]. Second, whereas such ectopy is not limited to patients with LV dysfunction, it is heavily concentrated among them [48] (Fig. 39-2); the prognosis of these patients is influenced far more prominently by their de-

Fig. 39-2
A. Distribution of ventricular ectopic activity (VEA; noncomplex versus complex) among patients with ejection fractions ≤ 40 percent versus ≥ 40 percent. Complex VEA is rare in the group with the higher ejection fraction. *B*. Distribution of ejection fractions (≤ 40 percent versus ≥ 40 percent) in patients with noncomplex versus complex ventricular ectopic activity. An ejection fraction ≥ 40 percent is rare in the group with complex ventricular ectopic activity. (Adapted from the data of R. A. Schultze et al. *Am. J. Med.* 62:192, 1977 by N. Goldschlager. *Cardiology* (Vol. 2). Philadelphia: Lippincott, 1987. With permission.)

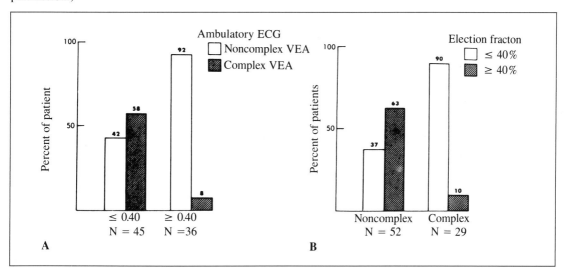

gree of LV dysfunction than by their ventricular dysrhythmias [19]. Conversely, in patients with LV ejection fractions of more than 0.40, mortality is low despite frequent VPCs; in one study, the 1-year mortality of postinfarction patients with an ejection fraction of 0.40 or more and a median VPC frequency of more than 100 per hour was 0 percent [37]. Most distressing is the fact that antiarrhythmic therapy of these postinfarction ventricular arrhythmias has never been shown to reduce the incidence of either sudden death or overall cardiac mortality. An early report that electrophysiologic testing of survivors of acute myocardial infarction could predict subsequent ventricular tachycardia and sudden death [49] raised hope that this technique would allow effective, directed prophylaxis

against these fatal sequelae; however, the results of later investigations have not been as encouraging [50, 51]. This therapeutic nihilism can be tempered somewhat by observations of the efficacy of invasive electrophysiologic studies for guiding therapy of recurrent ventricular tachycardia and out-of-hospital cardiac arrest in patients without recent myocardial infarction [52, 53].

In the absence of direct scientific evidence to support any recommendations for the evaluation and treatment of myocardial electrical instability after acute myocardial infarction, the following suggestions appear to constitute a rational approach to the problem (Fig. 39-3):

1. Routine ambulatory electrocardiographic monitoring of survivors of acute myocardial

Fig. 39-3

Management strategies for patients surviving acute myocardial infarction. MI = myocardial infarction; CHF = congestive heart failure; I,II = Killip class I or II; III,IV = Killip class III or IV; EF = ejection fraction; VT = ventricular tachycardia; VF = ventricular fibrillation; ETT = exercise tolerance test; cath = cardiac catheterization and coronary angiography; CABG = coronary artery bypass grafting; PTCA = percutaneous transluminal coronary angioplasty; med rx = medical therapy; EPS = electrophysiologic study.

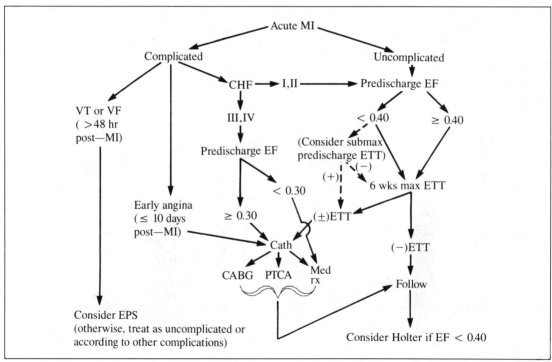

infarction with LV ejection fractions of more than 40 percent is not necessary.

2. Patients with sustained ventricular tachycardia discovered by any means more than 48 hours after acute myocardial infarction should be referred for programmed electrical stimulation in an attempt to direct therapy.

3. If survivors of acute myocardial infarction with an LV ejection fraction of less than 40 percent are to undergo ambulatory electrocardiographic monitoring, it should be with the intention of referring them for programmed electrical stimulation if runs of ventricular tachycardia are recorded. The documentation of frequent or complex ventricular ectopy during ambulatory electrocardiographic monitoring of these patients is likely, but it does not necessarily constitute an indication of antiarrhythmic therapy. If antiarrhythmic therapy is undertaken for the treatment of frequent ventricular ectopy, it should be with the understanding that there is no evidence that such treatment impacts favorably on survival; indeed, follow-up monitoring should be performed to determine that the drug chosen does not exert a proarrhythmic effect on the patient's ventricular ectopy.

Editorial Comments

Each physician should decide on a management strategy that is consistent and cost-effective. Unfortunately, there is such variance in how cardiologists approach acute coronary disease that consistency and cost-effectiveness seem to be relegated to a less important level. This situation is due in part to the still evolving concepts regarding acute care. However, some basic physiologic facts do not change. As Wolff and Karliner pointed out, maintenance of optimal myocardial oxygen supply and demand is always the overriding concern. All pharmacologic and mechanical interventions are designed to optimally reduce myocardial oxygen demand and improve myocardial flow. The 1970s witnessed attempts to control demand, and the 1980s comprised the

era of improved myocardial flow. In the final analysis, both are important. The combination of reduced heart rate, improved loading conditions, and augmented coronary blood flow likely serve the patient best. G.S.F.

References

1. Veterans Administration Coronary Artery Bypass Surgery Cooperative Study Group. Eleven-year survival in the Veterans Administration randomized trial of coronary bypass surgery for stable angina. *N. Engl. J. Med.* 311:1333, 1984.

2. Passamani, E., Davis, K. B., Gillespie, M. J., et al. A randomized trial of coronary artery bypass surgery. *N. Engl. J. Med.* 312:1665, 1985.

3. Vigilante, G. J., Weintraub, W. S., Klein, L. W., et al. Improved survival with coronary bypass surgery in patients with three vessel coronary disease and abnormal left ventricular function. *Am. J. Med.* 82:697, 1987.

4. O'Neill, W., Timmis, G. C., Bourdillon, P. D., et al. A prospective randomized clinical trial of intracoronary streptokinase versus coronary angioplasty for acute myocardial infarction. *N. Engl. J. Med.* 314:812, 1986.

5. Sasaguri, T., Itoh, T., Hirata, M., et al. Regulation of coronary artery tone in relation to the activation of signal transductors that regulate calcium homeostasis. *J. Am. Coll. Cardiol.* 9:1167, 1987.

6. Gibson, R. S., Boden, W. E., Theroux, P., et al. Diltiazem and reinfarction in patients with non-Q-wave myocardial infarction. *N. Engl. J. Med.* 315:423, 1986.

7. Ryan, W. F., Henning, H., and Karliner, J. S. Effects of morphine on left ventricular dimensions and function in patients with previous myocardial infarction. *Clin. Cardiol.* 2:417, 1979.

8. MIAMI Trial Research Group. Metoprolol in acute myocardial infarction (MIAMI): A randomized placebo-controlled international trial. *Eur. Heart J.* 6:199, 1985.

9. ISIS-1 (First International Study of Infarct Survival) Collaborative Group. Randomised trial of intravenous atenolol among 16,207 cases of suspected acute myocardial infarction: ISIS-1. *Lancet* 2:60, 1986.

10. Hjalmarson, A. International beta-blocker review in acute and postmyocardial infarction. *Am. J. Cardiol.* 61:26B, 1988.

11. Yusuf, S., Peto, R., Lewis, J., et al. Beta blockade during and after myocardial infarction: An overview of the randomized trials. *Prog. Cardiovasc. Dis.* 27:335, 1985.

12. DeWood, M. A., Spores, J., Notske, R., et al. Prevalence of total coronary occlusion during the early hours of transmural myocardial infarction. *N. Engl. J. Med.* 303:897, 1980.

13. Sherry, S. Recombinant tissue plasminogen activator (rt-PA): Is it the thrombolytic agent of choice for an evolving acute myocardial infarction? *Am. J. Cardiol.* 59:984, 1987.

14. Gruppo Italiano Per Lo Studio Della Streptochi-Nasi Nell'Infarto Miocardico (GISSI). Long-term effects of intravenous thrombolysis in acute myocardial infarction: Final report of the GISSI study. *Lancet* 2:871, 1987.

15. ISIS-2 (Second International Study of Infarct Survival) Collaborative Group. Intravenous streptokinase given within 0–4 hours of onset of myocardial infarction reduced mortality in ISIS-2. *Lancet* 1:502, 1987.

16. Rao, A. K., Pratt, C., Berke, A., et al. Thrombolysis in myocardial infarction (TIMI) trial—phase I: Hemorrhagic manifestations and changes in plasma fibrinogen and the fibrinolytic system in patients treated with recombinant tissue plasminogen activator and streptokinase. *J. Am. Coll. Cardiol.* 11:1, 1988.

17. Lee, G., Low, R. I., Takeda, P., et al. Importance of follow-up medical and surgical approaches to prevent reinfarction, reocclusion, and recurrent angina following intracoronary thrombolysis with streptokinase in acute myocardial infarction. *Am. Heart J.* 104:921, 1982.

18. Gorgels, A. P. M., Vos, M. A., Letsch, I. S., et al. Usefulness of the accelerated idioventricular rhythm as a marker for myocardial necrosis and reperfusion during thrombolytic therapy in acute myocardial infarction. *Am. J. Cardiol.* 61:231, 1988.

19. Multicenter Postinfarction Research Group. Risk stratification and survival after myocardial infarction. *N. Engl. J. Med.* 309:331, 1983.

20. DeBusk, R. F., Blomqvist, G., Kouchoukos, N. T., et al. Identification and treatment of low-risk patients after acute myocardial infarction and coronary-artery bypass graft surgery. *N. Engl. J. Med.* 314:161, 1986.

21. Stone, P. H., Raabe, D. S., Jaffe, A. S., et al. Prognostic significance of location and type of myocardial infarction: Independent adverse outcome associated with anterior location. *J. Am. Coll. Cardiol.* 11:453, 1988.

22. Krone, R. J., Friedman, E., Thanavaro, S., et al. Long-term prognosis after first Q-wave (transmural) or non-Q-wave (nontransmural) myocardial infarction: Analysis of 593 patients. *Am. J. Cardiol.* 52:234, 1983.

23. Gibson, R. S., Beller, G. A., Gheorghiade, M., et al. The prevalence and clinical significance of residual myocardial ischemia 2 weeks after uncomplicated non-Q-wave infarction: A prospective natural history study. *Circulation* 73:1186, 1986.

24. Phibbs, B. "Transmural" versus "subendocardial" myocardial infarction: An electrocardiographic myth. *J. Am. Coll. Cardiol.* 1:561, 1983.

25. Elwood, P. C., Cochrane, A. L., Burr, M. L., et al. A randomized controlled trial of acetyl salicylic acid in the secondary prevention of mortality from myocardial infarction. *Br. Med. J.* 1:436, 1974.

26. Aspirin Myocardial Infarction Study Research Group. A randomized, controlled trial of aspirin in persons recovered from myocardial infarction. *J.A.M.A.* 243:661, 1980.

27. Canner, P. L. Aspirin in coronary heart disease. *Isr. J. Med. Sci.* 19:413, 1983.

28. Marcus, A. J. Aspirin as an antithrombotic medication. *N. Engl. J. Med.* 309:1515, 1983.

29. Topol, E. J., Califf, R. M., George, B. S., et al. A randomized trial of immediate versus delayed elective angioplasty after intravenous tissue plasminogenactivator in acute myocardial infection. *N. Engl. J. Med.* 317:581, 1987.

30. Volpi, A., Maggioni, A., Franzosi, M. G., et al. In-hospital prognosis of patients with acute myocardial infarction complicated by primary ventricular fibrillation. *N. Engl. J. Med.* 317:257, 1987.

31. Nicod, P., Gilpin, E., Dittrich, H., et al. Late clinical outcome in patients with early ventricular fibrillation after myocardial infarction. *J. Am. Coll. Cardiol.* 11:464, 1988.

32. Mukharji, J., Rude, R. E., Poole, K., et al. Risk factors for sudden death after acute myocardial infarction: Two-year follow-up. *Am. J. Cardiol.* 54:31, 1984.

33. DeBusk, R. F., and Dennis, C. A. "Submaximal" predischarge exercise testing after acute myocardial infarction: Who needs it?. *Am. J. Cardiol.* 55:499, 1985.

34. Smeets, J. P., Rigo, P., Legrand, V., et al. Prognostic value of thallium-201 stress myocardial scintigraphy with exercise ECG after myocardial infarction. *Cardiology* 68:67, 1981.

35. Gibson, R. S., Watson, D. D., Craddock, G. B., et al. Prediction of cardiac events after uncomplicated myocardial infarction: A prospective study comparing predischarge exercise thallium-201 scintigraphy and coronary angiography. *Circulation* 68:321, 1983.

36. De Feyter, P. J., van Eenige, M. J., Dighton, D. H., et al. Prognostic value of exercise testing, coronary angiography and left ventriculography 6-8 weeks after myocardial infarction. *Circulation* 66:527, 1983.

37. Gottlieb, S. H., Ouyang, P., and Gottlieb, S. O. Death after acute myocardial infarction: Interrelation between left ventricular dysfunction, arrhythmias and ischemia. *Am. J. Cardiol.* 61:7B, 1988.

38. Killip, T., and Kimball, J. T. Treatment of myocardial infarction in a coronary care unit: A two

year experience with 250 patients. *Am. J. Cardiol.* 20:457, 1967.

39. Warnowicz, M. A., Parker, H., and Cheitlin, M. D. Prognosis of patients with acute pulmonary edema and normal ejection fraction after acute myocardial infarction. *Circulation* 67:330, 1983.

40. Braunwald, E., and Kloner, R. A. The stunned myocardium: Prolonged, postischemic ventricular dysfunction. *Circulation* 66:1146, 1982.

41. Stack, R. S., Phillips, H. R., Grierson, D. S., et al. Functional improvement of jeopardized myocardium following intracoronary streptokinase infusion in acute myocardial infarction. *J. Clin. Invest.* 72:84, 1983.

42. Mathey, D. G., Schofer, J., Sheehan, F. H., et al. Improved survival up to four years after early coronary thrombolysis. *Am. J. Cardiol.* 61:524, 1988.

43. Cohn, J. N., Archibald, D. G., Ziesche, S., et al. Effect of vasodilator therapy on mortality in chronic congestive heart failure: Results of a Veterans Administration cooperative study. *N. Engl. J. Med.* 314:1547, 1986.

44. CONSENSUS Trial Study Group. Effects of enalapril on mortality in severe congestive heart failure: Results of the cooperative north Scandinavian enalapril survival study. *N. Engl. J. Med.* 316:1429, 1987.

45. Schuster, E. H., and Bulkley, B. H. Early postinfarction angina: Ischemia at a distance and ischemia in the infarct zone. *N. Engl. J. Med.* 305:1101, 1981.

46. Wilson, W. W., Gibson, R. S., Nygaard, T. W., et al. Acute myocardial infarction associated with single vessel coronary artery disease: An analysis of clinical outcome and the prognostic importance of vessel patency and residual ischemic myocardium. *J. Am. Coll. Cardiol.* 11:223, 1988.

47. Taylor, G. J., Humphries, J. O., Mellits, E. D., et al. Predictors of clinical course, coronary anatomy and left ventricular function after recovery from acute myocardial infarction. *Circulation* 62:960, 1980.

48. Schulze, R. A., Strauss, H. W., and Pitt, B. Sudden death in the year following myocardial infarction: Relation to ventricular premature contractions in the late hospital phase and left ventricular ejection fraction. *Am. J. Med.* 62:192, 1977.

49. Greene, H. L., Reid, P. R., and Schaeffer, A. H. The repetitive ventricular response in man: A predictor of sudden death. *N. Engl. J. Med.* 299:729, 1978.

50. Richards, D. A., Cody, D. V., Denniss, A. R., et al. Ventricular electrical instability: A predictor of death after myocardial infarction. *Am. J. Cardiol.* 51:75, 1983.

51. Marchlinski, F. E., Buxton, A. E., Waxman, H. L., and Josephson, M. E. Identifying patients at risk of sudden death after myocardial infarction: Value of the response to programmed stimulation, degree of ventricular ectopic activity and severity of left ventricular dysfunction. *Am. J. Cardiol.* 52:1190, 1983.

52. Mason, J. W., and Winkle, R. A. Electrode-catheter arrhythmia induction in the selection and assessment of antiarrhythmic drug therapy for recurrent ventricular tachycardia. *Circulation* 58:971, 1978.

53. Wilber, D. J., Garan, H., Finkelstein, D., et al. Out-of-hospital cardiac arrest: Use of electrophysiologic testing in the prediction of long-term outcome. *N. Engl. J. Med.* 318:19, 1988.

IX
Administrative Decisions in the Coronary Care Unit

40
Administration of the Referral Comprehensive Coronary Care Unit

Galen S. Wagner, Margaret B. Munster, Wanda M. Bride, and Robert M. Califf

During the early days of coronary care, patients with symptoms suggesting an acute myocardial infarction were transferred into a specialized nursing area called a coronary care unit (CCU) from either a hospital emergency area or another impatient area; they were later transferred out to either a general medical or "step down" area. More recently, systems of "comprehensive coronary care" have evolved. They extend from the time the patient or bystander first contacts an emergency medical transport service through posthospital enrollment in a rehabilitation program. Patients are often transported via ambulance or helicopter from their local hospital emergency area where intravenous thrombolytic therapy has been initiated to a referral medical center. There they may undergo angiography in an interventional catheterization laboratory prior to entering a referral CCU. Patients who respond to reperfusion therapy and quickly stabilize may then be "reverse referred" from that CCU back to their local hospital for maximal continuity and entry into rehabilitation. This chapter presents an idealized plan for administration of such a referral comprehensive coronary care unit, the CCCU.

CCCU Leadership Team

The CCCU leadership team is comprised of the medical director of the CCU, nursing director of the CCU, coordinator of emergency medical transport services, director of the interventional catheterization laboratory, and director of cardiac rehabilitation/reverse referral program. This leadership team should meet monthly, with their minutes providing dynamic guidelines for the operation of the CCCU. Each member of this team has his or her specific job descriptions, and one of them should function as the coordinator for the CCCU leadership team.

The *director* of the CCU is usually a young cardiologist with an active ongoing clinical practice and research in coronary care. This individual is the principal investigator for a variety of clinical research protocols. He or she schedules house staff and senior staff physicians for the unit and takes a leadership role in the day-to-day continuing education of both physicians and nurses. The *nursing director* of the CCU is responsible for the scheduling of all of the nursing personnel and coordination of unit operations. This person should also work with each of the nurses in their own career development, which might include participation in scholarly projects relating to coronary care. Both the nursing and medical directors are responsible for the coordination of CCU activities and personnel. As a team, they should provide orientation, continuing education, direction, and feedback to all personnel on the unit. One or the other should be available for consultation for any problems that may arise in the day-to-day unit management.

The *coordinator of the emergency medical transport service* works closely with all of the emergency medical services that transport patients to and from the CCU. They may include both ground and air transport systems. The *director of the interventional catheterization laboratory* has administrative responsibility for that area and the physicians and nurses who care for the patient between the time of arrival in the hospital from the emergency transport service until admission to the CCU. The *director of the cardiac rehabilitation/reverse referral program* is responsible for the patient education and activity prescription that begins in the CCU, intensifies in the step-down area, and continues through either referral to an outpatient rehabilitation program or reverse referral back to the local hospital. This team should be continually developing and revising guidelines for optimal movement of the patients through the various phases of the CCCU.

Telecommunications

Modern telecommunication systems are important for facilitating patient entry into the CCCU. The high risk previously prepared patient can have direct access to the local CCU nurse, and the local physician can have direct access to a consultant interventional cardiologist. Such telecommunication systems are also required to provide the continuing link between local and referral physicians during the patient's stay on the referral CCU.

Patients known to be at high risk of acute myocardial infarction should be trained in the use of a transtelephonic electrocardiographic monitor and autoinjectable medications [1, 2]. They should be able to telephone to their local hospital CCU to transmit symptoms and rhythms. The CCU nurse receiving the call should decide whether an acute ischemic event might be in progress, follow a protocol for facilitating the patient's use of the appropriate autoinjectable medication, maintain continuous communication with the patient, and arrange transport to the hospital. This aspect of the CCCU should be directed by the coordinator of the emergency transport system.

Also, the director of the interventional catheterization laboratory should be responsible for having a physician continuously on call to receive consultation from referring personal or emergency room physicians. From a telecommunications center in their office or home, this "on call" interventional cardiologist can assist in the vital decision-making process when the patient first presents with symptoms of acute coronary insufficiency.

The patients in the CCCU should not lose their vitally important contact with their personal physician. That individual should not only be aware of the patient's course but also have input into the ongoing plans for therapy. The CCCU leadership team should develop a telecommunication system to facilitate this vital doctor–patient relationship. From either the local hospital CCU or a private clinic the personal physician should be able to "round" with their patients in the referral CCU. Via telephone from the patient's bedside there can be direct visualization and communication for review of electrocardiographic, echocardiographic, enzymatic, and angiographic results. In this way, the day-to-day treatment plan can be the joint effort of the personal physician and the consultants in the referral CCU. This transmission could be videotaped locally for later review by those personal physicians who could not be available at the designated "rounding time." This communication can also be used to plan the optimal time for reverse referral back to the patient's own local CCU as soon as he or she is stable, wishes to return, and a bed is available. The medical director of the CCU is responsible for ensuring that the personal physician and the patient do not "lose each other" during the referral CCU experience.

Function of the Referral CCU

The high levels of both patient instability and turnover require that there be sufficient numbers of staff so that there is neither undue fatigue nor too diffuse responsibility. There must be optimal rounding time so that there is not too little staff communication on the one hand or too little time for attention to the individual patient needs on the other. Usually, this requires that "work rounds," "teaching rounds," and "personal physician rounds" be made each day. Work rounds should be made about 7:30 a.m., immediately after conclusion of the report by the outgoing night time nursing staff. The leader of this work rounds should be the CCU resident, with the nurses and interns as key participants. Cardiology fellows may participate only if they are an intimate part of the day-to-day working team. Usually 5 to 10 minutes are required for greeting, evaluating, communicating with, and planning for the continuing care of the patients. No more than 1.5 hours should be required, and 1 hour would be optimal.

Teaching rounds should be directed by a member of the senior physician staff (either the CCU director or designate). The group may view radiographic results via telecommunications at each patient's bedside during the rounds. Each new patient on the service should be briefly presented by the most junior member of the team (student or intern usually) at the bedside. No more than 5 minutes should be required for even a complex presentation. The attending physician should review the current plan for each of the patients and make certain to identify which of the members of the ward team is responsible for carrying out each aspect of that plan. The attending physician should also be responsible for moving this teaching activity along so that it takes no more than 2 hours. These rounds should be "thinking ward rounds" [3]. The attending physician should make certain that the group understands the pathophysiology of each patient's problem. Differing opinions should be identified and an individual assigned to bring back reference sources for resolution. Often "nickel bets" are useful to focus these responsibilities and clarify the varying points of view [4].

Each attending physician should conduct personal physician rounds via telecommunications either during or after teaching rounds. The personal physician should be prepared to receive a telephone call at a certain time on days when important decisions are required, such as consideration of interventional procedures, initiation or discontinuation of life support systems, and time of reverse referral. It should be remembered that, when possible, the final decision rests with the personal physician and that all other physicians are consultants.

Patient's Point of View

The patients should feel that they are under the care of a team committed to minimizing the damage due to acute coronary insufficiency and maximizing the speed of safe return to health and function. They should feel that they are still under the overall care of their personal physician, and the time spent out of their own community should be kept to a minimum. The patient should have a clear understanding of all procedures that are contemplated and the potential cost-benefit ratio of each. The personal physician should continually feel responsible for the patient throughout the CCCU experience, even though some of the day-to-day decisions must be made primarily by specialists from either the referral interventional laboratory or the CCU. The personal physician should be able to continue involvement through telecommunication each day. There should be an understanding that a specialist should do only those things that cannot be done by the patient's personal physician. The CCCU leadership team should continually strive to create a unified system with all parts working smoothly and in concert.

Acknowledgment

This work was supported in part by research grant HL-17670 from the National Heart, Lung, and Blood Institute, National Institutes of Health, Bethesda, Maryland.

References

1. Capone, R. J., Grodman, R. S., and Most, A. S. Transtelephonic surveillance of cardiac arrhythmias. *J. Cardiovasc. Med.* 6(1):57, 1981.
2. Capone, R. J., Visco, J., Curwen, E., and VanEvery, S. The effect of early prehospital transtelephonic coronary intervention on morbidity and mortality: Experience with 284 postmyocardial infarction patients in a pilot program. *Am. Heart J.* 107:1153, 1984.
3. Stead, E. A. Thinking ward rounds are useful. *Med. Times* 95:706, 1967.
4. Ellis III, G. J. The profit of losing a nickel. *Ann. Intern. Med.* 69:990, 1968.

41
Ethical and Legal Dilemmas in the Coronary Care Unit

JOHN J. PARIS AND FRANK E. REARDON

The high-technology medicine available in today's coronary care unit (CCU) not only provides near miraculous benefits for some patients, it also creates new and troublesome ethical and legal dilemmas for patients and practitioners. Standards for access to and discharge from the CCU, "do not resuscitate" orders, determination of death, organ retrieval, advanced directives, decision-making capacity, and substantive and procedural guidelines for termination of treatment in incompetent patients are among the problems. Those issues, along with the emerging question of withholding nutrition and fluids, are discussed in this chapter.

In one of the first and most important studies of the public policy implications of intensive care delivery, Knaus and colleagues [1] at George Washington University Medical Center identified two principal roles for intensive care: "life support of organ system failure in critically ill patients or close monitoring of stable non-critically ill patients in case the need for life support suddenly occurs." From their study they determined that there is little evidence that the widespread use of such services has resulted in improved survival or quality of life for a substantial portion of the patients presently admitted to intensive care units (ICUs). In fact, they concluded that approximately 25 percent of the total ICU therapy is used for patients who are either at low risk of needing unique ICU services or are too

This chapter is adapted from J. J. Paris, and F. E. Reardon. Dilemmas in intensive care medicine: An ethical and legal analysis. *J. Intens. Care Med.* 1:75, 1986.

acutely and chronically ill to benefit from them.

The implications of their study, which confirmed the findings of others who examined the indications and outcomes of intensive care medicine [2–4], pointed to the need for more vigorous ICU and CCU admission and discharge standards. One attempt in that direction was undertaken at Sloan–Kettering Cancer Center, where it was early recognized that many patients admitted to the ICU were surviving their acute episodes only to die shortly thereafter from their underlying cancer. Rather than subject these patients and their families to the trauma of spending the final days in an ICU, the medical staff adopted a policy of formally classifying all hospital patients according to the underlying prognosis of their disease. As Turnbull and associates [5] reported, those patients whose short-term prognosis was poor and for whom no definitive therapy existed were not considered candidates for transfer to the ICU regardless of the acute problems that might develop.

To limit the inappropriate institution of other invasive "lifesaving" therapy, similar prognosticators were developed for patients suffering from advanced cystic fibrosis [6], severe burns [7], and nontraumatic coma [8]. In addition, work has begun on establishing quantitative predictive models such as the Acute Physiology and Chronic Health Evaluation (APACHE) scale developed by Knaus and colleagues [9] as an objective measure of the severity of illness of ICU patients. By design, however, the APACHE I and II scales are more appropriate for predicting outcomes for populations of ICU patients than for prognosticating for individuals. That task, at least in the initial stages, remains notoriously uncertain [10] and varied [11].

The remarkable growth of the hospice movement from only one program in 1974 to more than 1600 programs in 1985 [12] is another phenomenon in the attempt to limit inappropriate care of the critically ill. Many of these programs, though, are still in the fledgling stage and are available to only a small fraction of the nation's terminally ill patients. Most critically and terminally ill patients continue to be cared for in institutions in which aggressive intervention and treatment of acute episodes are the norm.

There are many reasons for this general practice of maximal response to crises in the seriously ill patient. Several were identified by Angell [13]: (1) the current fee for service reimbursement schedule, which rewards physicians preferentially for performing tests and procedures; (2) the ever present specter of malpractice; and (3) the American propensity to believe that every problem has a solution, often a technical one. The last factor leads to the familiar request of patients and families to "do everything possible," which is all too often translated into what Thurow [14] perceptively characterized as using every known experimental technique on the outside chance that the procedure just might work.

This process, which Fuchs [15] labeled "the technological imperative," when combined with the other forces now operative in our society, has produced a health care system in crisis: The cost of care has risen beyond our ability or at least our willingness to pay for it. Among the measures to control and limit the rising costs and thereby curb the demands for "rationing" of health care, Angell [13] suggested that we reexamine the proposition that in health care, as in other commodities, more is better. She insisted that, far from being beneficial, much of the medical care now provided in the United States is unnecessary. Much medical care is of no demonstrated value to those who receive it, and some is positively harmful. She cited among the unnecessary items the aggressive treatment of terminally ill patients for whom treatment other than palliative care is no longer appropriate.

As Ramsey [16] noted, it is imperative to distinguish between treatments that will benefit the patient and those that are useless and false remedies. For the patient who has truly entered the dying process, comfort and company, not further and futile attempts at treatment, are the appropriate care. Ramsey's comment forces us into the difficult but nonetheless important distinctions of medical ethics, distinctions whose origin can be traced back to the earliest formulations of the Hippocratic Corpus.

There we find the antidote to the notion that the physician's duty is to do everything possible to prolong life. As Admundsen's [17] historical analysis established, "The treatise entitled *The Art* in the Hippocratic Corpus defines medicine as having three roles: doing away with the sufferings of the sick, lessening the violence of their diseases, and refusing to treat those who are overmastered by their diseases, realizing that in such cases medicine is powerless."

The best contemporary restatement of the standards for appropriate care of the sick is found in the report of the President's Commission for the Study of Ethical Problems in Medicine and Biomedical and Behavioral Research [18]. That report, formulated by a multidisciplinary commission of ethicists, physicians, lawyers, theologians, and academics, has already had enormous impact on hospital policies, regulatory directives, court opinions, and the direction of medicine.

Many of the topics in the report responded to the concerns, fears, and worries of physicians, nurses, and patients, particularly those in the highly sophisticated setting of the CCU. The Commission approached its task primarily from the perspective of ethics, the traditions of medicine, and issues of human choice. Only secondarily did the Commission turn to the more narrow and necessarily limited perspective of law for its contributions to the development of standards and formation of public policy. The result is a balanced, sensitive, humane, and strikingly sensible approach to complex, difficult ethical dilemmas, an approach that is helpful to practitioners and patients alike.

Several of the issues reviewed by the Commission are of particular interest to those involved with intensive care medicine: "do not resuscitate" (DNR) orders, brain death, living wills, and decision-making for the incompetent patient.

DNR Orders

No issue vexes medical personnel more frequently or more seriously than hospital resuscitation practices. Nurses, physicians, and families regularly find themselves at odds over the topic; yet until recently the subject remained unaddressed and unresolved. All the while there has been a decided drift in the delivery of medical care to dying patients to the point that, in the words of Lawler [19], "Today very few people 'die'; they 'arrest.'"

The response to that "arrest" has undergone a profound shift during the 1970s and 1980s. Much of the credit for that change goes to the landmark 1974 American Medical Association Report on Standards for Cardiopulmonary Resuscitation [20], which set standards and initiated a massive and highly effective cardiopulmonary resuscitation (CPR) training program. The report declared:

The purpose of cardiopulmonary resuscitation is the prevention of sudden, unexpected death. Cardiopulmonary resuscitation is not indicated in certain situations, such as in cases of terminal irreversible illness where death is not unexpected or where prolonged cardiac arrest dictates the futility of resuscitation efforts. Resuscitation in these circumstances may represent a positive violation of an individual's right to die with dignity.

That thoughtful and carefully formulated statement has been all but forgotten as paramedics, nurses, and physicians trained in the new lifesaving techniques respond like firefighters, answering an alarm with "crash carts" and portable defibrillators to "code blues." In the words of Dr. Mitchell Rabkin, President of Boston's Beth Israel Hospital, "When the bell rings, you run!"

That response pattern soon led to attempted resuscitations for virtually all in-hospital deaths regardless of individual medical history and prognosis. As Lampton and Winship [21] reported, "Many medical staffs adopted universal, hospital-wide policies stating that CPR would be instituted on all patients experiencing sudden and unexpected cardiopulmonary arrest." They observed that, "Ultimately, it appears that many persons view CPR as a mandatory activity for all patients dying in a hospital." In an insightful and humane essay, Spenser [22] noted that that tendency has evolved into a fixed policy of attempting to overcome the death of all patients unless the physician has written a specific "no-code" order. Consequently, physicians find themselves in the position of having to write a negative, inhibiting-type order to protect their terminally ill patients from unwanted intrusions into their dying.

A further complication in this litigation-conscious era is that physicians are now looking to the courts and the legal profession for guidance and protection on the proper treatment of the dying patient. They are also asking families to share the burden of responsibility for such decisions to a degree that Spenser observed would have been unthinkable a few years ago.

How we got ourselves into this predicament and possible resolutions of it were the subject of a 2-year study by the President's Commission. Dr. Mitchell Rabkin provided the most complete explanation to the Commission. Rabkin testified that before his institution's well known 1976 "Orders Not to Resuscitate" directive [23] was in effect "a significant percentage of patients who died received cardiopulmonary resuscitation upon their *quietus* even though it was acknowledged that the resuscitation efforts for many would be useless." In his words, "the emergency code was called, and all of the troops—cardiologists, anesthetists, nurses, respiratory therapists, and others—responded in full."

The folly of that policy was symbolized for Rabkin when he came across a nurse standing in the corridor, weeping, outside the room of a patient, an octogenarian with widespread terminal cancer. The patient had stopped breathing, and a staff member called the code. A horde of professionals was applying intravenous medication and electrical current to stimulate the heart, and the anesthetist was ventilating the patient through an endotracheal tube just inserted—all to no avail, of course. "Why can't they just let him die in peace?" wept the nurse. The answer was straightforward and suggested in the 1976 Beth Israel directive [23]:

Both as a standard of medical care and a statement of philosophy, it is the general policy of hospitals to act affirmatively to preserve the life of all patients, including persons who suffer from irreversibly terminal illness. It is essential that all hospital staff understand this policy and act accordingly.

That pro-life policy, good in itself, was so rigidly interpreted that a DNR order could be entered only after (1) it was determined that the patient was irreversibly and irreparably ill and death was imminent (within 2 weeks); (2) an ad hoc committee of senior physicians and nurses concurred in that evaluation; and (3) the informed choice of the competent patient (or the family of an incompetent patient) was given. If in the judgment of the responsible physician the patient would be unable to cope psychologically with the consent stipulation, no order could be written. Here a misplaced emphasis on patient autonomy and informed consent pressured the dying patient into the trauma of a code/no-code choice as a final discretionary decision.

Several years' experience with those stringent stipulations and the increasing realization that these ill-considered resuscitation efforts in no way represent an affirmative act to preserve life led the medical staff to rewrite the DNR policy. In addition to the hospital's own experiences was the fact that a Massachusetts appellate court ruled that DNR decision-making should rest with the physician acting in accordance with the standards of good medical practice and the wishes of the patient or the patient's family [24].

That ruling led numerous Massachusetts hospitals to establish formal DNR policies or to reconsider existing procedures. The 1981 Beth Israel Hospital guidelines [25] omit the attempt to define the candidates for DNR orders; they leave that determination to the judgment of the attending physician. The 1981 policy specifies the process by which such possibilities are to be considered and orders written. It also eliminates the need for a bureaucratic ad hoc committee and substitutes the notification of the chief of service that such an order has been given.

In a dramatic shift from the previous emphasis on individual autonomy and "informed consent," the new guidelines state [25]:

If, in the opinion of the attending physician, the competent patient might be harmed by a full discussion of whether resuscitation would be appropriate in the event of an arrest, the competent patient should be spared the discussion; therefore, if the physician and the Chief of Service deem a DNR order appropriate and the family members are in agreement that the discussion might harm the patient and the resuscitation is not appropriate, a DNR order may be entered by the physician.

This new policy, which recognizes the difference between an automaton and an autonomous patient, conforms to Spenser's [22] insight that explanations of DNR orders to dying patients "are thoughtless to the point of being cruel except for the extremely unlikely case where the patient himself inquires."

Rabkin et al. [23] reported that the new Beth Israel policy has allowed more open discussion among caregivers on the appropriateness of orders not to resuscitate a given patient. Concomitantly, quasiorders (e.g., "Walk, don't run," "Page but don't stat page" or emergency page, and "Do not intubate if a code is called") have declined. Not only do partial orders such as these place unwarranted burdens on the hospital staff, but they are, in Goldenring's explicit phrasing, "an ethical fraud" [26].

Under the 1981 guidelines, a code can be called and answered as a well considered affirmative act to benefit the patient. As such, when a code is issued, staff can respond knowing that they will not be deliberately imposing a final useless indignity on the end of life.

Guidelines for Resuscitation Decisions

In its report the President's Commission [18] devoted an entire chapter to resuscitation decisions for hospitalized patients. The Commission noted that, among the general hospital population where virtually all deaths were attended by resuscitation efforts, only 3 percent of the attempts were successful. Furthermore, one in 20 patients who survived resuscitation sustained severe brain damage, and about one in four had some serious permanent injury. Consequently, the Commission concluded that the reflex resuscitation efforts presently attempted in hospitals are frequently a misguided adventure that injures the patient and violates the patient's control over his or her life.

In response, the Commission called for a reevaluation of resuscitation practices by hospitals, health care providers, and especially treatment areas (e.g., cardiac care units) where many patients are at risk for cardiac arrest and where CPR frequently is automatically attempted without appropriate prior deliberation.

In the advanced technical setting of an acute care hospital, the physician/patient/family relationship has been expanded to include health teams, rotating residents, triple shifts of nurses, and many other allied health professionals. Decisions that were once commonly agreed on and easily effected directly by the physician now involve a large, diverse, and frequently unknown cadre of caregivers—hence the emerging need for explicit policies and guidelines for procedures, including DNR orders.

Prior deliberation in such cases would (1) ensure that the patient's rights and decisions regarding self-determination are respected, (2) guarantee that medical interventions serve the patient's best interest, (3) allow adequate evaluation of resource allocation and equity considerations, and (4) reduce nurse/physician/family misunderstandings of resuscitation practices.

To protect both the patient and the caregivers, hospital policies should require appropriate communication with the patient (or the family) about the resuscitation decision. If a DNR order is deemed appropriate, that order should be written in the patient's chart, along with the rationale and supporting documentation.

There is an ongoing dispute over the extent to which the competent patient should or must be involved in the decision to write a DNR order [27]. Clearly, if the patient expresses an explicit desire for or against resuscitation, and the patient's comprehension of the medical situation is not questionable, that decision should be honored. The difficulty arises from the fact that most seriously ill patients have not directly expressed any opinion on the subject. Furthermore, as the President's Commission noted, many of these patients are unwilling to make a decision. How then should the decision-making process for such patients be approached?

In its 1976 directive, Beth Israel Hospital followed the standard that has now been adopted by the Commission: The focus is on patient autonomy and informed consent, which means that patients must make their preferences known. To spur patients to make a decision, the Commission believed that because "it is necessary to have some operative policy while the patient is being encouraged to make a choice, the patient should be informed about what that will be" [18].

That pressure, particularly on a dying patient—who is already overwhelmed with a deteriorating physical condition and attendant fears—strikes us as being entirely misplaced and inappropriate. Nor is the threat of such a mandate and its negative impact on decision-makers lessened by a footnoted reminder that "other care-giving professionals, religious advisors, or family members are in a good or better position to discuss the issue and convey the information (as is the attending physician)" [18]. Undue and misplaced pressure on the dying patient is not allayed by changing the bearer of the message.

Although Miles and co-workers [28] rightly placed the question of resuscitation within the context of the patient's total medical care and prognosis, their insistence on a frank but not overly technical discussion of resuscitation with the patient might well exacerbate the patient's plight. Among the nontechnical factors they believe the patient should understand is that "resuscitation may be followed by the need for life support including intratracheal tube, tracheotomy, respiratory ventilator assistance, arterial lines and monitoring, and continuous intravenous medication, all for an indeterminate period."

Such an approach to CPR decision making might be modified if compared with the 1974 and 1980 standards for CPR issued by the National Conference of the American Heart Association with Siegler's [29] reminder that "the principal ethical grounds for making a decision not to resuscitate a patient should be the sound medical judgment that the patient's death from the primary disease is imminent and that further treatment for the primary disease is futile." Finally, the emphasis by Miles and co-workers on the process of patient involvement in decision-making will not affect the outcome of resuscitation efforts appreciably. Siegler [29] graphically summarized the situation as follows.

Our CPR policies are enmeshed in rules, regulations, and procedures that minimize discretion and maximize bureaucratic bumbling. Some believe that placing the burden for such decisions on patients by invoking autonomy and self-determination will resolve the matter, but let me assure such legalists that the resolution will exist only on paper and not on hospital wards.

One attempt to meet the practical problem noted by Siegler—designed to protect both dignity and the personal values of the dying patient—is found in the work of the University of Massachusetts DNR Task Force. Its earlier focus on autonomy and informed consent was modified to reflect the clinical reality noted by Siegler and the respect for the dying patient highlighted in the 1981 Beth Israel policy. At the urging of several senior physicians, the University of Massachusetts draft guides [30] were changed from:

Physicians may enter Do Not Resuscitate (DNR) Orders after obtaining the patient's informed consent.

to:

Physicians may enter Do Not Resuscitate (DNR) Orders for competent patients who are irreversibly, terminally ill after the patient has been informed of his/her condition and agrees that no further aggressive therapy is appropriate.

If in the attending physician's judgment it would be inappropriate or unnecessarily burdensome to the dying patient to raise the topic of possible aggressive medical response to cardiopulmonary arrest, the physician would make the treatment recommendation to the family.

At this stage it is important to keep in mind Inglefinger's admonition that "a physician who merely spreads an array of vendibles in front of the patient (or family) and then says, 'Go ahead and choose, it's your life,' is guilty of shirking his duty, if not malpractice" [31]. The physician certainly should explain the patient's condition to the family and the realistic options available. However, Inglefinger reminded us that it is the physician's responsibility to recommend a specific course of action instead of merely asking the family to choose among them. In addition, the physician is not asking the family to substitute its judgment for that of the patient but, rather, is asking them to reflect the patient's own choice as close as is humanly possible.

A frustrating situation may arise if in the physician's judgment there is no further treatment that can benefit the irreversibly dying patient, yet the family, through ignorance, misunderstanding, fear, or guilt, demands that "everything possible" be done. Conversely, the problem may be insistence by the family on a DNR order for a patient who the physician believes has a good opportunity of recovery.

In these situations an intrainstitutional consultation or ethics committee should assess the case. Perhaps a simple airing of the issues or the benefit of consultation can dispel the disagreement. Sometimes a change of physician may be in order. Alternatively, the review committee may decide to petition a court to appoint a legal guardian to protect the patient's interests.

Another problem that frequently arises in major hospital settings is the elderly dying patient who has outlived all family and friends. Rather than unreflectively resuscitating all such patients or overusing the complex and somewhat costly role of legal guardian, the Commission noted that decisions against resuscitation might continue to be made as they customarily have been—by consultation with a disinterested physician, professional staff consensus, or by an institutionally designated patient advocate. These decisions are well within the scope of common medical practice and should not be elevated to the role of moral dilemma or judicial problem. Decisions that are more complex or uncertain might, of course, demand more formal institutional review or legal guardianship. Hence, as in almost all of its recommendations, the Commission is firm in its stance that rarely, if ever, is decision-making about life-sustaining care improved by resort to courts.

The President's Commission concluded by reminding us that the only court ever to address the issue ruled that: "The question (DNR) is not one for judicial decision, but one for the attending physician, in keeping with the highest traditions of his profession." It is, in the court's words, "a question peculiarly within the competence of the medical profession of what measures are appropriate to ease the imminent passing of an irreversibly, terminally ill patient in light of the patient's history and condition and the wishes of her family" [24].

The possibility that the highly invasive, costly, and often violent resuscitation procedures available in acute care settings might not be appropriate to a particular patient should be considered as a positive and prospective part of the delivery of high quality medical care. Such decisions should not be made arbitrarily, hastily, or casually. Nor should they depend on the personal fears or predilections of the physician. Rather, they should reflect a careful consideration of the patient's medical condition, prognosis, and values.

Furthermore, the writing of a DNR order does not diminish the physician's continuing responsibility to provide active medical care

to the patient. As the Minnesota Medical Society's Guidelines make clear, "DNR orders are compatible with maximal therapeutic care. The patient may be receiving vigorous support in all other therapeutic modalities and yet justifiably be considered a proper subject for the DNR order" [32].

DNR orders, which have been described in some detail because of the practical impact they have in the CCU, are but a part of the issues about treatment. Two other issues—brain death and living wills—raise troublesome legal and political implications that are out of proportion to the moral consensus on the topics.

Brain Death

One of the primary charges of the President's Commission was the formulation of a standard definition of death. Thirty years ago the definition of death was uniformly agreed on and easy to assess: When the heart and breathing stopped, the patient was dead. Two technologic developments have challenged that understanding: the advent of artificial life support systems and the possibility of organ transplantations. The first allows the revival of patients whose hearts or breathing have stopped. If the patient has suffered no more than a few minutes of oxygen deprivation, he or she can resume a normal life. If, alternatively, the patient undergoes prolonged oxygen deprivation (15 to 20 minutes) and brain cells are destroyed, the patient will be unable to maintain heart action and breathing without mechanical respiratory assistance. Neurologic examinations provide the basis to assess the extent of brain cell destruction and to distinguish patients who have suffered neocortical damage from those who have lost all brain functioning, including that of the brainstem. The first are in a persistent vegetative state. The overwhelming majority of these patients never regain mental functions of any type. Others may recover brain functioning after days to weeks in a sleep-like coma and have periods of wakefulness during which their eyes open and move. There may even be rare instances of consciousness recovery after months of coma, or, as in one case [33], almost 2 years after the initial trauma. All of these patients, including those such as Paul Brophy [34] or Nancy Jobs [35], who have suffered overwhelming destruction of the higher brain centers, continue to have functions of, and circulation to, the brain. They are clearly alive.

In contrast, brain-dead patients have little or no blood flow to the brain. Clinical examinations reveal no evidence of any brain function. The pupils do not respond to light, nor is there eye movement. Spontaneous respiration ceases because of the permanent destruction of the vital respiratory centers in the lower brainstem, and the patient depends on mechanical respiratory support. Because cardiac functioning is not dependent on neural regulation from the brain, heartbeat can continue indefinitely in a respirator-supported brain-dead patient, although heart stoppage usually occurs within a few days. There are, however, published cases of confirmed brain-dead children being maintained for 1 month or more, and Parisi et al. [36, 37] reported the case of a 49-year-old man who survived 74 days in a brain-dead condition before the court-ordered removal of his respirator resulted in death.

With the ability to sustain patients through ventilator assistance came the realization that organs of brain-dead individuals could be kept "fresh" for transplant purposes. However, before the organs can be harvested, the individuals must be dead. Physicians and society then faced two critical questions: First, when is a person dead? Second, is it legitimate to ventilate the cadaver to preserve the organs? Moralists quickly answered "yes" to the second question. The first, however, proved more problematic.

The issue of brain death was sharply focused with the advent of cardiac transplant surgery. As is true with many medicomoral topics, the courts were the first to publicly confront the problem. In the celebrated case of *Tucker v Lower* (1972), a Virginia court had to determine if the physicians who removed brain-dead Bruce Tucker from a respirator and then transplanted his heart into a patient dying from cardiac failure were guilty of wrongful determination of death [38]. The judge instructed the jury in a new definition of death: "In determining the time of death you may consider the following elements . . . among them the time of complete and irreversible loss of all function of the brain." The jury took less than 1 hour to return a verdict of not guilty.

To clarify the issue for physicians and families and to obviate the costly, burdensome, and often traumatic process of court battles, various states, led by Kansas in 1970, enacted brain-death statutes. To date, some 37 states and the District of Columbia have done so. In several of the nonstatute states, including Massachusetts and New York—major medical areas—courts have acknowledged the propriety of removing life-sustaining machinery from patients who meet the brain-death criteria [39, 40].

To provide for greater uniformity on this subject and to avoid the situation of the same body being alive in one state and dead in the next—and the even more paradoxical situation of a body being alive or dead in the same state, depending on an extrinsic factor such as a signed anatomic gift card [40]*—the President's Commission was charged by Congress with developing a uniform determination of death statute.

From the outset, the President's Commission was determined to take "extreme caution" [41] when formulating public policy in this area. Proposed changes in the existing laws were designed to produce a minimal shift in the definition as well as a maximal acceptance among laypersons, scientists, and clinicians. To that end, the Commission took a conservative posture in its hearings, findings, and final report. It evaluated, but did not accept, the philosophical understandings of death as the loss of personality or personal identity. It likewise studied and rejected the proposal that death be defined as the permanent loss of higher functioning. In its under-

---

*Judge ruled that a 23-year-old woman had suffered a total and irreversible cessation of all brain function and would be dead for anatomic gift purposes had she signed an anatomic gift card. Because she had not done so, however, the judge ruled that she was not legally dead.

standing those who, like Karen Ann Quinlan, survive in a persistent vegetative state are not dead.

The Commission adopted as its position the widely accepted brain-death standard; that is, death is established when "all functions of the brain including the brainstem have permanently and irreversibly ceased" [41]. Thus even if life continues in individual cells or organs, without the complex integration of the entire system a person cannot properly be regarded as being alive. It proposed the following Uniform Determination of Death Act: "An individual who has sustained either (1) irreversible cessation of all circulatory and respiratory function, or (2) irreversible cessation of all functions of the entire brain, including brainstem, is dead. A determination of death must be made in accordance with accepted medical standards" [41].

Despite the opposition of the radical right-to-life forces and of a small but influential band of Orthodox Jews [42–44] who share their belief that only destruction of the brain can be entertained as a possible definition of death, there is no longer any doubt as to what are the medically accepted standards. The "Guidelines for the Determination of Death," a landmark document summarizing currently accepted medical practices, was published in 1981 [45]. Signed by the nation's leading authorities in neurology, neurosurgery, critical care, and legal medicine, the document represents "a consensus that is truly a remarkable achievement, [one] of which the medical profession can be proud" [46]. That document endorsed the Uniform Determination of Death Act.

The one remaining moral dilemma that some physicians continue to perceive is the need for family permission to remove the respirator from brain-dead patients. A classic statement of that problem is seen in the case of a 4-year-old girl who was brain-dead as the result of meningitis. The physicians approached her parents, informed them of the girl's diagnosis, told them that her condition was hopeless, and recommended removal of the extraordinary life-support system. Given that moral choice, the parents opted for continued treatment. They did so in the hope of a

"miracle." The hospital, fearful of opposing the parents' wishes and unwilling to face the adverse publicity of a court proceeding to override the parents' decision, kept the child in the pediatric ICU until several months later when she succumbed to kidney failure.

As William Curran, Professor of Legal Medicine at Harvard Medical School and member of the original Harvard ad hoc committee on brain death [47] has repeatedly emphasized, the determination of brain death is a technical medical issue, one that does not involve patient consent or family approval. Once the medical staff has made a well informed determination of brain death, the patient is dead. The only moral issue remaining is the proper disposition of the corpse.

Not only is there no need to ask family permission to remove the respirator, to do so is highly inappropriate; it is to give a purported moral choice when, in fact, none exists. Furthermore, to do so, as happened with the meningitis victim, is to open the family to unnecessary feelings of ambivalence, anxiety, and guilt, feelings that may result in moral paralysis or a steadfast denial of death. Those emotions, in turn, may result in a decision to continue medical intervention in hopes of a miracle.

An approach more attuned to the reality of the situation would have been to inform the meningitis victim's family of her condition: "She is brain-dead; there is no possibility of recovery and no possibility of restoration." Physicians might have allowed the family some time to adjust and then presented them with available options: "You may see her before we remove the respirator; you may hold her in your arms while the respirator is shut off; or you may choose to remember her as she was." The family is thereby not asked to make a decision on the termination of what is now a futile intervention. Furthermore, this approach avoids the sense that the family is being asked to sign a "death warrant." It also saves them from the possible guilt of thinking they did not do everything possible to save the patient's life.

An alternative approach used by Pitts might be even better [48]. Following the Harvard ad hoc directive that the decision and the responsibility for declaring death and turning off the respirator belong to the physician, Pitts informs the family that the evidence suggests the patient is brain-dead. He then explains that several tests, including one for apnea, will be done to confirm that diagnosis. The family is asked if it wants to see the patient before these tests are done. After the family has gone, the tests, the last of which is for apnea, are performed. In that controlled situation when the respirator is removed, if the patient is unable to breathe, death is pronounced. The physician then informs the family that the evidence was correct: The patient is dead. There is no question of removing a respirator; none is in use.

Organ Retrieval

Because of the way in which health care professionals now handle brain-death cases, the potential for organ retrieval is often lost. The Centers for Disease Control estimated that no more than 15 percent of the 20,000 persons who might be organ donors actually do so [49]. That fact, coupled with the rapid advances being made in transplantation technique and the effectiveness of powerful new immunosuppressive drugs such as cyclosporine is creating a large gap between the supply and demand for organs.

It is estimated that between 6000 and 10,000 people nationwide are being maintained on dialysis while awaiting kidney transplant, yet in 1982 only 3691 cadaver kidney transplants were performed [50]. Similar shortages of hearts and livers are marked by the now familiar televised pleas of family and friends to help save the life of a loved one by locating a potential donor. In an attempt to overcome these perennial shortages, Caplan identified the problem as being not a limitation of potential donors or even the willingness of families to consent to donation but, rather, the reluctance of physicians and other health care providers to undertake the emotionally charged task of asking the families of the neomorts for the organs [51]. It is particularly true in the case of the young trauma victim in which

death itself comes as a shock to the family. This reticence is compounded when physicians and administrators fear adverse legal and financial consequences from their involvement with organ procurement.

Because the major factors hindering the efficacy of organ procurement from cadaver donors are physician- or hospital-based, Caplan has proposed legislation that would, in brain-death cases, require hospitals to ask family members to donate the organs of the newly deceased. To assure the family and the public that the determination of death was being made independently of the desire for organs, the request for organs would be made by someone other than the patient's physician.

A policy of "required request" has now been enacted in California, Oregon, and New York. These statutes, which went into effect 1 January 1986, mandate that a certificate indicating that organ donation had been requested and the family's response must be attached to the death certificate for anyone meeting organ donation criteria.

Although there have as yet been no data on the response to these enactments, it is hoped that once physicians are free of potential legal liability and are no longer pressured by the law into asking families to consider organ donations the ethical dilemmas created by chronic organ shortages will be mitigated.

Advance Directives

A problem more common in the CCU than brain death is what to do with the critically ill patient who is unable to make personal preferences known because of physical condition, age, or medication. The well documented legal history of informed consent and the summary of that development in the report *Making Health Care Decisions* [52] make clear that the primary responsibility of caregivers in this area is to ascertain as much as possible what the individual, if competent, would choose. The decision should reflect the individual's preferences, choices, and values as closely as possible.

That decision can be made, of course, by

learning the patient's values and discovering what the patient would have done for others in similar situations. The clearest and most convincing evidence would be the individual's direct testimony on the extent and duration of medical treatment. Ideally, the attending physician would explore and learn it over the course of the illness. Frequently, however, trauma or a sudden deterioration of the patient's condition precludes such conversations.

To provide for such contingencies, while remaining aware that in our litigious society many physicians do not act without some definitive directive from the patient, many people now establish an advance directive, or "living will." This document specifies the limitations on treatment desired by the patient in case of incapacitation and an irreversibly terminal condition [53]. Some 35 states, led by California, now have statutory regulations that govern such documents. In several other states, including New York, Massachusetts, and Florida, courts have recognized that even in the absence of a statute the prior oral or written statements of presently incompetent patients should be taken as evidence of what the patient would have wanted. The most explicit ruling in this area was given in *John F. Kennedy Memorial Hospital v Bludworth* [54]. In this case the Florida Supreme Court ruled that, in the absence of a statute recognizing a written living will, the prior written directive of an irreversibly comatose 81-year-old man that he not be maintained by artificial life-sustaining measures was "persuasive evidence" of the person's intention and should be given "great weight" by the decision-maker.

Furthermore, the Florida Supreme Court, in a ruling that reversed an earlier appellate court decision, stated there was no need for the family and physicians to seek prior court authorization for the decision to terminate treatment. All that is required of the decision-makers (the family) is that they act in a manner consonant with what the patient would have desired.

Because it is difficult to anticipate the degree of impairment and the specific forms of therapeutic interventions that might be proposed for the patient, those who write advance directives are well advised to name a proxy familiar with their values and desires to make specific treatment decisions for them. Even in jurisdictions where living-will legislation has not been enacted, such written directives help to ensure a greater likelihood that the individual's wishes will be known and followed. Many hospitals have adopted a practice of placing such directives in the patient's medical chart. Such statements can be relied on to assist in the traditional physician–patient (proxy) relationship without the need for third-party intervention in the decision-making process.

Although the report by the President's Commission provides detailed directions for the formulation of such directives, the actual statement need not be complex or drafted by an attorney. One can simply write what he or she wants in such circumstances. If the person wishes a prewritten form, the best and most readily available is Bok's "Directions for My Care" [55].

I wish to live a full and long life, but not at all costs. If my death is near and cannot be avoided, and if I have lost the ability to interact with others and have no reasonable chance of regaining this ability, or if my suffering is intense and irreversible, I do not want to have my life prolonged. I would then ask not to be subjected to surgery or resuscitation. Nor would I then wish to have life support from mechanical ventilators, intensive care services, or other life prolonging procedures, including the administration of antibiotics and blood products. I would wish, rather, to have care which gives comfort and support, which facilitates my interaction with others to the extent that this is possible, and which brings peace. In order to carry out these instructions and to interpret them, I authorize _____ to accept, plan, and refuse treatment on my behalf in cooperation with attending physicians and health personnel. This person knows how I value the experience of living, and how I would weigh incompetence, suffering, and dying. Should it be impossible to reach this person, I authorize _____ to make such choices for me. I have discussed my desires concerning terminal care with them, and I trust their judgment on my behalf. In addition, I have discussed with them the following specific instructions regarding my care:
Date _____ Signed _____
Witnessed _____ and by _____

Patients with Inadequate Decision-Making Capacity

Although it is relatively easy to make medical decisions for those who have provided clear directives for their care, the overwhelming majority of patients with impaired decision-making capacity will not have done so. They present the greatest dilemmas to health care providers. The first of those dilemmas is how to determine that the patient has become so incapacitated that he or she is no longer a competent decision-maker.

When confronted with this situation, many physicians' initial impulse is to call for a psychiatric consultation or seek a court order to declare the patient incompetent [56]. In most cases, neither of those approaches is appropriate. As the President's Commission emphatically noted, "'decision making incapacity' is not a medical or a psychiatric diagnostic category; it rests on a judgment of the type an informed layperson might make—that the patient lacks sufficient ability to understand a situation and to make a choice in light of that understanding" [18]. More specifically, the physician would want to ascertain that the patient understands his or her condition, the treatment options (including nontreatment), and the consequences of each option and is able to make a reasoned choice.

This choice need not be what the physician would consider reasonable, rational, or medically appropriate. The patient's decision need only reflect a reasoned choice among the options. As the Massachusetts Appeals Court stated in *Lane v Candura* [57]—a case involving an admittedly confused 78-year-old woman's refusal to have her gangrenous leg amputated—what must be determined is whether the "areas of forgetfulness and confusion cause or relate in any way to impairment of her ability to understand that in rejecting the treatment she is, in effect, choosing death over life."

Once it has been determined that the patient lacks adequate decision-making capacity, the need for a surrogate or proxy arises. Generally the surrogate should be a family member or a friend who knows the patient's interests and values—and ideally the patient's actual wishes—and can address them. If there has been no prior discussion of issues and the surrogate is unable to assess what the incompetent individual would have chosen, the surrogate must use a "best interests" test, which examines the patient's welfare and well-being. The President's Commission spelled out several factors that should be considered in such a determination, factors that the California Court of Appeals in the *Barber and Nejdl* [58] case adopted as normative: "relief of suffering, the preservation or restoration of functioning; the quality as well as the extent of life sustained . . . and the impact of a decision on the incapacitated patient's loved ones." The caveat is that the "quality of life and impact on family should be viewed exclusively from the perspective of the patient" [58].

One attempt to ensure that the process has produced an objective, disinterested, and publicly accountable decision is to take the issue to court [59]. That route, however, is terribly costly, cumbersome, traumatic, and uncertain. The personal predilections of judges, the highly diverse formulations of the law, and the fact that judges are poorly equipped for and not fond of handling such issues makes that route fraught with potential peril for patients, physicians, hospitals, and society [60, 61].

Furthermore, even court approbation does not protect a hospital and physicians from explosive societal repercussions. This point is illustrated by the Bloomington Baby Doe case, in which a family physician's decision not to treat a Down's syndrome infant with an esophageal fistula was approved by three courts, including the Indiana Supreme Court. Those repercussions proved we need a better way to resolve these problems than inflexible bureaucratic regulations [62].

Decision-Making Process

Whatever the process, good decision-making must consider three factors: the physician, the patient, and the community. Although we have long since surpassed the era of paternalistic physician and the passive patient [63], the physician continues to have a primary role and responsibility. The physician must make the diagnosis, provide the prognosis, and, after forming a professional judgment on the range of options, must make a recommendation. Here, once again, we are reminded of Inglefinger's [30] admonition that a physician who merely presents options to an uncounseled patient and expects a decision is guilty of, at least, shirking duties and, at most, malpractice.

Given the recommendation, the patient or proxy must then address the subjective values that will determine whether the proposal offers a proportionate benefit. Here the entire range of factors, e.g., cost, burden, pain, anticipated outcome, dislocation, family structure, and personal plans, comes into play. The patient, or the person acting on behalf of the patient, must plumb these points and then choose.

Although the combination of patient–family choice is generally final, a third factor—the community—must be considered. With the change in attitude from the strong paternalism of "the doctor knows best" to the elevation of autonomy into a near absolute, individual's sometimes forget that their actions and decisions have implications for, and impact on, others. Consequently, society, in its role of protecting individuals and the common good, places constraints and limits, both positive and negative, on individual rights [64].

Several examples of those constraints have emerged as ethical problems in health care delivery. A reflection on their resolution provides an insight into how we perceive ourselves as a people. For example, from the Johns Hopkins case [65] to the Bloomington Baby Doe dispute, many persons believe that parents should have the right to deny life-saving corrective surgery to a Down's syndrome infant because a retarded child would be a burden on the family [66, 67]. Now, however, a strong consensus has emerged in our society that such an infant may not be denied the necessary surgery simply because of its mental handicap [68]. Similarly, Elizabeth Bouvia, the quadriplegic who wanted to starve herself to death under medical supervision at Califor-

nia's Riverside General Hospital, has been definitively told by the courts that she has no right to impose her desires on the hospital and the medical staff.

An example of the restriction on one's right to positive claims would be the denial of a family request to have a rapidly deteriorating critically ill patient remain in or moved to the CCU to satisfy their demand that "everything possible be done." Use of that facility must rest on the medical staff's professional assessment of the usefulness of the CCU to the patient and the comparative merit of others' claims for that scarce resource [69]. To hold otherwise would transform the physician from a professional charged with making informed and sometimes difficult judgments into one who simply strives to fulfill family demands no matter how misplaced or misguided.

Perhaps the most succinct statement of the physician's professional role is found in a discussion on termination of treatment decisions in the Vatican's *Declaration on Euthanasia* [70]:

For such a decision to be made, account will have to be taken of the reasonable wishes of the patient and the patient's family, as also of the advice of the doctors who are especially competent in the matter. The latter may in particular judge that the investment in instruments and personnel is disproportionate to the results foreseen; they may also judge that the techniques applied impose on the patient strain or suffering out of proportion with the benefits which he or she may gain from such techniques.

Here an institution highly protective of the sanctity of life is indicating not only that there are limitations to the burdens an individual must undergo to preserve life, but there are limits that can and ought to be made by physicians concerning what may legitimately be offered to, or demanded for, such patients.

RESPONSIBILITY FOR THE DECISION

It is clear that the judgments concerning burden and benefit to the patient are value judgments. They are judgments in which, all things considered, the continuance of life is either called for or not worthwhile to the patient. Such judgments are the onerous prerogative of those who are primarily responsible for the welfare of the incompetent patient—the family or other surrogate. When the surrogate exercises this prerogative in a way that is questionably no longer in the best interests of the patient, especially by allowing the patient with a good prognosis to go untreated, society has the duty to intervene. That intervention can take many forms, e.g., legislation, criminal prosecution, or neglect hearings. The purpose of such proceedings is to guarantee that the primary decision-maker acts responsibly, in a manner that should be able to sustain public scrutiny. The public accountability and review, which guarantees that the values of society are respected and adhered to, can be invoked short of judicial intervention.

One approach to achieving that goal is found in the report *Deciding to Forego Life-Sustaining Treatment* [18]. In the opinion of the President's Commission, "routine judicial oversight (of medical decision making) is neither necessary nor appropriate." The remoteness from the clinical situation and the inability to keep pace with the ongoing fluctuations in the patient's condition, particularly in an intensive care setting, are strong arguments in support of that thesis. The Commission favored having the surrogate's decision in difficult cases reviewed by an in-place, broadly based, multidisciplinary hospital bioethics committee, which would be familiar with both the medical setting and community standards. That consultative body, which would have the ongoing charge of establishing standards of treatment and issuing guidelines for the institution, would provide a framework for impartial but sensitive review of difficult choices. It would also guarantee that the patient's interests were being considered without the formality and intensely adversarial character of a court proceeding, or worse, the persuasive fear and distrust generated by anonymous tipsters in the CCU.

If, after all this, irreconcilable disagreement persists, the President's Commission recommended referral to the court to appoint a legal guardian empowered to evaluate the options and make a decision "in the best interest" of the patient. The decision, of course, would be subject to judicial scrutiny as a last resort. Such an approach ensures that the decision-maker has received the most reliable information available, that the decision is within the range of acceptable options, and that those uncomfortable with it have had an opportunity to discuss their reservations with a concerned and disinterested representative of the public. It also insulates the agonizing and often tragic choices from the glare of publicity, the distortion of public posturing, and the costly tangled involvement of court proceedings.

The implementation of bioethics committees as mediating institutions was greatly enhanced in January 1984, when the Department of Health and Human Services, in response to the criticism of its revised, proposed Infant Doe Regulations [71], adopted the suggestion of the American Academy of Pediatrics [72]: The resolution of treatment-issue decisions for seriously ill newborns should be made in each hospital by a multidisciplinary infant care review committee [68].

SUBSTANTIVE GUIDELINES

The procedural aspects of good decision-making ensure that patient autonomy, physician responsibility, and societal values are considered. They do not produce the decision; they do not guarantee its character. Furthermore, the range of ethically acceptable options, the complexity of individual cases, and the variable situation of institutions and specific patients precludes prepackaged solutions to ethical dilemmas.

Nonetheless, there are some agreed-on norms and guidelines that are helpful when resolving difficult ethical questions. The most practical and readily available source for the clinician is Jonsen et al.'s *Clinical Ethics* [73], a superb short text in which an ethicist, a physician, and an attorney lay out some of the more agreed-on principles and illustrate them with brief case studies. That text could well join other reference works as standard equipment in every CCU. Interestingly, the best summary of the ethical norms is found not in discursive philosophical texts but in the major court opinions issued since *Quinlan.* Three of them—*Superintendent of Belchertown State School v Saikewicz* [58], *Barber v Superior Court* [74], and *In the matter of Claire Conroy* [75]—illustrate the emerging consensus of law and ethics on the appropriate care that is due an incompetent, terminally ill, or irreversibly comatose patient.

In *Saikewicz,* the Massachusetts Supreme Court ruled that the court could determine that a 67-year-old, profoundly retarded (IQ 10), institutionalized man with acute myelogenous leukemia would, if competent, opt for nontreatment. The argument was that the administration of chemotherapy, which for the nonretarded patient might be endured in the hope of a remission, would inexplicably change the character of Joseph Saikewicz's life from a peaceful routine into a bewildering nightmare of pain, fear, and physical restraint. As such, it would surely constitute "extraordinary" treatment. If the patient had no obligation to undergo such treatment, the physician had no moral obligation to provide it nor the judge to order it.

When forming this opinion, the Supreme Court gave judicial support to the distinction between ordinary and extraordinary means: "We should not use *extraordinary* means of prolonging life or its semblance when, after careful consideration . . . it becomes apparent that there is no hope of recovery for the patient" [74]. Furthermore, the court concurred with *Quinlan* in adopting the thesis of both Ramsey [16] and Kubler-Ross [77] that the distinction between "curing the ill and comforting and easing the dying" can and ought to be distinguished. It accepted the thesis that physicians ought not to treat the hopeless and the dying as though they were curable. In the court's view, they should recognize that the dying need comfort more than treatment. These positions, buttressed by recent developments in the law on informed consent and respect for the right of privacy, were the basis for the court's authorization of the withholding of chemotherapy for Saikewicz.

In an interesting turn, the court reversed the thesis that the value of life is lessened or cheapened by a decision to refuse treatment. It ruled that the value of life is diminished by the failure to allow a competent human being the right of choice and the right of privacy (i.e., the right to be left alone).

The more difficult problem is the attribution of these rights to the incompetent. There are those who argue strenuously that the state must always provide treatment for the incompetent or risk devaluing their dignity and worth. The Supreme Court rejected that proposition and, in a precedent-shattering contribution to the developing trend in the law, ruled that "the principles of equality and respect for all individuals require that a choice exist for incompetents as well as competents. To do otherwise would be to treat wards of the state as persons of lesser status or dignity than others" [74].

Having recognized the right of an incompetent to refuse life-prolonging treatment, the court was faced with the awesome task, in a case of first impression, of framing an adequate rationale to explain how that right may be exercised. It did so with an interesting yoking of the long-standing legal doctrine of substituted judgment with a Rawlsian reconstruction of the mental world of a "rational" incompetent.

Substituted judgment, a doctrine first articulated in English law over 150 years ago, deals with the authorization of gifts from the estate of incompetents [78]. The English court reasoned it could be done by "donning the mental mantle of the incompetent," i.e., what we might reasonably conclude the individual would do if he or she could understand the situation.

That theory of respect for the integrity and autonomy of all persons finds renewed vigor in John Rawls' highly influential *A Theory of Justice* [79], in which he wrote that maintaining the integrity of the person means that we act toward him "as we have reason to believe he would choose for himself if he were capable of reasoning and deciding rationally." It does not mean that we can impute preferences that the patient never held. However, as is true in the case of Saikewicz where no preferences have been made, the task is to ask how the patient would act if she or he could perceive the present situation.

Applying the substituted judgment theory to Saikewicz, the Supreme Court concluded that the probate court, the guardian *ad litem*, the physicians, and the staff operated in the best interests of Joseph Saikewicz (i.e., they chose what appeared to be the least detrimental alternative available). That choice, they argued, is what Saikewicz himself would have chosen if he were capable of doing so.

The California Court of Appeals in *Barber* refined and developed the ethical standards found in *Saikewicz*. Reflecting on the moral propriety of the physicians who honored the family request to remove the intravenous feeding tube from the irreversibly comatose Clarence Herbert, the court confronted a host of medical-ethical questions: Is the physician bound by the Hippocratic oath to do everything possible to save life? When, if ever, is it appropriate to stop treatment? What is the difference between killing or letting die, acts of omission or commission, withholding or withdrawing treatment? How does one distinguish ordinary from extraordinary means? Is not use of an intravenous feeding tube always ordinary? Who decides for the incompetent patient? Must there be a legal guardian? Is a court order necessary?

In the course of its 25-page opinion, the California Court of Appeals addressed all of these issues. In doing so, it adopted as normative nearly all of the recommendations on what constitutes appropriate care of the terminally ill or reversibly comatose patient that were proposed in the report by the President's Commission *Deciding to Forego Life-Sustaining Treatment.*

Here, for the first time, a court equated the termination of intravenous feeding with the removal of a respirator or any other medical intervention [80–82]. Each intervention, it declared, is a medical treatment and, as such, is to be used only if it benefits the patient. If the intervention merely sustained biologic function, it is not a treatment but a useless and futile gesture, one that the physician need not continue. As the court phrased it, "there is no duty to continue (life-sustaining machinery) once it has become futile in the opinion of qualified medical personnel" [58].

The court discarded the traditional "ordinary–extraordinary" language in favor of the increasingly common usage of "proportionate–disproportionate" "benefit–burden" to the patient. That approach, which was strongly advocated by the Commission, shifts the emphasis from the technique used to the condition of the patient. In the court's words:

Thus, even if a proposed course of treatment might be extremely painful or intrusive, it would still be proportionate treatment if the prognosis was for complete cure or significant improvement in the patient's condition. On the other hand, a treatment course which is only minimally painful or intrusive may nonetheless be considered disproportionate to the potential benefits if the prognosis is virtually hopeful for any significant improvement in condition.

Finally, bringing to completion a trend in the law that was first articulated in *Quinlan,* the court noted that in the case of incompetents, the surrogate, if unable to ascertain the patient's actual choices, should be guided by the patient's best interests. These, as previously noted, would include factors such as relief from suffering, the preservation or restoration of functioning, the quality as well as the extent of the life sustained, and the impact of the decision on the family.

In words that it is hoped will sweep away much of the fear and misapprehension of physicians in such cases, the court held that, without evidence of malevolence, the family is the proper surrogate for the incompetent patient. Furthermore, there is no need for the surrogate to seek prior judicial approval before a decision to withdraw treatment can be made. Such judicial involvement, the court concluded, is not only unnecessary but may be unwise.

The New Jersey Supreme Court, in *The Matter of Claire Conroy* [75], further refined the standards articulated in *Barber* on the withholding or withdrawing of medical treatments, including nutrition and fluids, from incompetent seriously ill patients who, even with treatment, will probably die within approximately 1 year.

After observing that there was no doubt that, if competent, an individual in Miss Conroy's condition would have the right to have a nasogastric tube withdrawn, the New Jersey Supreme Court declared the same right should be accorded the incompetent. It then articulated three tests to guide the substitute decision-maker. The first—"subjective standard"—would apply if the patient had previously communicated wishes by a written living will, an oral directive, or a durable power of attorney.

The other two tests—"limited objective" and "purely objective"—are "best interests" tests to be used if there had been no prior directives from the patient. Here the New Jersey court wished to avoid the naive pretense that it could discern the mind-set of the now incompetent patient, or worse, the position of the New York Court of Appeals in *Storer* which precluded any humane cessation of treatment for persons who had never expressed their desires about life-sustaining treatment, and who are now suffering a prolonged and painful death.

The limited objective test would allow the termination of treatment for someone in Claire Conroy's situation if there were some trustworthy evidence, such as life-style, attitudes, and values, that the patient would not want treatment or feeding continued because "it would involve too heavy a burden of unavoidable pain and suffering."

Even in the absence of any reliable evidence, or indeed of any evidence at all, treatment may be withheld or withdrawn if the purely objective test is satisfied. Under this standard "the net burdens of the patient's life with treatment" would "clearly and markedly outweigh the benefits derived from life." It would be true if the patient were suffering from such severe pain that the administration of life-sustaining treatment or feeding would be inhumane. Here the court cautioned that it expressly denied authority under this third test to remove life support from any patient either on a "quality of life" basis other than

extreme pain or on the grounds that the patient's "value to society" was negligible.

In a commentary on this case, Curran [83] observed that the importance of this decision "on the medical obligation to the dying cannot be overstated." Here, for the first time in American jurisprudence, a supreme court approved the removal of nutrition and hydration as well as other forms of life support and reinforced the legitimacy of allowing surrogates who, in good faith and without a conflict of interest, determine that the patient's best interests will not be served by prolonging a painful, hopeless existence. A similar decision has subsequently been rendered in Massachusetts in the celebrated *Brody* case [34].

The court's position on *Conroy,* however, is not new or strikingly novel in the perspective of medical ethics. Kelly [84], commenting on the morality of the removal of intravenous feeding from a terminally ill, pain-racked cancer patient, agreed that "the patient or his relative may licitly ask that the artificial feeding by discontinued and the physician may accede to this request."

A similar perspective was presented in a landmark review [85] by ten highly experienced physicians from the nation's most prestigious medical centers who, based on their clinical experiences, affirmed the propriety of introducing levels of care for the hopelessly ill patient. When the patient slips into the final stage of the disease, physicians asserted the moral legitimacy of foregoing treatment, including artificial nutrition and fluids, that would serve only to prolong the death process.

Essays by Kelly and the physician group address one problem of acute concern for the intensivist but left unresolved in *Conroy.* What is the appropriate treatment of the patient in a persistent vegetative state? If this patient had made no prior statement on the subject, he or she would not meet the purely objective test in *Conroy* because, by definition, the patient experiences no sensations and hence has no pain or suffering.

Wanzer and colleagues [85] believed that in such cases, if the family agrees, "it is morally justifiable to withhold antibiotics and artificial nutrition and hydration, as well as other forms of life-sustaining treatment, allowing the patient to die." Kelly [84] went even further. In a comment that is instructive and surprisingly current, Kelly wrote: "Apart from very special circumstances, the artificial means (oxygen and intravenous feeding) not only need not but should not be used, once the coma is reasonably diagnosed as terminal (irreversible)." His reasoning is important and enlightening for today's analysis of such situations: "Their use creates expense and nervous strain without conferring any real benefit."

Kelly's reasoning was adopted by the Massachusetts Supreme Court in a landmark ruling in *Brophy v. New England Sinai Hospital* [86] when it authorized the removal of a feeding gastrostomy from a 43-year-old patient who had been maintained for 2 years in a persistent vegetative condition. In what was the first instance of a court-authorized removal of nutrition and fluids from a nondying patient, the Massachusetts court held that "We recognize a general right in all persons to refuse medical treatment [including nutrition and fluids] in appropriate circumstances."

In June 1987 the New Jersey Supreme Court in *In re Peters* [87] authorized the removal of a life-sustaining feeding tube from an elderly nursing home patient who had previously expressed her desire not to be sustained in an irreversible condition. In the companion case of *In re Jobes* it approved [88] the removal of a feeding jejunostomy tube from a young woman who had been in a persistent vegetative condition for some 5 years. In a second companion case, *In re Farrell* [89], the New Jersey Supreme Court held that a competent patient suffering from advanced ALS (Lou Gherig's disease) could decline the placement of a life-prolonging feeding tube.

In the course of these rulings the New Jersey Supreme Court (contrary to the opinion of the Massachusetts court in *Brophy,* which specifically exempted the institution from an obligation to participate in the removal of an artificial feeding system) ruled that the nursing home where Nancy Jobes was being treated must continue to care for her despite its opposition to the removal of the feeding jejunostomy. The court did so because the patient or her family had the right to choose among med-

ical alternatives, including the placement or cessation of an artificial feeding system.

Summary

The high-technology medicine available today not only provides near-miraculous benefits for some patients, it also creates challenging and troublesome ethical and legal dilemmas for patients, families, and practitioners. Fortunately, with the work of the President's Commission and the subsequent report on Life-Sustaining Technologies and the Elderly [90] by the Office of Technology Assessment, we have begun the process of moral reflection and analysis necessary to meet these challenges. The task before us now is to continue this reflection so that we might come to understand, as others have tried since the time of Hippocrates, the appropriate duties and limits of medicine.

Editorial Comments

Paris and Reardon's thoughtful comments should be carefully studied by all physicians who manage patients. Coronary care provides numerous opportunities for physicians to consider ethical and legal dilemmas. Very often it is the attending physician in the coronary care unit, with his or her detailed knowledge of pathophysiology and natural history of disease coupled to a special relation to the patient, who is in the best position to help resolve these difficult issues. G.S.F.

References

1. Knaus, W., Draper, E., and Wagner, D. P. The use of intensive care: New research initiatives and their implications for national health policy. *Milbank Mem. Fund Q.* 61:561, 1983.
2. Schroeder, S. A., Showstack, J. A., and Roberts, H. E. Frequency and clinical description of high-cost patients in 17 acute-care hospitals. *N. Engl. J. Med.* 300:1306, 1979.
3. Thibault, G. E., Mulley, A. G., and Barnett, G. O. Medical intensive care: Indications, interventions, and outcome. *N. Engl. J. Med.* 302:938, 1980.

4. Zook, C. J., and Moore, F. D. High-cost users of medical care. *N. Engl. J. Med.* 302:996, 1980.

5. Turnbull, A. D., Goldiner, P., Silverman, D., and Howland, W. The role of an intensive care unit in a cancer center. *Cancer* 37:82, 1976.

6. Davis, P. B., and di Sant'Angnese, P. A. Assisted ventilation for patients with cystic fibrosis. *J.A.M.A.* 239:1851, 1978.

7. Imbus, S. H., and Zawacki, B. E. Autonomy for burned patients with survival is unprecedented. *N. Engl. J. Med.* 297:308, 1977.

8. Levy, D. E., Bates, D., Cardonna, J. J., and Niall, E. F. Prognosis in nontraumatic coma. *Ann. Intern. Med.* 94:293, 1981.

9. Knaus, W. A., Zimmerman, J. E., Wagner, D. P., et al. APACHE—acute physiology and chronic health evaluation: A physiologically based classification system. *Crit. Care Med.* 9:591, 1981.

10. Rodman, G. H., Etlint, T., Civetta, J. M., et al. How accurate is clinical judgement? *Crit. Care Med.* 6:127, 1978.

11. Pearlman, R. A., Inui, T. S., and Carter, W. B. Variability in physician bioethical decision making: A case study of euthanasia. *Ann. Intern. Med.* 97:420, 1982.

12. McCann, B. A., and Liffring, K. The hospice project. In K. Gordner (ed.), *Quality of Care for the Terminally Ill.* Chicago Joint Commission on Accreditation of Hospitals, 1985. P. 36.

13. Angell, M. Cost containment and the physician. *J.A.M.A.* 254:1203, 1985.

14. Thurow, L. Medicine versus economics. *N. Engl. J. Med.* 313:611, 1985.

15. Fuchs, V. R. Who shall live? In *Health, Economics and Social Voice.* New York: Basic Books, 1974. P. 41.

16. Ramsey, P. *The Patient as Person.* New Haven: Yale University Press, 1970.

17. Admundsen, D. The physicians' obligation to prolong life: A medical duty without classical roots. *Hastings Cent. Rep.* 8:23, 1978.

18. President's Commission for the Study of Ethical Problems in Medicine and Biomedical and Behavioral Research: *Deciding to Forego Life-Sustaining Treatment.* Washington, DC: US Government Printing Office, 1983.

19. Lawler, J. The ethical dilemma of resuscitation. *Lamp* 33:27, 1976.

20. National Conference Steering Committee: Standards for cardiopulmonary resuscitation (CPR) and emergency cardiac care (ECC). *J.A.M.A.* 227:837, 1974.

21. Lampton, L. M., and Winship, D. H. The no-code blue issue: Missouri is not Massachusetts. *Mo. Med.* 76:259, 1979.

22. Spenser, S. S. Code or no code: A non-legal opinion. *N. Engl. J. Med.* 300:138, 1979.

23. Rabkin, M. T., Gillerman, G., and Rice, N. R. Orders not to resuscitate. *N. Engl. J. Med.* 295:364, 1976.

24. Dinnerstein, 380 NE2d 134,135 (Mass App 1978).

25. *Guidelines: Orders Not to Resuscitate.* Boston: Beth Israel Hospital, 5 March 1981.

26. Goldenring, J. Code or no code decisions (Correspondence). *N. Engl. J. Med.* 300:1058, 1978.

27. Hashimoto, D. M. A structural analysis of the physician-patient relationship in no-code decision making. *Yale Law J.* 93:362, 1983.

28. Miles, S. H., Cranford, R. E., and Schulty, A. L. The do not resuscitate order in a teaching hospital. *Ann. Intern. Med.* 96:660, 1982.

29. Siegler, M. Does everything include CPR? *Hastings Cent. Rep.* 12:28, 1982.

30. University of Massachusetts Medical Center: *Do Not Resuscitate Policy.* Worcester: University of Massachusetts Medical Center, 1982.

31. Inglefinger, F. Arrogance. *N. Engl. J. Med.* 303:1507, 1980.

32. Minnesota Medical Association. Do not resuscitate (DNR) guidelines. In *President's Commission for the Study of Ethical Problems in Medicine and Biomedical and Behavioral Research. Deciding to Forego Life-Sustaining Treatment.* Washington, DC: US Government Printing Office, 1983. Pp. 499–500.

33. Paris, J. J., and Cranford, R. E. Brain death, pro-life and Catholic confusion. *America* 345, 1982.

34. Rust, M. Removal of tube barred. *Am. Med. News* Nov. 1:1, 1985.

35. Rust, M. Quinlan lawyer files artificial feeding suit. *Am. Med. News* Nov. 1:1, 1985.

36. Parisi, J. E., Kim, R. C., and Collins, G. H. Brain death with prolonged somatic survival. *N. Engl. J. Med.* 306:14, 1982.

37. Correspondence. *N. Engl. J. Med.* 306:14, 1982.

38. But when did he die? Tucker v. Lower and the brain death concept. No. 2831 (Ct Law & Eq, Richmond, VA, May 25, 1972). *San Diego Law Rev.* 12:424, 1975.

39. *Commonwealth v Golston,* 373 Mass 249, 366 NE2d 744 (1977), cert. denied 434 US 1039 (1978).

40. *Bacchiochi v Johnson Memorial Hospital,* No 256126 (Superior Court, Hartford, CT, 13 March 1981).

41. President's Commission for the Study of Ethical Problems in Medicine and Biomedical and Behavioral Research. *Summing Up.* Washington, DC: Government Printing Office, 1983.

42. Committee for Pro-Life Activities, National Conference of Catholic Bishops: *Definition of Death Legislation, Resource Paper.* Washington, DC, April 1983.

43. Byrne, P. A., O'Reilly, S., and Quay, P. M. Brain death: An opposing viewpoint. *J.A.M.A.* 242:1985, 1979.

44. Rosner, F., and Bleich, J. D. *Jewish Bioethics*. New York: Hebrew Publishing, 1979.
45. Guidelines for the determination of death. *J.A.M.A.* 246:2184, 1981.
46. Barclay, W. R. Editorial guidelines for the determination of death. *J.A.M.A.* 246:2194, 1981.
47. Harvard Medical School: Ad hoc committee to examine the definition of brain death report: A definition of irreversible coma. *J.A.M.A.* 205:337, 1968.
48. Pitts, L. H. Maintenance of a cadaver donor for multiple organ procurement. Read before National Institutes of Health Conference, Washington, DC, 21 January 1984.
49. Kotata, G. Organ shortage clouds new transplant era. *Science* 221:32, 1983.
50. Caplan, A. Organ procurement: It's not in the cards. *Hastings Cent. Rep.* 14:9, 1984.
51. Caplan, A. Ethical and policy issues in the procurement of cadaver organs for transplantation. *N. Engl. J. Med.* 311:981, 1984.
52. President's Commission for the Study of Ethical Problems in Medicine and Biomedical and Behavioral Research: *Making Health Care Decisions*. Washington, DC: US Government Printing Office, 1983.
53. Paris, J. J., and McCormick, R. A. Living will legislation, reconsidered. *America* Sept 5:86, 1981.
54. *John F. Kennedy Memorial Hospital v Bludworth*, 432 So2d 611 (Fla Cir 1983), rev'd 452 So2d 921 (Fla 1984).
55. Bok, S. Directions for my care. *N. Engl. J. Med.* 295:367, 1976.
56. Perk, M., and Shelp, E. E. Psychiatric consultation making moral dilemmas in medicine. *N. Engl. J. Med.* 307:618, 1982.
57. Lane v Candura, 6 Mass 377,576 NE2d 1232 (1978).
58. Barber v Supreme Court, 195 Cal 484 (1983).
59. Baron, C. H. Medical paternalism and the rule of law: A reply to Dr. Relman. *Am. J. Law Med.* 4:337, 1979.
60. Paris, J. J. Court intervention and the diminution of patients' rights: The case of Brother Joseph Fox. *N. Engl. J. Med.* 303:876, 1980.
61. Rothenberg, L. S. The empty search for an imprimatur, or Delphic oracles are in short supply. *Law Med. Health Care* 20:115, 1982.
62. Committee on the legal and ethical aspects of health care for children: Comments and recommendations on the "Infant Doe" proposed regulations. *Law Med. Health Care* 11:203, 1983.
63. Colline, J. Should doctors tell the truth? *Harpers* 155:320, 1927.
64. Callahan, D. Shattuck lecture: Contemporary biomedical ethics. *N. Engl. J. Med.* 302:1228, 1980.
65. Gustafson, J. Mongolism, parental desires and the right to life. *Perspect. Biol. Med.* 524:429, 1973.
66. Shaw, A., Randolph, J. G., and Manard, B. Ethical issues in pediatric surgery: A national survey of pediatricians and pediatric surgeons. *Pediatrics* 60:588, 1977.
67. Todres, I. D., Krane, D., Howell, M. C., et al. Pediatricians' attitudes affecting decision making in defective newborns. *Pediatrics* 60:197, 1977.
68. Office of the Secretary, Department of Health and Human Services: Nondiscrimination on the basis of handicap: Procedures and guidelines relating to health care for handicapped infants. *Fed. Register* 49:1622, 1984.
69. Schwartz, W. B, and Aaron, H. J. Rationing health care: Lessons from Britain. *N. Engl. J. Med.* 310:52, 1983.
70. Sacred congregation for the doctrine of the faith declaration on euthanasia, Vatican City, 1980. In *President's Commission for the Study of Ethical Problems in Medicine and Biomedical and Behavioral Research. Deciding to Forego Life-Sustaining Treatment*. Washington, DC: US Government Printing Office, 1983. App. C. Pp. 300–307.
71. Office of the Secretary, Department of Health and Human Services: Nondiscrimination on the basis of handicap. *Fed. Register* 48:846, 1983.
72. Committee on Bioethics, American Academy of Pediatrics: Treatment of critically ill newborns. *Pediatrics* 72:556, 1983.
73. Jonsen, A. R., Siegler, M., and Winslade, W. J. *Clinical Ethics*. New York: Macmillan, 1982.
74. *Superintendent of Belchertown State School v Saikewicz*, 370 NE2d 417 (Mass 1977).
75. *In the matter of Claire Conroy*, 486 A2d 1209 (NJ, 1985).
76. Paris, J. J. Withholding of life-supporting treatment from the mentally incompetent. *Linacre Q.* 8:237, 1978.
77. Kubler-Ross, E. *On Death and Dying*. New York: Macmillan, 1969.
78. Ex parte Whitebread in re Hinde, a lunatic. *English Rep.* 35:878, 1816.
79. Rawls, J. *A Theory of Justice*. Cambridge, MA: Harvard University Press, 1971.
80. Lynn, J., and Childress, J. F. Must patients always be given food and water? *Hastings Cent. Rep.* 13:17, 1983.
81. Paris, J. J., and Fletcher, A. B. Infant Doe regulations and the absolute requirement to use nourishment and fluids for the dying infant. *Law. Med. Health Care* 11:210, 1984.
82. Paris, J. J., and Reardon, F. E. Court responses to withholding or withdrawing artificial nutrition and fluids. *J.A.M.A.* 253:2243, 1985.
83. Curran, W. J. Defining appropriate medical

care: Providing nutrients and hydration for the dying. *N. Engl. J. Med.* 313:940, 1985.

84. Kelly, G. The duty of using artificial means or preserving life. *Theol. Stud.* June 11:203, 1950.

85. Wanzer, S. H., Adelstein, S. J., Cranford, R. E., et al. The physician's responsibility toward hopelessly ill patient. *N. Engl. J. Med.* 310:955, 1984.

86. *Brophy v. New England Sinai Hospital,* 398 Mass. 147, 497 N.E.2d 626 (1986).

87. *In re Peters,* 108 N.J. 365, 529 A.2d 419 (1987).

88. *In re Jobes,* 108 N.J. 480, A.2d 434 (1987).

89. *In re Farrell,* 108 N.J. 335, 529 A.2d 404 (1987).

90. United States Congress, Office of Technology Assessment. *Life-Sustaining Technology and the Elderly.* Washington, DC: U.S. Government Printing Office, 1987.

Index

Index